AF668009

ACS(I)
Textbook of
CUTANEOUS AND AESTHETIC SURGERY

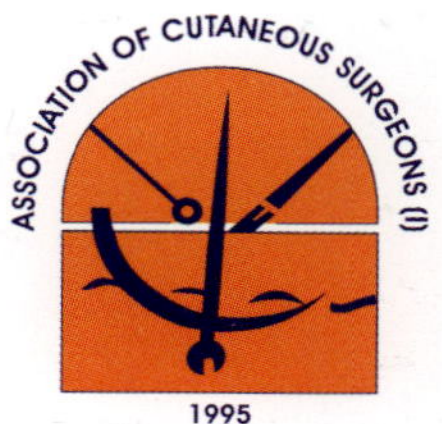

Under the Aegis of Association of Cutaneous Surgeons (I)

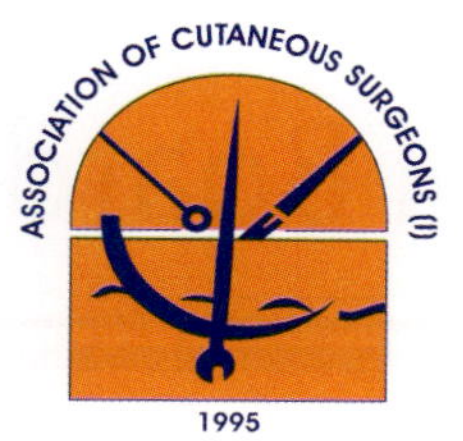

ACS(I)
Textbook of
CUTANEOUS AND AESTHETIC SURGERY

Volume 1

Second Edition

Editor-in-Chief

Mysore Venkataram DVD MD DNB DipRCPath (Lond) FRCP (Glasgow) FISHRS
Consultant: Dermatologist-Dermatopathologist-Hair Transplant Surgeon
Director: Venkat Charmalaya-Centre for Advanced Dermatology and Postgraduate Teaching Centre
Bengaluru, Karnataka, India
Treasurer: Dermatologists and Aesthetic Surgeons League (DASIL)
Editor-in-Chief of Journal of Cutaneous and Aesthetic Surgery, 2007-2010
President of Indian Association of Dermatologists, Venereologists and Leprologists, 2015
President of Association of Hair Restoration Surgeons, India, 2013
President of Association of Cutaneous Surgeons of India, 2010–2013

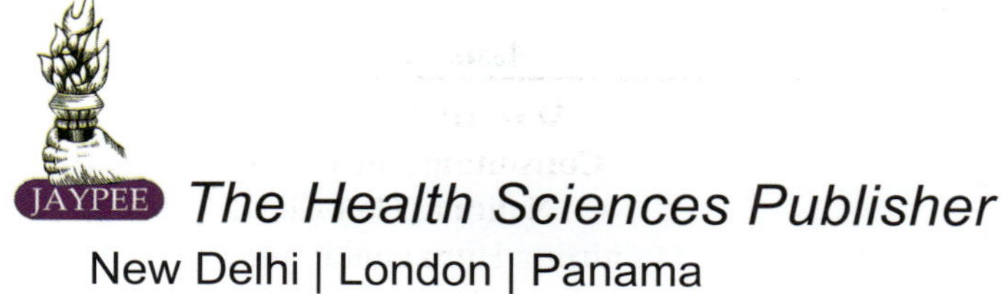

The Health Sciences Publisher
New Delhi | London | Panama

Editorial Board

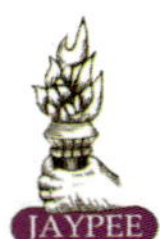

Jaypee Brothers Medical Publishers (P) Ltd

Headquarters
Jaypee Brothers Medical Publishers (P) Ltd.
4838/24, Ansari Road, Daryaganj
New Delhi 110 002, India
Phone: +91-11-43574357
Fax: +91-11-43574314
E-mail: jaypee@jaypeebrothers.com

Overseas Offices
J.P. Medical Ltd.
83, Victoria Street, London
SW1H 0HW (UK)
Phone: +44-20 3170 8910
Fax: +44(0)20 3008 6180
E-mail: info@jpmedpub.com

Jaypee-Highlights Medical Publishers Inc.
City of Knowledge, Bld. 235, 2nd Floor, Clayton
Panama City, Panama
Phone: +1 507-301-0496
Fax: +1 507-301-0499
E-mail: cservice@jphmedical.com

Jaypee Brothers Medical Publishers (P) Ltd.
17/1-B, Babar Road, Block-B, Shaymali
Mohammadpur, Dhaka-1207
Bangladesh
Mobile: +08801912003485
E-mail: jaypeedhaka@gmail.com

Jaypee Brothers Medical Publishers (P) Ltd.
Bhotahity, Kathmandu, Nepal
Phone: +977-9741283608
E-mail: kathmandu@jaypeebrothers.com

Website: www.jaypeebrothers.com
Website: www.jaypeedigital.com

Inquiries for bulk sales may be solicited at: jaypee@jaypeebrothers.com

ACS(I) Textbook of Cutaneous and Aesthetic Surgery (Volume 1)

First Edition: **2012**

Reprint: **2013**

Second Edition: **2017**

ISBN 978-93-5270-033-2

Printed at: Sanat Printers

Contributors

Mysore Venkataram DVD MD DNB DipRCPath (Lond) FRCP (Glasgow) FISHRS
Consultant: Dermatologist-Dermatopathologist-Hair Transplant Surgeon
Director: Venkat Charmalaya-Centre for Advanced Dermatology and Postgraduate Teaching Centre
Bengaluru, Karnataka, India
Treasurer: Dermatologists and Aesthetic Surgeons League (DASIL)
Editor-in-Chief of Journal of Cutaneous and Aesthetic Surgery, 2007-2010
President of Indian Association of Dermatologists, Venereologists and Leprologists, 2015
President of Association of Hair Restoration Surgeons, India, 2013
President of Association of Cutaneous Surgeons of India, 2010–2013

Aarti Sarda
Consultant Dermatologist, Wizderm Clinics
Kolkata, West Bengal, India

Abdul Latheef EN MD DVD MSc APPLIED PSYCHOLOGY
Associate Professor, Deparment of Dermatology
Calicut Medical College
Calicut, Kerala, India
E-mail: drlatheef.skin@yahoo.com, drlatheef90@gmail.com

Abhishek DK De MD FAGE
Consultant Dermatologist
Associate Professor, Calcutta National Medical College
Kolkata, West Bengal, India

Ajay R Hariani MS MCh (Plastic Surgery)
Vasudhan Cosmetic and Laser Surgery
BCJ Asha Parekh Hospital
Mumbai, Maharashtra, India
E-mail: ajayhariani@gmail.com

Alka Goel MD DNB MNAMS
Ex-Assistant Professor, Department of Dermatology
Chacha Nehru Bal Chikitsalya
(Affiliated to Maulana Azad Medical College)
New Delhi, India

Aman Dua MBBS MD (Dermatology)
Consultant Dermatologist
Ludhiana, Punjab, India

Amrendra Kumar
Dermamclinix, E/13, Defence Colony
Ring Road, New Delhi, India
E-mail: dr.amrendra07@gmail.com

Ankur Talwar MD (Dermatology)
Assistant Professor, Hind Institute of Medical Sciences, Lucknow
Consultant Dermatologist, Talwar Skin Institute
Lucknow, Uttar Pradesh, India

Aniketh Venkataram MBBS MS Mch (Plastic Surgery) FDAFPRS
Consultant Plastic, Aesthetic and Hair Transplant Surgeon
Venkat Charmalaya, Centre for Advanced Dermatology
Bengaluru, Karnataka, India
E-mail: anikethv@gmail.com

Anil Abraham MD
Professor and Head
Department of Dermatology
St John's Medical College Hospital
Bengaluru, Karnataka, India
E-mail: docanilabe@yahoo.co.in

Anil Ganjoo MD
Sr. Consultant Dermatologist and Laser Surgeon
Skinnovation Laser Klinik
New Delhi, India
E-mail: drganjoo1965@yahoo.co.in

Anil kumar Garg MS MCh
Diplomate of American Board of Hair Restoration
Director, Rejuvenate Hair Transplant Centre
Indore, Madhya Pradesh, India
E-mail: anilgarg61@yahoo.com

Anirudha Gulanikar DVD DNB
Associate Professor
Department of Dermatology
MGM Medical College
Aurangabad, Maharashtra, India
E-mail: agulanikar@hotmail.com

Anjali Pal MD Dermatology
Consulting Dermatologist
Dr Marwah's Skin and Laser Centre
Mumbai, Maharashtra, India

Anurag Tiwari DVD DNB
Director and Consultant Dermatologist
Center for Skin Disease and Laser Treatment
Bhopal, Madhya Pradesh, India

Apratim Goel MD DNB
Director of Cutis Skin Studio
Consultant Cosmetic Dermatologist and
Laser Surgeon Goel's Cutis Skin Mumbai, Maharashtra, India
E-mail: cutisgoel@gmail.com

Archana Singal
Professor, Department of Skin and STD
UCMS and GTB Hospital
New Delhi, India

Arika Bansal MD (Dermatology and Venereology)
Diplomate ABHRS (American Board of Hair Restoration Surgeons)
Diector, Eugenix Skin and Hair Sciences
Gurugram, Haryana, India

Arijit Coondoo
Professor, Department of Dermatology
KPC Medical College and Hospital, Kolkata, West Bengal, India
E-mail: acoondoo@gmail.com

Balaji AP MD DVL
Consultant Dermatologist
Ganesh Nagar
Vellore, Tamil Nadu, India

Banani Choudhury MD DNB MNAMS
Jaslok Hospital and Research Center
Skin Secrets
Mumbai, Maharashtra, India
E-mail: malavikakohli@gmail.com

Behroze M Deputy MD
Clinical Assistant to Dr Satish Savant
Mumbai, Maharashtra, India

Bhanu Prakash MD DHM PGDMLE
Professor, Department of Dermatology
Vydehi Institute of Medical Sciences and Research Center
Whitefield, Bengaluru, Karnataka, India
E-mail: drbhanuprakash@rediffmail.com

Biju Vasudevan MD FRGUHS
Assistant Professor
Department of Dermatology
Command Hospital
Pune, Maharashtra, India
E-mail: biju.deepa@rediffmail.com

BS Gill
Junior Resident
Department of Dermatology
Institute of Naval Medicine, INHS Asvini
Mumbai, Maharashtra, India

BS Shivaswamy MS
Professor and Head
Department of General Surgery
Bangalore Medical College and Research Institute
Bengaluru, Karnataka, India

Chaithra Shenoy MBBS MD FRGUHS
Cutis Academy of Cutaneous Science
Bengaluru, Karnataka, India
E-mail: chaithrashenoy@gmail.com

Chander Grover
Assistant Professor, Department of Skin and STD
UCMS and GTB Hospital
New Delhi, India

Chandrashekar BS MD DNB
Chief Dermatologist, Cutis Academy of Cutaneous Sciences
Bengaluru, Karnataka, India

CR Srinivas MD FRCP (Glasg)
Professor and Head, Department of Dermatology
Venereology and Leprosy
PSG Institute of Medical Sciences and Researches
Coimbatore, Tamil Nadu, India

C Shanmuga Sekar MD
Associate Professor
Department of Dermatology
PSG Hospitals
Coimbatore, Tamil Nadu, India

Davinder Parsad MD
Professor, Department of Dermatology
PGIMER
Chandigarh, India

D Dinesh Kumar
Consultant Dermatologist
Dr. Dinesh Skin and Hair Clinic
Chennai, Tamil Nadu, India

Dhanashree Bhide MD
Associate Consultant
KEM Hospital
Pune, Maharashtra, India

Dhepe Niteen V MD FAAD Fellow ASDS ASLMS EADV ISHRS IADVL ACSI
Medical Director
SkinCity, The Postgraduate Institute of Dermatology
1st Floor , Nucleus Mall, Church Road, Opp. Commissioner Office
Camp, Pune, Maharashtra, India.
E-mail: niteendhepe@skincityindia.com

Dilip Kachhawa MD
Associate Professor
Department of Dermatology
Dr SN Medical College
Jodhpur, Rajasthan, India

Dipali Rathod
Assistant Professor
Department of Dermatology
Institute of Naval Medicine, INHS Asvini
Mumbai, Maharashtra, India

Divya Gorur MD FRGUHS
Assistant Professor
Bangalore Medial College and Research Institute
Bengaluru, Karnataka, India

Ekta Romi MBBS DDV FCPS
Associate Consultant Dermatologist
Department of Dermatology and
Venereology, KEM Hospital
Pune, Maharashtra, India

Feroze Kaliyadan MD DNB MNAMS
Assistant Professor
Dermatology Department
King Faisal University, Saudi Arabia
Associate Professor
Dermatology Department
Amrita Institute of Medical Sciences
Kochi, Kerala, India

Firas Al-Niami MSc MRCP EBDV
Consultant Dermatologist
Guy's Hospital
London, United Kingdom

GR Rajput
Junior Resident, Department of Dermatology
Institute of Naval Medicine, INHS Asvini
Mumbai, Maharashtra, India

Harsh S Tahiliani MD
Consultant Dermatologist
Mumbai, Maharashtra, India
E-mail: drharshst@gmail.com

Harish Prasad BR MBBS MD (Dermatology) FRGUHS
Dermatosurgery (BMCRI)
We acknowledge help of Dr Harish Prasad in Proof Reading four Chapters

Harvinder Singh Marwah MD DVD DNB
Marwah's Skin and Laser Centre
Mumbai, Maharashtra, India
E-mail: drmarwah@hotmail.com

Imran Majid MBBS MD
Consultant Dermatologist
Cutis Institute of Dermatology
Srinagar, Jammu and Kashmir, India

Indrashis Podder MD
Sagar Dutta Hospital
Kolkata, West Bengal, India

Jaishree Sharad DDV Fellow in Cosmetic Dermatology (Florida) Fellow in Dermatologic Laser Surgery (Bangkok)
Cosmetic Dermatologist
Skinfiniti Aesthetic Skin and Laser Clinic
Navi Mumbai, Maharashtra, India
E-mail: jaishree19@gmail.com

Jayashree venkataram DGO MRCOG
Consultant Liposuction Surgeon
Venkat Charmalaya-Centre for Advanced Dermatology
and Postgraduate Teaching Centre
Bengaluru, Karnataka, India
E-mail: jayashreesampada@gmail.com

Jayakar Thomas MD DD PhD MNAMS FAAD FRCP (Edin, Glasgow, London, Ireland) FIAD
Professor and Head, Department of Dermatology
Sree Balaji Medical College, Chennai, Tamil Nadu, India
E-mail: jayakarthomas@gmail.com

Jyoti Gupta MD (Dermatology)
Dermaclinix, New Delhi, India
E-mail: jkgarg12@gmail.com

Kabir Sardana MD DNB MNAMS
Professor of Dermatology and STD
Dr Ram Manohar Lohia Hospital and
Post Graduate Institute of Medical Education and Research
New Delhi, India

KC Nischal MD
Associate Professor, Department of Dermatology
Adichunchanagiri Institute of Medical Sciences
Bellur, Karnataka, India
E-mail: kc_nischal@yahoo.com

Kanika Sahni MD
Assistant Professor, Department of Dermatology
All India Institute of Medical Sciences
New Delhi, India
E-mail: kanika_sah@yahoo.co.in

Kavish Chouhan MBBS MD
Consultant Dermatologist and Hair Transplant Surgeon
Director-Dermaclinix-the Complete Skin and Hair Solution Center
All India Institute of Medical Science, New Delhi, India

Kavya M MD (DVL)
Assistant Professor
Department of Dermatology, Venereology and Leprosy
Mandya Institute of Medical Sciences
Mandya, Karnataka, India

Keerthi Velugotla
Consulting Dermatologist
MS Skin Center
Bengaluru, Karnataka, India

KH Satyanarayana Rao MD PGDMLE PGDHHM Dip. STD/HIV (Bangkok)
Consultant Dermatologist
Central Government Health Scheme Polyclinic
Bengaluru, Karnataka, India
E-mail: konanurrao@gmail.com

Koushik Lahiri DVD
Consultant Dermatologist, Apollo Gleneagles Hospital
Rita Skin Foundation and WIZDERM Greenwood Nook
Kolkata, West Bengal, India
E-mail: dermakoushik@gmail.com

Kshama Talwar
Consultant Dermatologist
Talwar Skin Institute
Lucknow, Uttar Pradesh, India
E-mail: kshama.talwar@gmail.com

Krishan Mehra
Junior Resident
Department of Dermatology
Institute of Naval Medicine, INHS Asvini
Mumbai, Maharashtra, India

Krupa Shankar DS MD DVD
Academic Coordinator
Department of Dermatology
Manipal Hospital
Bengaluru, Karnataka, India
E-mail: dermakrupa@yahoo.com

KT Ashique DDVL
Consultant Dermatologist
Al Shifa Hospital, Perinthalmanna
Malappuram, Kerala, India
E-mail: drashique@gmail.com

Kuldeep Saxena MBBS DDV DAM (USA)
Cosmozone Hair Transplant
Center Gwalior, Madhya Pradesh, India

Lakshyajit D Dhami MS MCh (Plastic)
Professor of Aesthetic Surgery
Vasudhan Cosmetic and Laser Surgery
Hinduja and Nanavati Hospital
Mumbai, Maharashtra, India
E-mail: dhami@drdhami.com

Madura C
Consultant Dermatologist and
Dermatosurgeon, Cutis Academy
Bengaluru, Karnataka, India

Madhulika Mhatre
Consultant Dermatologist
Wockhardt Hospitals, Mulekar Vitiligo Clinic
Mumbai, Maharashtra, India

Malavika Kohli MD DVD DNB
Consultant Dermatologist
Director, Skin Secrets, Mumbai
Jaslok Hospital and Research Centre
Breach Candy Hospital Trust, Mumbai, Maharashtra, India

M Kumaresan MD (Dermatology)
Diplomate in American Board of Hair Restoration Surgery
Professor, Dermatology, PSGMSR
Coimbatore, Tamil Nadu, India
E-mail: dr_kumaresh@yahoo.co.in

Manas Chatterjee MD DNB (Dermatology)
Senior Adviser, Professor and Head
Department of Dermatology
Institute of Naval Medicine, INHS Asvini
Mumbai, Maharashtra, India

Manjit Sandhu Tahiliani DVD
Consultant Dermatologist
Mumbai, Maharashtra, India
E-mail: manjitsandhu88@gmail.com

Manjot Marwah MD
Consulting Dermatologist, National Hair Clinic
Hamirpur, Himachal Pradesh, India
E-mail: drmanjotmarwah@hotmail.com

Manoj GK MD
Senior Consultant Anesthesiologist
Fortis Hospital, Bengaluru, Karnataka, India

Masuma Molvi Manasawala
Cutis Skin Studio
Mumbai, Maharashtra, India

Milind N Naik MD
Ophthalmic and Facial Plastic Surgery
LV Prasad Eye Institute
Hyderabad, Telangana, India
Orbito-Facial Fellow, UCLA, Los Angeles (2006-07)
E-mail: milnaik@gmail.com

MK Shetty MD
Consultant Dermatologist and Cosmetic Laser Physician
Dr Shetty's Medical and Aesthetic Skin Solutions Prestige Delta
Bengaluru, Karnataka, India
E-mail: your_dermatologist@hotmail.com

Maya Vedamurthy MD MAMS FRCP (Edin)
Consultant Dermatologist
RSV Skin and Laser Centre
Apollo Hospitals, Chennai, Tamil Nadu, India

Mukta Sachadev MD
Senior Consultant Dermatologist
Department of Dermatology
Manipal Hospital
Bengaluru, Karnataka, India

Munish Paul MD
Consultant Dermatologist
Skin Laser Center, New Delhi, India
E-mail: paul_munish@yahoo.com

Murali Chakravarthy MD DA DNB FIACTA FICC
Chief Consultant
Department of Anesthesia
Critical Care and Pain Relief
Fortis Hospital
Bengaluru, Karnataka, India
E-mail: mailchakravarthy@gmail.com

Narendra Gokhale MD
Consultant Dermatologist
Indore, Madhya Pradesh, India

Narendra Patwardhan MD DV (London) DVD
Shreeyash Hospital, Pune, Maharashtra, India
Ex President: AHRS India
Ex Vice President: IADVL
Ex President: IADVL (Maharashtra)
Ex President: ACS(I)
E-mail: ngpatwardhan@gmail.com

Nicholas Collier MD
Senior Consultant Dermatologist
Department of Dermatology, Manipal Hospital
Bengaluru, Karnataka, India

Nidhi S Tandon MD
Consultant Dermatologist, SkinArt Clinic
Lucknow, Uttar Pradesh, India

Nilesh Goel MD
Consultant Dermatologist
SkinArt Clinic, Lucknow, Uttar Pradesh, India

Nirav V Desai MBBS DNB (Dermatology)
Consultant Dermatologist
Surat, Gujarat, India

Niti Khunger MD DDV DNB
Professor
Consultant Dermatologist
VM Medical College and Safdarjung Hospital
New Delhi, India
Ex-President: Association of Cutaneous Surgeons ACS(I)
Associate Editor: Journal of Cutaneous and Aesthetic Surgery
Author: Chemical Peels

Omprakash HM MD
Consultant Dermatologist
Vikram Hospital, Mysore, Karnataka, India
E-mail: drhmomprakash@yahoo.com

Parimalam Kumar MD DD DNB
Senior Assistant Professor
Department of Dermatology
Stanley Medical College
Chennai, Tamil Nadu, India
E-mail: drparimalam@gmail.com

Partha Mahapatra
Junior Resident
Department of Dermatology
Institute of Naval Medicine, INHS Asvini
Mumbai, Maharashtra, India

Pradeep Kumari DNB FCPS DVD MBBS
Asia Institute of Hair Transplant
Pune, Maharashtra, India
E-mail: drgahlotpradeep@gmail.com

Pradyumna Vaidya MBBS DVD DNB
Consultant Dermatologist
Skin and Laser Clinic
Pune, Maharashtra, India
E-mail: drpvaidya@gmail.com

Pawan Raj R MD FRGUHS (Dermatosurgery)
Cutis Academy of Cutaneous Sciences
Bengaluru, Karnataka, India
E-mail: pavanraj.r@gmail.com

Prangya Parimita Rana
Fellowship Trainee
Venkat Charmalaya
Centre for Advanced Dermatology
Bengaluru, Karnataka, India

Rachana Shilpakar MD
Consultant Dermatologist
Department of Dermatology and Aesthetic Medicine
MS Skin Centre
Bengaluru, Karnataka, India

Rachita Dhurat
Department of Dermatology
Lokmanya Tilak Municipal
Medical College and General Hospital
Mumbai, Maharashtra, India
E-mail: rachitadhurat@yahoo.co.in

Rachita Narad MD
Consultant Dermatologist
Kanpur, Uttar Pradesh, India
E-mail: drnarad_rachita@yahoo.in

Ragini Ghiya MD
Consultant Dermatologist and Hair Transplant Surgeon
Siddharth Clinic
Surat, Gujarat, India
E-mail: drraginighiya@gmail.com

Ragunatha S MD
Associate Professor
Department of Dermatology, Venereology and Leprosy
Sri Siddhartha Medical College
Tumkur, Karnataka, India
E-mail: drragus@yahoo.co.in

Raghunatha Reddy R MD DNB FRGUHS (Dermatosurgery)
Professor
Consultant Dermatologist and Dermatosurgeon
Dr Raghu's Mathapitha Polyclinic
Bengaluru, Karnataka, India

Rajat kandhari MD
Senior Resident
VM Medical College and Safdarjung Hospital
New Delhi, India
E-mail: rkandhari@gmail.com

Rajesh M Buddhadev MD
Senior Consultant
Dermatologist and Aesthetic Dermatosurgeon
President, NU Skin World
Surat, Gujarat, India
E-mail: buddhadev1@gmail.com

Rajetha Dami Setty MD (Dermatology)
Additional Medical Director
Oliva Chain of Hair and Skin Clinics
Hyderabad, Telangana, India
E-mail: drrajethadamisetty@gmail.com

Rashmi Sarkar MD MNAMS
Associate Professor Department of Dermatology
Maulana Azad Medical College and Lok Nayak Hospital,
New Delhi, India
E-mail: rashmisarkar@gmail.com

Rasya Dixit MD MBBS
Sri Sai Pinnacle Ashoka Avenue
KR Garden, Murugeshpalya, Bengaluru, Karnataka, India
E-mail: Dr.rasya@gmail.com

Reena Rai MD
Professor
PSG Institute of Medical Science and Research
Coimbatore, Tamil Nadu, India
E-mail: drreena_rai@yahoo.co.in

Rekha Sheth MD DVD
Consultant Dermatologist
Yuva Skin & Hair Clinics LLP
Mumbai, Maharashtra, India

Revanta Saha
Dermatologist
Venkat Charmalaya, Centre for Advanced Dermatology
#3437 1st 'G' cross, 7th main, Subbanna Garden, Vijayanagar
Bengaluru, Karnataka, India

R Jayashree
PSG Institute of Medical Science and Research
Coimbatore, Tamil Nadu, India
E-mail: drreena_rai@yahoo.co.in

S Sacchidanand MBBS MD (DVL) DVD DHA FRCP (Glasgow)
Director of Medical Education
Department of Medical Education
Government of Karnataka
Bengaluru, Karnataka, India

Sadhana Deshmukh DNB
Forever Yooung Skin Hair Body Aesthetics Clinic
Maharashtra, India

Sandeep Sattur MS MCh (Plastic Surgery) Consultant Hair Transplant
Surgeon Hairrevive-Centre for Hair Restoration and
Skin Rejuvenation, Mumbai, Maharashtra, India
E-mail: drsattur@hairrevive.com

Sandeep Savant MD DDV
Mumbai, Maharashtra, India
E-mail: drsandeepsavant@gmail.com

Sangeeta Varma MD
Senior Consultant in Kaya Skin Clinic and Apollo Clinic, Sector 14
Gurgaon, Haryana, India
E-mail: Sangvarma@yahoo.com

Sanjay Sane MS
Consulting Foot Surgeon
Diabetic Foot Clinic
Maharashtra Medical Foundation's
Joshi Hospital
Pune, Maharashtra, India
E-mail: sane@doctor.com

Sanjay Singh MD
Gautam Nagar, New Delhi, India
E-mail: sanjaysinghsnmc007@gmail.com

Sanjeev Aurangabadkar MD
Consultant Dermatologist and Laser Surgeon
Skin and Laser Clinic
Hyderabad, Telangana, India
E-mail: sanjeev.aurangabadkar@gmail.com

Sanjeev Gupta MD DNB MNAMS
Professor and Head
Department of Dermatology
MM Institute of Medical Sciences and Research
Ambala, Punjab, India
E-mail: Sanjeevguptadr@gmail.com

Sanjeev Mulekar MD
Consulting Dermatologist
National Centre for Vitiigo and Psoriasis
Riyadh, Saudi Arabia

Satish S Savant MD FAMS FCPS DVD DDV
Head, Department of Skin and STD
Dr Balabhai Nanavati Hospital and Medical Research Centre
West Mumbai, Maharashtra, India
E-mail: drsatishsavant@yahoo.co.in

Savita Yadav MD
Department of Dermatology
All India Institute of Medical Sciences
New Delhi, India

Savitha AS MD DNB FRGUHS (Dermatosurgery)
Assistant Professor
Department of Dermatology
Sapthagiri Institute of Medical Sciences and Research Institute
Bengaluru, Karnataka, India
*E-mail:*drsavithasomaiah@gmail.com

SDN Guptha MD
Consultant Dermatologist
Sri Satya Sai General Hospital
Bengaluru, Karnataka, India
E-mail: sdnguptha@gmail.com

Seema Garg
Consultant
Rejuvenate Hair Transplant Centre
Indore, Madhya Pradesh India
E-mail: nilgarg61@yahoo.com

Shashikumar BM MD (DVL) FIADVL (Dermatopatho)
Associate Professor
Department of Dermatology
Venereology and Leprosy
Mandya Institute of Medical Scinces
Mandya, Karnataka, India

Shehnaz Arsiwala MD DDV
Renewderm Skin
Hair Laser, Aesthetic Center
Mumbai, Maharashtra, India
E-mail: drshenaz@gmail.com

Shilpa K MD
Assistant Professor
Bangalore Medical College and Research Institute
Bengaluru, Karnataka, India

Shyamanta Barua MD
Assistant Professor
Assam Medical College and Hospital
Dibrugarh, Assam, India
E-mail: drshyamanta@gmail.com

Sidharth Sonthalia MD DNB MNAMS
Consultant Dermatologist
SKINNOCENCE, The Skin Clinic
Gurugram, Haryana, India
E-mail: sidharth.sonthalia@gmail.com

Silonie Sachdeva MD
Consultant Dermatologist
Carolena Skin and Laser Centre
Jalandhar, Punjab, India
E-mail: siloniederm@yahoo.com

Sindhu Potla MD (DVL) FRGUHS
Consultant Dermatologist
Cutis Clinic
Bengaluru, Karnataka, India
E-mail: sindhupotla9@gmail.com

Sitara GL
Consultant Dermatologist
Venkat Charmalaya, Centre for Advanced Dermatology
Bengaluru, Karnataka, India

Smriti Naswa MD
Consultant, Department of Skin
Government Medical College and SSG Hospital
Vadodara, Gujarat, India

Somesh Gupta MD DNB MNAMS
Professor
Department of Dermatology and Venereology
All India Institute of Medical Sciences
New Delhi, India
E-mail: someshgupta@hotmail.com

Sonam Vimadalal MBBS DDVL
Consultant Dermatologist
Dr. Malavika Kohli and Associates
Skin Secrets
Mumbai, Maharashtra, India
E-mail: sonam_v7@yahoo.com

Subhodip Mitra
Consultant
Department of Dermatoglogy
Vydehi Institute of Medical Sciences and Research Center
Bengaluru, Karnataka, India

Subodh Jane MD FRGUHS
Amravati, Maharashtra, India
E-mail: dr.subodhjane86@gmail.com

Subodh Sirur MBBS DVD DNB
Consultant Dermatologist
Wockhardt Hospital, Apolo Spectra
Mahatma Gandhi Memorial Hospital
Mumbai, Maharashtra, India

Sujala S Aradhya
Consultant Dermatologist and Dermatosurgeon
Sujala Polyclinic and Laboratory
Bengaluru, Karnataka, India

Sujay Khandpur MD DNB MNAMS
Additional Professor
Department of Dermatology and Venereology
All India Institute of Medical Sciences
New Delhi, India
E-mail: sujay_khandpur@yahoo.com

Sujit Shanshanwala
Department of Dermatology
Lokmanya Tilak Municipal
Medical College and General Hospital
Mumbai, Maharashtra, India
E-mail: shanshanwal.sujit@gmail.com

Sunaina Hameed MD
Medical Director and Consultant Dermatologist Skin
Health Advanced Dermatology Center
Bengaluru, Karnataka, India

Suresh Talwar MD
Senior Consultant Dermatologist, Talwar Skin Institute
Lucknow, Uttar Pradesh, India
E-mail: drsureshtalwar@gmail.com

Sushil Tahiliani MD DV & D
Consultant Dermatologist
Mumbai, Maharashtra, India
E-mail: drsushiltt@gmail.com

Swapnil Shah
Consultant Dermatologist
Solapur, Maharashtra, India
E-mail: drswapnilshah@gmail.com

Swati Mogra MBBS
Postgraduate Student, Dermatology
Department of Dermatology
Manipal Hospital
Bengaluru, Karnataka, India
E-mail: swatimogra@gmail.com

Swati Mutha MBBS DDV
Consulting Dermatologist
Dr Malavika Kohli and Associates
Skin Secrets, Mumbai, Maharashtra, India

Tanvi Gupta
Dermatologist, The Skin Clinic
Gwalior, Madhya Pradesh, India

T Salim MD DNB
Medical Director and Clinical Head
Cutis Institute of Dermatology and Aesthetic Sciences
Calicut, Kerala, India

TS Nagesh
Professor, Department of Dermatology
Venereology and Leprosy, SIMS and RC
Bangaluru, Karnataka, India

TS Vidya MD FRGUHS (MED Cosmetology)
Skin and Cosmetic Clinic
Bengaluru, Karnataka, India
E-mail: vidyaderma@gmail.com

Uday Kelkar DIM MD (Microbiology)
Senior Chief Medical Officer Senior Administrative Grade
In-Charge Laboratories
Central Govt. Health Scheme, Pune
Ministry of Health and Family Welfare
Government of India
Pune, Maharashtra, India
E-mail: udakelkar@gmail.com

Umashankar Nagaraju MD
Hon General Secretary, ACS(I)
Professor, Department of Dermatology
Rajarajeshwari Medical College and Hospital
Bengaluru, Karnataka, India
Consultant Dermatologist and Cutaneous Surgeon
Apollo Hospitals, Bengaluru, Karnataka, India
E-mail: usdermavision@gmail.com

Vaishalee Kirane DVD DNB
Dermatologist and Trichologist
Ruby Hall Clinic, Aditya Birla Hospital and Joshi Hospital,
Pune, Maharashtra, India
E-mail: vaishaleepk@gmail.com

Vani Yepuri
Consultant Dermatologist
Venkat Charmalaya
Centre for Advanced
Dermatology, Bengaluru, Karnataka, India

Venura Samarasinghe MRCP
Specialist Registrar
The Dermatology Centre
Salford Royal NHS Foundation Trust
Salford, Manchester, UK
E-mail: venuras1@hotmail.co.uk

Vikram Lele M Tech (IITM)
CTO, Mediverse Technologies LLP
New Delhi, India

Vinay Saraf MD DVD
Senior Consulting Dermatologist
Dr Balabhai Nanavati Hospital and Research Centre
President: ACS(I) (2000-2002)
Editor: ADSI' Manual of Dermatologic Surgery
Vitiligo Monograph and Color Atlas
Author: Chemical Peels on Facial and Nonfacial
Areas in Asian Skin

Vishal Chugh MD
Fellow in Dermatosurgery
Bangalore Medical College and Research Institute
Bengaluru, Karnataka, India
E-mail: drvishalchugh@rediffmail.com

Vishal Madan MD FRCP
Consultant Dermatologist, Laser and Mohs Surgeon
Salford Royal NHS Foundation Trust
Honorary Senior Lecturer, University of Manchester
President, British Medical Laser Association

Vishwanath Jigjinni MS FRCS
Hon Plastic Surgeon
Ruby Hall Clinic and Jehangir Hospital
Pune, Maharashtra, India
E-mail: plasticsurgeon1@hotmail.com

Vivek Nair MD
Consultant Dermatologist
Dr Nair's Skin Clinic,
Gurugram, Haryana, India
E-mail: viveknair2010@gmail.com

Yashwant Tawade MD DVD DDV
Professor and Head
Department of Dermatology Gynecology and Venereology
KEM Hospital, Pune, Maharashtra, India
E-mail: yashtawade@gmail.com

YS Marfatia MD
Professor and Head
Department of Skin-VD Medical College
SSG Hospital Vadodara, Gujarat, India
E-mail: ym11256@gmail.com

Akshitha Shetty MBBS MD
Yuva Skin & Hair Clinics LLP
Mumbai, Maharashtra, India

Shreya Pagariya Golchha MBBS DVD
Yuva Skin & Hair Clinics LLP
Mumbai, Maharashtra, India

Preface to the Second Edition

The most satisfying aspect of editing and authoring a book is when a second edition becomes due, very soon after the first edition. *ACSI Textbook of Cutaneous and Aesthetic Surgery* got sold out within months of its release, and several reprints had to be brought out. The preparation for the second edition began in 2016 and it is most satisfying that this edition is being brought out at the World Congress of Cosmetic Dermatology in May 2017 at Bengaluru, Karnataka, India as a thoroughly revised and enlarged version.

It was Charles Darwin who said, *"It is not the most intellectual of the species that survives; it is not the strongest that survives; but the species that survives is the one that is able to adapt to and to adjust best to the changing environment in which it finds itself."* This applies cogently to the dermatologist and to the subject of dermatosurgery. The subject has changed drastically and expanded exponentially, and the dermatosurgeon has had to adapt to this change. This change can be seen in this second edition. It has expanded from 66 chapters to 152 chapters; the number of authors has expanded from 105 to 147. New topics and new sections have been added apart from a thorough revision of the existing chapters. We hope the readers will receive these changes with enthusiasm.

While things change, certain things remain the same. Dermatosurgery continues to represent a Theseus' paradox: *"This is my grandfather's axe. My father replaced the shaft, and I put a new head on it. It's my grandfather's axe."*

I have, therefore, no hesitation in reproducing the following paragraphs from the preface to the first edition:

"Writing a book is an experience—exhilarating at times, excruciating at others. And, in a multiauthored book, it is even more so, as deadlines are chased furiously and frenetically. Despite the highs and the lows, I must say the experience has been something to cherish—it has been my privilege to have been the Editor-in-Chief for this effort—and on behalf of the editorial board, I thank each author for his contribution. It truly has been a **great work done by a number of smaller things together!**"

I was indeed fortunate to have an experienced editorial board of senior dermatosurgeons, available at all times for counsel and advice. My heartfelt gratitude to each one of them. And I record with a touch of pride and happiness the splendid work done by my young team of deputy and assistant editors, who toiled for long hours in correcting proofs, and drafts. The book would not have been possible without their long endeavors. In particular, the **Associate Editor**, **Manjot Marwah** has made a singular contribution and I place on record my appreciation and thanks to her.

Lastly, an effort of this size is never possible without the support and understanding from the family—my wife Dr Jayashree, my son Aniketh (both of whom contributed as authors) and daughter Ankitha (who supported silently)—my heartfelt thanks to them.

Jaypee Brothers Medical Publishers (P) Ltd. has done an outstanding work in bringing this book out on time—in particular, my thanks to Shri Jitendar P Vij (Group Chairman), Mr Ankit Vij (Group President), Ms Chetna Malhotra Vohra (Associate Director-Content Strategy), Ms Nikita Chauhan (Development Editor), and the production team—my gratitude to them.

It is my fond hope that this edition too will be well received and appreciated by the readers and *the grandfather's axe shall improve further*!

Mysore Venkataram

Preface to the First Edition

Dermatosurgery has been passing through interesting times, as disease dermatology paves the way for desire dermatology, as illness gets replaced by wellness and patients are replaced by clients—today's interventional dermatology seeks to dominate over armchair dermatology of yesterday. What we now have is a youthful, vibrant, fast-changing subspecialty. Change has been so striking over the last decade that, in some ways, dermatosurgery represents a Theseus' paradox: "*This is my grandfather's axe. My father replaced the shaft, and I put a new head on it. It's my grandfather's axe.*"

Despite the rapid progress, there have been few books in this field, specially focusing on brown skin, and the need for a comprehensive book, encompassing all the aspects of cutaneous surgery, lasers and aesthetics, has long been felt. Sensing this need, the Association of Cutaneous Surgeons (I) decided to bring out this book.

The rapidly changing profile, range and scope of the subject, with multitudes of procedures being performed, necessitated a multiauthored book. Fortunately, our association is blessed with the talent that was needed for authoring the chapters—the result is what you see; an exhaustive compilation with 66 chapters, including nearly 33 subchapters, by as many as 105 authors. Every aspect of cutaneous surgery has been comprehensively dealt with, keeping in mind the recent advances.

The brown skin has many peculiarities and variations—in fact, it defies any classification! Pigmentation response, healing and scarring reactions, aging changes are all different in the brown skin. Similarly, the epidemiological situations are also different; vitiligo surgery is more relevant than skin cancer surgery! The textbook aptly seeks to address these challenges and requirements.

Our effort has been to keep the book comprehensive, yet simple; to make the book all- inclusive, yet reader-friendly; exhaustive and yet relevant—to the beginner and the expert, the novice and the connoisseur. We hope that we have succeeded in achieving this objective.

Writing a book is an experience, exhilarating at times, excruciating at others. And, in a multiauthored book, it is even more so, as deadlines are chased furiously and frenetically. Despite the highs and the lows, I must say the experience has been something to cherish—it has been my privilege to have been the Editor-in-Chief for this effort—and on behalf of the editorial board, I thank each author for his contribution. It truly has been a **great work done by a number of smaller things together!**

I was indeed fortunate to have an experienced editorial board of senior dermatosurgeons, available at all times for counsel and advice. My heartfelt gratitude to each one of them. And I record with a touch of pride and happiness the splendid work done by my young team of deputy and assistant editors, who toiled for long hours in correcting proofs, and drafts. The book would not have been possible without their long endeavors.

Lastly, an effort of this size is never possible without the support and understanding from the family—my wife Dr Jayashree, my son Aniketh (both of whom contributed as authors) and daughter Ankitha (who supported silently)—my heartfelt thanks to them.

M/s Jaypee Brothers Medical Publishers have done an outstanding work in bringing it out on time—in particular, my thanks to Mr Jitendar P Vij (CEO), Ms Sunita Katla (PA to CEO), Ms Shagufta Khan (Exec. Asst. to MD), Mr Sumit Kumar and Mr Ram Murti (Graphic Designers), Ms Geeta Srivastava and Laxmidhar Padhiary (Proofreaders) and Mr Venugopal (Branch Manager). My gratitude to them.

I earnestly hope that the book will be appreciated by the readers, and welcome comments and feedback. My earnest hope is that book will serve as an instrument in furthering progress in the field, and *the grandfather's axe shall improve further!*

Mysore Venkataram

Contents

Volume 1

Section 1: Basic Principles of Cutaneous Surgery

Section 2: Standard Cutaneous Surgical Techniques

Section 3: Special Cutaneous Surgical Procedures

Vitiligo Surgeries

Section 5: Laser, Lights and Other Technologies

Section 6: Miscellaneous Topics

Section 5: Laser, Lights and Other Technologies

Section 6: Miscellaneous Topics

Section 1

Basic Principles of Cutaneous Surgery

Section Outline

- Skin: Basic Aspects
- Applied Surgical Anatomy in Relation to Facial Rejuvenation
- Regional Anatomy
- Wound Healing
- Wound Management
- Bandages in Dermatosurgery
- Universal Precautions for a Dermatosurgeon
- Dermato Surgical Instruments
- Wound Closure Materials and Techniques in Dermatosurgery
- Setting Up a Dermatosurgery Unit
- Disinfection and Sterilization
- Local Anesthesia
- Tips and Tricks for Using Local Anesthesia for Dermatosurgical Procedures
- Tumescent Local Anesthesia
- Nerve Blocks in Dermatosurgery
- Hemostasis in Dermatologic Surgery
- Antithrombotic Therapy and Dermatosurgery
- Management of Dermatosurgical Emergencies
- Pharmacology of Analgesic and Anxiolytic Drugs used in Dermatosurgery
- Pain Management in Dermatosurgery
- Antibacterial Agents in Dermatosurgery

Chapter 1

Skin: Basic Aspects

Shashikumar BM

Key Messages 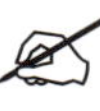

- Knowledge of basic anatomy is important to understand further applied anatomy.
- Understanding physiology and anatomy of melanocyte helps to understand pigmentation response.
- Epidermal layers and their turnover, dermis and its responses play vital role in explaining resurfacing techniques.

INTRODUCTION

Skin is the largest organ of body and it ensheaths all other organs. It plays a major role in defense (immunity), synthesis (vitamin D), homeostasis (temperature regulation, water and electrolyte balance) and aesthetics (complexion, wrinkles and baldness). Dermatosurgery and aesthetic surgery deal with the surgical aspects of skin and its appendages. However, this subject is now driven by aesthetics, the wellness component rather than diseases, the illnesses. Better understanding of basic features gives an edge with regard to safety and efficacy while performing dermatosurgical procedures. While detailed anatomy can be found in a textbook of dermatology, this chapter briefly presents structural and embryological aspects of skin and its appendages. Applied anatomy of head and neck is considered in detail in the next chapter and details of each region are elaborated in respective chapters on different dermatosurgical procedures.

EMBRYOLOGY

Skin is made up of three layers, namely (1) epidermis, (2) dermis and (3) hypodermis or subcutis (Fig. 1 and Table 1). It consists of cells, connective tissues and special appendages which are derived from ectoderm, neuroectoderm and mesoderm.

Development of skin goesthrough three phases: Specification (0–2 months), morphogenesis (2–5 months), differentiation (5–9 months).1 It is regulated by various signaling pathways like Notch, Wnt, Sonic Hedgehog (Shh), bone morphogenetic proteins and fibroblast growth factors, many of which play a vital role in aging later in life.[2] Skin starts developing by 3 weeks of intrauterine life with formation of a single layer of cells derived from ectoderm lateral to neuroectoderm. At 4 weeks, it is composed of two layers: outer periderm or epitrichial layer and inner, stratum germinativum. Tonofilaments (12–16 weeks) and keratohyalin granules (16–21 weeks) appear later with completion of cornification by 24 weeks. At 8–11 weeks, middle layer starts forming adding layers to skin. Basal lamina is secreted by basal cells and matures to form dermoepidermal junction as in adults by 12 weeks.[3]

Early attempt to form hair follicle is seen at 9 weeks of intrauterine life at eyebrows, upper lip and chin. There is aggregation of mesenchymal cells close to ectoderm leading to elongation of ectodermal cells (pregerm stage). These elongated cells also increase in number and start projecting down into mesenchyme. Simultaneously, the underlying collection of mesenchymal cells increases in number forming rudimentary hair papilla (hair germ stage). The short nubbins ectodermal downgrowths form slanting columns of cells with basal cells reorienting themselves perpendicular to the long axis of growth (hair-peg stage). The advancing tips of these downgrowths become bulbous and form a cup enclosing the aggregates of mesenchymal cells (bulbous hair-peg stage). These cells in the lower layers of hair bulb are matrix cells, which form outer and inner sheaths and hair. As the matrical cells proliferate and cornify, they are pushed up to form hair. The junction of matrical cells and cornified cells is the Adamson's fringe. At 16 weeks, three bulges are seen on the posterior aspect of these columns. Arrector pilorum muscle attaches to lower most bulge, middle bulge differentiates into sebaceous glands and upper most bulge forms apocrine gland. These apocrine glands persist in axilla, areola, periumbilical and anogenital areas, and regress to form anlage in other sites. Earliest hairs emerge from follicular openings in eyebrow region at 17 weeks. By 20 weeks, entire body except palms, soles, terminal phalanges, glans and labia minora are covered by hairs. Under the influence of maternal hormones, sebum secretion starts by 15th week. Thus, hair follicle grows from a close interaction of ectoderm with mesenchyme—an interaction which occurs through life during each hair cycle.[4]

Eccrine glands also develop as ectodermal downgrowths into dermis sans aggregation of mesenchymal cells. They first appear in palms and soles and start secreting by 6th month of intrauterine life.[4]

Nail development is earliest recognized in first trimester as a quadrangular area on tips of fingers and toes dorsally and is delineated by lateral and proximal shallow grooves. The primordial nail structure is made of three layers: (1) surface, (2) intermediate and (3) germinative layers. Intermediate and germinative layers grow proximally and form nail matrix. Nail plate starts to form by 14 weeks and by 20 weeks, it covers the nail bed completely. At the same time, granular layer is also lost from the nail matrix. Among all epithelial derivatives, nail plate is the first structure to cornify.

Table 1: Layers of the skin.

Skin layer	Description
Epidermis	Outer most layer, serving as the barrier lined by stratified squamous epithelium
Dermis	Lies beneath epidermis separated by dermoepidermal junction. Consists of supporting matrix, cells and vessels
Subcutis	Deeper layer consists of loose connective tissue and fat

Dermis also starts developing parallel with formation of nerves by 5 weeks, vessels, both vascular and lymphatic by 12 weeks, delicate collagen by 12 weeks and mature collagen by 16 weeks and elastic fibers by 24 weeks. Subcutis develops from aggregation of mesenchymal cells around blood vessels with accumulation of fat.

Summarizing the development, epidermis, pilosebaceous apocrine units, eccrine glands and nails are derived from ectoderm; melanocytes, nerves and sensory receptors from neuroectoderm and dermis, blood vessels, lymphatic channels, cells like Langerhans cells, fibrocytes, mast cells, macrophages, subcutis, and muscles are derived from mesoderm.

EPIDERMIS

Epidermis is the outermost layer of the skin and is composed of stratified squamous epithelium. From below upwards, it consists of four layers: (1) stratum basale, (2) stratum spinosum, (3) stratum granulosum, and (4) stratum corneum (Figs. 2A and B). Stratum lucidum is an additional thin, homogenous hyalinized layer present only in palms and soles. Total renewal time for epidermis is 39 days; 13 days for proliferation, 12 days for migration and 14 days for shedding.[4]

The epidermis is mainly composed of keratinocytes (80%). The "brick-like" shape of keratinocytes is provided by a cytoskeleton made of keratin intermediate filaments. As the epidermis differentiates, the keratinocytes become flattened. Other cells in the epidermis are the melanocytes, Langerhans cells and Merkel cells. Melanocytes are found in the basal layer of the epidermis as well as in hair follicles. Melanocytes, derived from neural crest

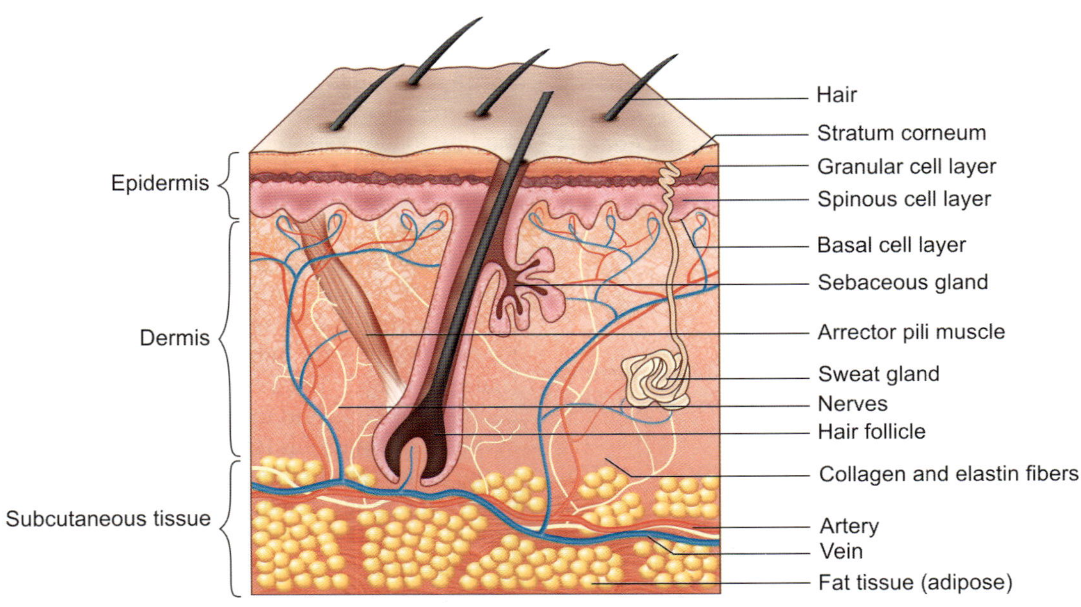

Fig. 1: Structure of skin.

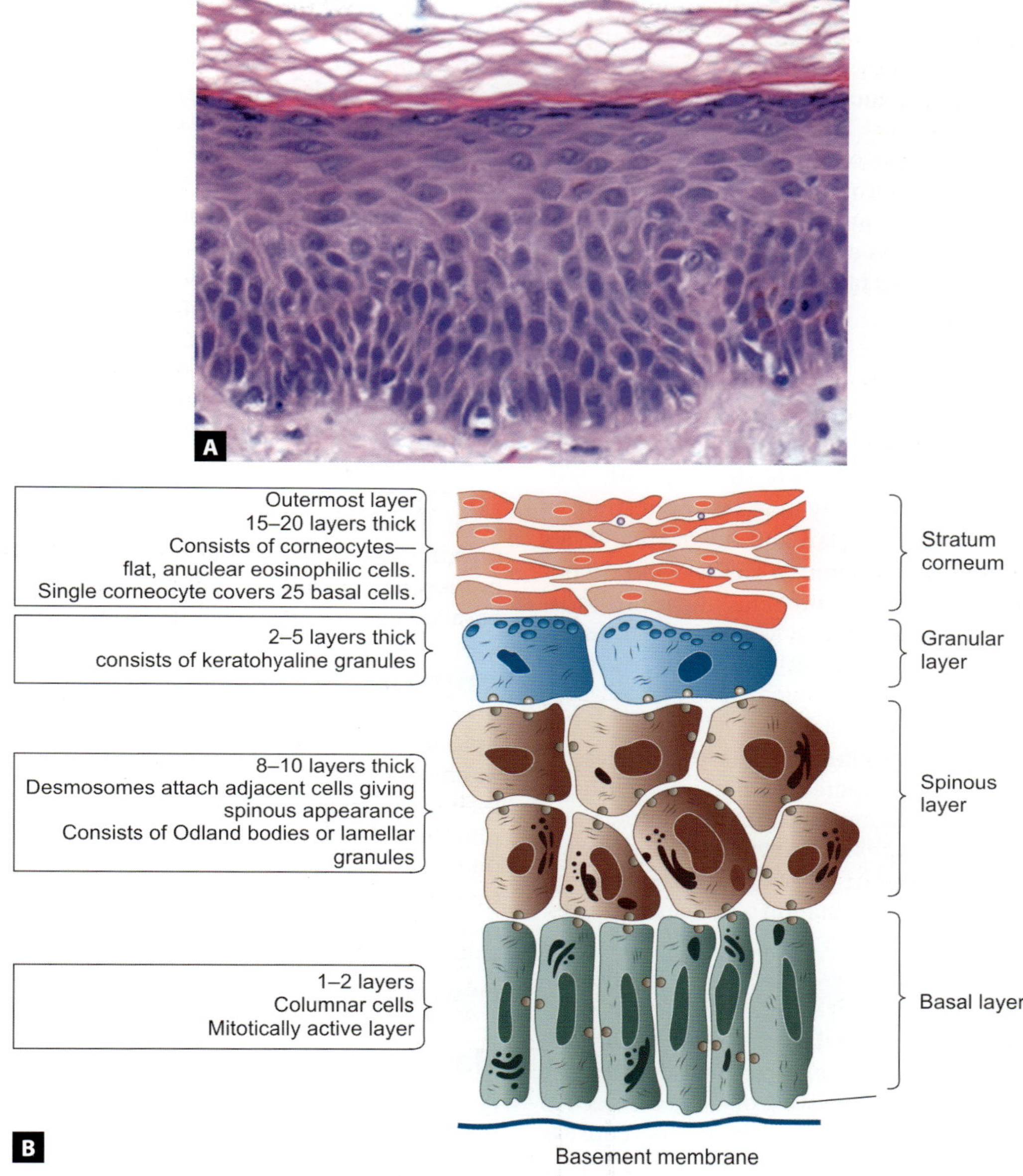

Figs. 2A and B: (A) Structure of epidermis: Uppermost layer—stratum corneum, stratum granulosum, stratum spinosum, stratum basalis; (B) Layers of the epidermis.

cells, primarily function to produce a pigment, melanin. Melanin accumulates in organelles called melanosomes that are incorporated into dendrites anchoring the melanosomes, which are transferred into the surrounding keratinocytes. The ratio of melanocytes to keratinocytes is approximately 1:36, and may vary in different regions like hair and exposed skin. Absolute numbers of melanosomes are the same among the sexes and various races. Differing pigmentation among individuals is related to melanosome size, amount of melanin and its aggregation pattern, rather than cell number.[2]

Skin is thickest on the palms and soles of the feet (1.5 mm thick), while the thinnest skin is present on the eyelids and in the postauricular region (0.05 mm). Dermal thickness too varies in different parts of face: eyelid (5-6 mm), cheek (1.0-2.0 mm), and forehead 2.0 mm (nose 2.0 mm). Male skin is generally thicker than female skin in all anatomic locations. Children have relatively thin skin, and likewise elderly people too have thin tskin. This thinning with aging is primarily a dermal change, with the loss of elastic fibers, epithelial appendages and ground substance, though epidermis too undergoes some thinning.[3]

Applied Anatomy

- Knowledge of cell turnover helps to understand the principle of several procedures, such as chemical peels and laser resurfacing.

- Knowledge of the barrier in skin is important for application of topical preparations.
- Cell adhesion and renewal play an important role in several treatments, such as resurfacing and post-resurfacing procedures.
- Knowledge of thickness of skin in different areas is vital in ensuring optimum choice of treatments and outcomes after such treatments. Levels of peels are determined by thickness and penetration of different ablative lasers too varies in depth.

SKIN TYPES

Depending on tanning and burning responses, six types of skin have been recognized by Fitzpatrick and Parrish scale (Table 2). They also correlate roughly with skin color and have been used widely in assessing responses to resurfacing techniques. Indian and Asian skin varies greatly in color, presents in different shades, and do not always conform accurately to this classification. Most Indians and Asians belong to type 3–5 of Fitzpatrick scale.[5]

Applied Anatomy

Excessive stimulation of melanocytes in the process of wound healing can lead to increased melanin synthesis resulting in hyperpigmentation—a common complication of all resurfacing procedures in brown skin. Hence, it is important to prime the skin with sun protection and depigmenting creams before initiation of such procedures.

DERMIS

The dermis is composed of two layers: (1) the superficial papillary dermis and (2) the deeper reticular dermis. The papillary dermis is thinner, consisting of loose connective tissue containing capillaries. The reticular dermis consists of thicker collagen fibers, elastic fibers, larger blood vessels and other appendages. There is a network of closely interlaced elastic fibers, and coarse bundles of collagen fibers arranged in layers parallel to the surface. The reticular layer also contains resident cells, such as fibroblasts, nerve endings, lymphatics and epidermal appendages.

Another important component of the dermis is the ground substance, an amorphous material that fills spaces between the fibrillar and cellular components of the dermis, imparting turgidity and resilience. The dermal matrix consists of glycosaminoglycans (mainly hyaluronic acid and dermatan sulfate) and glycoproteins. With aging, there is a decrease in these substances and the synthetic variant of hyaluronic acid is widely used as a filler in rejuvenation treatments.

The fibroblast is the major cell type of the dermis. These cells produce and secrete procollagen and elastic fibers. These collagen fibers provide tensile strength and are important in wound healing. Collagen constitutes 70% of the weight of the dermis. Elastic fibers constitute less than 1% of the weight of the dermis, but play an important functional role in defining elasticity of skin. Both tensile strength and elasticity are important concepts in excisions and wound healing.

Fibronectin, the major filamentous glycoprotein component of the dermal matrix, is also produced by the fibroblasts. Fibronectin ensheaths collagen and elastin bundles and also helps in attachment of keratinocytes to the basal lamina, a role which is important in wound healing.[6]

EPIDERMAL APPENDAGES

Epidermal appendages are derived from ectoderm as epidermal downgrowths during embryonic stage. It includes eccrine and apocrine glands with their ducts and pilosebaceous unit comprising sebaceous gland and hair, they all act as reservoir of epidermis. The keratinocytes from the adnexa migrate to the skin surface and cause re-epithelialization after an injury. Injury over the face heals faster when compared to back, vowing to the presence of more adnexal structures on the face.

Hair Follicle

Embryologically, hair is derived from both epidermis and dermis. They are distributed all over the body surface in varying density with most numerous on the scalp and face and absent on the palms, soles, dorsa of the terminal phalanges, labia minora, clitoris and glans penis.

Types of Hair

- Lanugo hair (Latin: Lana-wool): Seen in fetus; they are soft, fine and lightly pigmented.

Table 2: Fitzpatrick skin types.

Skin types	*I*	*II*	*III*	*IV*	*V*	*VI*
Skin color	Pale white or freckled skin	White skin	Olive skin	Light brown	Bark brown	Black
Tanning ability	Always burns, never tans	Burns easily, tans poorly	Mild burn, gradually tans	Burns minimally, tans easily	Rarely burns, tans easily	Never burns, always tans
Hair	Red, blonde	Blonde, red, light brown	Dark blonde	Brown, dark brown	Dark brown	Black
Eyes	Blue, gray, green	Blue, gray, green, hazel	Brown, blue, gray, green, hazel	Hazel, brown	Brown	Brown

Table 3: Three phases of hair cycle.

Phase	*Description*	*Duration*	*Percentage of hair*
Anagen	Active growth phase	3–5 years	84%
Catagen	Regression phase	3 weeks	2%
Telogen	Resting phase	3 months	14%

- Vellus hair (Latin: Vellus-fleece): The fine hair that cover most of the body of youngsters and adults.
- Terminal hair: Long coarse pigmented hairs with larger diameters, distributed over the eyebrows, eyelashes, scalp, beard, axillae and pubis. Terminal hair are the only hair to possess a medulla.

Human hair growth is cyclical and shedding is asynchronous. Hair cycle has three phases and is affected by various endogenous and exogenous factors (Table 3).

At any given point of time, follicles are found in all three phases of hair growth. This is extremely important for laser hair removal, because follicles in the anagen phase are susceptible to destruction, whereas resting follicles are more resistant. This explains why multiple treatments of an area may be necessary to ensure adequate hair removal. The intervals at which laser has to be performed depends on the length of the anagen phase which would vary from area to area.[7]

Hair follicles show considerable morphological and functional heterogeneity. Hairs differ from site to site in shaft length, thickness, curl, color and androgen sensitivity. Hair grows on an average 0.4 mm per day.[8] Terminal hairs grow longer and diameter exceeds 0.03 mm, whereas villous hairs diameter is less than 0.003 mm. In androgenetic alopecia, there is miniaturization of hair with the formation of villous-like hair which are depigmented, small and measure less than 0.003 mm in diameter. The scalp hair of white people is round whereas in black it is oval and has curvature just above the bulb which causes hair to curl. Caucasian hair follicles are oriented obliquely to the skin surface, whereas the hair follicles of black skin are oriented almost parallel to the skin surface. Asians have vertically oriented follicles that produce straight hairs. These anatomic variations are an important consideration in avoiding alopecia when making incisions in the scalp. Hair color depends on the degree of melanization and distribution of melanosomes within the hair shaft. Melanosomes are large in blacks and small and aggregated in whites. Red hair is characterized by spherical melanosomes. Melanocytes are decreased in gray hair.

Androgens are responsible for the follicular heterogeneity. Follicles over the body are either very sensitive (axilla and inguinal hair), mildly sensitive (beard hair), or insensitive to androgens (eyebrow).

Hair bulge is now known to be an important site for biotechnologist; stem cells are now produced from hair bulb and have great importance in future in organ transplant and artificial skin production.

Hair naturally grows in 1–4 hair follicular groupings called follicular units. This arrangement has become the basis of follicular unit transplantation, which is the redistribution of naturally occurring follicular groupings from the occipital donor region into the bald region of the recipient sites.[9,10]

Sebaceous Glands

Sebaceous glands are derived embryologically from upper portion of hair follicle as an outgrowth. It is a lipid producing gland that arises from the hair follicle at the junction of infundibulum and the isthmus. Sebaceous glands are associated with hair follicles all over the body. A sebaceous gland and the associated hair follicle are termed as pilosebaceous unit. The sebaceous glands exude lipids by disintegration of entire cells, a process known as holocrine secretion. Sebaceous glands of various sizes are distributed over the entire surface of the body with the exception of palms, soles and the dorsa of the feet. The glands may also be found in certain non-hairy sites, including the eyelids (meibomian glands), the nipples (Montgomery's glands), buccal mucosa and vermillion border of the lip (Fordyce spots) and around the genitals (Tyson's glands).[4]

Although sebaceous glands are well developed at birth, they regress soon and mature at puberty under the influence of androgens. Acne and acne form eruptions are common during this age. The hair and the sebaceous glands and the adipose cells are the site for the skin stem cells. This can be utilized for the development of stem cell therapy in dermatology.

Sweat Glands

There are thought to be over 2.5 million on the skin surface and they are present over the majority of the body. They are located within the dermis and are composed of coiled tubes, which secrete a watery substance. They are classified into two different types: (1) Eccrine and (2) apocrine.

Eccrine Sweat Glands

They are the only true sweat glands. Eccrine sweat glands are composed of a secretory portion, an intradermal duct and an upper intraepidermal part, called acrosyringium. The acrosyringium has a unique symmetrical and helicoidal course. Eccrine glands are found all over the skin especially on the palms, soles, axillae and forehead with exception of oral lips, clitoris, labia minora and external auditory canals.[4] Eccrine glands play a major role in thermoregulation and electrolyte balance. They are under psychological and thermal control. Sympathetic (cholinergic) nerve fibers innervate eccrine glands. A well-acclimatized person can perspire as much as several liters per hour and 10 L/day. In addition to secreting water and electrolytes, the sweat gland excretes heavy metals, drugs and organic compounds, and macromolecules.

Apocrine Glands

Apocrine glands are larger, the ducts of which empty out into the hair follicles. They are present in the axillae, anogenital region, areolae, periumbilical region, external auditory canals (ceruminous glands) and on the eyelids (Moll's glands). [4] They become active at puberty, producing an odorless protein-rich secretion which when acted upon by skin bacteria gives out a characteristic odor. These glands are under the control of sympathetic (adrenergic) nerve fibers.

BLOOD AND LYMPHATIC VESSELS

The dermis receives a rich blood supply through two intercommunicating plexuses. Branches from superficial artery plexus present at the junction of papillary and reticular dermis form capillary loops in the papillae of the dermis, each with a single loop of capillary vessels, one arterial and one venous. The veins drain into mid-dermal and subcutaneous venous networks. Dilatation or constriction of these capillary loops plays a direct role in thermoregulation of the skin. Lymphatic drainage of the skin occurs through abundant lymphatic meshes that originate in the papillae and feed into larger lymphatic vessels that drain into regional lymph nodes.[4]

NERVE SUPPLY

The skin has rich innervations, with the hands, face and genitalia having the highest density of nerves. Pain, itch and temperature sensation is detected by free sensory nerve ending. Pressure and vibration sensation is mediated by Pacinian corpuscles and touch sensation is by Meissner's corpuscles present in the dermis. The autonomic nervous system supplies the motor innervation of the skin: Adrenergic fibers innervate blood vessels, hair erector muscles and apocrine glands, while cholinergic fibers innervate eccrine sweat glands. Cutaneous nerves follow the route of blood vessels to the skin. The area supplied by a single spinal nerve, or single segment of the spinal cord, is termed as dermatome. Adjacent dermatomes may overlap considerably and are of importance to note when performing field blocks with local anesthesia.[4]

To have excellent cosmetic results, sound knowledge of surgical anatomy of skin is must. It will also help in reducing complications during or after the dermatosurgery. Important anatomical landmarks, anatomical relations and points are considered, which will help in excellent results and minimize complications.

REFERENCES

1. Chu DH. Structure and development of skin. In: Wolff K, Goldsmith LA, Katz SI, Gilcrest BA, Paller AS, Leffell DJ (Eds). Fitzpatrick's Dermatology in General Medicine, 7th edition. New York: McGraw Hill; 2007;pp. 57-72.
2. McGrath JA, Uitto J. Structure and function of the skin. In: Griffiths C, Barker J, Bleiker T, Chalmers R, Creamer D (Eds). Rook's Textbook of Dermatology, 9th ednition. Oxford: Blackwell Publishing; 2016;pp. 2.1-2.48.
3. McGrath JA, Eady RAJ, Pope FM. Anatomy and organization of human skin. In: Burns T, Breathnach S, Cox N, Griffiths C (Eds). Rook's Textbook of Dermatology, 7th edition. Oxford: Blackwell Publishing; 2004;pp. 3.1-3.84.
4. Jakubovic HR, Ackerman AB. Structure and function of skin: Development, morphology, and physiology. In: Moschella SL, Hurley HR (Eds). Dermatology, 3rd edition. Philadelphia: WB Saunders; 1992;3-87.
5. Sachdeva S. Fitzpatrick skin typing: applications in dermatology. Indian J Dermatol Venereol Leprol. 2009;75:93-6.
6. Chu DH. Structure and development of skin. In: Wolf K, Goldsmith LA, Katz SI, Gilcrest BA, Paller AS, Lefell DJ (Eds). Fitzpatricks Dermatology in General Medicine, 7th edition. New York: Mc Graw Hill; 2007. pp. 5772.
7. Prost-Squarcioni C. Histology of skin and hair follicle. Med Sci. 2006;22:131-7.
8. Thappa DM. Structure and functions of the skin. In: Valia RG, Valia AR, (Eds). Textbook and Atlas of Dermatology, 3rd edition. Mumbai: Bhalani Publishing House 2008; pp. 7-40.
9. Savant SS, Gore D. Applied anatomy for dermatosurgeons. In: Savant SS, AtalShah R, Gore D (Eds). Textbook and Atlas of Dermatosurgery and Cosmetology, 1st edition. Mumbai: ASCAD; 1998. pp. 311.
10. Robinson JK. Anatomy for procedural dermatology. In: Robinson JK, Hanke CW, Siegel DM, Fratila A (Eds). Surgery of the Skin: Procedural Dermatology, 3rd edition. Philadelphia: Elsevier Mosby; 2015. pp. 227.

Chapter 2

Applied Surgical Anatomy in Relation to Facial Rejuvenation

Mukta Sachdev, Sunaina Hameed, Keerthi Velugotla

Key Messages

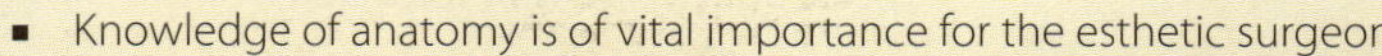

- Knowledge of anatomy is of vital importance for the esthetic surgeon.
- Different concepts such as cosmetic units, relaxed skin tension lines (RSTLs), subcutaneous muscular aponeurosis, angiosomes should be understood properly.
- Knowledge of vascular supply and nerve supply will prevent serious surgical events.

INTRODUCTION

Surgical techniques for facial rejuvenation have evolved tremendously over the last few decades. This is partly due to the better understanding of the relevant anatomy of the head and neck area. Enhanced surgical options are now available that have expounded on previous work on the geographic composition of the face and the changes they undergo with ageing. Proper surgical rejuvenation of the face can restore the original anatomy, giving the face a natural younger appearance that reflects the patient's appearance prior to the extended effects of gravity. A thorough familiarity with the surgical anatomy allows the surgeon freedom in performing surgical and semi-surgical procedures in a safe and efficient manner. On the other hand, unfamiliarity with the facial anatomy can limit a surgeon's confidence, his technique and ability to manipulate tissue, which can affect the surgical outcome.

An understanding of anatomy is also important to appreciate the likely spread of infection. It is also important to be aware of the variations in facial anatomy, especially in relation to certain facial muscles, when treating all esthetic patients.

Regional Anatomy

Facial anatomy can be divided into 13 anatomic regions (Fig. 1): (1) Frontal region, (2) Orbital region, (3) Infraorbital region, (4) Zygomatic region, (5) Nasal region, (6) Lips and mouth, (7) Mental branches region, (8) Buccal region, (9) Parotidomasseteric region, (10) Auricular region, (11) Temporal region, (12) Submental region and (13) Submandibular region.

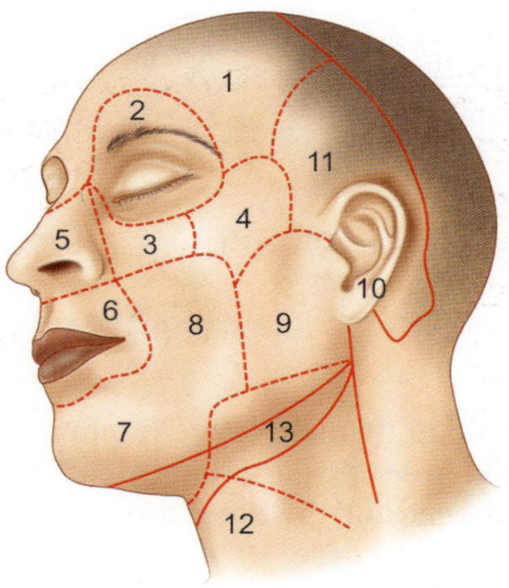

Fig. 1: Regions of the face: (1) Frontal region; (2) Orbital region; (3) Infraorbital region; (4) Zygomatic region; (5) Nasal region; (6) Lips and mouth; (7) Mental branches region; (8) Buccal region; (9) Parotido-masseterical region; (10) Auricular region; (11) Temporal region; (12) Submental region and (13) Submandibular region.

Cosmetic Units of the Face

The face can be divided into cosmetic units, also known as facial esthetic units (Fig. 2).[1] These cosmetic units share similar color, texture, thickness and mobility of the skin.

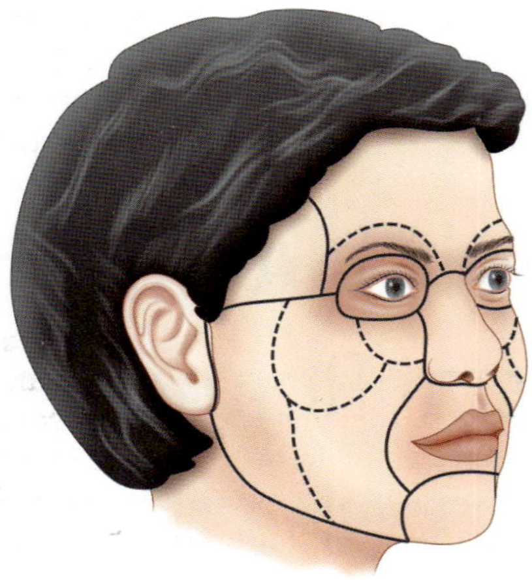

Fig. 2: Cosmetic units of the face.

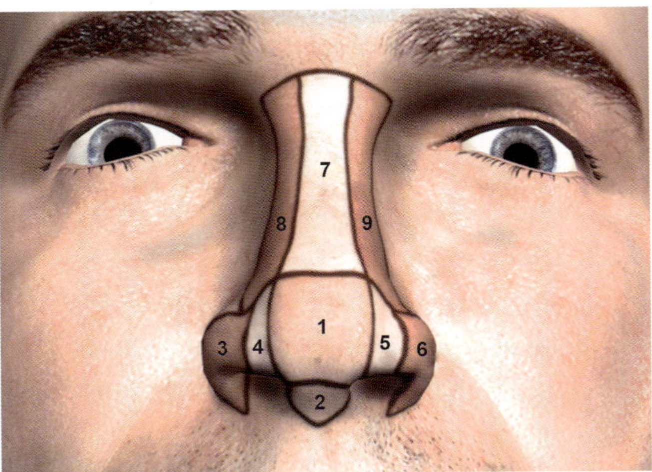

Fig. 3: Cosmetic units of nose: (1) Tip subunit; (2) Columellar subunit; (3) Right alar base subunit; (4) Right alar side wall subunit; (5) Left alar side wall subunit; (6) Left alar base subunit; (7) Dorsal subunit; (8) Right dorsal side wall subunit; (9) Left dorsal side wall subunit.

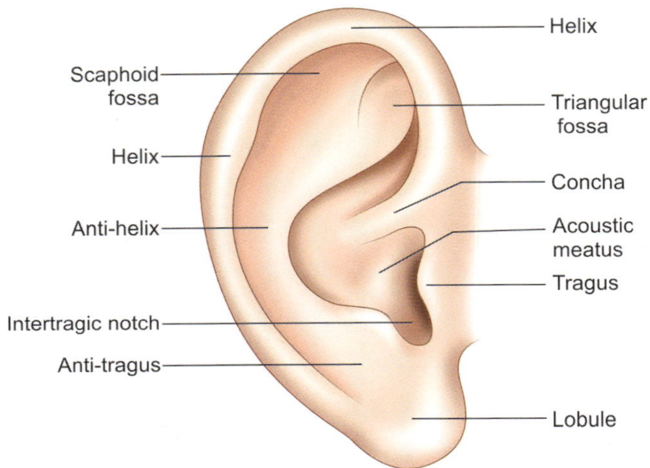

Fig. 4: Ear surface concha, antitragus, acoustic meatus.

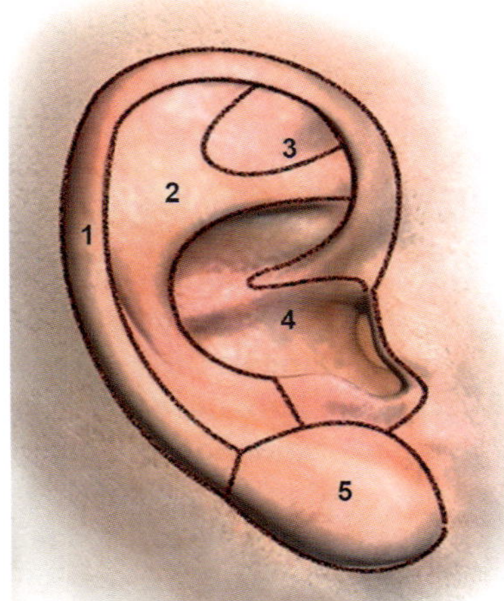

Fig. 5: Subunits: 1- Helix, 2-Antihelix, 3-Triangular fossa, 4- Acoustic meatus, 5-Lobule.

These cosmetic units include the forehead, the temple, the cheeks, the nose, the periorbital area, the lips, and the chin.[2] The forehead and the cheek have additional areas of variation in skin thickness.

This principle of facial units has been refined in recent years with the subunit principle.[3] Subunits are topographic units with a predictable contour from person-to-person. By placing incisions at the boundaries of these subunits, final scars are visually minimized because the eye is expecting a contour change.

Nose

Nose is the most prominent part in midface and even small alterations are noticed easily. It is important to know that skin is thinnest at rhinion and thickness increases toward the tip of nose. Nose tip and ala shows thick sebaceous skin. The nose is a three-dimensional organ and can be divided into nine subunits (Fig. 3). This concept is relevant in different procedures such as reconstruction and resurfacing. Venous drainage communicates with cavernous sinus via ophthalmic veins, ethmoid veins connects with the superior sagittal sinus. Rarely ascending infection can cause thrombosis in these sinuses.

Adequate antibiotic coverage must be given when procedure is done in this area.

Ear

The external ear is composed of skin and cartilage with the supporting nerves and blood vessels. The auricular cartilage provides a framework for the entire ear except the lobule. The landmarks on the ear are shown in Figures 4 and 5.

During surgeries on the ear, the following should be noted:

- Resection in pre- and posterior auricular areas can cause sensory denervation of ear.

- Field block of the skin around periphery of the auricle provides adequate anesthesia.
- Deep infiltration just in front of the ear may result in temporary paralysis of the facial nerve.
- Deep freezing during cryosurgery should be avoided as it can lead to necrosis of the cartilage.
- Strict asepsis must be observed to avoid perichondrial infection.

Lips

It is an expressive and visible structure in facial anatomy and has profound impact in social life, which explains the popularity of lip enhancement.

Size (full or thin), curvature (sinuous or straight) and eversion (turning out or in) are important characteristics which need to be assessed in lips. The upper lip extends from the base of the nose superiorly to the nasolabial folds laterally, and to the free edge of the vermilion border inferiorly. The lower lip extends from the superior free vermilion edge superiorly, to the commissures laterally, and the mandible inferiorly. In the upper lip vermilion-skin border, two paramedian elevations of the vermilion form the cupid bow. The philtrum is located between the paramedian elevations of the upper lip vermilion and the columella above. The labiomental crease passes horizontally in an inverted U-shape across the lower lip, which intraorally corresponds to the depth of the gingivolabial sulcus (Fig. 6).

Architecture of the Ideal Lip

Though there are significant variations, an ideal upper lip projects approximately 2–3 mm beyond the lower lip. The upper lip forms about one-thirds of the total lip volume while the lower lip forms about two-thirds of the total lip volume. Other desirable features include a well-defined philtrum, cupid's bow and philtral columns (Fig. 7). These concepts are important during counseling for lip augmentation.

Eye

The eyelids are a complex structure with multiple subunits. Palpebral (Pretarsal and preseptal subunits) and orbital (which encircles the eyebrow and extends to the junction of the cheek). Additional components of the eyelid include the superior palpebral fold, the palpebral fissure, the medial limbus and the medial canthus (Fig. 8).

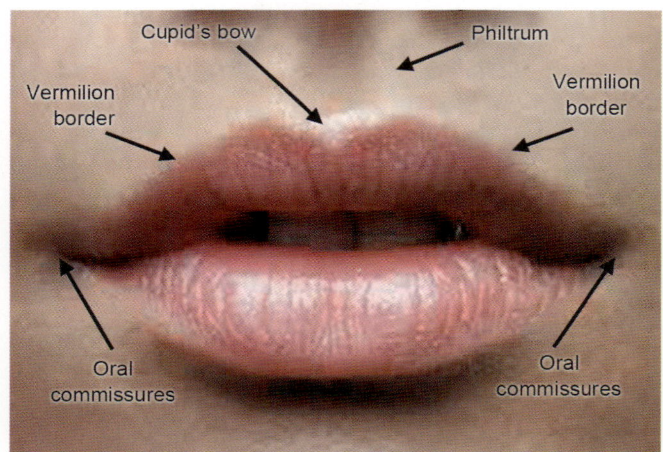

Fig. 6: Lip structure.

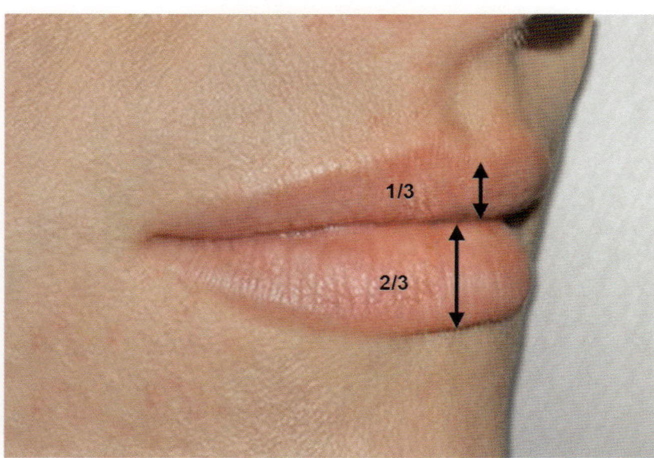

Fig. 7: Lip architecture.

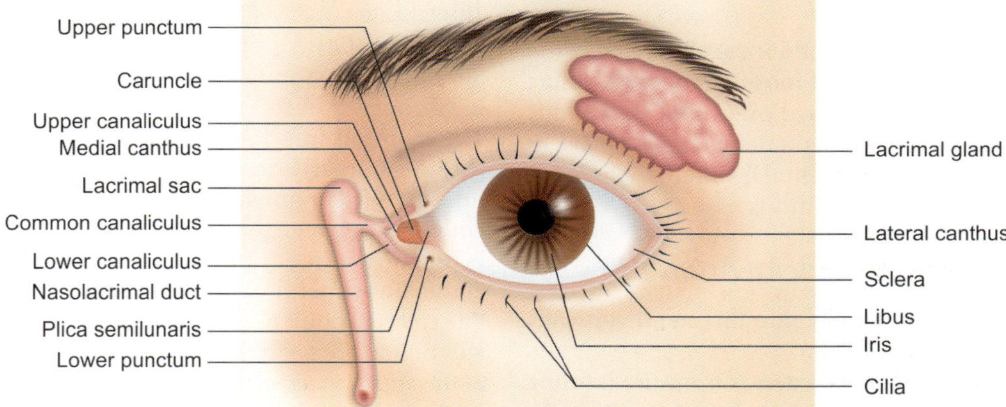

Fig. 8: Anatomy of eyelids.

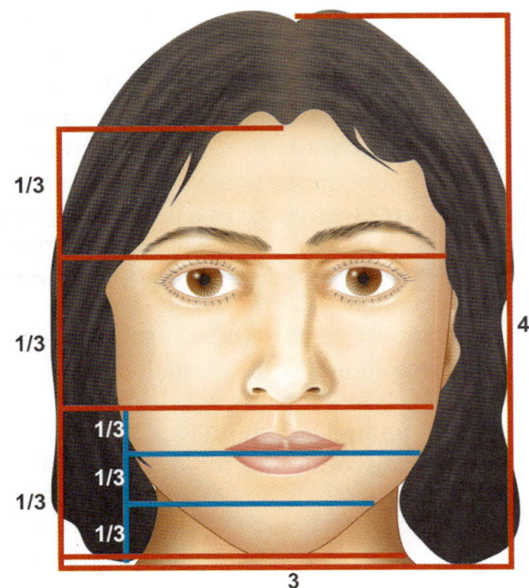

Fig. 9: Horizontal divisions of face, dividing it into upper, middle and lower part.

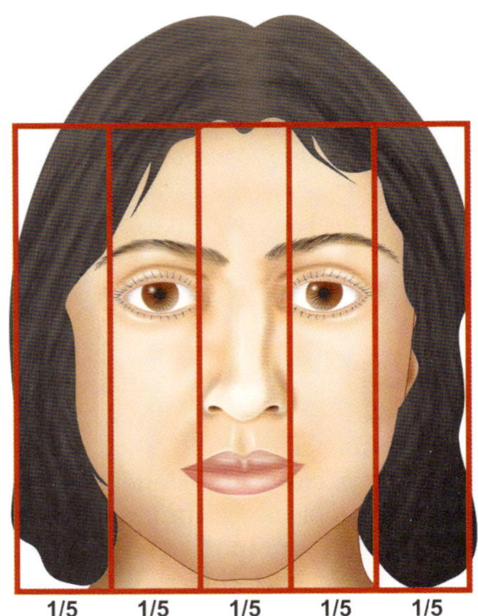

Fig. 10: Vertical division of the face.

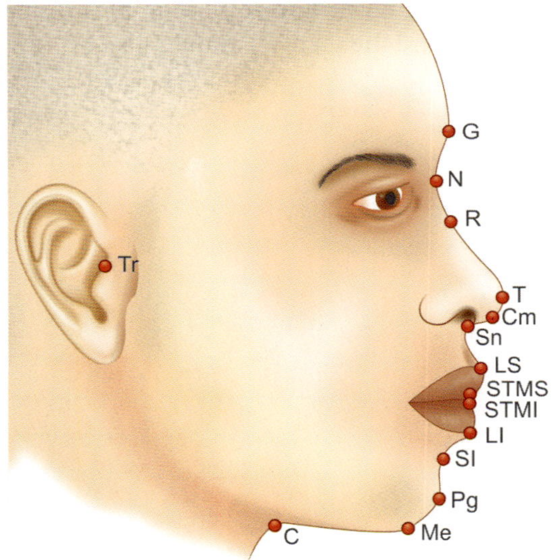

Fig. 11: Important soft tissue cephalometric points of the face (*see* text for abbreviations).

The skin of the eyelids is the thinnest of the body. The subcutaneous tissue consists of loose connective tissue. Fat is very sparse in preseptal and preorbital skin and is absent from pretarsal skin. Subcutaneous tissue is absent over the medial and lateral palpebral ligaments, where the skin adheres to the underlying fibrous tissue.

Facial Proportions and Facial Analysis

The face is divisible horizontally into three and vertically into five.

The upper horizontal third extends from the hairline to the glabella, the middle third extends to the subnasale, and the lower third extends to the menton. The lower third of the face may be subdivided further into thirds, from the subnasale to stomion, stomion to mentolabial sulcus, mentolabial sulcus to menton[3] (Fig. 9).

The face can also be divided into fifths based on the lateral projection of the helix to the lateral canthus, lateral canthus to medial canthus, intercanthal distance and so forth (Fig. 10). The face is usually 5 eye widths across.[3] The width to height ratio of the head is typically 3:4.

Soft tissue cephalometric analysis is important in planning and evaluating most facial reconstructive and cosmetic work. The major soft tissue cephalometric points are described in Figure 11.

The glabella (G) is the most prominent point in the midsagittal plane of the forehead. The nasion (N) is the deepest depression at the root of the nose in the midsagittal plane. The rhinion (R) represents the junction of the bony and cartilaginous dorsum and is usually the maximum on the nose. The tip (T) is the most anterior projection of the nose. The columella point (Cm) is the most anterior soft tissue point on the columella. The subnasale (Sn) is the junction of the columella with the upper cutaneous lip. The labrale superius (LS) represents the mucocutaneous junction of the upper lip at the midsagittal plane. Similarly, the stomion superioris (STMS) represents the lower border of the upper lip at the midsagittal plane. The stomion inferioris (STMI) and the labrale inferius (LI) are similarly described for the lower lip. The sulcus inferioris (SI) represents the deepest depression in the concavity between the lip and the chin. The pogonion (Pg) is the most anterior point on the chin. The menton (Me) is the lowest point on the contour of the soft tissue chin. The cervical point (C) represents the junction between the submental area and the neck. The tragion (Tr) is the point at the superior aspect of the tragus.[3]

Crumley and Lancer described appropriate projection of the nose and nasal tip.[4,5] A ratio of 5:4:3 should apply,

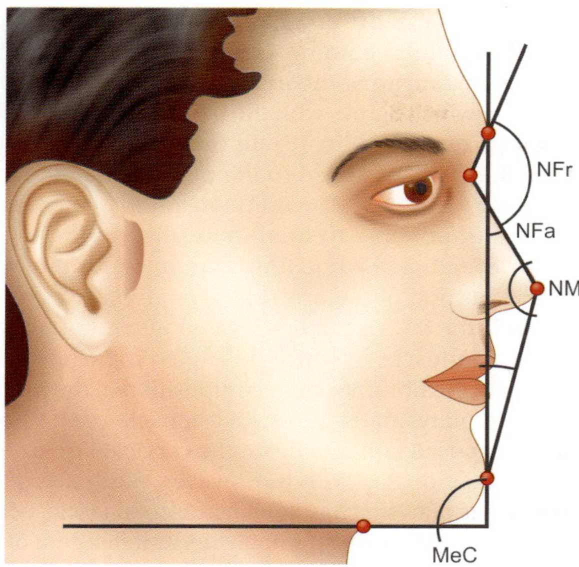

Fig. 12: Esthetic triangle of Powell and Humphreys (*see* text for abbreviations).

respectively, to a line from the nasion to the nasal tip, a line from the nasion to the alar crease, and a perpendicular line joining the other two.

The Frankfort horizontal plane is defined as the horizontal line extending from the superior border of the external auditory canal to the inferior border of the infraorbital rim.[3] The Hinderer's lines are two intersecting lines, one drawn from the nasal ala to the tragus, and the other drawn from the lateral canthus of the eye to the corner of the lips. The area in the upper outer quadrant of this intersection is defined as the malar prominence.[3]

The golden ratio denoted by the symbol phi (ϕ), also known as divine proportion is term used in esthetics in relation to ideal human beauty. Proportions in the face which are referred to as being beautiful are intimately related to golden ratio.[4,6,7] Marquardt devised a mathematical model (phi mask) using ϕ as the central measurement to map out facial proportions and aesthetically "ideal" shapes and sizes.[8] However, studies suggest the limitations of the use of golden ratio as a parameter in esthetics.[9,10]

The esthetic triangle of Powell and Humphreys allows relative comparisons of the soft tissue profile to be made from a variety of lateral facial representations, including photographs and soft tissue films (Fig. 12). This information is useful when one is using dermal filler implantation for chin or cheek augmentation or for filling the nasion. A vertical line dropped from the glabella to the pogonion defines the vertical anterior facial plane. A line from the nasal tip is then drawn to the nasion. A line from the glabella to the nasion meets this nasal line and creates the nasofrontal angle (NFr). The nasofacial angle (NFa) is between the anterior facial plane and the line tangent to the dorsum of the nose. The nasomental line is drawn from the nasal tip to the pogonion and creates the nasomental angle (NM). A line drawn from the cervical point to the menton intersects the anterior facial plane and creates the mentocervical angle (MeC). In Caucasians, typical "ideal" ranges are nasofacial angle equal to 30–40°, nasomental angle equal to 120–130°, nasofrontal angle equal to 115–130°, mentocervical angle equal to 80–95°. Standard values for other races have not been defined.[3]

Racial differences must be appreciated, especially in relation to nasal anatomy. For instance, the African nose has thicker skin, a smaller nasal spine, and less cartilage support than the Caucasian nose.

Relaxed Skin Tension Lines

Skin is anisotropic, which means skin tension and properties vary in different directions.[3] Although of historical importance, Langer's lines do not correspond to our current understanding of the direction of tension in the skin. Borges (1973) described the relaxed skin tension lines (RSTLs), which are the lines of skin tension present when the skin is in a relaxed state. The lines are parallel to the dermal collagen bundles and perpendicular to muscle contraction. In most cases, the RSTLs follow the wrinkles of the face. However, there are few areas, such as the glabellar creases and the temple, where strong muscle action can create creases in a different direction from that of the RSTLs. For example, in the temple, the RSTLs run approximately vertically rather than horizontally with the "crow's feet".

Experimental studies have demonstrated that it requires as much as twice the tension to close a wound made perpendicular to the RSTLs compared to one made along them.[11] Incisions made parallel to the RSTLs generally heal favorably. The lines of maximal extensibility run perpendicular to the RSTLs and represent the directions in which the skin can be advanced most easily. On the other hand, Langer's lines were determined based on the biopsy procedures on cadavers, and give a worse cosmetic result than with RSTL.

Superficial Musculoaponeurotic System

The superficial musculoaponeurotic system (SMAS) is a continuous fibromuscular layer investing and interlinking the muscles of facial expression.[12] In plastic and reconstructive surgery, a superficial musculoaponeurotic system is generally considered a landmark for subdividing the superficial from the deep region. The first description was published in 1974 by Mitz and Peyronie,[13] who gave a detailed explanation of it within the parotid and cheek region. The SMAS is thought to have multiple fibrous extensions through the different subcutaneous layers to the skin, allowing them to move together as a unit.

The characteristics used by Tessier and his students[14] to describe the SMAS are as follows:

- It divides the subcutaneous fat into two layers
- Fibrous septae extend from the SMAS to the dermis

- Fat without septae lies between the deep facial muscles and the SMAS
- Major vessels and nerves are initially deep to the SMAS and smaller branches perforate it, whereas the subdermal plexus is superficial to it
- The network of the SMAS acts as a distributor of force for the various facial muscles.

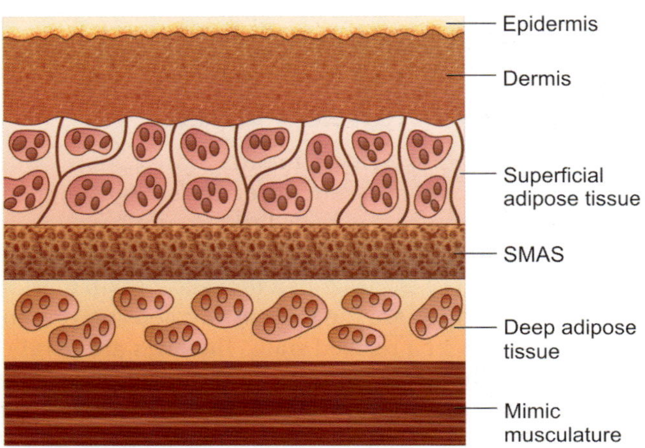

Fig. 13: The SMAS in the parotid and cheek area, in relation to subcutaneous layers are described by Mitz and Peyronie.

However, Gardetto et al.[15] in their study on fetal, neonatal and adult anatomy, concluded that other than the parotid region, no SMAS exists in the buccal, oral and neck region, which agrees with the basic criteria of Tessier, or Mitz and Peyronie (Fig. 13). In the parotid region, the SMAS is thick and attached to the parotid sheath. But it becomes very thin and discontinuous in the cheek area, where it is impossible to identify or dissect it. Toward the lower eyelid, a few fine fibers are in continuity with the lateral portion of the orbicularis oculi muscle. In the upper neck, the SMAS can be elevated in continuity with the platysma muscle, in which it is noted to be muscular, in contrast to the fibromuscular composition in the parotid region. The platysma is a skin-like muscle of the neck, which is proposed either to lie on the cervical fascia, or to come into relationship with it. However, Gardetto's study shows that the platysma has its own muscular fascia, which develops around it during prenatal life, independent of the cervical fascia. The platysma, accompanied by its fascia, divides the subcutaneous tissue at the neck into two layers. Thaller et al.[16] and Jost et al.[17] had described the SMAS as a primitive platysma muscle, being a large muscle sheet that covers the neck and the lower part of the face, which degenerates during evolution and is therefore called the fibrous platysma (Fig. 14).

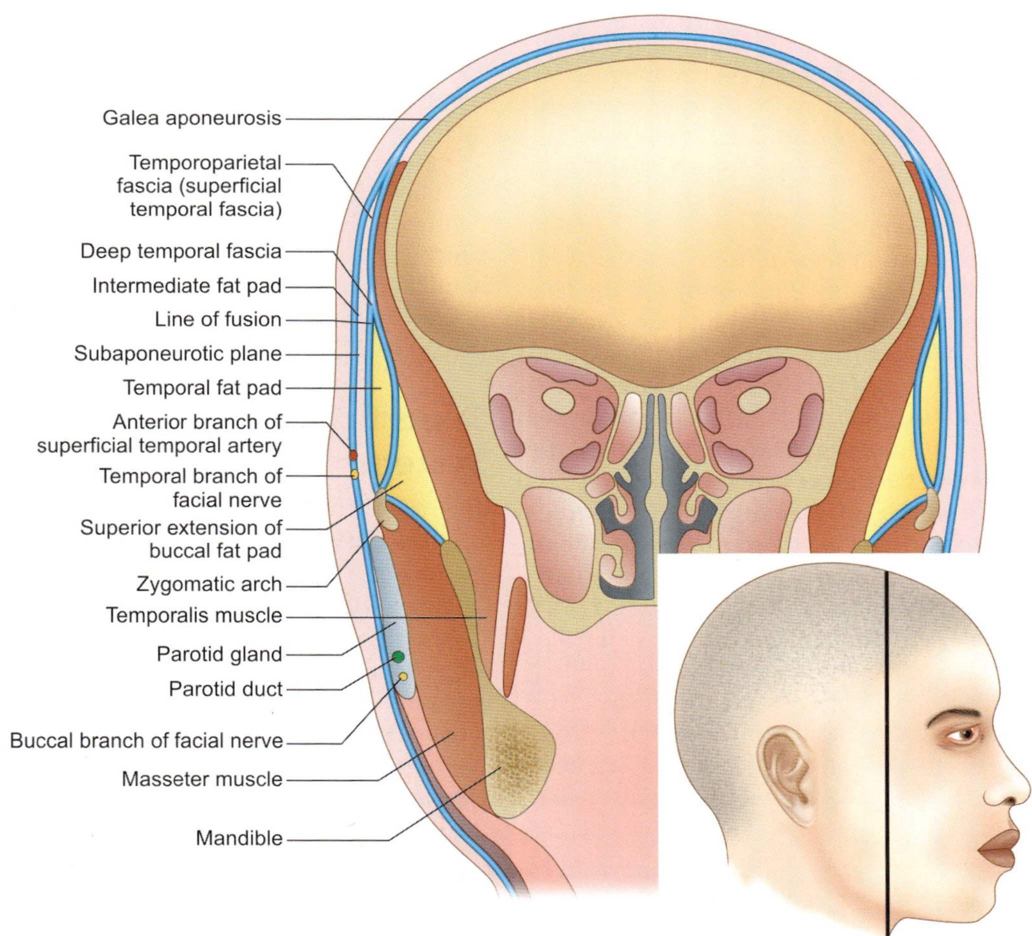

Fig. 14: Full face view of the superficial musculoaponeurotic system (SMAS) on cross-section.

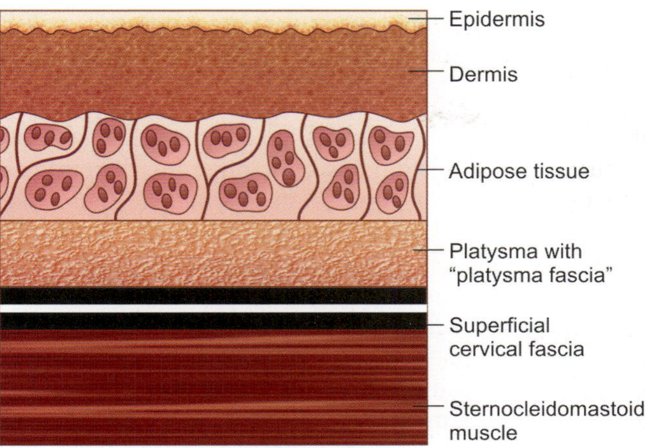

Fig. 15: The subcutaneous layers in the sternocleidomastoid region.

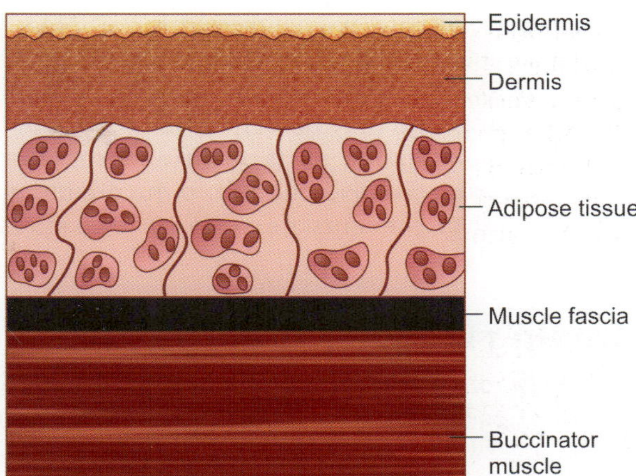

Fig. 16: The subcutaneous layers in the buccal region.

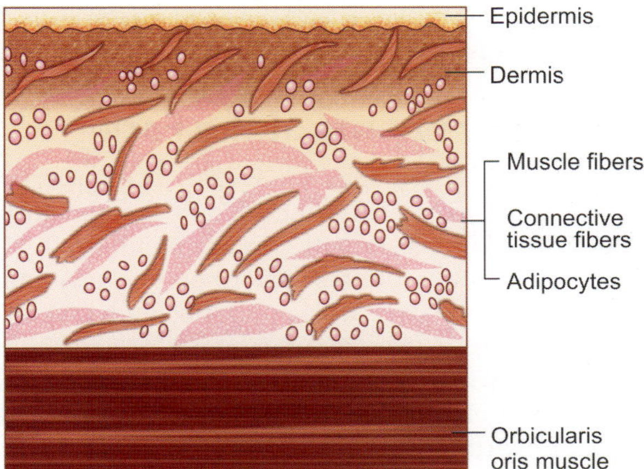

Fig. 17: The subcutaneous layers in the oral region.

There is no evidence of continuity between the SMAS and the temporoparietal fascia.[18] The SMAS above the zygoma is a more substantial layer than the fragile fibrous network seen in the midface. In the scalp, the SMAS is represented by the fibrous galea aponeurotica, which then splits to ensheathe the frontalis, the occipitalis, the procerus, and some of the periauricular muscles. In the region of the lip and nose, a fascial layer does not exist.

Part of the complexity of these fascial layers is the difference in embryologic development between the muscles of the lower face and those of the mid and upper face. Ghassemi et al. describe two variations of SMAS.

Type I SMAS exist in the forehead, parotid, zygomatic, and infraorbital areas is composed of network of small fibrous septae that traverse perpendicularly between fat lobules to the dermis and deeply to the facial muscles or periosteum.

Type II SMAS consists of a dense mesh of collagen, elastic, and muscle fibers and is found medial to the nasolabial fold, in the upper and lower lips.[19]

SMAS in Sternocleidomastoid Region

The platysma is situated directly under the skin, separated from the corium by a narrow space filled with adipose tissue and loose connective tissue. The sternocleidomastoid muscle is situated beneath the platysma and is enclosed by the superficial layer of the cervical fascia. The fascia of the platysma and the sternocleidomastoid muscle glide on a small layer of smooth connective tissue (Fig. 15).[15]

SMAS in the Buccal Region

The muscle fibers from the buccinator muscle intermingle with the orbicularis muscle. In fetal dissection, a thick fat pad is situated between the buccinator muscle and corium. The adipose lobules are separated by strong connective-tissue septa, the fibers of which arise from a thick fascia unsheathing the buccinator muscle (Fig. 16).[8]

SMAS in the Oral Region

The deep fibers of the orbicularis oris insert into the maxilla and mandible and into the skin of the nasal septum. Adjacent to these deep muscle fibers, a broad layer consisting of muscle fibers and connective tissue fibers can be found. Both are intermingled and directly connected to the corium. Groups of adipose tissue cells are embedded in a crisscross network of muscle fibers and corial connective tissue (Fig. 17).[15]

Applied Anatomy

In addition to its usefulness as a deep layer to tighten in aging face surgery, the SMAS serves as a guide to the depth of key neurovascular structures. In the lower face, the facial nerve branches are deep to the SMAS and enter the muscles of facial expression on their undersurface. This is true, with the exception of the deep facial muscles: the levator anguli oris, the buccinator, and the mentalis, which are all innervated on their surface. Similarly, in the lower face, vessels and sensory nerves originate deep to the SMAS and their terminal branches run with it superficially. In the upper face, the important neurovascular structures arise from their deeper origins and course within the SMAS. The infratrochlear and supratrochlear neurovascular pedicles lie within the SMAS over the frontalis muscle.[12] The SMAS as a guiding structure may be helpful in reconstructive surgery for facial palsy or face-lifting procedures. Particularly during the dissection from the preauricular region, the SMAS prevents necrosis in the skin and subcutaneous tissue.[15]

Retaining Ligaments of the Face

There are several very strong retaining ligaments in the face known as fasciocutaneous and osteocutaneous ligaments (Fig. 18).

The fasciocutaneous attachments are multiple and exist at sequential facial planes. These attachments emanate from the dermis and attach to the underlying SMAS. The fasciocutaneous ligaments are particularly strong over the forehead, eyes, nose, lip, and chin areas. They are of intermediate strength over the lateral cheek and neck areas and tend to be relatively loose over the medial cheek and temple areas.[12]

The *osteocutaneous ligaments* are the strongest of the ligament attachments and exist between the periosteum and the overlying skin. These stout ligaments emanate from the periosteum of the zygoma and mandible and are termed the zygomatic cutaneous ligaments (McGregor patch) and the mandibular cutaneous ligaments.[12]

The mandibular ligament arises from the parasymphyseal mandibular body and inserts into the skin inferior to the insertion of the depressor anguli oris (DAO), interdigitating with the platysma, which lies deeper to the DAO.

The fasciocutaneous masseteric ligaments pass from the region of the anterior border of the masseter muscle toward the dermis.

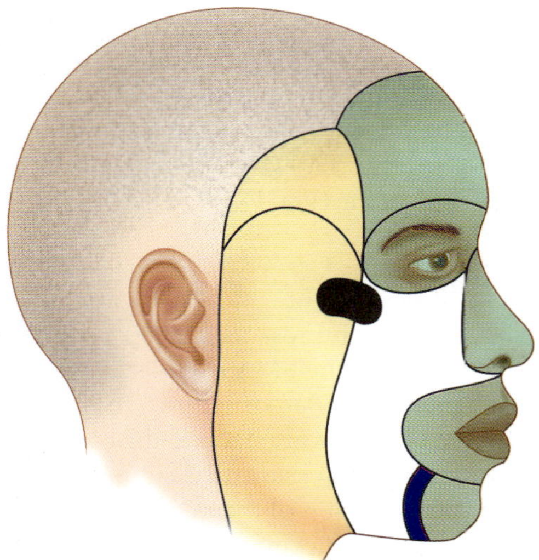

Fig. 18: The retaining ligaments of the face. The fasciocutaneous ligaments are represented by the green, pink and yellow areas, while the osteocutaneous ligaments are in black and blue.

Applied Anatomy

With age, these ligaments become lax, leading to the inferomedial migration of the malar fat pad and formation of the nasolabial fold. Knowledge of retaining ligaments is crucial as the desired aesthetic outcome depends on the surgical release of appropriate ligaments.[20] Their close relation to the facial nerve branches enables the surgeon to avoid accidental nerve injury during aesthetic surgery. The cutaneous insertion of the zygomatic muscles (i.e. levator labii superioris and levator labii anguli oris) determines the nasolabial crease.[21] Conversely, the depressor anguli oris superiorly and the mandibular ligaments inferiorly determine the boundaries of the labiomandibular crease, which similarly is converted into a fold (the jowl) as a result of the laxity of the masseteric ligaments that occur with age.[22] The anterior limit of the jowl is the mandibular ligament. The masseteric ligament also approximates the mid-cheek furrow of ageing and the posterior boundary of the mimetic muscles.[23]

Fat Compartments of the Face

Rohrich et al. noted that fat within the superficial subcutaneous layer of the face is not located in one confluent layer but is actually compartmentalized.[24] The borders of the compartments are formed by fascial septae that travel from the deep fascia or periosteum and insert into the dermis. These compartments provide a new method of viewing the aging face and neck as resulting from variable changes in volume and position in the various compartments.

The *malar fat pad* is composed of three separate compartments: Medial, middle and lateral temporal cheek fat. The forehead is similarly composed of three anatomical units including central, middle and lateral temporal cheek fat. Orbital fat is noted in three compartments determined by septal borders. Jowl fat is the most inferior of the subcutaneous fat compartments. Facial ageing is in part, determined by how these compartments change with age (Fig. 19).[24]

Malar fat compartments: Medial cheek fat is lateral to the nasolabial fold. This compartment is bordered superiorly by the orbicularis retaining ligament and the lateral orbital compartment. Jowl fat lies inferior to this fat compartment.

Middle cheek fat lies superficial in its mid-portion. This fat compartment is found anterior and superficial to the parotid gland. At the superior portion, the zygomaticus major muscle is adherent. The zone where the medial fat abuts with the middle cheek fat corresponds to the location of the parotidomasseteric ligaments. The lateral temporal-cheek compartment lies immediately superficial to the parotid gland and connects the temporal fat to the cervical subcutaneous fat. The lateral temporal-cheek fat pads span the entire face from the forehead to the cervical area.[25]

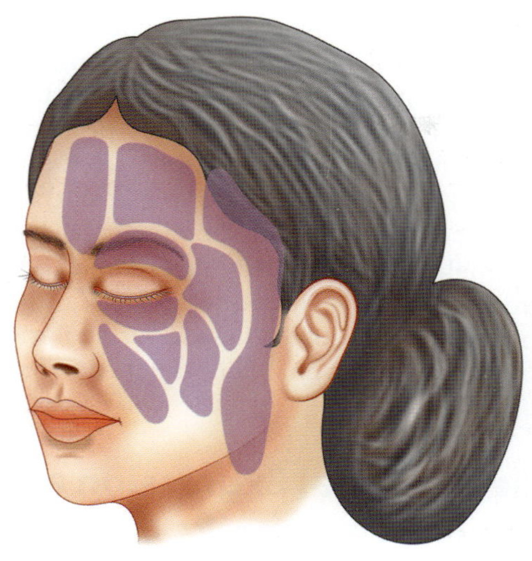

Fig. 19: Fat pads of the face.

A confluence of septa occurs at this location where three compartments meet, and forms a dense adherent zone where the zygomatic ligament has been described.

Forehead and temporal fat compartments: The subcutaneous fat of the forehead is composed of three compartments. The central compartment is located in the midline region of the forehead. The inferior border is at the nasal dorsum. The middle temporal fat compartments lie on either side of the central forehead fat. The inferior border is the orbicularis retaining ligament. The lateral temporal-cheek compartment has been previously described.

Orbital fat compartment: Three subcutaneous fat compartments exist around the eye. The most superior compartment is bounded by the orbicularis retaining ligament as it courses around the superior orbit. The orbicularis retaining ligament is a truly circumferential structure that spans the superior and inferior orbits and blends into the medial and lateral canthi. The inferior orbital fat is a thin, subcutaneous layer that lies immediately below the inferior lid tarsus. Its inferior boundary is the orbicularis retaining ligaments. The superior border of the lateral orbital fat compartment is the inferior temporal septum, the inferior border is the superior cheek septum. The zygomatic major muscle is adherent to this compartment as well, along with the middle cheek fat compartment.

Nasolabial fat compartment: This lies anterior to the medial cheek fat and overlies the jowl fat. The orbicularis retaining ligament is the superior border, and the zygomaticus major muscle is adherent to the inferior border.

Jowl fat compartment: Jowl fat adheres to the depressor anguli oris muscle. The medial boundary of this compartment is the lip depressor muscle, and the inferior boundary is determined by a membranous fusion of the platysma muscle. The fusion point between these two muscles occurs at the region of the mandibular retaining ligament.

Applied Anatomy

Volume loss in the fat compartments occurs with ageing, and leads to changes in facial contour, including deepening of the jowl and the nasolabial fat. The zygomatic major muscle provides an important area of fixation of three different fat compartments, and surgical dissection becomes much easier once this muscle is transitioned.

Ligaments may be formed where septal barriers and fat compartments meet. This is apparent in the zygomatic area, where the inferior orbital, lateral orbital, and middle cheek compartments meet. This is a highly vascular area that corresponds to the zygomatic ligament. This fusion area represents an area of risk to the facial nerve, due to the tethering function where several compartments merge. Similar fusion planes occur in many regions of the face, both in transverse and vertical directions. For instance, in the area beneath the ear, the lateral temporal cheek fat compartment abuts with the postauricular fat compartment. The greater auricular nerve is at risk by improper transition of the subcutaneous plane at this point. Also, the transition zones between the subcutaneous fat compartments are highly vascular.

The deep layers of facial fat include the suborbicularis, the retro-orbicularis, and buccal fat pads. This deep fat is required for the anteriorly projecting midface. A fat compartment surrounds the levator anguli muscle, and there exists a fat compartment beneath the lip levator muscles. Descent of this fat compartment leads to marionette lines. A tenet of facial anatomy is that fat is noted both above and below most facial muscles, probably to facilitate the necessary gliding mechanism.[24]

Knowledge of the fat compartments gives a better insight into mid and lower face ageing. Malar fat pad ptosis occurs with age, which leads to a cascade of changes, like the deepening of the nasolabial fold, jowl prominence, and diminished midface projection. It also allows excess traction to be placed in the lower eyelid.[22]

Buccal fat pad: It is positioned between the masseter muscle anteriorly and the buccinator muscle posteriorly. Therefore in order to approach the buccal fat pad through an intraoral approach, the buccinator muscle must be pierced. It is a unique form of fat in a three-dimensional structure called syssarcosis, whose main function is to provide a surface for the gliding motion of the muscles of mastication.[26] It was first accurately described by Bichat in 1801. Its weight is approximately 8 grams and does not vary with the overall degree of adiposity of the subject. It has three main extensions: Buccal, pterygoid, and temporal.

The buccal extension is the most important from an esthetic standpoint. It extends anteroinferiorly from the main body in a globular mass with a convex lateral face, covering most of the buccinator. Two surgically vulnerable structures, the facial nerve and the parotid duct, lie in close proximity to the buccal extension. The buccal rami of the facial nerve that exit the anterior border of the parotid gland lie on the surface of the masseter muscle, tightly bound by the thin sheet of parotid masseteric fascia. An extension of this fascia envelops the buccal fat pad; thus, the buccal extension has facial nerve fibers immediately lateral to it. The parotid duct runs immediately superior to the buccal extension before diving through the fibers of the buccinator to enter the oral cavity.[26] The blood supply of the buccal fat pad is from the branches of the facial artery. The nerve supply is from the buccal branch of the mandibular nerve. The buccal fat pad may be used for free fat grafts, or can be removed incrementally to effect a change in cheek contour.

The surgical approach may be external or through an intraoral approach. The buccal rami of the facial nerve are at risk in an external approach.

Fat Compartments of the Neck

There are two distinctly separate depots of fat in the submental region of the neck that must be taken into consideration when planning rejuvenation procedures for the ageing neck. *The submental fat pad (or submandibular fat compartment)* is the more superficial one, which lies directly anterior to the platysma in the subcutaneous plane. The anterior boundary of this compartment, previously without name, has been labeled the "submental septum". The posterior boundary of the submental fat compartment is created by a septum that arises from the platysma at a point superficial to the hyoid.[27] *The subplatysmal fat pad* lies more deeply in the neck, residing behind and posterior to the platysma.

Applied Anatomy

Herniation and protrusion of the subplatysmal fat pad in the ageing neck are predicated upon the type of anatomic variant of the platysma (*refer* below to "Platysma and its aponeurosis") present in an individual, and whether or not there is a significantly wide enough separation of the two muscle sheets inferior to the mentum. In those individuals with excessive amounts of submental fat in the subplatysmal layer, the loss of platysmal muscle tone permits the subplatysmal fat pad to herniate through the free borders of the platysm and establish a central fullness of submental fat in between vertical columns of neck bands, which contributes to the "turkey gobbler" neck deformity.[27] Suborbicularis fat of the lower lip is different from the submentalis fat pad. A prominent labiomental crease is often noted in mature individuals and may be related to how this fat compartment behaves with age. The subplatysmal fat must be excised directly and not suctioned, as there are numerous vessels that can be ruptured with a suction cannula.[28]

Loss of volume of deep medial cheek fat leads to pseudoptosis and is an additional determinant of the nasolabial fold. Augmentation of deep medial fat has four effects: (1) it increases anterior projection (not addressed by lateral redraping alone); (2) it diminishes the nasolabial fold; (3) the V-deformity is corrected; and (4) a youthful cheek with natural boundaries is recreated. The term "malar fat" is probably a misnomer: This region is composed of both distinct superficial and deep fat compartments. Submentalis and suborbicularis oris fat play a role in the formation of the labiomental hollow and ageing lip respectively.[29]

Muscles of Facial Expression and Anatomical Landmarks

The muscles of the face can be divided into two groups: (1) the muscles of facial expression, and (2) the muscles of mastication. The muscles of facial expression are unique; in the sense, they do not act in isolation but have complex anatomic and physiologic interactions. Most facial muscles insert directly into the skin and soft tissue, thereby facilitating "expression". Emotions and facial animations are conveyed and understood by the coordinated action of these muscles. The muscles of facial expression are connected to the overlying skin through a series of fibrous septae and an intervening fascial layer known as the SMAS. Thus when the underlying muscle contracts, the overlying skin moves with it (Fig. 20). The muscles of mastication, such as the masseter and temporalis, have bony attachments and function to move the jaw in a way similar to muscles elsewhere on the body.

Frontalis Muscle

The frontalis is the largest muscle of the upper face. The frontalis begins superiorly at the frontal scalp where the fibers originate from the galea aponeurotica, a fascial plane of the scalp that lies beneath the fat. The fibers of the frontalis extend vertically downward where they mesh with the skin and muscles at the eyebrow and glabella, finally inserting into the supraciliary ridge of the frontal bone. The muscle can appear as a single belly, or as two halves. Its function is to raise the eyebrows. This muscle is supplied by the temporal branches of the facial nerve.

Applied Anatomy

As this muscle interdigitates with the muscles of the glabellar complex, it is difficult to treat this muscle in isolation using botulinum toxin A, for fear of eyebrow ptosis or failure to efface the lines completely. The forehead lines must always be treated in conjunction with the frown for harmonious results. A high lateral injection into the frontalis can modulate a severe lateral brow elevation. The injections should be symmetrical as asymmetric injections result in asymmetric eyebrows.

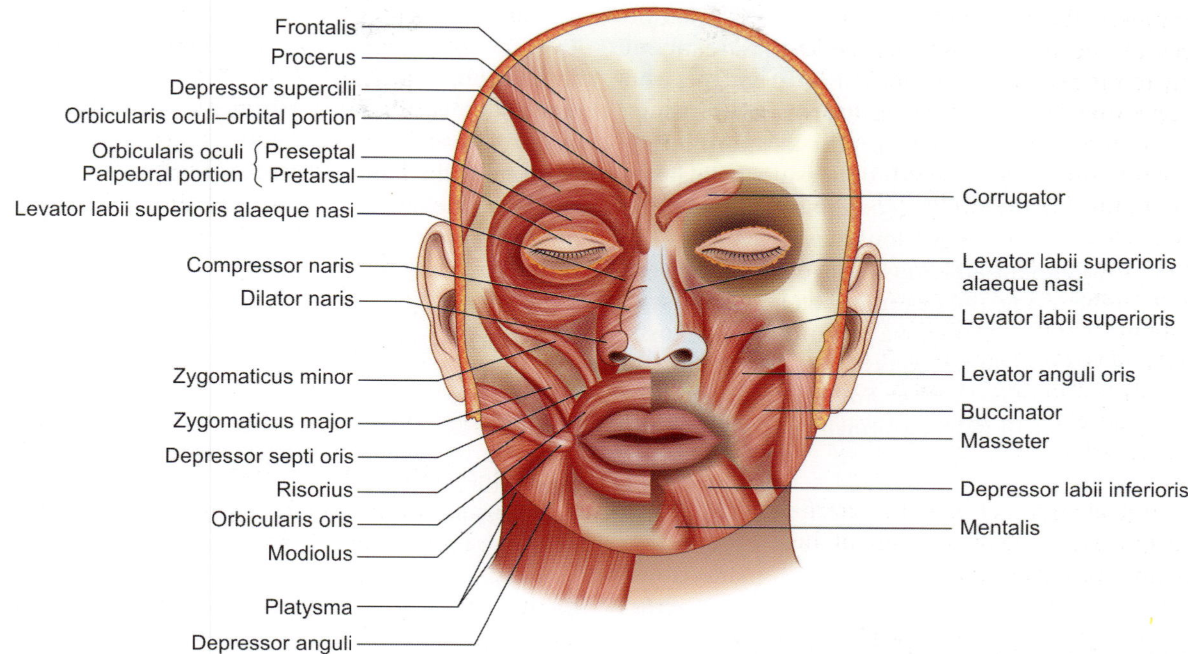

Fig. 20: Facial musculature.

Muscles in the Glabellar Complex

The primary muscles of the glabellar complex are the corrugator supercilii, the procerus and the depressor supercilii. In addition, the medial fibers of the orbicularis oculi and the frontalis also contribute, as fibers from these muscles may interdigitate with those of the corrugator. The corrugator is a bilateral muscle deep to the frontalis, superficial to the periosteum, and placed directly on the frontal bone of the upper medial orbits. It acts as a brow adductor, meaning it moves the brow downward and medial. The corrugator muscle has a transverse head and an oblique head. The transverse head of the corrugator is supplied by the temporal branch of facial nerve, and the oblique head is supplied by the zygomatic branch of the facial nerve.[30] The procerus is a flat muscle on the bridge of the nose. It is a vertical muscle which acts as a brow depressor, i.e. it depresses the medial head of the eyebrows, resulting in transverse lines on nasal dorsum.[31]

Applied Anatomy

It is important to assess the brow position to rule out pre-existing asymmetries and ptosis. In women, consider whether the brows have been plucked or tattooed. Avoid injecting too low to the superior rim of the orbital bone, and use caution with lateral brow injections. Inject perpendicular to the muscle, when treating the procerus, and inject deep into the belly of the corrugators, reaching almost to the periosteum. When injecting the corrugators, the belly of the muscle can be more easily palpated if the patient actively elevates the eyebrows immediately after frowning. Use your nondominant hand to raise the medial eyebrows before injecting into the corrugators. This allows the muscle fibers of the orbital portion of the orbicularis oculi and the lower muscle fibers of the frontalis to rise above the supraorbital rim while the adherent corrugator supercilii remains in place against bone.[32] Injecting too high may place the toxin in the frontalis muscle leading to medial brow ptosis. Do not completely paralyze the muscle as that can lead to 'spocking' of the lateral eyebrows and a "quizzical" look. Botulinum toxin injections into these muscles last 3–4 months.

Orbicularis Oculi

The orbicularis oculi is a circular sphincter-like broad and thin muscle which encircles the eyes. The muscle fans out from the ligamentous attachment superiorly to about the level of the eyebrow where it inserts into the skin and frontalis, and inferiorly to the level of the lower orbital rim, to encircle the globe 360°. It is composed of a palpebral portion (which covers the eyelid), an orbital portion (which surrounds the orbit) and a lacrimal portion (a small portion at the medial side of the orbit). The palpebral portion is further divided into the preseptal and pretarsal portion. The palpebral portion acts both voluntarily, and involuntarily, to close the eyelids, and the orbital portion depresses the lateral brow.

Applied Anatomy

The lateral vertical fibers of this muscle contract to form the crow's feet. Botulinum toxin A can remove these wrinkles. However, the injection sites must be kept well lateral, approximately 1–1.5 cm from the orbital rim. Duration of effect is usually less than that observed in other areas of the upper face, typically 3 months. As the muscle fibers insert directly into the dermis, the injections must be superficial and intradermal. Botulinum toxin A treatment should be approached with greater caution in patients who have undergone recent blepharoplasty or visual/refractive procedures like laser-assisted in situ keratomileusis (LASIK) procedures.[31] Prior to injection, evaluate lid laxity using the snap test. Laxity indicates potential for developing an ectropion, and lower lid injections may be avoided. The area below the zygomatic arch must be avoided, to prevent inadvertent injection to the zygomaticus major muscle, which has the potential to cause lip and cheek ptosis. Recruitment of the horizontal fibers of the orbicularis oculi following treatment of corrugator and procerus produce "lateral recruitment lines" just above the brow in the midline in midpupillary region.[33]

Nasalis

The nasalis is shaped roughly like an upside-down horseshoe, with the upper part traveling transversely across the nasal dorsum (also known as the compressor naris), and two lower arms traveling vertically down the sides of the nose (also known as the dilator naris). Bunny lines on the sides of the nose are caused by contraction of the transverse portion of the nasalis. This portion arises from the maxilla and runs diagonally across the bridge of the nose. It expands into a thin aponeurosis and is continuous with that of the muscle on the opposite side and with the aponeurosis of the procerus.

Applied Anatomy

Due to its connection with the procerus, bunny's lines must always be treated in conjunction with the glabellar complex, for harmonious results. The injections should be superficial. Treatments may be less effective in patients who have had rhinoplasty.[31] Do not inject too low, or one can paralyze the levator labii alaeque nasi and the levator labii superioris, which can cause drooping of the upper lip. Vigorous or downward massage can also lead to the same complication.

Levators of the Upper Lip

These include the levator labii alaeque nasi, levator labii superioris, depressor septi muscle, the levator anguli oris, zygomaticus minor, zygomaticus major and the risorius muscle. The depressor septi muscle attaches to the midline upper lip and runs up the columella of the nose. The levator labii alaeque nasi inserts bilaterally to the medial portion of the upper lip and runs superiorly up along the side of the nose to originate from the skull at the level of the inner canthus. The levator labii superioris extends upwards and attaches to the bone at the level of the lower orbital rim in the mid-pupillary line. The zygomaticus major and minor muscles extend upwards at an oblique angle from the upper lip and attach just below the lateral portion of the orbital rim. Inserting into the lateral aspect of the upper lip is the levator anguli oris, which originates superiorly at the canine fossa. Lastly, the risorius muscle also inserts at the lateral portion of the upper lip and travels obliquely upward toward the ear. As several muscles come together to insert at the lateral commissure of the lips, this area is known as the modiolus, and can be thought of as a dense, fibromuscular interface that acts as a scaffold for the various muscles to pull on.[34]

Applied Anatomy

Paralysis of the upper poles of these muscles can be an unintended consequence of injecting too low in the lateral canthal area when treating crow's feet. The patient may note difficulty raising the lip to smile. The muscles in this area form the midface musculature and help in performing functions such as eating, speaking and emotional expression. None of the lip levator muscles are targets for botulinum toxin injections, even though they contribute toward the creation of the nasolabial fold. This is because inadvertent paralysis of these muscles can alter a patient's smile, which is an unacceptable complication which has no antidote.

Orbicularis Oris

This is a major muscle of the lower face. This is a circular flat sphincteric muscle that encircles the mouth.

Applied Anatomy

Contracture of the upper, horizontally oriented fibers that travel along the upper lip is responsible for the vertical rhytides seen above the upper lip. However, complete paralysis of the muscle with botulinum toxin A is not advisable as it would interfere in the normal actions of chewing, sipping, speech impairment (especially when pronouncing "b" and "p"), whistling and sucking. Therefore, only very small amounts of the toxin must be used. Due to the frequent and often unavoidable use of this muscle, the effect of the botulinum toxin lasts for only 2–3 months. Musicians, singers and public speakers are not good candidates. The injections must always be symmetrical. Avoid treating the midline of the upper lip to prevent flattening of the cupid's bow, which can paradoxically give the appearance of an ageing mouth. Keep injections superficial and massage laterally.[32]

Depressors of the Lower Lip

There are two depressors of the lip: (1) the depressor anguli oris and (2) the depressor labii inferioris. These muscles insert superiorly into the lateral and medial orbicularis oris respectively, and originate inferiorly at the border of the mandible. The depressor anguli oris muscle is responsible for pulling down the corners of the mouth.

Applied Anatomy

Hyperactivity of these muscles with age results in sad face appearance. While injecting the depressor anguli oris, care must be taken not to inject too medially (into the depressor labii inferioris) in order to avoid speech difficulties and altered smile.[31]

Mentalis Muscle

This muscle originates from the mandible, covers the chin, and inserts into the skin of the lower lip. The mentalis raises the chin and is responsible for protrusion of the lower lip.

Applied Anatomy

This muscle allows for the puckering and pouting of the lower lip which expresses emotions like sadness, disdain or doubt. It is also responsible for the creation of the mental crease in some patients. As one ages, the contraction of the mentalis along with loss of collagen and subcutaneous fat in the chin, leads to the dimpled appearance of the chin (popply chin) or the "peach pit" deformity. While some authors suggest a single injection of botulinum toxin in the lower midline mass of the muscle, others suggest injections at two sites, slightly away from the midline, and near the jawline.[31] Avoid injecting too high (into the orbicularis oris) to prevent lip incontinence and drooling. Avoid injecting too laterally into the depressor labii inferioris.

Platysma

This muscle has been dealt with separately, further ahead in the chapter.

The muscles of mastication are the *Masseter, the temporalis muscle, the lateral pterygoid and the medial pterygoid*. The masseter originates at the inferior border and medial surface of the zygomatic arch. This quadrangular muscle then inserts on the lateral surface of the ramus of the mandible and its coronoid process. When contracted, the masseter shortens and thickens, elevating and protruding the mandible and closing the jaws. The temporalis originates in the temporal fossa and inserts deep to the masseter on the coronoid process of the mandible. The medial pterygoid originates on the pterygoid plate, palatine bone, and tuberosity of the maxilla and inserts on the mandible deep and anterior to the masseter. These redundant masticatory muscles are sufficiently separated to allow injection into the masseter without inadvertently injecting additional muscles.[35]

Applied Anatomy

Hypertrophy of the masseter muscle can lead to the appearance of a heavy or bulky jaw. In women, especially, a square jawline is considered unfeminine. The muscle must be palpated (by asking the patient to clench their teeth) to confirm true muscular hypertrophy. When in doubt, an MRI can be performed to rule out other soft tissue masses. Masseter hypertrophy could be caused due to dental malalignment and chronic bruxism among other causes. However, most of the time, it is idiopathic.

Botulinum toxin injections are safer to surgical resection of the masseter.[36] The injections are made below an imaginary line drawn from the corner of the mouth to the tragus. The injections are made perpendicularly at 2–3 points, into the most prominent and bulkiest portion of the muscle. Above the masseter and just below the muscles of the midface lie their motor nerves. The zygomatic, buccal, marginal mandibular and cervical branches of the facial nerve cross the masseter. Overlying the masseter posteriorly is the parotid gland and its duct. The facial artery and vein also cross the masseter at its anteroinferior corner and then course superiorly and anteriorly.[35] Lower dilutions of botulinum toxin must be used to avoid diffusion in this area. Injections to the deep portions of the muscle is advisable to avoid the facial artery and branches of the facial nerve. This muscle is best approached using electromyographic guidance. Patients must be advised to clench their teeth vigorously after treatment. Results may take 3–8 weeks to be noticeable, however the improvement may last for 5–8 months. Weakened mastication resulting in malocclusion can result from overzealous masseter muscle treatment and should be avoided.

Applied Anatomy of Facial Vasculature

Facial vasculature has already been discussed in detail in the preceding chapter. This chapter will confine itself to the anatomic considerations to be kept in mind while performing soft tissue augmentation using dermal fillers. Some of the rare, but feared complications of soft tissue augmentation include skin necrosis due to interruption of the vascular supply to the area by direct injury to the vessel, compression of the area around the vessel, or obstruction of the vessel by the filler material.[37] This process is associated with prolonged blanching and possibly pain at the site of injection, followed later by a dusky discoloration. Ultimately, an eschar of necrotic skin develops over an ulcer. The nose and the glabella are high-risk areas. This is because of the limited collateral circulation, and the superficial location of the supratrochlear and supraorbital arteries.[27] Inadvertent intraarterial injection of filler material around the eye can lead to occlusion of the central retinal vessels and potentially blindness.[28]

Direct arterial embolization of filler material will generally cause an immediate skin blanching that may appear in a geographic distribution; pain may vary from severe to minimal.

Conversely, *venous occlusion* can occur if excessive amounts of filler are placed in a small area, leading to venous congestion. This is associated with persistent dull, aching pain and swelling, with the development of a violaceous discoloration of the affected area, with pain being out of proportion to simple bruising.[38] A comprehensive knowledge of anatomy of the facial vasculature can help avoid these complications.

Supratrochlear Artery

The supratrochlear artery, a branch of the ophthalmic artery, predominantly supplies this region. It exits the medial orbit and courses upward, supplying blood to the nasal root and the inferior central forehead. At the glabellar region, this artery is at particularly high-risk of necrosis following dermal filler injections. A dusky purple discoloration is noted in the central forehead, extending to the nasal side walls and up to the nasal tip. Although, the initial symptoms often occur immediately after the injection cases of delayed onset of symptoms have also been reported.[39] Rare cases of visual impairment and blindness have also been reported.[40] These complications are believed to result from retrograde spread of intravascularly injected material into the ophthalmic artery. The injected material then enters other distal branches and blocks blood supply to the retina and cornea.

In order to minimize the risk of glabellar necrosis, inject smaller volumes of filler at a time, place the filler superficially (at the level of deep dermis or high subcutaneous fat), and use a reflex maneuver to aspirate prior to injection.

Superior and Inferior Labial Arteries

The superior and inferior labial arteries both branch off the facial artery at the angle of the mouth. The arteries course between the mucosa and the orbicularis oris muscle, anastomosing at the midline with branches from the contralateral side. The superior labial artery provides blood supply to the upper lip, with terminal branches supplying the nasal alae and septum. The inferior labial artery provides blood supply to the lower lip and part of the superior chin.

These arteries are at potential risk during soft tissue augmentation of perioral areas and the lips.[41]

Angular Artery

After the facial artery gives-off the inferior and superior labial branches, it courses with tortuous curves along the medial cheek as the angular artery.[41] This artery provides to the nasal ala, sidewall, and dorsum. The angular artery continues upward toward the medial canthus, where it anastomoses with the dorsal nasal artery. This anastomosis provides a link between the internal and external carotid systems. The intravascular injection of filler into this artery can occur during soft tissue augmentation of the nasolabial fold or the nasal tip.[42] Injection directly into the vessel or compression of them due to large volumes of filler is possible particularly at the alar groove, where the coming together of embryonic fusion planes may not allow for the accommodation of filler volume and tissue distension.[43] Impending necrosis following filler injection to the nasolabial groove will present with violaceous or dusky reticulated appearance to the upper lip, the nasolabial fold, as well as the alar groove and areas of the nose (Fig. 21).[44]

Angiosome

The concept of angiosome was introduced by Taylor and Palmer in 1987. An angiosome is a composite segment of bone, muscle, nerve, and overlying skin, supplied by a common source vessel (Fig. 22).[45] These segments form the theoretical basis for the design of complex tissue flaps. A flap that is based on the source vessel of a single angiosome can frequently incorporate some tissues from an adjacent angiosome; nutrient blood will be supplied to the adjacent

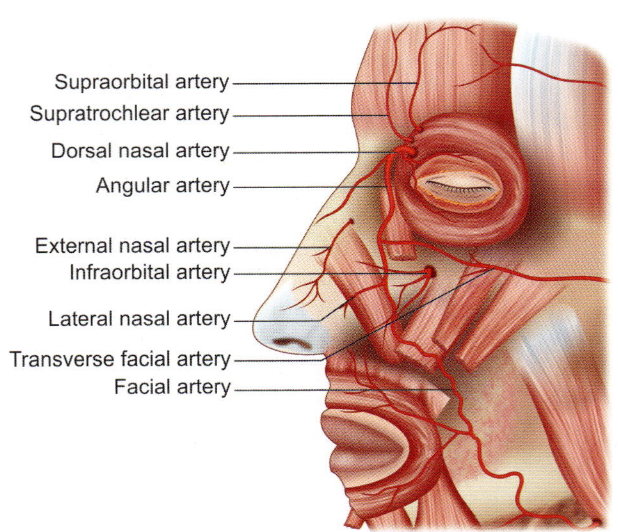

Fig. 21: Facial vasculature.

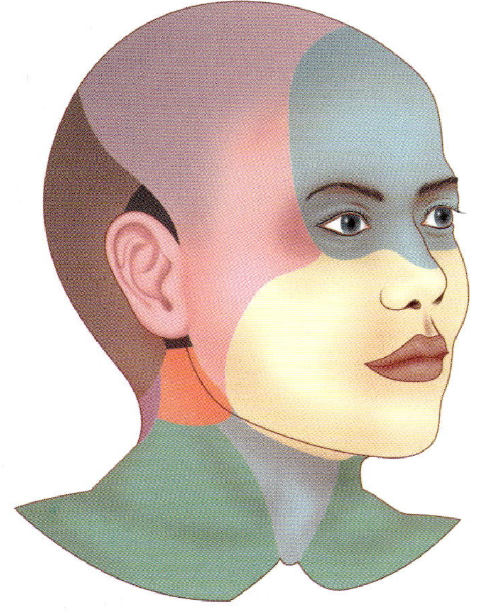

Fig. 22: Angiosomes of the face.

angiosome through collateral channels.[45] Most of the skin and subcutaneous tissue is supplied by branches of the external carotid system. The exception to this rule lies within a mask-like region of the face, which includes the eyes, the upper nose, and the central forehead. This central region serves as an anastomotic link between the internal (ophthalmic artery) and external (facial, superficial temporal arteries) carotid systems.

Cutaneous Vascular Plexus

The cutaneous tissues and their nutrient vessels form a stack of interconnected vascular tissue planes called the vascular plexus, consisting of the fascial plexus, the subcutaneous plexus, and the subdermal plexus. The nerve *fascial plexus* (at the level of deep muscle fascia) derives its blood supply from small vessels that branch off the septocutaneous and musculocutaneous arteries as they penetrate the muscular fascia, and from retrograde flow from the overlying subcutaneous plexus. By including the fascial plexus in the design of the fasciocutaneous flap, tissue survival may be improved.[45] Overlying the fascial plexus is the subcutaneous plexus, a significant network of vessels corresponding to the level of the superficial fascia SMAS.

The subdermal, or cutaneous, plexus is the most significant of the horizontal vascular layers and has a primary role in the distribution of blood to other regions of the cutaneous system.[45] The *subdermal plexus* lies at the junction between the reticular dermis and the underlying subcutaneous fat. Clinically, this level corresponds with the phenomenon of dermal bleeding, which is often seen at the leading edge of skin flaps. Superficial to these major subcutaneous plexus lie the dermal plexus and the closely associated *subepidermal plexus*.[45] These layers perform two primary functions: (1) the dermal plexus provides thermoregulation, (2) whereas the capillary beds of the subepidermal plexus provide nutrients to the skin.

Applied Anatomy of Nerve Supply to the Face in Relation to Nerve Blocks

Regional nerve blocks which are used in dentistry may result in inconsistent and imperfect analgesia when needed for facial esthetic surgery. Dermatologists and plastic surgeons must know how to perform accurate and reproducible nerve blocks to provide effective anesthesia. Certain procedures like dermabrasion, deep chemical peels and ablative laser resurfacing techniques may require full face anesthesia. Other procedures like dermal filler injections to tear trough or laser resurfacing for periorbital and perioral rhytids require effective perioral and periorbital anesthesia support. Cosmetic surgeons who have a thorough understanding of facial anatomy, sensory nerve supply to the face, and important anatomical landmarks for the safe administering of regional blocks, stand at a huge advantage. Limitation of this knowledge may force the surgeon into more expensive and often riskier venues, such as the operating room and general anesthesia.

Sensory Dermatomes of the Head and Neck

The main sensory innervation of the face is derived from the trigeminal nerve and the upper cervical nerves. The *trigeminal nerve* is named for its three sensory branches called the ophthalmic nerve (O), the maxillary (Mx) and the mandibular (Md) nerve (Fig. 23).

The *ophthalmic nerve* supplies the cornea, iris, lacrimal gland and conjunctiva, eyelids, eyebrow, forehead and upper lateral nose. It divides into three branches: (1) the frontal, (2) nasociliary, and (3) lacrimal. The frontal nerve divides into the supratrochlear and supraorbital nerves which provide sensation to the forehead and anterior scalp.[46]

The *maxillary nerve* appears at the infraorbital foramen as the *infraorbital nerve*. Its terminal branches supply the nasal ala, the lower eyelid and upper lip. Its other branches supply sensation to the skin on the side of the forehead *(zygomaticotemporal nerve)* and the skin on the prominence of the cheek *(zygomaticofacial nerve)*. These branches need to be anesthetized to carry out procedures on the upper lip, mid face, nasolabial fold and temples.[46]

The *mandibular nerve* supplies the teeth and gums of the mandible, the temporal region, part of the external ear, the lower lip and the chin. The *inferior alveolar nerve* is the largest branch, exits at the mandibular foramen, traverses the mandibular canal, to finally exit at the mental foramen, where it divides into the *incisive and mental nerves*. The *mental nerve* supplies the skin and mucosa of the lower lip. The *buccal branch* supplies the skin over the buccinator muscle.[46]

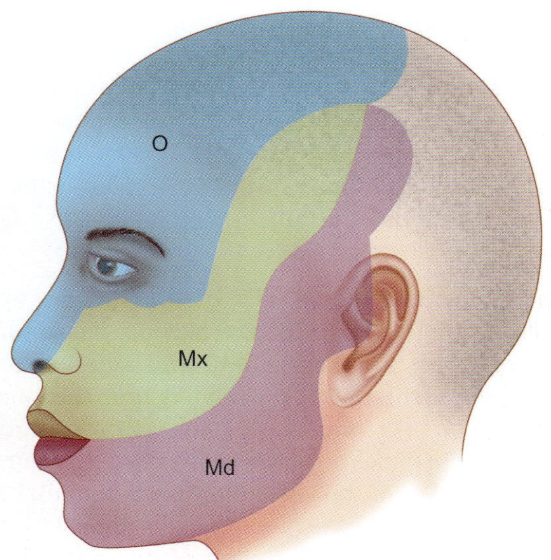

Fig. 23: Sensory innervation of the face. (O: Ophthalmic nerve; Mx: Maxillary nerve; Md: Mandibular nerve).

A set of the seven blocks can anesthetize the entire face.[46]

Infraorbital nerve: The infraorbital foramen is located on a line dropped from the medial limbus of the iris. If the patient stares straight ahead, the infraorbital foramen is located 4–7 mm below the orbital rim on that line. The alveolar branch of the infraorbital nerve supplies sensation to the anterior gingival and maxillary teeth. This nerve can be blocked using two transcutaneous and one intraoral technique. However, the intraoral method and perpendicular transcutaneous method do not allow the practitioner to know that he has entered the foramen. For this he must use the transcutaneous nasolabial approach. This approach has a point of injection medial to the upper nasolabial groove a few millimeters lateral to the alar groove. The injection point for the infraorbital nerve is in the center of the small triangle lateral to the alar rim and medial to the nasolabial fold. With your left index finger on the infraorbital rim, ask the patient to look straight ahead. Holding the syringe like a pen, you advance the needle to bone toward the designated point about 4–7 mm down from the rim. Then inject 1–2 cc of anesthetic. It is advisable to use a 28-gauge 1.5 inch needle, which is bent at a 45° angle, to facilitate the transcutaneous technique. The transcutaneous perpendicular technique involves injecting directly into the foramen at the anatomical landmark.

While the transcutaneous route is preferred by plastic surgeons, most dermatologists are comfortable employing the transoral route, which is equally effective when performed properly. To perform this anesthesia, elevate the lip and insert a half inch 30-gauge needle in the vestibular sulcus between the canine and the first premolar tooth, and direct superiorly toward the infraorbital foramen. Bending the needle at a 45° angle upwards can facilitate the insertion. Use the nondominant hand to palpate the infraorbital rim to avoid injecting superior to the orbit.[47] Inject 2–4 mL of anesthetic and feel the bolus below the infraorbital nerve to confirm the correct placement.

Area of anesthesia: Include the nose (entire side wall, ala and base of the columella), cheek, lip and lower eyelid. Lateral to the commissure, numbness extends for 1–1.5 cm. After a bilateral injection, lip filling procedures using dermal fillers, can be carried out.

Mental nerve: The mental nerve usually exits from a foramen below the apex of the second bicuspid. The variability of this foramen is 6–10 mm anterior or 6–10 mm posterior to this point. After exiting from the foramen, it divides into 2–3 branches. These branches provide sensation to the pink lip, the vermillion to the labiomental fold, and the skin of the chin. Because the mental nerve courses directly below the mucosa in the area of the lower canine tooth, surgical traction often makes the upper nerve fascicles visible or palpable in this area. The mental nerve can be blocked at the mental foramen or a few centimeters after it leaves the foramen submucosally. To block it at the foramen, locate the second lower bicuspid. Use the thumb of one hand to pull out the lower lip, lateral to the lower canine tooth. The nerve is visible submucosally about 85% of the time.[46] Place the needle tip vertically down in the buccal sulcus, near the base of the second premolar tooth, and inject 2–4 mL.[47]

Alternatively, the mental nerve can also be blocked using a transcutaneous approach.

Area of anesthesia: This injection only anesthetizes the lower lip down to the labiomental fold. To anesthetize the chin as well, perform the mental plus block. Here an end branch of the mental nerve and the terminal branches of the myelohyoid need to be blocked. This can be done immediately after the mental block by an anterior premandibular injection anterior to the vestibule in front of the anterior teeth.[46]

Supraorbital, supratrochlear and infratrochlear nerves: The supraorbital notch, rarely the foramen, is easily palpable at the supraorbital rim just above the medial limbus. The *supraorbital nerve* exits the foramen, traverses the lower corrugator muscles, and then splits into the medial and lateral branches. The medial branches proceed cephalad on the surface of the frontalis to supply the skin of the forehead medially and the anterior scalp for many centimeters. The lateral branches, under the frontalis muscle, supply the lateral forehead. The *supratrochlear nerve* supplies sensation to the mid forehead. It can be found under the medial centimeter of the eyebrow. The *infratrochlear nerve* is a branch of the nasociliary that runs along the medial orbital wall and leaves the orbit below the trochlea to supply the skin in the medial eyelids, the side of the nose above the medial canthus, the conjuctiva, and lacrimal apparatus.

The block is performed by injecting along the supraorbital rim from lateral to medial. Stretch the eyebrow laterally and pierce the lateral part of the middle third of the eyebrow. The supraorbital notch is readily palpated in most patients, and is approximately 27 mm lateral to the glabellar midline.[47] The supratroclear nerve exits a foramen approximately 17 mm from the midline, while the infratrochlear nerve exits a foramen below the trochlea.[47] Aim the needle at the supraorbital notch (which is palpable). After injecting 1–2 cc prior to the notch under the muscle, the needle moves medially about 10 millimeters along the rim, and another 1 cc is deposited at the supratrochlear notch (which is not palpable).

Another 1 cc is deposited as the needle advances toward and touches the nasal bones.[46]

Area of anesthesia: The forehead, the upper eyelid and a few millimeters of the frontoparietal scalp.

Zygomaticotemporal nerve: This nerve is a terminal branch of the zygomatic nerve. It emerges through a foramen which is posterior to the zygoma on the lateral orbital rim, around 1 cm below the level of the lateral canthus.[46] From behind the patient, a 27-gauge 1.5 inch needle must be inserted behind the concave portion of the lateral orbital rim. This is about 10–12 mm behind and just below the zygomaticofrontal suture (which is palpable). Accurate blocking of this nerve requires skill and experience, and some practicing on a model skull.[47]

Area of anesthesia: This nerve provides sensory innervation to a fan-shaped area posterior to the lateral orbital rim, extending into the hair. This may assist in the injection of dermal fillers for volume augmentation at the temples or to fill out rhytides on the lateral temporal area.

Zygomaticofacial nerve: This nerve exits through a foramen in the inferior lateral portion of the lateral orbital rim at the zygoma. By palpating the portion and injecting just lateral to the palpating finger with 1–2 mL of local anesthetic, this nerve is successfully blocked.

Area of anesthesia: The zygomaticofacial block is always done right after the zygomaticotemporal block.[46] The anesthesia is achieved in a triangular area on the cheek prominence. This block is useful before carrying out cheek augmentation procedures using dermal fillers.

A "horseshoe" pattern subcutaneous tumescent facial block has also been described.[48] This is performed on each side of the face beginning at the temporal hairline and extending sequentially to the preauricular area, jawline, and chin. This requires the infiltration of tumescent local anesthesia utilizing lidocaine 0.2% with epinephrine 1:1,000,000.[48] Injections are given slowly with a 30-gauge 1 inch needle attached to a 10 mL syringe. A total volume of 25–50 mL of tumescent local anesthesia is required to complete this part of the procedure, and the block requires 20 minutes of slow infiltration for completion.

Advantages: General anesthesia or intravenous sedation is not necessary. Infusion pumps can be avoided. Thorough cutaneous anesthesia is achieved. Post-anesthesia recovery is complete. The anesthetic effect lasts for many hours postoperatively.[48]

Disadvantages: The procedure time is lengthened for the patient and the staff. Also, the patient is required to undergo multiple needle injections which may not be accepted by all patients.

Surgical Anatomy of the Midface

The contour of the cheek, unlike other esthetic units of the face, is defined primarily by soft tissue. This soft tissue is framed by the malar complex above and the mandible below, but its shape is largely determined by the parotid gland, the facial musculature, and the buccal fat. Ageing of the middle third of the face affects the periorbital region, the cheeks and the nose. Dermatochalasis and gravity lead to laxity of the eyelid skin, resulting in decreased lid tone as evidenced from the "snap test". The orbital septum may weaken over time leading to protrusion of upper and lower-lid fat compartments in some (leading to eyebags), and loss of periorbital subcutaneous tissue in others (leading to "sunken eye" appearance). The cheeks show volume loss due to atrophy of the buccal fat pad, leading to appearance of prominent malar eminences. The supporting mechanisms of the nasal tip become inelastic, leading to nasal tip ptosis and an apparent elongation of the middle third of the face.[49]

The *malar complex* is a key component of facial form, but its curves are not easily analyzed. The most prominent part of the malar eminence can be determined using the Hinderer's method of analysis. One line is drawn from the lateral commissure of the lip to the lateral canthus. Another line is drawn from the inferior aspect of the ala to the superior tragus. The area posterior and superior to the intersection of these lines should be the most prominent part of the malar eminence. All dermal filler implantations for cheek and midface volume augmentation must be done in this area.

The key elements to the midface that contribute structurally to the anatomy of the *submalar triangle* include the buccal fat pad, the masseter muscle, the zygomatic bone, and the nasolabial fold.[50] The superior border of the submalar triangle is defined by the malar prominence. With age, there is a loss of the inherent deep anatomic substructure of the midface, which manifests itself as a predictable change in surface anatomy, comprising a roughly triangular flattening that is confined within the relatively constant landmarks of the face, which make up the boundaries of the submalar triangle. Changes also occur posterior to the submalar triangle and inferior to the zygomatic arch overlying the insertion of the masseter muscle. The combined loss of volume in both the submalar triangle and the infrazygomatic area gives rise to a cadaver-like appearance.

Applied Anatomy

While volume loss in the submalar triangle can be successfully remedied by filler injections using poly-L-lactic acid, fat transfer, liquid silicone injection, submalar facial prostheses, and free facial grafting; attempts to correct volume loss in the infrazygomatic area, using the same techniques, have been less than successful.[50]

The *midfacial muscles* include levator alae nasi, levator labii superioris, zygomaticus major, zygomaticus minor and risorius. An analysis of 50 hemifacial cadaver dissection by Pessa et al.[51] revealed that the zygomaticus minor was noted in only 36% and the risorius was present in only 6% of the cadavers. Although, the zygomaticus major was always present, two distinct forms of this muscle were found to exist: (1) a single muscle was noted in 66% and (2) a true double or bifid variant was noted in only 34% of cadavers.

In relation to botulinum toxin injections, the reciprocating action of opposing mimetic muscles in the midface can prove to be more complicating and challenging than in the upper face. In the upper face, the muscles are easily distinguishable due to various topographic landmarks. However in the midface, there is an interdependence of superficial and deep muscles for facial expression, which also are adjacent to some of the muscles surrounding the mouth, that function in articulation of sounds, mastication, and deglutition. These muscles of facial expression are interlaced with, and even form the SMAS and many of them perform complimentary, and at times, unrelated functions. The muscles around the mouth (which includes midface and lower face muscles), act in a complex and synergistic manner. They allow us to smile, laugh, whistle, blow, chew, suck on a straw, grimace, pucker and pout. They also facilitate the action of chewing and swallowing. During treatment of the midface, the upper lip levators are easily affected by the slightest diffusion of the toxin, leading to complications like ectropion, lip ptosis, cheek ptosis, a frozen smile or an asymmetric smile. This is why, some authors believe that botulinum toxin injections to the midface are best performed under electromyographic guidance. Overall, in the midface, better, safer and longer lasting cosmetic results can be achieved with soft tissue implants and fillers, or resurfacing techniques.[52]

Applied Anatomy of the Stenson's Duct

The parotid duct enters the mouth at the level of the second upper molar. It is vulnerable to trauma during midface and cheek augmentation, especially in patients receiving large volumes of filler for significant degrees of HIV lipoatrophy. These patients have minimal subcutaneous tissue, making the duct vulnerable to inadvertent injury, where it lies superior to the masseter muscle. An accidental needle puncture can result in a draining fistula, due to the larger caliber needle that is often used to inject subcutaneously for this condition, such as the 25 or 27-gauge needles used for poly-L-lactic acid or calcium hydroxyl-apatite.[41]

The Platysma and Its Aponeurosis

The platysma is composed of two separate broad flat sheets of muscle which originates from the clavicle, first rib, and acromion and blends as a thin muscular sheet into an aponeurosis that covers the parotid gland and inserts below the zygomatic arch. It is confluent with the orbicularis oculi, zygomaticus major, orbicularis oris, and the sternocleidomastoid musculature. It interdigitates with the depressor anguli and its platysma counterpart from the other side of the neck.

Its anterior fibers from both sheets of muscle on either side of the neck interdigitate with each other in various patterns at or near the symphysis menti of the mandible. The posterior fibers pass over the lower border of the body of the mandible superficial to the marginal mandibular branch of the facial nerve, artery and vein. Even the submandibular gland lies deep to the platysma. The upper fibers of the platysma (pars mandibularis) then insert into the lower border of the body of the mandible, and into the skin and subcutaneous tissue of the lower part of the face. Some platysmal fibers (pars labialis) also interdigitate and blend into the muscles around the angle of the mouth (orbicularis oris and risorius), the chin (mentalis), and the depressors of the lower lip, especially the depressor anguli oris.[53]

There are three anatomic variations of the platysma based on the pattern of decussation of its interlacing fibers as it approaches the submental region (Figs. 24A to C).

- Type I variation is seen in 75% of the individuals, where the fibers of the platysma interdigitate with its counterpart on the opposite side of the neck 1–2 cm below the chin.
- Type II variant is seen in 15% of the individuals, where the decussation of the fibers occurs at the level of the thyroid cartilage, and becomes a unified sheet of muscle from there on up over the entire submental region.
- Type III variant is seen in 10% of all individuals, which is seen as two separate straps of platysma that run parallel to each other up the neck, attaching to the mandible and skin, without decussating its fibers.

Men generally have a thicker platysma than women, and in some individuals, the platysma may even be absent. Many anatomists and plastic surgeons now believe that the SMAS is actually the platysma aponeurosis.[54] Laxity of the platysma with age creates platysma banding and can accentuate submandibular gland ptosis.

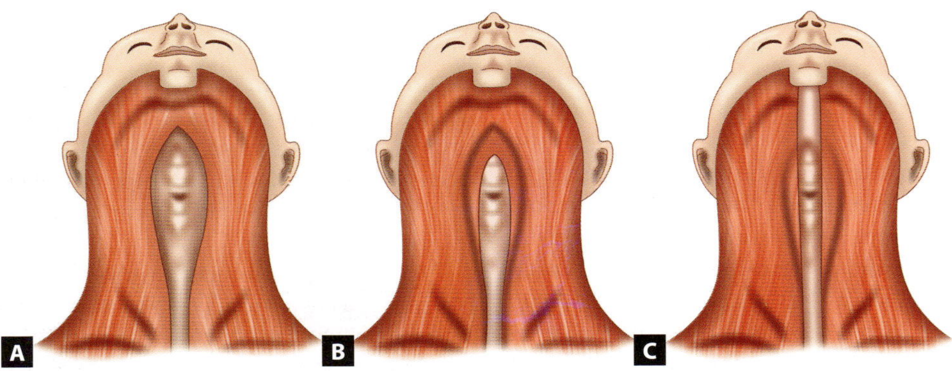

Figs. 24A to C: Decussation and de-decussation of the anterior fibers of the platysma.

The nerve supply to the platysma is by the cervical motor branch of the facial nerve. This nerve emerges from the junction of the platysma where it crosses over the sternocleidomastoid muscle, known as "Erb's point". Cervical branches from the carotid artery supply the platysma. This artery is located in the deeper layers of the neck, between the sternocleidomastoid muscle and the thyroid cartilage. Two large veins which should be avoided with any injection in this area are: (1) the anterior jugular vein, running vertically on either side of the thyroid cartilage, and (2) the external jugular vein running vertically on the anterior surface of the sternocleidomastoid muscle.[28]

Functions and Applied Anatomy of the Platysma

The platysma is a depressor of the lower lip innervated by the cervical branch of the facial nerve. With maximum contraction, it pulls the skin overlying the clavicle upwards, and wrinkles the skin of the neck in an oblique direction, increasing the diameter of the neck. The platysma is also active during sudden, rapid and deep inspiration. Contracting the platysma can increase negative pressure in the superficial jugular veins of the neck, facilitating venous circulation.[53]

When the platysma becomes less elastic with age, it separates anteriorly and can be appreciated clinically as two or more divergent bands or folds of skin that extend from the lower margin of the mandible to the medial aspect of the clavicles. These anterior neck bands often tighten and become more visible, especially when the patient turns the head from side to side, as they speak or gesticulate. Vertical bands and cords develop as a result of a hyperactive platysma attempting to support the ptotic structural changes which are characteristic of a senescent neck. These thick vertical muscle bands are very distressing to patients. The length of the platysma band between chin and sternal notch shortens as the neck ages. This is why surgical procedures that tighten the bands together, but do not release the inferior aspect of the platysma band at the thyroid cartilage, may create an even tighter band. This is why botulinum toxin A may inhibit muscle activity and allow lengthening and softening of the bands.[28] In other individuals, the anterior edges of the fibers eventually lose muscle tone, separate over time and protrude anteriorly, which along with fat herniation, causes the "turkey neck" deformity.

Careful injections of botulinum toxin to the platysmal bands can help relax horizontal neck lines. This procedure works best on younger patients with good skin elasticity. It is also beneficial in preparing a patient for submental liposuction, because by relaxing the neck bands, a more even draping of the anterior neck skin can be achieved in the postoperative period after liposuction. Botulinum toxin cannot however, correct fat herniation. Injecting the superior mandibular fibers of the platysma with botulinum toxin can affect the corners of the mouth, lower lip and chin, because of the interdigitation of platysmal fibers into the mimetic muscles of the lower face (Box 1).

Box 1: Salient points.

- Important danger points include temporal artery and nerve at the temple and facial artery near mandible
- Facial nerve blocks are performed at supraorbital, infraorbital and mental foramen for respective nerves
- Always preserve cosmetic units of the face
- Place incisions along RSTLs.

ACKNOWLEDGMENT

The material on lips, ears and eyes was contributed by Dr A Gulanikar and his contribution is gratefully acknowledged.

REFERENCES

1. Gonzalez-UlloaM, Castillo A, Stevens E, et al. Preliminary study of the total restoration of the facial skin. Plast Reconstr Surg. 1954;13:151-61.
2. Burget GC, Menick FJ. The subunit principle in nasal reconstruction. Plast Reconstr Surg. 1985;76:239-47.
3. Larrabee WF, Makielski KH, Henderson JL. Skin and soft tissue. In: Merritt J (Ed). Surgical anatomy of the face, 2nd edition. Philadelphia: Lippincott Williams & Wilkins; 2004; 46-9.
4. Prendergast PM, Facial proportions. In: Erian A, Shiffman MA (Eds). Advanced Surgical Facial-rejuvenation. Springer, Berlin: Heidelberg, 2012. pp. 15-22.
5. Crumley RJ, Lanser M. Quantitative analysis of nasal tip projection. Laryngoscope. 1988;98(2):202-8.
6. Ricketts RM. Esthetics, environment, and the law of lip relation. Am J Orthod. 1968;54(4):272-89.
7. Ricketts RM. The biologic significance of the divine proportion and Fibonacci series. Am J Orthod. 1982;81(5):351-70.
8. Marquardt SR. Dr Stephen Marquardt and the golden decagon of human facial beauty. Interview with Dr Gottlieb. J Clin Orthod. 2002;36(6):317-8.
9. Bragatto FP, Chicarelli M, Kasuya AV, et al. Golden proportion analysis of dental-skeletal patterns of class II and III patients pre and post Orthodontic-orthognathic treatment. J Contemp Dent Pract. 2016;17(9):728-33.
10. Anand S, Tripathi S, Chopra A, et al. Vertical and horizontal proportions of the face and their correlation to phi among Indians in Moradabad population: a survey. The Journal of the Indian Prosthodontic Society. 2015;15(2):125-30.
11. Larrabee WF. A finite element model of skin deformation I-III. Laryngoscope. 1986;96:399-419.
12. Larrabee WF, Makielski KH, Henderson JL. Superficial musculoaponeurotic system. In: Merritt J (Ed). Surgical Anatomy of the Face, 2nd edition. Philadelphia: Lippincott Williams & Wilkins; 2004;50-6.
13. Mitz V, Peyronie M. The superficial musculoaponeurotic system (SMAS) in the parotid and cheek area. Plast Reconstr Surg. 1976;58:80-8.
14. Tessier P. The conjunctival approach to the orbital floor and maxilla in congenital malformation and trauma. J Maxillofac Surg. 1973;1:3-8.

15. Gardetto A, Dabernig J, Rainer C, et al. Does a superficial musculoaponeurotic system exist in the face and neck? An anatomical study by the tissue plastination technique. Plast Reconstr Surg. 2003;111:664-72.
16. Thaller SR, Kim S, Patterson H, et al. The submuscular aponeurotic system (SMAS): a histologic and comparative anatomy evaluation. Plast Reconstr Surg. 1990;86:690-6.
17. Jost G, Wassef M, Levet Y. Subfascial lifting. Esthetic Plast Surg. 1987;11:163-70.
18. Gosain AK, Yousif NJ, Madiedo G, et al. Surgical anatomy of the SMAS: a reinvestigation. Plast Reconstr Surg. 1993;92:1254-63.
19. Ghassemi A, Prescher A, Riediger D, et al. Anatomy of the SMAS revisited. Aesthetic Plast Surg. 2003;27(4):258-64.
20. Alghoul M, Codner MA. Retaining ligaments of the face: review of anatomy and clinical applications. Aesthetic Surg J. 2013;33(6):769-82.
21. Pessa JE, Brown F. Independent effect of various facial mimetic muscles on the nasolabial fold. Aesthetic Plast Surg. 1992;16:167-71.
22. Pessa JE, Garza PA, Love VM, et al. The anatomy of the labio-mandibular fold. Plast Reconstr Surg. 1998;101:482-6.
23. Truswell W, Truswell WH. Relevant surgical anatomy for rejuvenation of the ageing face. In: Truswell WH (Ed). Surgical Facial Rejuvenation: a roadmap to safe and reliable outcomes, 1st edition. New York: Thierne Medical Publishers, Inc; 2008;9-23.
24. Rohrich RJ, Pessa JE. The fat compartments of the face: anatomy and clinical implications for cosmetic surgery. Plast Reconstr Surg. 2007;119:2219-31.
25. Pendergast PM. Anatomy of the face and neck. In: Shiffman MA, Di Guiseppe A, editors. Cosmetic Surgery. Berlin-Heidelberg: Springer-Verlag; 2012. pp. 29-45.
26. Larrabee WF, Makielski KH, Henderson JL. Cheeks and neck. In: Merritt J (Ed). Surgical Anatomy of the Face, 2nd edition. Philadelphia: Lippincott Williams & Wilkins; 2004;50-6.
27. Hatef DA, Koshy JC, Sandoval SE, et al. The submental fat compartment of the neck. Semin Plast Surg. 2009;23:288-91.
28. Hoefflin SM. Anatomy of the platysma and lip depressor muscles. A simplified mnemonic approach. Dermatol Surg. 1998;24:1225-31.
29. Rohrich RJ, Pessa JE, Ristow B. The youthful cheek and deep medial fat compartment. Plast Reconstr Surg. 2008;121:2107-12.
30. Knize D. Muscles that act on glabellar skin: a closer look. Plast Reconstr Surg. 2000;105:350-61.
31. Carruthers J, Fagien S, Matarasso SL. Consensus recommenda-tions on the use of Botulinum toxin type A in facial aesthetics. Plast Reconstr Surg. 2004;114:1-22.
32. Benedetto AV, Lahti JG. Measurements of the anatomical position of the corrugator supercilii. Derm Surg. 2005;31:923-7.
33. Petrus GM, Lewis D, Maas CS. Anatomic considerations for treatment with botulinum toxin. Facial plastic surgery clinics of North America. 2007;15(1):1-9.
34. Benedetto AV. Facial anatomy and the use of Botulinum Toxin. In: Benedetto AV (Ed). Botulinumtoxin in Clinical Dermato-logy, 1st edition. London: Taylor & Francis. 2006;201-53.
35. Benedetto AV. Muscle contouring with Botulinum Toxin. In: Benedetto AV (Ed). Botulinum Toxin in Clinical Dermatology, 1st edition: London: Taylor & Francis; 2006;201-53.
36. Bas B, Ozan B, Muglali M, et al. Treatment of masseteric hypertrophy with botulinum toxin: a report of two cases. Med Oral Pathol Oral Cir Bucal. 2010;15:649-52.
37. Schanz S, Schippert W, Ulmer A, et al. Arterial embolization caused by injection of hyaluronic acid (Restylane). Br J Dermatol. 2002;146:928-9.
38. Glaich AS, Cohen JL, Goldberg LH. Injection necrosis of the glabella: protocol for prevention and treatment after use of dermal fillers. Dermatol Surg. 2006;32:276-81.
39. Souza Felix Bravo B, Klotz De Almeida Balassiano L, Roos Mariano Da Rocha C, et al. Delayed-type necrosis after soft-tissue augmentation with hyaluronic acid. The Journal of Clinical and Aesthetic Dermatology. 2015;8(12):42-7.
40. Silva MT, Curi AL. Blindness and total ophthalmoplegia after aesthetic polymethyl methacrylate injection: case report. Arq Neuropsiquiatr. 2004;62:873-4.
41. Cohen JL, Brown MR. Anatomic considerations for soft tissue augmentation of the face. J Drugs Dermatol. 2009;8:13-6.
42. Grunebaum LD, Dayan S, Mandy S, et al. The risk of alar necrosis associated with dermal filler injection. Dermatol Surg. 2009;35:1635-40.
43. Hirsch RJ, Lupo M, Cohen JL, et al. Delayed presentation of impending necrosis following soft tissue augmentation with hyaluronic acid and successful management with hyaluroni-dase. J Drug Dermatol. 2007;6:325-8.
44. Hirsch RJ, Cohen JL, Carruthers JD. Successful management of an unusual presentation of impending necrosis following a hyaluronic acid injection embolus and a proposed algorithm for management with hyaluronidase. Dermatol Surg. 2007;33:357-60.
45. Larrabee WF, Makielski KH, Henderson JL. Vascular Patterns of the face. In: Merritt J (Ed). Surgical anatomy of the face, 2nd edition. Philadelphia: Lippincott Williams & Wilkins. 2004;50-6.
46. Niamtu J, Carruthers J. Pain control in cosmetic facial surgery. In: Carruthers J and Carruthers A (Ed). Soft Tissue Augmentation, 1st edition. New Delhi. 2006;11-8.
47. Zide BM, Swift R. How to block and tackle the face. Plast Reconstr Surg. 1998;101:840-51.
48. Hanke CW. The tumescent facial block: tumescent local anesthesia and nerve block anesthesia for full face laser resurfacing. Dermatol Surg. 2001;27:1003-5.
49. Tan SR, Glogau RG. Filler Esthetics. In: Carruthers J, Carruthers A (Eds). Soft Tissue Augmentation, 1st edition. New Delhi. 2006;11-8.
50. Tobias GW, Binder WJ. The Submalar Triangle. Its anatomy and clinical significance. Facial Plast Surg Clin of N America. 1994;2:255-64.
51. Pessa JE, Zadoo VP, Adrian EK, et al. Variability of the mid facial muscles: analysis of 50 hemifacial cadaver dissections. Plast Reconstr Surg. 1998;102:1888-93.
52. Benedetto AV. Cosmetic uses of Botulinum toxin A in mid face. In: Benedetto AV (Ed). Botulinumtoxin in clinical dermatology, 1st edition. London: Taylor & Francis. 2006;152-200.
53. Benedetto AV. Cosmetic uses of Botulinum toxin A in the lower face, neck and upper chest. In: Benedetto AV (Ed). Botulinum toxin in clinical dermatology, 1st edition. London: Taylor & Francis. 2006;201-53.
54. Hoefflin SM. The platysma aponeurosis. Plast Reconstr Surg. 1996;97:1080-8.

Chapter 3

Regional Anatomy

Madura C, Balaji AP

Key Messages 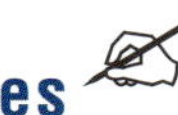

- The working knowledge on anatomy and its applied aspects are important in planning surgeries and to avoid complications.
- Knowing the surface anatomy, RSTLs, blood and nerve supply, understanding the variations in soft tissue structures and locating important danger zones at various regions are the highlights of chapter.
- The knowledge on regional anatomy makes dermatosurgeon more confident and competent.

INTRODUCTION

The knowledge on regional anatomy makes a dermatosurgeon more competent in performing surgical procedures. The anatomy and its applied aspects are important in planning surgeries. There exist significant variations in the skin of each region and with relationship to underlying structures, expected functional alterations and skin tension lines. The working knowledge on surface landmarks (to locate important structures), soft tissue planes and neurovascular distribution at various regions is equally important. Lastly, the lymphatic drainage is critically important while treating cutaneous malignancy. This chapter describes brief anatomy pertaining to dermatologic surgery of scalp, ear, neck, tarso, hand, feet and external genitalia with more emphasis on applied aspects.

BASIC SKIN STRUCTURE

Skin has epidermis, dermis, and appendages. Each region has unique properties. The epidermis varies in thickness of 0.04 mm on the eyelids and genitalia to 1.5 mm on the palms and soles.[1] Understanding of the relative thickness of the skin in various regions helps the surgeon while planning a repair. The dermis is a connective tissue network of collagen and elastin fibers embedded in a ground substance. It is responsible of skin stretchability, a major factor in wound closure. The areas like scalp and back are relatively inflexible and lack elasticity, even a small degree of skin rotation can cause protrusion at the pivot point unlike face which has significant elasticity. The stretchability is tested by lifting and stretching the skin between index and thumb to check the elasticity of the skin before wound closures. It is important to note that in anatomic sites, such as back of the hand or elbow, the skin is easily movable but quite inelastic.

SKIN BIOMECHANICS

Intrinsic elasticity of the skin is an important characteristic to understand during wound closure. This is explained by load-extension response of skin. The load-extension response is the ability of skin to stretch/extend to the applied load/pull. Langer stated “skin does not stretch proportionally with applied load; it shows nonlinear load extension to simple tension. The load-extension response can be divided into three phases. The first phase of initial extension is characterized by the high compliance of the tissues where small loads produce large extensions. The second phase represents a progressive, but nonlinear, stiffening of the tissue with increasing extension. This ability of skin to stretch over time is called creep. Mechanical creep occurs when the skin is stretched at a constant force beyond its inherent extensibility and it contributes to skin deformation. The stretching achieved during mechanical creep does not retract intraoperatively. The third, terminal phase is one in which the stiffness of the tissues is greater and the load-extension response becomes linear. Therefore, if the skin is still stretched there is breakage of collagen fibers and results in almost complete relaxation of dermis called stress relaxation, however, after

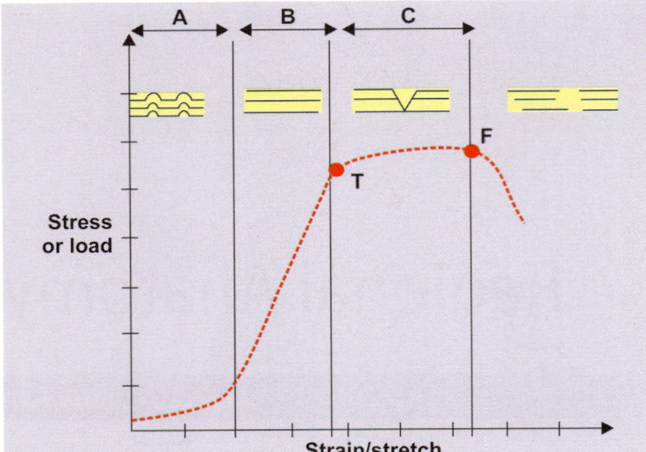

Fig. 1: Stress versus strain relationship of skin. (A) Toe region: Considerable extension occur with little force, there is initial deformation of randomly arranged collagen fibers; (B) Elastic region: Rapid extension with increasing force and collagen deformation occurs in direction of applied force; (C) Plastic region: Little extension with increased force and collagen brakes with further applied force.

this point additional undermining will not reduce closure tension, but will make skin plastic and increase the risk of hematomas or nerve damage. The wounds closed under tension will stretch-back (subsequent spreading of scars) at 12 weeks. Before planning any excision surgery, one must be aware of stretch-back phenomenon (Fig. 1 and Box 1).[3-7]

Relaxed Skin Tension Lines

In 1881, Langer first described the concept of lines of minimal tension and called Langer's lines or lines of cleavage. These lines of minimal tension are thought to correlate with the orientation of collagen bundles and elastic tissue in the dermis. Stretching of the collagen in the direction of the pull of the underlying muscles produces these lines. He considered the skin to be less extensible in the direction of the lines of tension than across them. The lines of skin tension result from the movement of underlying muscles. A correlation exists between skin crease lines and Langer's lines.[3,4] Where skin crease lines are present, Langer's lines will generally run parallel to these skin creases. If incisions and excisions are performed parallel to these lines, the wound tension is decreased and scarring is minimized. The pattern of relaxed skin tension line (RSTL) is described separately for each region.

Dermatomes

Dermatome is the area of skin with sensory supply derived from specific spinal nerves (Figs. 2A to C). It signifies the area anesthetized when specific nerves are blocked.

Box 1: Applied aspects.

- The stress versus strain relationship of skin explains intraoperative tissue expansion in closing the wound using the rule of halves.[2] Each suture progressively reduces the tension across the wound as the surgeon takes advantage of tissue creep
- This feature can be applied in closing a wound, intraoperative by placing temporary retention sutures (pulley stitch) for about 15 minutes for the mechanical creep to occur
- This load extension is maximum across Langer's lines
- Highly vascularized anatomical regions withstand tension better than poorly perfused ones, which may undergo necrosis
- On areas of less elasticity (scalp, upper back, and deltoid region) the results are esthetically compromised by scar spreading.

Scalp[8-15]

Scalp is a soft tissue envelope of the cranial vault, it extends from the external occipital protuberance and superior nuchal lines posteriorly, supraorbital margins anteriorly, and zygomatic arches laterally. Scalp is anatomically less complex but has innate characteristics like rich blood supply and hair follicles. A working knowledge of scalp anatomy is briefed in this section.

Scalp is divided into five layers, from superficial to deep as skin, subcutaneous tissue, galea aponeurotica, loose connective tissue, and periosteum (Fig. 3). The first three layers are bound together and glide as a single unit along the loose areolar tissue over the pericranium, which is adherent to the calvaria (Box 2).[8-10]

Skin of the Scalp

It is hair-bearing and contains numerous sebaceous and sweat glands. It has relatively a thin epidermis and a variably thicker dermis. The dermis is thinnest over the forehead about 3 mm and thickest over the occipital area approximately measuring 8 mm. The dermis contains a rich network of nerves, vascular, and lymphatic vessels. Langer's lines tend to be longitudinal on the scalp (Ref. Figs. 12A to C).

Connective Tissue (Superficial Fascia)

The superficial fascia is an inelastic, fibro-fatty layer connects skin to the underlying aponeurosis and it is 4–7 mm thick, thickest at the vertex. This layer is also called as dense connective tissue layer as interwoven sheets of connective tissue (fibrous septae) separate the subcutaneous fat into small compartments. It is highly-vascularized, provides a passage way for nerves and blood vessels to the other scalp layers. Subcutaneous fat is divided into multiple small compartments by fibrous septa which bind down the scalp skin firmly to the muscles and aponeurosis, making dissection in this plane difficult and bloody. There are also vertically oriented reticular fibers present that form strong attachments with the dermis above, and galea below. These vertical fibers in essence bind the first three layers of the scalp together.

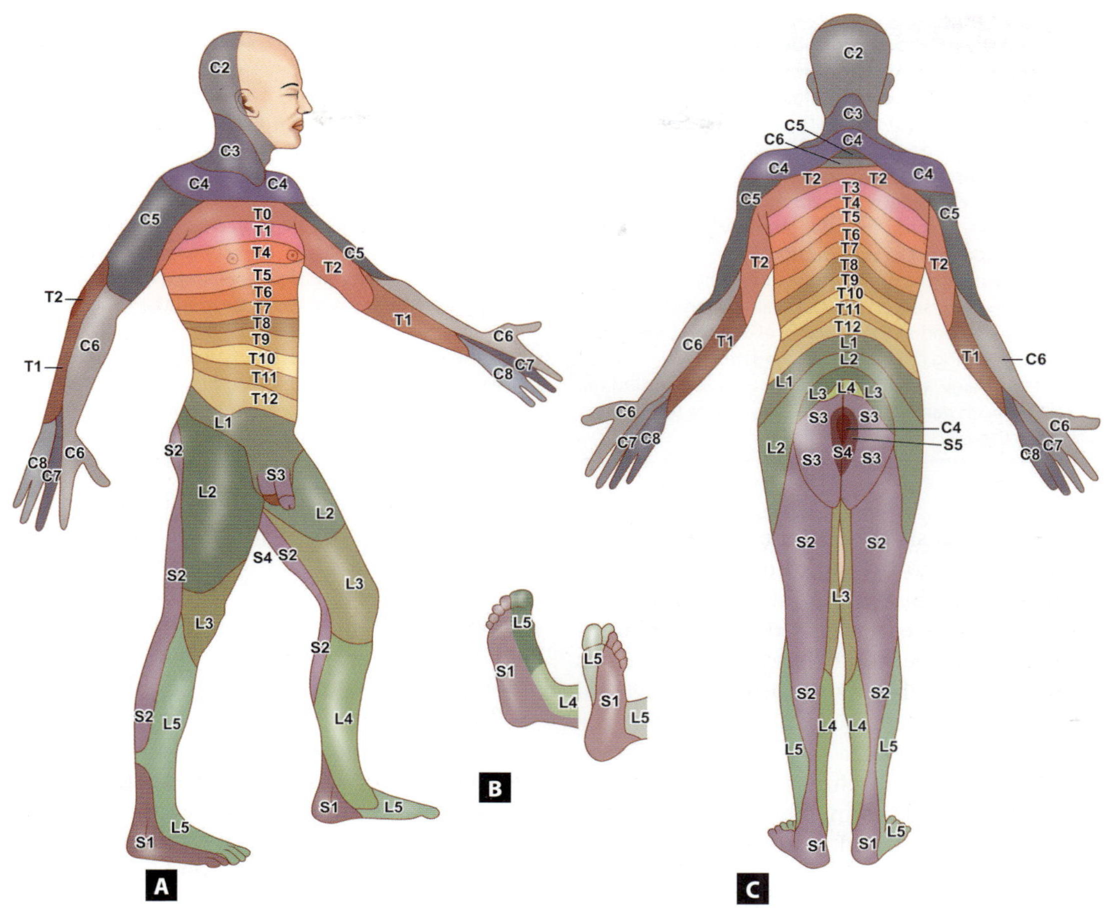

Figs. 2A to C: Dermatomes: (A) Anterolateral view; (B) Inferior view; and (C) Posterior view.
Source: Gray's anatomy for students.

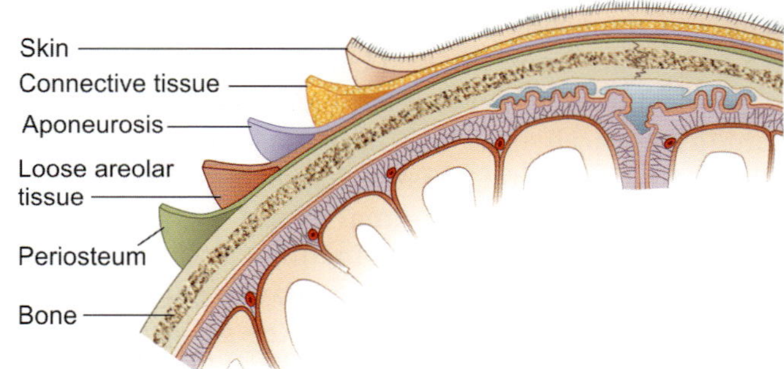

Fig. 3: Layers of scalp.
Source: Grant's Atlas of Anatomy, 13th edition.

Epicranial Aponeurosis (Galea Aponeurotica)

The galea aponeurotica is the strongest layer of the scalp. It is made of dense fibrous tendinous sheet, measuring 1–2 mm in thickness. It extends from the superior occipital line to approximately 2 cm below the frontal hairline on the forehead where it interdigitates with the superficial muscular aponuerotic system (SMAS). Posterolaterally,

Box 2: Applied aspects of surgical layers of scalp (first three layers are called surgical layers of scalp).

- The incisions on the scalp should be closed vertically following relaxed skin tension lines, except for in the occipital area where incisions are best horizontal, paralleling the skin crease lines (Figs. 12A to C) Scalp incisions must be at an angle and parallel to the hair follicles to minimize their transection and to avoid localized scarring alopecia.
- The sheets of connective tissue in second layer bind the blood vessels to the dermis and fibrous septa in such a way that vasoconstriction and vasospasms are prevented when a vessel is cut. This is the reason behind the profuse bleeding that can be observed during surgery or following scalp trauma.
- The third layer galea is substantially stronger than the overlying skin and its site to secure retaining sutures which is anchored deep throughout this fascia. Also during artificial hair implantation, galea is the anchoring point.
- Wounds superficial to the aponeurosis gape less because aponeurosis holds the skin tight. Traumatic wounds that extend to the galea will tend to gape open widely and bleed profusely because the pull of the frontalis muscle anteriorly and occipitalis muscle posteriorly will separate the laceration widely.
- The galea is resistant to stretch; the top of the galea is strongly adherent to the subcutaneous layer, making dissection between these two layers extremely difficult and bloody.
- In deeper wounds, galea must be reapproximated properly by grabbing a large bite of galea with the suture needle; this minimize tension on the overlying skin, and results in good scar.[8]

Box 3: Points to remember on subgaleal layer.

- The subgaleal layer is important from a surgical standpoint and lends itself to easy avascular dissection during surgical procedures.
- In addition, the blood supply to the scalp runs in the subcutaneous tissues, thus surgical dissection of the subgaleal space does not compromise the blood supply to scalp tissue in any way.
- The emissary veins connect surface of scalp to the brain, therefore infections in the subgaleal space may dangerously communicate with the surface of the brain via this connection.
- As this space extend beneath the orbicularis oculi and into the eyelids and root of the nose, injury/surgery on the scalp or forehead may result in the pooling of blood in the upper eyelids and sometimes lower eyelids as well, causing the black eyes or edema.
- Subcutaneous hemorrhage and inflammation in closed wound in second layer causes much pain with little swelling due to unyielding reticulum of fibrous tissue.

Box 4: Anatomic surgical considerations.

- The scalp laxity determines the possible extent of scalp excisions. It depends on glidabilty and elasticity. The ability of the scalp to slide over the pericranium contributes to scalp laxity (determined by subgaleal space with loose fibroareolar tissue). The ability of the tissue to stretch (scalp can stretch to full capacity along Langer's lines) contributes to scalp elasticity.
- Both of these factors are subjected to individual variations either in loose fibroareolar tissue or in content of elastic tissue, this explains why some scalps are tight and some are loose and stretch better. Excessive removal of tissue beyond the capacity of stretching will lead to plastic scalp.
- Scalp undermining must be in proper plane. Extensive undermining, especially when done blindly, can be associated with traumatized blood vessels and nerves, increased scaring in the undermined area, and open up tissue planes that may increase infection rates,[17] however, the rich vascular plexus makes defects of the scalp to heal quickly, even by secondary intention.

the epicranial aponeurosis attachment extends from the superior nuchal line to the superior temporal line. Laterally, it continues as the temporal fascia. Anteriorly, the subaponeurotic space extends to the upper eyelids due to the lack of a bony insertion. There are blood vessels present in the galea, which extend into the subgaleal layer below, or the superficial vascular plexus of the subcutaneous layer above. Galea provides an insertion site for the occipitofrontalis muscle. It is connected to the pericranium by loose areolar connective tissue, resulting in a largely avascular space and is an optimal site for undermining of the scalp. This avascular space also allows the aponeurosis to recruit mobility, carrying the hair-bearing skin with it.[8]

Subgaleal Layer or Loose Areolar Tissue

The subgaleal layer connects the epicranial aponeurosis to the pericranium and allows the superficial three layers of the scalp to move over the pericranium. It is a space containing loose areolar tissue largely avascular. Scalp flaps are elevated along this avascular plane; however, certain emissary veins traverse this layer, which connects the scalp veins to the diploic veins and intracranial venous sinuses. The easy gladability of scalp is due to property of subgaleal space that allows easy approximation of wide wounds, however in areas where it is absent closure is difficult (Boxs 3 and 4).[11,12]

Pericranium

The pericranium is the periosteum of the skull bones. Along the suture lines, the pericranium becomes continuous with the endosteum. A subperiosteal hematoma, therefore, forms in the shape of the skull bones.

Nerve Supply

The motor innervation of the scalp comes from facial nerve. Sensory innervation comes from the trigeminal nerve (area of scalp anterior to the auricles) or the cervical nerves C2 and C3 (area of scalp posterior to the auricles). These nerves run in the second or subcutaneous layer of the scalp. The six sensory nerves includes: (1) supratrochlear, (2) supraorbital (branches of the ophthalmic division of the trigeminal nerve), (3) zygomaticotemporal (branch of the maxillary division of the trigeminal nerve), (4) auriculotemporal nerve (branch of the mandibular division of the trigeminal nerve), (5) lesser occipital (branch of the C2) and (6) greater occipital nerves (branch of the posterior ramus of the C2) (Fig. 4 and Box 5).[13,14]

Blood Supply

The scalp has a rich vascular supply. The major blood supply of the scalp is from five paired main arteries, two pairs come from internal carotid system anteriorly (supraorbital and supratrochlear arteries) and the remaining three from the external carotid system posteriorly (occipital, postauricular, and superficial temporal arteries). A minimal blood supply comes from the bone perforators of meningeal arteries. The large arteries lie in subcutaneous layer, held in place by the connective tissue bundles of the scalp, and send penetrating branches superiorly into the skin. The blood vessels anastomose freely in the scalp. The arteries of the scalp run centripetally, that is the larger trunks of the arteries start laterally, running in a central and medial fashion, becoming smaller as they enter a system of free anastomosis towards the medial aspect of the scalp. Any transaction of arteries on peripheral scalp may grossly limit blood supply to areas both adjacent to and remote from the locus of transection.[14,15] The midline scalp possesses a relative watershed zone where perfusion may be less predictable. This centripetal distribution and a fact that the scalp does not have musculocutaneous perforators together are important from surgical point of view for surgical flap survival (Figs. 5 and 6 and Box 5).

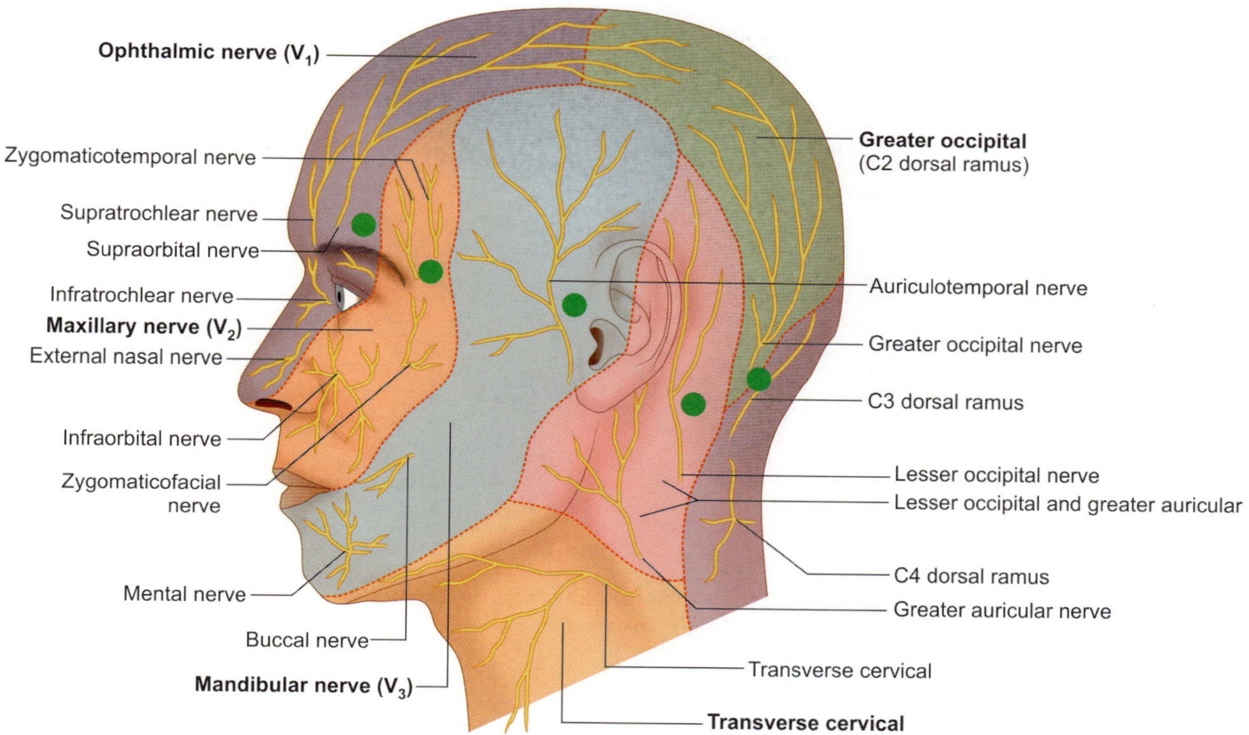

Fig. 4: Sensory innervation of the scalp lateral view. Supratrochlear nerve supplies the scalp in the medial plane at the frontal region, up to the vertex. Supraorbital nerve supplies the scalp at the front, lateral to the supratrochlear nerve distribution, up to the vertex. Zygomaticotemporal nerve supplies the scalp over the temple region. Auriculotemporal nerve supplies the skin over the temporal region of the scalp. Lesser occipital supplies the scalp over the lateral occipital region. Greater occipital nerve supplies the scalp in the median plane at the occipital region, up to the vertex.
Source: Drake, Vogl, Mitchell. Grants atlas of anatomy. 2005.

Box 5: Applied aspects on neurovasculature of scalp.

- All nerves and vessels of the scalp originate below the level of the brow as it is extended circumferentially around the scalp following centripetal distribution. This anatomical location of the arteries and nerves of the scalp makes central scalp surgeries easy with minimal neurovascular trauma.
- There is relative loss of vascular network and decrease in midline anastomoses with aging, that can affect wound healing, especially for deeper defects.
- The incisions in the peripheral scalp can transect nerve trunks and result in large areas of permanent hypoesthesia, a complication that can be avoided or explained to the patient if one is familiar with the anatomical locations of these nerves.
- Knowledge of anatomy of nerves is important during scalp blocks. Infiltrating local anesthetic around the scalp's periphery (through which all the sensory nerves traverse) can produce total scalp anesthesia.
- The lymphatic drainage of scalp is diffuse, scalp lacks lymph nodes and there are no barriers to lymph flow contributing to the significant spread of pathology that may be seen in this location.

Venous Drainage

The scalp has superficial and deep venous drainage. The superficial drainage (superficial temporal, occipital, posterior auricular, supraorbital and supratrochlear veins) follows the arteries (Fig. 5). The deep component of the skull is drained by the pterygoid venous plexus. The veins of the scalp connect to the diploic veins of the skull via valve less emissary veins. This establishes a connection between the scalp and the dural venous sinuses (Box 5).

Lymphatic Drainage

There are no lymph nodes in the scalp, but multiple lymphatic vessels drain the scalp to local regional lymph node chains in centrifugal pattern. The region posterior to the auricle drain into the posterior auricular (mastoid) and occipital lymph nodes, which then drain into the superficial cervical nodal chains. The regions anterior to the auricle drain into the preauricular and parotid lymph nodes, which further drain into the submandibular and deep cervical nodes.[16]

Muscles of the Scalp

The occipitofrontalis muscle consists of two occipital bellies and two frontal bellies. The occipital bellies arise from the superior nuchal lines on the occipital bone. The frontal bellies originate from the skin and superficial

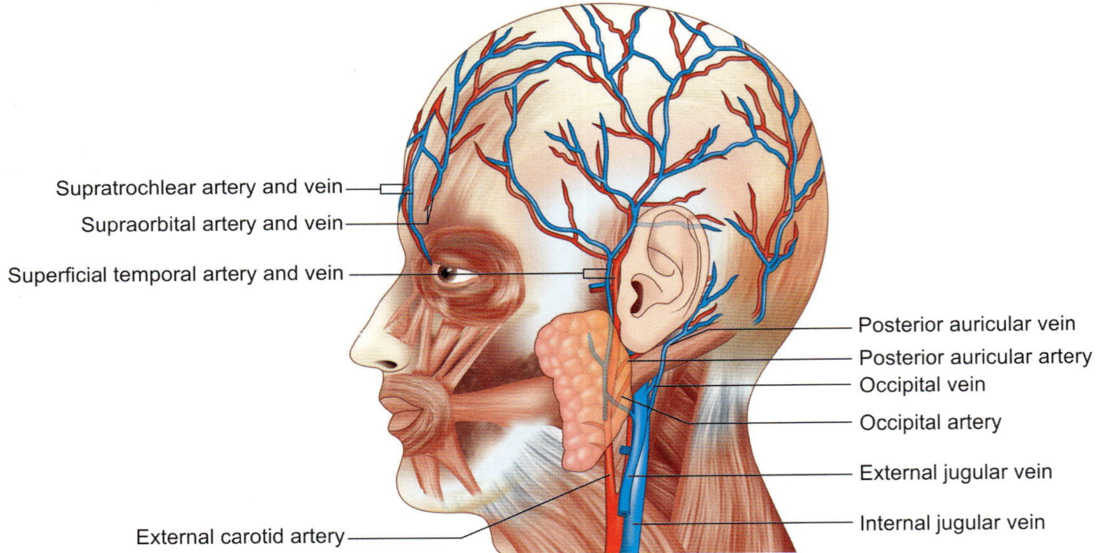

Fig. 5: Arterial and venous system of scalp in lateral view.
Source: Gray's anatomy for students.

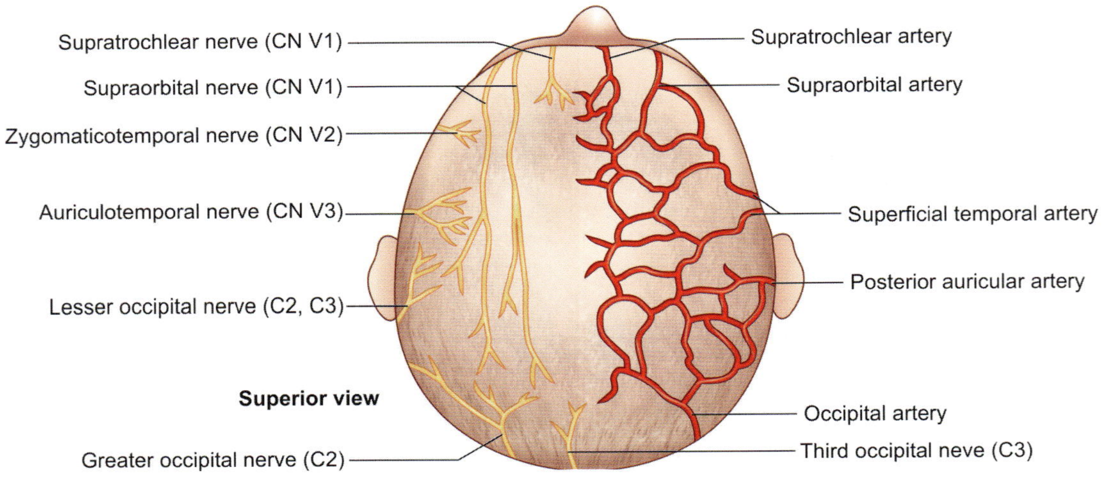

Fig. 6: Neurovascular supply of scalp in superior view from the midline anterior to posterior, the arteries are as follows: Supratrochlear artery, supraorbital artery, superficial temporal artery, posterior auricular artery and occipital artery.
Note: Midline anastomoses are rare. Area anterior to the ear is trigeminal distribution and posterior to the ear is cervical distribution.
Source: Textbook of Grant's atlas of anatomy, 13th edition.

fascia of the upper eyelids. The occipital and frontal bellies insert into the epicranial aponeurosis. The galea connects the two muscles, and is referred as one structure, the occipitofrontalis muscle. Each occipital belly is innervated by the posterior auricular branch of the facial nerve, and each frontal belly is innervated by the frontal branch of the facial nerve. The frontal bellies can raise the eyebrows (Fig. 7).

Ear[8,13,14,18]

The external ear or auricle is organ of cosmesis (Fig. 8). It has both functional and cosmetic importance. It mainly protects the internal ear and localizes and directs the sound waves into the ear. The auricle or pinna is formed by complex cartilaginous framework with lot of depressions and elevations covered by skin. The important landmarks are (Fig. 8) helix, antihelix, tragus, antitragus, lobule, and concha. The skin is avidly attached to cartilage all over except on helix. The layers of ear are anterior surface of epidermis, dermis, perichondrium, cartilage, fat, posterior dermis, and epidermis (from anterior to posterior surface). The lobule does not contain cartilage. The external ear does not contain muscle.

Ear has a rich blood supply from anterior and posterior auricular artery and sensory nerve supply comes from cranial nerves V, VII, X, and C2 C3 of cervical plexus. The sensory nerves are as follows (Figs. 9A and B).

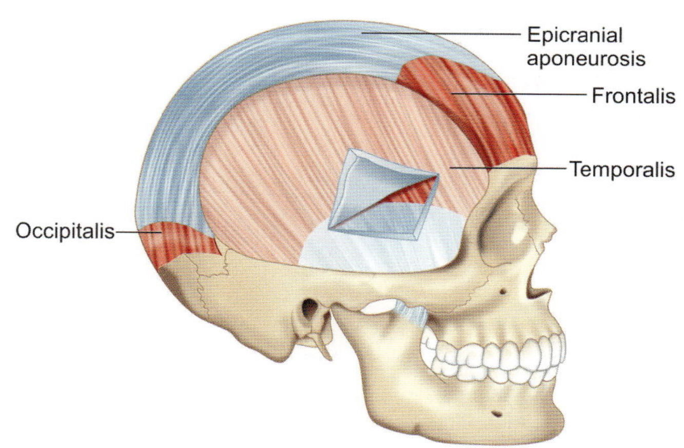

Fig. 7: Figure demonstrating the occipitalis, frontalis, and temporalis muscles of the scalp
Source: Textbook of Grant's atlas of anatomy, 13th edition.

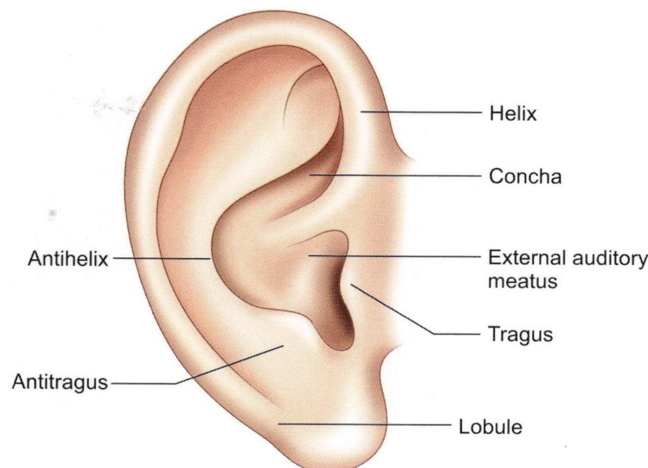

Fig. 8: Surface anatomy of the ear

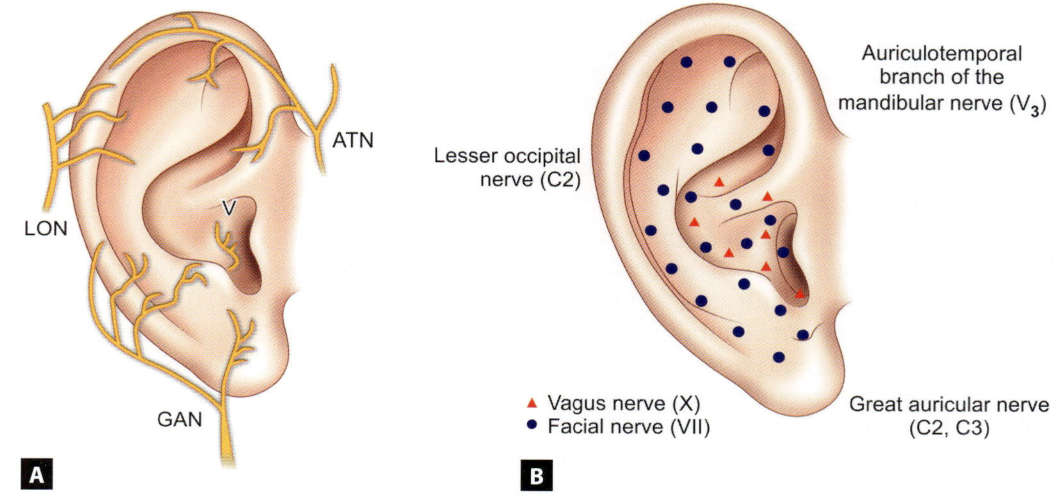

Figs. 9A and B: Sensory innervation of the external ear.
(ATN: Auriculotemporal nerve; GAN: Greater occipital nerve; LON: Lesser occipital nerve; V: Vagus nerve)
Source: Gray's anatomy for students.

- The greater auricular nerve is a branch of the cervical plexus. It innervates the posteromedial, posterolateral, and inferior auricle (lower two-thirds both anteriorly and posteriorly)
- The lesser occipital nerve innervates a small portion of the helix.
- The auricular branch of the vagus nerve innervates the concha and most of the area around the auditory meatus.
- The auriculotemporal nerve originates from the mandibular branch of the trigeminal nerve, innervates the anterosuperior and anteromedial aspects of the auricle. The lymphatics drain to superficial, deep cervical, and mastoid lymph nodes (Box 6).

Box 6: Anatomic surgical considerations.

- As lobule has no underlying muscle, the wound closure is parallel to the force of gravity.
- The level of undermining is subdermal in helix.
- Excision surgeries around the ear with unopposed tension may affect the free margins (helices or lobule) of the ear and distort these structures. Wound closure in these locations often require flap and/or graft placement to lessen the risk.[18]
- Simple excision and closure of skin lesions over the edge of the pinna may distort the curve of the pinna, with a noticeable defect. Wedge excision or autoflaps for keloids are preferred.
- The retroauricular and preauricular area make good match for harvest of the free grafts.

NECK[8,10,13,14,19-22]

The neck is the exposed part of body, long and supple with functions as full range of movements. The neck extends between lower margin of the mandible to upper margin of manubrium sternum. The neck is the vulnerable region encompassing important vital structures. The dermatologic surgeon must be familiar with the anatomy of the neck, and be knowledgeable and cautious while operating on this vital area with danger zones.

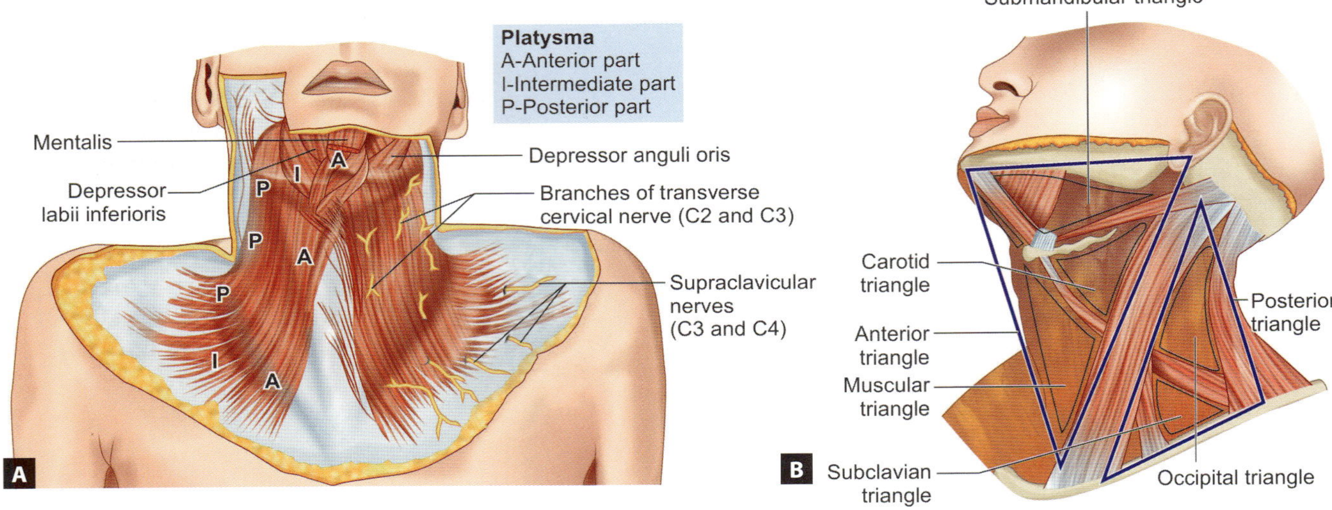

Figs. 10A and B: (A) Superficial muscles of neck anterior (platysma) and (B) Lateral view (shows sternocleidomastoid muscle and triangles of the neck). Submental triangle (borders: hyoid bone, mandible, anterior belly of the digastric muscle, midline), submandibular triangle (borders: anterior and posterior bellies of the digastric muscle, mandible), carotid triangle (borders: SCM, posterior belly of the digastric muscle, superior belly of the omohyoid muscle, stylohyoid muscle), muscular triangle (borders: hyoid bone, SCM, superior belly of the omohyoid muscle, midline posterior triangle), posterior triangle (borders: SCM, trapezius muscle, clavicle).

Surface Anatomy

The superficial landmarks of the neck are the hyoid, larynx, and trachea in midline anteriorly, vertebral column posteriorly and the sternocleidomastoid muscle (SCM) laterally, that becomes more prominent on turning neck to one side. It divides neck into anterior and posterior triangles. A platysmal muscle becomes more prominent on clinching the jaws (Figs. 10A and B). Adam's apple is most prominent part on anterior neck. The thyroid cartilage is below hyoid bone and cricoid cartilage is below Adam's apple at C6. The emergency laryngectomy is done between these two points.[19]

Skin and Subcutaneous Tissue

The skin covering the anterior and side of the neck is thin, quite elastic, and can readily be raised into folds, which contain the platysma muscle. In these respects it differs from the skin over the nape of the neck, which is very dense, with thick dermis and adherent and more freely supplied with nerves, but not nearly so well-supplied with blood vessels.

Skin Tension Lines

Relaxed skin tension lines typically lie in a transverse direction on the neck. The placement of excision lines in this orientation is essential, as vertical incisions have a tendency toward scar contracture (Figs. 12A to C).

Muscles of the Neck

The key cutaneous muscles of the neck are the platysma and SCM (Figs. 10A and B). The platysma lies immediately below skin. It is an extremely thin muscle that is superficial in the neck and arises from the fascia of the muscles of the chest and shoulders and passes upward over the clavicles and neck toward the lower face. It originates inferiorly from the pectoralis and deltoid fascia. The fibers ascend upwards and at the mandible some fibers insert directly into bone under the mandible, its only bony insertion. The other fibers blend into the modiolus, the depressor anguli oris, the lower lip, the depressor labials inferioris and mostly continue to ascend above the mandible where they blend into the SMAS. In the midline of the neck the platysma is absent except when the fibers from each side decussate (intertwine) with the other side under the chin. It is innervated by the cervical branch of the facial nerve. It functions to depress the corner of the mouth and to depress the mandible during deep inspiration but is probably more important as a mimetic muscle to express horror or disgust. It also assists in venous return.

As part of aging, its medial fibers attenuate or thicken to create platysmal bands. It is responsible for wrinkles of the neck. Superficial cervical fascia, a loose connective tissue separates platysma and sternocleidomastoid from underlying structures. This plane allows platysma to glide easily over sternocleidomastoid and enables effective minimally invasive suture lifting of platysma.[20] The SCM is prominent landmark in neck. The muscle extends from the medial clavicle to the postauricular area and divides the neck into anterior and posterior triangles. It protects underlying structures. The carotid pulsations are noted along anterior edge of SCM at C6 vertebra.

Triangles of Neck

The anterior triangle is divided into four triangles by small muscles into submental, submandibular, carotid, and muscular triangles (Figs. 10A and B). The submental triangle contains submental lymph nodes. Submandibular triangle is marking for danger zone for facial artery. The key components of the carotid triangle include the internal and external carotid arteries, the internal jugular vein, vagus, and hypoglossal nerves.[21] The important structures in posterior triangle include spinal accessory nerve, greater auricular nerve, lesser occipital nerve, and transverse cervical nerve. The spinal accessory nerve (CN XI) innervates the sternocleidomastoid and trapezius muscles. It is located immediately below the SMAS fascia within the posterior triangle and emerges at the posterior border of the SCM at a point known as Erb's point. As it is covered only by skin and superficial cervical fascia, it is vulnerable to injury during surgery in the posterior triangle, transection of which results in a winging of scapula and difficulty with arm abduction (Fig. 11). Erb's point is located by turning the head away and is defined by an imaginary line connecting the middle of the angle of the mandible to the mastoid process, intersecting the posterior border of the SCM (Fig. 11).[14,21,22]

The external carotid artery and the thyrocervical trunk are the main blood supply to the face and neck. The venous system of the neck includes the internal jugular veins, the external jugular veins, and the anterior jugular veins. The superficial venous drainage of the anterior neck is located deep to the platysma muscle.

Applied Aspects

- The skin of the neck is relatively loose with transverse creases and wrinkles. Elective incisions are easily placed in these lines. Because of the concave shape of the neck, vertical incisions have a tendency toward scar contracture with web formation, which may have functional as well as cosmetic implications.
- Adam's apple is most prominent part on anterior neck. The thyroid cartilage is below hyoid bone and cricoid cartilage is below Adam's apple at C6. The emergency laryngectomy is done between these two points.
- The carotid pulsations are noted along anterior edge of SCM at C6 vertebra.
- Incisions on anterior neck must be superficial to avoid damage to the important underlying structures.
- Nape of neck is the site for carbuncle seen at the lower part of the back of the neck in median line. The skin is thick and dense deeper incision is required during excision. Wide unplanned excisions can lead to contractures.
- The botulinum toxin injections must be specifically injected into the platysmal bands, in the deep dermal layer. Transverse neck lines are injected more superficially as diffusion of toxin to the strap muscle or deeper muscles of the neck can cause dysphagia, dysphonia, dysarthria or life-threatening breathing difficulties.[10,14,16.]
- Platysma is the superficial muscle of the anterior neck. When performing surgery in this area, one should be mindful of suturing the platysma carefully as irregularities in this muscle may pull unevenly on a healing scar.
- Cervical branch of the facial nerve supplies motor innervation to the platysma muscle. This is important because skin incisions over the angle of the mandible can distort the mouth, if careful observation to muscular innervation is not considered.
- Neck and face drain into submandibular, submental, occipital, and superficial cervical lymph nodes.

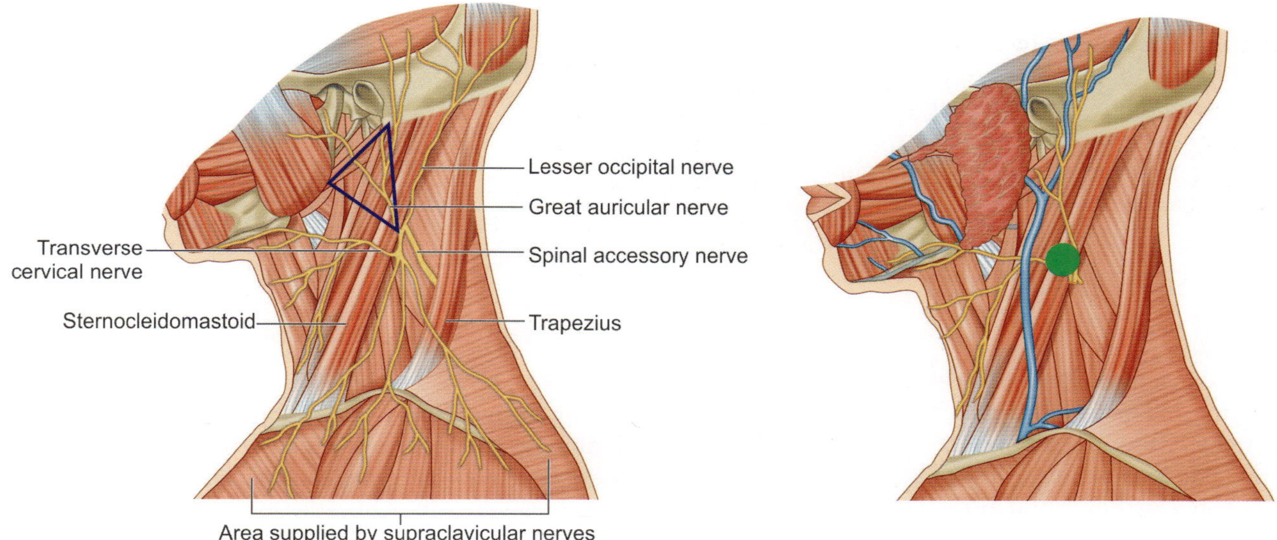

Fig. 11: Innervation of the neck and marking of Erb's point (lateral view). The spinal accessory nerve exits behind the sternocleidomastoid. Three important sensory nerves, the greater auricular, the transverse cervical and the lesser occipital nerves, that supply sensation to the neck and ear emerge 2 cm above and 2 cm below Erb's point.

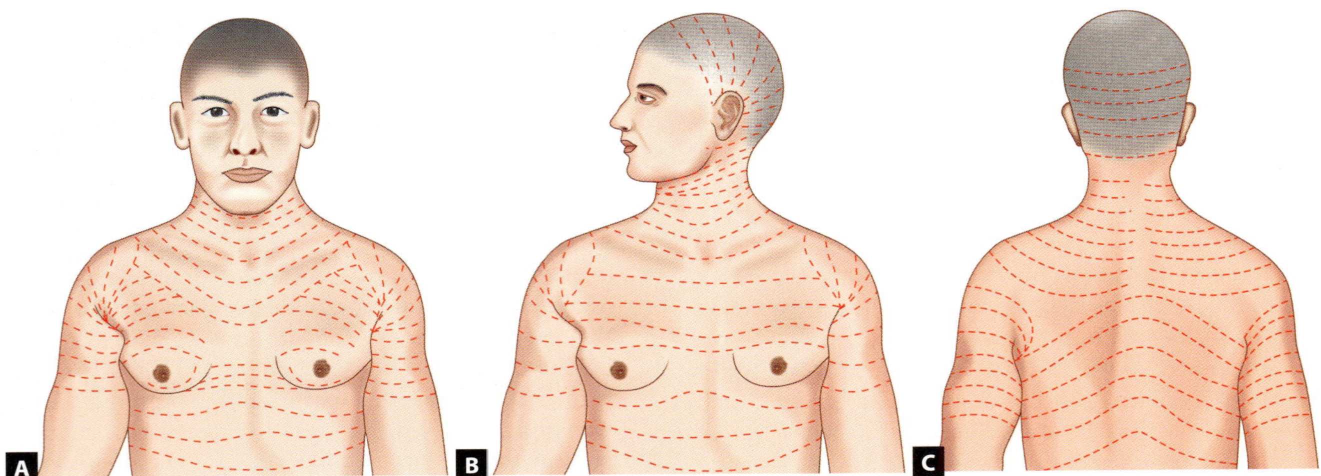

Figs. 12A to C: Relaxed skin tension line of the torso, neck and head.

Understanding the anatomy of lymphatic drainage of the head and neck is crucial to locating and working up a suspected malignancy or metastasis.

- Erb's point is the site where the accessory nerve exits from the SCM to cross the posterior triangle. Extreme care must be observed during surgery in the area 2 cm above and below this point to avoid inadvertent nerve injury (Fig. 11).
- The marginal mandibular nerve is vulnerable to injury especially during neck rejuvenation (liposuction of neck and platysma repair or SMAS plication). It crosses the mandible in the vicinity of the facial artery and vein, as well as at the posterior angle of the mandible. Injury can be avoided by suctioning in the midfat over the nerve, and avoiding over the mandibular ramus.

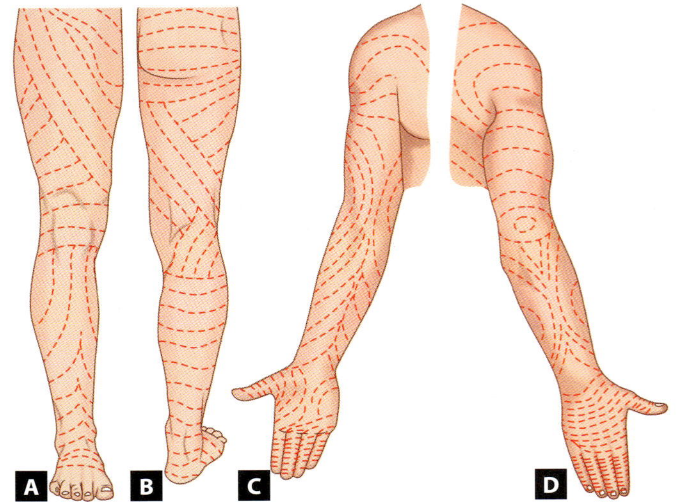

Figs. 13A to D: Relaxed skin tension line of the extremities.

TARSO[8,13,14]

The regional anatomy of tarso includes trunk and its extremities with special surgical considerations. The dermatosurgery is only restricted to skin and subcutaneous tissue in these areas. We must be well-versed with the RSTL's, important areas such as danger zones and surgical anatomy of axilla and breast.

Relaxed Skin Tension Lines (Figs. 12 and 13)

Relaxed skin tension lines are oriented transversely across the trunk and extremity, placing sutures along these lines reduce wound tension. Pinch test is a simple test to identify skin tension lines. Pinch the planned surgical site of skin between thumb and index finger, if pinch produces straight lines it is parallel to skin tension lines, if it produces S-shaped curve, pinch lines are across skin tension lines. The areas like anterior chest, abdomen, upper arms, and back pose difficulty in evaluating pinch test. On pendulous structures like breast and abdomen, where action of muscle is not prime concern, closure should be parallel to the force of gravity.[14] Over the joints like nape of neck, elbow, wrist, knee and ankle, wound closure must be perpendicular to the primary action of the underlying joint or muscle. This avoids wound contracture especially over joints and hence do not affect joint mobility.

Anatomic Surgical Consideration

The torso, arms, and legs are cylindrical structures and create varied forces unlike face. The mobile joints of limbs create added tensile forces. The wound closures are associated with large dog ears and also pose more tension during closure. The skin varies in thickness, thickest on the back. The skin is slightly redundant on flexures compared to extensors. The shoulder, arm, and chest are high-risk area for keloid formation.[23] Thickness of the dermis varies from less than 0.5 mm to more than 5 mm. The dermal

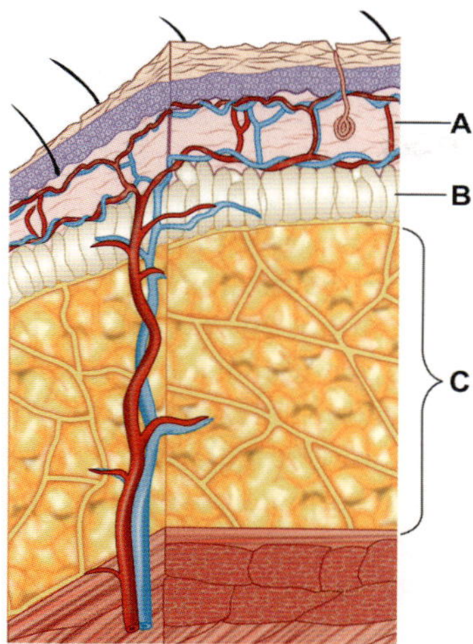

Fig. 14: Subcutaneous fat layers from dermis to muscle. (A: Apical layer; B: Mantle layer; C: Deeper layer).

grafts can be harvested from areas of thick dermal tissue (lower back and thigh), for smaller harvest medial arm or postauricular regions is a choice. In some areas of limbs, superficial blunt dissection and undermining are recommended to avoid damage to vessels and nerves. In joint areas, neurovascular bundles lie deep to the muscle fascia. The undermining must be deep subcutaneous on the trunk. Remember, the blood supply is less in the trunk and extremities when compared to the face. Distribution of hair and appendages also vary. The medial aspect of arm and groin forms the less common but important site for full thickness graft harvest, as they are comparatively in covered areas and also laxity is more and easy closure.[24] Split thickness grafts are harvested from anterolateral thigh, because of ease of harvest on the rounded contour, the harvest is of even thickness and lastly large size can be harvested because of large surface area of thigh.

Blood supply to the tarso and limbs are less compared to face. Preserving a 1:1 length to base ratio will maximize the blood flow to the donor skin. Knowledge of lymphatic drainage is important plan base of the flap inferiorly whenever possible.

Subcutaneous Fat

The apical, mantle, and deep layers are three layers of subcutaneous fat. Apical layer is a periadnexal (thecal) layer and it lies just beneath the reticular dermis, it is yellow in appearance (Fig. 14). It surrounds sweat glands and hair follicles, vascular and lymphatic channels. Mantle layer is a superficial fat consisting organized layer of fat cells composed of more columnar-shaped lipocytes. It is separated from the deep layer of fat by a fascia-like layer of fibrous tissue. It acts as shock absorber and contributes to the skin's ability to resist trauma. Deep layer lies between mantle layer and muscle fascia. The thickness of this layer depends on the sex, genes, and diet of the individual. The fat cells are arranged in pearls, and are gathered into globules. These globules are then packed together in lobules separated by fibrous septa and then arranged between tangential and oblique fibrous planes. The tangential planes are much thicker and run parallel to the underlying muscle fascia, but they are of little consequence when performing liposuction. Oblique planes are thinner and interconnect the tangential fibrous layers. Though thinner, they are of a cosmetic importance because the vertical arrangement of subcutaneous fat from skin to muscle fascia is the cause of cellulite.[25,26] The deep fat layer is the zone for liposculpture. The apical and mantle layers represent the "no man's zone" of liposuction. Damage to these layers increases the risk of postoperative complication such as seroma or dermal necrosis (Box 7).

Box 7: Applied aspects of subcutaneous fat.

- In the submental region, the fat immediately beneath the platysma must be removed and the fat between the digastric muscles and beneath the superficial layer of the deep, or the investing fascia of the neck should not be removed, as it can cause permanent depression.
- In abdomen, subcutaneous fat is divided by superficial campers fascia and the deeper Scarpa fascia. The deep fascia overlays the musculoaponeurosis, and covers the small arteries and veins along the surface of the anterior rectus sheath. Liposuction is performed between these fascial layers in the abdomen.
- The neurovascular structures are deeper to fascia and muscle in thigh and abdomen.
- In hips, the subcutaneous fat is divided into superficial and the deep. The superficial fascial system (SFS) encases the superficial fat, is light yellow and dense, whereas the deeper fat is usually darker and less well-structured.
- Zones of adherence are sites where the SFS connects to the underlying muscle fascia which are different for men and women and responsible for the android and gynecoid appearance of hips. The gluteal crease represents another zone of adherence. The zones of adherence should not be violated with a liposuction cannula.
- The lower leg is also a site for harvesting fat. The major vessels and nerves are beneath the investing fascia of the superficial fat of the legs. The lateral knee should never be liposuctioned, as it is an area of insertion of thigh musculature.
- Owing to low vascularity of donor sites (lateral thigh and abdomen), they are sites of fat harvest during autologous fat transfer.[27]

Breast

Breast tissue has fibroglandular tissue with rich vascularity. It lies over a pectoral muscle. It extends from just below the clavicle to the axilla and across to the sternum. The fibroglandular tissue is encircled by a thin layer of connective tissue called fascia. The deep layer of this fascia lies on pectoralis muscle, and the superficial layer is just beneath the skin. Nipple and areola are a part of pendulous structure and lacks support, differs from normal skin by being pigmented and rich in montgomery glands. The epidermis and dermis are thin with fine fat layer beneath. The dermatosurgeon must be well-aware of this while performing vitiligo surgery, in assessing depth of dermabrasion and also when creating recipient pits in mini punch grafting, owing to thinner skin of areola. The RSTL is curved and wound closures to be planned accordingly

(Figs. 12A to C). The vascularity of the breast is more and tumescence anesthesia must be given adequately. The retromammary space is the site for placing implanters and fillers (Fig. 15). The breast tissue lies on pectoralis major and minor muscle, which form the basis for botulinum toxin injection for breast lift.[8,13]

Axilla

It is a pyramidal interval between the arm and the chest wall. The anterior and posterior axillary folds are formed by pectoralis major and latissimus dorsi, respectively. It contains the axillary vessels and the brachial plexus, branches of the intercostal nerves and lymph nodes with fat and loose areolar tissue. The long thoracic nerve and intercostobrachial nerve are most superficial, damage to which must be avoided. The axilla is rich in sweat glands, they are concentrated most in the central elliptical area of approximately 4–5 centimeters. It is important to note that a tail of breast tissue called the "axillary tail of Spence" does extend into the axilla. This is important because this could be mistaken for abscess or excess fat accumulation, which does not require an intervention from dermatosurgeon. The axilla is more prone for hematoma and seroma after any surgical intervention, due to inability to compress the axillary cavity. This can increase the risk of postoperative infections, delay healing and may lead to the formation of hypertrophic scars and irregularities on the skin surface. Proper compressive bandages avoid this complication.[28,29]

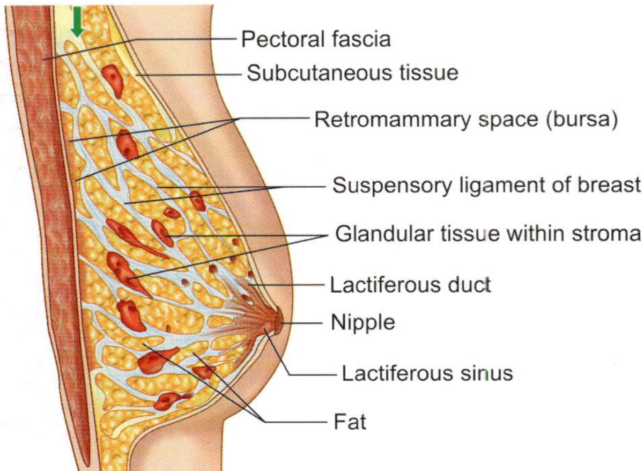

Fig. 15: Lateral section of the breast showing skin subcutaneous fat with glandular tissue retromammary and pectoral fascia. The implanters or the fillers are placed in retromammary space during breast augmentation.

HAND[8,13,14,22,30]

Hand is an important functional part with unique structure. Dermatologic surgery of the hand is generally limited to surgery of the skin and subcutaneous tissue. The vital structures like nerves, arteries, veins, ligaments, and tendons, sit superficially below a thin layer of skin and fat. Anatomy of the hand is complex, should be carefully considered to preserve function and cosmesis.

Surface Anatomy

The hand has dorsal and ventral surface and a radial and ulnar aspect. The five digits are named or numbered from radial to ulnar side. The fingers are divided into distal, middle, and proximal phalanges, thumb has only two phalanges. The phalanges are attached to the metacarpals. The palm has named creases. There are two volar muscular prominences, thenar radially and hypothenar on the ulnar aspect (Figs. 16A and B).

Structure of Skin

There is a great disparity in the character of skin and soft-tissue envelope covering the dorsum of the hand and that

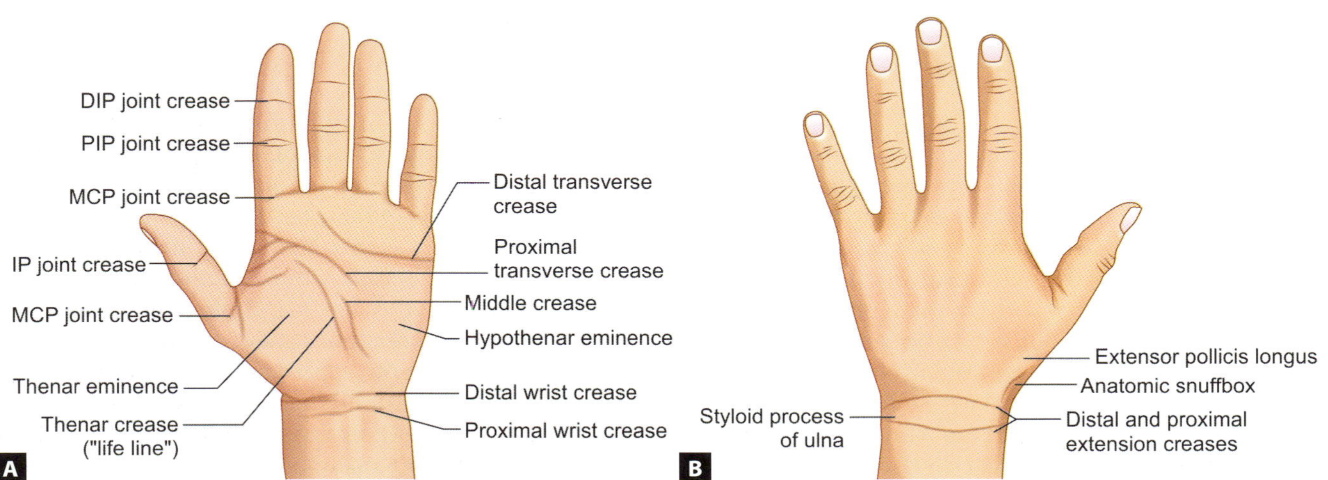

Figs. 16A and B: Surface anatomy of hand: (A) Left palm; (B) Left hand.
(DIP: Distal interphalangeal; PIP: Proximal interphalangeal; MCP: Metacarpophalangeal; IP, Interphalangeal).
Source: Gray's anatomy for students.

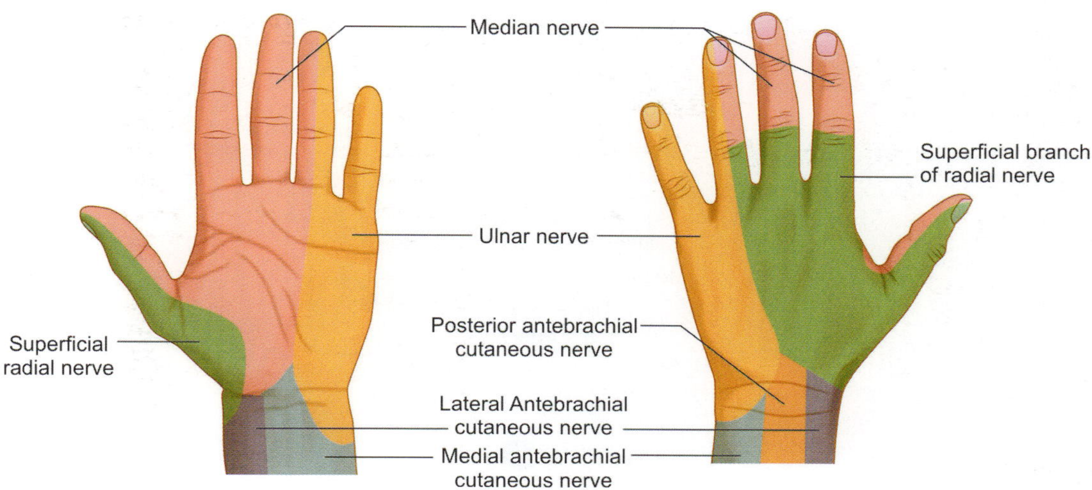

Fig. 17: Sensory distribution of hand. (The radial nerve supplies the radial aspect of the dorsal two-thirds of the hand but notably not the distal aspects of the index, middle, or ring fingers. The ulnar third of the dorsal surface is supplied by the ulnar nerve, with the exception of the distal ring and little fingers. The ulnar nerve also supplies the palmar third to the hand on the ulnar aspect. The median nerve is responsible for the remainder of the sensation, most of which is on the palmar aspect of the hand).
Source: Gray's anatomy for students.

covering the palm. The dorsal skin is thin and pliable, anchored to the investing fascia by loose areolar tissue. Palmar skin in contrast is characterized by a thick dermal layer and a heavily cornified epithelial surface. The skin of palm is laden with high concentration of sensory end organs and sweat glands. The skin is not as pliable as dorsal skin and it is held tightly to the fibrous palmar fascia by diffusely distributed vertical fibers between fascia and dermis at palmar creases. Stability of palmar skin is critical for hand function.

Deeper Anatomy[30]

There are 20 intrinsic muscles of the hand that includes thenar muscles (action of thumb), hypothenar (action of little finger), lumbricals and interossei, responsible for dexterity of hand. The motor supply of intrinsic muscles of the hand and flexors are supplied by the ulnar nerve and median nerve, while all of the extensors are supplied by the radial nerve (Fig. 17).

Nerve Supply of Hand

Sensory innervation of hand is by a combination of the ulnar, median, and radial nerves (Fig. 17). Ulnar nerve supplies medial one-third of hand, median supplies lateral two-thirds and the radial nerve supplies the radial aspect of the dorsal two-thirds of the hand. Knowledge of sensory innervation is important, when regional or digital anesthesia is being considered (Fig. 17).

At the wrist, median nerve is located between the tendons of palmaris longus (PL) and the flexor carpi radialis (FCR) tendon. The PL tendon becomes more prominent on approximating thumb with ring finger with slight flexion at wrist, the median nerve passes just deep and lateral to PL tendon. It is located 2.5 cm proximal to the wrist crease between PL and FCR tendon. The ulnar nerve runs between the ulnar artery and flexor carpi ulnaris (FCU) tendon. The nerve is deeper to the tendon of the FCU and lies medial to the artery. It branches 1 cm distal to the ulnar styloid to give dorsal cutaneous branch of the ulnar nerve to supply skin of the back of the hand. The ulnar nerve is located under the tendon of the FCU muscle close to its distal attachment just above the styloid process of the ulna (Figs. 18A and B).

The superficial branch of the radial nerve (SRN) runs along the medial aspect of the brachioradialis muscle, and then passes between its tendon and radius to pierce the fascia on the dorsal aspect. It branches to give digital branches just above the styloid process of the radius that pass superficially over the anatomic "snuff box". The nerve is located, 3 cm proximal to the radial styloid, with wrist held in slight dorsiflexion. It is at this site the nerve can be easily accessed for biopsy (Figs. 19A and B).

To block radial nerve, it requires a more extensive infiltration because of its less predictable anatomic location and division into multiple, smaller, and cutaneous branches.

Digital Nerve Supply

The sensory innervation of digits comes from palmar and dorsal digital nerves that run medially and laterally in the fingers. The palmar digital nerves are branches of ulnar and median nerves, they supply sensation to the volar skin, interphalangeal joints of all five digits and also the dorsal distal aspect of the finger, including the fingertip and nail bed. The ulnar side of the fourth finger receives innervation from the dorsal nerve. The dorsal nerves originate from the radial and ulnar nerves. They innervate the nail beds of the

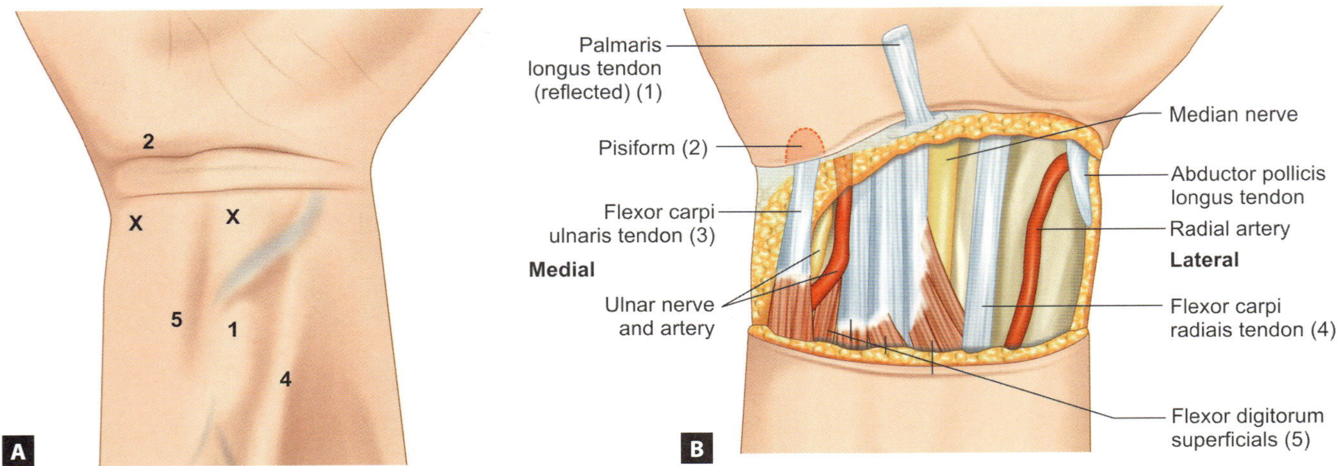

Figs. 18A and B: Surface anatomy of ulnar and median nerve. (A) The nerve can be accessed at the proximal crease of the wrist at the marked points; (B) Anterior view of right hand and wrist.

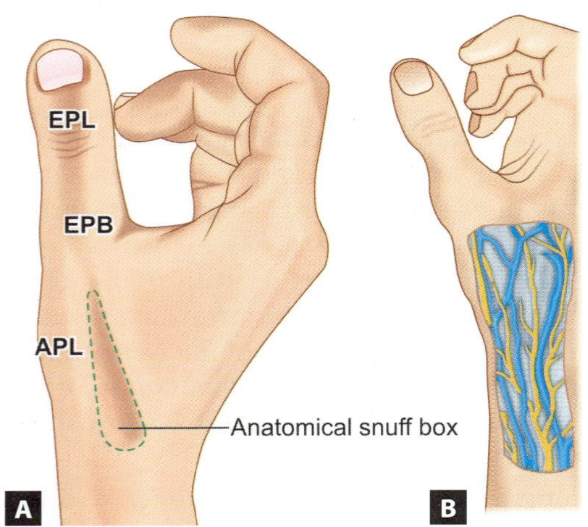

Figs. 19A and B: Shows location of radial nerve in anatomical snuff box at the level of radial styloid and location of radial cutaneous nerve that runs along the radial border of forearm. (It is located 3 cm proximal to the radial styloid for nerve biopsy).
(EPL: Extensor pollicis longus; EPB: Extensor pollicis brevis; APL: Abductor pollicis longus).

thumb and small fingers, as well as the dorsal aspect of all five fingers up to the distal interphalangeal joints (Figs. 20A to C).

The hand has rich blood supply, derived from superficial and deep palmar arch system formed by the radial and ulnar arteries. The superficial palmar arch lies directly deep to the palmar fascia. It gives rise to the volar common digital arteries and interosseous arteries. Distal in the palm, the common digital arteries bifurcate into the proper digital arteries. In the palm, the arteries lie volar to the corresponding nerves, a relation that is reversed in the digits. At the digits, the neurovascular bundle always lies volar to the ligament of Cleland. This pattern gives protection to the bundle and can serve as a guide for their surgical dissection. Common digital arteries arise from the superficial palmar arch to form proper digital arteries at the webs. The palmar aspect of the digits receives arterial flow through these proper digital arteries. The dorsum of each digit, distal to the proximal interphalangeal (PIP) joint, is vascularized by dorsal branches of the proper digital arteries. The deep palmar arch lies at the base of the metacarpals deep to the flexor tendons. It is the major blood supply to the thumb and radial half of the index finger by the first metacarpal artery. Veins generally follow the deep arterial system as venae comitantes. A superficial venous system also exists at the dorsum of the hand and contributes to the cephalic and basilic vein in the upper extremity.

Applied Anatomy

Knowledge of the anatomy is crucial for a dermatologic surgeon. Always assess the motor and sensory status prior to surgery on hand and note any deficits so they cannot be attributed to the procedure. As neurovascular bundles lies together, during digital anesthesia always withdraw the plunger of syringe to ensure that a vessel has not been entered. No vessel should be ligated in hand surgeries. During infiltration anesthesia, the dorsal approach is the preferred method because it is less painful than the palmar approach.[30] Tourniquet is the best way to achieve hemostasis in digits. Under no circumstance should hemostasis be achieved with ligature (Box 8).

FOOT[8,13,14,21,27,30-32]

The foot is a part of body which is in regular contact with the ground and serves important function of locomotion. Plantar skin is unique in several ways. It is markedly thickened and glabrous with numerous eccrine glands and absent apocrine and pilosebaceous units. The only relevant anatomic landmark, pertaining to cutaneous surgery is highlighted.

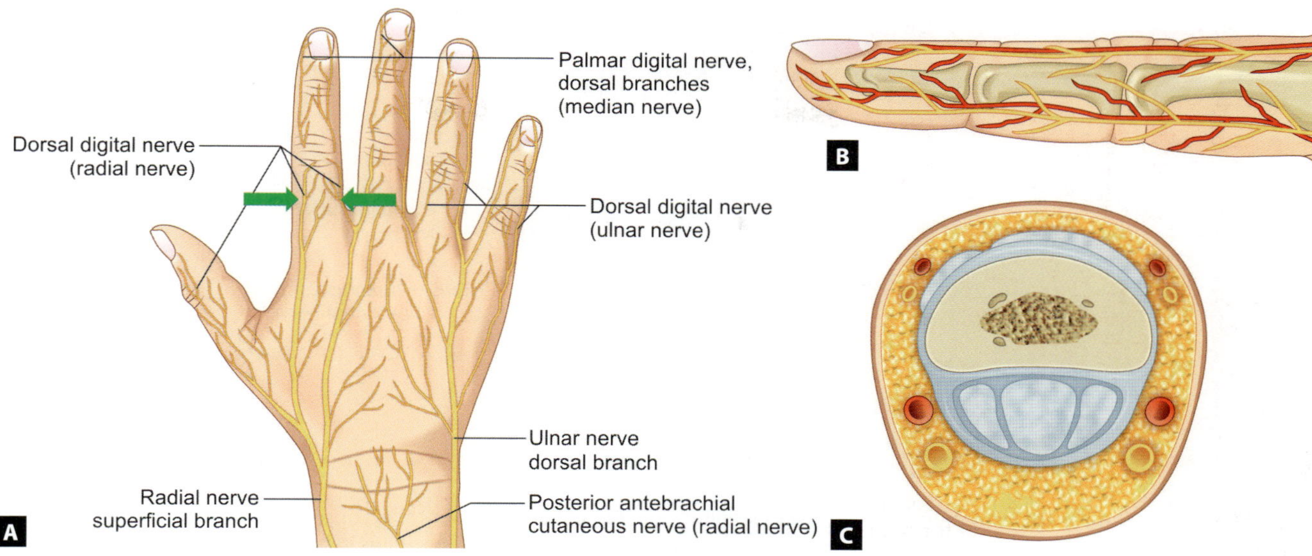

Figs. 20A to C: (A) Cutaneous nerve supply of dorsum of hands; (B) Dorsal and palmar digital arteries and nerves run together; and (C) They are located alongside the phalanges at the 2, 4, 8 and 10 o'clock positions.

Box 8: Surgical anatomic consideration of hand.

- Plan the excisions, by keeping in mind the loose dorsal skin and fascia of the hand that becomes tight when on full flexion. Avoid undue tension on wound edges or else it can cause wound dehiscence, unsightly scarring and contractures.
- The surgical incisions must be along relaxed skin tension lines and creases to minimize skin contractures. Palmar incisions must be parallel to flexion creases or at an angle of 45° or less, to avoid functionally bad, painful thick scars. Transverse dorsal incisions are preferred on the dorsum of the hand. Avoid longitudinal cuts on digits that may impair joint mobility. Curvilinear lazy "S" incisions over the dorsal surface of the digits not only prevents scar contracture but also minimizes the risk of injury to longitudinal structures of the digit.[21]
- As dorsal surface of the hand has relatively less fat and also veins lie more superficially and extensor tendons run just under the thin skin and are therefore at risk from both the scalpel and cryosurgery. Punch biopsies must be safely performed in this area by applying pressure to penetrate the skin and later on not to put too much downward pressure to reach the subcutaneous tissue and this minimizes injury to underlying vessels.
- As the palmar skin is inelastic and is fixed to palmar fascia and positioned on the concave side, its more prone for contractures. Hence excisions on palms may prove impossible to close, it must be handled only by a suitably trained specialist hand surgeon.
- Biopsy should be deeper as the palmar skin is thick. Superficial biopsy reveals only thick stratum corneum. The flexor tendons are close to the skin of palm and also there is no laxity.
- Deep dermal sutures are usually impossible to use as there is no depth to the dermis. In addition, although the epidermis may be very tough, the skin is actually torn very easily by a tightly pulled suture. Sutures need to be left in for longer duration to ensure[28] adequate healing, and this makes stitch marks more likely to be visible.
- Plane of neurotoxin injection is into deep dermis and it should be avoided in subcutaneous tissue as it causes diffusion into intrinsic muscles of the hand causing weakness. The needle should be at an oblique angle as perpendicular injections can result in back flow from the injection tract because of thick skin.

Surface Anatomy

The foot has dorsal and the plantar aspect with five toes numbered from medial to lateral and subdivided into distal, middle, and proximal phalanges. The foot can be divided into the rear foot, midfoot, and forefoot. The important joint landmarks are ankle joint, distal interphalangeal joints, the PIP joints, and the metatarsal phalangeal (MP) (Figs. 21A and B).

Skin of the plantar and the dorsal foot vary tremendously, in terms of thickness, and the amount of subcutaneous fat. The plantar skin is thicker, tighter, and more fixed than the dorsal skin. It is particularly thick at the ball big toe and the heel. The plantar skin has a well-developed stratum corneum with many sweat glands. The superficial fascia has abundant fibrous fatty tissue and is firmly attached to the underlying deep fascia by connective tissue septa. The cutaneous nerves and vessels lie within the superficial fascia. The plantar aspect of the foot is well-vascularized.

Musculature

In general, the muscles of the leg (and the foot and ankle) are divided into the anterior group of extensor muscles (dorsiflex the ankle) a posterior group of flexor muscles, and a lateral group of muscles (eversion of foot) derived from the extensors. The plantar muscles of the foot consist of the intrinsic muscles of the hallux and minimus, lumbricals, interossei, and short digital flexors. The tendons of the

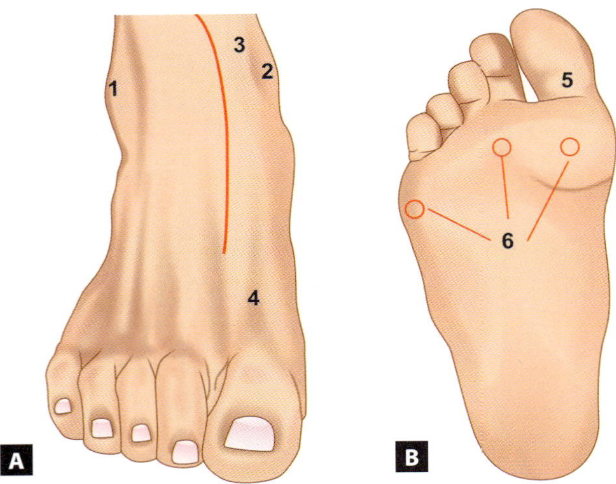

Figs. 21A and B: Surface anatomy of foot. (1) Lateral malleoli, (2) Medial malleoli, (3) Tibialis anterior, (4) Extensor hallucis longus tendon, (5) Ball of great toe. Red line indicates dorsalis pedis artery, (6) Head of metatarsal bone.

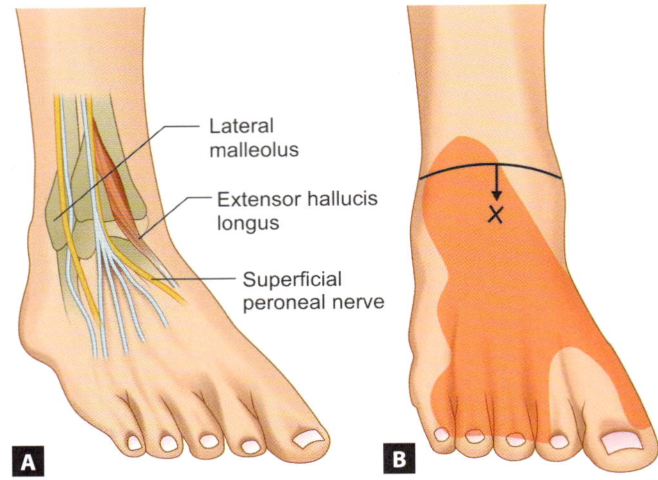

Figs. 22A and B: Location of superficial peroneal nerve and its sensory distribution, it lies in between the midpoint of medial malleolus and lateral malleolus. It is localized by palpating the extensor hallucis longus tendon and the lateral malleolus.

muscles of the leg are bound down by localized thickenings of the deep fascia, forming retinacular bands that prevent bowstringing of the tendons. The tendons that cross the ankle joint are all deflected from a straight course and held down by the retinacula.

Vascular Supply

The dorsalis pedis and the plantar arteries are main arterial supply to the foot. The posterior tibial artery terminates as medial and lateral plantar arteries. The lateral plantar arteries continues as plantar arch, it gives off three perforating and four plantar metatarsal branches and numerous other branches that supply the skin, fascia, and muscles of the sole. The blood supply to skin of feet is by two sources, one by the perforating musculocutaneous arteries and other by direct cutaneous blood vessels. The perforating musculocutaneous arteries supply muscle and overlying skin and end in the subdermal plexus. The direct cutaneous vessels supply specific and larger areas of the skin and end in subdermal plexus. Thus, the subdermal arterial plexus forms the major blood supply to the skin and it is important to know that any area of skin is not solely dependent on one artery. This is also responsible for tiny skin bleeders encountered during skin surgery. Venous blood drains the entire thickness of the dermis into the subdermal venous plexus. Plantar digital and dorsal digital veins arise from plexuses and unite into four plantar metatarsal veins. These connect by perforating veins with dorsal veins and continue to form the deep plantar venous arch, which accompanies the plantar arterial arch. From the venous arch, medial and lateral plantar veins run with their corresponding arteries, communicate with the great and small saphenous veins and form the posterior tibial veins behind the medial malleolus.

Sensory Innervation

Motor and sensory innervation to the foot is supplied by five nerves. The dorsal aspect of the foot is innervated by three nerves (superficial peroneal, deep peroneal, and saphenous nerves) that run on the anterior side of the lower leg and ankle. The volar aspect of the foot is innervated by two nerves (posterior tibial and sural nerves) that run on posterolateral aspect of the ankle.[31]

The superficial peroneal nerve innervates most of the dorsum of the foot and the dorsal aspect of each of the toes and web spaces, with the exception of the lateral portion of the great toe and the medial side of the second toe, and corresponding web space. The nerve passes subcutaneously on the anterolateral side of the ankle. The superficial peroneal nerve (L4-S1) is located lateral to the extensor digitorum longus (Figs. 22A and B).

The deep peroneal nerve (L4-L5) is located deeper in the ankle, lateral and slightly behind the extensor hallucis longus, it extends the toes. It supplies lateral portion of the great toe and medial side of the second digit, as well as the first web space. This area is referred as "flip-flop" region because it innervates the area surrounding the thong of a sandal. It can be located by having the patient dorsiflex the foot and great toe and it lies between anterior tibial tendon and the extensor hallucis longus tendon approximately 1 cm superior to the medial malleolus (Figs. 23A and B).

The saphenous nerve (L3-L4) is just anterior to the medial malleolus alongside of the saphenous vein, provides sensation to the skin on anteromedial side of the leg and medial side of foot. It can be located between the medial malleolus and the anterior tibial tendon (Figs. 24A and B).

The posterior tibial nerve is the largest in the ankle and branches into the medial and lateral plantar nerves in the foot, supplying sensation to the entire volar surface, as well

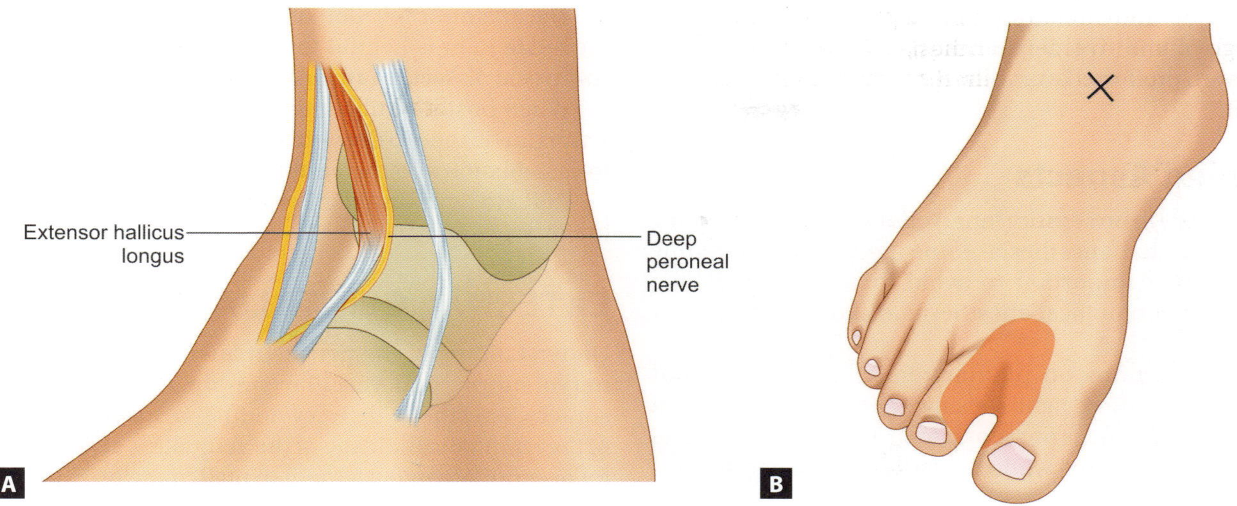

Figs. 23A and B: Shows location of deep peroneal nerve and its sensory distribution. It runs lateral to the dorsalis pedis artery.

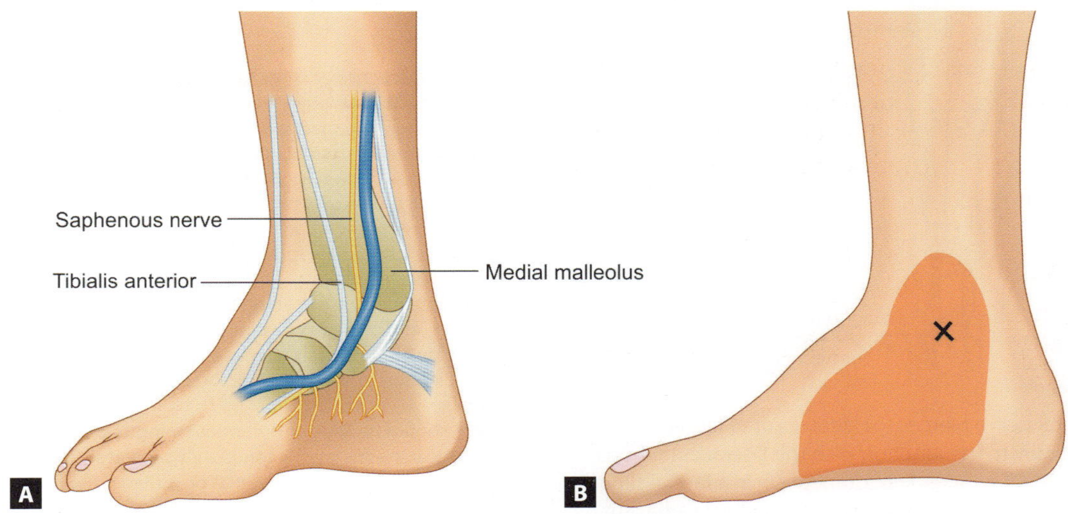

Figs. 24A and B: Shows location of saphenous nerve and its sensory distribution. It is located anterior to the medial malleolus.

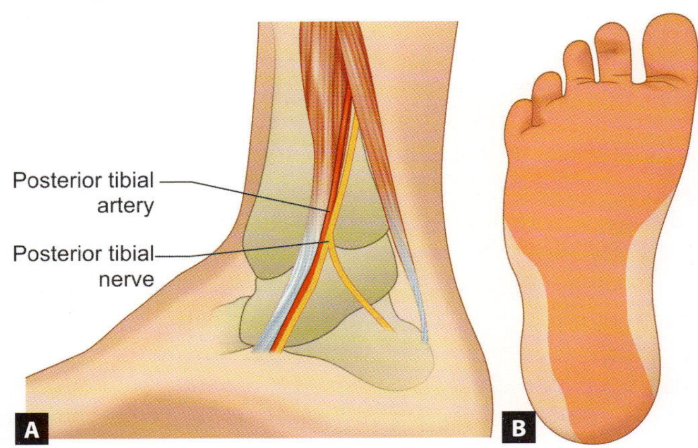

Figs. 25A and B: Location of posterior tibial nerve, it lies posterior to the artery and anterior to the Achilles tendon and its sensory distribution.

as providing motor innervation to the intrinsic muscles of the foot. It runs deep to the posterior tibial artery. The nerve can be located posterolateral to the artery at the level of the medial malleolus (Figs. 25 and 26).

Sural Nerve

The sural nerve (S1-S2) is located superficially in subcutaneous plane between the lateral malleolus and the Achilles tendon. It supplies sensation on posterolateral leg, lateral foot and 5th toe. The sural nerve has relatively constant course and is on average 7.4 × 0.1 cm posterior to the distal tip of the fibula, where it can be palpated[32] (Fig. 26).

Digital nerves (dorsal and ventral) of the toes are the terminal branches of the tibial, peroneal, and sural nerves. The presence of fibrous tissue (prevents spread of anesthetics) and limited space in this region cannot inject enough volume to achieve anesthesia within the toe, hence blocks are preferred over infiltration anesthesia (Figs. 27A and B).

Applied Aspects

The knowledge on sensory innervations aids in performing ankle or digital anesthesia. Knowing vascular anatomy of the foot is important to avoid these vessels during administration of local anesthesia to avoid intravascular injections.

The injections on plantar region are painful and difficult due to thick, tight, sensitive, and tightly bound skin to the fascia that does not separate easily. Therefore, dorsal approach is preferred while injecting into plantar region.

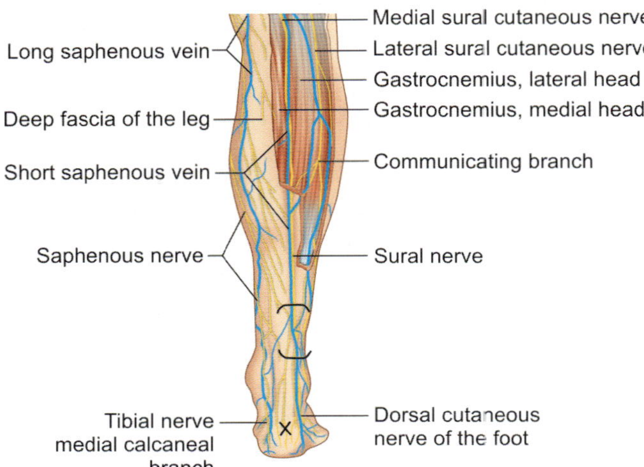

Fig. 26: The sural nerve pierces the deep (crural) fascia in the proximal calf distally to the junction with the lateral cutaneous sural nerve. Distally, it courses subcutaneously in a fascial sling between the deep crural fascia and superficial fascia adjacent to the short saphenous vein and lateral to the Achilles tendon. Marked site shows the site for sural nerve biopsy.

The anatomic location of the sural nerve at the level of the ankle joint is helpful for the incision placement and soft-tissue dissection and also to access it for biopsy.

When posterior tibia nerve is blocked, there is loss of sympathetic tone to the vascular supply of the foot leading to vasodilation and increased bleeding during surgery.

Rules to be followed in wound closure of feet are given in Box 9.

EXTERNAL GENITALIA

Understanding of the pertinent anatomy of genital skin, nerve supply and vascular supply will facilitate safe surgery, anesthetic delivery and hemostasis. Knowledge of the lymphatic drainage of the genitalia is also necessary for appropriate management of malignancies.

Male Genitalia[8,13,21]

The scrotum is a fibromuscular pouch. Scrotal skin is unique as it contains smooth muscle called dartos muscle,

Box 9: Rules to be followed in wound closure in feet.

- Place incisions along relaxed skin tension lines and along flexion and extension creases and plantar crease lines (Fig. 28). Do not injure the neurovascular bundles of the foot as they are relatively superficial because of the paucity of the subcutaneous fat.
- Follow nerve pathways in the overlying skin to avoid damaging them. Curved or oblique incisions can compensate for the resulting scar contraction.
- Avoid placing incisions along bony prominences or weight-bearing surfaces, as it causes more pain.
- Adequate hemostasis is by means of tourniquet to keep a bloodless field. Ligation of vascular structures should be avoided as much as possible.
- There should be little or no undermining or angled dissection until the subcutaneous layer is completely separated. This will preserve as much blood supply to the skin as possible.
- Avoid inadvertent trapping of underlying structures while suturing. Dog ear commonly occur on the dorsal foot and they remodel well; hence, these redundancies are not corrected.

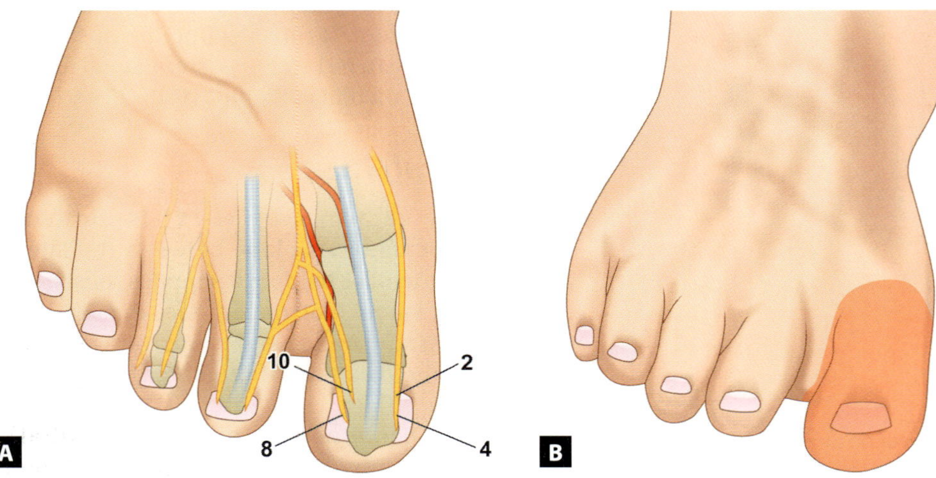

Figs. 27A and B: Dorsal and ventral digital nerves and sensory supply.

which is responsible for the rugosity of scrotal skin. The skin, smooth muscle, and fascial layers cover the contents of the scrotum (the testes, epididymides, and the cord). Its penile part does not contain any muscle (Figs. 29A and B).

The scrotal and perineal skin has a uniquely rich blood supply. Branches of the external and internal pudendal arteries supply the scrotal wall. The external pudendal arteries (two on each side) continue as the anterior scrotal arteries, and send branches to the dorsum penis. The anterior surface of the scrotum is vascularized by the superior external pudendal artery which also arterializes the base of the penis. The posterior surface of the scrotum is arterialized by the superficial perineal artery which is a branch of the internal pudendal artery. If these vessels are occluded, the viability of the scrotal skin and perineum is jeopardized. The penile skin, which is vascularized by the dorsolateral and ventrolateral branches of the superficial external pudendal artery, has cross-connections with the scrotal branches of the internal pudendal artery. General venous drainage of the scrotum is through pelvic venous plexuses that empty into the internal iliac vein and the anterior scrotal veins. As with the penile skin, the lymphatic drainage of the scrotum is to the inguinal nodes.

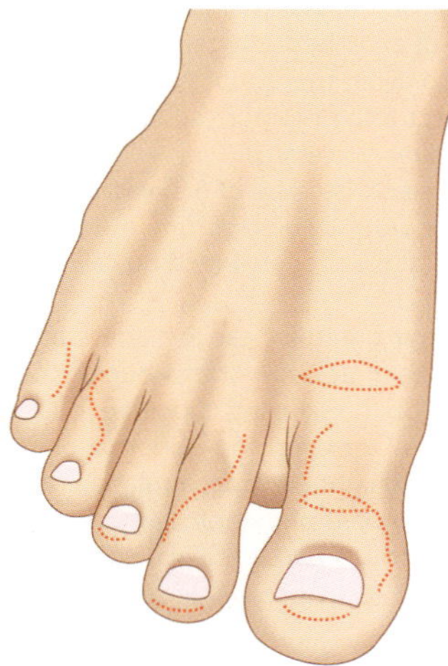

Fig. 28: Excision line planning on foot based on relaxed skin tension line and joints movements.

The skin and dartos of the scrotum are largely supplied posteriorly by the posterior scrotal nerves, and branches of the pudendal nerve which supply the sensory innervation to the external genitalia. The perineal branches of the posterior femoral cutaneous nerves expand laterally toward the scrotum. Its anterior and upper part is supplied by the ilioinguinal and genitofemoral nerves, the ilioinguinal nerve originating from the lumbar plexus and descending through the superficial inguinal ring to form the anterior scrotal nerves. The genitofemoral nerve supplies both the skin and the cremaster muscle.

The penis consists of a root and a body. The body is formed by the union of the corpus cavernosa and the corpus spongiosum. The two corpora are bounded by a thick fascia called the tunica albuginea. Buck's fascia, a tough fascial sheath, binds all the components. The skin surrounding the body of the penis is very loose and becomes redundant at the prepuce (foreskin), but it is particularly immobile over the corona and glans. The penis is innervated by autonomic (sympathetic and parasympathetic) and somatic (sensory and motor) nerves. The dorsal nerve of the penis is one of the two terminal branches of the pudendal nerve (the other one reaches the scrotum). The dorsal arteries of the penis lie immediately lateral to the deep dorsal vein. Lateral to the arteries lie the dorsal nerves.[8] All these components form the dorsal neurovascular bundle of the penis.

Female External Genitalia[33-38]

The external genitalia consist of the mons pubis, labia majora and minora, vestibule, and clitoris. The mons pubis consists of skin and subcutaneous tissue overlying the pubic symphysis. The labia majora are prominent

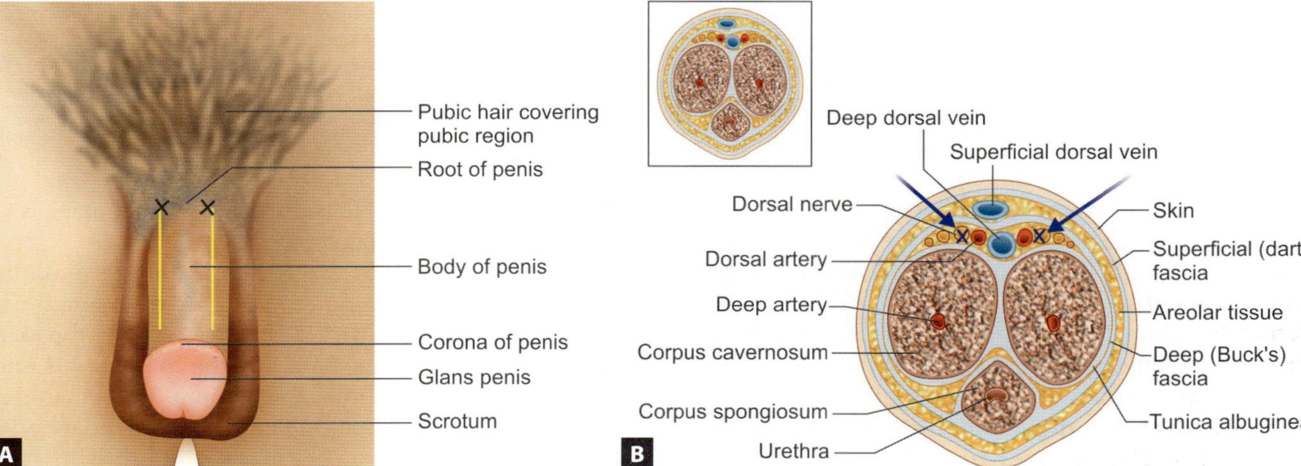

Figs. 29A and B: Male genital anatomy and applied aspects. It shows the location of dorsal penile nerves beneath Buck's fascia at the 1 and 11 o'clock positions.

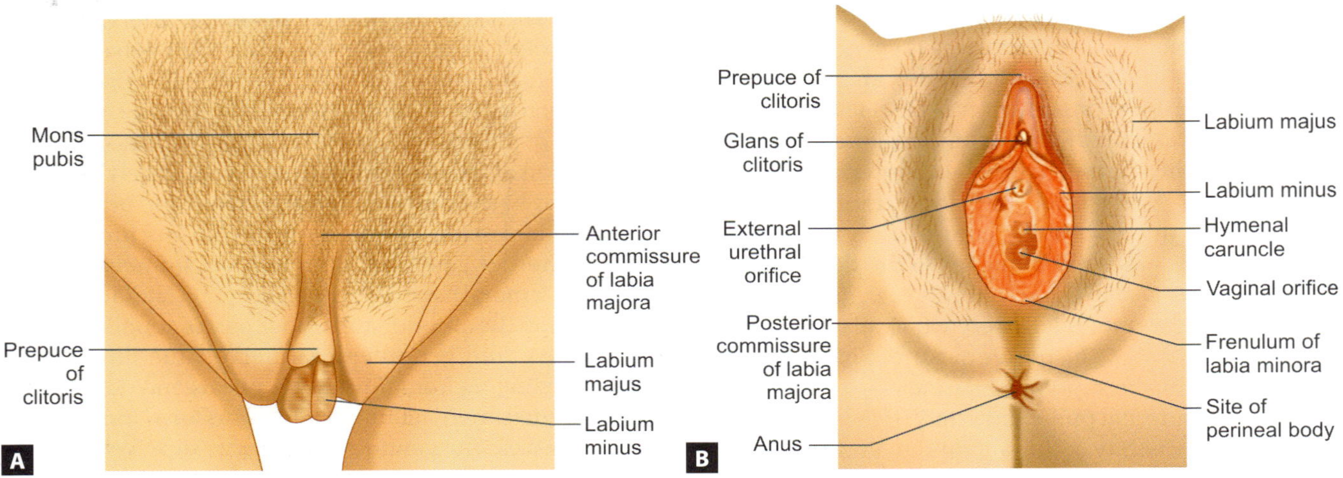

Figs. 30A and B: Female external genitalia (A) Anterior view; (B) Antero-inferior view (Lithotomy position).

longitudinal folds of skin supported by underlying fat. They are homologous to the male scrotum. The skin overlying the outer aspect is pigmented and hair bearing. The labia are united anteriorly and posteriorly at the commissures (Figs. 30A and B).

The labia minora, smaller folds within the pudendal cleft of the labia majora, surround the vaginal vestibule. Posteriorly, the labia minora unite as the frenulum of the labia (fourchette). Anteriorly, the labia split into the superior (lateral) and inferior (medial) portions. The superior portions pass above the clitoris to form the prepuce, and the inferior portions pass below the clitoris, forming the frenulum of the clitoris. The clitoris is the homolog of the male penis.

The labia majora are composed essentially of two layers: Skin and subcutaneous tissue. The skin that covers the lateral face is thick with hyperpigmentation and thick curly hair, with numerous sebaceous and sweat glands. The medial surface is instead covered by a thinner skin, translucent with a minor presence of hairs, of rosy color until it becomes a mucosa. The labia minora are two skinfolds, flattened, free of fat, medial in respect to the labia majora, and delimiting the vaginal vestibule, and they are separated from the interlabial grooves. The anterior extremity runs anteriorly towards the clitoris and the posterior extremity runs towards the perineum.

The blood supply and drainage of the external female genitalia occurs mostly via branches of the internal iliac vessels. Majority of the venous drainage follows the same pattern, terminating in the internal iliac vein. Portions of the anterolateral aspects of the labia majora drain into the external iliac vein. The lymphatics of the female genitalia drain to both superficial and deep nodes. The lymphatics from the lower portion of the vagina join those from the vestibule and labia to drain into the superficial inguinal lymph nodes. The perianal region, extending up the anal canal to the dentate line (marker of transition from cutaneous to mucosal epithelium), drains to the superficial femoral nodes. Proximal to the dentate line, drainage is to the deeper pelvic lymph nodes.

The nerve supply of the female external genitalia also comes from two distinct sources. The ilioinguinal (L1) and genitofemoral (L1, L2) nerves supply the skin and subcutaneous tissue overlying the mons pubis and anterolateral portions of the labia majora. The remainder of the female genitalia is supplied by the pudendal nerve (S2, S3, S4).

The surgical anatomic consideration of genitalia is summarized in Box 10.

Box 10: Surgical anatomic consideration of genitalia.

- Small procedures on the external genitalia can be performed with local infiltration of anesthetic, larger procedures require blocks. As a rule, it is best to avoid the use of epinephrine when injecting the penis. Avoid direct infiltration of the foreskin, as this can result in tissue necrosis on rare occasion.
- Scrotal skin is thin and because of rich vascularity, bleeds profusely, always suture the wounds on scrotum. It heals excellently. Always dress the wounds as reactionary bleeding can occur to avoid patient getting panic.
- Biopsy on external genitalia can be adequately sampled using a punch or snip technique. A sharp punch tool combined with adequate tension on the skin and subcutaneous tissue helps ensure the least distortion of the overlying epidermis or mucosa. Hemostasis can be achieved with light electrocoagulation or pressure.
- Sutures should be placed perpendicular to the natural skin tension lines. In the penis, this is perpendicular to the long axis to prevent traction during erection. Absorbable sutures are preferable from a patient perspective.
- The Bartholin's glands are located bilaterally at the base of the labia minora and drain through 2–2.5 cm long ducts that empty into the vestibule at about the 4 o'clock and 8 o'clock positions. The glands are usually the size of a pea and rarely exceed 1 cm. They are not palpable except in the presence of disease or infection.
- The ageing process and, more importantly, the endless variation in the anatomy of the labia minora, may generate concern in women when evaluating the appearance of their own external genitalia. An increasing number of women seek to improve the shape or size of their labia minora or majora and they should be approached with sensitivity and extreme professionalism by the physician.

SUMMARY

A good understanding of the anatomy, circulation, innervation, function and cosmesis is important before performing a surgical procedure. It not only aids in planning surgical procedures but also to reduce complications and give optimum results.

REFERENCES

1. Farmer ER, Hood AF. Pathology of the skin. Norwalk, CT: Appleton & Lange; 1990. pp. 3-29.
2. Marcus J, Horan DB, Robinson JK. Tissue expansion: past, present, and future. J Am Acad Dermatol. 1990;23:813-25.
3. Fung YC. Biomechanics in mechanical properties of living tissues. Springer-Verlag: New York; 1981.
4. Barbenel JC. Skin biomechanics. In: Payne PA (Ed). Concise encyclopaedia of biological and biomedical measurement systems. Pergamon Press: Oxford; 1991. p. 347.
5. Wan Abas WAB, Barbenel JC. The response of human skin to small tensile loads in vitro. Eng Med. 1982;11:43.
6. Gibson T, Stark HL, Evans JH. Directional variation in extensibility of human skin in vivo. J Biomech. 1969;2:201-4.
7. Larrabee WF Jr. A finite element model of skin deformation. I. Biomechanics of skin and soft tissue: a review. Laryngoscope. 1986;96:399-412.
8. Agur AMR, Lee MJ, Grant JC. Grant's Atlas of Anatomy, 13th edition. Baltimore, Md: Lippincott Williams & Wilkins; 2013.
9. McMinn NH, Hutchings RT, Logan BM. Color Atlas of Head and Neck Anatomy, 2nd edition. Baltimore, Md: Mosby-Wolfe; 1995. pp. 161-3.
10. Snell RS. Clinical anatomy for medical students, 5th edition. Boston, Mass: Little Brown & Co; 1990. pp. 659-61.
11. Dzubow LM. Facial flap: biomechanic and regional applications. Norwalk, CT: Appleton & Lange; 1989.
12. Chayen D, Nathan H. Anatomical observations on the subgaleotic fascia of the scalp. Acta Anat.1974;87:427-8.
13. Drake RL, Vogl W, Mitchell AWM. Gray's Anatomy for Students, 1st edition. Churchill: Livingstone (Elsevier Science); 2005. pp. 898-936.
14. Roenigk HH, Ratz JL, Roenigk RK. Roenigk's Dermatologic Surgery. In: Roenigk RK, Ratz JL, Roenigk HH (Eds). Current techniques in procedural dermatology, 3rd Edition. New York, London: Informa Healthcare; 2007.
15. Seery GE. Surgical anatomy of the scalp. Dermatol Surg. 2002;28:581-7.
16. Moore K. Clinically oriented anatomy, 2nd edition. Baltimore, MD: Williams & Wilkins; 1985. p. 855.
17. Nouri K. Complications in Dermatologic Surgery. Philadelphia, PA: Saunders Elsevier. 2008;16:65.
18. Tromovitch TA, Stegman SJ, Glogau RG. Flaps and Grafts in Dermatologic Surgery. Chicago, IL: Yearbook Medical Publishers; 1989.
19. Bernstein G. Surface landmarks for the identification of key anatomic structures for the face and neck. J Dermatol Surg Oncol. 1986;12:722-6.
20. Labbe D, Franco RG, Nicolas J. Platysma suspension and platysma plasty during neck lift. Anatomical study and analysis of 30 cases. Plast Reconstr Surg. 2006;117(6):2001-7.
21. Robinson JK. Basic cutaneous surgery concepts. In: Robinson JK, Arndt KA, LeBoit PE, Wintroub BU (Eds). Atlas of cutaneous surgery. Philadelphia: Saunders; 1996. pp. 1-4.
22. King RJ, Motta G. Iatrogenic spinal accessory nerve palsy. Ann R Coll Surg Engl. 1983;65:35-7.
23. Datubo-Brown DD. Keloids: a review of literature. Br J Plast Surg. 1990;43(1):70-7.
24. Kim S, Chung SW, Cha IH. Full thickness skin grafts from the groin: donor site morbidity and graft survival rate from 50 cases. J Korean Assoc Oral Maxillofac Surg. 2013;39(1):21-6.
25. Salasche SJ, Bernstein G, Senkarik M. Surgical anatomy of the skin. Norwalk, CT: Appleton & Lange; 1988.
26. Swanson NA. Atlas of cutaneous surgery, 1st edition. Boston, Massachusetts: Little Brown and Company; 1987.
27. McCurdy JA Jr. Five years of experience using fat for leg contouring (Commentary). Am J Cosmet Surg. 1995;12(3):228.
28. Botting J, Schofield J. Anatomical hazards and pitfalls. In: Brown's Skin and Minor Surgery: A Text & Colour Atlas, 5th edition. Taylor & Francis Group; 2015.
29. Swinehart JM. Treatment of axillary hyperhidrosis: combination of the starch-iodine test with the tumescent liposuction technique. Dermatol Surg. 2000;26:392-6.
30. Dinehart SM. Topical, local, and regional anesthesia. In: Wheeland R (Ed). Cutaneous surgery. Philadelphia: WB Saunders; 1994. pp. 105-10.
31. Spektor M, Kelly J. Regional anesthesia of the thorax and extremities. In: Roberts Hedges (Ed). Clinical procedures in emergency medicine, 5th edition. Philadelphia, PA: Saunders Elsevier; 2010. pp. 528-30.
32. Eastwood DM, Irgau I, Atkins RM. The distal course of the sural nerve and its significance for incisions around the lateral hindfoot. Foot Ankle. 1992;13(4):199-202.
33. Yavagal S, de Farias TF, Medina CA, et al. Normal vulvovaginal, perineal, and pelvic anatomy with reconstructive considerations. Semin Plast Surg. 2011;25(2):121-9.
34. Neill S, Lewis F. Ridley's the vulva, 3rd edition. Hoboken: Wiley-Blackwell; 2009.
35. Puppo V. Embryology and anatomy of the vulva: The female orgasm and women's sexual health. Eur J Obstet Gynecol Reprod Biol. 2011;154(1):3-8.
36. Dickinson RL. Atlas of human sex anatomy, 2nd edition. Baltimore: Williams & Wilkins; 1949.
37. Stenchever MA. Comprehensive gynecology, 4th edition. St. Louis: Mosby, 2001. pp. 482-6, 645-6.
38. Hill DA, Lense JJ. Office management of Bartholin gland cysts and abscesses. Am Fam Physician. 1998;57:1611-6, 1619-20.

Chapter 4

Wound Healing

CR Srinivas, C Shanmuga Sekar

Key Messages

- Wound healing includes three phases: inflammatory, proliferative and remodeling.
- Neutrophils play a role in the initial inflammatory stage of the wound process.
- Macrophages function to remove residual bacteria, foreign bodies and remaining necrotic tissue in the late inflammatory phase.
- Platelets, which are the initial cells in healing process, release several important mediators which are responsible for the initiation and progression of wounds through the subsequent phases of wound healing.
- Mast cells are increased in numbers in keloids and hypertrophic scars.
- Transforming growth factor-β (TGF-β) is the main inflammatory mediator responsible for the recruitment of neutrophils to start the inflammatory phase of wound healing.
- Vascular endothelial growth factor (VEGF) is responsible for the neoangiogenesis in the later stages of wound healing.
- Matrix metalloproteinases (MMPs) are zinc-dependent endopeptidases which degrade the extracellular matrix and help in wound remodeling.

DEFINITION

Dorland's medical dictionary defines wound as "disruption in the normal continuity of the body structure". Even though the conventional definition specifies a wound as disruption of skin layer, wounds secondary to dermatology procedures can be superficial. The healing process depends on local wound factors, systemic mediators, the underlying disease and the type of injury. Chronic wounds are the result of an inadequate repair process that is unable to restore anatomic and functional integrity in an appropriate length of time.[1]

PHASES IN WOUND HEALING

The three phases in wound healing are (Figs. 1A to D):

1. Inflammatory phase
2. Proliferative phase
3. Remodeling phase

Inflammatory Phase

The initial phase after cutaneous injury is dominated by inflammatory reactions mediated by cytokines, chemokines, growth factors and their actions on cellular receptors.

The first step in this phase is **vascular response and hemostasis**.[2] Hemostasis consists of two phases: (1) formation of fibrin clot; and (2) coagulation. Following tissue injury, hemostasis occurs to minimize hemorrhage. When the blood vessels constrict, platelets are activated by binding to the exposed collagen in the extracellular matrix. The platelets then release various factors; such as fibronectin, thrombospondin and von Willebrand factor, which promote further platelet activation and aggregation.[3] The activated factors result in the formation of a fibrin matrix which functions as a provisional matrix to stabilize the wound site. The aggregated platelets then become trapped in the fibrin matrix, thus forming a stable clot within the provisional matrix.

Platelets release several important mediators which are responsible for the initiation and progression of wounds through the subsequent phases of wound healing. The degranulation of alpha granules and dense bodies causes release of mediators such as platelet-derived growth factor (PDGF) and transforming growth factor-β (TGF-β). Transforming growth factor-α (TGF-α) and PDGF recruit various cells, such as neutrophils and macrophages to enter the wound. Platelet-derived growth factor (PDGF) also recruits fibroblasts to the wound and activates

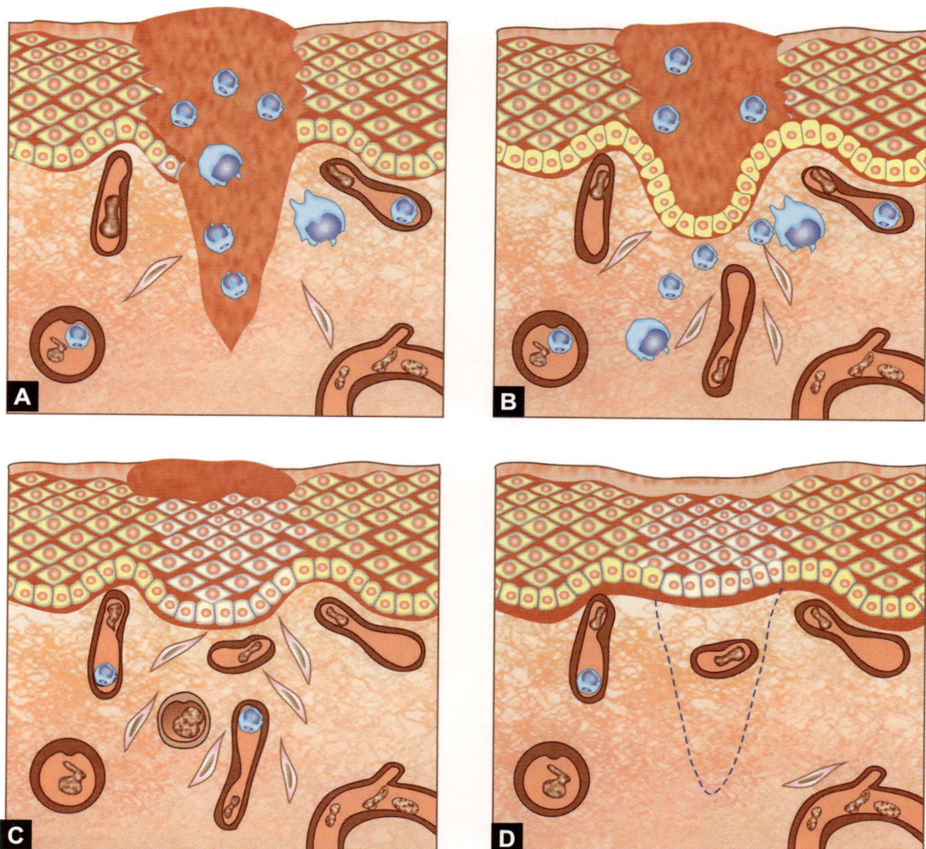

Figs. 1A to D: (A) Inflammatory phase—The wound is rinsed by blood and filled with blood-collagen and fibrin constituents. (B) Proliferative phase—Resorption of blood-collagen and re-epithelialization. (C and D) Maturation and remodeling phase—Growth of new epithelial cell.

the production of collagen and glycosaminoglycans by fibroblasts, which are important for the repair of the extracellular matrix.[4,5]

The next phase of wound healing is **inflammation**, which begins within the first 24 hours after an injury. The vasoactive substances released by the damaged cells and clot breakdown mediate this response. The dilated capillaries become leaky and, thus, allow the efficient movement of neutrophils from the vasculature to the site of injury. Leucocyte migration occurs by diapedesis and margination. As various chemical signals are released from the wound site, the endothelial cells in the nearby vessels are activated and begin to express specialized cell adhesion molecules (CAMs) called selectins. These CAMs cause the neutrophils to bind to the endothelial cell surface by a process called pavementing. The adherent neutrophils begin to roll along the endothelial cell lining and then by a process called diapedesis, they squeeze through the cell junctions that have been made leaky by the mast cell mediators.[6,7]

The primary function of the neutrophils is phagocytosis of any foreign materials and to kill bacteria by the powerful battery of enzymes and reactive oxygen species, which they can generate. The neutrophils actually initiate the first stage of the proliferative phase by releasing IL-1 and tumor necrosis factor (TNF-α) to begin the activation of fibroblasts and epithelial cells.

During the inflammatory phase, activated macrophages also play a key role in the regulation of wound healing. Wound macrophages are derived from fixed tissue monocytes that originate from circulating monocytes. The macrophages function to remove residual bacteria, foreign bodies and remaining necrotic tissue. Macrophages also secrete a number of growth factors and cytokines, such as PDGF, TGF-β, TNF-α, fibroblast growth factor (FGF), insulin like growth factor-1, and IL-6, which then recruit fibroblasts and endothelial cells to the wound site for matrix deposition and neovascularization. The macrophages also produce tissue inhibitors of matrix metalloproteinases which inhibit the enzymatic destruction of tissues.[8] The result of the inflammatory phase is a clean wound bed.

Proliferative Phase

The proliferative phase is characterized by fibroblast proliferation and collagen deposition to provide a stable extracellular matrix at the wound site. Within a few days after wounding, the fibroblasts start synthesizing collagen. Deposition of collagen gradually enables the skin integrity to be restored. The new extracellular matrix consists of collagen, proteoglycans and fibronectins. In addition, angiogenesis occurs such that new blood vessels replace the previously damaged capillaries and provide nourishment for the matrix.

The hallmark of proliferation stage is formation of granulation tissue. Granulation tissue consists of a dense network of blood vessels and capillaries, elevated cellular density of fibroblasts and macrophages and randomly organized collagen fibers. Fibroblasts migrate into the wound in response to mediators released from the platelets and macrophages and move through the extracellular matrix. The fibroblasts also secrete matrix metalloproteinases (MMPs), which facilitate their movement through the matrix and help with the removal of damaged matrix components. Once the fibroblasts have entered the wound, they produce collagen, proteoglycans and other components.

Neoangiogenesis is stimulated by angiogenic factors secreted by keratinocytes at the wound site. Endothelial cells are activated by TNF-α and basic FGF (bFGF) to initiate angiogenesis. The newly formed blood vessels invade the matrix and promote blood flow to support the high metabolic activity in the newly deposited tissue. Angiogenesis is regulated by a combination of local stimulatory factors, such as vascular endothelial cell growth factor (VEGF) and antiangiogenic factors, such as angiostatin, endostatin, thrombospondin and pigment epithelium-derived growth factor.[9] Local factors that stimulate angiogenesis include low oxygen tension, low pH and high lactate levels.[10]

Remodeling Phase

The last phase of wound healing is the remodeling phase in which granulation tissue matures to form a scar. The tissue remodeling phase starts as early as a few days after injury and lasts up to 2 years. The capillaries aggregate to form larger blood vessels and cell density and overall metabolic activity of the wound decrease. The collagen fibers become organized resulting in increased tensile strength of the wound. Initially, there is an increased deposition of type III collagen, also referred to as reticular collagen, that is gradually replaced by type I collagen, the dominant fibrillar collagen in skin.[11] As the wound continues to remodel, changes in collagen organization increase the tensile strength to a maximum of about 80% of normal tissue.[9]

An important group of proteinases are matrix metalloproteinases (MMPs) which play a central role in wound healing as they degrade certain constituents of provisional wound tissue, such as collagen I, III, IV, and VII.[12] They also facilitate epithelial cell migration into the wound, angiogenesis and overall tissue remodeling. Matrix metalloproteinases (MMPs) are secreted by epidermal cells and modulate tissue inhibitors of metalloproteinases (TIMPs) as well as degrade other growth factors.[13,14] Similarly, a disruption in the balance between MMPs and their inhibitors has been reported in diabetic and venous stasis ulcers.[15] In addition, MMPs can be found in increased levels in chronic wounds.[16] MMP expression is regulated by TGF-β. Transforming growth factor-β also minimizes matrix degradation by downregulating protease secretion and stimulating synthesis of TIMP.

The process of collagen synthesis and degradation usually continues for a long time as the matrix strives to achieve the original highly organized structure that was present before the wound injury. The scar tissue is always weaker than the normal surrounding matrix and can only achieve about 80% of the tensile strength that was present initially. If matrix synthesis is greater than degradation, then a hypertrophic scar may form. Conversely, if matrix degradation is greater than synthesis or if synthesis is inhibited by pharmacologic agents such as steroids or cancer chemotherapeutic agents, the scar becomes too weak and wound dehiscence can occur.

FACTORS RESULTING IN CHRONICITY OF WOUND

These include both local and systemic factors as shown in Table 1.

Table 1: Factors affecting wound healing and resulting in chronicity of wound.

Local factors	*Systemic factors*
Oxygenation	Age and gender
Infection	Sex hormones
Foreign body	Stress
Venous sufficiency	Ischemia
	Diseases: diabetes, keloids, fibrosis, hereditary healing disorders, jaundice, uremia
	Obesity
	Medications: glucocorticoid steroids, nonsteroidal anti-inflammatory drugs, chemotherapy
	Alcoholism and smoking
	Immunocompromised conditions: cancer, radiation therapy, AIDS Nutrition

WOUND HEALING IN DERMATOLOGICAL AND ESTHETIC CONDITIONS AND PROCEDURES

Keloids and Hypertrophic Scars

The presence of TGF-β isoforms, receptors and activity modulators, rather than the mere presence or absence of TGF-β, may have a major role in the development of both keloids and hypertrophic scarring.[17] Similar results were detected with co-culturing of keloid derived keratinocytes and fibroblasts,[18] suggesting that keratinocytes might have an important role in keloid and hypertrophic scar pathogenesis by producing signals that stimulate the fibroblasts in the underlying dermis to proliferate or produce more extracellular matrix (ECM). Increased numbers of mast cells have been reported during the active period of hypertrophic and keloid scar formation.[19] Clinically, the release of histamine by these cells contributes to the common patient complaint of itchiness. In addition, the vasodilatory effect of histamine may promote erythema and leakage of plasma proteins into the regional tissues.

The major effectors of ECM degradation and remodeling belong to a family of structurally-related enzymes called MMPs. The levels of MMP expression in normal cells are low and allow healthy connective tissue remodeling. Several MMPs have been shown to mediate the breakdown of type I and III collagen, the most abundant types of collagen in the skin ECM.[20] Specifically, MMP-2 and MMP-9 activity persists after wound closure and seems to play a potent role in the remodeling process.[21] Interestingly, hypertrophic scars and keloids were found to have high levels of MMP-2 and low levels of MMP-9.

Decorin, a small proteoglycan with one dermatan sulfate sugar chain, is normally prevalent in the dermal ECM. Decorin is able to bind and neutralize TGF-β, thus minimizing the stimulatory effects of this cytokine on collagen, fibronectin and glycosaminoglycan production.[22] The low levels of decorin found in hypertrophic scarring may thus account for their irregular collagen organization as well as increased ECM production.

Other abnormalities seen in keloids include delayed apoptosis of myofibroblasts and prolongation of scar maturation.

Acne Scars

The pathogenesis of acne is currently attributed to multiple factors such as increased sebum production, alteration of the quality of sebum lipids and rogen activity, proliferation of *Propionibacterium acnes* (*P. acnes*) within the follicle and follicular hyperkeratinization.[23]

The inflammatory process occurs in the infundibular region which result in follicular rupture and perifollicular abscess formation. These initiate a cascade of wound healing events. Holland et al. found that the inflammatory reaction at the pilosebaceous gland was stronger and had a longer duration in patients with scars than those without; in addition, the inflammatory reaction was slower in those with scars than patients who did not develop scars. They showed a strong relationship between severity and duration of inflammation and the development of scarring, suggesting that treating early inflammation in acne lesions may be the best approach to prevent acne scarring.[24]

Fibroblasts and keratinocytes produce enzymes including those that determine the architecture of the MMPs and tissue inhibitors of MMPs. As a consequence, an imbalance in the ratio of MMPs to tissue inhibitors of MMPs results in the development of atrophic or hypertrophic scars. Inadequate response results in diminished deposition of collagen factors and formation of an atrophic scar while, if the healing response is too exuberant, a raised nodule of fibrotic tissue forms hypertrophic scars.[25]

WOUND HEALING AFTER PROCEDURES

Cryosurgery

Freezing of tissue with liquid nitrogen results in blister formation in a span of 2–3 days. Rupture of the blister results in eschar formation. Post-procedural depigmentation can occur in dark skinned patients.

Chemical Peeling

Chemical peels are utilized to produce damage to the epidermis and superficial dermis. This results in epidermalregeneration and postinflammatory neocollagen formation.

Dermabrasion

Dermabrasion creates a partial thickness wound to heal by secondary intention. In partial thickness wounds, the adnexal structures are preserved and act as a reservoir for epidermal proliferation. Transforming growth factor-β, keratinocyte growth factor and epidermal growth factor stimulate re-epitheliazation from both the appendageal structures and epithelial cells.

Fractional Lasers

The mechanisms of the action of laser resurfacing include tissue ablation, immediate collagen shrinkage, and dermal collagen remodeling.[26] Fractional laser may result in macroscopic epidermal regeneration. Collagen contraction induced by fractional reticular dermal ablation was thought to be the underlying factor leading to clinically observed skin tightening.[27] The improvement resulting from the ablation process may be seen soon after the epidermal regeneration phase is complete, whereas the clinical benefit arising from the dermal remodeling process normally starts months after treatment and continues over years after the initiation of the cutaneous wound healing cascade. A recent in vivo study in human skin revealed that neocollagenesis was persistent for a minimum of 3 months after a CO_2 ablative fractional resurfacing treatment as confirmed by a constant upregulation of the heat shock protein 47 expression.[28]

Platelet-Rich Plasma and Platelet-Rich Fibrin in Wound-Healing

Platelet-rich plasma (PRP) is used in various clinical disciplines and is considered to improve tissue regeneration due to the presence of essential growth factors and cytokines. PRP is autologous form of concentrated platelets and growth factors occurring naturally in the body. Platelet rich plasma can be made either by centrifugation or filtering whole blood with anticoagulant to obtain a formulation of platelets and plasma with supraphysiologic concentrations of platelets.[29]

PRP contains bioactive molecules which plays an important role in wound healing. These include platelet-derived growth factor (PDGF), transforming growth factor (TGF), platelet factor 4 (PF4), interleukin (IL) 1, platelet-derived angiogenesis factor (PDAF), vascular endothelial growth factor (VEGF), epidermal growth factor (EGF), platelet-derived endothelial growth factor (PDEGF), epithelial cell growth factor (ECGF), and insulin-like growth factor (IGF). These molecules, along with other bioactive molecules, have diverse functions in the local regeneration environment, such as proliferation, migration, cell differentiation and angiogenesis.[30]

In addition to platelets and their products, the natural wound response requires the presence of a fibrin matrix, which enhances the delivery of growth factors.[31] PRF is an immune and platelet concentrate that collects on a single fibrin membrane.[32] The PRF membranes simultaneously support the development of the three keys to healing and soft tissue maturation, namely angiogenesis, immunity, and epithelial cover.

PRP is also used in the management of acne scars, facial rejuvenation in skin ageing and in the treatment of alopecia.

Wound Dressing

The various wound dressings and their clinical applications are enlisted in Table 2.[33]

Table 2: Wound dressing.

Product	*Indications and action*	*Advantages*	*Disadvantages*	*Use*	*Examples*
Antimicrobials Mupirocin	Wounds infected with gram positive organisms Prevents bacterial protein and cell wall synthesis	Very effective against staphyloco-ccus, especially MRSA Do not damage healthy tissue	Costly	Can be applied daily	T-bact (Glaxo), Bactroban, Mupibact
Retapamulin	Effective against staphylococcus aureus and pyogenes inhibit bacterial protein synthesis	Effective against mupirocin and fucidin-resistant staphylococcus	Costly		Retral (Ajanta pharma)
Silver-impregnated dressings	Deep burns skin sloughing disorders (toxis epidermal necrolysis and Stevens Johnson syndrome). donor sites and meshed skin grafts	Effective for wounds infected both with gram negative and gram positive organisms, esp-MRSA and vre and fungi also	Argyria costly	Change every 5–7 days	Acticoat (Smith and Nephew), Silvel (Datta phatrma), Biatalnag (Coloplast) Actisorb (Johnson and Johnson) Aquasel ag (Convatec)
Foams	Pressure ulcers and lower limb ulcers with min to mod exudates	Absorbent Occlusive Thermal Insulation	Opaque Malodorus discharge	Change every 3 days	Alleyn (Smith and Nephew), lyofoam (Convatec), 3 m foam dressing (3 m Health Care), biatain foam dressing (Coloplast)
Films	Partial thickness Wounds with minimal exudates, pressure ulcers, grafts	Transparent Occlusive moisture retentive protection from contamination Easy to inspect wounds	No absorption Fluid trapping skin stripping not for infected wounds	Leave on till 7 days or when fluid leaks or secretions collect underneath	Tegaderm (3 m Healthcare), bioclusive (Johnson and Johnson), Opsite (Smith and Nephew), dermasite (Dermasciences), comfeel film (Coloplast)
Hydrogels	Dry wounds Painful wounds mainly pressure sores, lower limb ulcers, skin tears and surgical wounds	Moisture retentive Nontraumatic removal	May overhydrate	Change in 1–3 days	Intrasite gel (Smith and Nephew), Solosite (Smith & Nephew), restore (Hollister)
Hydrocolloids	Wounds with min to mod exudates like pressure ulcers and venous stasis ulcers	Absorbent Occlusive protection from contamination	Opaque Fluid trapping maldorous discharge	Left on till 7 days	Duoderm (Convatec), comfeel (coloplast), 3 m tegasorb (3 m Health Care), restore (Hollister), Nuderm (Johnson and Johnson).

Contd...

Contd...

Product	Indications and action	Advantages	Disadvantages	Use	Examples
Alginates	Pressure sores, Diabetic ulcers, infected wounds, Lower extremity ulcers with moderate to heavy exudates Mild hemostasis	Highly absorbent Hemostatic Non-toxic, non-allergenic	Fibrous debris	Left on till soaked with exudate	Kaltostat (Convatec), Algiderm (Bard), Kalginate (De Royal).
Enzymatic debridement	For necrotic Sloughy wounds	Digest necrotic matter Without harming normal tissue	Papain in Nonselevtive and may be painful No absorbing action, so need a secondary dressing	Minimum daily use	Collagenase Santyl (Healthport), Accuzyme (Healthport), salutyl (Elder pharma), Debridace (Virchow Healthcare)
Growth factors	Useful in small non-healing wounds	Accelerate healing of chronic wounds	Not indicated in Necrotic wounds, Daily cancerous growths require a secondary dressing with gauze	To be applied	Plermin (Dr. Reddy's lab), Eugraf (Lupin), Epigrof (Marksons), Regen D (Bharat Biotech)

Biolologic and Synthetic Skin Substitutes

One of the current options for the treatment of chronic wounds is the use of skin substitutes, which can be either synthetic (generated by tissue engineering) or of human origin, such as allografts (derived from cadaver skin) and xenografts (derived from animal skin). Skin substitutes are a heterogeneous group of biological and/or synthetic elements that enable the temporary or permanent occlusion of wounds.[34]

Goals for treating acute and chronic wounds with skin substitutes are to provide temporary coverage or permanent wound closure, to reduce postoperative contracture, to improve function, to reduce healing time and to decrease morbidity from more invasive treatments such as skin grafting.

Properties of the Ideal Dermal-epidermal Substitute[34]

- Hypoxia tolerant
- Broad availability
- Presence of dermal and epidermal components
- Rheology comparable to the skin
- Resistance to infection
- Suitable cost/effectiveness
- Easy to prepare
- Low antigenicity
- Easy to store
- Resistance to shear

Skin substitutes can be categorized according to whether they are acellular or cellular. Acellular products, such as cadaveric human dermis with removed cellular components, contain a scaffold or matrix of hyaluronic acid, collagen, or fibronectin. Cellular products contain living cells such as fibroblasts and keratinocytes within a matrix. These cells can be autologous, allogeneic, or from another species. Skin substitutes can also be divided into three major categories: dermal replacement, epidermal replacement and dermal/epidermal replacement. They can also be used as either permanent or temporary wound coverings.[35]

Box 1: Tips for optimizing wound healing.

- Asepsis promotes wound healing
- Proper apposition of wounds, proper hemostasis and removal of necrotic debris after surgical excisions promotes healing
- Avoidance of tension, elimination of dead space also promotes healing
- Use of occlusive dressings hastens healing. Film dressings are useful on face. Hydrocolloid dressings on exudating wounds. Foam dressings reduce pain
- Honey releases cytokines, exerts osmotic effect and produces hydrogen peroxide.
- Skin substitutes are the latest development in the management of chronic wounds

Future of Bioengineered Skin Substitutes

At the present time, the most advanced skin substitutes lack the properties of normal skin and dermal appendages. They lack glands, pilosity and specialized cells for the perception of cold, heat, pain, pressure, and vibration.[36] Skin pigmentation is discrepant. The ideal substitute should contain all three components involved in dynamic skin reciprocity—cells, ECM, and bioactive molecules. Future constructs should induce an environment that helps wounds heal quickly without scarring so that skin regenerates, preserves its function and cosmesis.

Some tips for optimizing wound healing are listed in Box 1.

CONCLUSION

Current limitations in the treatment of chronic wounds are due to the incomplete understanding of the molecular mechanisms hindering repair. The success of novel therapies depends upon a comprehensive knowledge of the underlying pathophysiology and correction of pathogenic factors. Advances in molecular and cellular biology, as well as in material sciences, have expanded research and it is expected that these findings, along with a better understanding of the molecular aspects of tissue repair will lead to the development of enhanced therapeutic modalities.

REFERENCES

1. Schreml S, Szeimies RM, Prantl L, et al. Wound healing in the 21st century. J Am Acad Dermatol. 2010;63:866-81.
2. Kirsner RS, Eaqlstein WH. The wound healing process. Dermatol Clin. 1993;11:629-40.
3. Cho J, Mosher DF. Role of fibronectin assembly in platelet thrombus formation. J Thromb Haemost. 2006;4:1461-9.
4. Bennett NT, Schultz GS. Growth factors and wound healing: biochemical properties of growth factors and their receptors. Am J Surg. 1993;165:728-37.
5. Rumalla VK, Borah GL. Cytokines, growth factors, and plastic surgery. Plast Reconstr Surg. 2001;108:719-33.
6. Frenette PS, Wagner DD. Adhesion molecules—part 1. N Engl J Med. 1996;334:1526-9.
7. Frenette PS, Wagner DD. Adhesion molecules—part II: Blood vessels and blood cells. N Engl J Med. 1996;335:43-5.
8. Cross KJ, Mustoe TA. Growth factors in wound healing. Surg Clin N Am. 2003;83:531-46.
9. Goldberg SR, Diegelmann RF. Wound healing primer. Surg Clin North Am. 2010;90:1133-46.
10. Bhushan M, Young HS, Brenchley PE, et al. Recent advances in cutaneous angiogenesis. Br J Dermatol. 2002;147:418-25.
11. Clore JN, Cohen IK, Diegelmann RF. Quantitation of collagen types I and III during wound healing in rat skin. Proc Soc Exp Biol Med. 1979;161:337-40.
12. Baker EA, Leaper DJ. Proteinases, their inhibitors, and cytokine profiles in acute wound fluid. Wound Repair Regen. 2000;8:392-8.
13. Chen WY, Rogers AA, Lydon MJ. Characterization of biologic properties of wound fluid collected during early stages of wound healing. J Invest Dermatol. 1992;99:559-64.
14. Vaalamo M, Leivo T, Saarialho-Kere U. Differential expression of tissue inhibitors of metalloproteinases (TIMP-1,-2,-3, and -4) in normal and aberrant wound healing. Hum Pathol. 1999;30:795-802.
15. Cowin AJ, Hatzirodos N, Holding CA, et al. Effect of healing on the expression of transforming growth factor beta(s) and their receptors in chronic venous leg ulcers. J Invest Dermatol. 2001;117:1282-9.
16. Wysocki AB. Fibronectin in acute and chronic wounds. JET Nurs. 1992;19:166-70.
17. Lu L, Saulis AS, Liu WR, et al. The temporal effects of anti-TGF-beta1, 2, and 3 monoclonal antibody on wound healing and hypertrophic scar formation. J Am Coll Surg. 2005;201:391-7.
18. Lim IJ, Phan TT, Song C, et al. Investigation of the influence of keloid-derived keratinocytes on fibroblast growth and proliferation in vitro. Plast Reconstr Surg. 2001;107:797-808.
19. Smith CJ, Smith JC, Finn MC. The possible role of mast cells (allergy) in the production of keloid and hypertrophic scarring. J Burn Care Rehabil. 1987;8:126-31.
20. Ghahary A, Ghaffari A. Role of keratinocyte fibroblast cross-talk in development of hypertrophic scar. Wound Repair Regen. 2007;15:S46-53.
21. Fujiwara M, Muragaki Y, Ooshima A. Keloid-derived fibroblasts show increased secretion of factors involved in collagen turnover and depend on matrix metalloproteinase for migration. Br J Dermatol. 2005;153:295-300.
22. Armour A, Scott PG, Tredget EE. Cellular and molecular pathology of HTS: basis for treatment. Wound Repair Regen. 2007;15:S6-17.
23. Kurokawa I, Danby FW, Ju Q, et al. New developments in our understanding of acne pathogenesis and treatment. Exp Dermatol 2009;18:821-32.
24. Holland DB, Jeremy AH, Roberts SG, et al. Inflammation in acne scarring: a comparison of the responses in lesions from patients prone and not prone to scar. Br J of Dermatol. 2004;150:72-81.
25. Chivot M, Pawin H, Beylot C, et al. Acne scars: epidemiology, physiopathology, clinical features and treatment. Ann Dermatol Et Venereol. 2006;133:813-24.
26. Ross EV, McKinlay JR, Anderson RR. Why does carbon dioxide resurfacing work? A review. Arch Dermatol. 1999; 135:444-54.
27. Rahman Z, MacFalls H, Jiang K, et al. Fractional deep dermal ablation induces tissue tightening. Lasers Surg Med. 2009; 41:78-86.
28. Hantash BM, Bedi VP, Kapadia B, et al. In vivo histological evaluation of a novel ablative fractional resurfacing device. Lasers Surg Med. 2007;39:96-107.
29. Weibrich G, Hansen T, Kleis W, et al. Effect of platelet concentration in platelet-rich plasma on peri-implant bone regeneration. Bone 2004; 34: 665-71
30. Conde ME, Fernando SME, Suarez FR. Platelet rich plasma: applications in dermatology. Actos Dermosifiliogr 2015;106: 104-11.
31. Anitua E, Sanchez M, Nurden AT, et al. Autologous fibrin matrices: a potential source of biological mediators that modulate tendon cell activities. J Biomed Mater Res A 2006; 77:285-93.
32. Choukroun J, Diss A, Simonpieri A, et al. Platelet-rich fibrin (PRF): A second-generation platelet concentrate. Part IV: Clinical effects on tissue healing. Oral Surg Oral Med Oral Pathol Oral Radiol Endod. 2006;101:56-60.
33. Sarabahi S. Recent advances in topical wound care. Indian J Plast Surg 2012;45:379-87.
34. Ferreira MC, Paggiaro AO, Issac C, et al. Skin substitutes. A current concept and a new classification. Rev Bras Cir Plast 2011;26:696-702.
35. Vyas KS, Vasconez HC. Wound healing: Biologicals, Skin Substitutes, Biomembranes and Scaffolds. Healthcare 2014;2: 356-400.
36. Auger FA, Lacroix D, Germain L. Skin substitutes and wound healing. Skin Pharmacol Physiol 2009;22:94-102.

Chapter 5

Wound Management

Manas Chatterjee, BS Gill, GR Rajput

Key Messages 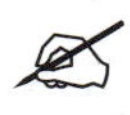

- Proper wound management includes wound cleaning, dressings and debridement.
- Management of wounds depends on the type of wound and is affected by general and local factors.
- Moist environment aids wound healing.
- Various types of dressings such as occlusive, semiocclusive dressings, biological dressings such as grafts, are available.

INTRODUCTION

A wound is a break in the continuity of skin/soft tissues. It is defined as a separation or discontinuity of the skin, mucous membrane or tissue caused by physical, biological or chemical insult. Proper wound care is important in dermatosurgery to ensure safe and effective outcomes. While the previous chapter dealt with wound healing, its pathogenesis and factors affecting healing, this chapter deals with management of wounds.

WOUNDS CLASSIFICATION

Types of Cutaneous Wounds[1]

Type I: Those having superficial loss of tissue involving epidermis and superficial (papillary) dermis. Heal by epithelialization with negligible granulation and contraction.

Type II: Involving full thickness of dermis up to subcutaneous tissue.

Type IIA: Without significant tissue loss, heal with epidermization and minimal granulation tissue with some contracture.

Type IIB: Substantial tissue loss, heal by granulation/contraction.

In addition, wounds can be classified in different ways. They may be *Open* (incisions, lacerations, abrasions, puncture wounds, penetration wounds and gunshot wounds) and *Closed* (contusions, hematomas). Surgical wounds can be classified as *Clean*, *Clean contaminated* (a wound involving normal tissue colonized with microorganisms), *Contaminated* (a wound containing foreign or infected material) and *Infected* (a wound with presence of pus). In dermatosurgery, a more relevant classification is classification in to *acute* and *chronic wounds*.

1. **Acute wounds:** These wounds of less than 4 weeks occur with incisional wounds, excisional surgical wounds and traumatic skin injury including burns. These wounds are characterized by definite orderly progression of inflammation, granulation tissue formation and healing through activation of mitogen-activated protein kinase pathways and activator-protein 1. There is no underlying healing defect and when large, these wounds are best dealt within the hospital settings.
2. **Chronic wounds:** Chronic wound is classified as one that fails to heal within four weeks and shows no sign of improvement within eight weeks. These wounds suffer from impairment of inflammation, angiogenesis, re-epithelialization and wound remodeling, leading to the apparent loss of capacity to heal. Leg ulcers, pressure sores are examples. These wounds are best dealt within the community rather than in hospitals to reduce cost of care and dependency.

The pathophysiology of wound healing has been dealt with in detail in the preceding chapter on wound healing and the reader should refer to it.

The most common types of wound seen by a dermatosurgeon are chronic wounds (trophic ulcers due

Box 1: Wound assessment.

- Wound bed color or tissue type
- Exposed bone, tendon or muscle
- Exudate: Color and amount
- Wound odor
- Clinical infection or spreading infection
- Measurement: Linear, tracing on grided acetate films and counting number of grids, photography, computerized planimetry in research settings
- Depth can be measured using sterile probe or spatula, volume of fluid under an occluding membrane
- Condition of surrounding skin for callus (tissue breakdown or ulceration underneath), cellulitis, eczema or maceration
- Pain assessment: Pain related to change of dressing or bathing, or constant as in case of ischemia or neuropathy
- Primary factor delaying healing: Diabetes mellitus, malnutrition, systemic steroid use and others
- Investigation of primary pathology: Doppler
- Research studies use laser Doppler assessment of blood flow, ultrasound measurement of depth, optical coherence tomography, wound pH, and direct measurement of arterial and venous pressures.
- Assessment of chronic wounds: TIME system[4,5] [**T**issue (viability, as necrotic tissue, slough or eschar delay healing and need removal), **I**nfection/**I**nflammation (infection needs treatment), **M**oisture (balance important as too much and too little moisture are both bad), **E**dge (if non-progressive or undermined may be debrided or grafted]

Box 2: Factors affecting wound healing.

General factors

- Age
- Underlying illnesses or disease: Amino acid deficiencies (histidine, tryptophan), diabetes or immunocompromise (correction of iron, B-complex deficiencies in addition to others mentioned below to be considered for chronic wounds) (correction of anemia, malnutrition, infections)
- Medications such as corticosteroids, anticoagulants, nonsteroidal anti-inflammatory, colchicine and antineoplastic pharmacotherapy delay wound healing[6-8]
- Conditions predisposing to ulceration such as varicose veins, hypertension, leprosy
- Effect of the injury on healing (e.g. devascularization)
- Skin disorders such as epidermolysis bullosa require special care of wounds including of anemia, malnutrition, infection and pruritus

Wound factors

- Rest to injured oragan
  - Adequate rest ensures faster healing
- Organ or tissues Injured
- Rest-adequate rest ensures faster healing
- Extremity location due to lesser blood supply
- Extent of injury
- Nature of injury (for example, a laceration will be a less complicated wound than a crush injury)
- Contamination or infection
- Time between injury and treatment (sooner is better)

Local factors

- Hemostasis and debridement
- Use of electrosurgery
- Timing of closure
- Formation of biofilms (can lead to chronicity of wounds)

to leprosy, diabetes, and venous and arterial leg ulcers) in addition to postoperative wounds.

WOUND ASSESSMENT[2]

Proper wound assessment is the key to proper wound management; the factors that need to be assessed are shown in the Box 1.

FACTORS THAT AFFECT WOUND HEALING AND THE POTENTIAL FOR INFECTION[3]

Factors affecting healing include general factors, local factors and wound factors and are shown in the Box 2. These have been dealt with in the preceding chapter and need to be carefully considered during management.

Wound Management

History of Wound Management and Use of Natural Products

In some ways, the early history of medicine is dominated by the care of wounds, especially those injuries caused in battles. In Mesopotamia (2100 BC), after cleaning a wound with beer, a bandage with wine and turpentine was applied. In Ancient Egypt, a natural product such as honey became common in wound management; after irrigating a wound with wine, physicians would then cover the wound with fat and honey. In Greece, during the time of Homer, wounds were covered and treated with herbs, whereas infected wounds were healed by dropping scrapings from bronze spears into them.

Four hundred years later, Hippocrates taught that wounds should be washed with wine, bandaged and then saturated with more wine. Galen, of ancient Rome, cleaned wounds with vinegar but nevertheless believed that suppuration ("*pus bonum et laudabile*") was necessary for healing. This belief prevailed for many centuries.

When gunpowder was first used in battle, boiling oil was used as wound treatment, with the aim "to inactivate" the gunpowder effect within gunshot wounds. This practice was abandoned when, in 1542, Ambroise Paré performed one of the first cohort studies to demonstrate that egg yolk and turpentine were better than boiling oil for treatment of gunshot wounds.

In 1867, the first antiseptic dressings were introduced by Lister, who soaked lint and gauze in phenol and then applied them to wounds. In general, before twentieth century, it was believed that wound heal best when left open and dry as advocated by Pasteur. However in 1958, Odland observed that a blister healed faster when left unbroken. In 1962, Winter showed in swine that superficial wounds kept moist healed faster by two times. Hinman and Maibach repeated this study in humans with similar results. These studies transmuted wound care by bespeaking importance of moist wound healing.

There are limited data on natural products, such as yogurt (which seems to help in controlling wound odor), tea tree oil and potato peelings; however, there is a great interest in the use of honey for wound healing. Although science and technology march ever forward, we must not fail to exploit the potential of natural products, because they may represent a hope for modern medicine.[9]

Techniques of Wound Management

Different techniques of wound management include wound cleaning, closure, dressings, use of antimicrobials, use of agents which promote wound healing, etc. These vary depending on the different wound and host factors mentioned in Box 2.

Wound Cleansing[10]

Wound cleansing is done to remove foreign material or debris present in the wound. It includes wound irrigation and debridement.

Irrigation:[11] Irrigation helps in cleansing and removal of superficial debris. It should be noted that swabbing is not helpful. Solutions used for irrigation include potable tap water, saline, boiled and cooled water or distilled water.[12] Solutions used should be at body temperature. Povidone-iodine solution can be used as it can maintain bactericidal activity even at low concentration. It should be used in low concentration only, as it is toxic in high concentrations. Its effect on wound healing is not clearly established, but there is some evidence to suggest a beneficial effect on chronic wounds.[13,14] As iodine can cause contact dermatitis, it should be used with caution.

However, due to their cytotoxic effects, higher concentration povidone-iodine-based antiseptics and hydrogen peroxide should no longer be used in any wound to prevent infection. Both solutions alter the migration and proliferation of skin fibroblast, fundamental cells in the proliferative phase of wound healing and the matrix metalloproteinase release by the dermal fibroblasts, thus making the wound bed a harsh environment for adequate healing. Chlorhexidine too is not without its own concerns. First, the required bactericidal concentration varies widely among microorganisms. For example, methicillin-resistant *Staphylococcus aureus* only requires a concentration of 0.002%, while gram-negative organisms might require a bactericidal concentration of 1%. Hexachlorophene is tissue toxic and tends to be painful to apply on open wounds.

As a precaution, hands must be washed before changing dressings and irrigation. Equipment needed for irrigation is simple and consists of a 50 cc syringe with 18 G needle for wound irrigation which produces about a pressure of 8–10 psi. Amount used should be at least 100–300 cc with continued irrigation until all visible particles are removed. A general rule of thumb is to use 50–100 cc per cm of wound length.

Debridement: If irrigation alone is ineffective in removing contaminants from a wound, the wound should be lightly scrubbed. Gentle scrubbing may be useful in wounds older than 3–4 hours, even if they are clean, as it removes a glycoprotein matrix that may cover the wound and allows bacterial colonization. Debridement of devitalized tissue is paramount to reducing risk of infection. Scalpel excision of wound margins can be used in grossly contaminated wounds. Debridement is more relevant for infected wounds and hence more information is provided on debridement later in this chapter.

Management of Infected Wounds[2]

Infection is said to have occurred when bacterial numbers in wound overwhelm the immune response and clinical signs of infection appear. Risk of infection can be reduced by proper hand washing, infection control, wound cleansing and debridement. Protection of wounds from exogenous sources of contamination is important. Prevention of infection can enhance wound healing and reduce hospital stay and cost. In presence of systemic and clinical signs of infection, systemic antimicrobial therapy should be considered. Culture swab is required only if clinical signs of spreading infection are present such as pyrexia, heat, redness, swelling or pain. One must review antibiotic choice and duration when swab results are available. Changing of dressing daily or alternate days, depending on exudate is important. If purulent material or foul odor is present, more frequent cleansing and possibly debridement are required.

Topical antimicrobials: Topical antiseptic agents are commonly used, but suffer from certain disadvantages. They have been shown to retard wound healing.[15,16] Topical antibiotics, particularly neomycin and gentamicin are frequent causes of contact dermatitis. However, certain topical antimicrobial agents are useful and are mentioned below:

- Silver dressings, e.g. silver sulfadiazine: Silver compounds are widely used in burn care, being effective against *Staphylococcus aureus* and *Pseudomonas aeruginosa*, in a concentration as low as 10 mmol/L and possibly having an effect by enhancing epithelialisation.[17]
- Povidone-iodine in low concentration as described above.
- Honey[18] stimulates tissue growth and epithelialization, as well as reducing inflammation and infection, debriding and deodorizing wounds.[19] It is also effective against antibiotic resistant bacteria, including methicillin-resistant *Staphylococcus aureus*.[20]
- Cane sugar containing sucrose, which is not metabolized outside the gastrointestinal tract, prevents bacterial growth by decreasing available water, and it has also been claimed to stimulate granulation tissue.[21]
- Metronidazole which acts against anaerobes.

- Newer anti-infective biomaterials, antimicrobial biocides and novel types of antimicrobial agents such as rapamycin are now available.[22]

Topical antibiotics in general should not be used for prolonged periods. Systemic antibiotics should be preferred where there is clinical sign of infection.

Wound Closure[3,4,23]

Wound closure has definite role in management of clean wounds-clean wounds should be closed immediately to allow healing by primary intention. A closed dressing exposes the wound continuously to proteinases, chemotactic, complement and growth factors in the surrounding fluid, which may be otherwise lost in case the wound is left exposed. The electrical gradient required for stimulation of fibroblasts and epithelial cell migration is maintained and further trauma to the wound is avoided by this physical barrier. However, contaminated and infected wounds should not be closed but left open to heal by secondary intention. In treating clean contaminated wounds and clean wounds that are more than 6–8 hours old, one must manage with surgical toilet, the wound left open and then closed 48 hours later. This is called delayed primary (or tertiary) closure. Table 1 shows different types of wound closure and their characteristics.

Table 1: Indications and key points to consider for each closure type.

Intention (Closure)	*Unique characteristics*	*Key points*
Primary	Clean, minimal contaminated, mostly shearing forces 6–8 hours old	May close with tape, staplers, and sutures
Secondary	Noncosmetic animal bites Abscess cavities, ulcers	No sutures Delayed skin coverage, graft
Tertiary	Too contaminated to close	Clean, debride, and observe 4–6 days before suturing

Negative Pressure Wound Therapy

Negative pressure wound therapy (NPWT) or vacuum-assisted closure (VAC) has played a major role as a bridge to reconstruction. It is a significant, clinically proven advancement in wound care that promotes active wound healing at the cellular level through negative pressure. Pressure used is negative pressure or sub-atmospheric pressure (100–125 mm Hg) in a continuous or intermittent manner. The intermittent negative pressure is delivered at wound site through a porous dressing, which applies mechanical forces known as macro strain (physical response) and micro strain (biological response) and subsequently removes exudates by an electromechanical pump.

PRIMARY WOUND REPAIR[3]

Primary closure requires that clean tissue is approximated without tension. Primary closure is done by suturing, wound adhesives or staples. Injudicious closure of a contaminated wound will promote infection and delay healing. These have been dealt with in detail in the chapter on sutures.

Body hair entangled in sutures and staples or buried inside the wound can alter the healing process and increase the risk of infection. It is important to understand that routine hair removal by shaving before suturing can lead to poor outcomes. If hair has to be removed, scissors or clippers should be used. It has also been shown that use of clean non-sterile gloves are not inferior to sterile gloves in terms of infection control.

The hair apposition technique (HAT) for scalp wounds and lacerations should be considered for the repair of scalp lacerations that are non-crush injuries less than 10 cm long with regular wound edges, minimal contamination, without evidence of underlying skull fractures and with an intact galea in patients with hair strands longer than 3 cm. These techniques are associated with less scarring, fewer overall complications, shorter procedural time, lower pain scores, and substantially lower costs than standard suturing and stapler techniques. The HAT technique consists of twisting together three to seven strands of hair on either side of the wound. The two bundles of hair are then interlocked in a 360° revolution and a small drop of tissue adhesive can be applied. The hair is not tied. This same process is repeated as needed for the entire length of the wound. The glue will break down and the hair will unravel by itself after 7–10 days.[24]

TISSUE ADHESIVES (2-OCTYL CYANOACRYLATE)[25]

The commonly used wound adhesives include 2-butyl cyanoacrylate and 2-octyl cyanoacrylate.

2-Octyl cyanoacrylate use is often correlated with laceration repair, which is certainly a popular application. However, it is also widely used for operative incision repair. Sutureless pediatric circumcisions, cleft lip repair and upper eyelid blepharoplasties are a few innovative surgical incision closures that have been facilitated with the use of 2-octyl cyanoacrylate. It is most commonly used in dermatology to hold in place punch and suction blister grafts. Cosmetic results with 2-octyl cyanoacrylate equals those of sutures. Tips on use of 2-octyl cyanoacrylate are in Box 3. More details can be found in the chapter on wound and closure materials.

Contraindications for Use of Tissue Glue

These include:

- A person with a history of allergy to cyanoacrylates
- Animal bite wound

Box 3: Tips on technique of using 2-octyl cyanoacrylate.

- Maintaining everted skin apposition with fingers or forceps during application to improve apposition
- Using multiple thin applications, with the first layer protecting the skin from the exothermic reaction of the layers above it
- Allowing the adhesive to dry between applications
- Advising the patient not to scrub the site where the adhesive is applied so that the cyanoacrylate does not get rubbed off

Box 4: Recommendations for use of tissue glue.

- Useful in wounds with edges less than 5 mm apart, clean, sharp edges, nonmobile areas and laceration less than 5 cm in length
- Not useful in wounds near eye, on mucous membrane or mucosal surfaces, wet wounds or those exposed to body fluids, or in areas with dense hair, wounds under significant tension

- Stellate crush injury
- Partial-thickness facial laceration in a patient with diabetes
- Decubitus ulcers
- Nonsurgical puncture wounds.

In addition, 2-octyl cyanoacrylate should be used carefully on the oral mucosa, hands, feet, or joints, where repetitive movement and washing may cause the adhesives to slough prematurely.

Follow-up

Close attention should be paid when closing wounds near surrounding structures that could become encased in or stuck to the glue. In such a case, petroleum jelly or acetone can be used, which weakens the polymerization. Using water and alcohol, which speed up the exothermic reaction that polymerizes 2-octyl cyanoacrylate, is to be avoided.

Patients who have had 2-octyl cyanoacrylate applied to their wounds should be monitored for allergic-type reactions. Generally, it takes 7–14 days for 2-octyl cyanoacrylate to flake off and prolonged retention, either on the surface or within the edges of the wound, could lead to allergic reactions.

Complications

Inflammation, tissue necrosis, granulation tissue formation and wound breakdown can occur, when cyanoacrylates are implanted subcutaneously. The process causing the toxicity is thought to be related to the byproducts of degradation, viz. cyanoacetate and formaldehyde. Recommendations for use of tissue glue are in Box 4.

WOUND: SECONDARY HEALING[3]

To promote healing by secondary intention, perform wound toilet and surgical debridement.

Box 5: Tips for surgical wound debridement.

- Systematically perform wound toilet and surgical debridement, initially to the superficial layers of tissues and subsequently to the deeper layers
- After scrubbing the skin with soap and irrigating the wound with saline, prepare the skin with antiseptic keeping in mind what has been mentioned earlier in this chapter
- Do not use antiseptics within the wound
- Debride the wound meticulously to remove any loose foreign material such as dirt, grass, wood, glass or clothing
- With a scalpel or dissecting scissors, remove all adherent foreign material along the wound edge with a thin margin of underlying tissue and then irrigate the wound again
- Continue the cycle of surgical debridement and saline irrigation until the wound is completely clean
- Leave the wound open after debridement to allow healing by secondary intention
- Pack it lightly with damp saline gauze and cover the packed wound with a dry dressing
- Change the packing and dressing daily or more often if the outer dressing becomes damp with blood or other body fluids
- Large defects will require closure with flaps or skin grafts but may be initially managed with saline packing
- During debridement, one must excise only a very thin margin of skin from the wound edge

- Surgical wound toilet involves cleaning the skin with antiseptics, irrigation of wounds with saline and surgical debridement of all dead tissue and foreign matter. Dead tissue does not bleed when cut.
- Wound debridement involves removal of dead and devitalized tissues, debris, to promote healing.

Types of Debridement

Debridement is the removal of necrotic debris which accumulates on the surface of or around a wound which may impair healing by forming a physical barrier to re-epithelialization, as well as acting as a focus for infection. Different types of debridement are described below:

Surgical debridement: It is a rapid and selective form of debridement used for wounds with a significant amount of necrotic tissue (Box 5).

Autolytic debridement: This involves debridement by autolysis of necrotic tissue by body enzymes and moisture. It occurs after the use of dressings that maintain fluid contact with necrotic tissue such as films, hydrogels and hydrocolloid dressings in dry wounds, and foams, alginates or hydrofibers in more sloughy wounds. These dressings exploit the presence of endogenous collagenases and proteases present in a wound to break down necrotic tissue. Care must be taken to protect surrounding normal tissue.

Mechanical debridement: Moist dressing is applied to a wound and then removed after drying. Hydrotherapy is another form of mechanical debridement. The latter can also be done under pressure in a whirlpool.

Enzymatic debridement: They enhance granulation tissue formation and epithelialization. Studies in animal models have shown the effectiveness of collagenase in wound debridement.[26] Streptokinase/streptodornase and proteolytic enzymes derived from antarctic krill have also been shown to be effective in wound debridement;[27] papain is also used in some countries.

High-pressure water irrigation: Hydrocision (Regd) or pressurized irrigation (Versajet, Smith and Nephew) is the new tool in surgical debridement and cleaning of the wound with either high or low pressure, razor thin stream of water, saline or antibiotic solution and is serving as a better alternative compared to the above methods. High pressure irrigation is effective in removing bacteria, particulate matter and necrotic debris from the wounds, thus lowering the rate of infection compared to low pressure irrigation. The only concern is that there is a risk of bacteria being driven into soft tissue by the high pressure. It is particularly useful in concavities of pressure sores and joint spaces and in tight spaces. It is indicated for use in necrotic wounds and deep burns also. Since it preserves the viable dermal tissue, it allows rapid wound healing with better cosmetic outcome.

Maggot therapy (*biosurgery*): Maggots are used for treatment of chronic wounds refractory to conventional treatment. *Lucilia sericata* is the commonly used maggot. Up to 1,000 maggots are introduced into the wound and left for 1–3 days before a dressing change. They facilitate healing by secretion of proteolytic enzymes that liquefy necrotic tissue, maggot digestion of necrotic tissue and MRSA and b-hemolytic streptococcus, increase in wound pH secondary to larval excretion of ammonia and calcium carbonate and secretion of allantoin and urea. Movement of maggots stimulate granulation tissue. Maggots effectively separate necrotic from living tissue, thereby making subsequent surgical debridement unnecessary or much easier.[29,30]

WOUND DRESSINGS

Wound dressings protect the surface of wounds and prevent bacterial, fungal and viral (herpes group of viruses most commonly) contamination of healing wounds. Occlusive dressings help in creating a moist environment, which has a beneficial effect on wound healing through accumulation of endogenous growth factors and other biological effects on angiogenesis, generation of granulation tissue and re-epithelialization. Though rate of tissue bacterial colonization are slightly higher, it has been shown to be non-significant in terms of prevention of re-epithelialization.[31,32]

Properties of an Ideal Dressing

- Able to maintain a good moisture balance at the wound bed but not too much to avoid maceration of surrounding tissue
- Easy to remove without damaging the wound or surrounding skin
- Impermeable to bacteria
- Prevents capillary loops penetrating into dressing material
- Capable of being sterilized
- Confer mechanical protection to the wound
- Non-toxic and non-allergenic
- Comfortable for the patient
- Conformability with patient lifestyle and requirements
- Cost-effective
- Have a long shelf life.

Wound dressings can help healing by different mechanisms. Functions of wound dressings are shown in Table 2.

Types of Dressings

Before a discussion on the various types of dressings is embarked upon, the conventional composite dressing needs to be understood, as it has stood the test of time. It composes of 4/5 layers:

- A layer of antibiotic ointment
- A contact layer of nonadhesive material such as paraffin gauze, silver sulfadiazine, framycetin/chlorhexidine tulle or iodine tulle. The last two if available obviates the need for the first layer
- An absorbent layer of dry gauze
- Outer securing layer of tape or roller bandage. Tackifiers such as tincture benzoin may be used to increase adhesion of dressing to the skin
- Sometimes, a fifth layer of gauze or cotton padding may interpose before the layer of tape or roller bandage.

Adhesive bandages such as Band-Aid® are pre-made composite dressings (Fig. 1).

Different types of dressings and their properties are shown in Table 3.

Dressings can also be classified into passive and interactive dressings. Passive dressings are simple products which only protect wound without interacting with it. Most modern dressing products are interactive dressings as they interact with the wound bed to provide optimum environment at the wound dressing interface.

Table 2: Functions of wound dressings.

Function	*Benefit*
Covering the wound	Protection from trauma and contamination from bacteria and foreign material and minimizes fluid and heat loss, provide contact with topical antibiotics, cosmetic acceptability of wound till it heals
Absorption of wound drainage	Keeps wound moist but not wet, minimizes maceration
Compression	Increases hemostasis, minimizes edema and hematoma formation, prevents dehiscence
Providing moist environment	Facilitates healing of acute wounds and reduces pain of chronic wounds
Immobilization	Assists re-epithelialization, reduces pain, promotes healing, improves resultant scar

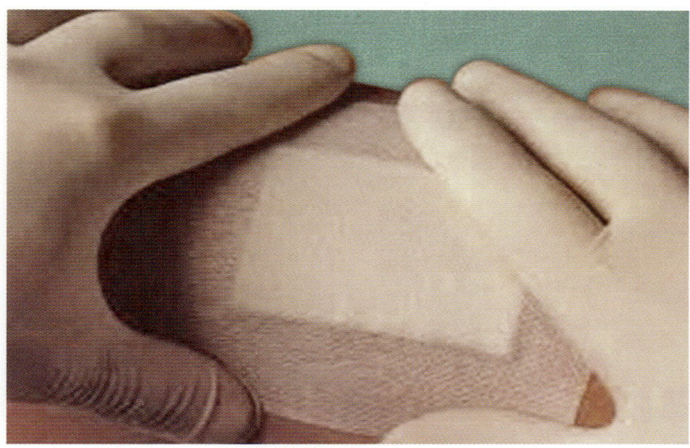

Fig. 1: Composite dressing.

Table 3: Different types of dressings.

Nonadherent fabrics	
Absorptive	Gauze Foams Alginates
Occlusive/moisture-retentive dressings	
Non-biologictraditional	Foams Polyurethane films Hydrocolloids Hydrogels Alginates
Non-biologic—new	Hydrofiber dressings Collagen dressings Hyaluronic acid dressings
Biologic grafts	Split-thickness skin grafts Full-thickness skin grafts Composite grafts
Biologic/biosynthetic—skin substitutes	Cultured epidermal grafts Dermal replacements Biocomposite skin substitutes
Odor absorbing dressings	
Biosynthetic dressings	

Appropriate Wound Dressings in Different Types of Wounds[33]

Each of the various types of dressing can be used in a specific setting and Table 4 shows different types of dressings and their role in different types of wound. It has been proved that moist environment is beneficial for healing. The moisture vapor transmission rate (MVTR) measures the moisture retentive property of a dressing. A dressing is moisture retentive if its MVTR is less than 840 $g/m^2/24$ hrs. The MVTR of hydrocolloids is less than 300 $g/m^2/24$ hrs, in contrast to gauze whose MVTR is 1200 $g/m^2/24$ hrs. MVTR is a useful tool for choosing dressing according to the wound type.[34]

Table 4: Types of dressings and their role in different types of wound.

Types of wound	Suitable dressings
Acute wound	
Abrasions, lacerations Catheter or cannula sites Burns	Films, hydrocolloids, foams Films Hydrocolloids, hydrogels, biosynthetic dressings
Donor sites of grafts Dermabrasion, chemical peels	Films, hydrocolloids Hydrogels
Surgical wounds	Films, hydrocolloids, hydrogels, alginates
Chronic wound	
Venous ulcer Heavy exudates Moderate exudates Mild exudates Malodorous	 Foams, alginates, hydrofibers Hydrocolloids, foams Hydrogels, hydrocolloids Foams, alginates, hydrocolloid charcoal
Arterial	Hydrogels
Neuropathic Moist Dry	 Hydrogels, alginates, hydrofibers Hydrogels, hydrocolloids
Pressure ulcers Stage I Stage II–III Stage IV	 Films, thin hydrocolloids Hydrocolloids, foams, hydrogels, debriding agents Alginates, hydrofibers, debriding agents
Fungating	Hydrocolloids, hydrogels, alginates, foams, charcoal

Different types of dressings are discussed in detail below:

Gauze is one of the most commonly used absorptive dressing. It is excellent at drawing fluid and exudates away from wound surface, but loses its efficacy when saturated. It is usually used to cover non-occlusive, non-adhering fabric dressing material and absorb discharge, which drains through them. It can also be used to cover occlusive dressing as secondary dressing to keep them in place. Wide mesh gauze is not to be placed in direct contact with wounds as it adheres to surface causing pain on removal, only exception is when mechanical debridement is warranted.

Semipermeable (Polyurethane) Films (Fig. 2)

Examples: Opsite, Tegaderm, etc.

These are often coated with adhesive to ease application. They are impermeable to bacteria and fluids, but are permeable to air and water vapor. One can inspect the wound without need for removal of these dressings. They can be left in situ for days at a time. They provide a moist environment, but are not good for large amount of exudate. They provide, however, no mechanical protection of the wound. Care needs to be taken during removal as new epithelium can be stripped off during removal.

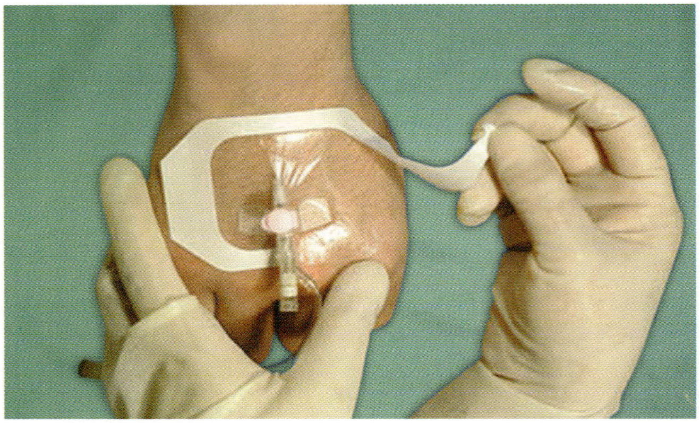

Fig. 2: Polyurethane films.

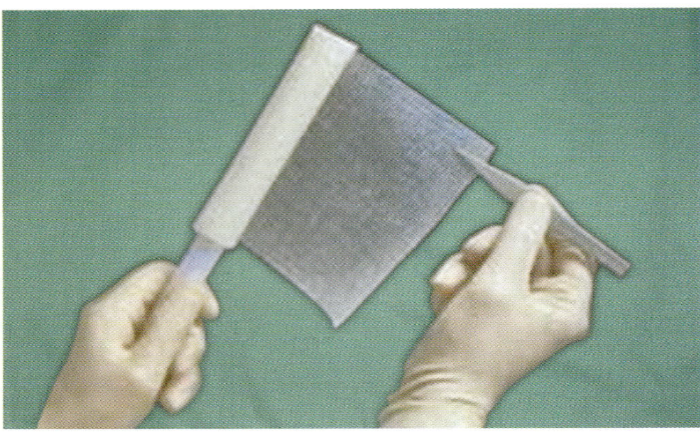

Fig. 3: Bactigras dressing.

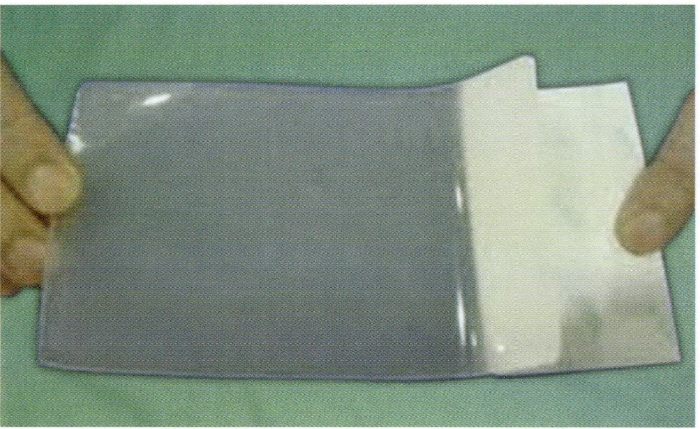

Fig. 4: Hydrogel wound dressing.

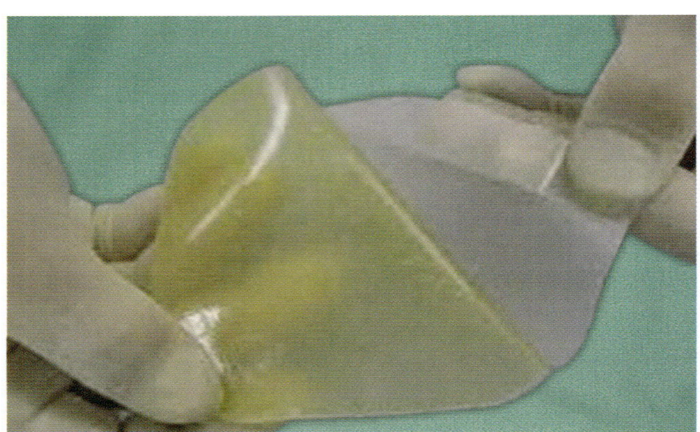

Fig. 5: Hydrocolloid dressing.

Low Adherence Dressings

Examples: Bactigras (Fig. 3), Jelonet, etc.
These provide a moist wound environment. They allow exudate to pass from wound to a secondary dressing and are low adherence and hence, good for fragile skin.

Hydrogels (Fig. 4)

Examples: Hi-zel and Sterigel.
They are formed of translucent, jelly-like non-adhesive matrices of insoluble polymers. They donate water to moisten the wound surface. However, their absorptive capacity is limited. These dressings are semi-permeable to gas and water vapor and are used as gel, sheets or impregnated in gauze. They require a secondary dressing to be applied over them. They have a cooling effect due to reduced temperature by about 5°C by water entrapment.Care needs to be taken to avoid maceration of surrounding skin. They are best suited for dry wounds or those with minimal exudates.

Hydrocolloids (Fig. 5)

Examples: Duoderm, Tegasorb
They are opaque mixture of adhesive absorbent polymers and gelling agents such as gelatin, pectin and sodium carboxymethyl cellulose. They adhere to wound edges and hence, allow the patient to bathe and shower. They have a polyurethane backing. Hydrophilic particles in the dressing interact with wound exudate to form a yellow gel. They provide an acidic environment, which is antibacterial and antiviral. Hydrocolloids help autolytic wound debridement and are good for difficult to dress areas such as heel, sacrum, etc. Care needs to be taken as they may cause increased amount of granulation tissue and maceration. They are not indicated for arterial/neuropathic ulcers, infected or heavily exuding wounds because of risk of periwound maceration. Another disadvantage is their tendency to produce malodorous exudates, which can be mistaken for infection.

Hydrofibers (Fig. 6)

Example: Aquacel.
These are carboxymethyl cellulose fibers in a non-woven sheet. They form a soft gel when exposed to heavily exudative wounds and are very highly absorptive. They require a secondary dressing as they absorb three times the amount of exudate than that of alginates, which are the highest in this class. They are indicated for pressure ulcers, lower limb ulcers and surgical wounds.

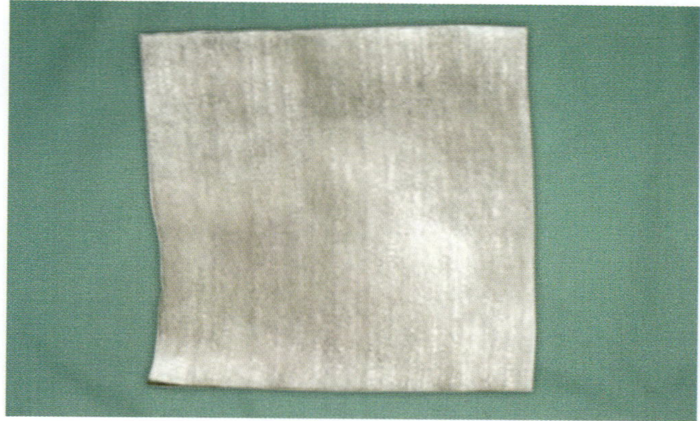

Fig. 6: Hydrofiber dressing.

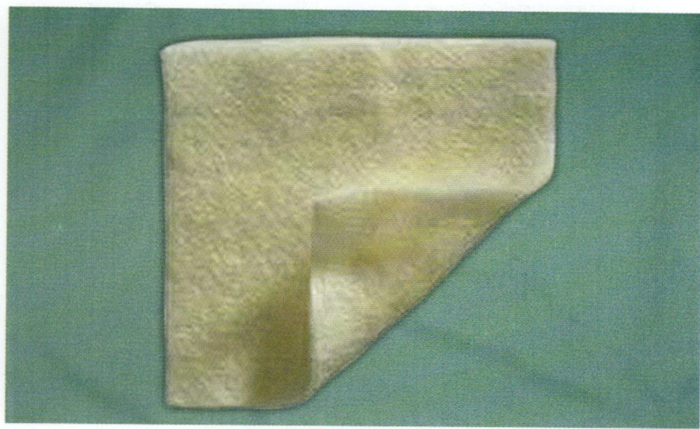

Fig. 7: Alginate dressing.

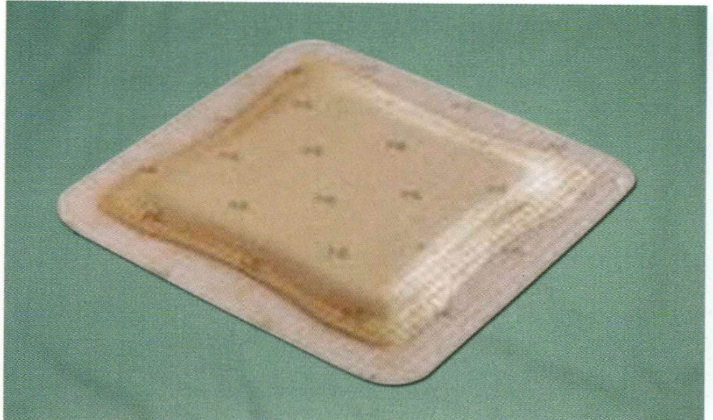

Fig. 8: Foam dressing.

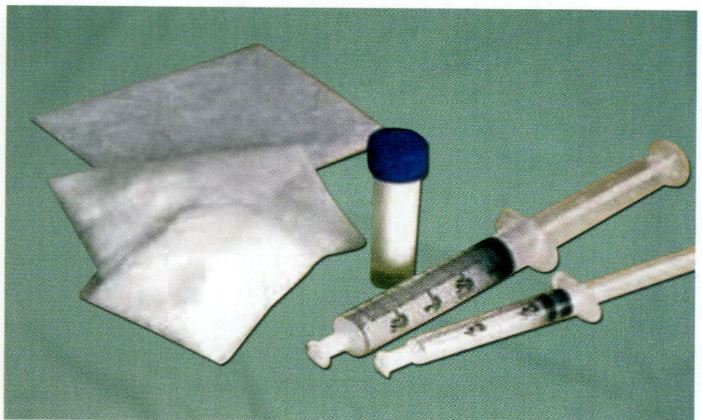

Fig. 9: Collagen sheets and particles.

Alginates (Fig. 7)

Example: Kaltostat.

They are made from brown seaweed and are highly hydrophilic. Alginates change from fibrous to gel form on absorbing water (up to 20 times their weight). Ingredients include calcium salts of alginic, mannuronic and guluronic acids. In sodium rich environment of wounds, calcium and sodium ions exchange and free calcium helps clotting. When placed over a moist wound, an ion exchange reaction occurs between calcium in the alginate and sodium in the wound fluid producing soluble calcium-sodium alginate—a gelatinous mass, which helps in maintaining moist environment and facilitates autolytic debridement. Secondary dressing is required to absorb exudates and this dressing needs to be changed daily. They conform to the shape of the wound and should be cut accordingly because if larger they can cause periwound maceration because of their tendency to absorb fluid across entire surface (lateral wicking).[34]

Foams (Fig. 8)

Examples: Allevyn and Mepilex.

These are absorbent, opaque polyurethane or silicone sheets. They are permeable to gas and water vapor and have a semi-permeable backing. They create a moist environment and provide thermal insulation to the wound. They are nonadherent, easy to apply and remove and are meant for highly exuding wounds. They can be layered in combination with other materials with overlying compression bandages. Their fluid absorption capacity varies with foam thickness; therefore, their MVTR ranges between 800 and 5000g/m^2/24 hours. They may be used for their cushioning effect but they are not a substitute for pressure relieving devices. Foams may produce excessive malodorous drainage necessitating frequent dressing change.[34]

Collagen Dressings (Fig. 9)

Examples: Kollagen and Catrix.

They are usually of human, porcine or bovine origin and are available as particle or sheet form. They accelerate wound healing by providing a collagenous matrix to enhance cell migration. Chemotaxis of fibroblasts and macrophages occurs providing a temporary scaffold to allow ingrowth of tissue. They absorb wound exudates to form a soft biodegradable gel over the wound surface, which maintains wound moisture.

Antimicrobial Dressings (Fig. 10)

Examples: Inadine and Iodosorb.

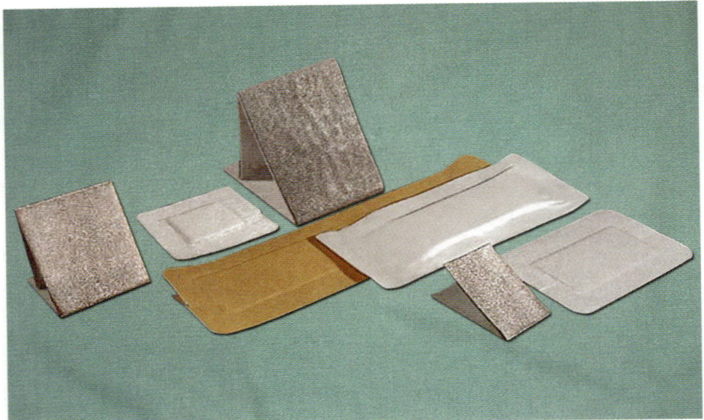

Fig. 10: Silver impregnated antimicrobial dressing.

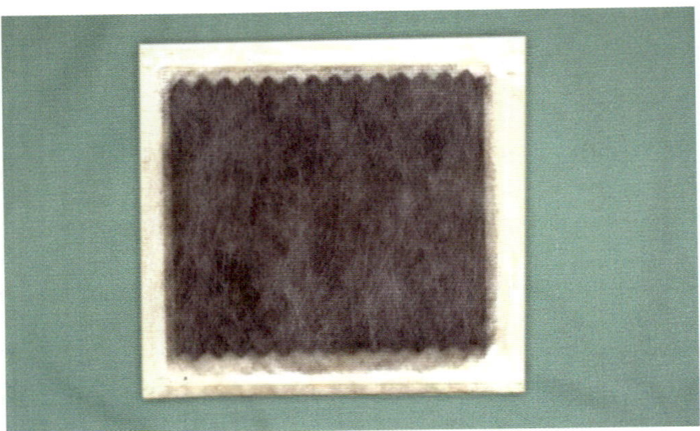

Fig. 11: Charcoal dressing.

They counter the effect of bacterial colonization on delays in wound healing. They are slow release iodine preparations (cadexomer iodine) with concentrations of the range of 0.001%. These low concentrations do not adversely affect wound healing. Care needs to be taken since thyroid function may be affected on long-term iodine dressings. Other antimicrobial dressing compounds include silver compounds. Silver impregnated dressings are bactericidal and maintain a moist environment to facilitate wound healing. They have broad spectrum action against bacteria such as vancomycin resistant enterococci and methicillin resistant *Staphylococcus aureus*, and fungi. Metronidazole gel in dressings is antibacterial for anaerobes. Silver nitrate and silver sulfadiazine release silver at concentration of 3200 ppm. Most pathogenic organisms are killed in vitro at concentration of 10–40 ppm. The newer nanochemistry technique has produced micro-fine particles which increase silver's solubility and produces silver ions concentration of 70–100 ppm.[34]

Odor Absorbing Dressings

Example: Clinisorb.
These are based on activated charcoal (Fig. 11). They are combined in other dressings for best effect.

Hyaluronic Acid Dressings

Example: Hyalofil.
They are made of biodegradable absorbent biopolymers that form a hydrophilic mesh. They accelerate granulation tissue formation and re-epithelialization. They also help to stabilize clot and attract inflammatory cells.

The latest types in dressings are those containing compounds or drugs. This could be local antiseptics (silver, other antiseptics, honey) and pain relieving drugs such as ibuprofen and morphine. They may be in the form of powders such as nanoflex powder dressings.

Biological Dressings—Skin Grafts

Skin grafts are biological dressings and are of different types:

Pinch and Split-thickness Grafts

Pinch grafts are small (2–3 mm^2) partial thickness skin removed under local anesthesia and placed as islands on venous and arterial ulcers. Split thickness grafts are usually meshed before application for large wounds.

In Vitro Prepared Skin Grafts

The possibility of expanding a small donor site up to 10,000-fold led to the application of cultured keratinocytes for grafting.[35] Autografts and allografts have been used clinically. Cultured epidermal autografts have also been used to treat Epidermolysis bullosa wounds,[36] wound beds of congenital naevi,[37] and chronic leg ulcers,[38] where repeated grafting from passaged cultures is a major advantage. Keratinocytes can also be suspended in fibrin. Use of allografts helps by producing growth factors and matrix proteins. Tissue engineered substitutes of epidermis, dermis or combined epidermis-dermis are available.

Use of bone marrow stem cells is an area of research.

Bandaging

Bandaging is an important component of wound care. Bandaging is particularly important in the setting of leg ulcers and venous ulcers.[39,40] Techniques of bandaging, different types, in different anatomical settings, their advantages and disadvantages are described separately.

WOUND MANAGEMENT IN SPECIAL SITUATIONS IN DERMATOSURGERY

Bleeding Control in Dermatosurgery

Bleeding must be controlled. If required, dermatosurgical wound hemostasis can be achieved by direct pressure, application of a tourniquet or blood pressure cuff inflated 20 mm Hg above the patient's systolic blood pressure, or with the use of topical or subcutaneous epinephrine. Epinephrine-moistened gauze (1:100,000) applied directly over the wound for 10 minutes helps to constrict small blood vessels and decrease the bleeding. Pressure should only be applied for 5 minutes when controlling bleeding over the nose tip, mucosa, penis, and earlobe. Hemostatic gelatin foam can also be used. Large nondigital vessels can be directly visualized and ligated with clamping or a figure-of-8 suture. The digital arteries should never be ligated or clamped, as they run parallel and in very close proximity to the digital nerve, and clamping both is almost inevitable. The blind clamping of any bleeding wound is strongly discouraged. Large extremity tourniquets are rarely needed, but when used they must be properly placed. Cotton gauze should be placed on the limb to provide some protection to the skin, and then an inflatable tourniquet or blood-pressure cuff can be inflated to 20 mm Hg higher than the patient's systolic blood pressure, not to exceed 250 mm Hg, to control distal arterial blood flow. The tourniquet should be inflated for no longer than 20 to 30 minutes, before it is deflated for 5 minutes. Total inflation time should not exceed 1 hour. For digital tourniquets, a stretched Penrose drain can be placed at the base of a previously exsanguinated digit or a commercial rubber ring tourniquet can be applied for a maximum of 30 minutes.

Dressings after Specific Dermatosurgical Procedures

While details can be found in individual chapters, a brief discussion is provided here.

- Minor wounds after excisions: Composite 4-layer dressing after minor surgery may be removed after one day for wound inspection. The edges of the wound have to be palpated to look for induration/swelling and if so, relevant sutures are to be removed and the hematoma evacuated by pressure to prevent infection/dehiscence. This can be followed by secondary suturing and dressing. In case of infection as evidenced by features of inflammation and discharge from the wound, pus culture is appropriate and antibiotics should be started/changed and dressings changed daily. If wound is progressing well, it may be redressed and removed after 7–10 days.
- If the procedure is of minor nature such as a biopsy or electrosurgery, dressing may be dispensed with or done for a day or two. Thereafter, topical antibiotic ointment should be adequate.
- A pressure dressing is required on donor area after procedures such as hair transplant and skin grafting.
- A bimodal dressing for differential pressure is recommended for liposuction.
- Following resurfacing procedures (dermabrasion, laser or radiofrequency), it is preferable to have an open dressing with zinc oxide paste and allow the wound to ooze out, wiping the wound with sterile wipes repeatedly for the first 24–48 hours till oozing stops.
- Pressure sores: Decubitus ulcers are best prevented. This is done by turning or shifting the susceptible patient every 2–3 hours, use of pressure relieving bed such as water air bed and education of relatives. Once ulcer develops, absorbent padding for incontinence, nutritional support, healing by secondary intention or grafting in addition to management of infection are required. Pressure on the ulcer must be avoided at all times.

Adjuvants in Wound Management

Several agents have been promoted as wound healing adjuvants. While evidence may be lacking for many of these agents, they are useful in special situations such as venous ulcers, non-healing leg ulcers, etc.

Pentoxifylline: Pentoxifylline increases fibrinolysis, decreasing blood viscosity, increasing red cell deformability and inhibiting platelet aggregation. The drug is useful in chronic venous leg ulcers.[41]

Prostaglandin E2 and I2, Iloprost and Calcium Channel Blockers such as Nifedipine: These have shown conflicting results in various studies. Some calcium channel blockers may help keratinocyte migration.[42] The serotonin antagonist, ketanserin has been shown to be of benefit when applied topically to diabetic foot and leg ulcers.[43,44]

Ascorbic Acid: High dose ascorbic acid has been beneficial in wound management.[45] It is a cofactor for proline hydroxylase necessary for collagen synthesis.

Zinc: Its precise role in wound healing is unclear at present. It has important antioxidant role in the skin. Systemic zinc is mainly useful in those who are zinc deficient. Topical zinc may be beneficial in wound healing through local actions reducing infection and promoting epithelialization.[46,47]

Oxygen and Nitrous Oxide: Nitric oxide has also been shown to regulate collagen synthesis, cell proliferation and wound contraction.[48] The inducible form (iNOS) is synthesized in the early stages of normal wound healing. Hyperbaric oxygen therapy increases wound nitric oxide levels, which is thought to promote healing of chronic wounds, particularly diabetic foot ulcers.

Vacuum assisted Closure: Negative pressure is used to assist wound closure, particularly deep wounds, chronic leg ulcers and diabetic ulcers.[49,50] Removal of wound fluid helps the process of healing.

Ultrasound: Low-frequency, noncontact ultrasound has been shown to improve wound healing, though this method is still to be completely validated.

Electrical Stimulation of Skin: These promote wound healing by stimulating fibroblast function, increasing transforming growth factor-β (TGF-β) expression and facilitate wound contraction. Pulsed stimulation is better than continuous.

Low Level Laser Therapy: The effect of He-Ne laser on tissue regeneration by monitoring collagen synthesis in wound granulation tissues in Swiss albino mice has been evaluated using analysis of laser induced fluorescence (LIF) and light microscopy techniques. There has been dose dependant increase in wound collagen levels in addition to improvement in other wound healing parameters.[51] Low-level Light Therapy with blue LED light also impacts wound healing.[52]

Photodynamic Therapy: Collagen-based scaffolding material, embedded with a liposomal formulation of metatetra (hydroxyphenyl) chlorin and photodynamic therapy on wound healing in mice has shown rapid improvement.[53]

Extremely Low Frequency Electromagnetic Fields (ELF-EMF): Data analysis supports three main effects of electromagnetic fields on the wound healing pathways: 1) an anti-inflammatory effect, by modulation of cytokine profile that induces the transition of the healing process from a chronic pro-inflammatory to an anti-inflammatory state; 2) a neoangiogenic effect, by increased endothelial cells proliferation and tubulization and production of fibroblast growth factor (FGF)-2; and 3) a re-epithelialization effect by stimulation of collagen formation.[54]

Growth Factors to Augment Wound Healing: The addition of exogenous growth factors in pharmacological amounts may have measurable effects in wound-healing models, but can be disappointing in the clinical arena.[55] Platelet-derived growth factor (PDGF) is the only growth factor which has been found useful clinically in diabetic ulcers.[56] Promising results of the first human gene therapy trial using PDGF have recently been reported.[57] There are recent reports on the role of epidermal growth factor (EGF) in animal models.[58] EGF, IL-1 and TGF-β have also shown encouraging results, though not replicated consistently. More recently, fibroblast growth factor receptor 1 oncogene partner 2 (FGFR1OP2), has been shown to significantly modulate fibroblast-driven wound closure in vitro and in vivo. The dynamic role of cytoskeleton in different experimental models may provide a novel platform for designing the therapeutic target of wound management.[59]

Topical Insulin: Many experiments on animals as well as humans have been performed but the usefulness of insulin in wound healing still remains speculative and safety issues still have to be addressed.

Topical insulin in combination with zinc in animal studies has been shown to heal wounds faster. It regulates wound inflammatory response by stimulating proliferation and migration of macrophages and keratinocytes in adjacent tissues.[34]

Wound Healing Promoters: Substances such as tretinoin, *Aloe vera* extracts, benzoyl peroxide, chamomilla extracts? (promotes granulation, epithelialization, alleviates pain, irritation, astringent, deodorant. Animal studies have proved beneficial effects of chamomilla, being anti-inflammatory/anti-mutagenic. Human studies are lacking/warranted), dexpanthenol (converted to pantothenic acid forming coenzyme A), tetrachlorodecaoxide solution (TCDO combines with hemoglobin, myoglobin and cytochromes releasing molecular oxygen), clostebol acetate (promotes protein synthesis), platelet rich plasma (PRP), topical vitamin E, etc. have been shown to promote healing.

Others: Infrared radiation, UVC radiation, warming devices have been used, though evidence to support their use is not available.

Triage-based Wound Care

Triage is the process of prioritizing patient care based on need and available resources. Clinicians in wound clinics triage daily because time and resources never seem to be sufficient.

Creation of a Wound Care Service

It is important that a wound care service outside of operation theaters is created to reduce load and increase patient accessibility. This kind of a service would be helpful in reducing costs and increasing wound healing rates, being manned by medical and paramedical personnel with a special interest and expertise in this important aspect of care. Specialists may be chosen depending on the major causes of wounds in the specific area, but must include a dermatologist, surgeon and wound care nurse, in addition to support staff. Interdisciplinary management of wounds is the new mantra. Home care wound management using telemedicine has also been possible.[60] In addition, self care taught properly is highly important in the management of wounds such as in leprosy. It is sustainable and can be carried out as part of routine work.

Future of Wound Care

These include tissue engineering techniques like stem cells and gene therapy for achieving wound closure. Stem cells have the ability to migrate to the site of injury or inflammation, participate in regeneration of damaged tissue, stimulate proliferation and differentiation of resident progenitor cells, secreting growth factors, remodeling of matrix, increasing angiogenesis, inhibiting scar formation and improving tensile strength of the wound. Stem cells hold good hope for exploitation in the form of gene transfer.[61-65]

CONCLUSION[2]

- A moist wound bed is needed for all stages of wound healing.
- Wound healing is affected by many factors: age, vascular state, nutritional state, comorbidity, some drug therapy, debris and infection.

- A systematic assessment of the wound is essential to evaluate healing and treatment efficacy.
- Regular wound reassessments are required.
- Infection control guidelines should be followed in the management of all wounds. Tetanus prophylaxis may be needed in contaminated wounds.
- Potable tap water may be used to wash and cleanse most chronic wounds.
- Cleansing solutions should be at body temperature to prevent wound cooling.
- There is insufficient evidence to determine if one type of dressing is superior to another.
- Clinical infection should be treated with systemic antibiotics, not topical antimicrobials.
- Routine wound swabs are not recommended.
- Topical antimicrobial dressings, where used, should be for short-term use only.
- The frequency of dressing changes, type and location of wound and patient acceptability, including impact on comfort and odor control are important factors in the choice of dressing for a particular wound.
- In the treatment of wounds, the new trend in the wound device market is to produce dressings containing compounds or drugs. This could be local antiseptics (silver, other antiseptics, honey) and pain relieving drugs such as ibuprofen and morphine. New treatments such as antitumor necrosis factor-alpha and *Lactobacillus plantarum* cultures have also been successfully used in hard to heal, atypical wounds. Knowledge of influencing factors such as smoking and biofilms on the healing process has also improved. Smoking results in delayed healing and increased risk of postoperative infection, whereas the role of biofilm is being debated, with thoughts on them delaying wound healing. Organizing models for optimal wound management are constantly being developed and refined.[66]

REFERENCES

1. Bennett RG.Fundamentals of cutaneous surgery. 1st ed. St Louis, MO: CV Mosby; 1988. P 778.
2. NHSSB Wound Management Manual. (2005). [online] Accessed from http://www.nhssb.n-i.nhs.uk/publi-cations/primary_care/Wound_Manual.pdf [Accessed in February 2012].
3. WHO Guidelines on Wound Management: Best practice guidelines in disaster situations. [online] Accessed from http://www.who.int/surgery/publica¬tions/Wound Management. pdf [Accessed in Febuary 2012].
4. Falanga V. Classifications for wound bed preparation and stimulation of chronic wounds. Wound Repair Regen. 2000;8:347-52.
5. Schultz G, Sibbald RG, Falanga V, et al. Wound bed preparation: a systematic approach to wound management. Wound Repair Regen. 2003;11:S1-28.
6. Singer AJ, Quinn JV, Thode HC Jr, et al. Determinants of poor outcome after laceration and surgical incision repair. Plast Reconstr Surg. 2002;110:429-35.
7. Howell JM. Current and future trends in wound healing. Emerg Med Clin North Am. 1992;10:655-63.
8. Marks JG Jr, Cano C, Leitzel K, et al. Inhibition of wound healing by topical steroids. J Dermatol Surg Oncol. 1983;9:819-21.
9. Petrosillo N. Natural products and wound management: a never-ending story. Clin Infect Dis. 2008;47:730-1.
10. Greenfield G, Johnston B. Wound Management. [online] Accessed from http://www.docstoc.com/docs/76010789/ Wound-Management [Accessed in February 2012].
11. Pronchik D, Barber C, Rittenhouse S. Low-versus high-pressure irrigation techniques in Staphylococcus aureus-inoculated wounds. Am J Emergency Med. 1999;17:121-4.
12. Fernandez R, Griffiths R. Water for wound cleansing. Cochrane Database Syst Rev. 2008;23:CD003861.
13. Kramer SA. Effect of povidone-iodine on wound healing: a review. J Vasc Nurs. 1999;17:17-23.
14. Eming SA, Smola-Hess S, Kurschat P, et al. A novel property of povidon-iodine: inhibition of excessive protease levels in chronic non-healing wounds. J Invest Dermatol. 2006;126:2731-3.
15. Brennan SS, Leaper DJ. The effect of antiseptics on the healing wound: a study using the rabbit ear chamber. Br J Surg. 1985;72:780-2.
16. Lineweaver W, Howard R, Soucy D, et al. Topical antimicrobial toxicity. Arch Surg. 1985;120:267-70.
17. Geronomus RG, Mertz PM, Eaglstein W. Wound healing: the effects of topical antimicrobial agents. Arch Dermatol. 1979;115:1311-4.
18. Robinson JK. Surgery of the Skin: Procedural Dermatology, 2e p 120.
19. Molan PC. Re-introducing honey in the management of wounds and ulcers—theory and practice. Ostomy Wound Manage. 2002;48:28-40.
20. Blaser G, Santos K, Bode U, et al. Effect of medical honey on wounds colonized or infected with MRSA. J Wound Care. 2007;16:325-8.
21. Chirife J, Herszage L, Joseph A. Microbiological basis for the use of sugar in treating infected wounds. Antimicrob Agents Chemother. 1983;23:766-73.
22. Martin C. Recent Developments in Wound Management: intelligent biomaterials to novel anti¬microbials. 24 September 2009, London, UK. IDrugs. 2009;12:695-8.
23. García-Gubern CF, Colon-Rolon L, Bond MC. Essential Concepts of wound management. Emerg Med Clin N Am. 2010;28:951-67.
24. Karaduman S, Yuruktumen A, Guryay SM, et al. Modified hair apposition technique as the primary closure method for scalp lacerations. Am J Emerg Med. 2009;27:1050-5.
25. 2-Octyl Cyanoacrylate Wound adhesives. [online] Accessed from http://emedicine.medscape.com/article/874047-overview#showall [Accessed in Febuary 2012].
26. Mekkes JR, Zeegelaar JE, Westerhof W. Quantitative and objective evaluation of wound debriding properties of collagenase and fibrinolysin/desoxyribonuclease in a necrotic ulcer animal model. Arch Dermatol Res. 1998;290:152-7.
27. Mekkes JR, Le Poole IC, Das PK, et al. In vitro tissue-digesting properties of krill enzymes compared with fibrinolysin/DNAse, papain and placebo. Int J Biochem Cell Biol. 1997;29:703-6.
28. Klein MB, Hunter S, Heimbach DM, et al. The versajet water dissection: A new tool for tangential excision. J Burn Care Rehabil 2007;26:483-7

29. Reames MK. The use of maggots in wound debridement. Ann Plast Surg. 1988;21:388-91.
30. Mumcuoglu KY. Clinical applications for maggots in wound care. Am J Clin Dermatol. 2001;2:219-27.
31. Winter GD, Scales JT. Effect of air drying and dressings on the surface of a wound. Nature. 1963;197:91-2.
32. Hutchinson JJ. Prevalence of wound infection under occlusive dressings: a collective survey of reported research. Wounds. 1990;1:23-33.
33. O'Toole EA, Mellerio JE. Wound healing. In: Burns DA, Breathnach SM, Cox N, Griffiths C, (Eds). Rook's Textbook of Dermatology, 8th edition, Oxford: Wiley-Blackwell; 2010;1419-27
34. Sujata Sarabahi. Recent advances in topical wound care. Indian Journal of Plastic Surgery May-August 2012;45: 379-87.
35. Green H, Kehinde O, Thomas J. Growth of cultured human epidermal cells into multiple epithelia suitable for grafting. Proc Natl Acad Sci USA. 1979;76:5665-8.
36. Collin B, Balderson D, Papini R, et al. Cultured autologous keratinocyte grafting of chronic erosions in three patients with epidermolysis bullosa. Clin Exp Dermatol. 2006;31:718-9.
37. Gallico GG, O'Connor NE, Compton CC, et al. Cultured epithelial autografts for giant congenital naevi. Plast Reconstr Surg. 1989;84:1-9.
38. Limova M, Mauro T. Treatment of leg ulcers with cultured epithelial autografts: clinical study and case reports. Osteotomy Wound Manage. 1995;41:54-60.
39. Hendricks WM, Swallow RT. Management of stasis ulcers with Unna's boots versus elastic support stockings. J Am Acad Dermatol. 1985;12:90-8.
40. Gohel MS, Barwell JR, Tayler M, et al. Long term results of compression therapy alone versus compression plus surgery in chronic venous ulceration (ESCHAR): randomized controlled trial. BMJ. 2007;335:83-7.
41. Jull A, Arroll B, Parag V, et al. Pentoxifylline for treating venous leg ulcers. Cochrane Database Syst Rev. 2007;3:CD001733.
42. Trollinger DR, Isseroff RR, Nuccitelli R. Calcium-channel blockers inhibit galvanotaxis in human keratinocytes. J Cell Physiol. 2002;193:1-9.
43. Martínez-de Jesús FR, Morales-Guzmán M, Castáeda M, et al. Randomized single-blind trial of topical ketanserin for healing acceleration of diabetic foot ulcers. Arch Med Res. 1997;28:95-9.
44. Quatresooz P, Kharfi M, Paquet P, et al. Healing effect of ketanserin on chronic leg ulcers in patients with diabetes. J Eur Acad Dermatol Venereol. 2006;20:277-81.
45. Taylor TV, Rimmer S, Day B. Ascorbic acid supplementation in pressure sores. Lancet. 1974;2:544-6.
46. Stromberg HE, Agren MS. Topical zinc oxide treatment improves arterial and venous leg ulcers. Br J Dermatol. 1984;111:461-8.
47. Rostan EF, DeBuys HV, Madey DL, et al. Evidence supporting zinc as an important antioxidant for skin. Int J Dermatol. 2002;41:606-11.
48. Sen CK, Khanna S, Gordillo G, et al. Oxygen, oxidants, and antioxidants in wound healing: an emerging paradigm. Ann NY Acad Sci. 2002;957:239-49.
49. Eginton MT, Brown KR, Seabrook GR, et al. A prospective randomized evaluation of negative-pressure wound dressings for diabetic foot wounds. Ann Vasc Surg. 2003;17:645-9.
50. Vuerstaek JDD, Vainas T, Wuite J, et al. State-of-the-art treatment of chronic leg ulcers: a randomized controlled trial comparing vacuum-asssisted closure (V.A.C.) with modern wound dressings. J Vasc Surg. 2006;44:1029-38
51. Prabhu V, Rao SB, Chandra S, et al. Spectroscopic and histological evaluation of wound healing progression following Low Level Laser Therapy (LLLT). J Biophotonics. 2012;5:168 84.
52. Adamskaya N, Dungel P, Mittermayr R, et al. Light therapy by blue LED improves wound healing in an excision model in rats. Injury. 2011;42:917-21.
53. Garrier J, Bezdetnaya L, Barlier C, et al. Foslip®-based photodynamic therapy as a means to improve wound healing. Photodiagnosis Photodyn Ther. 2011;8:321-7.
54. Costin GE, Birlea SA, Norris DA. Trends in wound repair: cellular and molecular basis of regenerative therapy using electromagnetic fields. Curr Mol Med. 2012;12:14-26.
55. Braund R, Hook S, Medlicott NJ. The role of topical growth factors in chronic wounds. Curr Drug Deliv. 2007;4:195-204.
56. Wieman TJ, Smiell JM, Su Y. Efficacy and safety of a topical gel formulation of recombinant platelet-derived growth factor-BB (becaplermin) in patients with chronic neuropathic diabetic ulcers: a phase III randomized placebo-controlled double-blind study. Diabetes Care. 1998;21:822-7.
57. Margolis D, Crombleholme T, Thom S, et al. Phase I gene transfer study of H5.020CMV.PDGF-b in venous leg ulcer. J Invest Derm. 2007;127:S55.
58. Kalay Z, Cevher SC. Oxidant and antioxidant events during epidermal growth factor therapy to cutaneous wound healing in rats. Int Wound J. 2011.
59. Lin A, Hokugo A, Nishimura I. Wound closure and wound management: A new therapeutic molecular target. Cell Adh Migr. 2010;4:396-9.
60. Terry M, Halstead LS, O'Hare P, et al. Feasibility study of home care wound management using telemedicine. Adv Skin Wound Care. 2009;22:358-64.
61. Hanson SE, Bentz ML, Hematti P. Mesenchymal stem cell therapy for nonhealing cutaneous wounds.Plast Reconstr Surg 2010;125:510-16.
62. Cha J, Falanga V. Stem cells in cutaneous wound healing. Clin Dermatol 2007;25:73-8.
63. Langer R. Biomaterials in drug delivery and tissue engineering: onelaboratory's experience. Acc Chem Res 2000;33;94-101.
64. Korbling M, EstronZ. Adult stem cells for tissue repair –a new therapeutic concept? N Eng J Med 2003;349:570-82.
65. Eming SA, Kreig T, Davidson JM. Gene therapy and wound healing. Clin Dermatol 2007;25:79-92.
66. Gottrup F, Jørgensen B, Karlsmark T. News in wound healing and management. Curr Opin Support Palliat Care. 2009;3:300-4.

Chapter 6

Bandages in Dermatosurgery

Umashankar Nagaraju

Key Messages 

- Bandage should be used only to hold in place the primary dressing which covers a wound.
- It should not be applied, so tightly that it stops circulation or so loosely that it allows the dressing to slip.
- Bandages are terminated by applying several overlying circular turns and fastening the ends securely.
- Compression bandage reduce effect of venous hypertension by reducing superficial venous pressure.

A bandage is primarily used to hold the dressing in place over a wound to create pressure over a bleeding wound for control of hemorrhage, to provide immobilization after a graft, and to provide support to surgery area. A dermatosurgeon needs to be familiar with different types of bandages, particularly in surgeries such as vitiligo surgery, hair transplantation, liposuction, etc. In particular, surgeries are performed for vitiligo lesions in different parts of the body and need proper immobilization for proper draft take.

Bandaging the wound is an art; the human body parts differ in shape and are capable of a wide range of movements due to joints. Due to variety of shapes and movements, there can be no universal bandaging technique. Following body shapes should be considered while selecting bandaging technique:

- Body shapes with blunt ends such as fingers, hands, forefoot, or head.
- Body parts with a tapered shape such as an arm, leg or trunk, where the circumference of the body part either increases or decreases.
- Joints which allow a hinge movement, such as the knee, elbow and ankle.
- Body parts with an almost constant circumference, such as the midfoot, middle of the hand, ankle and wrist.

GENERAL PRINCIPLES OF BANDAGING

- Bandage should be used only to hold in place the dressing which covers a wound.
- It should never be applied directly over a wound.
- A bandage should be applied firmly and fastened securely. It should not be applied so tightly that it stops circulation or so loosely that it allows the dressing to slip.

BANDAGE TECHNIQUES

There are four basic techniques with which nearly all parts of the body can be bandaged. These include **(A) triangular and cravat bandages, (B) roller bandages, (C) tailed bandages and (D) special bandages**.

Triangular and Cravat Bandages

These are easy to apply, quick and stay well. Hence, they are valuable in dermatosurgeries to place temporary bandages till the completion of surgery, e.g. to cover the donor sites in vitiligo surgeries or hair tranplantation. A square of sterile gauze material about 3 feet × 3 feet, or slightly more, is folded diagonally. The long side of the triangle is called the 'base', the point opposite the base is called the 'apex', and the points at each end of the base are called the 'ends'. This bandage may be used either as a triangle or as a cravat. Cravat (term derived from neck kerchief worn by boy scouts) is made from the triangle by bringing the apex to the base and folding it upon itself a sufficient number of times to obtain the desired width (Fig. 1).

Triangle of Forehead or Scalp (Fronto-occipital) (Figs. 2A to C)

This is used to hold dressings on the forehead or scalp.

a. Place middle of base of triangle so that edge is just above the eyebrows and bring apex backward, allowing it to drop over back of head (occiput). Bring ends of triangle backward above ears.
b. Cross ends over apex at occiput, carry ends around forehead, and tie them in a square knot.

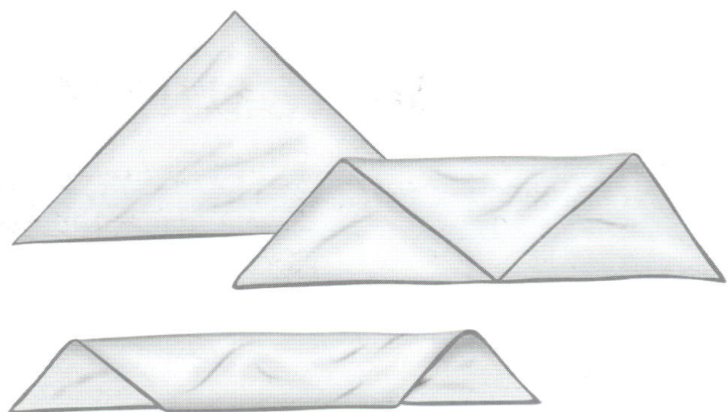

Fig. 1: Triangular and cravat bandages.

c. Turn up apex of bandage toward top of head. Tuck in behind crossed part of bandage.

Triangle of Chest or Back (Figs. 3A to C)

This bandage is used to hold dressings on burns or wounds of chest or back.

a. Drop apex of triangle over shoulder on injured side. Bring bandage down over chest (or back) to cover dressing, so that middle of base of bandage is directly below injury. Turn up a cuff at base.
b. Carry ends around and tie in a square knot, leaving one end longer than the other.
c. Bring apex down and tie to long end of first knot.

Triangle of Shoulder (Figs. 4A to D)

The triangle of the shoulder is used to hold dressings on wounds of the shoulder. Two bandages are required, one a triangle and the other a cravat or roller bandage.

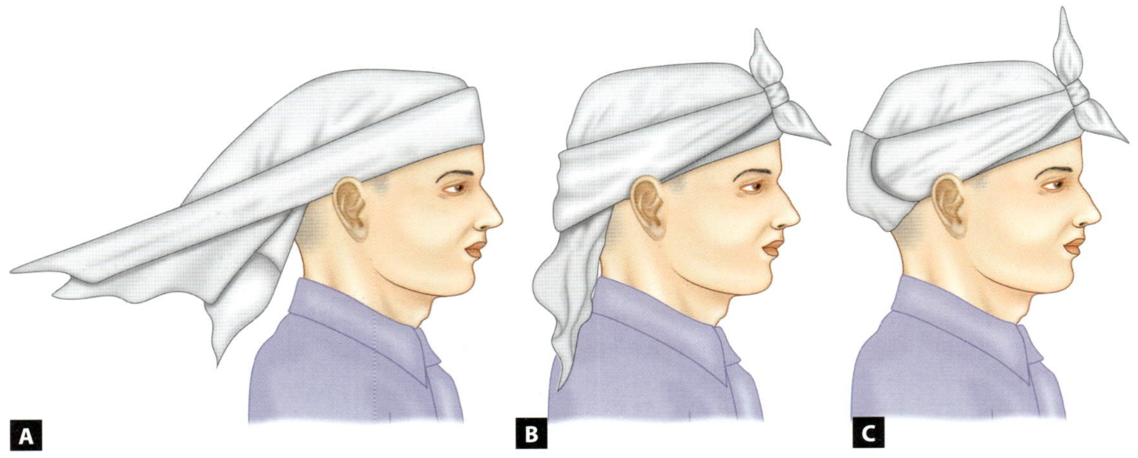

Figs. 2A to C: Triangle of forehead or scalp.

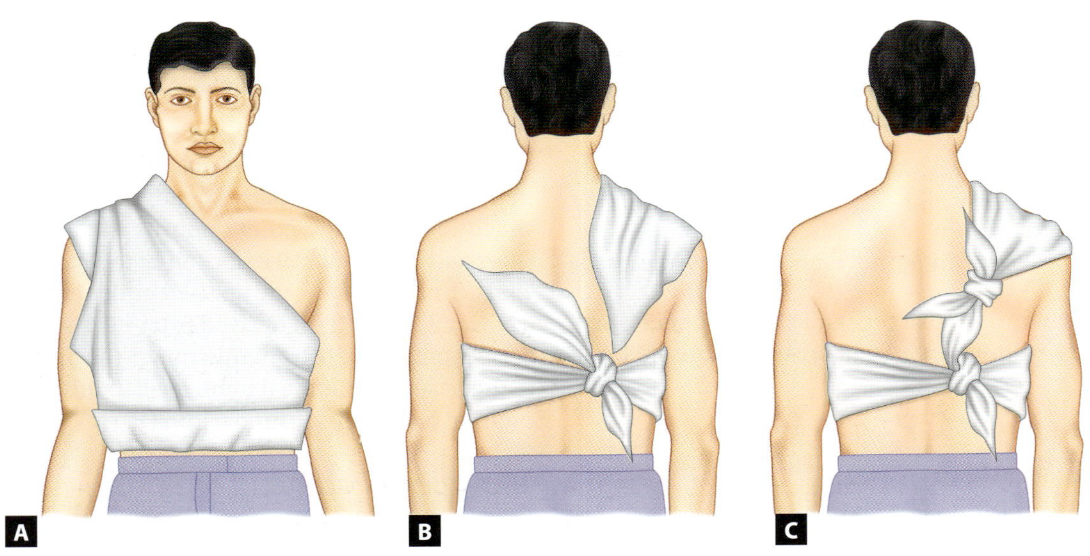

Figs. 3A to C: Triangle of chest bandage.

a. Place center of cravat or roller bandage at base of neck on injured side, and fasten just forward of opposite armpit.
b. Slide apex of open triangle under cravat at base of neck and place over dressing on injured shoulder and upper arm. Turn up cuff at base.
c. Bring ends around arm and tie.
d. Secure apex to cravat at neck by fastening with adhesive tape.

Triangle of Hip (Figs. 5A to C)

The triangle of the hip is used to hold dressings on the buttock or hip. It requires two bandages, one a triangle and the other a cravat or roller bandage.
a. Fasten cravat or roller bandage around waist.
b. Place base of triangle below buttock (gluteofemoral fold) and slide apex under cravat at waist. Fold base upward to form cuff and carry ends of base around thigh.
c. Tie ends of base with square knot. Fasten apex to waist cravat by an adhesive tape.

Triangle of Foot (Figs. 6A to E)

Triangle of foot is used to hold dressings of considerable size on the foot.
a. Center foot upon bandage at right angles to base, with heel well forward of base.
b. Carry apex of triangle over toes to ankle, and tuck excess fullness of bandage into small pleats on each side of foot.
c. Cross each half of bandage toward opposite side of ankle.
d. Bring ends of triangle around ankle.
e. Tie ends in square knot.

Triangle of Hand (Figs. 7A to E)

The triangle of the hand is used to hold dressings of considerable size on the hand.
a. Place middle of base of triangle well up on palmar surface of wrist.

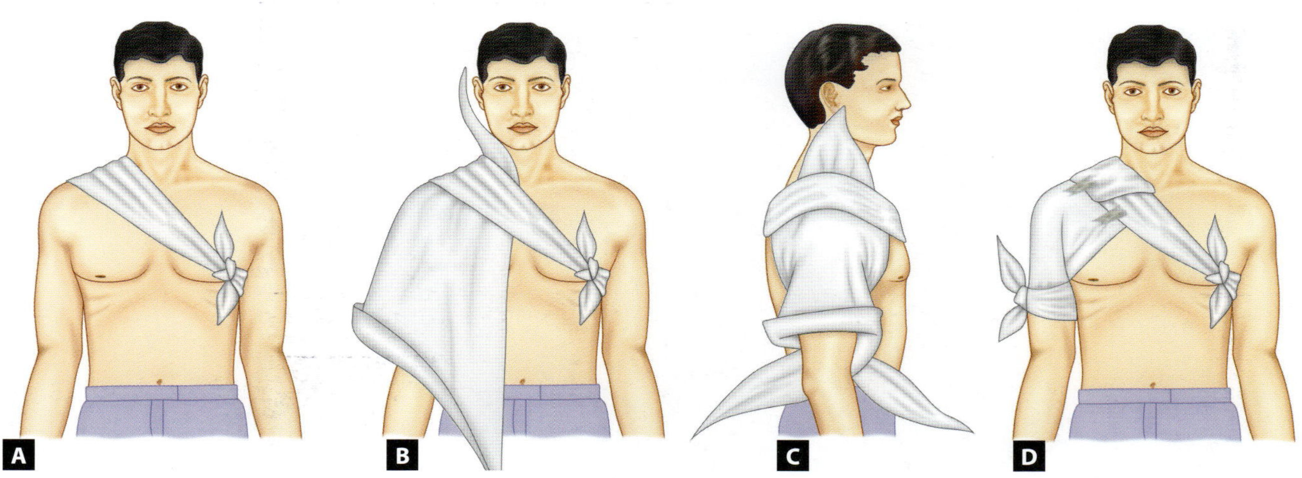

Figs. 4A to D: Triangle of shoulder bandage.

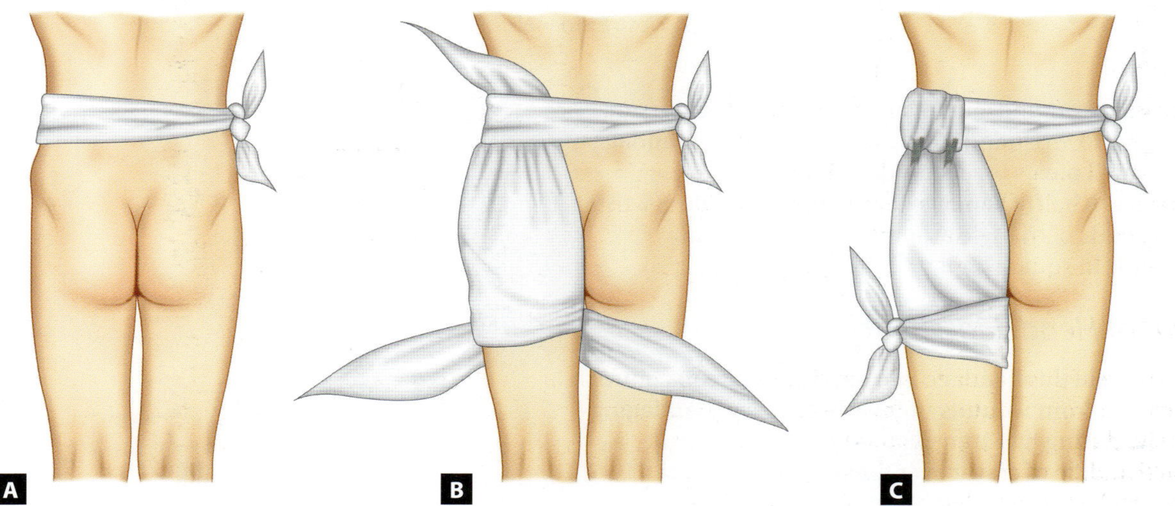

Figs. 5A to C: Triangle of hip bandage.

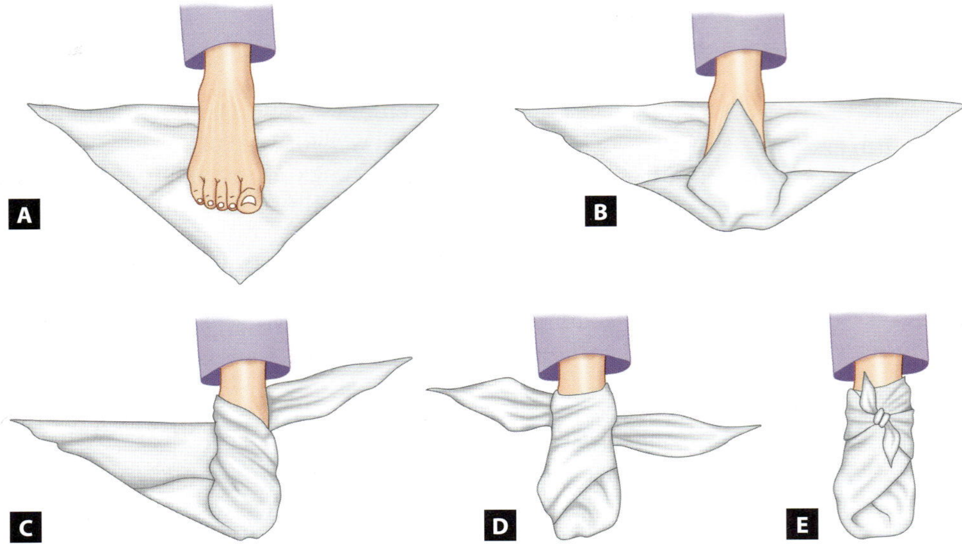

Figs. 6A to E: Triangle of foot bandage.

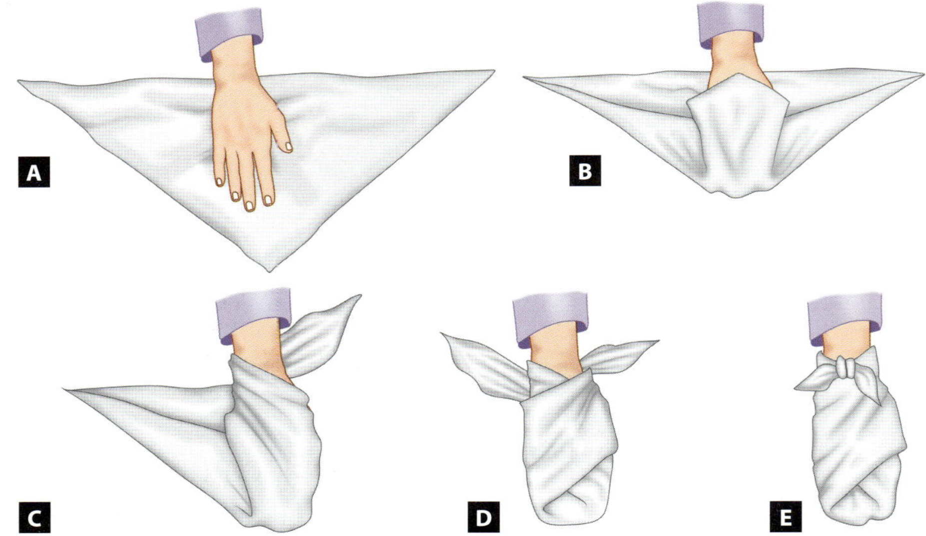

Figs. 7A to E: Triangle of hand.

b. Carry apex around ends of fingers. Cover back (dorsum) of hand to wrist and tuck excess fullness of bandage into small pleats on each side of hand.
c. Cross each half of bandage toward opposite side of wrist.
d. Bring ends of triangle around wrist.
e. Tie ends in square knot.

Cravat of Head (Figs. 8A to C)

The purpose of this bandage is to apply pressure to control hemorrhage from wounds of lower scalp, e.g. bandaging donor site during hair transplantation.

a. Place middle of cravat over dressing.
b. Pass each end completely around head.
c. Tie in square knot.

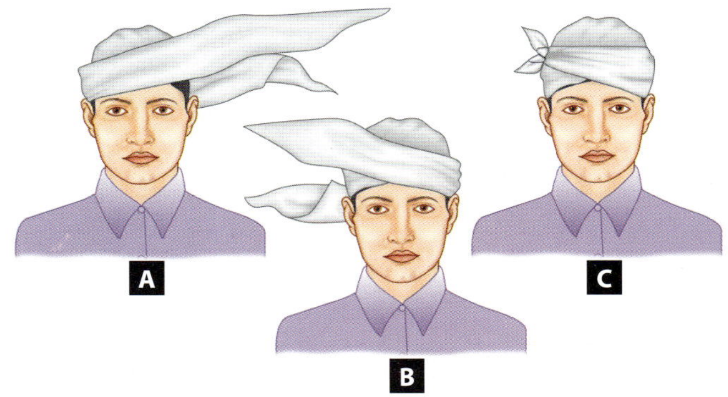

Figs. 8A to C: Cravat of head.

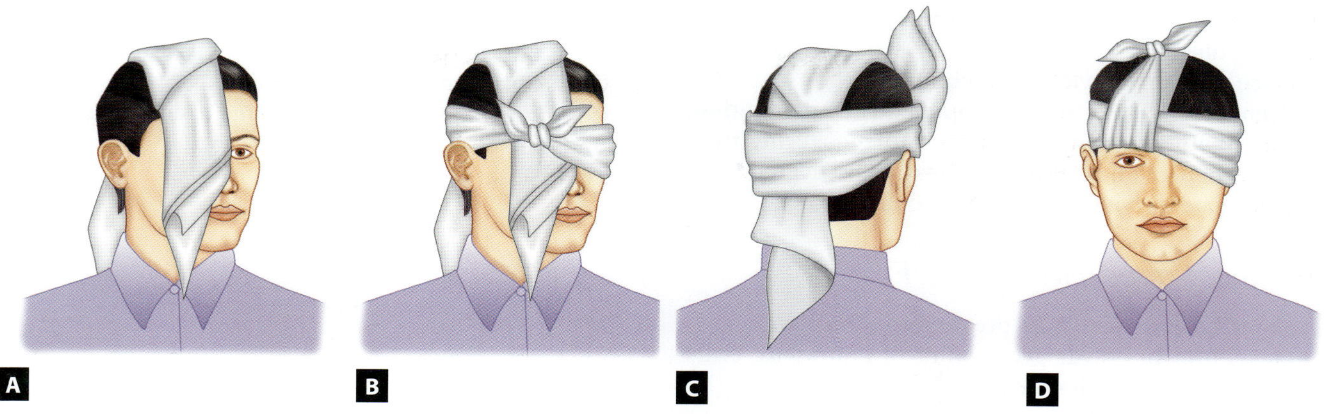

Figs. 9A to D: Cravat bandage of eye.

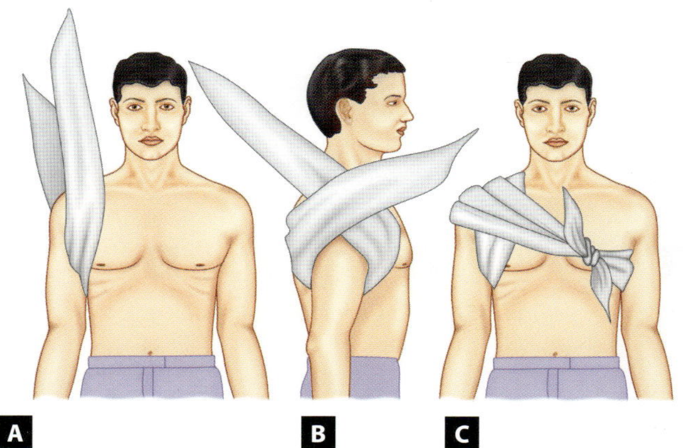

Figs. 10A to C: Shoulder-armpit cravat.

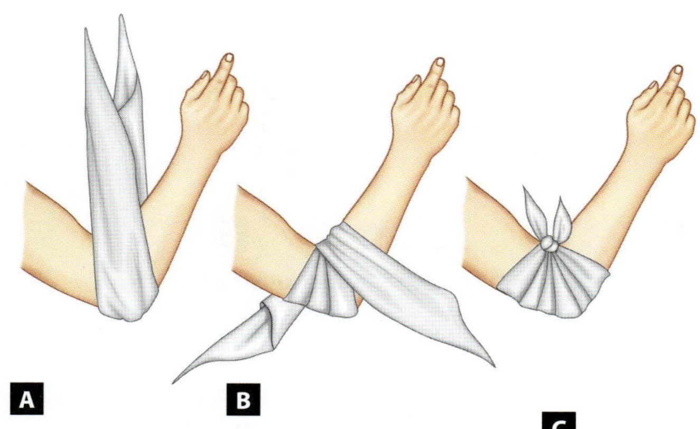

Figs. 11A to C: Cravat of elbow.

Cravat Bandage of Eye (Figs. 9A to D)

The cravat bandage of the eye is used to hold a dressing over the eye, e.g. following ptosis surgery. Two cravats are required.

a. Lay center of first cravat over top of head with the front end falling over uninjured eye.
b. Bring second cravat around head, over eyes and over loose ends of first cravat. Tie in front.
c. Bring ends of first cravat back over top of head, tying there and pulling second cravat up and away from uninjured eye.

Shoulder-Armpit Cravat (Figs. 10A to C)

The shoulder-armpit cravat (bisaxillary) is used to hold dressings in the axilla or on the shoulder.

a. Place cravat over dressing in axilla so the front end is longer than the back. Carry the ends upwards.
b. Bring ends across each other over top of shoulder.
c. Cross ends over back and chest respectively to opposite axilla. Tie ends just in front of uninjured axilla.

Cravat of Elbow (Figs. 11A to C)

The cravat of the elbow is used to hold dressings around the elbow.

a. Bend arm at elbow and place center of cravat at point of elbow (olecranon).
b. Bring ends up and across each other in overlapping spiral turns. Continue one end up arm and the other end down forearm.
c. Bring ends to front of elbow (antecubital fossa) and tie.

Cravat of Knee (Figs. 12A to C)

The cravat of the knee is used to hold dressings around the knee.

a. Place center of cravat over knee cap and let ends hang down each side of knee.
b. Cross ends underneath and continue several overlapping descending turns down calf and several overlapping ascending turns up thigh.
c. Bring ends together and tie under knee.

Cravat of Leg (Figs. 13A to C)

The cravat of the leg is used to hold dressings on the leg, e.g. in leg ulcers

a. Place center of cravat over dressing.
b. Begin ascending turns with upper end and descending turns with lower end, with each turn covering two-thirds of preceding turn until dressing is covered.
c. Terminate by tying both ends in square knot.

Cravat of Palms (Figs. 14A to F)

This bandage is used to hold dressings on the palm.

a. Lay center of cravat over center of palm with ends hanging down each side.
b. Bring the thumb end across back of hand, over palm and through hollow between thumb and palm.
c. Bring the other end across back of hand, toward base of thumb and obliquely across palm to base of little finger.
d. Cross both ends at back of hand.
e. Continue procedure, ends crossing first at back of hand and then over palm.
f. Tie in square knot at wrist.

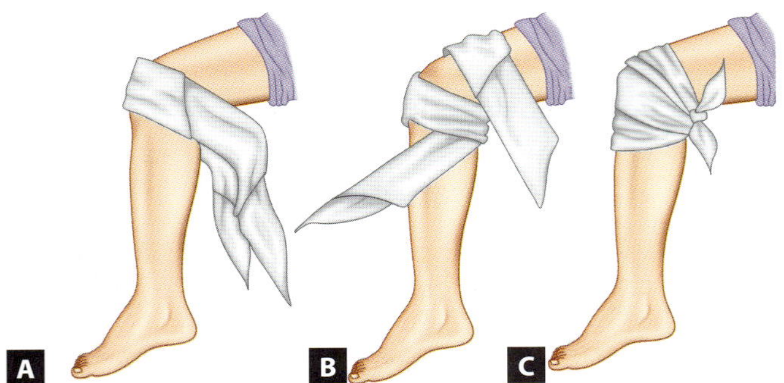

Figs. 12A to C: Cravat of knee bandage.

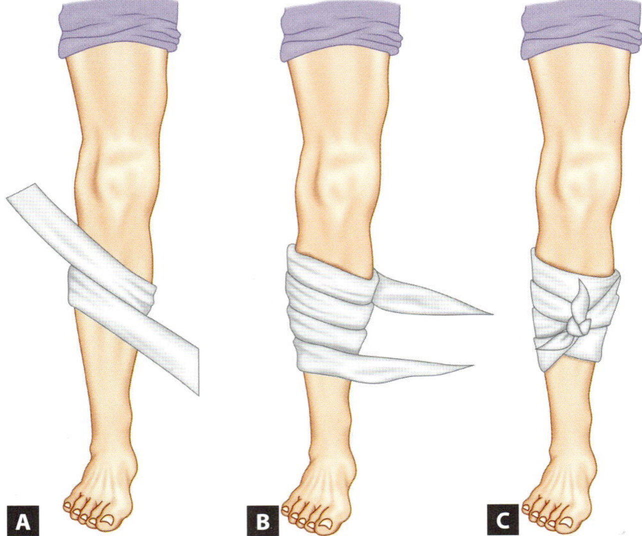

Figs. 13A to C: Cravat bandage of leg.

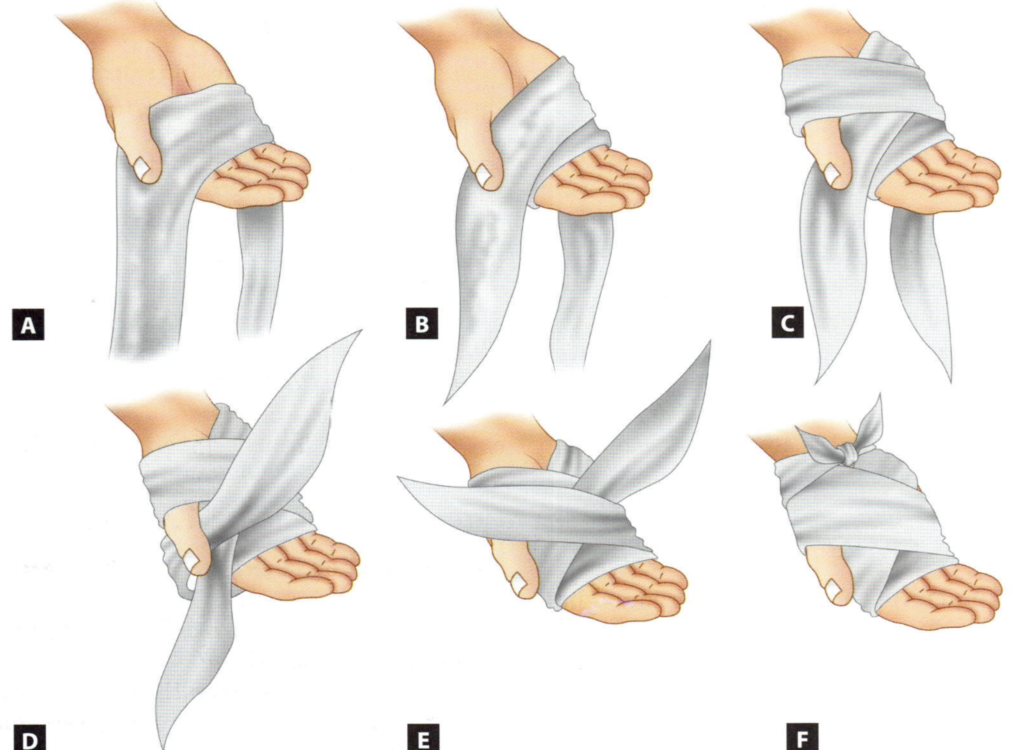

Figs. 14A to F: Cravat bandage of palm.

Roller Bandages

The roller bandages are used to hold dressings in place, to support surgery site and to create pressure for control of hemorrhage. Roller bandages are made from gauze, flannel, muslin, rubber or elastic webbing, the width and length depending upon the part to be bandaged.

Sizes Recommended (Fig. 15)

The sizes most frequently used are 2 inches width and 6 yards long for hand, finger, toe and head bandages; 3 inches wide and 10 yards long for extremities; and 4 inches wide and 10 yards long for thigh, groin, and trunk.

For convenience and ease of application, the strip of material is rolled into the form of a cylinder. Each bandage of this type should consist of only one piece, free from wrinkles, seams, selvage and any imperfections that may cause discomfort to the patient.

Applying the Roller Bandage

When a roller bandage is to be applied to a part, the roll should be held in the right hand so that the loose end is on the bottom.

The outside surface of the loose end is next applied to the part and held there with the left hand. The roll is then passed around the part by the right hand, which controls the tension and direction of the bandage. Two or three of the initial turns of a roller bandage should overlie each other to secure the bandage. In applying the bandage, it is often necessary to transfer the roll from one hand to the other.

Precautions to be taken while applying roller bandages:

- Roller bandages should be applied evenly, firmly and not too tightly. Excessive or uneven pressure will interfere with the circulation.
- In bandaging an arm or leg, the entire extremity (except the fingers or toes) should be covered to maintain uniform pressure. The fingers or toes should be left exposed so the circulation in these parts can be checked.
- An extremity should be bandaged in its final position, since bending will change the pressure of parts of the bandage.
- It is safer to use a large number of turns rather than a few too firmly applied turns to secure splints or dressings. This is particularly important in applying a wet bandage, or one that may become wet while securing a wet dressing.
- Bandage turns should overlap to completely cover the skin, since any uncovered skin may be pinched between turns. To prevent chafing and irritation when two parts are bandaged together, skin surfaces should be separated by absorbent material.

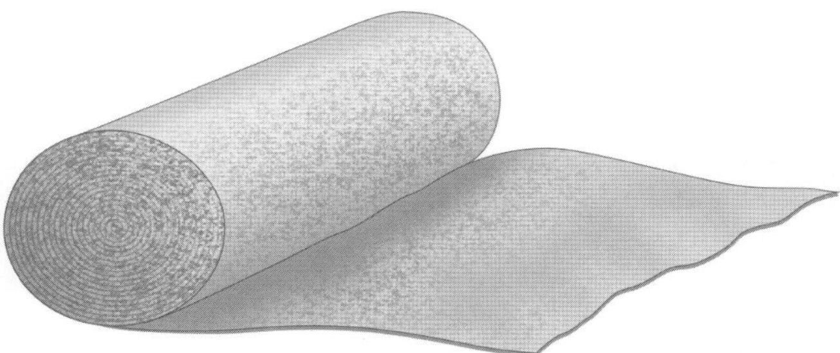

Fig. 15: Roller bandage.

Fastening the Bandage

Bandages are terminated by applying several overlying circular turns and fastening the ends securely. The ends may be tied or fastened with adhesive tape. Two methods of tying are (Figs. 16A to C):

a. The end of the bandage is folded back upon itself to form two ends which can be tied.
b. The end of the bandage is split lengthwise for a suitable distance and the split ends are then brought around in opposite directions and tied.
c. The square knot is the best type of knot for tying bandages. It holds firmly and can be easily unfastened.

Removing the Bandage

Bandage scissors are preferable when the bandage is to be removed by cutting. Interference with the underlying dressing and wound should be carefully avoided. Folds should be gathered up when the bandage is merely unwound.

Types of Roller Bandages Based on Site of Application

Circular Bandage (Fig. 17)

A circular bandage is used to cover cylindrical parts and to anchor bandages. As illustrated in Figure 17, a turn is made around the part and anchored. Similar succeeding turns are made, overlying each other completely. The bandage is then terminated and secured.

Spiral Bandage (Figs. 18A to C)

Spiral bandage covers a larger area than that covered by the circular bandage. It can be applied to the arm as well as to other cylindrical parts.

a. Anchor at wrist.
b. Apply succeeding spiral turns up the forearm, with each turn overlapping one-third of preceding turn.
c. Terminate and secure just below elbow.

Recurrent Bandage of Head with One Bandage (Figs. 19A to D)

This bandage is used to hold a dressing on the scalp.

a. Anchor bandage with several turns around the head, terminating behind head. At this point fold bandage upward, with assistant holding fold in place with two fingers.

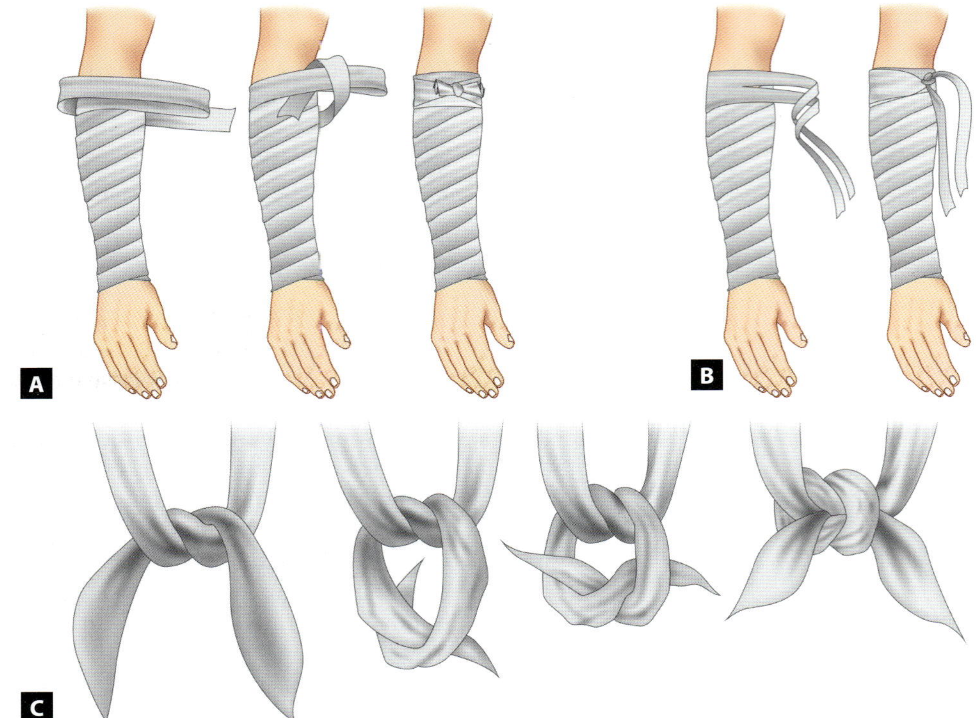

Figs. 16A to C: Fastening the bandage.

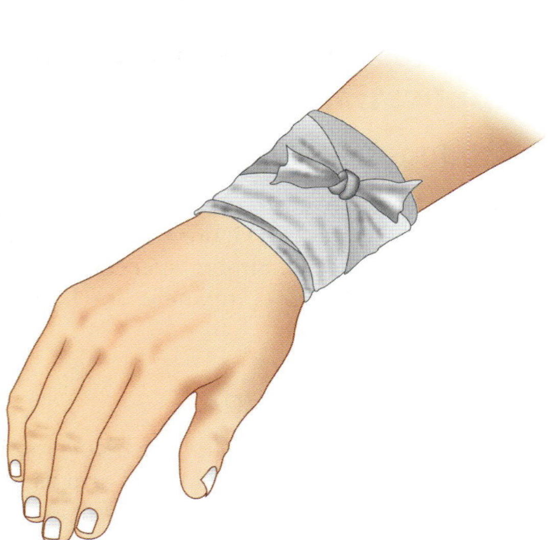

Fig. 17: Circular bandage.

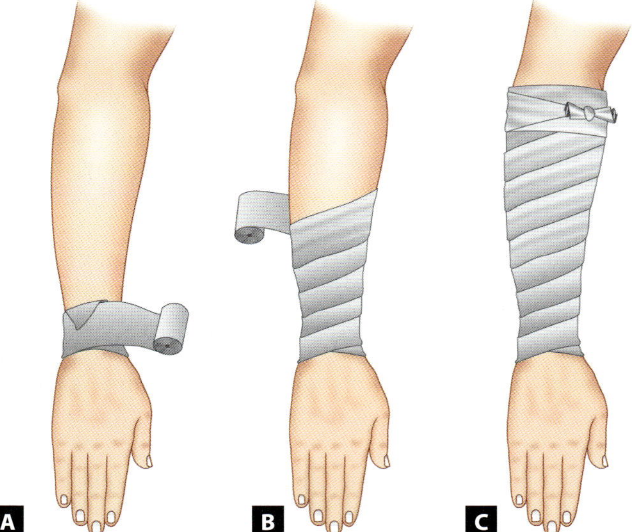

Figs. 18A to C: Spiral bandage.

b. Continue bandage over top of head to center of forehead. Fold bandage back at this point and hold it there with free hand. Carry bandage back to point held by assistant at rear of head.
c. Continue procedure until entire head is covered, turns alternating to the left and right of the center line and each turn overlying the outer half of the preceding turn.
d. Apply several circular turns around head, covering the ends of the initial turns, and secure.

Shoulder Bandage (Figs. 20A to D)

Shoulder bandage is used to retain dressings of the shoulder and axilla, e.g. following surgery for hidradenitis suppurativa.

a. Pad the axilla well and anchor by several circular turns around upper arm where surgery is performed.
b. Carry across back to axilla of opposite side; then across chest obliquely to top of primary turns.

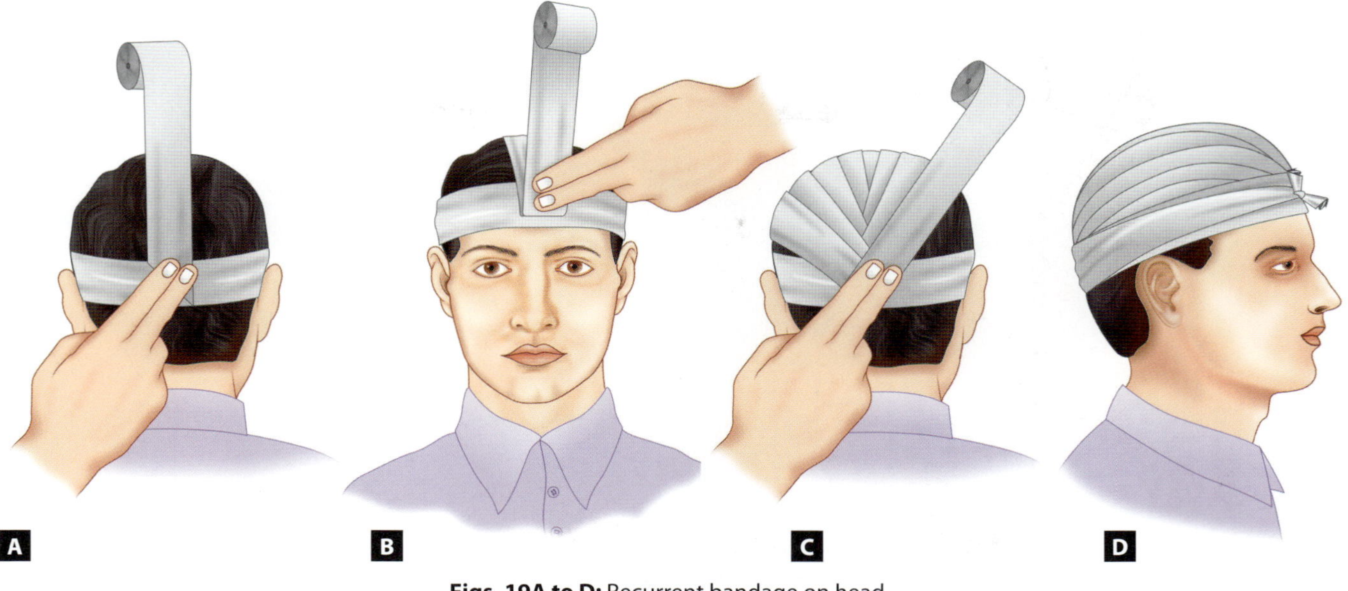

Figs. 19A to D: Recurrent bandage on head.

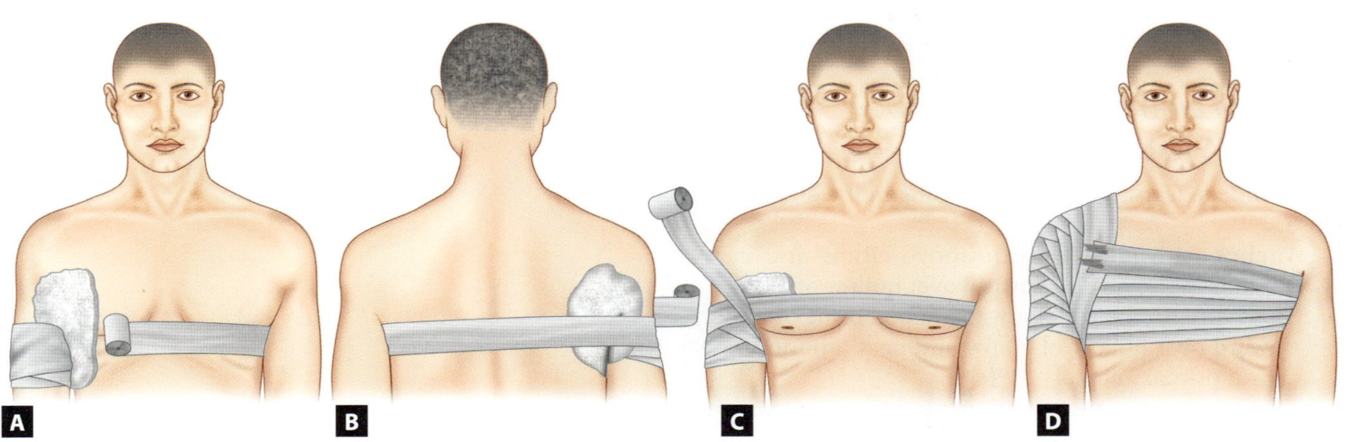

Figs. 20A to D: Shoulder bandage.

c. Carry around arm, axilla, and upward toward shoulder. Repeat procedure, each turn overlying about two-thirds of preceding turn.
d. Continue until entire shoulder is covered. The line crossings on the shoulder be straight and should pass over the point of the shoulder. Secure with adhesive tape.

Figure of Eight Bandage for Hand (Fig. 21)

This bandage is used to hold dressings on dorsum of hand or palm, e.g. flap rotation or tendon transfer.

a. Anchor bandage on hand with circular turns near ends of fingers. Carry obliquely across back of hand to thumb. Bring under thumb and across palm to back of hand.
b. Carry obliquely across back of hand to bottom of primary turn and across palm.
c. Follow with several similar turns, each one overlying about two-thirds of preceding turn on back of hand. After sufficient turns, terminate with circular turns around wrist and secure.

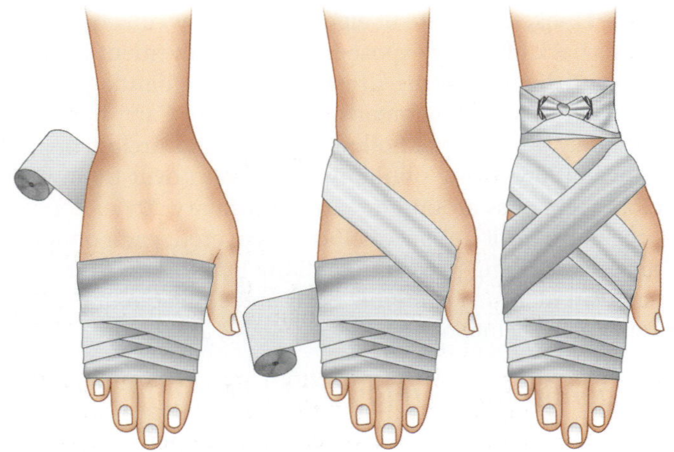

Fig. 21: Figure of eight bandage of hand.

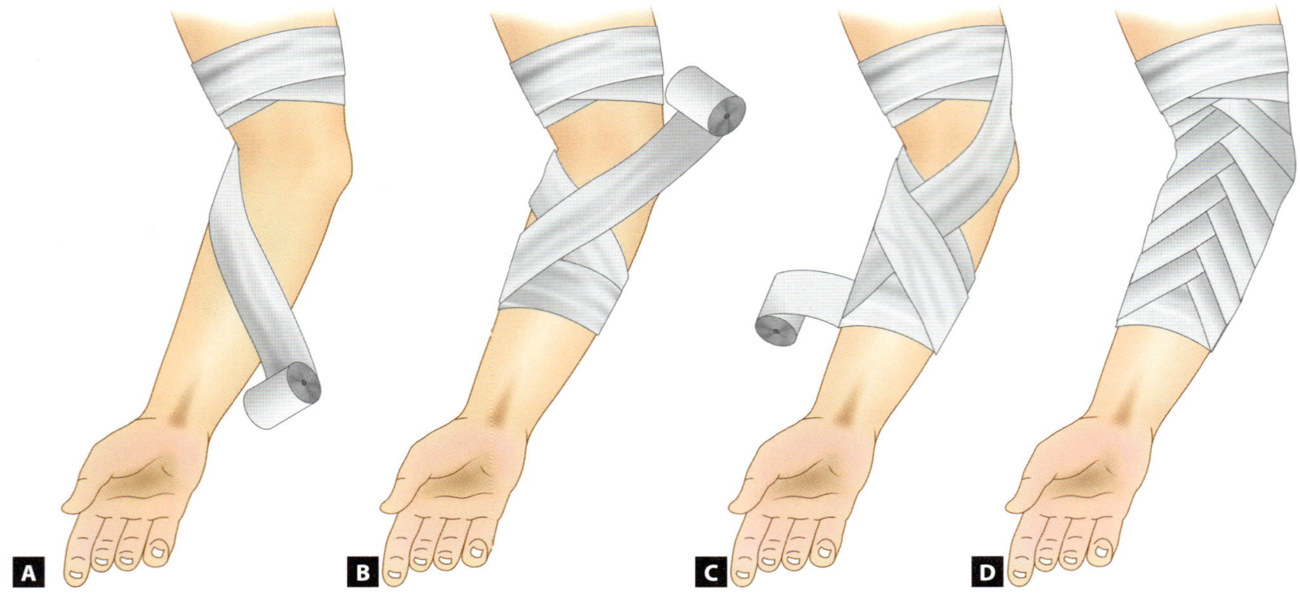

Figs. 22A to D: Figure of eight bandage of elbow.

Figure of Eight Bandage for Elbow (Figs. 22A to D)

This bandage is used to hold a dressing in the antecubital fossa.

a. Anchor with circular turn above elbow and carry bandage obliquely downward over hollow of elbow.
b. Circle forearm below elbow to anchor, bring obliquely upward over hollow of elbow and pass around upper arm at primary circle.
c. Repeat procedure with oblique turns progressing up forearm, each turn overlapping preceding turn by two-thirds.
d. Terminate at starting point and secure.

Front of Elbow Bandage (Fig. 23)

This bandage is also used to hold dressings on the antecubital fossa. Unlike the figure of eight of the elbow, this bandage leaves back of elbow exposed. It allows movement of joint without disturbing the dressing. Anchor bandage with circular turns around forearm below elbow. Carry bandage obliquely upward over hollow of elbow, and circle arm just above elbow. Bring obliquely downward over hollow of elbow and pass around forearm at primary circle. Repeat procedure until hollow of elbow is covered, each oblique turn overlapping preceding oblique by three-fourths and each circular turn overlying each preceding circular turn. Terminate at circular turns above elbow, and secure.

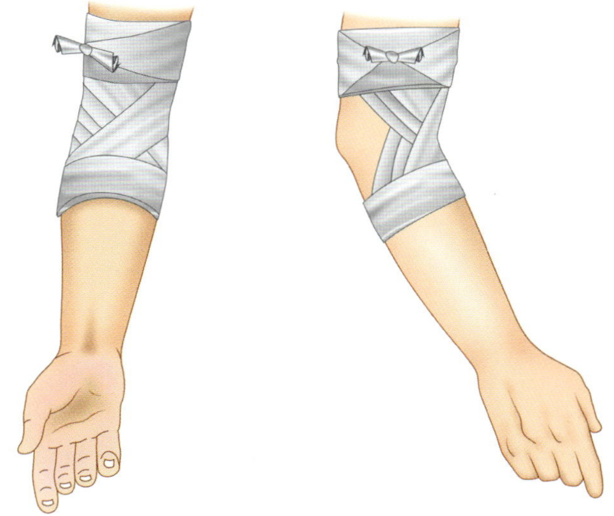

Fig. 23: Front of elbow bandage.

Finger Bandage (Figs. 24A to C)

The finger bandage secures dressing on finger.

a. Anchor bandage at wrist. Bring over back of hand and make one complete turn at base of injured finger over dressing. Make spiral turn to tip of finger to hold dressing while applying bandage.
b. Make another spiral turn back to base of finger.
c. Complete bandage with figure of eight, progressing from tip to finger base. Terminate with circular turns around wrist and secure.

Foot Roller Bandage (Figs. 25A to D)

The foot roller bandage is used to hold dressings on foot, e.g. plantar ulcers or following flap rotation.

a. Anchor around foot near base of toes. Carry obliquely across instep and around heel. Continue obliquely across instep, crossing preceding turn to base of large toe.

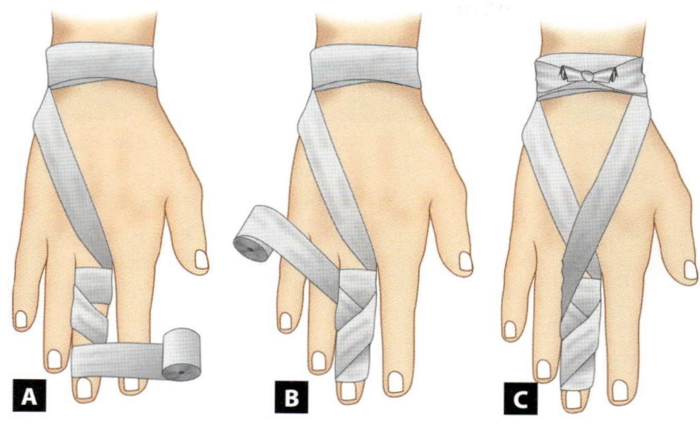

Figs. 24A to C: Finger bandage.

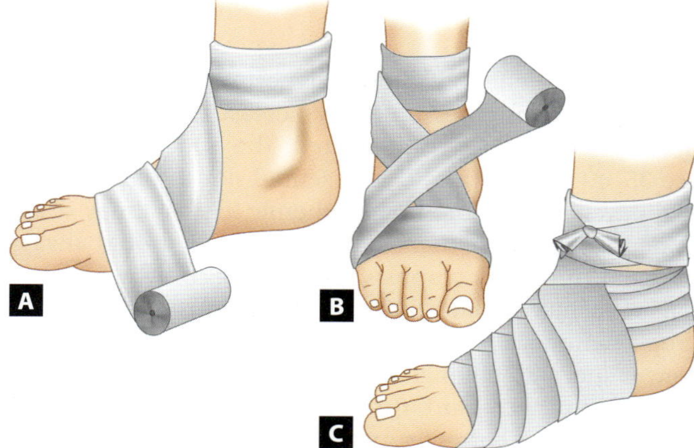

Figs. 26A to C: Figure of eight bandage of foot with heel exposed.

b. Repeat procedure, turns gradually ascending on both foot and heel, crossings being in line along middle of instep.
c. Continue procedure in above step.
d. Terminate above ankle and secure.

Figure of Eight Bandage of Foot (with Heel Exposed) (Figs. 26A to C)

This bandage is used to hold dressings on foot, e.g. plantar ulcers, flap rotation or melanoma excision.

a. Anchor just above ankle, bring bandage obliquely across instep to base of large toe, with turn around base of toes.
b. Continue obliquely across instep to point of beginning.
c. Repeat procedure, leaving heel exposed, with turns ascending until arch and instep are covered. Terminate at starting point and secure.

Tailed Bandages

Tailed bandages consist of the T-bandage, the double T-bandage, the four-tailed bandage and the many-tailed bandages (Figs. 27A to D). These bandages are used to secure dressings to parts which do not lend themselves to roller bandage applications.

a. The T-bandage is a T-shape bandage consisting of a vertical strip of material sewn or pinned to the center of a horizontal strip. This bandage may be used to secure dressing on scalp, ear, eye or perineum.
b. The double T-bandage may be made by sewing two vertical strips of material to the center of a horizontal strip and about 4 inches apart. The double T-bandage may be used to hold dressings on the chest, back or perineum, e.g. scrotal surgery, vitiligo grafts.
c. The four-tailed bandage is a piece of material 4–6 inches wide and about 30 inches long with each end cut about 12 or 14 inches down its middle, leaving the center piece about 12 or 14 inches in length. The four-tailed bandage is used to hold dressings on the jaw, nose, forehead, and the back of the head.

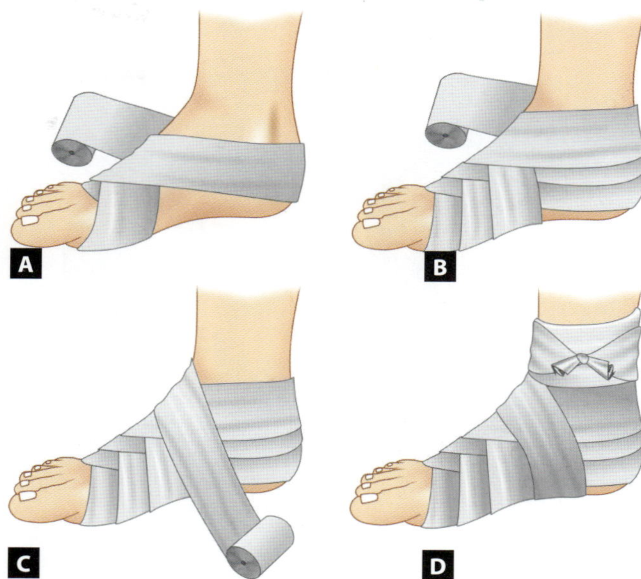

Figs. 25A to D: Foot roller bandage.

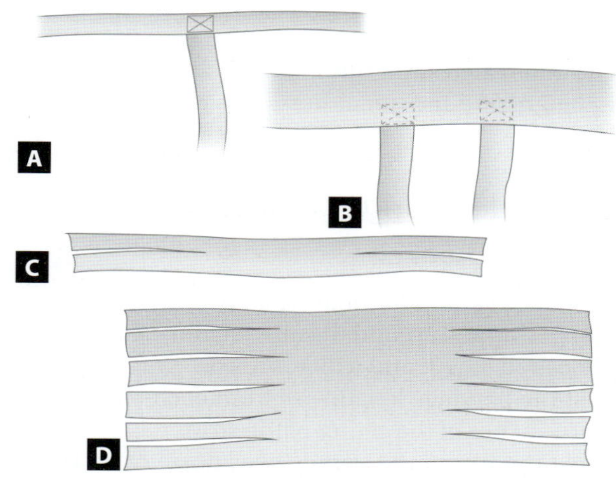

Figs. 27A to D: Tailed bandage.

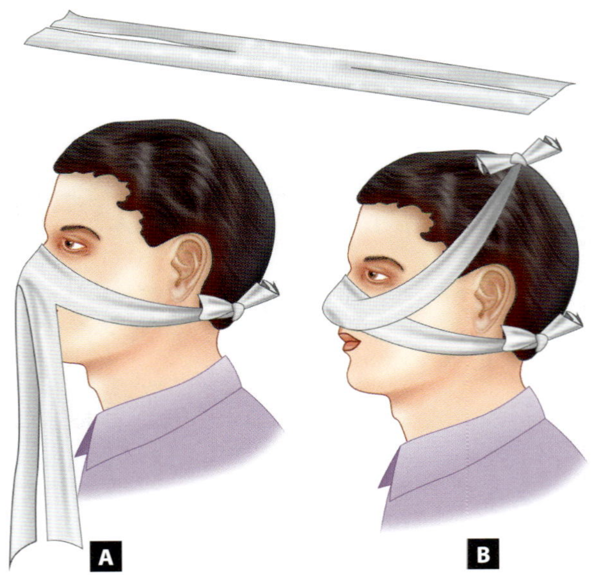

Figs. 28A and B: Four-tailed bandage of the nose.

d. The many-tailed bandage is similar in construction to the four-tailed bandage, except that the ends are cut into the desired number of tails about 16 inches in length and the uncut portion is about 20 inches in length.

Four-Tailed Bandage of the Nose (Figs. 28A and B)

This bandage is used for holding a dressing following any surgery performed around the nose. A four-tailed bandage of the desired length and width is used.

a. Split the bandage lengthwise from each end to within 3 or 5 inches of the center of the strip.
b. Place the top of the center over nose, carry the two upper ends under ears and around to nape of neck and tie.
c. Fold the bottom of the center under nose, carry the two lower ends above ears to top of head and tie.

Table 1: Different types of compression bandages and their indications

Types of bandage	Ankle pressure	Indication
Compression hosiery	15–35 mm Hg	Varicose veins, mild edema and prevention of venous ulcers, venous insufficiency
Single layer bandages	15–50 mm Hg (depending on technique)	Uncomplicated venous leg ulcers with or without lymphedema, venous insufficiency following thrombosis
Multilayer bandages	35–50 mm Hg	Uncomplicated and complicated venous leg ulcers and ulcers secondary to lymphedema

Special Bandages—Compression Bandaging

These reduce effect of venous hypertension by reducing superficial venous pressure. They increase the rate of wound healing, especially if multilayered. The optimal pressures are 35–40 mm Hg and it is essential not to deliver such high levels of pressure to an ischemic leg, as it may result in necrosis or gangrene. Doppler pressures should always be measured and compression dressings only used if the ankle brachial pressure index is greater than 0.8. Traditional crepe bandages do not provide adequate compression. Newer short stretch high performance bandages are more effective in this regard. Combining compression therapy with surgery to correct superficial venous reflux does not lead to improved healing rates compared with compression alone, but reduces ulcer recurrence and increases ulcer-free time. Table 1 shows different types of compression bandages and their indications.

Further details can be found in chapter 54 (Leg Ulcers).

RECOMMENDED READING

1. Bandaging and splinting, Chapter 2, Field Manual No.8-50, Department of the Army, Washington 25, DC, 1957; 1-39.

Chapter

7

Universal Precautions for a Dermatosurgeon

YS Marfatia, Smriti Naswa

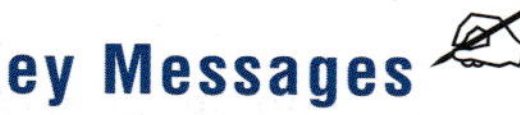

Key Messages

- It is not possible to evaluate every patient to be offered dermatosurgery for all transmissible blood-borne pathogens; thus universal precautions every time everywhere are the key to prevention of infection.
- Universal precautions encompass the following measures:
  - Hand hygiene breaks the chain of transmission of infection through person-to-person contact.
  - Personal protective equipment like gloves, masks, and gowns create a physical barrier to the source of microorganisms
  - Safe-handling and disposal of the sharps is of utmost importance; as most common form of occupational exposure to blood and the most likely to result in infection is needlestick injury.
  - Hospital waste should be properly collected and disposed off in respective colored bags.
  - Post-exposure prophylaxis protocols for HIV and HBV must be followed in cases of accidental exposure.

INTRODUCTION

Definition of Universal Precautions[1]

Universal Precautions are a simple set of effective practices designed to protect health workers and patients from infection with a range of pathogens including blood-borne viruses. These practices are used when caring for all patients regardless of diagnosis. They are applied universally.

Health care workers deal with blood every day. Blood is a very good culture medium and nidus for various pathogenic microorganisms, many of which are associated with high morbidity and mortality (Box 1). The importance lies in the fact that most blood exposures in health settings are preventable. Dermatosurgeons must take stringent precautions to prevent occupational exposure to blood borne pathogens. A thorough knowledge about strategies like universal precautions, immunization against hepatitis B, provision of personal protection and the management of exposures is a must for every health care physician.[1] Adherence to recommended practices decreases transmission of infectious agents. But observed adherence to universal precautions is not universal and varies from 43% to 89%.[2] Universal precaution guidelines were developed in response to HIV/AIDS epidemic and several guidelines have been published[2-4] (Box 2).

EPIDEMIOLOGY

Annual Infection of Healthcare Personnel with Blood-Borne Pathogens

There are approximately 35 million health workers worldwide, of whom approximately 3,85,000[5] experience percutaneous exposures to blood-borne pathogens annually; two million of those to HBV, 0.9 million to HCV and 1,70,000 to HIV. These injuries may culminate into 15,000 HCV; 70,000 HBV and 1000 HIV infections. Of the estimated 385,000 needlestick injuries occurring in hospitals each year, 23 percent occur in surgical settings.[6] Moreover about 90% of these infections occur in developing countries.[1] The most common cause of occupational exposure is needle-stick injury.[5] Among NaSH (National Surveillance System for Health Care Workers) hospitals in US, the operating room is the second most common environment in which sharps injuries occur, accounting for 27% of injuries, following 40% injuries in in-patient units. It is interesting to note that majority of such exposures occur from medical floors.[5] Table 1 lists the blood-borne pathogens against which universal precautions are necessary.[7] Universal

Box. 1: Do dermatosurgical procedures require mandatory pre-procedure testing of blood-borne pathogens like HIV, HBV and HCV?

1. The answer lies in what is the BASIS BEHIND APPLICATION OF UNIVERSAL PRECAUTIONS as quoted by WHO
   "It is not feasible, effective or cost-effective to test all patients for all pathogens prior to giving care in order to identify those who are infected and take precautions only with them. Knowing a patient is infected does not prevent occupational exposure to blood. Thus, decisions regarding the level of precautions to use are based on the nature of the procedure and not on the actual or assumed serological status of the patient."
2. Negative serology for infective pathogen does not rule out infection as the patient may be in WINDOW PERIOD.
3. No test is 100% specific and sensitive.
   Adaptation of universal precautions is essential irrespective of sero-status of patient.

Box 2: Key points about skin[20]

- Health care-associated pathogens frequently colonize areas of normal, intact patient skin, besides being recovered from infected or draining wounds.
- Normal skin sheds nearly 106 squamous cells per day, containing viable microorganisms (cutaneous microflora) which contaminate the patients' immediate environment including clothes, bed covers, furniture and others.
- Many studies have shown that hands or gloves of HCWs can be contaminated with pathogens like C. difficile, Gram-negative bacilli, enterococci or S. aureus even by touching intact skin of patients or while performing "clean procedures" on them.
- Following contact with contaminated environment or patients, microorganisms can survive on hands from 2 to 60 minutes.
- After detergent action of soaps/handrubs, 50–60% of the normal barrier function [measured as recovery of trans-epidermal water loss (TEWL)] recovers rapidly within 6 hours, but complete normalization of the function requires 5–6 days.

Table 1: List of blood borne pathogens.[7]

Viral	*Bacterial*	*Parasitic*
Human immunodeficiency virus (HIV)		
Hepatitis B virus (HBV)	Syphilis	Malaria
	Brucella	Toxoplasma
Hepatitis C virus (HCV)		Microfilaria
Hepatitis G virus (HGV)		
Epstein Barr virus (EBV)		
Cytomegalovirus (CMV)		
Human T lymphotropic viruses (HTLV-1 and HTLV-II)		
Ebola virus		
Zika virus (under investigation)		

Table 2: Universal precautions and Other Potentially Infectious Materials (OPIMs).[8]

Universal precautions apply to:	*Universal precautions do not apply to*:*
Semen	If the following body fluids are not blood-stained:
Vaginal secretions	Feces
Synovial fluid	Nasal secretions
Cerebrospinal fluid	Sputum
Pleural fluid	Sweat
Peritoneal fluid	Tears
Pericardial fluid	Urine
Amniotic fluid	Vomitus
	Saliva (except in the dental setting, where saliva is likely to be contaminated with blood)

* These are covered under "standard precautions" or "routine practices". These practices aim to protect against the transmission of all microorganisms through contact with all body fluids, excretions, mucous membranes, non-intact skin and soiled items in addition to precautions for blood. An example in this chapter is Ebola virus disease (vide supra).[8] For further details, refer to the Glossary section.

precautions apply to certain body fluids which harbor potentially infectious pathogens[8] which are listed in Table 2.

NEWER VIRUSES AFFECTING THE WORLD

Ebola Virus

Ebola virus disease (EVD), which was formerly known as Ebola hemorrhagic fever, is a severe illness with an average case fatality rate of 50%. The Ebola virus disease (EVD) outbreak in West Africa in 2014 has affected >8 countries in the world and by 22 March 2015, 10326 deaths have been reported by WHO worldwide.[9,10] Allaranga et al. had observed that almost one-tenth of all cases of EVD in Africa occurred in health care and laboratory workers. WHO reported that by October 27, 2014, a total of 521 health care workers had acquired EVD and 272 had died.[10]

The natural hosts of Ebola virus are the fruit bats of Pteropodidae family. Since India comes under the home range of these bats, there is a potential risk of Indian population being affected with the virus and its disease.[10]

In healthcare settings, Ebola is spread through direct contact with blood or body fluids of a person who is sick with Ebola or with objects (e.g. bathroom surfaces, medical equipment) that have been contaminated with infectious blood or body fluids (hence, the safe work practices to prevent Ebola spread come under standard precautions rather than universal precautions.[8] For details vide Glossary section). The virus can enter a person's body through broken skin or unprotected mucous membranes. For all healthcare workers caring for patients with Ebola, PPE that fully covers skin and clothing and prevents any exposure of the eyes, nose, and mouth is recommended.[11]

Key safe work practices recommended by CDC include the following:

- Promptly isolate EVD patient in a single room with a closed door and a private bathroom.

- Restrict entry of non essential healthcare workers or other visitors.
- Monitor the patient care area at all times.
- The healthcare workers should take sufficient time to don and doff PPE slowly and correctly without distraction, preferably in presence of a trained observer.
- Reinforce the need to keep hands away from the face during any patient care and to limit touching surfaces and body fluids.
- Frequently disinfect gloved hands by using an alcohol-based handrub (ABHR), particularly after contact with body fluids.
- Prevent needlestick and sharps injuries by adhering to correct sharps handling practices.
- Avoid unnecessary procedures involving sharps.
- Use needleless IV systems whenever possible.
- Immediately clean and disinfect any visibly contaminated PPE surfaces, equipment, or patient care area surfaces using a disinfectant wipe.
- Footwear should be closed-toe, soft-soled, washable, and have a closed back.
- Although airborne transmission of Ebola has not been documented to date, CDC recommends that all healthcare workers entering the room of a patient with Ebola wear respiratory protection which include a NIOSH-certified, fit-tested N-95 or higher respirator, or a PAPR.
- Double-gloving is an easy way to remove gross contamination by changing an outer glove during patient care and when removing PPE.
- Regularly clean and disinfect surfaces in the patient care area, even in the absence of visible contamination.
  - Only nurses or physicians should clean and disinfect surfaces in the patient care areas to limit the number of additional healthcare workers who enter the room.

Doffing

- Removing used PPE is a high-risk process that requires a structured procedure, a trained observer, a doffing assistant in some situations, and a designated area for removal to ensure protection.
- PPE must be removed slowly and deliberately in the correct sequence to reduce the possibility of self-contamination or other exposure to Ebola.

  For further details on Ebola virus disease visit.[11]

Zika Virus

Zika virus disease (ZVD) is caused by a flavivirus, the outbreaks of which have been recorded in Africa, the Americas, Asia and the Pacific. People with ZVD can have symptoms including mild fever, skin rash, conjunctivitis, muscle and joint pain, malaise or headache; lasting for 2–7 days. Zika virus is a cause of microcephaly and Guillain-Barré syndrome.[12]

Zika virus is primarily transmitted through the bite of an infected mosquito from *Aedes aegypti* in tropical regions. Sexual transmission of Zika virus is also possible. Blood transfusion as a mode is being investigated.[13]

Clinical symptoms and recent history of travel to an area with active Zika virus transmission can give a clue to the diagnosis, which can only be confirmed through laboratory tests on blood or other body fluids, such as urine, saliva or semen.[13]

Till the possibility of spread of Zika by blood is confirmed, it is advised to follow all universal precautions in probable or confirmed case of Zika. Though Zika is not present in India yet, the breeding grounds including the vector has ample presence. Hence, any recent travel to the places or a pregnant woman or child with suspected symptoms should be thoroughly tested.

Multi-Drug-Resistant Bacteria

The Indian Network for Surveillance of Antimicrobial Resistance (INSAR) group, India, in a study conducted at 15 tertiary care centers on 26,310 isolates of *S. aureus* found the prevalence of MRSA to be 41%. Along with this, MRSA had a high rate of resistance to ciprofloxacin, gentamycin, cotrimoxazole, erythromycin, and clindamycin.[14]

HCWs frequently become contaminated with MDR bacteria. Hayden et al. found that 62% of HCWs, who entered the room of patients known to be colonized with VRE contaminated their gloves or hands during care.[15]

Contaminated HCW hands, in turn, were capable of transmitting VRE to inanimate surfaces. In a study by Morgan et al. even after appropriate use of gloves and gown while caring for a patient on contact precautions, 1.7% to 4.2% of HCWs had an MDR bacterium on their hands without hand hygiene. This emphasizes the importance of hand hygiene after removal of gloves and gown.[16]

Overall, 8% of HCW room entries occurred with an HCW who had MDR bacteria on their hands. This highlights the importance of performing hand hygiene before room entry.

A greater risk of contamination was observed when HCWs performed a physical examination or remained in the room longer. Hence, universal use of gown and gloves for all patient contact in the ICU may be an answer to this problem.[16]

HCWs entering a room that had environmental contamination with MDR bacteria were over four times as likely to become contaminated with that organism, highlighting the importance of environmental cleaning.[16]

Although cosmetic surgeries are done in otherwise healthy individuals, basic procedures like skin biopsy might be required to be done bedside in ICU patients. Hence, universal precautions are of equal importance to these procedures as any other major/minor surgeries. Moreover, it is safe to do the dermatosurgeries in OTs specifically meant for these procedures (avoiding shared OTs). These measures assume more importance in public hospitals.

Modes of Occupational Exposure to Blood

1. Percutaneous injury (needle-stick or other sharps injury)
2. Mucocutaneous injury (splash of blood or other body fluids into the eyes, nose or mouth)
3. Blood contact with non-intact skin.

Factors Affecting Occupational Exposure[1]

The risk of infection for health workers depends on:
1. Prevalence of disease in the patient population
2. The nature and frequency of exposures—higher risk in:
   a. Operating, delivery and emergency rooms
   b. Laboratories
   c. Cleaners, waste collectors

Risk of Infection after Exposure has been explained in Table 3.

WHO SUGGESTS FOLLOWING INTERVENTIONS UNDER THE UNIVERSAL PRECAUTIONS[1]

1. Handwashing after any direct contact with patients
2. Wearing gloves for contact with body fluids, nonintact skin and mucous membranes
3. Wearing a mask, eye protection and a gown (and sometimes a plastic apron) if blood or other body fluids might splash
4. Covering all cuts and abrasions with a waterproof dressing
5. Preventing two-handed recapping of needles
6. Safe collection and disposal of needles (hypodermic and suture) and sharps (scalpel blades, lancets, razors, scissors), with required puncture- and liquid-proof safety boxes in each patient care area
7. Promptly and carefully cleaning up spills of blood and other body fluids
8. Using a safe system for health care waste management and disposal.

Table 3: Risk of infection with HIV, HBV and HCV after exposure by various modes.[1,17]

Virus	*Mode of exposure*	*Risk of infection*
HIV	Needle stick or cut exposure to HIV-infected blood	0.3%
	Exposure of the eye, nose, or mouth to HIV-infected blood	0.1%
	Non-intact skin	< 0.1%
	After a mucous membrane exposure	Approx. 0.09%
HBV	Single needle stick or cut exposure risk	6–30%
HCV	Needlestick or cut exposure risk	1.8% (range: 0-7%)
	After a mucous membrane exposure	Rare
	Intact/non-intact skin	None

Discussion of the steps included in universal precautions for a dermatosurgeon will be under following headings:
1. Hand hygiene
2. Personal protective equipment
3. Safe practices to use sharps and their disposal
4. Hospital waste management
5. Post-exposure prophylaxis (to HIV, HBV and HCV).

WHO promotes the slogan "CLEAN CARE, SAFER CARE" highlighting the importance of hand hygiene.

Appropriate handwashing can minimize microorganisms acquired on the hands by contact with body fluids and contaminated surfaces. Handwashing breaks the chain of infection transmission from person-to-person contact.[18] But, adherence of HCPs to recommended hand-hygiene procedures has been poor, ranging from 5% to 81%.[19]

HAND HYGIENE[18-20]

It is a general term that applies to handwashing, antiseptic handwash, antiseptic handrub, or surgical hand antisepsis. Detailed description of different hand wash chemicals can be found in chapter 4 (Sterilization and disinfection for dermatosurgeon).

Hand hygiene can be divided into 3 types according to the method and type of cutaneous microflora they affect (Table 4).

Handrub vs Handwash

Contents of Alcohol-based Handrubs with Optimal Antimicrobial Efficacy[19,20]

About 75–85% ethanol, isopropanol, or n-propanol, or a combination of these WHO-recommendation-formulations containing either 75% v/v isopropanol, or 80% v/v ethanol.

As per WHO, alcohol solutions containing 60–80% alcohol are considered to have efficacious microbicidal activity, with concentrations higher than 90% being less potent.[20]

Advantages of Handrub[20]

1. Elimination of the majority of germs (including viruses)
2. Waterless procedure: No need for any particular infrastructure (clean water supply network, washbasin, soap, hand towel).
3. Less time taken (20 to 30 seconds).

Table 4: Various types of hand hygiene[18-20]

S. No	Type of hand hygiene	Cutaneous microflora affected	Duration	Method	Remarks
1	Routine/social handwash	Likely to reduce transient flora	10–15 sec	Washing hands with plain (i.e. non-antimicrobial) soap and water	
2	Hygienic hand antisepsis Antiseptic handwash Antiseptic handrub	Reduces transient microbial flora without necessarily affecting the resident skin flora	15–30 sec	Treatment of hands with either an antiseptic handrub or antiseptic handwash	
				Antiseptic handwash: It is broad spectrum, but is usually less efficacious and acts more slowly than the hygienic handrub	
				Antiseptic handrub: These preparations are broad spectrum and fast-acting, and persistent activity is not necessary	
3	Surgical hand antisepsis Surgical hand scrub/wash Surgical handrub	Eliminates transient flora and reduce resident skin flora	Minimum 2–3 minutes	Surgical handscrub/presurgical scrub refers to surgical hand preparation with antimicrobial soap and water	Surgical hand antisepsis is required preoperatively by the surgical team before performing invasive procedures
				Surgical handrub refers to surgical hand preparation with a waterless, alcohol-based handrub	

4. Humectants are present in the handrub, thus no drying or irritation of skin.
5. Availability of the product at the point of care

Disadvantages not preferred over soaps and less efficacious if:[20]

1. the hands are soiled/dirty
2. when exposure to potential spore-forming organisms is strongly suspected or proven
3. after using the lavatory.

Indications for Hand Hygiene[20]

1. Before and after touching the patient
2. Before handling an invasive device for patient care, regardless of whether or not gloves are used
3. After contact with body fluids or excretions, mucous membranes, non-intact skin, or wound dressings
4. If moving from a contaminated body site to another body site during care of the same patient
5. After contact with inanimate surfaces and objects (including medical equipment) in the immediate vicinity of the patient
6. After removing sterile or non-sterile gloves.

Notes:

1. Use an alcohol-based handrub as the preferred means for routine hand antisepsis in all other clinical situations described above (1–6) **if hands are not visibly soiled** (in which case soap and water are advised)
2. Soap and alcohol-based handrub should not be used concomitantly.

ROUTINE/SOCIAL HANDWASHING[18]

It is usually limited to hands and wrists; the hands are washed with soap (plain or antimicrobial) and water.

Duration: Minimum 10–15 seconds (of rubbing the hands); duration of entire procedure—40–60 seconds.

Steps in Handwashing

1. Preparing for handwashing:
   a. Remove jewellery and watches before washing hands
   b. ensure that the nails are clipped short (do not wear artificial nails)
   c. Roll the sleeves up to the elbow.
2. Wet the hands and wrists, keeping hands and wrists lower than the elbows (permits the water to flow to the fingertips, avoiding arm contamination).
3. Apply soap (plain or antimicrobial) and lather thoroughly.
4. Use firm, circular motions to wash the hands and arms up to the wrists, covering all areas including palms, back of the hands, fingers, between fingers and lateral side of fifth finger, knuckles, and wrists. Rub for minimum of 10–15 seconds.
5. Repeat the process if the hands are very soiled.
6. Clean under the fingernails.
7. Rinse hands thoroughly, keeping the hands lower than the forearms.
8. If running water is not available, use a bucket and pitcher.
9. Do no dip your hands into a bowl to rinse, as this re-contaminates them.
10. Collect used water in a basin and discard in a sink, drain or toilet.
11. Dry hands thoroughly with disposable paper towel or napkins, clean dry towel, or air-dry them.

12. Discard the towel if used, in an appropriate container without touching the bin lids with hand.
13. Use a paper towel, clean towel or your elbow/foot to turn off the faucet to prevent recontamination.

Routine handwashing is illustrated in Figure 1.

HAND ANTISEPSIS/ DECONTAMINATION[18,20]

Hand antisepsis removes or destroys transient micro-organisms and confers a prolonged effect.

Hand hygiene technique with soap and water

Duration of the entire procedure: 40–60 seconds

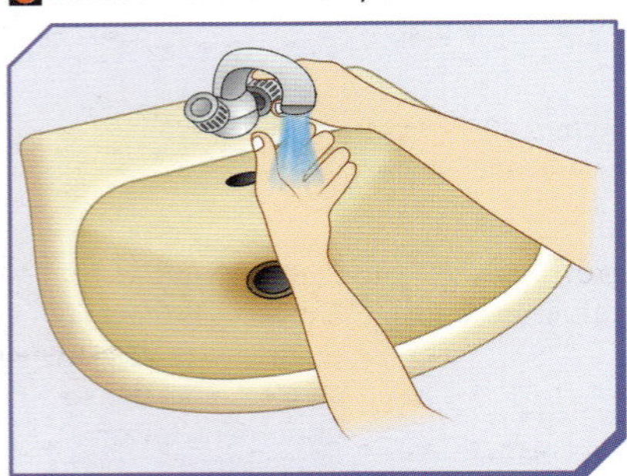

Wet hands with water

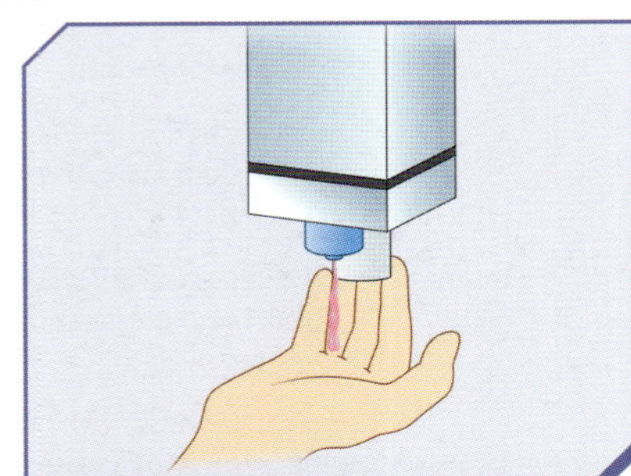

Apply enough scap to cover all hand surfaces

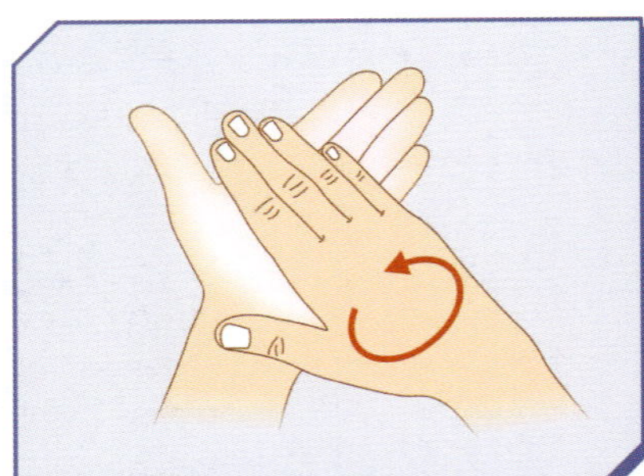

Rub hands palm to palm

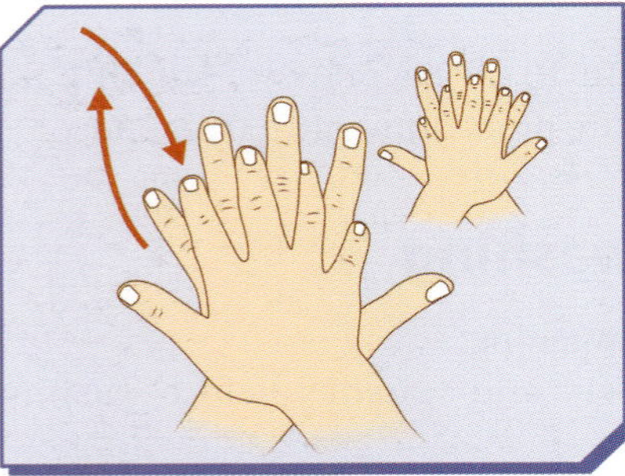

Right palm over left dorsum with interlaced fingers and vice versa

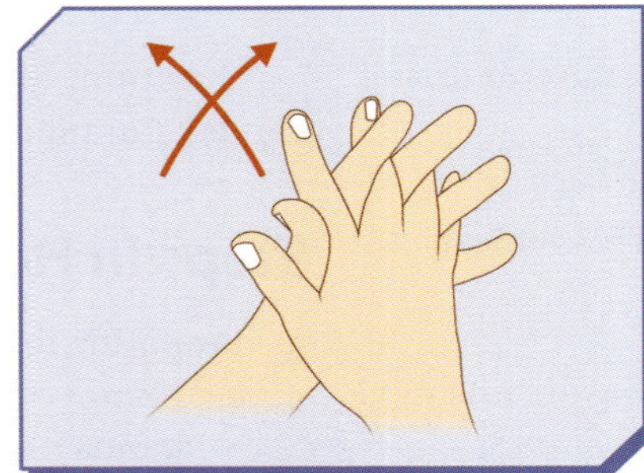

Palm to palm with fingers interlaced

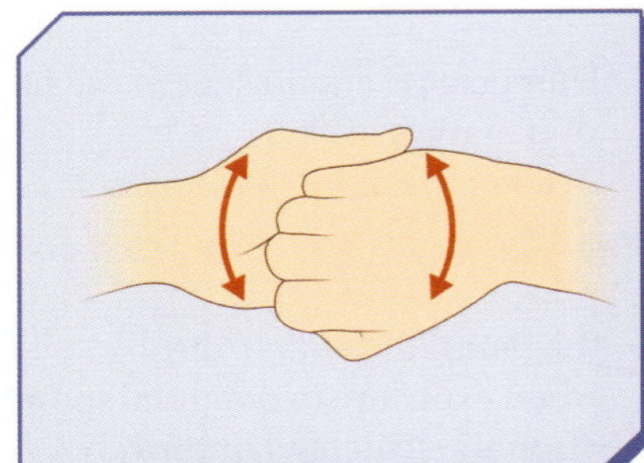

Backs of fingers to opposing palms with fingers interlocked

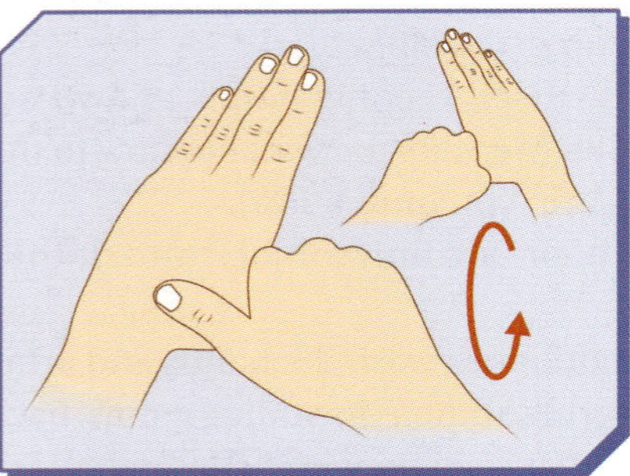

Rotational rubbing of left thumb clasped in right palm and vice versa

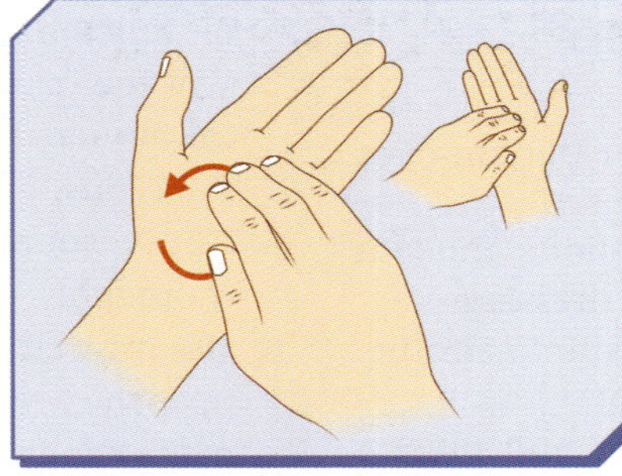

Rotational rubbing, backwards and forwards with clasped fingers of right hand in left palm and vice versa

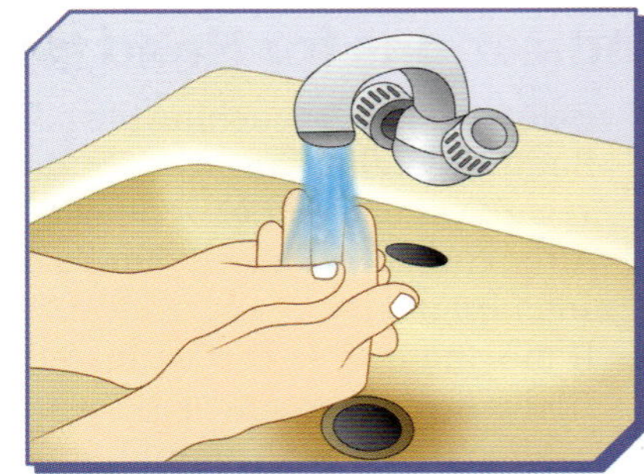

Rinse hands with water

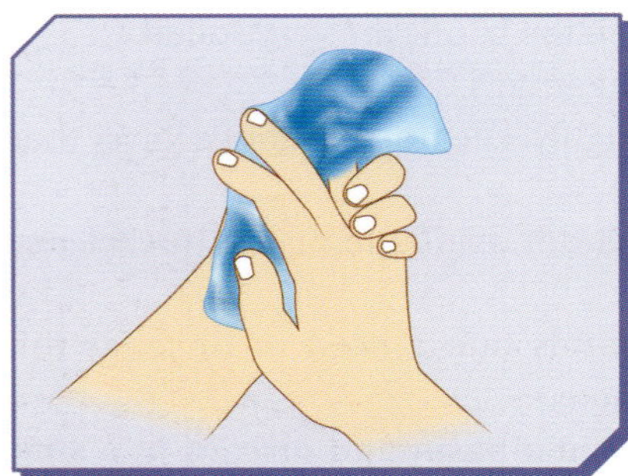

Dry thoroughly with a single use towel

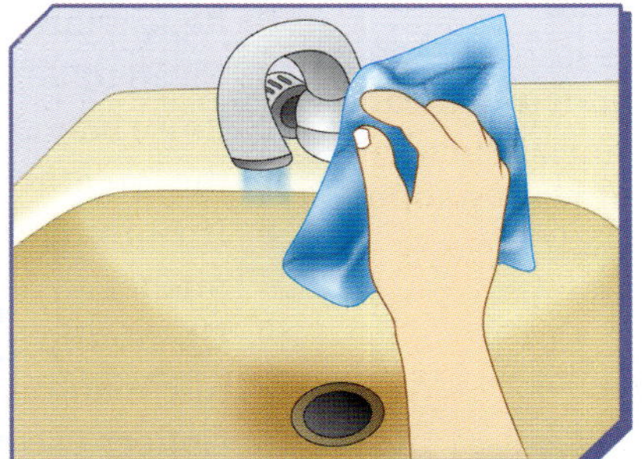

Use towel to turn off faucet

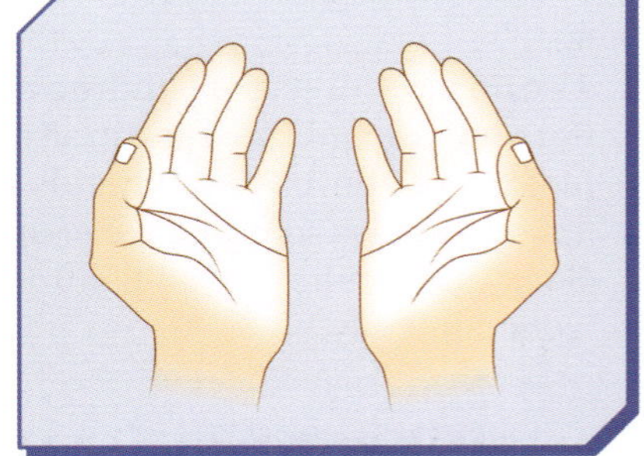

Your hands are now safe

Fig. 1: Routine handwashing with soap and water.

Courtesy: WHO Guidelines on Hand Hygiene in Health Care. World Health Organization, 2009. Reproduced with permission.[20]

Hand hygiene technique with alcohol-based formulation

Duration of the entire procedure: 20–30 seconds

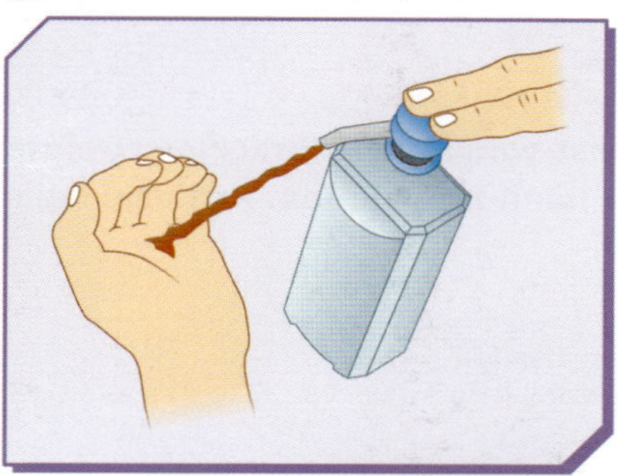

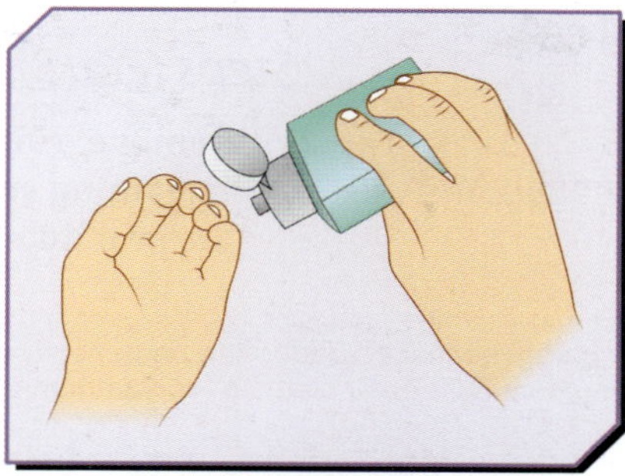

Apply a palmful of the product in a cupped hand, covering all surfaces

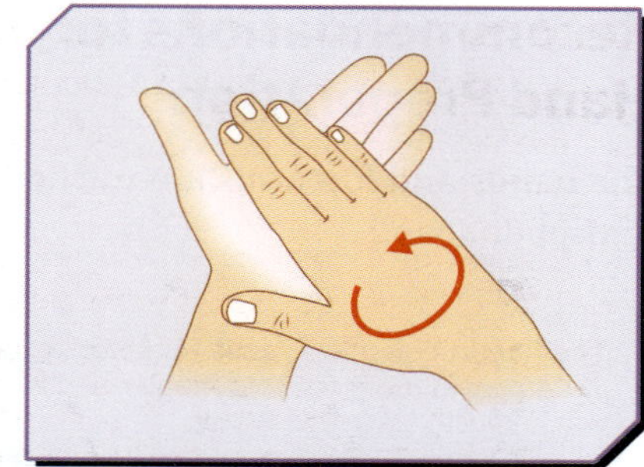

Rub hands palm to palm

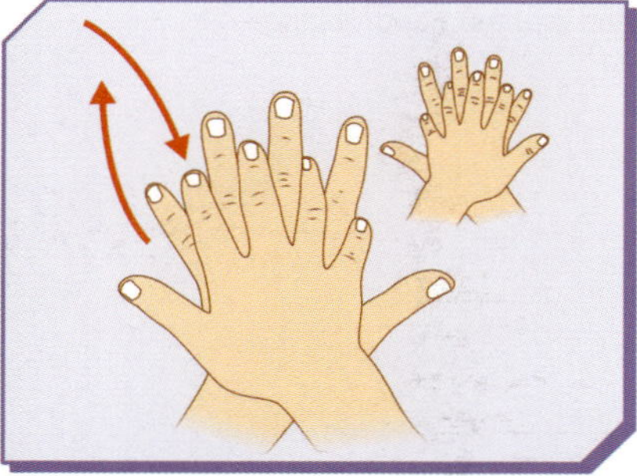

Right palm over left dorsum with interlaced fingers and vice versa

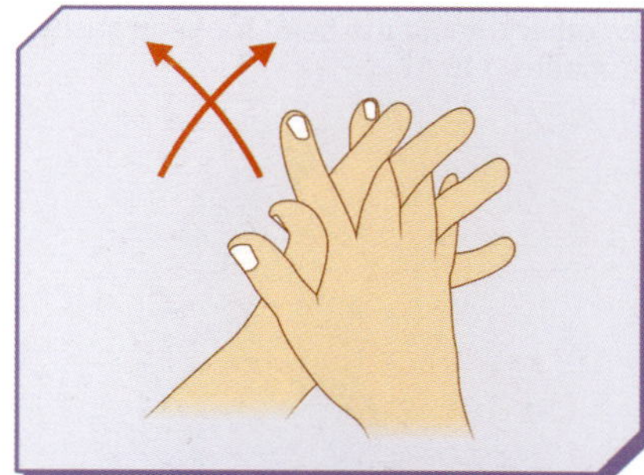

Palm to palm with fingers interlaced

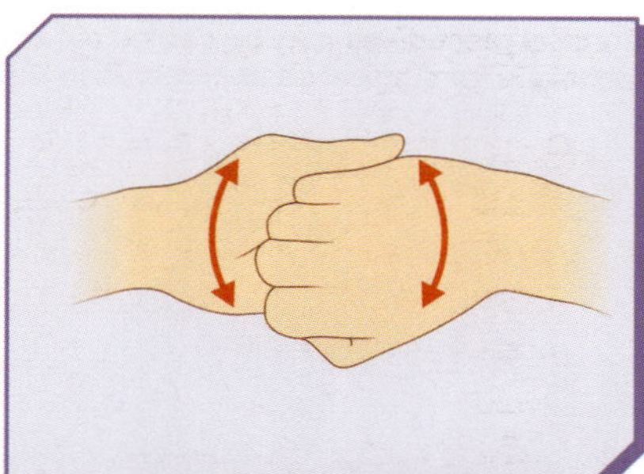

Backs of fingers to opposing palms with fingers interlocked

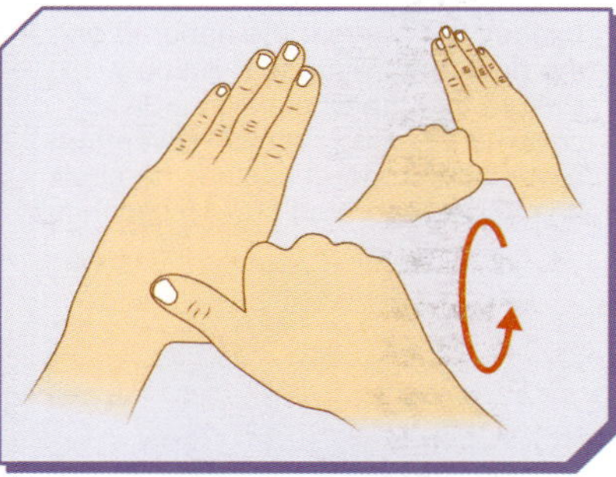

Rotational rubbing of left thumb clasped in right palm and vice versa

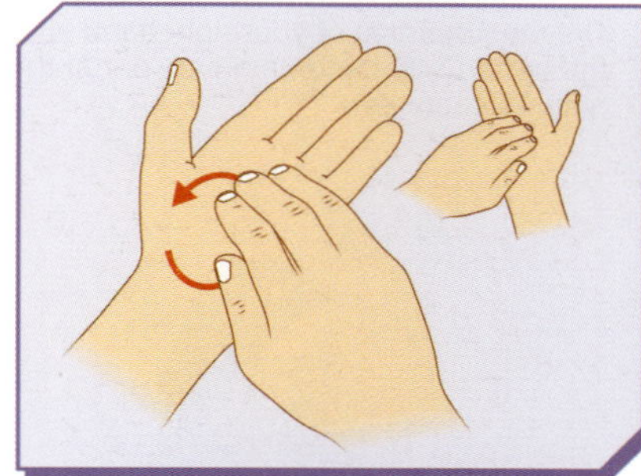

Rotational rubbing, backwards and forwards with clasped fingers of right hand in left palm and vice versa

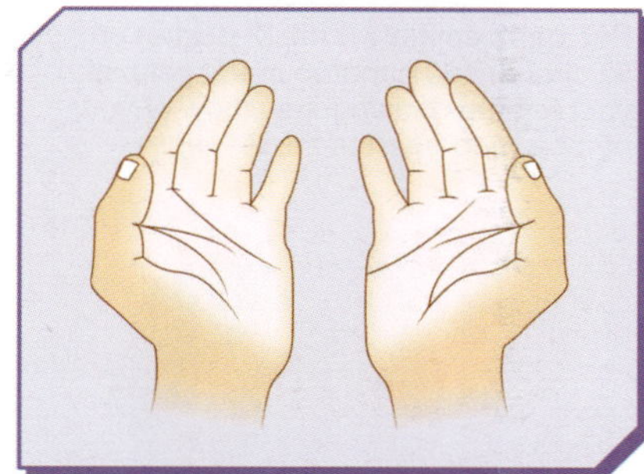

Once dry, your hands are safe

Fig. 2: Antiseptic hand hygienic technique with alcohol-based handrub.

Courtesy: WHO Guidelines on Hand Hygiene in Health Care. World Health Organization, 2009. Reproduced with permission.[20]

Specific antiseptics: recommended for hand antisepsis:

a. 2–4% chlorhexidine,
b. 5–7.5% povidone iodine,
c. 1% triclosan, or
d. 70% alcoholic handrubs.

Duration: 15–30 seconds

Immersion of hands in bowls of antiseptics is not recommended.

It may be carried out in one of the following two ways:

1. *Antiseptic handwash*: Wash hands and forearms with antimicrobial soap and water. (Details already discussed earlier).
2. *Antiseptic handrub*: Decontaminate hands with a waterless, alcohol-based hand gel or handrub. This is appropriate for hands that are not soiled with protein matter or fat (Fig. 2).

Steps

1. Apply the product to the palm of one hand. The volume needed to apply varies by product.
2. Rub hands together, covering all surfaces of hands and fingers, until hands are dry.
3. Do not rinse.

Note

1. When there is visible soiling of hands, they should first be washed with soap and water before using waterless handrubs gels or alcohol swabs.
2. If soap and water are unavailable, hands should first be cleansed with detergent-containing towelettes, before using the alcohol-based handrub, gel or swab.

SURGICAL HAND ANTISEPSIS

Recommendations for Surgical Hand Preparation[20]

The hands and forearms are washed thoroughly with an antiseptic soap.

Duration: minimum 2–3 minutes (Long scrub times (e.g. 10 minutes) are not necessary).

Steps (Fig. 3)

1. Remove rings, wrist-watch, and bracelets before beginning surgical hand preparation. Artificial nails are prohibited.

The handrubbing technique for surgical hand preparation must be performed on perfectly clean, dry hands.
On arrival in the operating theater and after having donned theater clothing (cap/hat/bonnet and mask), hands must be washed with soap and water.
After the operation when removing gloves, hands must be rubbed with and alcohol-based formulation or washed with soap and water if any residual talc or biological fluids are present (e.g. the glove is punctured).

Surgical procedures may be carried out one after the other without the need for handwashing, provided that the handrubbing technique for surgical hand preparation is followed (Images 1 to 17)

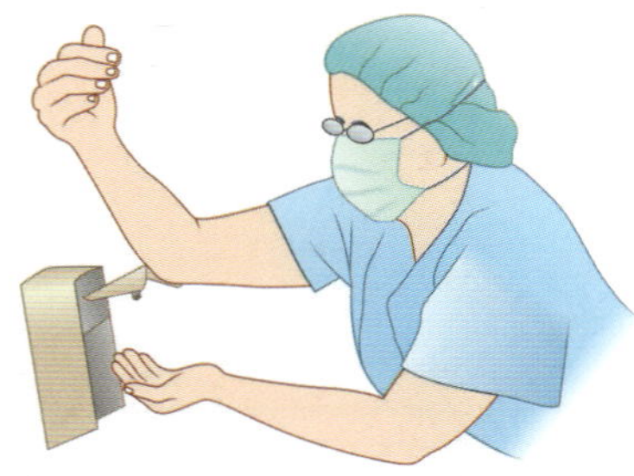

1
Put approximately 5 mL (3 doses) of alcohol-based handrub in the palm of your left hand, using the elbow of your other arm to operate the dispenser

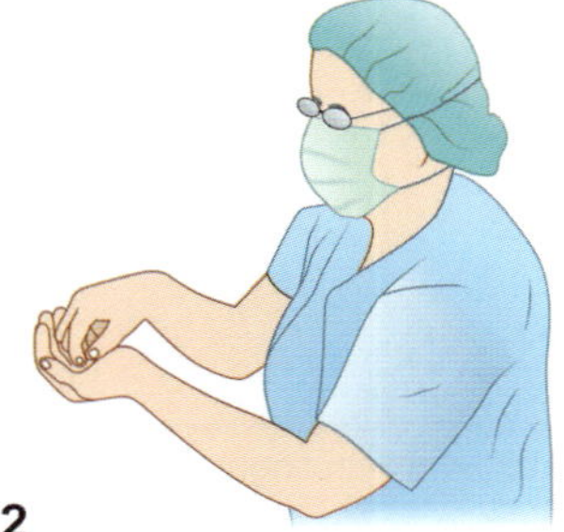

2
Dip the fingertips of your right hand in the handrub to decontaminate under the nails (5 seconds)

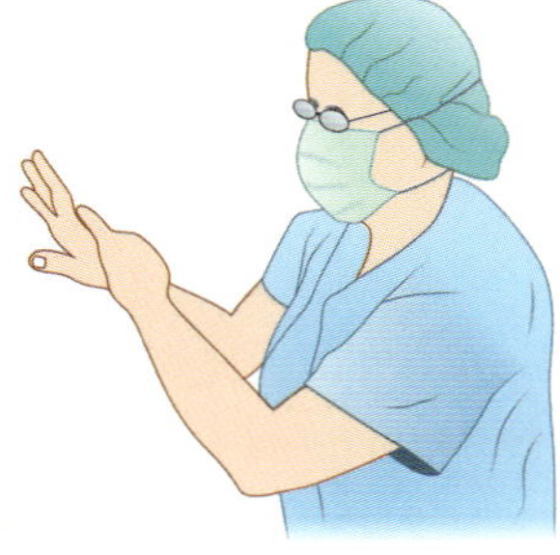

3
Images 3–7: Smear the handrub on the right forearm up to the elbow. Ensure that the whole skin area is covered by using circular movements around the forearm until the handrub has fully evaporated (10–15 seconds)

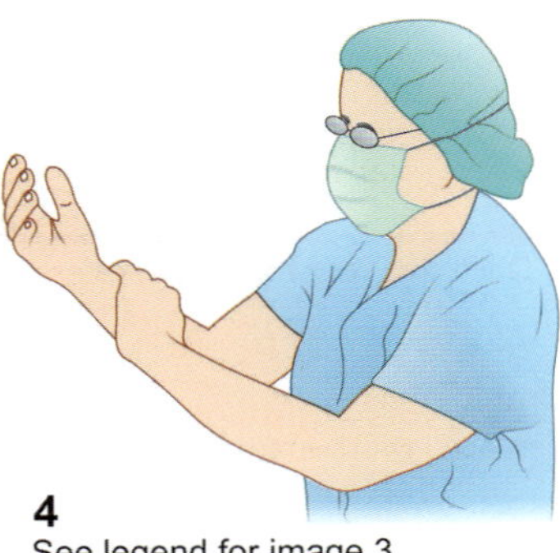

4
See legend for image 3

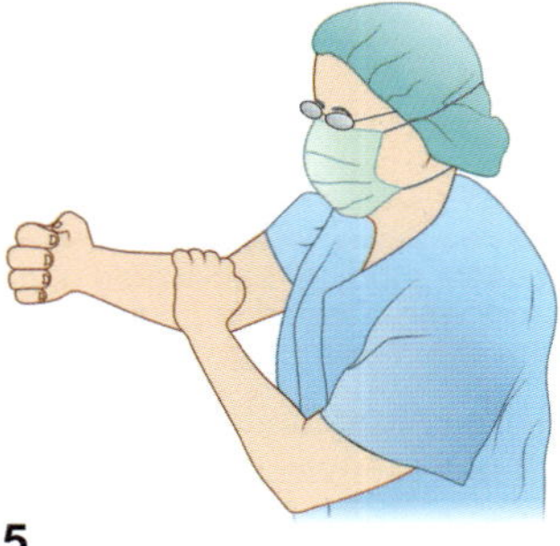

5
See legend for image 3

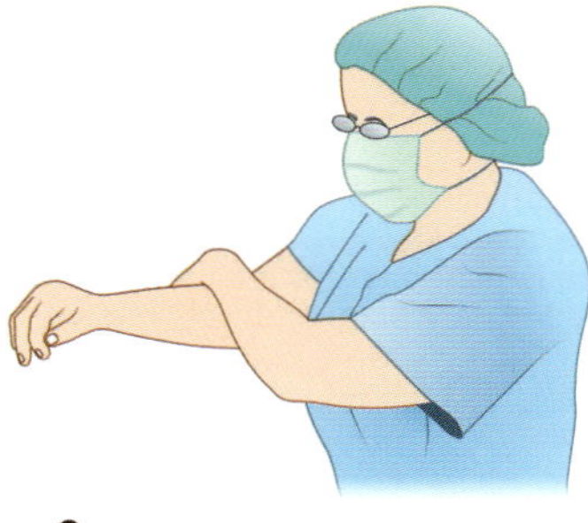

6
See legend for image 3

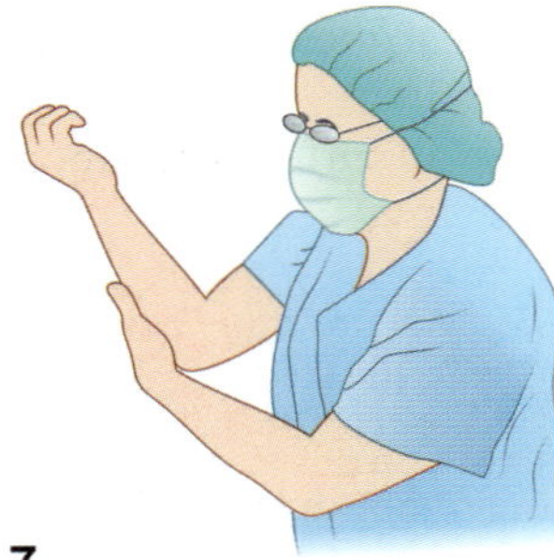

7
See legend for image 3

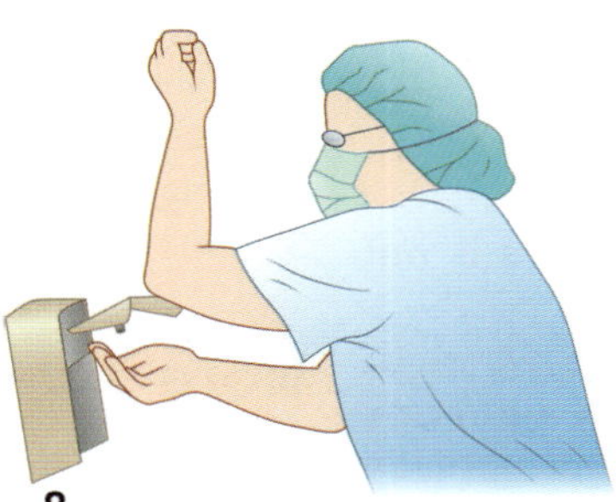

8
Put approximately 5 mL (3 doses) of alcohol-based handrub in the palm of your right hand, using the elbow of your other arm to operate the dispenser

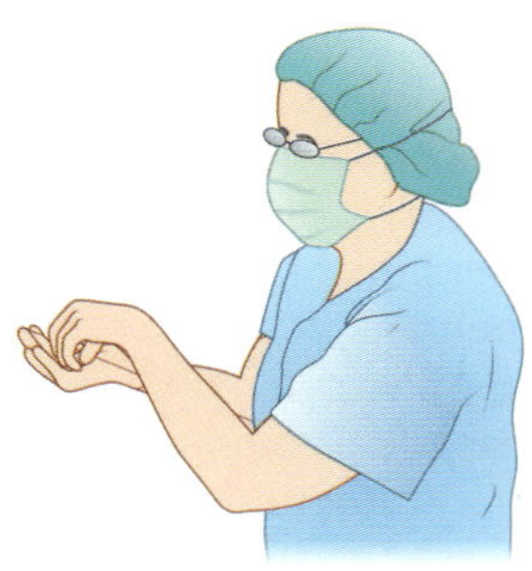

9
Dip the fingertips of your left hand in the handrub to decontaminate under the nails (5 seconds)

Contd...

Contd...

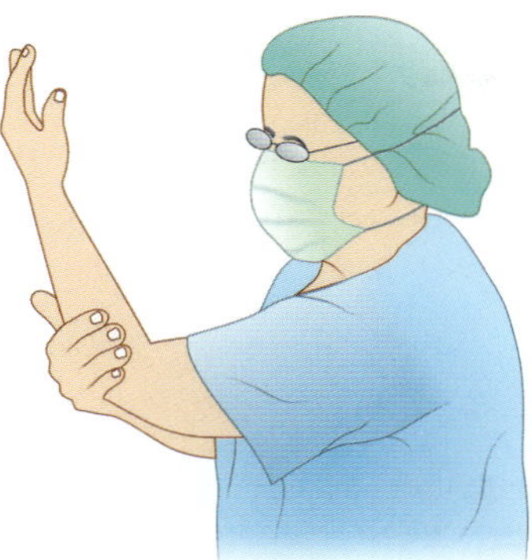

10

Smear the handrub on the left forearm up to the elbow. Ensure that the whole skin area is covered by using circular movements around the forearm until the handrub has fully evaporated (10–15 seconds)

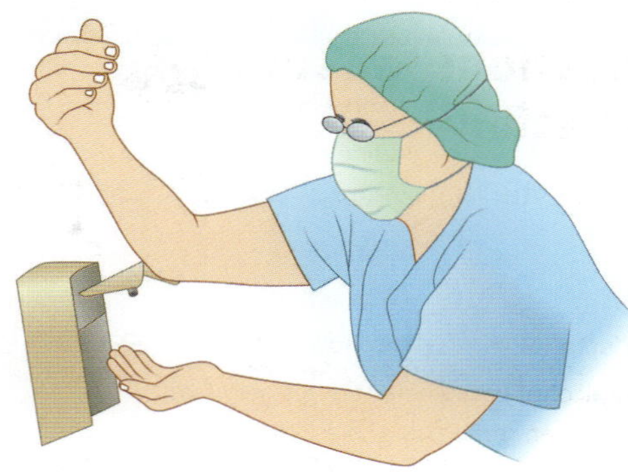

11

Put approximately 5 mL (3 doses) of alcohol-based handrub in the palm of your left hand, using the elbow of your other arm to operate the dispenser. Rub both hands at the same time up to the wrists, and ensure that all the steps represented in images 12–17 are followed (20–30 seconds)

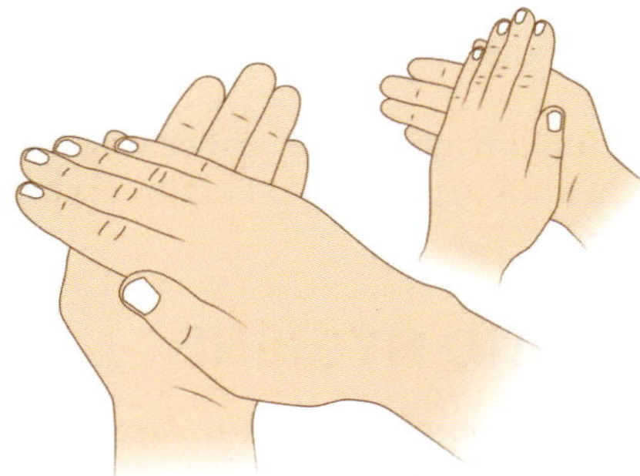

12

Cover the whole surface of the hands up to the wrist with alcohol-based handrub, rubbing palm against palm with a rotating movement

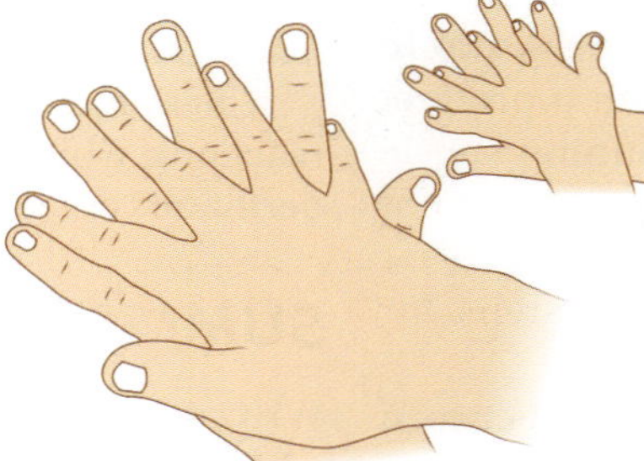

13

Rub the back of the left hand, including the wrist, moving the right palm back and forth and vice versa

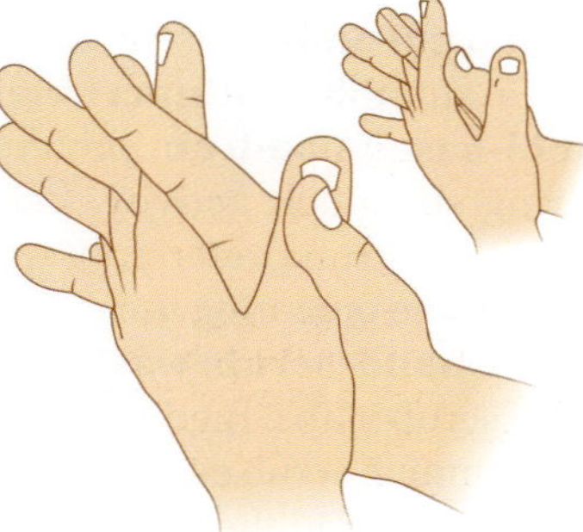

14

Rub palm against palm back and forth with fingers interlinked

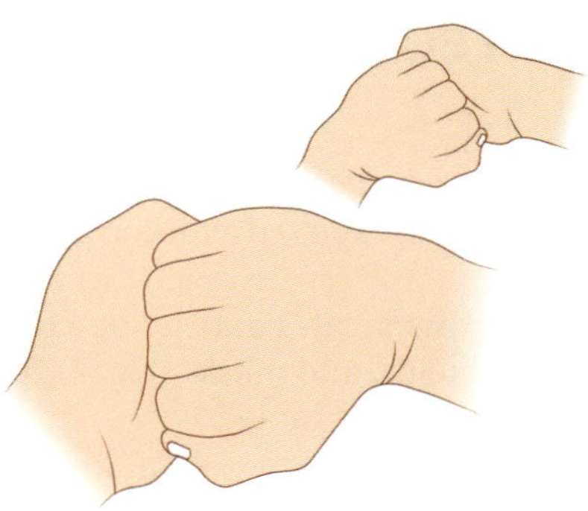

15

Rub the back of the fingers by holding them in the palm of the other hand with a sideways back-and-forth movement

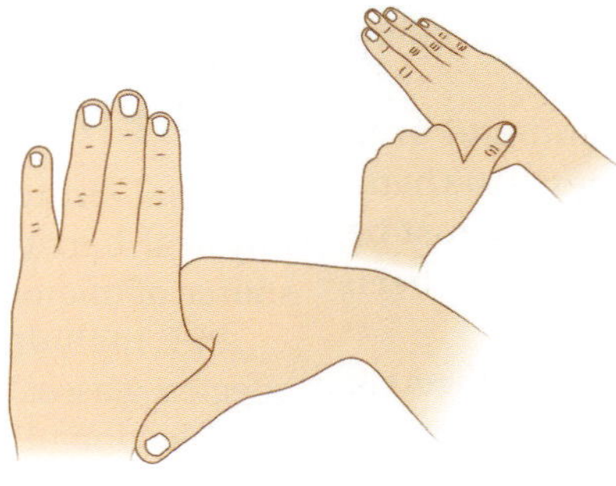

16

Rub the thumb of the left hand by rotating it in the clasped palm of the right hand and vice versa

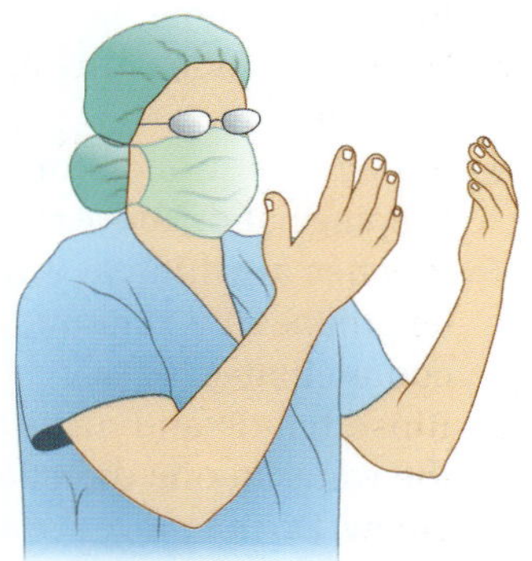

17

When the hands are dry, sterile surgical clothing and gloves can be donned

Repeat the above-illustrated sequence (average duration 60 seconds) according to the number of times corresponding to the total duration recommended by the manufacturer for surgical hand preparation with an alcohol-based handrub

Fig. 3: Illustration of surgical handwash.

Courtesy: WHO Guidelines on Hand Hygiene in Health Care. World Health Organization, 2009).[20]

Table 5: Chemicals causing contact dermatitis.

Irritant contact dermatitis (ICD)	*Allergic contact dermatitis (ACD)*
(In decreasing frequency)	Quaternary ammonium compounds
Iodophors	Iodine or iodophors
Chlorhexidine	Chlorhexidine
Chloroxylenol	Triclosan
Triclosan	Chloroxylenol
Alcohol-based products	Alcohols
ICD and ACD due to alcohol-based handrubs are very rare	

2. Sinks should be designed to reduce the risk of splashes.
3. If hands are visibly soiled, wash hands with plain soap before surgical hand preparation. Remove debris from underneath fingernails using a nail cleaner, preferably under running water.
4. Brushes are not recommended for surgical hand preparation.
5. Surgical hand antisepsis should be performed using either a suitable **antimicrobial soap or suitable alcohol-based handrub**, preferably with a product ensuring sustained activity, before donning sterile gloves. (Hand rub preferred if quality of water is not assured in the operating theatre).
6. **Surgical hand scrub/wash:** Procedural steps for surgical scrub with a medicated soap:
   a. Start timing. Scrub each side of each finger, between the fingers, and the back and front of the hand for 2 minutes.
   b. Proceed to scrub the arms, keeping the hand higher than the arm at all times. This helps to avoid recontamination of the hands by water from the elbows and prevents bacteria-laden soap and water from contaminating the hands.
   c. Wash each side of the arm from wrist to the elbow for 1 minute.
   d. Repeat the process on the other hand and arm, keeping hands above elbows at all times. If the hand touches anything at any time, the scrub must be lengthened by 1 minute for the area that has been contaminated.
   e. Rinse hands and arms by passing them through the water in one direction only, from fingertips to elbow. Do not move the arm back and forth through the water.
   f. Proceed to the operating theatre holding hands above elbows.
   g. At all times during the scrub procedure, care should be taken not to splash water onto surgical attire.
   h. Once in the operating theatre, hands and arms should be dried using a sterile towel and aseptic technique before donning gown and gloves.
7. **Surgical hand rub:** When using an alcohol-based surgical handrub product with sustained activity, follow the manufacturer's instructions for application times. Apply the product to dry hands only.

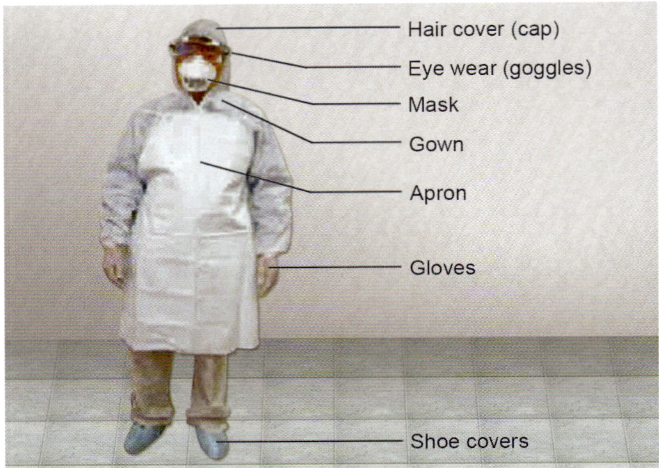

Fig. 4: Full personal protective equipment.[18]

Note: Do not combine surgical hand scrub and surgical hand rub.

Chemicals used for hand hygiene may cause adverse reactions, which include both irritant and allergic contact dermatitis as shown in Table 5.

SUMMARY OF HAND HYGIENE

WHO describes it as "My five moments for hand hygiene"; which states that HCWs should clean their hands:[20]

1. before touching a patient,
2. before clean/aseptic procedures,
3. after body fluid exposure/risk,
4. after touching a patient, and
5. after touching patient's surroundings

PERSONAL PROTECTIVE EQUIPMENT

Personal Protective Equipment (PPE) helps create a physical barrier between the exposed worker and the source of microorganisms.[8]

PPE includes gloves, gowns, lab coats, shoe covers, goggles, glasses with side shields, and masks (Fig. 4).[8]

Selection of protective barriers (Table 6).

GLOVES

Gloves are PPE for hands and may be made of materials like vinyl, latex, nitrile, etc.[22]

Key Points to be Remembered about Gloves

1. Gloves are for single-patient and single-procedure use only.

Table 6: Suggested PPE as per type of exposure (NACO).[21]

Type of exposure	*Examples*	*Protective barriers*
Low risk		
Contact with skin with no visible blood	Injections; Minor wound dressing	Gloves helpful but not essential
Medium risk		
Probable contact with blood; splash unlikely	Insertion or removal of intravenous canula; Handling of lab oratory specimens; Large open wounds dressing; Venepuncture, handling blood spills	Gloves, gowns and aprons may be necessary
High risk		
High chances of contact with blood, infected body fluid as well as splashing; uncontrolled bleeding	Major surgical procedures (e.g. oral surgery), endoscopy, vaginal delivery, uncontrolled bleeding	Gloves Water proof Gown or Apron Eye wear Mask

2. Technique for removing gloves should be a **glove-to-glove or skin-to-skin technique** to prevent contamination of hands.
3. Gloves often create a moist environment that facilitates the growth of microorganisms.
4. Gloves must be changed when:
   a. They become heavily soiled
   b. Between two patients
   c. Going from dirty to clean area in the same patient
5. Hand hygiene is of foremost importance in safe practices and the use of gloves does not replace the need for hand hygiene. Hands should be properly washed before the gloves are put on and after their removal.
6. Heavy duty rubber gloves should be worn for cleanings instruments, handling soiled linen or when dealing with spills

WHO describes method to don (Fig. 5A) and remove (Fig. 5B) gloves in a proper fashion.

GOWNS

Gowns must always be used especially when a splash of blood/body fluids is anticipated. Gowns can be either reusable or disposable.[18]

The steps of gown donning and removal are as follows:

Gown Donning[22] (Fig. 6)

1. Perform hand hygiene.
2. Put gown on, opening to the back.
3. Fasten both the neck and waist ties.

Gown Removal[22]

1. Unfasten ties and peel gown away from neck.
2. Slip fingers of one hand under the wrist cuff and pull hand inside.
3. With inside hand, push sleeve off with the other arm.
4. Fold dirty-to-dirty and roll into bundle (do not shake).
5. Discard in hamper.
6. Perform hand hygiene.

FACE PROTECTION

Face protection is an effective barrier to protect a worker's eyes, nose or mouth from splashes or aerosolized body fluids.[18]

Different types of face protection are a mask with safety glasses, a fall face shield, or a mask with an attached visor.[22]

Wearing a Mask and Safety Goggles[22] (Fig. 7)

1. Place mask over nose, mouth and chin
2. Fit flexible nose piece of mask over nose bridge
3. Secure on head with ties or elastic
4. Adjust to fit
5. Then position goggles over eyes and secure to the head using the ear pieces or headband
6. Adjust to fit comfortably.

BOOTS/SHOE COVERS

Boots/shoe covers are used to protect the wearer from splashes of blood, body fluids, secretions and excretions over feet. If using personal shoes, shoe covers should be worn so as to cover the shoes adequately.[18]

OCCLUSIVE BANDAGE

All skin defects like cuts and scratches must be covered with water-proof dressing before patient care.[7]

Overall the following steps should be followed while donning and removing PPE (Table 7):

Adverse Reactions to Gloves

Adverse reactions to latex glove are common. The allergy to latex can be prevented by the following measures: [23, 24]

1. Use of powder-free, low protein latex, and/or non-latex gloves
   a. Non-latex gloves include those containing neoprene (polychloroprene polymer), styrene butadiene block polymer, styrene ethylene butadiene co-polymer, nitrile (butadiene co-polymer), etc.

The purpose of this technique is to ensure maximum asepsis for the patient and to protect the healthcare worker from patient's body fluid. To achieve this goal, the skin of the healthcare worker remains exclusively in contact with the inner surface of the glove and has no contact with the outer surface. Any error in the performance of this technique leads to back of asepsis requiring a change of gloves.

A. How to don sterile gloves

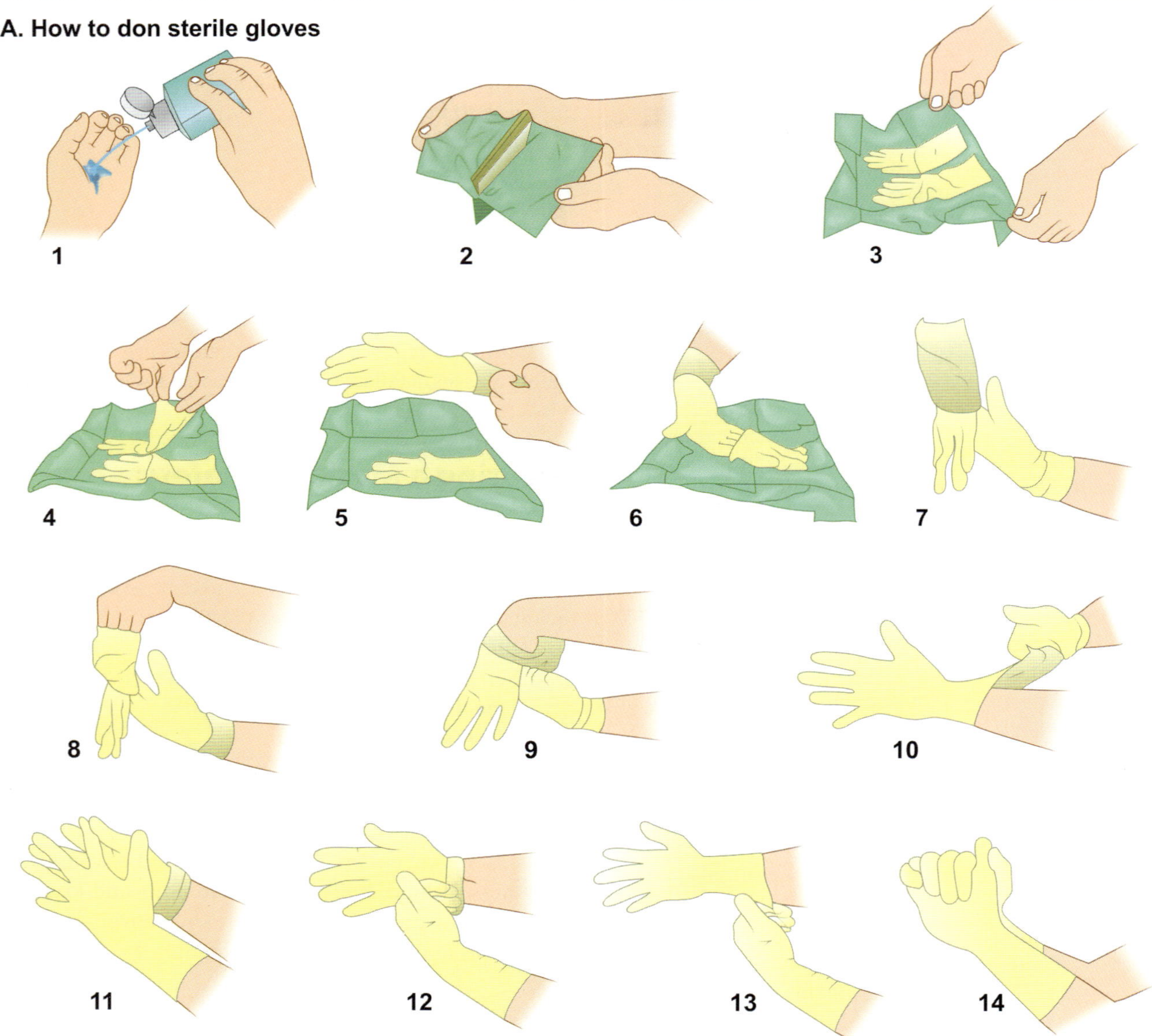

1. Perform hand hygiene before and "aseptic procedure" by hand rubbing or hand washing.
2. Check the package for integrity. Open the first non-sterile packaging by peeling it completely off the heat seal to expose the second sterile wrapper, but without touching it.
3. Place the second sterile package on a clean, dry surface without touching the surface. Open the package and fold it towards the bottom so as to unfold the paper and keep it open.
4. Using the thumb and index finger of one hand, carefully grasp the folded cuff edge of the glove.
5. Slip the other hand into the glove in a single movement, keeping the folded cuff at the wrist level.

6–7. Pick up the second glove by sliding the fingers of the gloved hand underneath the cuff of the glove.

8–10. In a single movement, slip the second glove on to the ungloved hand while avoiding any contact/resting of the gloved hand on surfaces other than the glove to be donned (contact/resting constitutes spaces until the gloves fit comfortably).

11. If necessary, after donning both gloves, adjust the fingers and interdigital spaces until the gloves fit comfortably.

12–13. Unfold the cuff of the first gloved hand by gently slipping the fingers of the other hand inside the fold, making sure to avoid any contact with a surface other than the outer surface of the glove (lack of asepsis requiring a change of glove).

14. The hands are gloved and must touch exclusively sterile devices or the previously disinfected patient's body area.

Contd...

Contd…

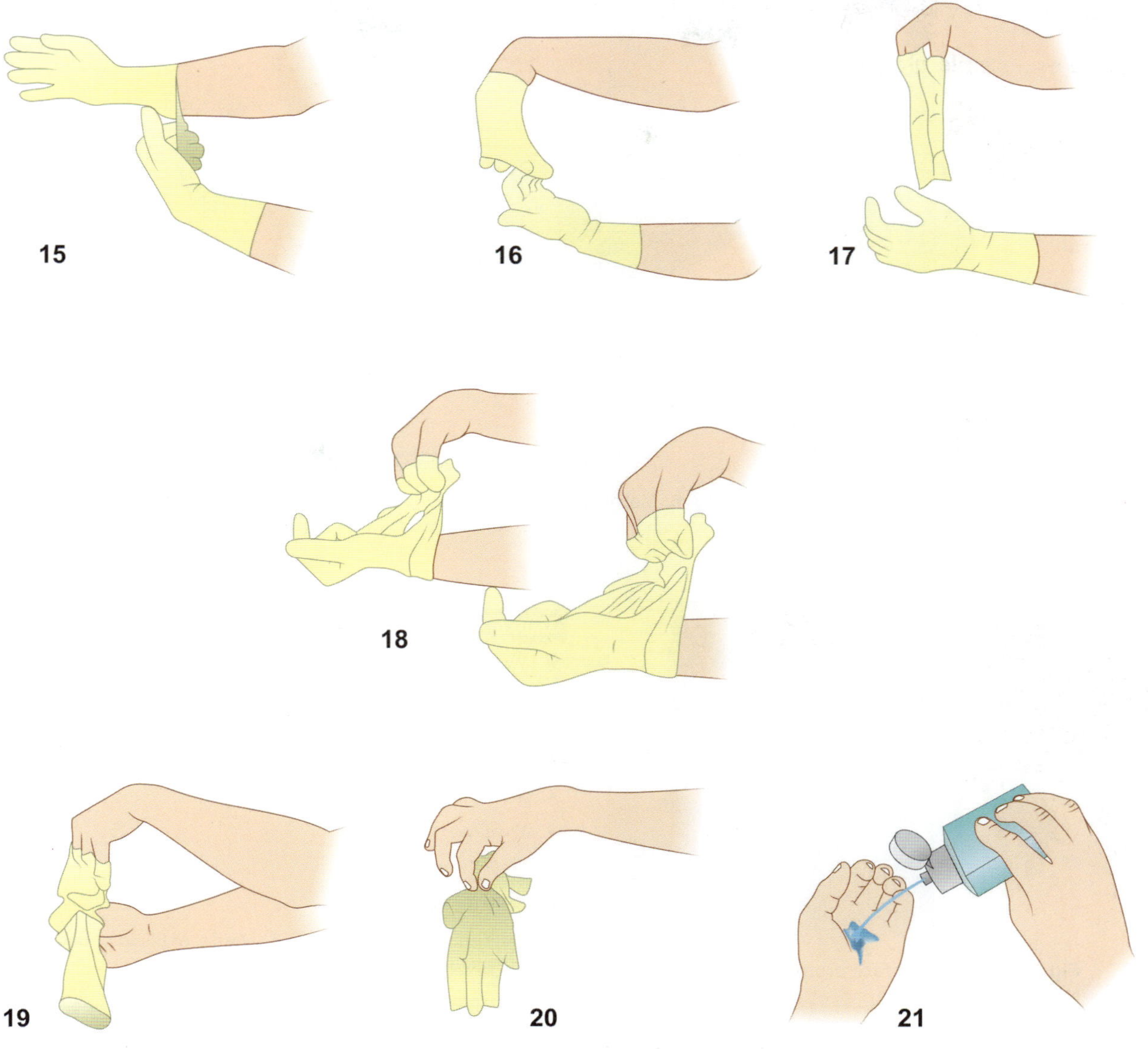

15–17. Remove the first glove by peeling it back with the fingers of the opposite hand. Remove the glove by rolling it inside out to the second finger joints (do not remove completely).

18. Remove the other glove by turning its outer edge on the fingers of the partially ungloved hand.

19. Remove the glove by turning it inside out entirely to ensure that the skin of the healthcare worker is always and exclusively in contact with the inner surface of the glove.

20. Discard gloves.

21. Perform hand hygiene after glove removal according to the recommended indications.

NB: Donning surgical sterile gloves at the time of a surgical intervention follows the same sequences except that:

- It is preceded by a surgical hand preparation;
- Donning gloves is performed after putting on the sterile surgical gown;
- The opening of the first packaging (non-sterile) is done by an assistant;
- The second packaging (sterile) is placed on a sterile surface other than that used for the intervention;
- Gloves should cover the wrists of the sterile gown.

Figs. 5A and B: (A) How to don sterile gloves; (B) How to remove sterile gloves.[20]

Courtesy: WHO Guidelines on Hand Hygiene in Health Care. World Health Organization, 2009.[20]

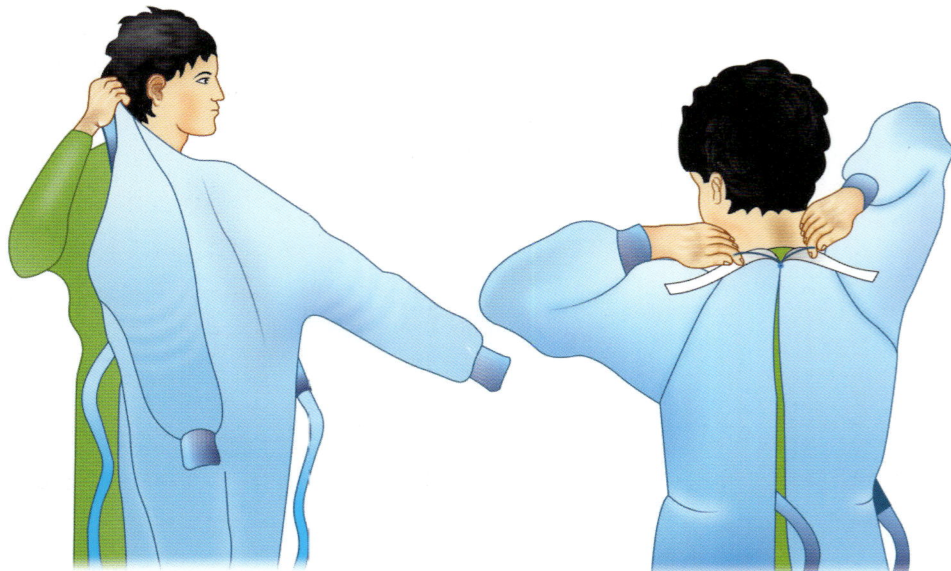

Fig. 6: Method to don gown.[22]

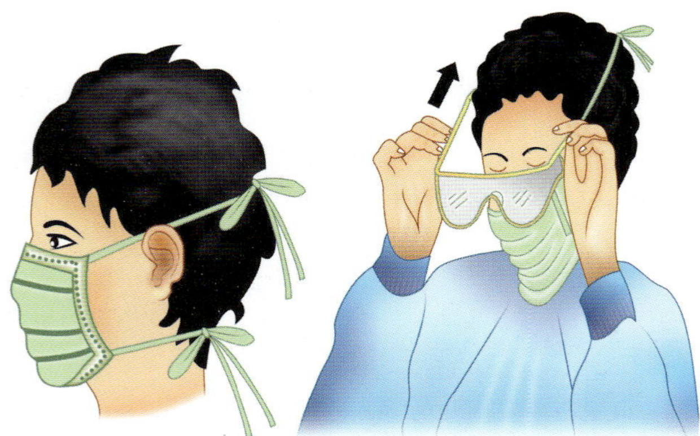

Fig. 7: How to wear face protection.[22]

b. Important to note: Vinyl gloves are not as effective as latex gloves against viral penetration (hence should not be used by dermatosurgeon; can be used by hospital kitchen workers etc.)

2. Good housekeeping practices to remove latex-containing dust from the workplace including:
   a. avoiding contact with eyes and face,
   b. handwashing after glove removal
   c. use of HEPA vacuum cleaners
3. Use of glove-liners
4. Attention to hand care and minimizing occlusion (prevents nonimmune irritant contact dermatitis)
5. OSHA guidelines suggest employers/hospitals to provide workers with education programs and periodic screening questionnaires related to latex allergy
6. "Hypoallergenic" gloves are usually made from latex so latex-sensitive workers should be careful while using them.

Table 7: Steps to wear and remove PPE.[18]

Steps to wear PPE
▪ Wash hands.
▪ Wear scrub suit or old set of thin clothes before entering the designated changing room or area.
▪ Wear boots or shoe covers with trousers tucked inside.
▪ Wash hands.
▪ Wear cap.
▪ Wear the mask.
▪ Wear the gown.
▪ Wear an impermeable apron if splashes of blood or body fluids are expected.
▪ Wear protective eye wear/goggles.
▪ Wash hands and dry them.
▪ Wear gloves with gown sleeve cuff tucked into glove.
Steps to remove PPE
Following the steps for removal of PPE in proper order is crucial as it prevents the HCP to get infected with contaminated PPE. The steps are:
▪ Remove gloves.
▪ Remove gown.
▪ Perform hand hygiene.
▪ Remove eye protection.
▪ Remove mask.
▪ Remove boots and place in appropriate container.
▪ Perform hand hygiene.

7. Latex proteins are water soluble. Manufacturing processes like washing, chlorination etc can reduce the burden of latex protein antigen.

SAFE PRACTICES TO USE SHARPS AND THEIR DISPOSAL

A dermatosurgeon has to come in contact with various sharps in his practice like disposable syringes and needles, scalpel, blade, hollow bore needles of IV cannula, suture needles and even instruments of electrosurgical/radiofrequency devices.

The most common form of occupational exposure to blood and the most likely to result in infection is needle-stick injury. The most common causes of needle-stick injury are two-handed recapping and the unsafe collection and disposal of sharps.[1]

Risk of Various Sharps Causing Injuries in a Hospital Set-up

Seven to 50% of exposures during operative procedures have some type of blood exposure to healthcare personnel (HCP) and in 2% to 15% of these exposures; the cause is a percutaneous injury, usually from a suture needle.[5]

Aggregate data from NaSH indicate that 6 devices are responsible for nearly 80% of all injuries.

Overall, hollow-bore needles are responsible for 56% of the injuries[5] (Table 8).

Unpublished data by CDC suggests that likelihood of injuries from sharp devices is[5]

1. After use and before disposal of a sharp device–in 40%
2. During use of a sharp device on a patient–41%
3. During or after disposal–15%

Hollow-bore Needle vs Solid Sharp Injuries[5]

Injuries from hollow-bore needles (e.g. needles used for blood collection or IV catheter insertion), are associated with an increased risk for HIV transmission because these devices are likely to contain residual blood. While solid sharps, such as suture needles and scalpels, generally deliver a smaller blood inoculum, especially if they first penetrate gloves or another barrier. Therefore, these may have lower risk for HIV transmission.

Table 8: Risk of various sharps causing percutaneous injuries in hospital set-up as per CDC.[5]

Type of sharps/devices causing percutaneous injuries	*Contribution in injuries in hospital set-up as per NaSH percentage*
Disposable syringes	30%
Suture needles	20%
Winged steel needles	12%
Scalpel blades	8%
Intravenous (IV) catheter stylets	5%
Phlebotomy needles	3%

According to CDC, in December 2001, out of the documented percutaneous exposures to HCPs which resulted in HIV seroconversion, 90% were due to hollow bore needles.[5]

GUIDELINES FOR SAFE PRACTICES BY CDC

Measures of safe practices and safe handling of sharps is dually advantageous and help protect both the healthcare provider and patient from exposure to the other's blood.

Work Practices to Prevent Sharp Injuries through the Use and Handling of a Device[5]

1. Before the beginning of a procedure that involves the use of a needle or other sharp device:
   a. Necessary equipment for performing a procedure available within arm's reach
   b. Adequate lighting and space to perform the procedure
   c. Sharps in a procedure tray should always point away from the operator
   d. Place sharps disposal container as close to the point-of-use as appropriate for immediate disposal of the sharp
   e. Obtain assistance from other staff or a family member to assist in calming or restraining the patient if the patient is likely to be uncooperative, combative, or confused.
   f. Inform the patient of what the procedure involves and explain the importance of avoiding any sudden movement that might dislodge the sharp.
2. During a procedure that involves the use of needles or other sharp devices:
   a. Double gloving.
   b. Maintain visual contact with the procedure site and location of the sharp device.
   c. When handling an exposed sharp, take care to avoid injury to oneself and other staff.
   d. Do not hand-pass exposed sharps from one person to another; use a predetermined neutral zone or tray for placing and retrieving used sharps. Verbally announce when sharps are being placed in a neutral zone.
   e. Use instruments, rather than fingers, to grasp needles, retract tissue, and load/unload needles and scalpels.
   f. Use alternative cutting methods such as blunt electrocautery and laser devices when appropriate.
   g. Use round-tipped scalpel blades instead of pointed sharp-tipped blades.
   h. Use of blunt suture needles is preferred.

   i. If the procedure necessitates reusing a needle multiple times on the same patient (e.g. giving local anesthesia), recap the needle between steps using techniques enumerated in next subsection.
3. During clean-up following a procedure:
   a. Visually inspect procedure trays and other surfaces like patient beds containing waste materials and sharps left inadvertently after the procedure.
   b. Transport reusable sharps in a closed container that has been secured to prevent the spillage of contents.
4. During disposal:
   a. Visually inspect the sharps container for hazards caused by overfilling.
   b. Make sure the sharps container being used is large enough to accommodate the entire device.
   c. Avoid bringing the hands close to the opening of a sharps container; never place hands or fingers into a container to facilitate disposal of a device.
   d. Keep the hands behind the sharp tip when disposing the device.
   e. If disposing of a sharp with attached tubing (e.g., winged steel needle), be aware that the tubing can recoil and lead to injury.
5. After disposal:
   a. Visually inspect sharps containers for evidence of overfilling before removal. If a sharps container is overfilled; take help of safety assistants, obtain a new container and use forceps to remove protruding devices and place them in it.
   b. Keep filled sharps containers in a secure area.
6. Improperly disposed sharps:
   a. If an improperly disposed sharp is encountered in the work environment, handle the device carefully, keeping the hands behind the sharp at all times.
   b. Use a mechanical device to pick up the sharp if it cannot be performed safely by hand.

Safe Recapping Procedures[25]

In situations where recapping is considered necessary, safe approaches are needed to be followed. The bottom line remains that the workers should never move an exposed needle tip towards an unprotected hand.

Following are some options (though they need to be further investigated for their safety potential):

1. Single-handed scooping
   a. Recapping by laying the cap on a flat surface and scooping it onto the tip of a syringe held in one hand
   b. Must keep the free hand away from the sheath and well behind the exposed needle.
2. Recapping devices:
   a. Some devices permit **single-handed recapping** by parking a needle cap on a flat surface.
   b. Some devices are designed to protect the hand that holds the cap during **two-handed recapping** procedures.

OTHER SHARPS[7]

1. Safe handling of sharps:
   a. Extreme care should be used to avoid auto-inoculation.
   b. All chipped or cracked glassware should be discarded in appropriate containers.
   c. Broken glass should be picked up with a brush and pan. Hands must never be used.
   d. The disposable needles should never be manipulated, bent, broken, recapped or removed from syringes.
   e. The used sharps should never be passed directly from one person to another.
   f. One should always dispose of his/her own sharps
   g. Used needles should be discarded in puncture-proof rigid containers (plastic or cardboard boxes) after disinfection in 0.5–1% freshly prepared sodium hypochlorite solution (common bleach).
   h. If a needle shredder is available, only the needles or the needles along with syringe nozzle may be shredded depending upon the type of the shredder
   i. Sharp disposal containers should be sent for disposal **when three-fourth full.**
2. Safe handling of specimens (blood etc.):
   a. Specimens, especially blood and body fluids should be collected in pre-sterilized screw-capped plastic containers properly sealed to prevent spillage or leakage.
3. Safe handling of blood/body fluid spills:
   a. In case of a spill of blood/body fluid in the OT, the area should be flooded with a disinfectant solution, e.g. freshly prepared 0.5–1% sodium hypochlorite solution and left for 30 minutes.
   b. After wearing gloves, the area should be covered with paper towels or gauze sponges to absorb the liquid followed by a thorough wash with soap and water.
   c. All contaminated materials should be disposed of as infectious waste.

HEALTH CARE WASTE MANAGEMENT AND DISPOSAL[26]

"Biomedical waste" means any waste, which is generated during the diagnosis, treatment or immunization of human beings or animals or in research activities pertaining thereto or in the production or testing of biological.

The waste disposal follows the rule of "Decontaminate-Disinfect-Dispose" (Table 9).

Notes:

1. Color coding of waste categories with multiple treatment options shall be selected depending on treatment option chosen.

Table 9: Categories of biomedical waste and color-coding and type of container for their disposal [as per the Biomedical Wastes (Management & Handling) Rules, by Ministry of Environment & Forests, India].[26]

Category no.	Waste category	Color coding and type of container	Treatment and disposal
1	Human anatomical waste (human tissues, organs, body parts)	Yellow (Plastic bag)	Incineration*/deep burial
3	Microbiology and biotechnology waste (wastes from laboratory cultures, vaccines, human and animal cell culture used in research, toxins, dishes and devices used for transfer of cultures)	Yellow (Plastic bag)	Yellow–incineration*
		Red (Disinfected container/plastic bag)	Red–local autoclaving/microwaving
4	Waste sharps (needles, syringes, scalpels, blades, glass, etc. that may cause puncture and cuts. This includes both used and unused sharps)	Blue/White translucent (Plastic bag/ puncture-proof container)	disinfection (chemical treatment**/ auto claving/microwaving and mutilation/shredding
5	Discarded medicines and cytotoxic drugs	Black (Plastic bag)	Incineration*/destruction and drugs disposal in secured landfills
6	Soiled waste (Items contaminated with blood, and body fluids including cotton, dressings, soiled plaster casts, lines, beddings, other material contaminated with blood)	Yellow (Plastic bag)	Yellow–incineration*
		Red (Disinfected container/plastic bag)	Red–local autoclaving/microwaving
7	Solid waste (wastes generated from disposable items other than the waste sharps, such as tubings, catheters, intravenous sets etc).	Red (Disinfected container/plastic bag)	Red–disinfection by chemical treatment** autoclaving/ microwaving
		Blue/White translucent (Plastic bag/puncture-proof container)	Blue/white translucent–disinfection by chemical treatment** autoclaving/ microwaving and mutilation/ shredding##
8	Liquid waste (waste generated from laboratory and washing, cleaning, house-keeping and disinfecting activities)	-	Disinfection by chemical treatment** and discharge into drains.

#- Only categories relevant to dermatosurgical practices are included.
** Chemicals treatment using at least 1% hypochlorite solution or any other equivalent chemical reagent. It must be ensured that chemical treatment ensures disinfection.
Mutilation/shredding must be such so as to prevent unauthorized reuse
*There will be no chemical pretreatment before incineration. Chlorinated plastics shall not be incinerated.

Table 10: Chemical disinfectants effective in inactivating HIV.

Solution	Strength of solution (in %)	Minimum time of contact for effective disinfection (in minutes)
Sodium hypochlorite solution*	1%	30
Ethanol	70%	3–5
2-propranol (isopropyl alcohol)	70%	3–5
Povidone iodine	2%	15
Formaline	4%	30
Glutaraldehyde (CIDEX)	2%	30
Hydrogen peroxide	6%	30

*Contains 10,000 ppm of chlorine. Household bleach contains 4–5% of available chlorine that may be diluted to form 1% available chlorine. Minimum contact time recommended is 30 minutes.

2. Waste collection bags for waste types needing incineration shall not be made of chlorinated plastics
3. Category 8 (liquid) does not require containers/bags.
4. Category 3, if disinfected locally, need not be put in containers/bags.

CHEMICAL DISINFECTANTS EFFECTIVE IN INACTIVATING HIV (TABLE 10)[27]

Post-Exposure Prophylaxis

Definition: Post-exposure prophylaxis (PEP) is short-term antiretroviral treatment to reduce the likelihood of HIV infection after potential exposure, either occupationally or through sexual intercourse.[28]

POST-EXPOSURE PROPHYLAXIS OF HIV

Six steps of PEP as advised by NACO are:[29,30]

Step 1: First Aid in Management of Exposure (Table 11)

For the skin: If the skin is broken after a needle-stick or sharp instrument:

- Immediately wash the wound and surrounding skin with water and soap, and rinse. Do not scrub.
- Do not use antiseptics or skin washes (bleach, chlorine, alcohol, betadine).

  After a splash of blood or body fluids on unbroken skin:
- Wash the area immediately
- Do not use antiseptics:

For the eye:

- Sit in a chair, tilt head back and irrigate exposed eye immediately with water or normal saline with the help of a colleague.
- If wearing contact lens, leave them in place while irrigating, as they form a barrier over the eye and will help protect it. Once the eye is cleaned, remove the contact lens and clean them in the normal manner. This will make them safe to wear again.
- Do not use soap or disinfectant on the eye.

For the mouth:

- Spit fluid out immediately
- Rinse the mouth thoroughly, using water or saline and spit again. Repeat this process several times
- Do not use soap or disinfectant in the mouth
- Consult the designated physician of the institution for management of the exposure immediately.

Table 11: Dos and Don'ts after exposure with HIV-infected blood/OPIM.

Dos	Don'ts
Remove gloves, if appropriate	Do not panic
Wash the exposed site thoroughly with running water	Do not put pricked finger in mouth
Irrigate with water or saline if eyes or mouth have been exposed	Do not squeeze wound to bleed it
Wash the skin with soap and water	Do not use bleach, chlorine, alcohol, betadine, iodine or any antiseptic or detergent
Do consult the designated physician immediately as per institutional guidelines for the management of the occupational exposure	

Step 2: Establish Eligibility for PEP

- The risk of infection transmission is proportional to the amount of HIV transmitted, which depends on the nature of exposure (Exposure Code-EC) and the status of the source patient (Status Code-SC).
- A baseline rapid HIV testing of exposed and source person after informed consent must be done for PEP.
- However, initiation of PEP should not be delayed while waiting for the results of HIV testing of the source of exposure.

First PEP Dose within 72 Hours—Window of Opportunity

- Start treatment, ideally within **two hours** but certainly within 72 hours; PEP is not effective after 72 hours of exposure.
- If the risk is insignificant, PEP could be discontinued, if already commenced.

Assessing Risk of Transmission

- Exposure is defined under three categories based on the amount of blood/fluid involved and the entry port. (Table 12).

Assess Exposed Individual

- The exposed individual should be sent to experienced physician for assessment.

Table 12: Exposure code (EC).

Categories of exposure	Definition and example
Mild exposure	Mucous membrane/non-intact skin with small volumes, e.g.: - a superficial wound (erosion of the epidermis) with a plain or low calibre needle - contact with the eyes or mucous membranes - subcutaneous injections following small-bore needles.
Moderate exposure	Mucous membrane/non-intact skin with large volumes OR percutaneous superficial exposure with solid needle, e.g. a cut or needlestick injury penetrating gloves
Severe exposure	Percutaneous with large volume, e.g.: - an accident with a high-calibre needle (>18 G) visibly contaminated with blood - a deep wound (hemorrhagic wound and/or very painful) transmission of a significant volume of blood - an accident with material that has previously been used intravenously or intra-arterially

The wearing of gloves during any of these accidents constitutes a protective factor.

Note: In case of an Accidental Exposure to blood (AEB) with material such as discarded sharps/needles, contaminated for over 48 hours, the risk of infection is negligible for HIV, but still remains significant for HBV. HBV survives longer than HIV outside the body.

Table 13: HIV PEP evaluation.

Exposure code (EC)	Status of source (SC)		
	HIV+ and asymptomatic	HIV+ and clinically symptomatic	HIV status unknown
Mild	Consider 2-drug PEP	Start 2-drug PEP	Usually no PEP or consider 2-drug PEP
Moderate	Start 2-drug PEP	Start 3-drug PEP	Usually no PEP or consider 2-drug PEP
Severe	Start 3-drug PEP	Start 3-drug PEP	Usually no PEP or consider 2-drug PEP

Table 14: PEP regimens.[31]

	Preferred regimen	Alternate regimen
2-drug regimen (Basic PEP regimen) (*Strong recommendation, low-quality evidence)	Tenofovir (TDF) 300 mg once daily + Lamivudine (3TC) 150 mg twice daily or 300 mg once daily *	Tenofovir (TDF) 300 mg once daily + Emtricitabine (FTC) 200 mg once daily*
3-drug regimen ## (Expanded PEP regimen) (Consult expert opinion)	Lopinavir/ritonavir (LPV/r)** 400/100 mg twice a day or 800/200 mg once daily with meals Atazanavir/ritonavir (ATV/r)** 300 mg + 100 mg once daily	Raltegravir (RAL) 400 mg twice daily Darunavir/ritonavir (DRV/r)** 800 mg + 100 mg once daily or 600 mg + 100 mg twice daily
(Basic regimen plus a protease inhibitor) (Conditional recommendation, very low-quality evidence)		Efavirenz (EFV)# 600 mg once daily
Not recommended	ddI + d4T combination NNRTI such as Nevirapine should not be used in PEP because of ADR and hepatotoxicity in immunocompetent HCW	

#If protease inhibitor is not available and the 3rd drug is indicated, one can consider using Efavirenz (EFV 600 mg once daily). Monitoring should be instituted for side effects of this drug e.g. CNS toxicity such as nightmares, insomnia etc.

##The latest guidelines recommend three-drug regimen for everyone, for three reasons—simplified prescription; availability of less toxic and better tolerated medications; and this removes the need to obtain information about drug resistance risk. The two-drug regimen is now prescribed when there is non availability of third drug (in resource restricted set-ups) and where the risk of additional toxicity outweighs the benefit.

**Ritonavir requires refrigeration.

- Exposed individuals who are known or discovered to be HIV positive should not receive PEP.

Step 3

- Counselling for PEP
  - Exposed persons should be sent to experienced HIV care physician for appropriate counselling.

Note:

- Exposed person known or discovered to be HIV positive is not eligible for PEP and should be sent for assessment for initiation of ART
- It should be clear that PEP is not mandatory
- Document exposure
  - Documentation of exposure is essential. Special leave from work should be considered for a period of two weeks.

Step 4

- Prescribe PEP
- Deciding on PEP regimen
  - There are two types of regimens:
    1. Basic regimen: 2-drug combination
    2. Expanded regimen: 3-drug combination

The decision to initiate the type of regimen depends on the type of exposure and HIV serostatus of the source person (Table 13).

- Duration of PEP–4 weeks
- Seek expert opinion in case of:
  - Delay in reporting exposure (> 72 hours).
  - Unknown source
  - Known or suspected pregnancy, but initiate PEP
  - Breastfeeding mothers, but initiate PEP
  - Source patient is on ART
  - Major toxicity of PEP regimen.

Step 5

- HIV chemoprophylaxis (Table 14)[29-31]
- ARV drugs during pregnancy:
  - None of the current ARV drug regimens recommended for post-exposure prophylaxis are contraindicated for pregnant women.[31]

ARV Drugs during Breastfeeding

Breastfeeding should not contraindicate postexposure prophylaxis, but the risks and benefits of continuing breastfeeding while HIV transmission risk is unknown should be discussed with the mother.[31]

- Side-effects and adherence to PEP:
  - More side effects, most commonly nausea and fatigue, among HCP taking PEP than PLHAs taking ART.
  - Occur mainly at the beginning of the treatment and include nausea, diarrhea, muscular pain and headache.
  - Most side-effects are mild and transient.
  - Anemia and/or leucopenia and/or thrombocytopenia may occur during the month of treatment.
  - Side effects can be reduced through medications.
  - A complete blood count and liver function tests (transaminases) may be performed at the beginning of treatment (as baseline) and after 4 weeks.
  - Adherence: More than 95% adherence is important in order to maximize the efficacy of the medication in PEP. Recent evidence shows PEP uptake has been insufficient: only 57% of the people who initiated PEP have completed the full course.[28] To improve uptake and completion of PEP, WHO recommends providing the full 28-day course at first visit, rather than requiring patients to return multiple times for prescriptions.[28]

Step 6

- Follow-up of an exposed person:
  - Whether or not PEP is started, a follow up is needed to monitor for possible infections and to provide psychological support.
  - Exposed persons should have post-PEP HIV tests. HIV-test at 3 months and again at 6 months is recommended. If the test at 6 months is negative, no further testing is recommended.

POST-EXPOSURE PROPHYLAXIS OF HEPATITIS B

Routine Hepatitis B Immunization of All HCP[1,17]

- Routine immunization of all HCP (including nursing staff and sweepers, cleaners) comes under universal precautions.
- They should be vaccinated against the hepatitis B virus. The vaccination for Hepatitis B consists of 3 doses: initial, 1 month, and 6 months. Most (99%) seroconvert after completing the full course.

Efficacy of PEP for HBV

Percutaneous exposure from HBsAg positive blood:

- Multiple doses of HBIG initiated within 1 week- offers 75% protection
- Combination of HBIg with hepatitis B vaccine series- increase to 85–95% protection.

Recommendations for HBV post-exposure management (Table 15).

PEP for HBV during pregnancy and lactation.

HBIG and hepatitis B vaccine are not a contraindication to pregnancy and lactation.[17]

POST-EXPOSURE PROPHYLAXIS OF HEPATITIS C

Immune globulin and antiviral agents (e.g. interferon with or without ribavirin) are not recommended for PEP of hepatitis C. Because 15–25% of patients with acute HCV infection spontaneously resolve their infection, treatment of these patients during the acute phase could expose them

Table 15: Recommendations for HBV postexposure management.[17,32]

Vaccination and antibody response status of exposed workers	Treatment		
	Source HBsAG positive	Source HBsAG negative	Source unknown or not available for testing
Unvaccinated	HBIG (0.06 mL/kg IM) x 1 and Hep B vaccination series	Hep B vaccination series	Hep B vaccination series
Previously vaccinated			
Responder [i.e. with adequate levels of serum antibody to HBsAg (i.e. anti-HBs >10 mIU/mL)]	No treatment	No treatment	No treatment
Non-responder (i.e. serum anti-HBs < 10 mIU/mL)	HBIG (0.06 mL/kg IM) x 1 and revaccinate OR HBIG (0.06 mL/kg IM) x 2 (at the time of exposure and 1 month after exposure)	No treatment	If known high risk source, treat as if source is HBsAg (+)
Ab response unknown	Test-exposed person for anti-HBs Ab: 1. If adequate, no PEP necessary 2. If inadequate, administer HBIG x 1 and vaccine booster	No treatment	Test-exposed person for anti-HBs: 1. If adequate, no PEP necessary 2. If inadequate, give vaccine booster and recheck titer in 1–2 months

unnecessarily to the discomfort and side effects of antiviral therapy (interferon ± ribavirin).[17]

In the absence of PEP for HCV, recommendations for post-exposure management are intended to achieve early identification of chronic disease and, if present, referral for evaluation of treatment options.[17]

Recommended investigations following occupational exposure to HCV:[32]

- For the source, perform testing for anti-HCV
- Perform baseline and follow-up testing for anti-HCV and alanine aminotransferase (ALT) 4–6 months after exposures.
- Perform HCV RNA at 4–6 weeks if earlier diagnosis of HCV infection desired.
- Confirm repeatedly reactive anti-HCV enzyme immunoassays (EIAs) with supplemental tests.
- When HCV infection is identified early, the person should be referred for medical management to a specialist.

SUMMARY OF UNIVERSAL PRECAUTIONS[33]

- Handwashing:
  - After touching blood, bodily fluids, secretions, excretions and contaminated items
  - Immediately after removing gloves
  - Before contact with next patient.
- Gloves:
  - For contact with blood, bodily fluids, secretions and contaminated items
  - For contact with mucous membranes and non-intact skin.
- Masks, Goggles, Face Masks:
  - Protect mucous membranes of eyes, nose and mouth when contact with blood and bodily fluids is anticipated.
- Gowns:
  - Protect skin from blood or bodily fluid contact
  - Prevent soiling of clothing during procedures that may involve contact with blood or bodily fluids.
- Linen:
  - Handle soiled linens so that they do not touch skin/mucous membranes
  - Do not pre-rinse soiled linens.
- Patient Care Equipment:
  - Handle soiled equipment in a manner that prevents contact with skin or mucous membranes and to prevent contamination of clothing or the environment
  - Clean reusable equipment before reusing it.
- Environmental Cleaning:
  - Routine care, cleaning, and disinfection of equipment and furnishings in patient care areas.
- Sharps:
  - Avoid recapping used needles
  - Avoid removing used needles from disposable syringes
  - Avoid bending, breaking, or manipulating used needles by hand
  - Place used sharps in puncture-resistant containers.
- Patient Resuscitation:
  - Use mouthpieces, resuscitation bags, or other ventilation devices to avoid mouth-to-mouth resuscitation.
- Patient Placement:
  - Place patients who contaminate the environment or cannot maintain appropriate hygiene in private rooms.

CONCLUSION

Universal precautions every time, everywhere is the key to prevention of infection with blood borne pathogens and there is no substitute.

GLOSSARY

1. *Blood-borne Pathogens* means pathogenic microorganisms that are present in human blood and can cause disease in humans. These pathogens include, but are not limited to, hepatitis B virus (HBV) and human immunodeficiency virus (HIV).[34]
2. *Other Potentially Infectious Materials (OPIM)* means (1) The following human body fluids: semen, vaginal secretions, cerebrospinal fluid, synovial fluid, pleural fluid, pericardial fluid, peritoneal fluid, amniotic fluid, saliva in dental procedures, any body fluid that is visibly contaminated with blood, and all body fluids in situations where it is difficult or impossible to differentiate between body fluids; (2) Any unfixed tissue or organ (other than intact skin) from a human (living or dead); and (3) HIV-containing cell or tissue cultures, organ cultures, and HIV- or HBV-containing culture medium or other solutions; and blood, organs, or other tissues from experimental animals infected with HIV or HBV.[34]
3. *Occupational Exposure* means reasonably anticipated skin, eye, mucous membrane, or parenteral contact with blood or other potentially infectious materials that may result from the performance of an employee's dutie.[34]
4. *Source Individual* means any individual, living or dead, whose blood or other potentially infectious materials may be a source of occupational exposure to the employee.[34]
5. *Universal Precautions* is an approach to infection control. According to the concept of Universal Precautions, all human blood and certain human body fluids are treated as if known to be infectious for HIV, HBV, and other blood-borne pathogens.[34]

6. *Routine practices/Standard precautions* are a combination of universal precautions and body substance isolation (BSI- which includes guidelines for body secretions such as urine, vomitus, feces, or sputum are not controlled under universal precautions).[8] For further details visit.[35]

Abbreviations

AEB	Accidental Exposure to blood
ALT	Alanine AminoTransferase
ACD	Allergic Contact Dermatitis
CMV	Cytomegalovirus
EIAs	Enzyme Immunoassays
EBV	Epstein Barr Virus
EC1	Exposure Code
FDC	Fixed Dose Combination
HCW	Health Care Workers
HCP	Healthcare Personnel
HEPA	High Efficiency Particulate Air
HBV	Hepatitis B virus
HCV	Hepatitis C virus
HGV	Hepatitis G virus
HTLV	Human T lymphotropic Viruses
IV	Intravenous
ICD	Irritant Contact Dermatitis
MMWR	Morbidity and Mortality Weekly Reports
NACO	National AIDS Control Organization
NaSH	National Surveillance System for HCWs
OSHA	Occupational Safety and Health Administration
OPIM	Other Potentially Infectious Materials
PPE	Personal Protective Equipment
PEP	Post-exposure Prophylaxis
TEWL	Trans-Epidermal Water Loss

REFERENCES

1. World Health Organization (2003). AIDE-MEMOIRE for a strategy to protect health workers from infection with blood borne virus. World Health Organization 2003. [online] WHO website. Available from www.who.int/injection_safety/toolbox/docs/en/AM_HCW_Safety.pdf [Accessed on April, 2017].
2. Siegel JD, Rhinehart E, Jackson M, et al. 2007. Guideline for Isolation Precautions: Preventing Transmission of Infectious Agents in Healthcare Settings. [online] CDC website. Available from www.cdc.gov/ncidod/dhqp/pdf/isolation2007.pdf [Accessed April, 2017].
3. Centers for Disease Control and Prevention. Perspectives in Disease Prevention and Health Promotion Update: Universal Precautions for Prevention of Transmission of Human Immunodeficiency Virus, Hepatitis B Virus, and Other Blood Borne Pathogens in Health-Care Settings. MMWR Recommendations and Reports 2017. [online] CDC website. Available from wonder.cdc.gov/wonder/prevguid/p0000255/p0000255.asp [Accessed April, 2017].
4. Last JM. Universal Precautions. Encyclopedia of Public Health. 2002. [online] Encyclopedia website. Available from www.encyclopedia.com/doc/1G2-3404000889.html [Accessed April, 2017].
5. Centers for Disease Control and Prevention. Workbook for designing, implementing, and evaluating a sharps injury prevention program. 2008. [online] CDC website. Available from www.cdc.gov/sharpssafety/pdf/sharpsworkbook_2008.pdf [Accessed April, 2017].
6. Food and Drug Administration. Blunt-Tip Surgical Suture Needles Reduce Needlestick Injuries and the Risk of Subsequent Bloodborne Pathogen Transmission to Surgical Personnel: FDA, NIOSH and OSHA Joint Safety Communication. 2015. [online] FDA website. Available from www.fda.gov/MedicalDevices/Safety/AlertsandNotices/ucm305757.htm [Accessed April, 2017].
7. National Institute of Communicable Diseases and NACO. 1999. HIV Testing Manual: Laboratory Diagnosis, Biosafety and Quality Control. [online] NICD website. Available from www.nicd.nic.in/writereaddata/linkimages/194.doc [Accessed April, 2017].
8. Canadian Centre for Occupational Health and Safety. Routine Practices. 2011. [online] CCOHS website. Available from www.ccohs.ca/oshanswers/prevention/universa.html [Accessed April, 2017].
9. World Health Organization. Ebola Situation Report. 2015. [online] WHO website. Available from apps.who.int/iris/bitstream/10665/159060/1/roadmapsitrep_25Mar2015_eng.pdf?ua=1&ua=1 [Accessed April, 2017].
10. Daral S, Singh SK, Khokhar A. Ebola virus: Awareness about the disease and personal protective measures among junior doctors of a tertiary hospital in Delhi, India. 2015. [online] IJMEDPH website. Available from www.ijmedph.org/sites/default/files/IntJMedPublicHealth_2015_5_3_217_161524.pdf [Accessed April, 2017].
11. Centers for Disease Control and Prevention. Guidance on Personal Protective Equipment (PPE) To Be Used By Healthcare Workers during Management of Patients with Confirmed Ebola or Persons under Investigation (PUIs) for Ebola who are Clinically Unstable or Have Bleeding, Vomiting, or Diarrhea in U.S. Hospitals, Including Procedures for Donning and Doffing PPE. 2015. [online] CDC website. Available from www.cdc.gov/vhf/ebola/healthcare-us/ppe/guidance.html [Accessed April, 2017].
12. National Health Portal India. Zika virus disease. 2016. [online] NHP website. Available from www.nhp.gov.in/disease/communicable-disease/zika-virus-disease [Accessed April, 2017].
13. World Health Organization. Zika virus. (2016). [online] WHO website. Available from www.who.int/mediacentre/factsheets/zika/en/ [Accessed April, 2017].
14. Mathur P, Singh S. Multidrug resistance in bacteria: A serious patient safety challenge for India. J Lab Physicians. 2013;5(1):5-10.
15. Hayden MK, Bonten MJ, Blom DW, et al. Reduction in acquisition of vancomycin-resistant Enterococcus after enforcement of routine environmental cleaning measures. Clin Infect Dis. 2006;42(11):1552-60.
16. Morgan DJ, Rogawski E, Thom KA, et al. Transfer of multidrug-resistant bacteria to healthcare workers' gloves and gowns after patient contact increases with environmental contamination. Crit Care Med. 2012;40(4):1045-51.
17. Centers for Disease Control and Prevention. Updated US Public Health Service Guidelines for the Management

of Occupational Exposures to HBV, HCV, and HIV and Recommendations for Postexposure Prophylaxis. 2001/50(RR11);1-42. [online] CDC website. Available from www.cdc.gov/mmwr/preview/mmwrhtml/rr5011a1.htm [Accessed April, 2017].

18. World Health Organization. Practical Guidelines for Infection Control in Health Care Facilities. WHO Regional Office for South East Asia/WHO Regional Office for the Western Pacific 2004; SEARO Regional Publication No. 41: pp. 76-101, 2017. [online] WPRO website. Available from www.wpro.who.int/NR/rdonlyres/006EF250-6B11-42B4-BA17-C98D413BE8B8/0/practical_guidelines_infection_control.pdf.
19. Centers for Disease Control and Prevention. (2002). Guideline for Hand Hygiene in Health-Care Settings: Recommendations of the Health care Infection Control Practices Advisory Committee and the HICPAC/SHEA/APIC/IDSA Hand Hygiene Task Force. MMWR 2002;51(No. RR- 16):[3,22]. [online] CDC website. Available from www.cdc.gov/mmwr/PDF/rr/rr5116.pdf [Accessed April, 2017].
20. World Health Organization. WHO Guidelines on Hand Hygiene in Health Care 2009. Available from whqlibdoc.who.int/publications/2009/9789241597906_eng.pdf [Accessed April, 2017].
21. National AIDS Control Organization, Indian Nursing Council. Training Manual for Auxiliary Nurse Midwives (ANM). 2012. [online] NACO website. Available from naco.gov.in/sites/default/files/Website%20file%20ANM%20English.pdf. [Accessed April, 2017].
22. Centers for Disease Control and Prevention. Guidance for the Selection and Use of Personal Protective Equipment (PPE) in Healthcare Settings. 2016. [online] CDC website. Available from www.cdc.gov/ncidod/dhqp/pdf/ppe/PPEslides6-29-04.ppt [Accessed April, 2017].
23. Reddy S. Latex Allergy. American Family Physician. 2017. [online] AAFP website. Available from www.aafp.org/afp/980101ap/reddy.html [Accessed April, 2017].
24. Canadian Centre for Occupational Health and Safety. Latex Allergy. 2009. [online] CCOHS website. Available from www.ccohs.ca/oshanswers/diseases/latex.html [Accessed April, 2017].
25. Canadian Centre for Occupational Health and Safety. Needlestick and Sharp Injuries. 2005. [online] CCOHS website. Available from http://www.ccohs.ca/oshanswers/diseases/needlestick_injuries.html [Accessed April, 2017].
26. Ministry of Environment & Forests. The Biomedical Wastes (Management & Handling) Rules, Ministry Of Environment & Forests 1998/2000. 1998. [online] ENVFOR website. Available from envfor.nic.in/legis/hsm/biomed.html [Accessed April, 2017].
27. Ministry of Health & Family Welfare. Manual for Control of Hospital Associated Infections, National AIDS Control Organization. Government of India: Ministry of Health & Family Welfare; 1999. pp. 47-8.
28. World Health Organization. Post-exposure prophylaxis to prevent HIV infection. Fact sheet - 1 December 2014. [online] WHO website. Available from www.who.int/hiv/topics/prophylaxis/info/en/ [Accessed April, 2017].
29. UP State Aids Control Society. Post Exposure Prophylaxis (PEP)- NACO guidelines. 2016. [online] UPSACS website. Available from upsacs.nic.in/PEP.pdf [Accessed April, 2017].
30. NACO, Ministry of Health and Family Welfare. Antiretroviral Therapy Guidelines for HIV-infected Adults and Adolescents including Post-exposure Prophylaxis, NACO, Ministry of Health and Family Welfare, Government of India. 2007. [online] NACO website. Available from naco.gov.in/sites/default/files/1.%20Antiretroviral%20Therapy%20Guidelines%20for%20HIV-Infected%20Adults%20and%20Adolescents%20Including%20Post-exposure.pdf [Accessed April, 2017].
31. World Health Organization. Post-exposure prophylaxis for HIV. Supplementary section to the 2013 WHO consolidated guidelines on the use of antiretroviral drugs for treating and preventing HIV infection, Chapter 5 - Clinical guidelines across the continuum of care: HIV diagnosis and ARV drugs for HIV prevention. 2014. pp. 15-21. [online] WHO website. www.who.int/hiv/pub/guidelines/arv2013/December2014-ARVsupplement-chap5.pdf?ua=1 [Accessed April, 2017].
32. Beal J, Deitrick L, Janelle J, Orrick JJ (Eds). Pre-Exposure Prophylaxis (PrEP), Non-Occupational Post-Exposure Prophylaxis (nPEP) and Occupational PEP (oPEP). Florida/Carribean AIDS education and training center (FCAETC). 2015. [online] FCAETC website. Available from www.fcaetc.org/treatments/PrEPPEP.pdf [Accessed April, 2017].
33. National AIDS Control Organization. Operational guidelines for programme managers and service providers for strengthening STI/RTI services. National AIDS Control Organization. Ministry of Health and Family Welfare Government of India. October 2007. [online] NACO website. Available from http://naco.gov.in/sites/default/files/21%2C%20Operational%20Guidelines%20STI%20RTI.pdf [Accessed April, 2017].
34. Occupational Safety and Health Administration. Bloodborne pathogens, Appendix A. [Standard number:1910.1030]. Part Title: Occupational Safety and Health Standards. 2016. [online] OSHA website. Available from www.osha.gov/pls/oshaweb/owadisp.show_document?p_table=STANDARDS&p_id=10051#1910.1030(b) [Accessed April, 2017].
35. World Health Organization. Aide Memoire. Standard precautions in health care. 2007. [online] WHO website. Available from www.who.int/csr/resources/publications/EPR_AM2_E7.pdf [Accessed April, 2017].

Chapter

8

Dermatosurgical Instruments

Anirudha Gulanikar

Key Messages

- Proper knowledge of instruments is important to ensure optimal safety and surgical outcome.
- High-quality instruments, even if they are of high cost, should be preferred—they have longer shelf life and greater precision.
- Proper maintenance, cleaning and disinfection enhance safety.
- Proper training of staff is needed for proper care of instruments.
- Care should be taken to avoid injury to the surgeon during surgery.

Surgery or Cheirourgia, which is a Greek word—"cheir" meaning "hand" + "ergon" meaning "work", is the branch of medicine that deals with the physical manipulation of a bodily structure to diagnose, prevent, or cure an ailment. The history of surgical instruments can go back to stone ages. *Sushruta* is considered as the "founding father of surgery. Sushruta is known for one of the oldest known surgical texts in Sanskrit- The Sushruta Samhita and the instruments for cosmetic surgery. The Early modern era of surgery starts from Hippocrates, Celcus and Galen. The scientific surgery starts from John Hunter (1728-93). Joseph Lister developed antiseptic in surgery.

As surgical technology evolves continuously, so does the type and complexity of surgical instruments. Surgical instruments require special care and handling to maintain proper function and longevity. This is dependent solely on knowledge of the instruments and how they are used. The names are difficult, the differences are minute, and the uses and handling for each instrument even more obscure. The surgeon and the staff in operating room must be well trained with instruments they are handling.

While some of these are specific for each surgery (such as those for vitiligo surgery, hair transplantation, liposuction, etc.), others are common and basic. Such basic and common instruments have been discussed in this chapter, while specific instruments have been mentioned in the corresponding chapters.

SURGICAL EQUIPMENT

Operating Table

The installation of a high-quality surgical table is preferred. The table makes the patient more comfortable and provides easy access for the surgeon. The adjustability and dimensions of the table are important parameters to be considered. Powered tables with foot-operated or fingertip controls are the most desirable. Adjustments in back and foot elevation are essential for the patient's comfort. The tilt positioning of the table is important, because it enables the physician to change the angle of the table (Fig. 1). Both manual and automatic tables are available. Automatic tables are preferred for ease of maneuvering. Additional attachments to be considered include a U-shaped head arm rest for hair transplantation.

Trolley and Stands

The trolleys and stands with their adjustable heights allow for easy access to the instruments. A table unit with 4–6 wheels is the most maneuverable and stable, and can be moved during the procedure as per requirement and convenience (Figs. 2 and 3).

Waste Containers

Well-equipped surgical suites should include kick-bucket waste containers. These waste containers are made of either plastic (Fig. 4) or stainless steel with rubber baskets.

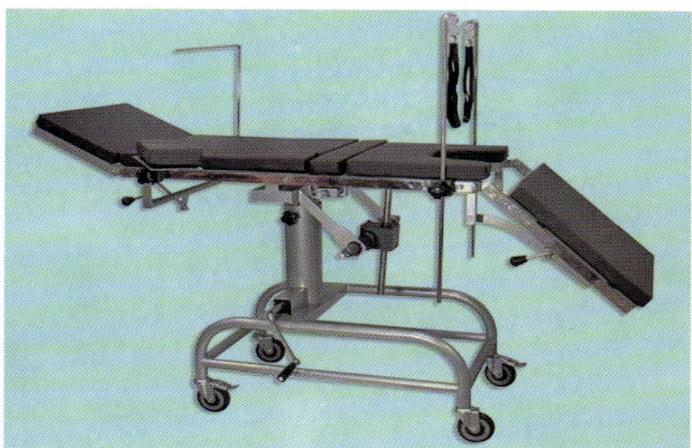

Fig. 1: Operating table.

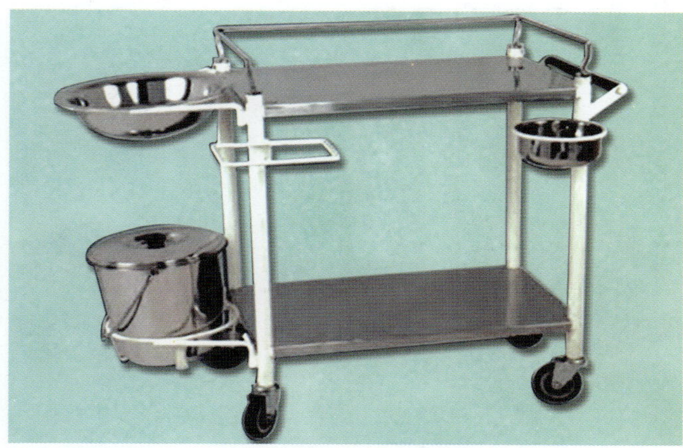

Fig. 2: Instrument trolley.

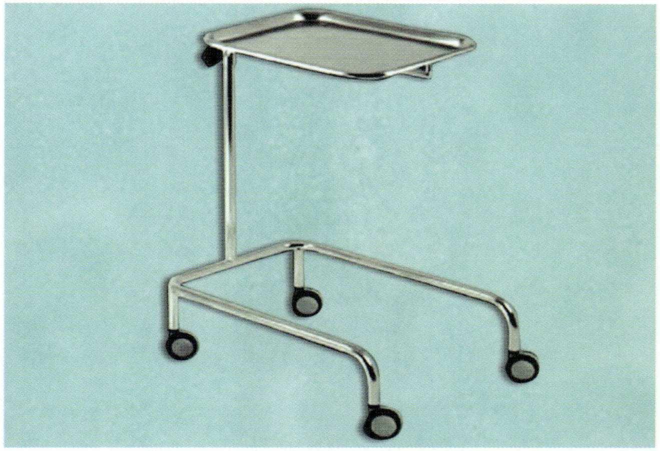

Fig. 3: Mayos trolley.

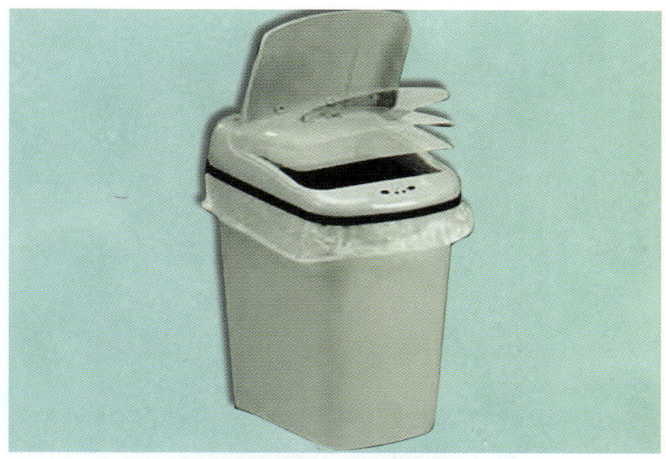

Fig. 4: Plastic waste disposal container.

They can be mounted on wheels, have a protective hard rubber, and steel rim that the staff can use to move the bucket with their feet during the procedure.

Monitoring Equipment

Monitoring equipment should be available, so that the staff can determine the patient's pulse, blood pressure, electrical cardiac activity and blood oxygen saturation at a glance. Pulse oximeters of different types are available. Digital pulse oximeters are small, which are attached to the patient's finger and show only pulse rate and oxygen saturation. These are adequate for most skin surgeries. Larger pulse oximeters show other parameters such as blood pressure (Fig. 5) and may be used for extensive surgeries such as liposuction. The data should be recorded by the attending personnel.

Medical Gases

Oxygen cylinders should be available, preferably more than one. Nitrous oxide and compressed air are the gases that are necessary only in larger theaters.

EMERGENCY EQUIPMENT

A major consideration in an office-based operating room should be the management of emergencies. All staff should be trained to use emergency equipment. The staff should also be trained in pediatric as well as adult basic and advanced life support. Adequate equipment must be immediately available.

The following equipments are essential:

- Stethoscope
- Blood pressure apparatus
- Thermometer
- Cardiac monitor and pulse oximeter
- Defibrilitor (Fig. 6)
- Laryngoscope with endotracheal tubes of various sizes (Fig. 7)
- Ambu bag with airways of various types and sizes
- Oxygen supply/cylinder
- Intravenous fluids and drugs for emergency treatment
- Availability of transportation from the operating room to an emergency facility.

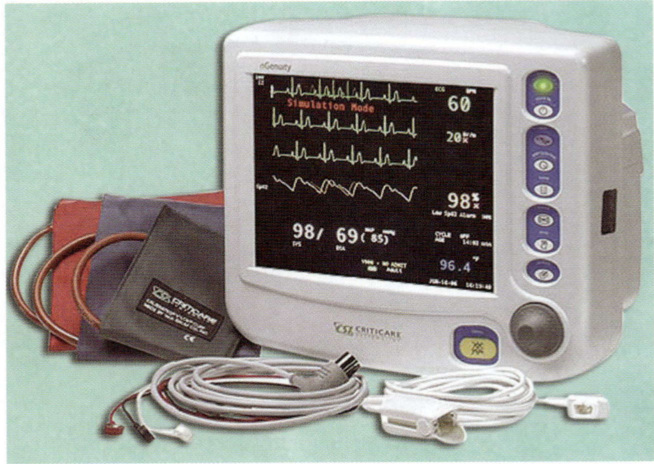

Fig. 5: Noninvasive blood pressure monitor (NIBP).

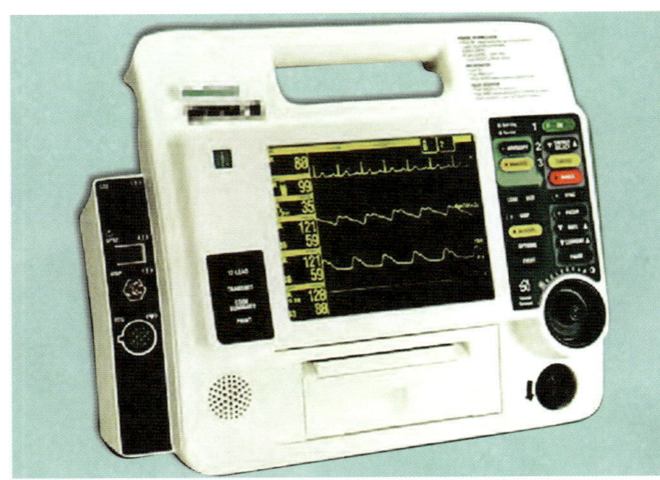

Fig. 6: Cardiac monitor and defibrillator.

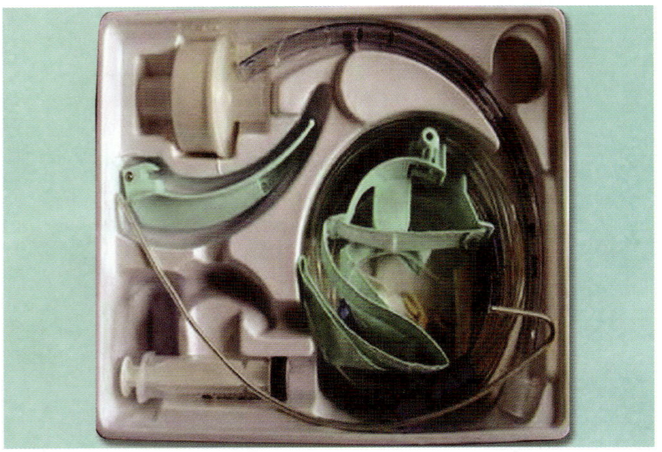

Fig. 7: Endotracheal intubation kit.

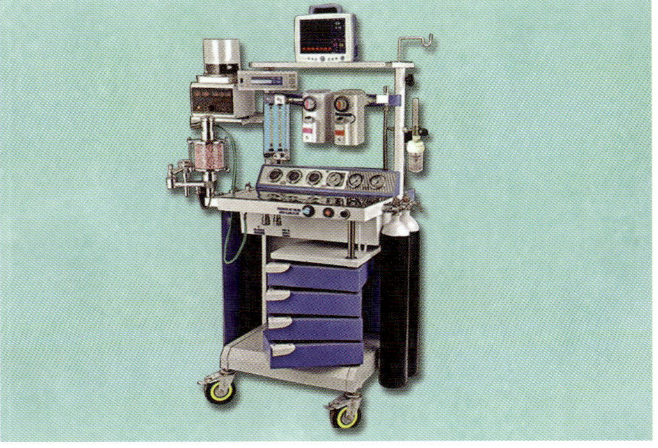

Fig. 8: Anesthesia Boyle's apparatus.

Even though general anesthesia is not chosen to perform dermatosurgical procedures, availability of Boyle's apparatus (Fig. 8) can be of additional help in case of serious emergencies. An emergency kit with all necessary equipment should be available and all operating theater staff should be familiar with this kit. The kit needs to be regularly checked by a senior staff.

BASIC SURGICAL INSTRUMENTS

Surgical instruments are one of the important factors in determining outcome of the dermatologic surgery. Surgical instruments of the highest quality should be preferred. Instruments made up of high-grade stainless steel are costly, but have a long life. To make them more effective in use and to have a longer life, some instruments have tungsten carbide inserts in the jaws of needle holders and blades.

Surgical instruments are precisely designed and manufactured tool and may either be disposable or reusable. They must be resistent to physical and chemical effects, body fluids, secretions, cleaning agents and sterilization, and hence most of them are made of high-quality stainless steel; chromium and vanadium alloys to ensure the durability of edges, springiness and resistance to corrosion.

Surgical instruments can be divided into groups:
1. Cutting and dissecting instruments.
2. Grasping, clamping instruments.
3. Artery forceps, mosquito forceps
4. Retractors and exposing instruments
5. Wound-closing instruments and materials
6. Special instruments used in nail surgery, vitiligo surgery, acne scar surgery and hair transplant surgery.

Scissors

Surgical scissors are available in various sizes and shapes, each suited for specific purpose. Specialized scissors should not be used for cutting suture, as it may result in loss of sharpness of the scissors. The jaws of the scissors may be straight or curved; and blunt or sharp. Serrations are added to one blade to avoid slipping, while trying to cut any thin tissue including skin. Curved scissors offer more directional mobility and visibility, while straight scissors have mechanical advantage when cutting tough tissues. Short-handled scissors are useful for fine work; while long-handled scissors give more reach and usually used to reach deeper areas such as cavities. Serrations are made on blade to prevent tissue slipping when cutting (Figs. 9 to 14).

Different types of scissors and their indications are mentioned in Box 1.

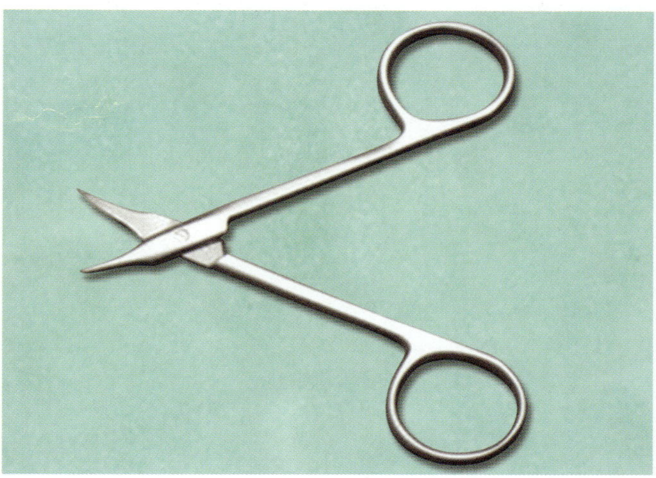

Fig. 9: Gradle scissor.

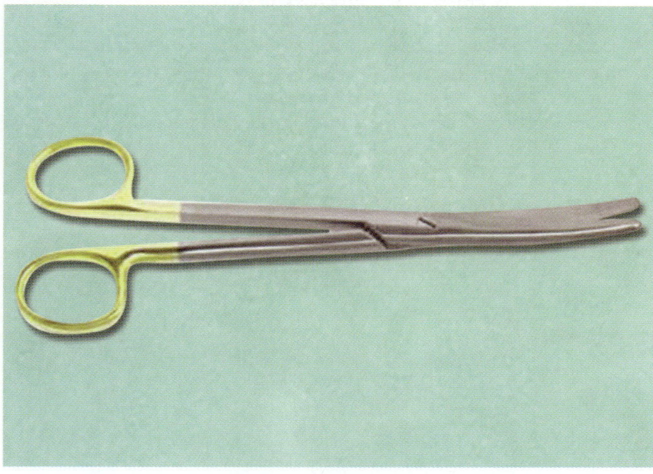

Fig. 10: Mayos scissor.

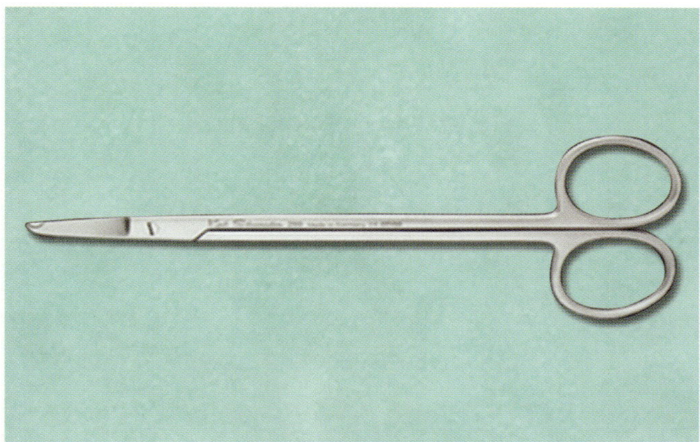

Fig. 11: Littures scissor.

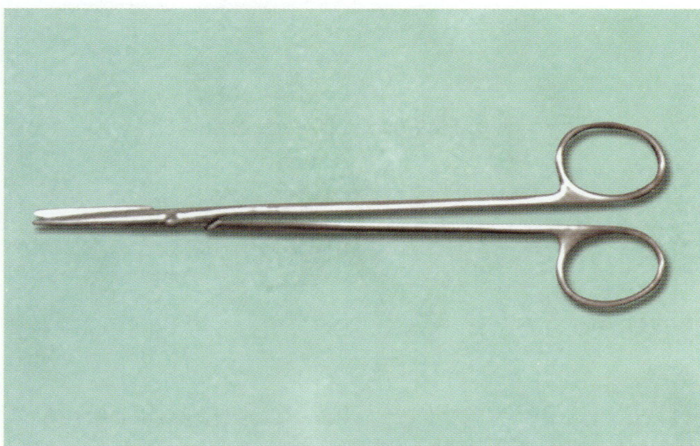

Fig. 12: Metzenbaum scissor.

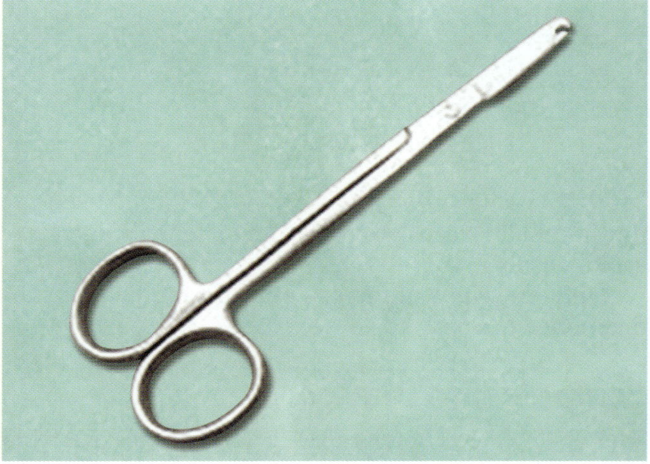

Fig. 13: Spencer's suture removal scissor.

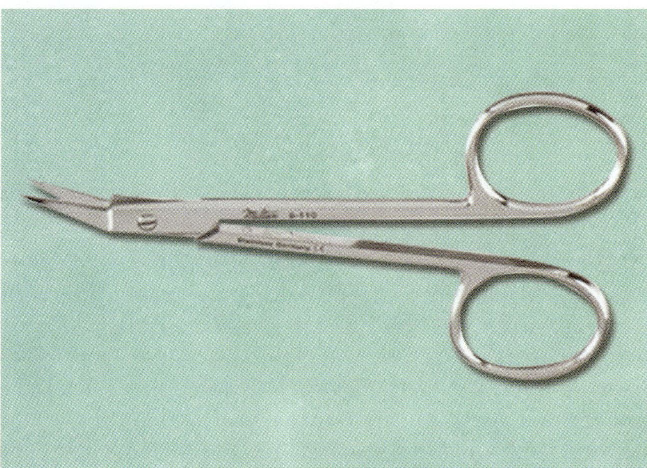

Fig. 14: O'Briens scissor.

Box 1: Types of scissors and their indications.

- Iris scissors are short-tipped and are useful for dissection and cutting
- Castroviejo's spring scissor is also used for fine work
- Horizontally curved and blunt-tipped scissors: For undermining example, Mayo's blunt tipped—undermining, blunt dissection
- Straight sharp-tipped scissors: For tough fibrotic tissues
- Straight blade scissors: For trimming flaps
- Beveled or sharper outer-edged scissors: For tissue dissection
- Littauer, Northbent, Shortbent, Spencers: For suture removal. They have concavity, which helps in elevating and cutting sutures. O'Briens suture cutting in delicate and tight areas
- Gradel scissors: Small scissors used for tiny dissection, have slightly curved, sharp blades, used for surgery around eye, sharp cutting.

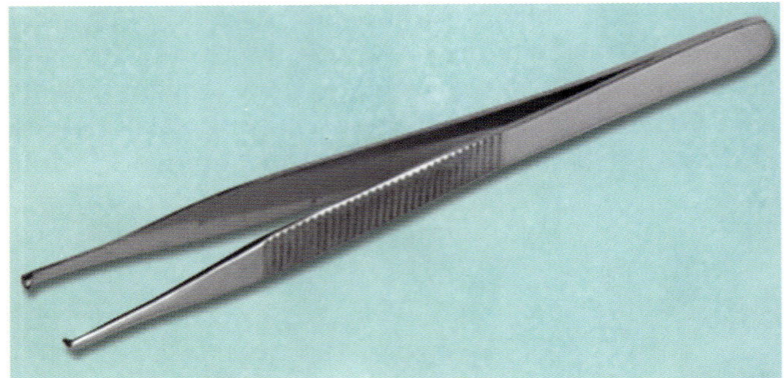

Fig. 15: Adson's forceps toothed.

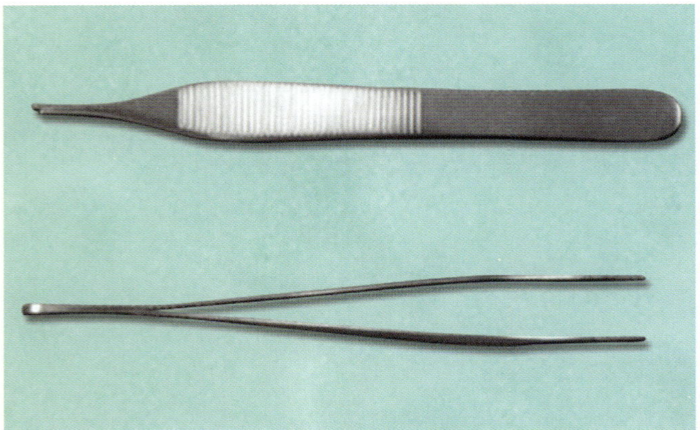

Fig. 16: Adson's forceps plain.

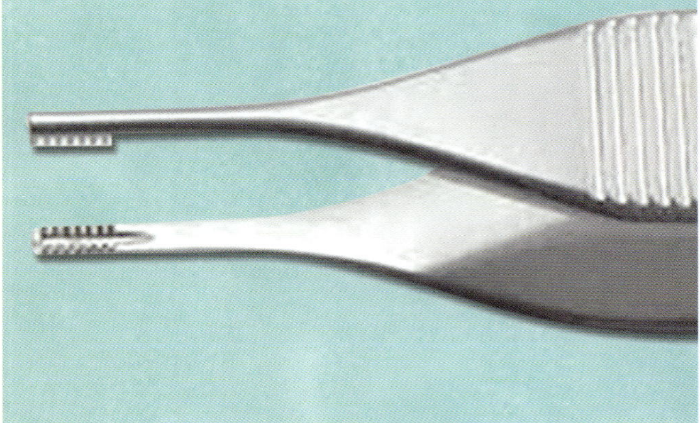

Fig. 17: Adson's Brown forceps.

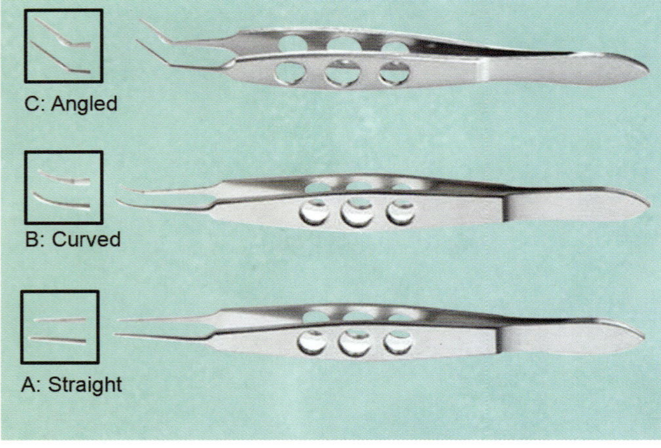

Fig. 18: Bishop-Harmon forceps.

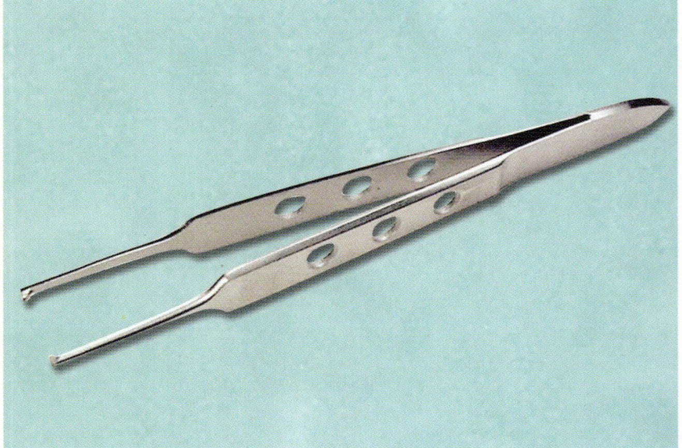

Fig. 19: Bishop-Harmon tissue forceps.

Forceps

Surgical forceps are the most utilized instruments in dermatosurgery. They hold the tissue in place during an operation or during insertion of another surgical instrument into a cavity. A variety of forceps are available for various surgical procedures. The choice of forceps depends on individual surgeon and the purpose. Forceps are available in various sizes and shapes (Figs. 15 to 29). Serrated forceps cause more tissue injury and hence, non-toothed forceps are preferred by many surgeons to avoid crushing.

Different types of forceps and their indications are mentioned in Box 2.

Scalpels and Blades

There is a wide variety of blades and handles available, but commonly used by many surgeons is handle no. 3. Handles are of two types—Bard-Parker and Beaver. Bard

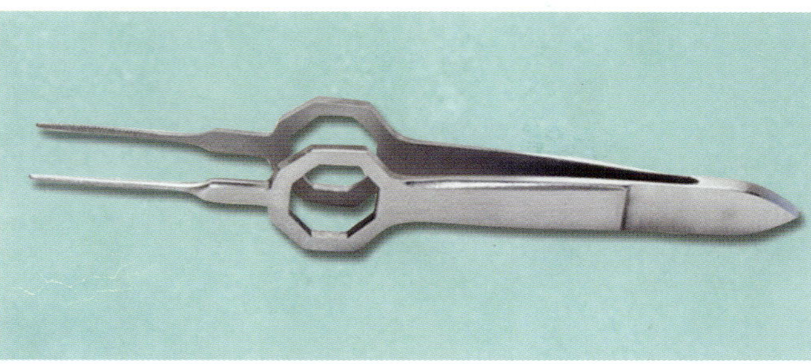

Fig. 20: Fosters tissue forcep.

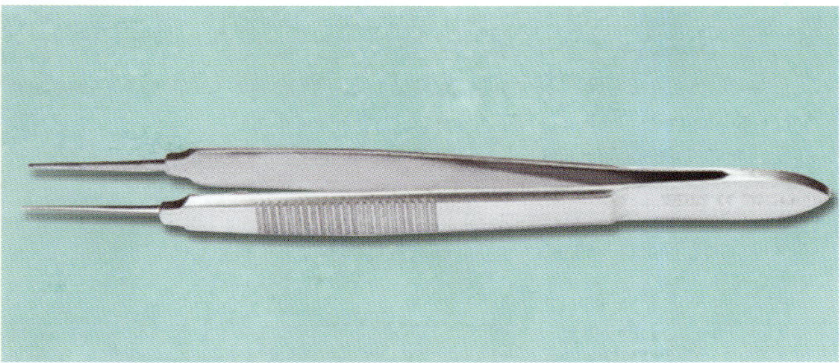

Fig. 21: Castroviejo forcep.

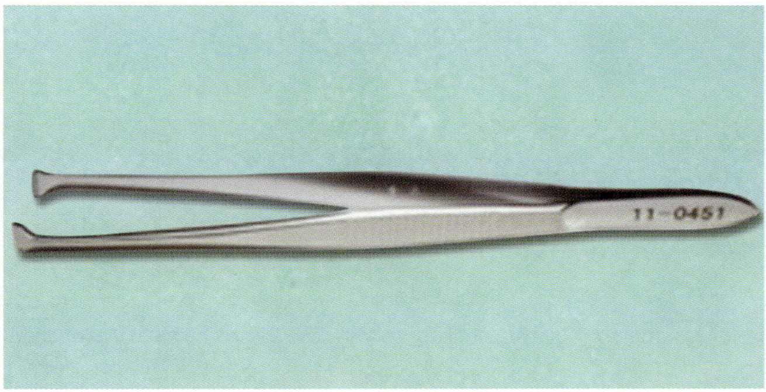

Fig. 22: Graefe's forcep.

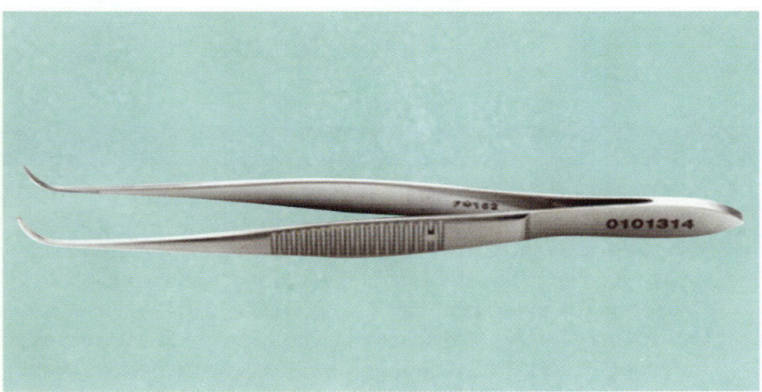

Fig. 23: Iris forcep.

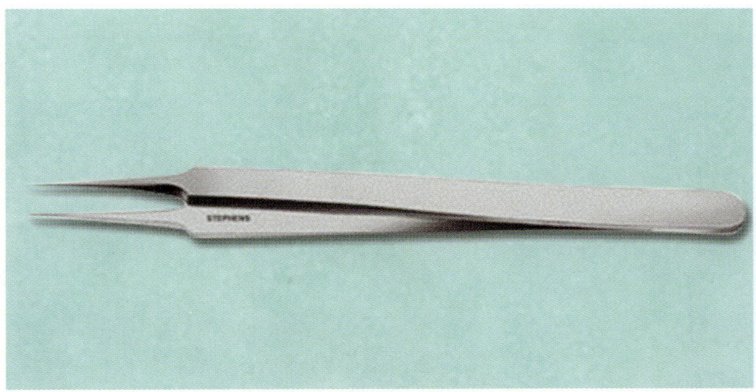

Fig. 24: Jewelers forcep (straight).

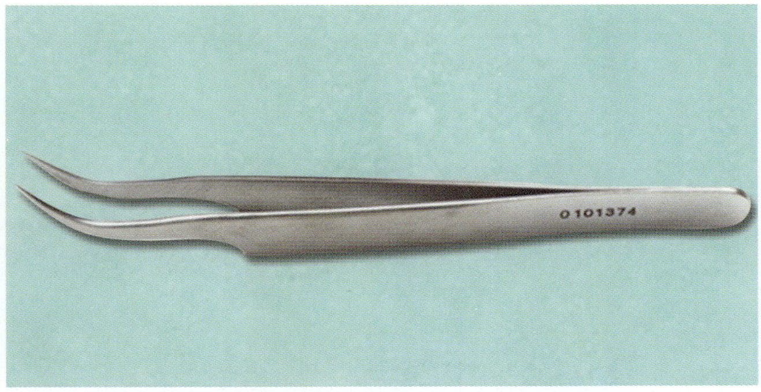

Fig. 25: Jewelers forcep (curved).

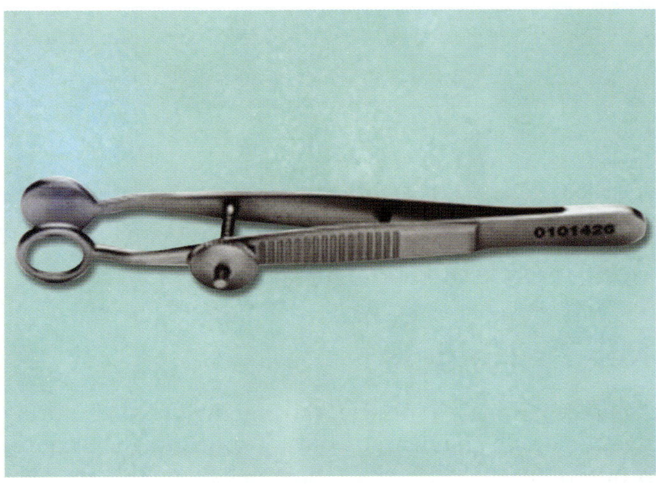

Fig. 26: Chalazion forcep.

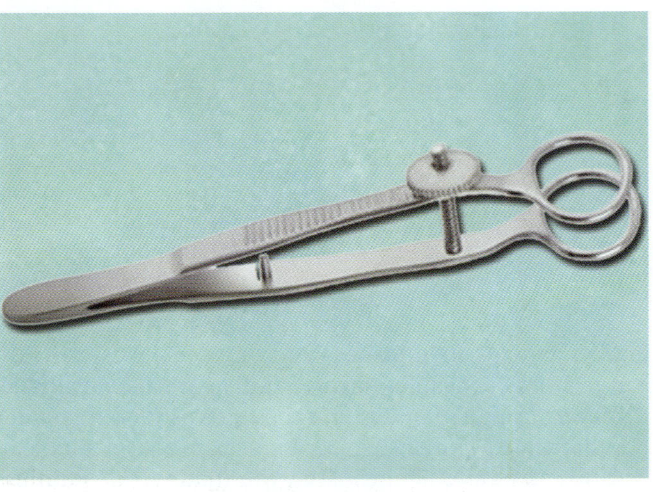

Fig. 27: Earlobe clamp.

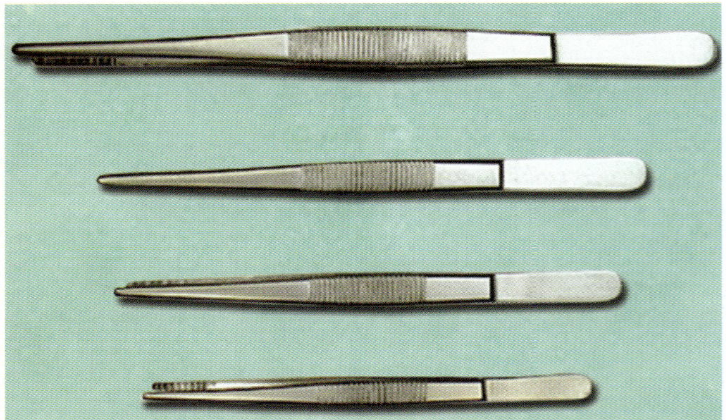

Fig. 28: Dressing forceps.

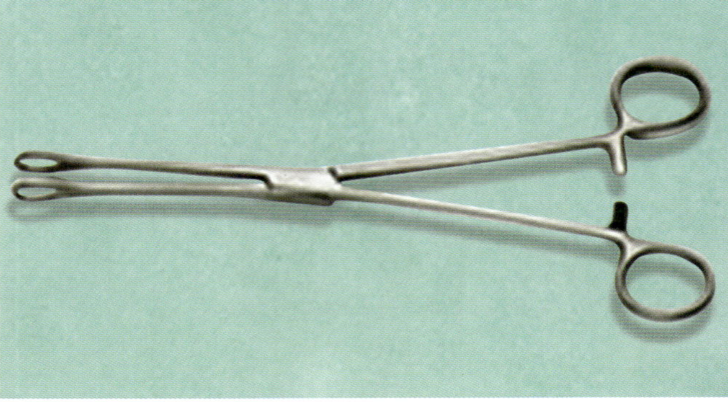

Fig. 29: Fosters forcep.

Box 2: Types of forceps and their indications.

- Adsons: The most versatile type, with broad handle and narrow teeth suitable for facial surgery and wound closure
- Adsons anatomical: Useful for tissue undermining and wound closure
- Bishop Harmon and Castroviejo small forceps: These are used for delicate work, microsurgery, eyelid surgery and thin skin
- Jewelers forceps: They are small and used for delicate work
- Graefe and Green forceps: They are useful to hold eyelid skin or cartilage
- Brown Adson forceps (like Adson but with 16 teeth): Tissue forceps are for holding and manipulating delicate tissues. These forceps have a wide, flat thumb grasp area that is commonly serrated. The jaws are short and the tips are narrow
- Foerster which may also be known as Foerster-Ballenger sponge forceps, are commonly used in surgical procedures to hold gauze squares that will absorb excess fluids and blood from the surgical site or hemostasis. The ratcheted locking mechanism of these finger ring forceps securely grip the gauze and hold it in place
- Chalazion forceps: Used for eyelid surgery, mucous cyst removal to achieve hemostasis
- Earlobe clamp: Surgery of ear, earlobe repair

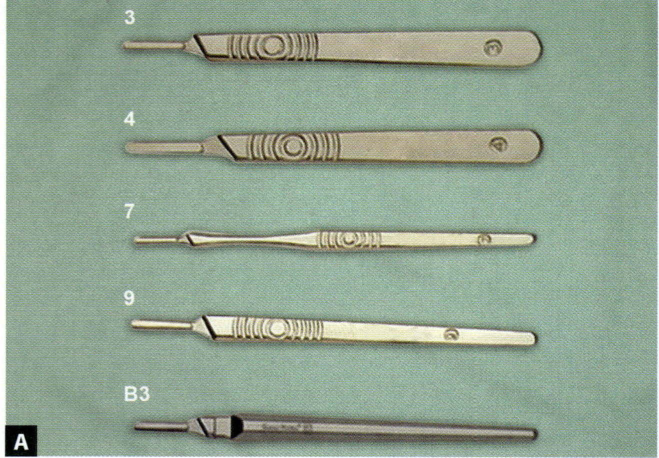

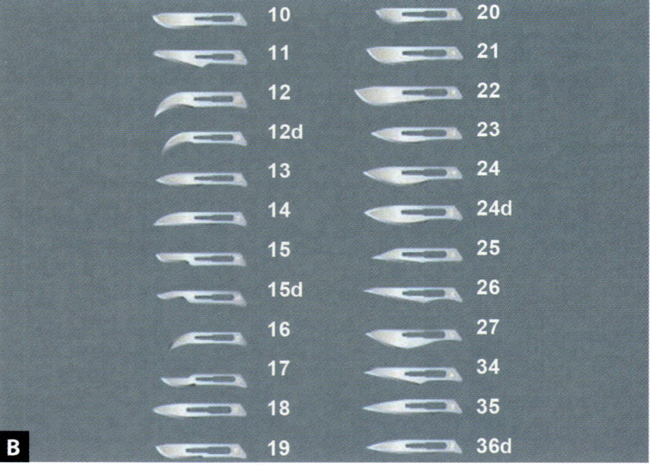

Figs. 30A and B: Scalpel blades and their handles.
Handle #3: For use with scalpel blades #10, #11, #12 and #15
Handle #4: For use with scalpel blades #20, #21, #22, #23 and #24
Handle #7: For use with scalpel blades #10, #11, #12 and #15
Handle #9: For use with scalpel blades #6, #9, #10, #11, #12, #15 and #16
Handle # B3: For use with 6, 9, 10, 11, 12, 12D, 13, 14, 15, D/15, 15T, 1

parker handles are the ones which are usually used in skin surgeries. Disposable plastic handles are also available. Different scalpel handles and their corresponding blades are shown in Figures 30 to 32. Blades are also available in various sizes and shapes. They are made from stainless steel, carbon steel or teflon-coated blades (Box 3).

Needle Holders

A needle holder is a surgical instrument to hold a suturing needle for closing wounds during suturing and surgical procedures. The parts of a simple needle holder are jaws, joint and handles. Most needle holders also have a clamp

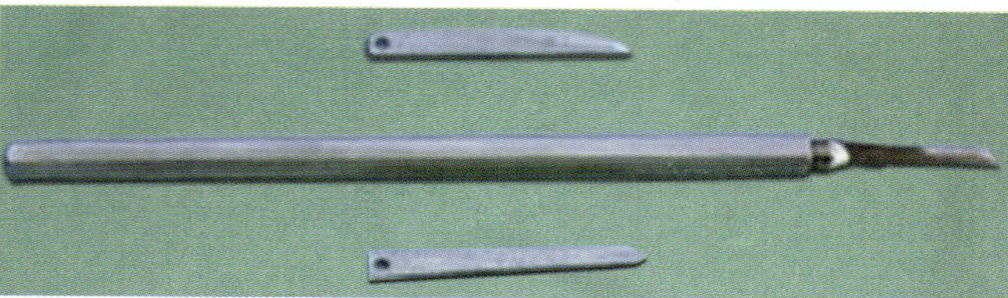

Fig. 31: Beaver scalpel handle with 64, 67 number blades.

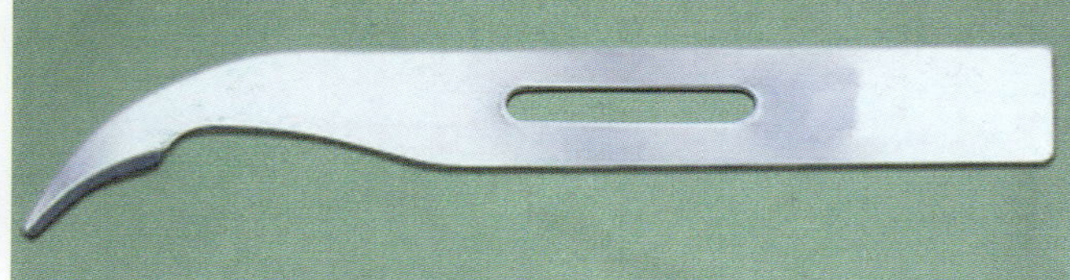

Fig. 32: Stich cutting blade.

Box 3: Blade numbers and their uses.

- Blade no. 15: It is the most commonly used in dermatosurgery and is ideal in performing skin biopsies where incision is less than 5 cm
- Blade no. 15d: It is useful in procedures where incision is less than 5 cm involving delicate areas like face
- Blade no. 11: It has a tapered sharp point and allows precise, vertical and acute angled incisions. It is useful to drain an abscess and to perform a shave biopsy
- Blade no. 10 and 21: They have wide convex belly, and are useful during excision of large lesions, in surgeries involving thick skin, like trunk and scalp, to make incisions longer than 5 cm and in wound debridement
- Blade no. 12: Sometimes used for suture cutting
- Blade 64 and 67 are small size and require Beaver handle. Number 64 blade has a round tip with sharp cutting edge and no. 67 blade has a sharp tip used for fine cutting, near delicate areas such as near eye, ear and ear canal surgery

Box 4: Uses of different needle holders.

- Crile wood needle holders (Fig. 33) are long, have blunt tips and are used for 3-0 or 2-0 suture needles
- Castroviejo needle holders (Figs. 34A and B) are small-jawed with a detachable spring handle and are used for 6-0 or 7-0 suture needles
- Ryder or Derf needle holders (Figs. 35A and B) are used for 4-0 or 5-0 suture needles
- Halsey needle holder—long delicate jaws for suture 5-0 or smaller (Fig. 36)
- Webster needle holder—for suture 6-0 or smaller (Fig. 37)
- Baumgartner needle holder and Collier needle holder—3-0 to 6-0 suture; has fenestrated jaws (Figs. 38A and B)

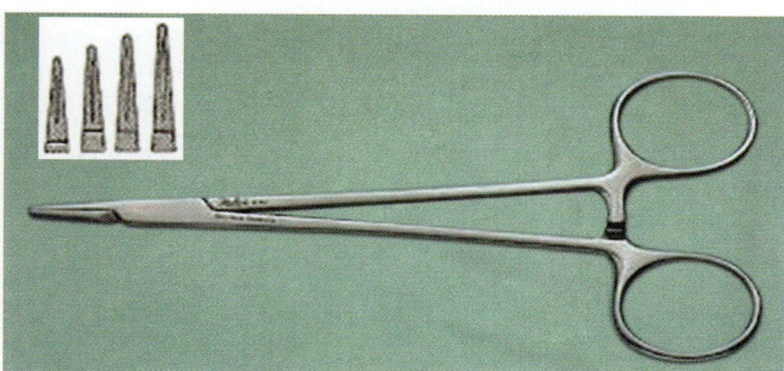

Fig. 33: Crile wood needle holder (curved and straight).

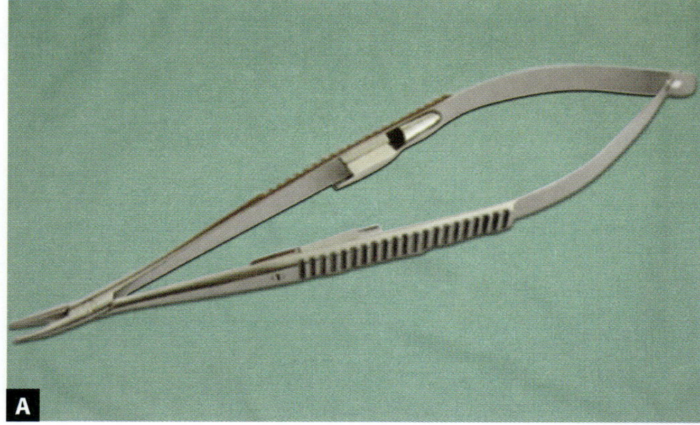

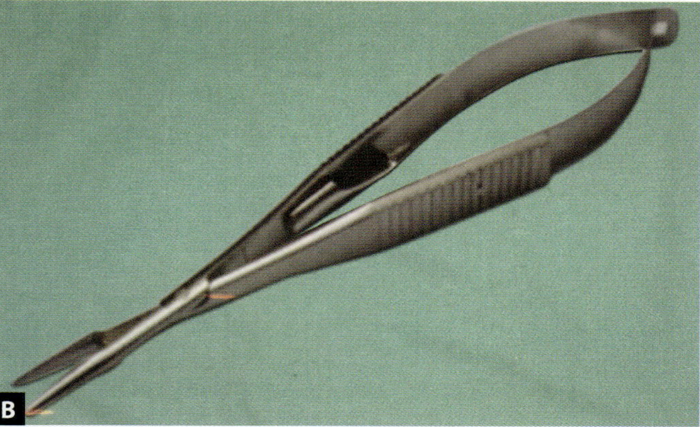

Figs. 34A and B: Castroviejo needle holders.

mechanism that locks the needle in place, allowing the user to maneuver the needle through various tissues. To maintain a firm grip on the needle, jaws are often textured and are short as compared to handles. Jaws may be smooth or firm toothed. The tips may also have a metal alloy for secure grasping.

The selection of a needle holder usually depends on the needle used and the anatomic site (Box 4).

Hemostats/Artery Forceps

Hemostat is a vital surgical tool used in almost every surgical procedure, usually to control bleeding. The hemostat has handles that can be held in place by the locking mechanism (Fig. 39). The locking mechanism is typically a series of interlocking teeth, a few on each handle that allows the user to adjust the clamping tension of the

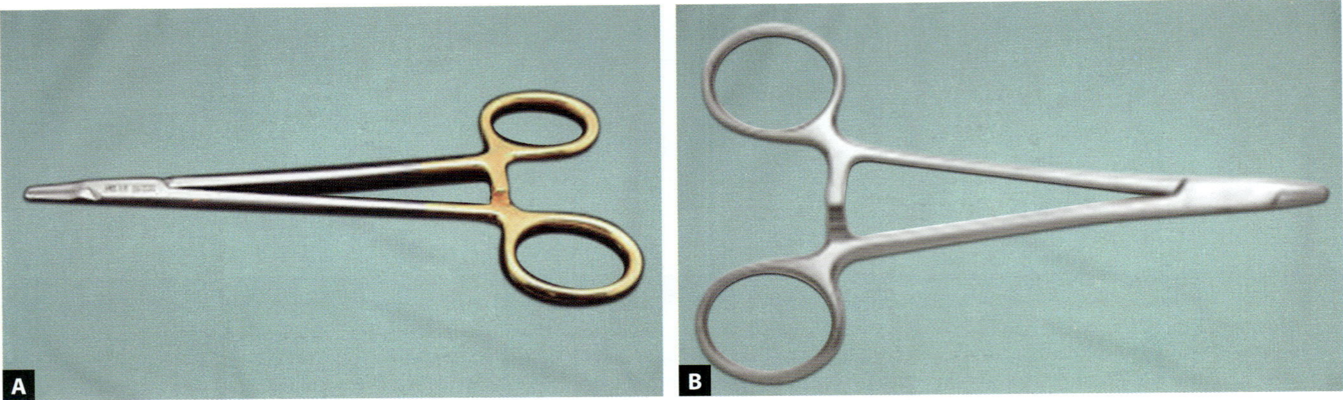

Figs. 35A and B: Ryder and Derf needle holders.

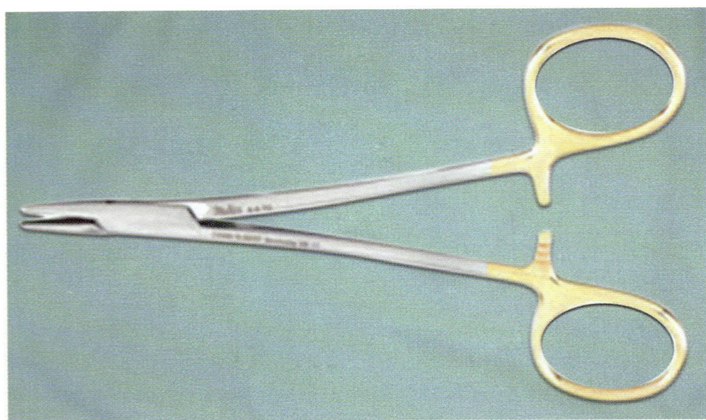

Fig. 36: Halsey needle holder.

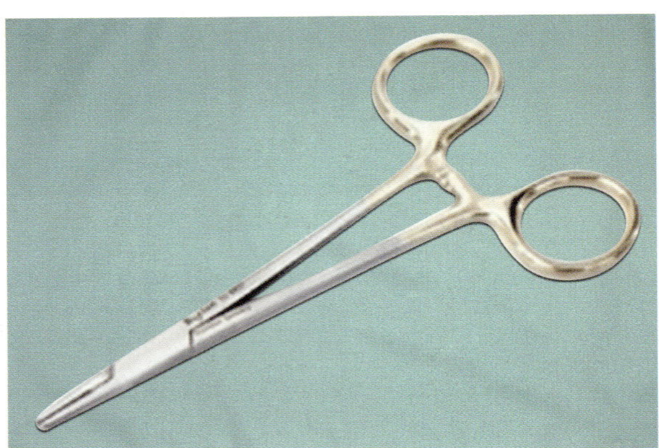

Fig. 37: Webster needle holder.

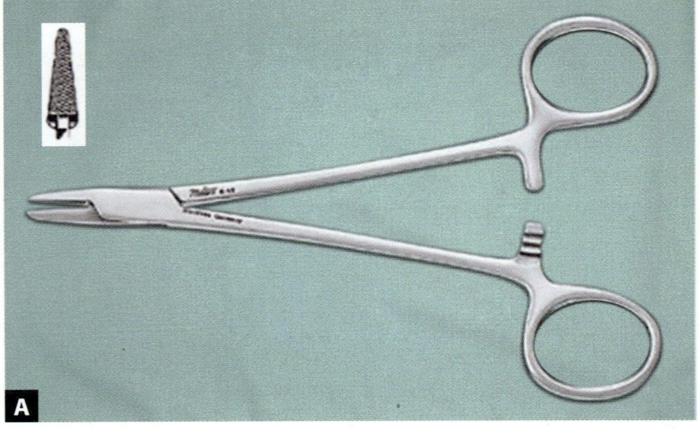

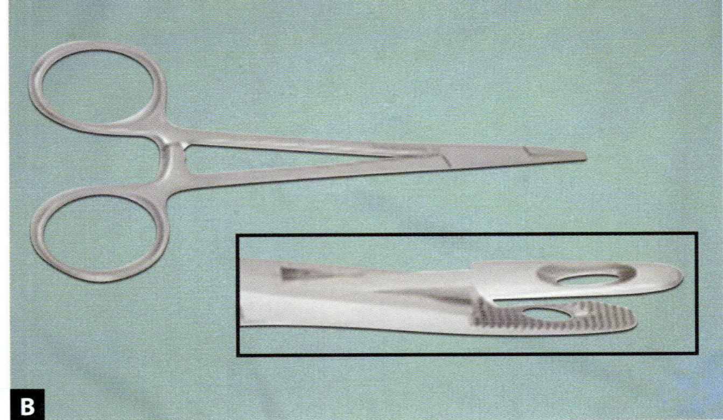

Figs. 38A and B: Baumgartner needle holder (A) and Collier needle holder (B).

pliers. Mosquito forceps (Figs. 40A and B) are nontraumatic with straight or curved jaws, whereas Kocher type has teeth (Fig. 41).

Retractors

A retractor (Fig. 42) is a surgical instrument, by which a surgeon can either actively separate edges of a surgical incision or wound, or can hold back underlying organs and tissues, so that body parts under the incision may be accessed. Types of retractors include double- and single-hooked with blunt and curved prongs. They are used to move skin flaps, when extensive undermining is required, to remove deep lesion and to displace vessels and nerves.

Skin Hooks

Skin hooks (Figs. 43A and B) are widely used in dermatologic surgery instead of forceps to avoid undue damage to skin edges as they are less traumatic. Skin hooks

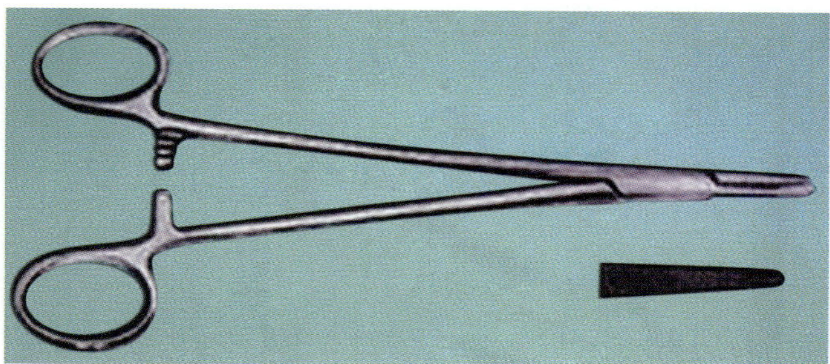

Fig. 39: Artery forceps.

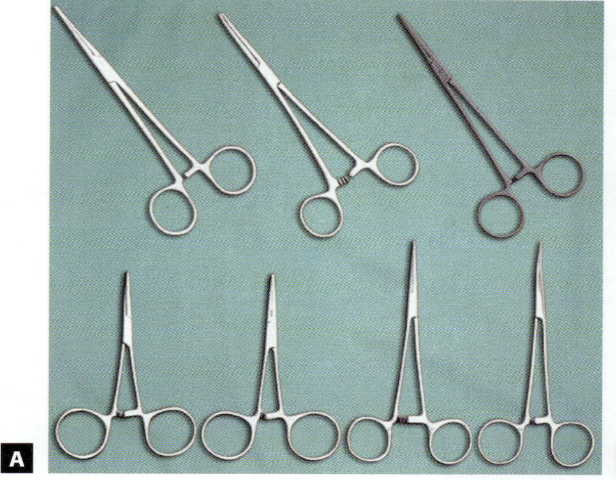

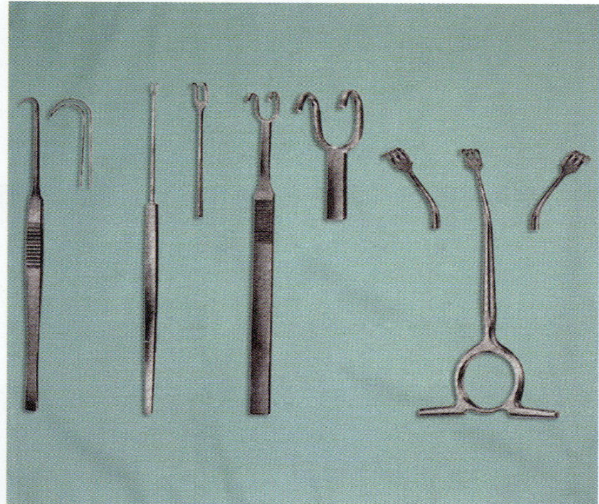

Figs. 40A and B: Mosquito artery forceps.

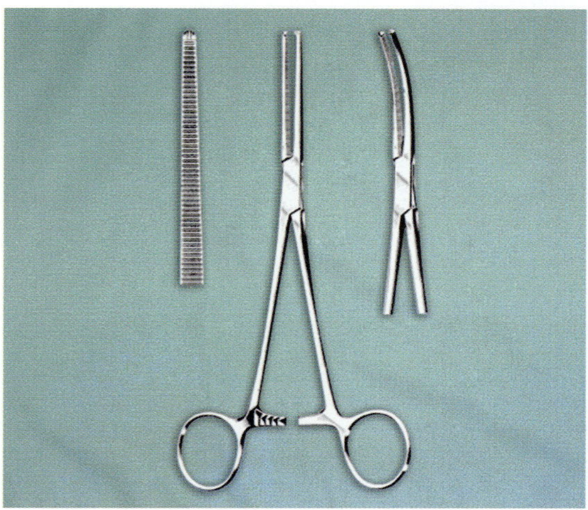

Fig. 41: Kocher artery forceps.

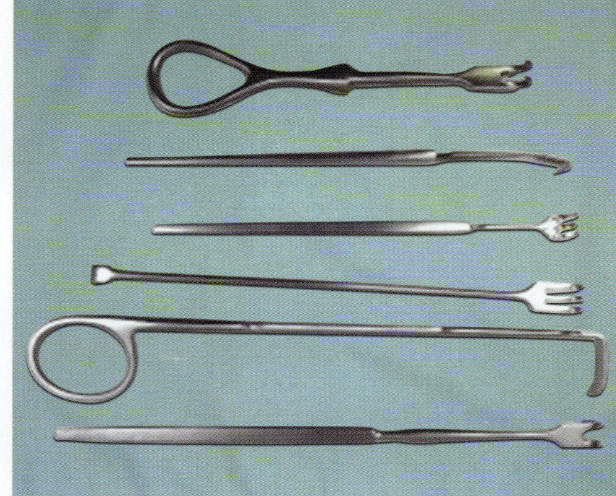

Fig. 42: Retractors—Army navy and cats paw.

with one, two or multiple teeth are available. They are used in donor dissection in hair transplant surgery, flap surgery, grafts, etc. (Box 5).

HOW TO HOLD SURGICAL INSTRUMENTS (FIG. 44 TO 47)

Scissors

When cutting the tissue is important to see that the tissue is correctly located between the two blades of the scissors. The surgeon's grip on the scissors must be proper. The grip is properly achieved by putting ring finger and thumb through the rings of the scissors and index finger placed near fulcrum on the shanks.

Forceps

The forceps should be held in the first three fingers as one would hold a pen, using the first three fingers. Grasp the forceps between thumb and middle finger and use index finger to stabilize. It is always advisable to grasp the dermis rather than epidermis to prevent injury to wound edge.

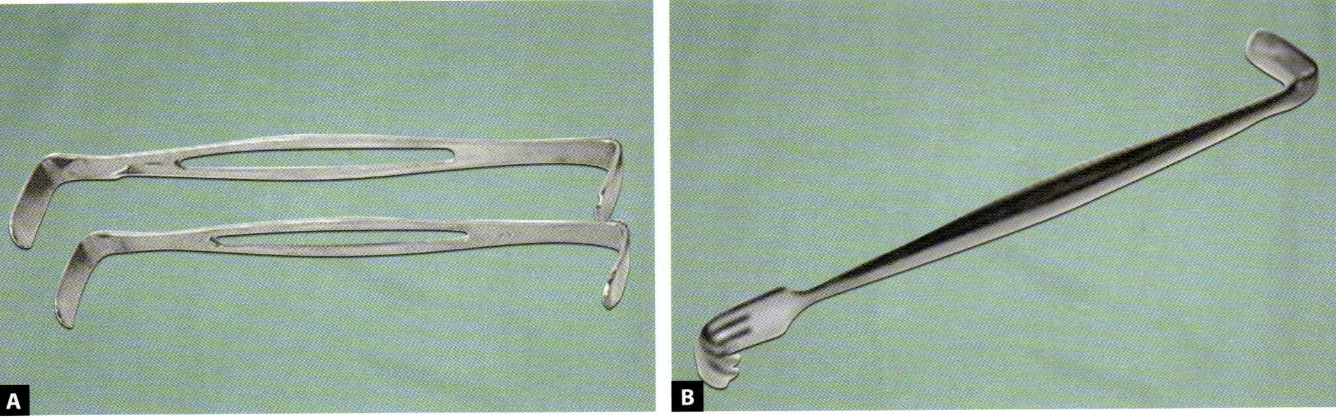

Figs. 43A and B: Skin hooks.

Box 5: Skin hooks and their uses.

- Gillies skin hook—large hook with long shaft; good for retracting scar tissue
- Tyrell iris skin hook—small hook for delicate procedures
- Frazier Skin hook—holds tongue, lips, and cheeks away from surgical area; Shepherd's crook design

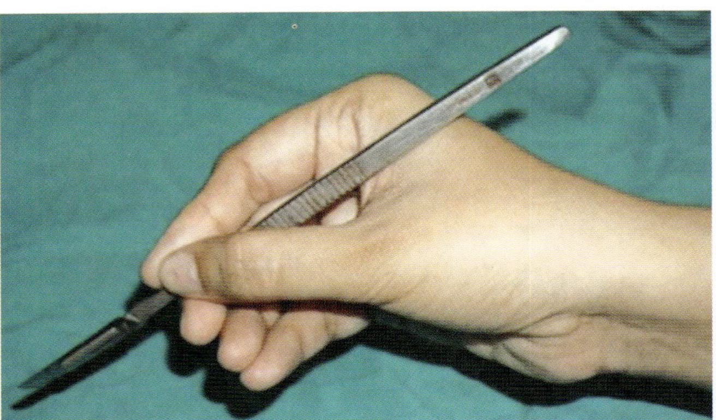

Fig. 44: Holding scalpel.

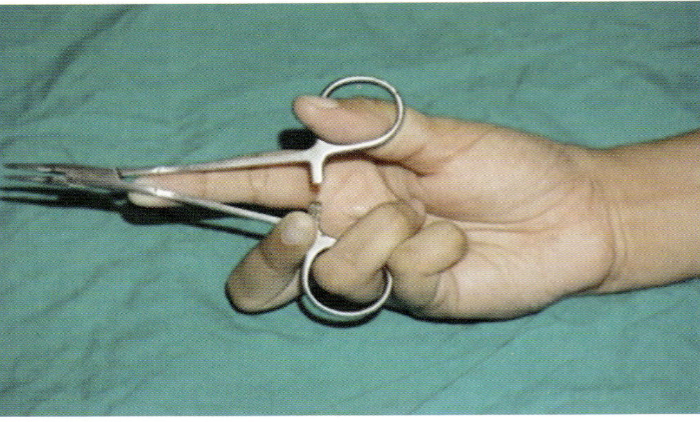

Fig. 45: Holding needle holder.

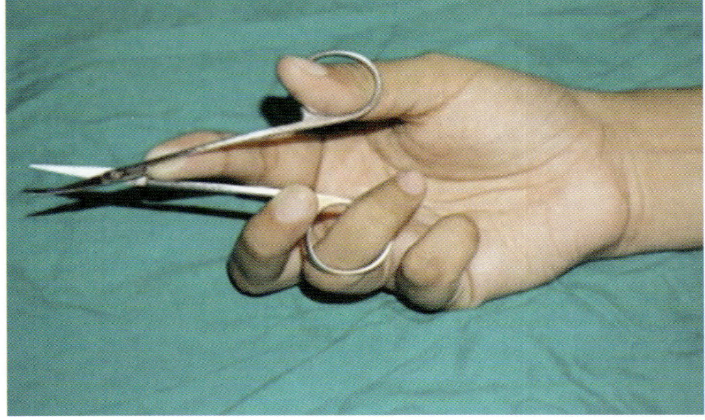

Fig. 46: Holding scissor.

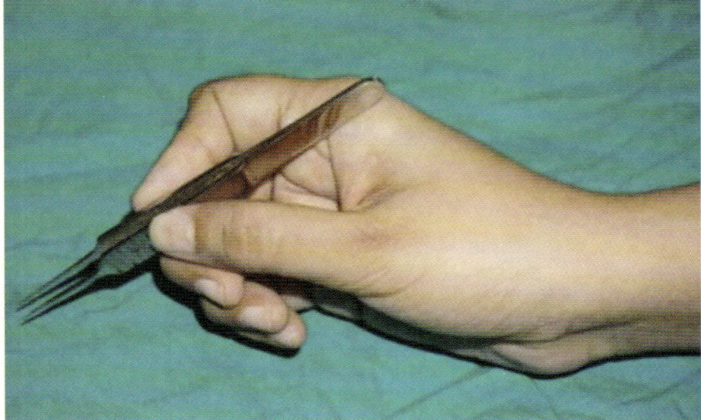

Fig. 47: Holding forcep.

Needle Holder

The needle holder should be held in a way that is comfortable and affords maximum control. Grasp the needle holder by partially inserting the thumb and ring finger into the loops of the handle. The index finger provides additional control and stability.

Box 6: Quality of instruments.

- The instrument should sustain repeated use and sterilization
- They should be from reputed manufacturer and of high-quality stainless steel
- Some instruments such as needle holder and scissors are available with special tungsten carbide alloy inserts. This material is hard and maintains precise cutting edge

Needle

Needle should be held just behind its midpoint. If the needle is held near the tip, it will point downward. If the needle is held near the thread end, it will point upward. It is approximately at junction of 2/3 and 1/3 portion of the needle.

Scalpel

Scalpel should be held like pen with handle resting on anatomical snuffbox. Before taking incision stabilize the skin with thumb on one side and fingers other side. Make incision with properly held scalpel.

Hemostat

Holding is same as scissors. Use tips of the jaw to hold vessels and secure the lock. Learn to release hemostat with single hand.

ARRANGEMENT OF INSTRUMENTS

The instruments should be arranged on a trolley, surgical stand, or surgical tray with pointed or sharp ends pointing away. The order of instruments should be predetermined and should be same every day for a particular surgery, so that the arrangement is familiar to the surgeon and assisting nurse. Separate specific trays may be prepared for each surgery. The height of the tray or trolley should be at a level comfortable to the surgeon/assisting nurse. Care should be taken to see that there is no admixture of clean and soiled instruments. Gauze or pads should be kept separately, so that they do not obscure sharp objectives.

Box 7: Precautions during surgery.

- Always work away from the surgeon's field
- Keep instruments in an orderly manner with all instruments pointing in the same direction
- Use properly fitting gloves
- Always use instruments to handle tissue; avoid exposure of hands to the surgical field
- Sharp objects such as needles or blades should be handled after mounting on another instrument such as forceps or needle holder and never with hand
- If hand needs to be entered into the operating field, introduce only one hand, after withdrawing all sharp instruments from the field of surgery
- Do not recap needles

MAINTENANCE OF INSTRUMENTS

Proper care and maintenance of instruments is important to enhance longevity. A trained nurse should clean the instruments. All instruments should be inspected daily during cleaning to check for any damage or wear and tear. In particular, fine forceps and fine scissors are prone to get damaged frequently and need special care.

The tips for instrument selection, and to avoid injury during use of surgical instruments are mentioned in the Boxes 6 and 7, respectively.

RECOMMENDED READING

1. Advanced Surgical Reconstructive Techniques. Dermatologic Clinics. 2005;23:44-5.
2. Bishop WJ. The early history of Surgery. Hale, London; 1960.
3. Bogle MA, Fisher VT, Joseph AK. Instruments and Materials. In: Robinson JK, Hanke CW, Siegel DM, Fratila A (Eds). Surgery of the skin: Procedural dermatology. 2nd edition. Edinburg: Mosby Elsevier; 2010. pp. 65-72.
4. Colleman W, Hanke CW, Thomas H, et al. Cosmetic Surgery of the Skin: Principles and Techniques, 2nd edition. USA: Mosby Publishers; 2005. pp. 7-17.
5. Roenigk RK, Roenigk HH Jr (Eds). Roenigk and Roenigk's Dermatologic Surgery: Principles and Practice, 2nd edition. New York: Marcel Dekker Publishers; 1996. pp. 192-205, 293-5, 313-5, 329-35.
6. Sawant S, Shan R, Gore D (Eds). Textbook and Atlas of Dermatologic Surgery and Cosmetology. Mumbai: ASCAD Publishers; 1998. pp. 3-23.

Chapter 9

Wound Closure Materials and Techniques in Dermatosurgery

Umashankar Nagaraju

Key Messages 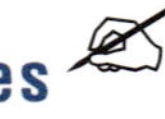

- Knowledge of proper wound closure materials is essential for ensuring rapid wound healing.
- Choice of suture materials is based on its properties: memory, elasticity, knot strength, tensile strength, tissue reaction and capability to be absorbed.
- A surgical wound attains progressively increasing cutaneous tensile strength after suture; 3–5% of original strength 2 weeks after suturing, 20% of the ultimate wound strength by 3rd week, 50% by 1 month.
- Important factors to be considered while choosing the suture material are the location of wound, static and dynamic wound tension, presence of wound infection and cost of suture material.
- Skin tapes, staples or wound adhesives are also useful in certain situations.

INTRODUCTION

The choice of an appropriate wound closure material and technique makes a large contribution for the best functional and cosmetic result. Various methods for mechanical wound closure include suture,[1] staples, tape and adhesive. All these promote primary wound healing.

HISTORY

Suture materials have undergone an evolutionary process over many decades. In olden era, sutures were made of plant materials (flax, hemp, and cotton) or animal materials (hair, tendons, arteries, muscle strips, nerves, silk, and catgut).[2] Interestingly, South Americans used large black ant sutures by coaxing insects to bite wound edges with their powerful jaws acting in a similar manner to Michel Clips. Subsequently, ant's body was twisted off leaving its head in place.[3,4] Needles were made of bone or metals such as silver, copper and aluminum bronze wire.

The earliest reports of surgical suture date back to 3000 BC in ancient Egypt, and the oldest known suture is in a mummy from 1100 BC. The first detailed description of a wound suture and the suture material used in it is by the Indian sage and physician Sushruta (Fig. 1), written in 500 BC. Galen of Pergamon, AD 150 (Fig. 2) comments for the first time on the use of catgut.[3] Catgut was made from the twisted intestine of herbivorous animals (usually sheep or goat) and even today it is widely used accounting for nearly half the usage of all sutures and ligatures. The origin of the word 'catgut' is not fully known, but it may have been an abbreviation of the word "cattlegut". Alternatively, it may have been derived from the word *kitgut* or *kitstring,* the word *kit,* meaning fiddle. The kit may have lead to the word cat, *kit* being the word for little cat. Certainly, it is not derived from cats!

The chemical industry introduced the synthetic threads in the early 1930s, which began the era of production of numerous synthetic absorbable and nonabsorbable sutures.[3]

SUTURES

Suture is a foreign body either natural or synthetic which may be monofilament or multifilament material used to close a surgical or accidental wound and to secure apposition of the edges and join tissues. Three vital properties of a suture material which affects its handling are memory, elasticity and knot strength. Tensile strength, tissue reaction and capability to be absorbed are other important characteristics of the suture material. The selection of the type of suture to be used depends on tissue type and anatomical location. Several suture materials have been developed today over its millennia of history and

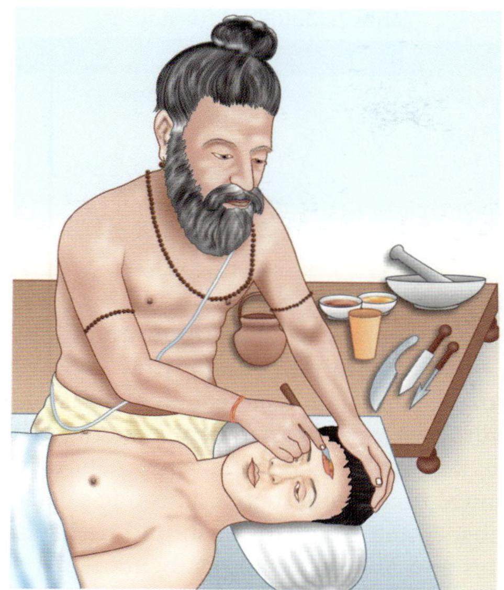

Fig. 1: Sushruta: Father of anesthesia and plastic surgeon.

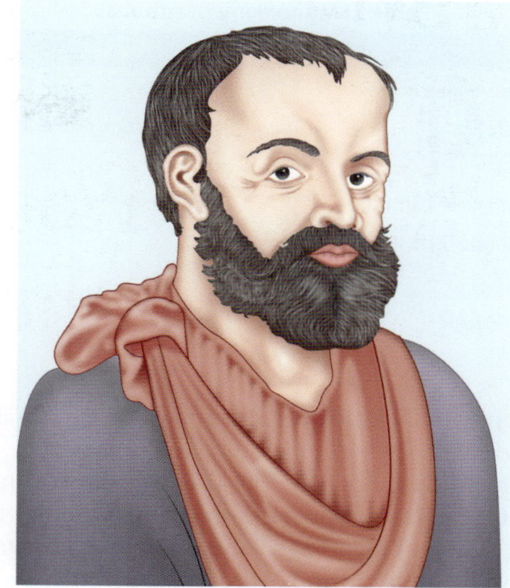

Fig. 2: Claudius Galen (129–200 AD).

each material presents advantages and disadvantages. An ideal suture material has great strength and knot security while remaining elastic with minimal tissue reactivity.[1]

Characteristics of an Ideal Suture

Ideal suture material should:[5,6]

- Be easy to handle
- Cause minimal tissue injury or tissue reaction (natural material elicits more tissue reaction than synthetic)
- Allow secure knots
- Have high tensile strength
- Not cut through tissue
- Be sterile and resistant to infection
- Have favorable absorption profile
- Be affordable.

No single material can provide all of these characteristics.

Properties of a Suture to be Assessed before Selection[6-9]

- *Tensile strength*: Measure of a material or tissue's ability to resist deformation and breakage.
- *Elasticity*: Ability of the material to regain its original form and length after deformation.
- *Plasticity*: Ability to deform without breaking and to maintain a new form after relief of the deforming force.
- *Capillarity*: Extent to which absorbed fluid is transferred along the suture.
- *Memory*: Inherent capability of suture to return to or maintain its original gross shape (related to elasticity, plasticity, and diameter). High memory sutures are stiff and require additional throws to be secured.
- *Knot strength*: Amount of force necessary to cause a knot to slip (related to the coefficient of static friction and plasticity of a given material). The knot is the weakest section of the suture. In general flat knots are more secure than sliding knots.
- *Pliability*: Ease of handling of suture material; ability to adjust knot tension and to secure knots.
- *Tissue reactivity*: This is an inflammatory response produced by implanted suture materials. In general natural and multifilament sutures have greater tissue reaction when compared to synthetic materials.
- *Absorbable*: Progressive loss of mass and/or volume of suture material.
- *Nonabsorbable*: Surgical suture material that is relatively unaffected by the biological activities of the body tissues and is therefore permanent unless removed.

Suture Size (as per the United States Pharmacopeia Classification System)[6]

Size refers to the diameter of the suture strand and is denoted as zeroes. The more zeroes characterizing a suture size, the smaller the resultant strand diameter (e.g. 4-0 or 0000 is larger than 5-0 or 00000). The smaller the suture, the less tensile strength of the strand. Modern sutures range from #5 (heavy braided suture for orthopedic use) to #11-0 (fine monofilament suture for ophthalmic use).

Tissue Response to Suture Materials

All sutures are foreign bodies and produce an inflammatory response in the host dermis. Natural suture materials evoke more inflammatory reaction than synthetic materials.[10] Peak inflammatory response is seen between 2nd day and 7th day with abundance of polymorphonuclear leukocytes, lymphocytes, and large monocytes in dermis.[11] Epithelial

Table 1: Monofilament sutures.

Absorbable	Nonabsorbable
Surgical gut-Plain chromic	Nylon
Polyglycolic acid	Polypropylene (Prolene)
Poliglecaprone 25	Hexafluoropropylene
Polytrimethylene carbonate	Polybutester
Polydioxanone (PDS II)	
Glycomer 631	
Polyglytone 6211	

Table 2: Multifilament sutures.

Absorbable	Nonabsorbable
Polyglycolic acid	Surgical silk
Polyglactin 910	Cotton
Polyglactin 910 rapide	Polyamide braided
Polyglactin 910 coated with antibacterial agent triclosan	Polyester

cells deeply invade the suture tracts between the 3rd day and 8th day.

A surgical wound never attains the same cutaneous tensile strength as of normal uncut skin. Two weeks after suturing, 3–5% of original strength will be achieved by a surgical wound. By the end of 3rd week, 20% of the ultimate wound strength is achieved and by 1 month, only 50% of wound strength is attained.[5]

Classification of Suture Materials

Suture materials can be classified in different ways;

a. Based on type of filament as monofilament and multifilament sutures.
b. Based on absorbability as absorbable and nonabsorbable.

a. Based on Type of Filament (Tables 1 and 2)

- *Monofilament suture*: It is made of a single strand and is relatively more resistant to harboring microorganisms.[6] Great care must be taken in handling and tying monofilament suture because crushing or crimping of this suture can nick or weaken the suture and lead to undesirable and premature suture failure.
- *Multifilament suture*: It is composed of several filaments twisted or braided together. It has increased capillarity and thus increases the absorption of fluid leading to form a tract for the entry of pathogens. Multifilament suture generally has greater tensile strength and better pliability and flexibility than monofilament suture.[6] This type of suture handles and knots well. It is less stiff but has a higher coefficient of friction. Do not pull them roughly through the tissues; their surfaces are not as smooth as monofilaments, so there is a dragging and sawing effect.[10]

b. Based on Absorbable Property (Tables 1 and 2)

- *Absorbable suture materials:* Sutures that lose the majority of their tensile strength within 60 days are considered absorbable.[12] Absorbable sutures[9,13,14] provide temporary wound support, until the wound heals. Absorption occurs either by proteolytic enzymatic degradation as seen in natural materials or by hydrolysis as seen in synthetic materials. Hydrolysis causes less tissue reaction than enzymatic degradation. Chemical treatments such as chromic salts lengthens the absorption time. These should be used as deep sutures and are placed into subcutaneous tissues to eliminate dead space and into the dermis to minimize tension during wound healing. Placing absorbable sutures too superficially may result in epithelization of the suture tunnels leading to permanent suture tracts and cyst formation. This can compromise the appearance of the scar.[5]

Factors influencing absorption:[6] Accelerated absorption may occur in patients with:

- Fever,
- Infection,
- Protein deficiency and
- In a body cavity that is moist or filled with fluid or if sutures become wet during handling prior to implantation.

Different Suture Materials and Their Properties

Absorbable Suture (Table 3)

Absorbable sutures include natural and synthetic sutures.

a. *Natural:* These include:

- *Catgut:* Catgut, commonly known as surgical gut, is chiefly made of collagen derived from naturally occurring purified connective tissue of intestinal submucosa of sheep or the intestinal serosa of cattle.[12] Weak spots produced during manufacture may cause uneven absorption of suture and premature rupture. In comparison with the other absorbable sutures, surgical gut sutures tend to lose their tensile strength and knot security rapidly.[15] Approximately, 60% of the tensile strength of surgical gut is lost in 4–5 days post-implantation and knot security is retained only for 2 weeks. For this reason, it is not wise to use this suture in patients predisposed to delayed wound healing.[9]

  Plain surgical gut is treated with an aldehyde solution to strengthen the suture and make it more resistant to enzymatic degradation. These are indicated in

Table 3: Absorbable sutures and their characteristics.[8]

Properties	*Catgut*	*Polyglycolic acid*	*Polyglactin*	*Polydioxanone*	*Polytrimethylene carbonate*	*Poliglecaprone*
Handling	Fair	Fair–good	Good	Poor	Good	Excellent
Knot security	Poor	Fair–good	Fair	Poor	Good	Good
Tensile strength	Low	High	High	Moderate	High	High
	Proteolysis by	Hydrolysis by	Hydrolysis by	Hydrolysis by	Hydrolysis by	Hydrolysis by
	60–90 d, unpredictable	90–120 d	60–90 d	180–210 d	180–210 d	90–120 d
Coefficient of friction	High	High	Medium	Low	Low	Low
Memory	Low	Low	Low	High	Low	Low
Tissue reactivity	High	Low–moderate	Low–moderate	Low	Low	Low
Uses	Mucosal tissues, vessel ligation	Buried	Commonly used in dermatological surgeries. Buried; Vicryl Rapide (Ethicon) in wounds requiring short-term dermal support	Buried; in wounds requiring long-term dermal support	Buried; in wounds requiring long-term dermal support	Buried
Other		Low elasticity Beige, violet, or green	Low elasticity Clear or violet	Clear or violet	Clear or green	High elasticity Clear

repairing rapidly healing tissues that require minimal support and for ligating superficial blood vessels.

Chromic surgical gut is a catgut soaked in chromic salts. This was introduced to enhance the tensile strength by increasing the resistance to degradation. Tensile strength varies depending on the chromic salt concentration.[12,15] Normally, tensile strength of chromic gut sutures is maintained for 10–14 days.

The tendency to fray during knot construction is the distinct disadvantage of surgical gut. Gut sutures have been banned in Europe and Japan owing to concerns regarding Bovine spongiform encephalopathy. It is no more used in dermatologic surgery today.

b. *Synthetic:* These include:

- *Polyglycolic acid or dexon*: It was the first available synthetic absorbable suture which was introduced in 1970.[1] This is an absorbable synthetic homopolymer of glycolic acid. It is available in both a monofilamentous and braided form. It is supplied as an uncoated or coated form. Coated polyglycolic acid suture is undyed or dyed green or violet which provides easier visibility.[9,13,14] Being synthetic, it elicits less inflammatory response than surgical gut. It is degraded by hydrolysis. Polyglycolic acid possesses good tensile strength and excellent knot security. After 2 weeks of implantation, 65% of the initial tensile strength remains with polyglycolic acid suture, in contrast to 0% of surgical gut suture.[5]
- *Polyglactin 910 (vicryl)*: Polyglactin 910 is the most widely used absorbable suture material in dermatologic surgery resulting in excellent cosmetic outcome. It is a synthetic braided multifilament copolymer consisting of 90% of glycolide and 10% of lactide. The suture is coated with calcium stearate, which permits easy tissue passage and precise knot placement.[6] It is degraded by hydrolysis and therefore yields only minimal tissue reaction. Vicryl is completely hydrolyzed by 60 days postimplantation.[16] It is an excellent option for soft tissue approximation and vessel ligation. Greater residual tensile strength and a faster absorption rate renders polyglactin 910 suture to be superior when compared to polyglycolic acid suture.[1,13]

  Variants[1,3]
  - *Vicryl Rapide®* irradiated with gamma rays to speed absorption.
  - *Vicryl Plus*, the only suture impregnated with triclosan for its antibiotic and anti-inflammatory effect.
- *Poliglecaprone 25 (Monocryl)*: It is a synthetic monofilament suture that is a copolymer of glycolide and e-caprolactone.[6] High tensile strength (50–60%) is maintained for 7 days which will be absorbed completely by 3 months. It offers better handling and knot security than most other monofilament sutures. Hence, it is useful for subcuticular closure and soft tissue approximations and ligations.
- *Polytrimethylene carbonate (Maxon)*: It is a synthetic monofilament absorbable suture. It retains 75% of original strength at 2 weeks of postimplantation. Complete absorption does not occur until 180–210 days.[15] Its advantages over other sutures are improved handling properties, lacks memory, passes easily through tissues and demonstrates superior strength.[14]

Maxon has proved to be an excellent addition to the armamentarium of the surgeon and is considered to be one of the best absorbable suture materials available so far.

- *Polydioxanone*: Polydioxanone (PDS II) is a polyester monofilament suture made of p-dioxanone. Stiffness which is one of the important disadvantages of monofilament has been addressed in PDS II thus making it more easy to handle.[1] Polydioxanone retains 74% of its tensile strength at 2 weeks postimplantation and takes 180 days to be completely absorbed.[15,17] Polydioxanone has also demonstrated minimal tissue reaction. Hence, it is a suture material of choice for wounds that require prolonged tensile strength.
- *Glycomer 631*: It is a synthetic absorbable monofilament similar to poliglecaprone 25 in characteristics but with prolonged strength akin to polytrimethylene carbonate. It passes through the tissue more easily but the knot security is inferior.[5]
- *Polyglytone 6211*: Polyglytone 6211 is a recently developed monofilament, absorbable, synthetic suture.[9,13] It is polyester of glycolide, caprolactone, trimethylene carbonate and lactide. It loses its tensile strength rapidly, mimicking surgical gut. However, absorption occurs via hydrolysis. Knot strength decreases to 50–60% of original strength at 5 days postimplantation.

Nonabsorbable Sutures (Table 4)

Nonabsorbable sutures maintain most of their tensile strength 60 days postimplantation.[12] These sutures should be just tight enough to approximate, not strangulate tissues.[14] Nonabsorbable sutures often cause less scarring because they provoke less immune response and thus are used where cosmetic outcome is important. They require manual removal postoperatively after a certain time.

Nonabsorbable sutures include natural and synthetic suture materials.

a. *Natural:* These include:

- *Surgical silk*: Silk is a natural suture material extruded by silk worm larvae of *Bombycidae* family during their cocoon production.[1,14] It is braided and black dyed, thus allows for easy handling and greater visibility. However, due to its braided configuration, silk is prone to get infected and can be infiltrated by tissue ingrowth.[12,15] Coating with wax or silicone helps to reduce tissue friction and capillarity.[5,6] Silk is a naturally occurring organic substance and evokes a significant inflammatory response, second only to catgut.[18] A special quality of silk is its ease of handling. Unfortunately, its tensile strength is very low. Although classified as a nonabsorbable material, silk suture becomes absorbed by proteolysis and is often undetectable in the wound site by 2 years. Due to its property of reactivity, it is rarely used for cutaneous closures; however, it is commonly used on mucosal and intertriginous areas as it is soft and pliable.
- *Surgical cotton*: It is made of twisted, long, stable cotton fibers.[6] Tensile strength is 50% in six months and 30–40% by two years. Surgical cotton is nonabsorbable and becomes encapsulated within body tissues.

b. *Synthetic:* These include:

- *Nylon*: It was introduced in 1940 as the first synthetic suture material.[1] Nylon suture materials are available in both mono (Ethilon/Monosof) or braided multifilament (Nurolon/Surgilon) forms. It is a polyamide polymer fiber which is chemically inert. Due to its property of elasticity, it is useful for surface (epidermal, superficial) closure. Monofilament nylon suture has a great deal of memory and its proclivity for knot slippage is known.[5] Multifilament braided nylon sutures exhibit decreased memory and they are associated with higher

Table 4: Nonabsorbable sutures and their characteristics.[8]

Properties	Silk	Nylon, Monofilament	Nylon, Multifilament	Polyester	Polypropylene	Polybutester
Handling	Excellent	Poor	Fair-good	Good	Poor	Good
Knot security	Excellent	Poor	Fair-good	Good	Poor	Fair-good
Tensile strength	Low	High	High	High	Moderate	High
Coefficient of friction	High	Low	High	High	Very low	Very low
Memory	Low	High	Medium	Medium	High	Low
Tissue reactivity	High	Low	Moderate	Low-moderate	Low	Low
Uses	Mucosal tissues, conjunctiva or intertriginous zones; to elevate or retract tissues	Percutaneous; buried if prolonged dermal support is needed	Minimal use in dermatologic surgery	Minimal use in dermatologic surgery	Widely used in dermatological surgeries. Percutaneous; buried if prolonged dermal support is needed; running subcuticular closures	Percutaneous; running subcuticular closures
Other	Black	Black, green, or clear		Green or clear	High plasticity Blue or clear	High elasticity Blue or clear

infection rate. The braided forms are coated with silicone. Nylon is quite pliable, especially when moist. Of note, a premoistened form is available for cosmetic plastic surgery. Nylon suture has good handling characteristics. It is hydrolyzed slowly, but remaining suture material is stable at two years, due to gradual encapsulation by fibrous connective tissue.[6]

- *Monofilament (Ethilon)*: It remains one of the most popular nonabsorbable sutures in dermatological surgery as a result of its high tensile strength, low tissue reactivity, high elasticity and low cost.[15]
- *Polypropylene (Prolene)*: It was developed in 1970 as a first synthetic nonabsorbable suture. It is a monofilament suture made of isostatic crystalline stereoisomer of a linear propylene polymer with few unsaturated bonds.[5,14] Its significant advantage is its high plasticity which allows it to expand to accommodate the wound edema. This decreases the risk of the suture cutting the tissue.[1] However, it leaves the stitches loose once the swelling subsides which is due to its properties of high memory and lack of elasticity. Polypropylene has a tensile strength more than nylon and can easily pass through tissues. This material is biologically inert and elicits minimal tissue reaction. It does not adhere to the tissues which makes it ideal for intradermal suture like subcuticular closure. As a result of its smooth surface, prolene may be smoothly implanted and removed without tugging of the skin. It is available as dyed or undyed form. This material is useful in contaminated and infected wounds, as it minimizes sinus formation and suture extrusion.[6] Because of smooth surface, knot security is decreased and it should be compensated for with extra throws.[12,15]
- *Hexafluoropropylene*: It is a newly developed nonabsorbable monofilament suture made of polyvinylidene fluoride and polyvinylidene fluoride-co-hexafluoropropylene.[14] It exhibits lack of adherence to tissues which makes it a possible choice for 'pull-out' sutures. Like polypropylene, it resists infection and elicits minimal tissue response. It is dyed blue.
- *Polyester*: Polyester[5] sutures are nonabsorbable synthetic braided multifilament sutures composed of polyethylene terephthalate. Due to its unique properties, such as minimal tissue reactivity, high tensile strength, good handling and lasting indefinitely in the body, it is ideal for face lifts. Other indications include prosthetic implantations and cardiovascular surgeries. Polyester sutures are available in both coated or uncoated forms.
- *Polybutester suture*: The newest advance in nonabsorbable sutures is Polybutester suture, which is a block copolymer that contains butylene terephthalate (84%) and polytetramethylene ether glycol terephthalate (16%).[19] It is the newest of the synthetic nonabsorbable sutures.[1] Being monofilamentous, it produces little inflammatory response and is less likely to harbor bacteria. High elasticity is one of its unique and advantageous characteristics. As previously discussed, high elasticity allows it to stretch with wound edema but return to its original length and form once swelling has subsided. Polybutester is able to stretch to 50% of its original length at a load of 25% of its knot breaking point.[15,20] This high degree of elasticity provides obvious clinical advantages, as it is less likely to cut through the skin during swelling and effectively approximates wound edges throughout the healing process.

Suture Selection

Important factors to be considered while choosing the suture material are the location of wound, static and dynamic wound tension, presence of wound infection or fever and cost of suture material.

Following are the general principles to be considered for suture selection.

a. Based on Tensile Strength

The tensile strength of the suture should never exceed the tensile strength of the tissue. As the wound heals, the relative loss of suture strength over time should be slower than the gain of tissue tensile strength. Esthetic concerns are at a premium in the anatomic regions of the head and neck.

- Eyelid, periorbital area, nose, pinna, lip, and vermillion—Sutures with less tensile strength and smaller sizes are preferred.
- The activity and mobility of the face, anterior and posterior neck, scalp, superior trunk, and nasal and oral mucosa require sutures with higher tensile strength.
- Major musculocutaneous flaps tend to be closed under significant tension and hence require maximal long-term tensile strength.

b. Based on Absorbable Property

Sutures are no longer needed when a wound has reached maximum strength. Therefore, consider nonabsorbable suture in skin, fascia and tendons (slowly healing tissues), while mucosal wounds (rapidly healing tissues) may be closed with absorbable sutures.

c. Based on Type of Filament

Special consideration of suture selection in infected wounds is imperative. Multifilament sutures are more likely to harbor contaminants than monofilament sutures; thus, monofilament sutures are generally preferable in potentially contaminated tissues. Use the smallest inert monofilament suture materials, such as nylon or polypropylene, in this setting.

d. Based on Size of Suture Material (Table 5)

Optimal suture size is generally the smallest size necessary to achieve the desired tension-free closure. If wound tension is high, smaller diameter sutures may actually

Table 5: Showing the preferred size of suture materials.[12,21]

Site	Suture size
Thin-skinned areas of low tension (eyelids and scrotum)	6–0
Face	5–0
Facial areas closed under some tension (forehead and other body areas)	4–0
Thick-skinned areas (scalp, back and scapular areas) closed under tension	3–0 or 2–0

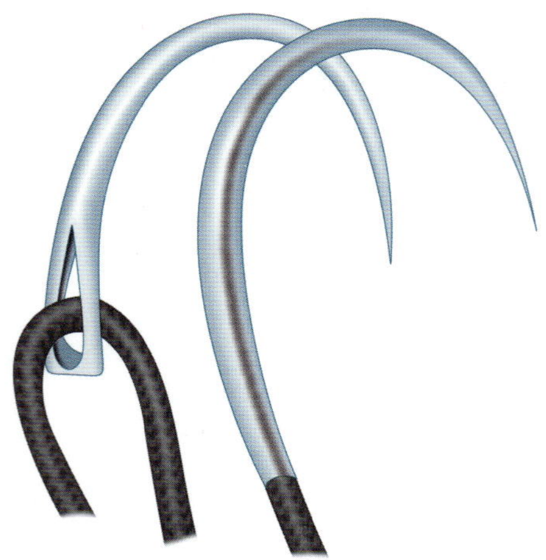

Fig. 3: Traumatic and atraumatic needles.

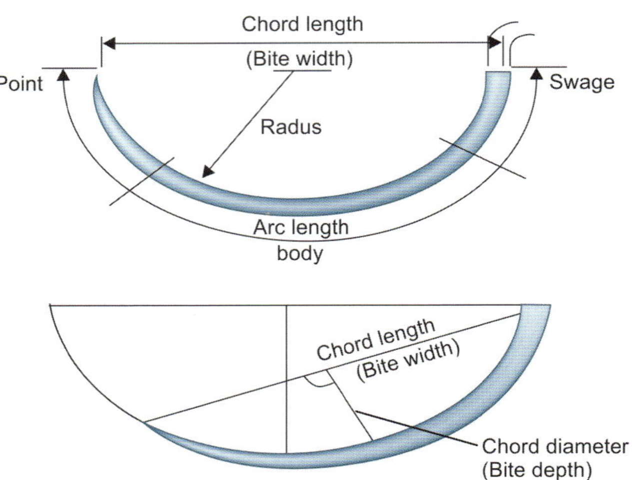

Fig. 4: Anatomy of needle.

injure tissues by cutting through them. Therefore, closely match the tensile strength of the suture and tissue.

NEEDLES

Surgical needles are made of stainless steel alloys, which have excellent resistance to corrosion.[22] Scientists have successfully used the concept of high nickel maraging stainless steels (S45500/SURGALLOY™)[19] to develop stainless steel wires with superior strength and ductility for use as surgical needles. Surgical needles made of a high nickel maraging stainless steel have a greater resistance to bending and breakage than stainless steels without nickel.

Based on this characteristic, surgical needles may be classified as traumatic or atraumatic.[2]

Traumatic needles are needles with eyes which are available without suture thread whereas atraumatic needles comprise an eyeless needle swaged to a specific length of suture thread (Fig. 3).

Wound closure and healing is affected by the initial tissue injury caused by needle penetration along with subsequent suture passage. Hence, proper selection of needle is necessary.

Ideal Surgical Needle Characteristics[6]

- High-quality stainless steel
- Smallest diameter possible
- Stable in the grasp of the needle holder
- Capable of implanting suture material through tissue with minimal trauma.
- Sharp enough to penetrate tissue with minimal resistance.
- Sterile and corrosion-resistant to prevent introduction of microorganisms or foreign materials into the wound.

Anatomy of Needle

Point

This portion of the needle extends from the tip to the maximum cross-section of the body.[6]

Body

This part of the needle incorporates most of the needle length (Fig. 4). The body of the needle is important for interaction with the needle holder and the ability to transmit the penetrating force to the point. The needle factors that affect this interaction include needle diameter and radius, body geometry, and stainless steel alloy. These components determine the needle-bending moment, ultimate moment, surgical-yield moment and needle ductility.[6,23]

Swage

The suture attachment end creates a single, continuous unit of suture and needle (Fig. 5).

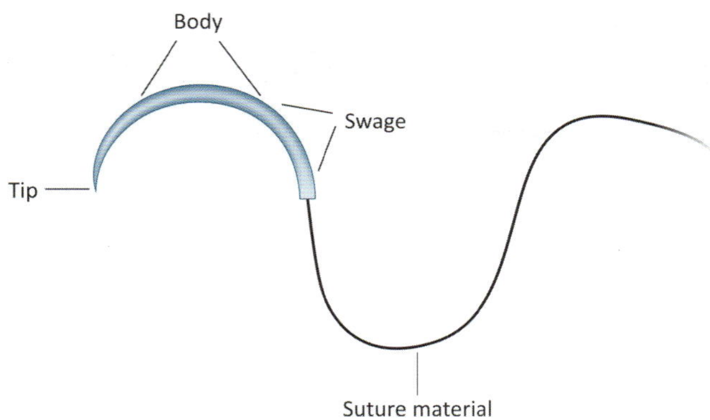

Fig. 5: Parts of swaged needle.

Advantages of Eyeless or Swaged Needles

- It minimizes the trauma on the sutured tissue as suture end of the swaged needle is smaller than the needle body. Moreover, in traumatic needle, the thread comes out of the needle's hole on both sides. When passing through the tissues, this suture may tear the skin to a certain extent, thus the name traumatic.[3,10]
- Unlike in eyed needle, suture is less likely to become unthreaded prematurely.
- Decreased handling helps maintain suture integrity.
- Time spent on threading the suture on the needle is avoided in atraumatic needles.
- Sutures are supplied in sealed packets after gamma ray sterilization. Hence, each patient has the benefit of a new, sharp, guaranteed sterile needle.
- Nearly all modern sutures feature swaged atraumatic needles.

Silicone Coating

Needles coated with silicone are available allowing easier tissue passage.[6]

Needle Measurements

Chord Length

This is the linear distance from the point of the curved needle to the swage (bite width).[6]

Needle Length

The distance measured along the needle from the point to the swage is termed needle length. It is the needle length and not the chord length (bite width), is the measurement supplied on suture packages.

Radius

This is the distance from the body of the needle to the center of the circle along which the needle curves (bite depth).

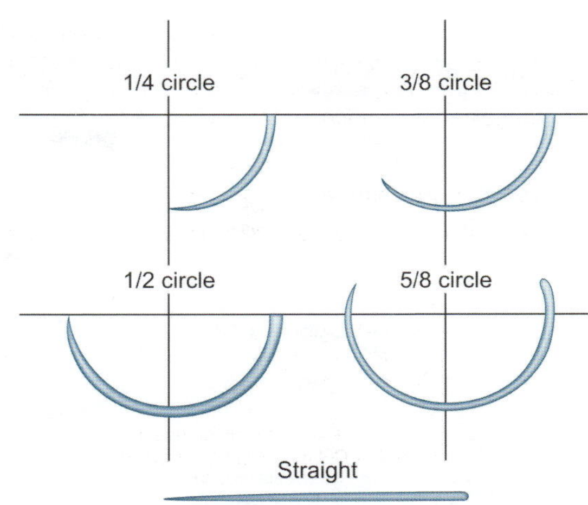

Fig. 6: Different shapes of curved needle.

Diameter

The gauge or thickness of the needle wire is considered the diameter.

Needle Types

Needles can be classified based on different criteria such as size, body type and on cross section.

a. *Based on size:* Different needle lengths are available for each suture size and the length required depends on the thickness of the tissue being sutured.[24] Always use the thinnest needle and the finest filament the wound can tolerate.
b. *Based on body types:* Surgical needles are available in various body shapes like straight needle, curved and compound curved of which curved needles are exclusively used in dermatosurgery.[6]

   Curved needle has a predictable path through tissue and requires less space for maneuvering than a straight needle. Body curvature is commonly a quarter inch, three-eighth inch, half inch or five-eighths inch circle (Fig. 6). The three-eighths inch circle is used most commonly for skin closure. It is shaped like a fish hook in case of subcutaneous sutures.[5] It is important to rotate the wrist when passing the curved needle through the tissue.
c. *Based on cross-section:* Needle may be either cutting or non-cutting (round-bodied). Cutting needles are commonly used in dermatosurgery since they are designed for penetration through dense, irregular, and relatively thick tissues like skin.

Commonly Used Cutting Needles in Dermatosurgery

- *Conventional cutting:*[6] This type of needle has three cutting edges (triangular cross-section that changes to a flattened body). The third cutting edge is on the

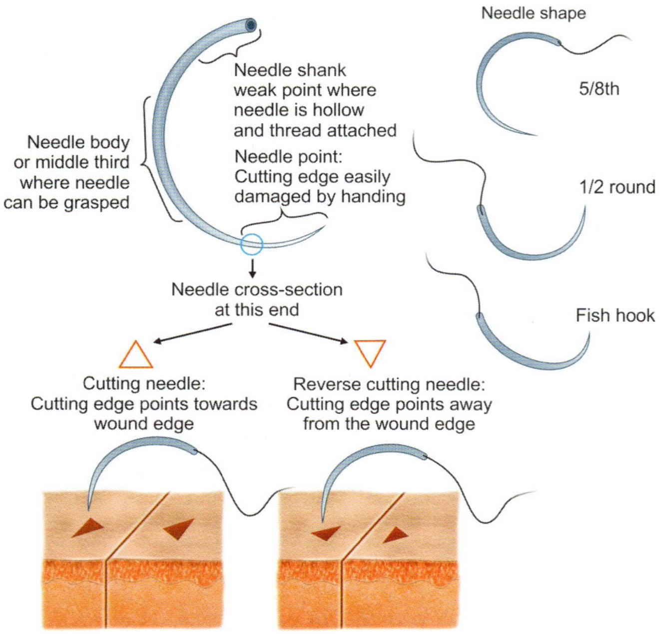

Fig. 7: Types of needles.

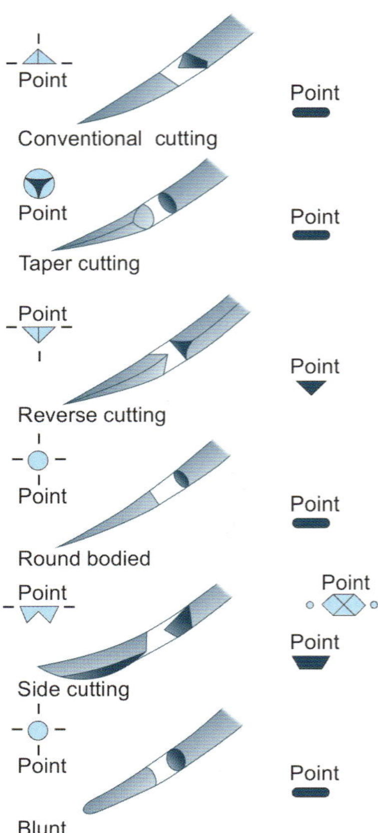

Fig. 8: Cross-section of different types of eyeless needle.

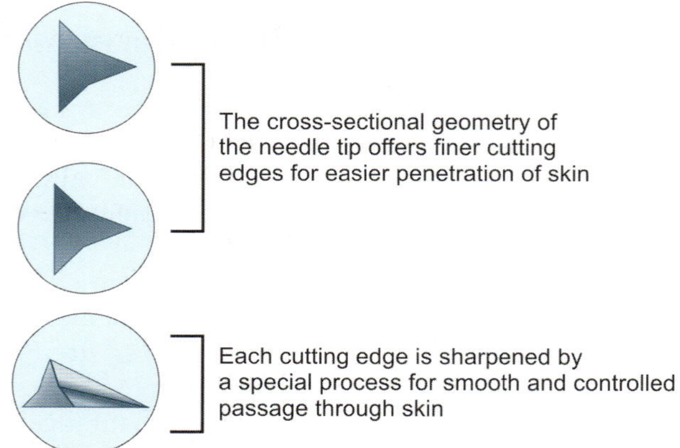

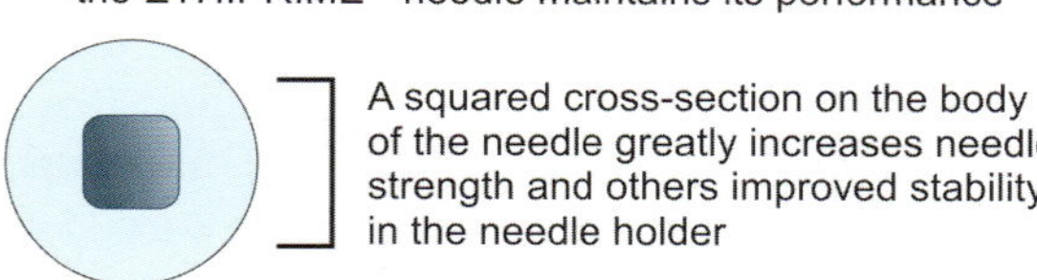

Fig. 9: SUB Q ethiprime® needle, special needle for cosmetic surgery.

inner, concave curvature (surface-seeking) and can cut through wound edge (Figs. 7 and 8).

- *Reverse cutting:*[6] The third cutting edge is on the outer convex curvature of the needle (depth-seeking). These needles are stronger than conventional cutting needles and have a reduced risk of cutting out tissue. The needles are designed to penetrate tough tissues like skin, tendon sheaths, oral mucosa. Reverse cutting needles are commonly used in cosmetic surgery, causing minimal trauma.
- *SUB Q needles* (Fig. 9):[3] These are the needles especially designed for cosmetic surgeons seeking excellence in skin closure. The cross-sectional geometry of the needle tip offers finer cutting edges for easier penetration of skin. Each cutting edge is sharpened by a special process for smooth and controlled passage through skin.

Needle and Needle Holder Interaction

Suture needles should be handled carefully. Avoid blunting the cutting point or bending the weaker end of the suture needle.[25,26] The stability of the needle within the needle holder affects needle control and performance. The jaws of the needle holder must be appropriate to the needle size to hold it securely and prevent rocking, turning and twisting.[6] The difference between the length of the handle and the jaw creates a mechanical advantage for exerting force through the needle point. The jaws of the needle holder contact a curved needle at one point on the outer curvature and two points along the inner curvature as shown in Figures 10A to C. The force against the needle creates a moment arm, which may flatten the curvature of the needle. The needle holder clamping moment must be less than the surgical yield of the needle which otherwise can bend and break the

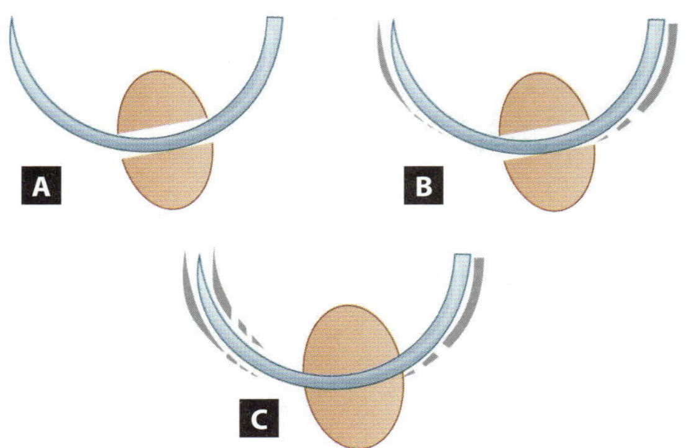

Figs. 10A to C: Interaction between the needle holder and suture needle.[6] (A) Needle holder of appropriate size for the needle; (B) Needle holder that is too large for the needle. Pressure applied by the needle holder leads to inadvertent straightening of the suture needle; (C) Needle holder that is too small for the needle. The needle rotates around the long axis of the needle holder.

needle. Repetitive injury by the needle holder also may cause the needle to break. A bent needle further increases soft tissue injury affecting cosmetic outcome.

Surgical Glove Selection

Surgeons who use sutures and needles should wear sterile surgical gloves without cornstarch. Cornstarch has been documented to promote wound infection, to cause serious peritoneal adhesions and granulomatous peritonitis and to be a well-documented vector of the latex allergy epidemic.[27]

Holes allow the transmission of blood-borne viral infections between the patient and the surgeon. FDA has laid down specific standards of criteria for surgical gloves. The use of the Biogel double-glove hole indication system is recommended to detect the location and presence of holes in the gloves, allowing the surgeon to change the gloves when a hole is detected.[28,29]

PRINCIPLES OF SUTURING

The technique of suturing cutaneous wounds is a millenium old. The goals of suturing are closing dead space, supporting and strengthening wounds until healing increases their tensile strength, approximating skin edges for an esthetically pleasing and functional result and minimizing the risks of formation of hematoma and infection.

Selection of proper suturing technique is important to ensure best cosmetic results in dermatologic surgery. The choice of suture technique depends on the type and anatomic location of the wound (e.g. eyes, vermilion border of the lips), the thickness of the skin, the degree of tension, and the desired cosmetic result.[23] Wound eversion is essential to maximize the likelihood of good epidermal approximation. Eversion is desirable to minimize the risk of scar depression secondary to tissue contraction during healing. Usually, inversion is not desirable and it probably does not decrease the risk of hypertrophic scarring in an individual with a propensity for hypertrophic scars. Suture material elicits a foreign body tissue reaction. During wound closure, meticulous aseptic technique is critical to minimize the risk of wound infection. Gentle handling of the tissue is also important to optimize wound healing.

Often, two layers are sutured:

1. Deep sutures below the surface to maintain the closure until the wound has fully healed and can support itself without widening of the scar.
2. Surface sutures to closely approximate the epidermal edges providing the best possible cosmetic result.

To obtain the best cosmetic results, it is important to have good quality instruments that are the correct size for the location and nature of the wounds being closed. The instruments also need to be correctly sterilized and handled carefully.

The basic suturing kit includes:

- Needle holder
- Fine suture cutting scissors
- Toothed tissue forceps or skin hook
- Appropriate suture material.

Techniques of Needle Holding and Suture Placement

The jaw of the appropriate needle holder is used to grasp the needle at its distal portion at the junction of anterior two-thirds and posterior one-third. The needle holder is tightened by squeezing it until the first ratchet catches. The needle holder should not be tightened excessively because damage to both the needle and the needle holder may result. The needle is held vertically and longitudinally perpendicular to the needle holder (Figs. 11 to 16).[23]

- As described earlier, incorrect placement of the needle in the needle holder may result in a bent needle, difficult penetration of the skin, and/or an undesirable angle of entry into the tissue.
- The needle holder is held by placing the thumb and the fourth finger into the loops and by placing the index finger on the fulcrum of the needle holder to provide stability (Fig. 12).
  Alternatively, the needle holder may be held in the palm to increase dexterity (Fig. 13).
- The tissue must be stabilized to allow suture placement. Depending on the surgeon's preference, toothed or untoothed forceps or skin hooks may be used to gently grasp the tissue. Excessive trauma to the tissue being sutured should be avoided to reduce the possibility of tissue strangulation and necrosis.
- The needle should always penetrate the skin at a 90° angle, which minimizes the size of the entry wound and promotes eversion of the skin edges (Figs. 14A to C).[30] The needle should be inserted 1–3 mm from the wound edge, depending on skin thickness. The depth and angle of the suture depends on the particular suturing

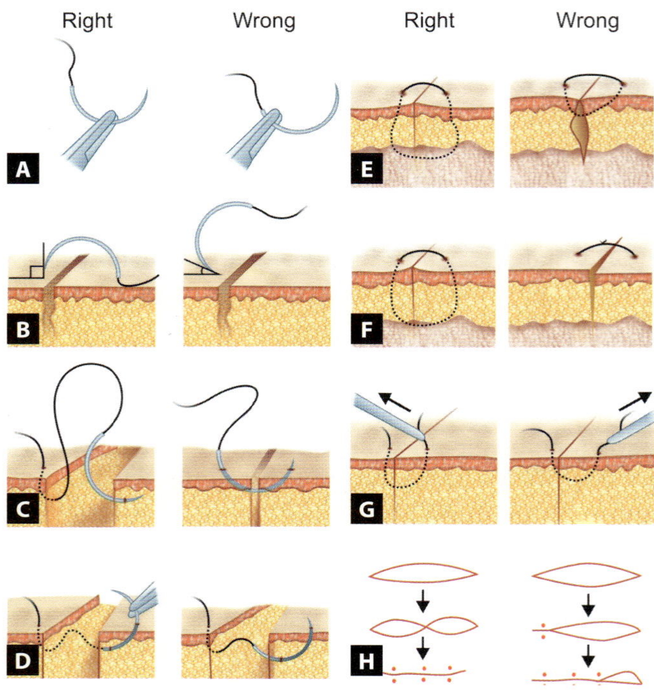

Figs. 11A to H: Techniques of needle holding and suturing.

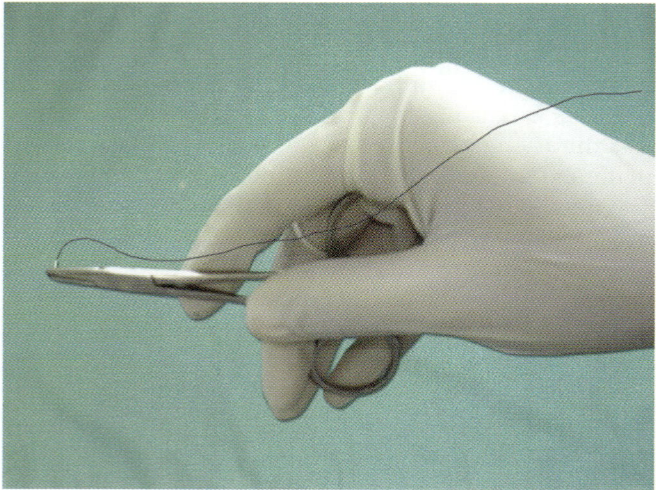

Fig. 13: Holding needle holder to increase dexterity.

technique. The needle should be driven in an arc that follows the curvature of the needle (Figs. 15A to C).

- Fine forceps are necessary for grasping the needle as it exits the tissue after a pass. Prior to removing the needle holder, grasping and stabilizing the needle is important. This maneuver decreases the risk of losing the needle in the dermis or subcutaneous fat and it is especially important if small needles are used in areas such as the back, where large needle bites are necessary for proper tissue approximation (Fig. 16).
- The needle tip is grasped with the needle holder and by rotating the needle holder in the same arc as the

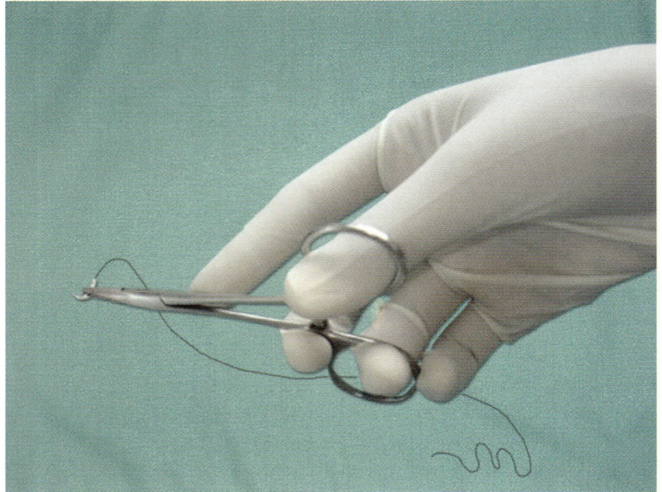

Fig. 12: Holding needle holder to provide stability.

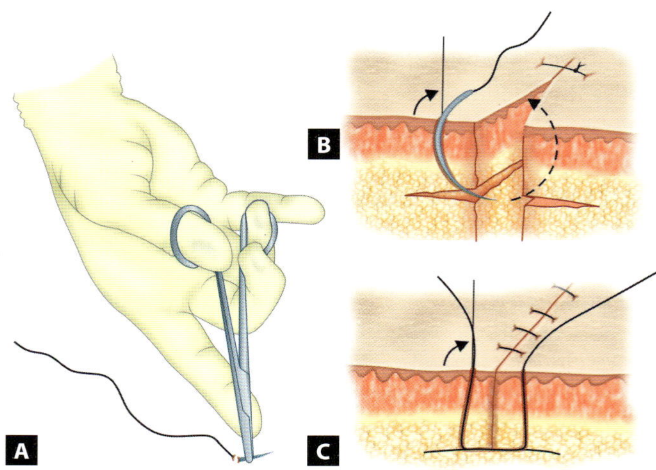

Figs. 14A to C: Basic Suturing. (A) Proper grip; (B) Angle of entry; (C) Angle of exit.

needle, the rest of the needle will emerge from the tissue and the attached suture material will follow.

- The needle must be repositioned in the jaws of the needle holder for penetrating the deep tissue of the opposing wound edge. The needle must penetrate the opposing side at precisely the same depth as the side from which it is emerged. The opposing wound edge is stabilized with forceps prior to penetration with the needle.
- In general, the two sides of the suture should become mirror images, and the needle should also exit the skin perpendicular to the skin surface.[31]

Key Precautions

- Avoid picking up the needles with your fingers. Always use needle holder and forceps to control them.
- Place needles with other sharp instruments in a kidney tray when not in use. Never pass them hand-to-hand.

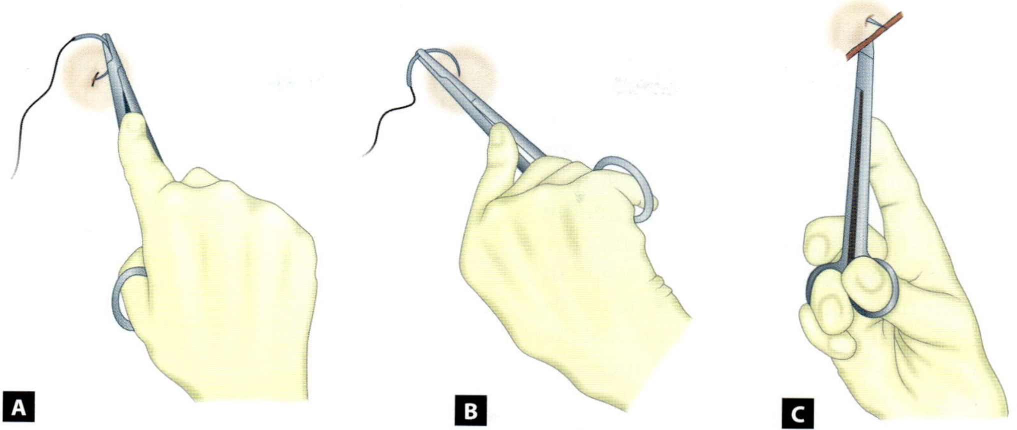

Figs. 15A to C: (A) Proper grip of the needle with hand-fully pronated; (B) Needle progressed along its arc by progressively supinating the hand; (C) Needle exits with fully supinated hand.

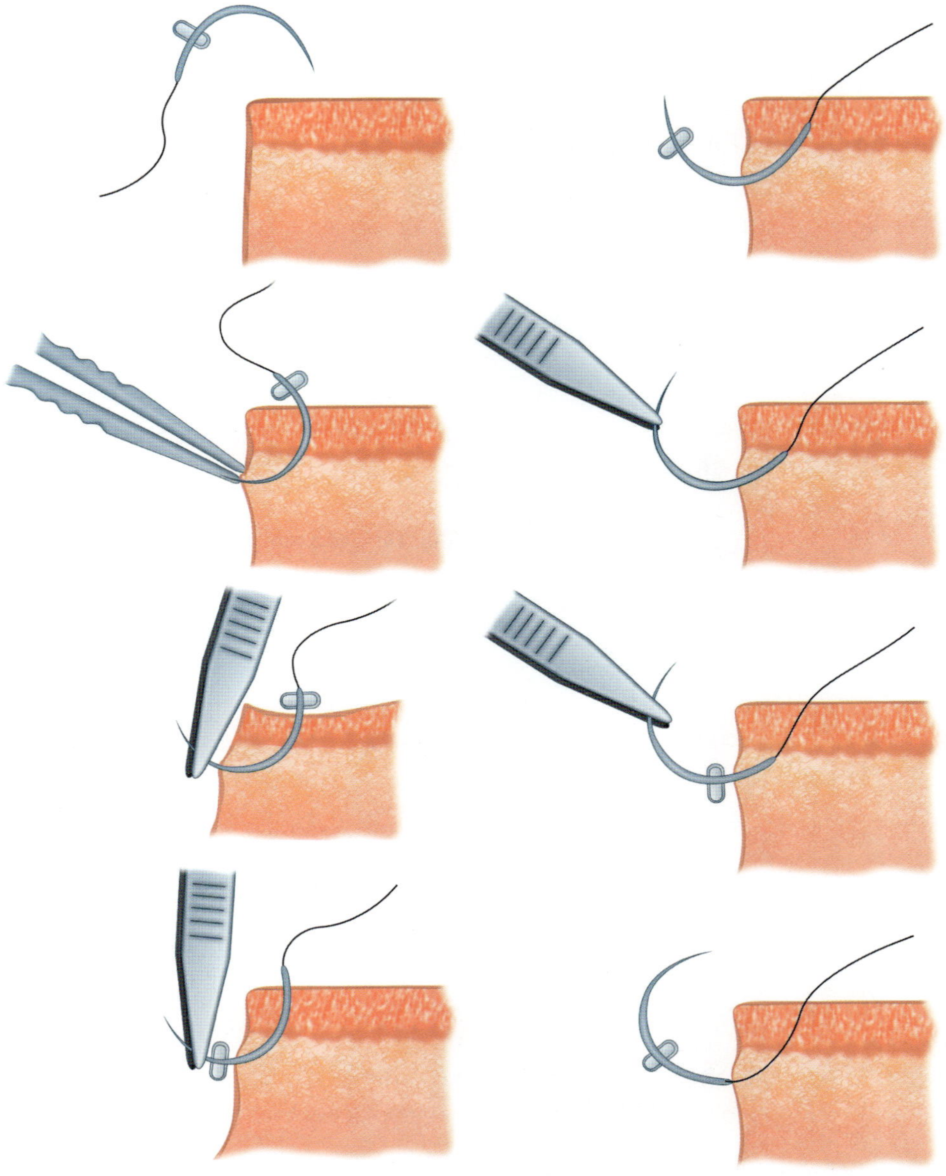

Fig. 16: Illustration showing exit of the needle with the help of fine forceps and needle holder.

Knot Tying

Once the suture is satisfactorily placed, it must be secured with a knot (Figs. 17 to 20). The instrument tie is used most commonly in cutaneous surgery. The square knot is traditionally used. First, the tip of the needle holder is rotated clockwise around the long end of the suture material for two complete turns. The tip of the needle holder is used to grasp the short end of the suture. The short end of the suture is pulled through the loops of the long end by crossing the hands, such that the two ends of the suture material are situated on opposite sides of the suture line. The needle holder is rotated counterclockwise once around the long end of the suture. The short end is grasped with the needle holder tip, and the short end is pulled through the loop again. First throw may get loosened while forming and tightening the second throw resulting in separation of skin edges. Rotate the threads clockwise or anticlockwise, to lock them. As the second throw tightens, it unlocks the trapped first throw without giving it a chance to slacken. An effective method of preventing slippage is to ask your assistant to compress the tightened first throw with a finger while you form and tighten the second throw, leading the tightening loop under the compressing finger (Fig. 21).

- The suture should be tightened sufficiently to approximate the wound edges without constricting the tissue. Sometimes, leaving a small loop of suture after the second throw is helpful. This reserve loop allows the stitch to expand slightly and is helpful in preventing the strangulation of tissue because the tension exerted on the suture increases with increased wound edema.[10,32] Depending on the surgeon's preference, 1–2 additional throws may be added.
- Knot should be placed on one side of the wound for all sutures and not on the wound.
- Properly squaring successive ties is important. That is, each tie must be laid down perfectly parallel to the previous tie. This procedure is important in preventing the creation of a granny knot, which tends to slip and is inherently weaker than a properly squared knot. When

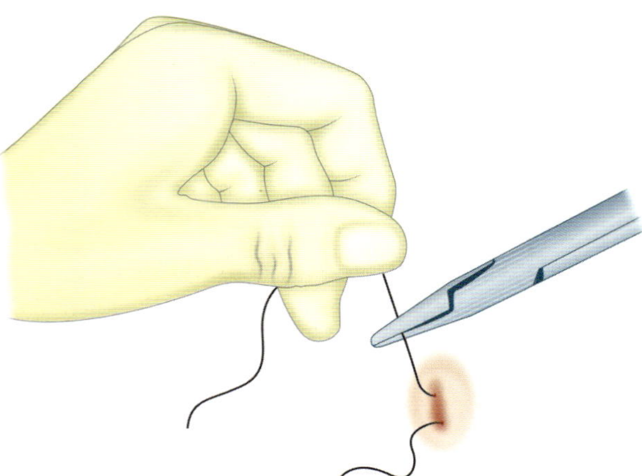

Fig. 17: Place the needle holder on the long thread.

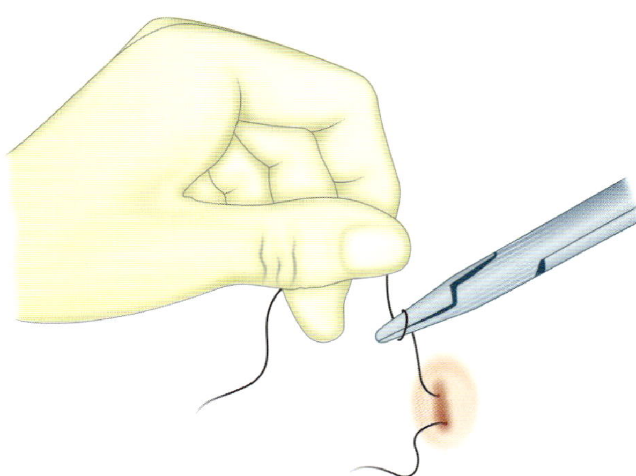

Fig. 18: Take a turn of the long thread around the needle holder.

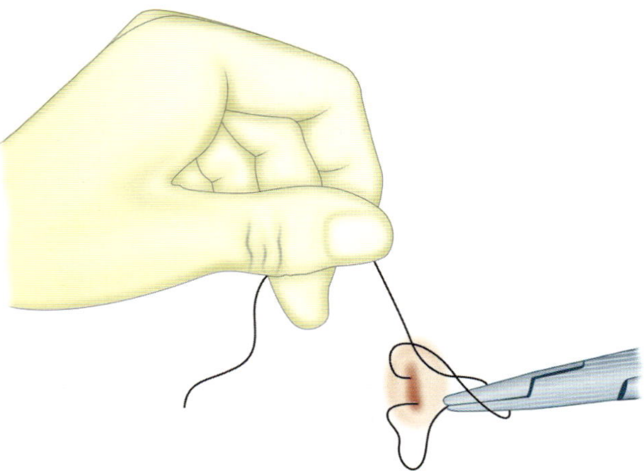

Fig. 19: Short end is grasped through the loop.

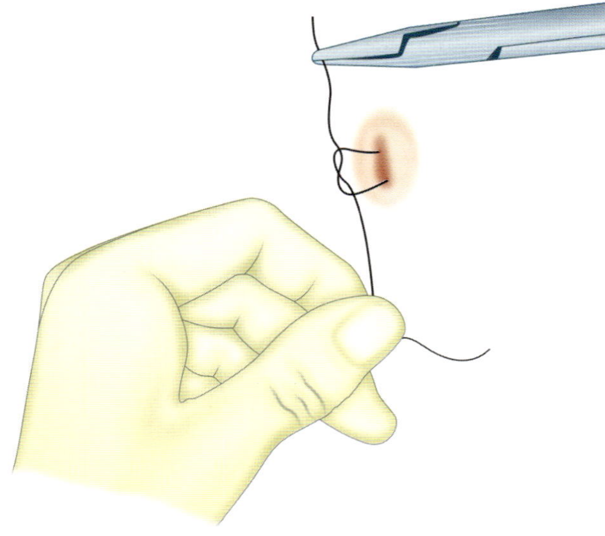

Fig. 20: Short end is pulled through the loop taking away from you while long end of the thread is drawn toward you.

the desired number of throws is completed, the suture material may be cut off with scissors, leaving one cm of suture on either side of the knot (if interrupted stitches are used) or the next suture may be placed.

SUTURING TECHNIQUES

Different suturing techniques exist. It can be interrupted, continuous/running or special sutures.

Tables 6 and 7 summarize the suturing patterns.

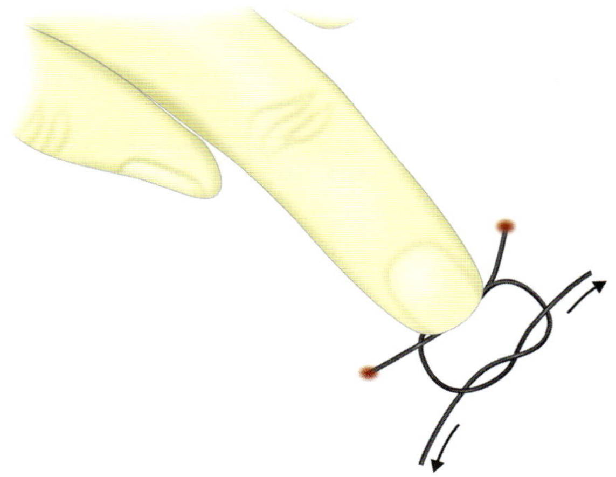

Fig. 21: Assistant compressing the tightened first throws with a finger while you form and tighten the second throw.

Interrupted Sutures

i. Simple Interrupted Sutures

The simple interrupted suture is the gold standard and the most commonly employed suture in cutaneous surgery.

Procedure: This suture is placed by inserting the needle perpendicular to the epidermis 1–2 mm from the skin edge, traversing the epidermis and the full thickness of the dermis, and exiting perpendicular to the epidermis on the opposite side of the wound. The two sides of the stitch should be symmetrically placed in terms of depth and width. In general, the final configuration of the suture should be flask shaped, that is, the stitch should be wider at its base (dermal side) than at its superficial portion (epidermal side) (Fig. 22).[10] Such configuration prevents wound inversion.[33]

Taking tissue bites at the same level on either side of the wound edges will also minimize the possibility of mismatched wound-edge heights (i.e. stepping). Distance between two sutures vary with the site of the wound and is approximately 3 mm on eyelid, 5 mm on face and 1–2 cm at other sites.[34] Proper tension is important to ensure precise wound approximation while preventing tissue strangulation. Tight sutures cause ischemia, delay healing and increase scarring.[30]

Table 6: Comparison of various interrupted sutures

Properties	*Simple interrupted sutures*	*Vertical mattress sutures*	*Half-buried vertical mattress sutures*	*Pulley sutures*	*Far-near near-far modified vertical mattress sutures*	*Horizontal mattress suture*
Tensile strength	Moderate	High	Moderate	High	Moderate	High
Advantages	Less potential for wound edema and impaired circulation. Allows expression of serum or blood from between sutures	Reduces dead space, maximizes wound eversion and minimizes wound tension	Eliminates two of four entry points of vertical mattress suture thus minimizes the scarring	Facilitates greater stretching of wound edges	Elevate the deeper tissue of the wound and evert the epidemis	Reduces dead space, evert wound edges and reduces wound tension
Disadvantages	May leave a series of cross-hatched linear scars More time needed to tie individual knots	Greater risk of cross hatching if not removed early	Risk of cross-hatching present but minimal	Risk of cross hatching if not removed early	Bites must be symmetrical or the wound will invariably misalign	Risk of strangulation of the dermal blood supply and edge necrosis is known if tied too tightly
Uses	To approximate the wound edges of uneven thickness	In closing high tension wounds	Used in cosmetically important areas like face	Useful when additional wound closure strength is desired	Useful when tissue expansion is desired	Used as stay stich to temporarily approximate wound edges. In thick glabrous skin (palms and soles)

Table 7: Comparison of various continuous and special sutures.

Properties	*Simple running sutures*	*Running horizontal mattress sutures*	*Running locked sutures*	*Dermal-subdermal sutures*	*Running subcuticular sutures*	*Running subcutaneous sutures*	*Half burried horizontal mattress sutures*	*Barbed sutures*
Tensile strength	Low	moderate	High	Low	Low	Low	Low	Moderate
Advantages	Useful for long wounds in which wound tension has been minimized Allows rapid reapproximation of wound edges Less scarring compared to interrupted sutures	Allows good skin eversion Results in smoother and flatter scars as compared to simple running sutures	Useful in wounds under moderate tension and in those demanding additional hemostasis	Reduces dead space and wound tension	Provides best cosmetic outcome as it precisely approximate the wound edges	Used to close deep portion of surgical defects under moderate tension	Used primarily to position the corners and tips of flaps	Quicker wound closing time Reduces the amount of scar tissue
Disadvantages	Risk of dehiscence if the suture material ruptures Not as strong as interrupted sutures	Time consuming	Can cause tissue strangulation if placed too tightly	Weaker than simple running sutures of skin	Does not provide significant wound strength Fails if the suture is cut in just one place	Risk of suture breakage resulting in formation of dead space beneath the skin surface	May result in depressed scar	Skin dimpling around the suture placement
Uses	In split and full thickness skin graft Over eyelids, ears, dorsa of hands and scalp wounds especially when good hemostasis is expected	In areas with a high tendency for inversion, such as face and neck	In areas with good vascularization like scalp	In wound closure following lipoma/large epidermal cyst excision	Valuable in areas where best cosmetic result is desired Useful in children when absorbable suture material is used	Subcutaneous closures	In M-plasties and V-Y closures	For face lift, breast reduction

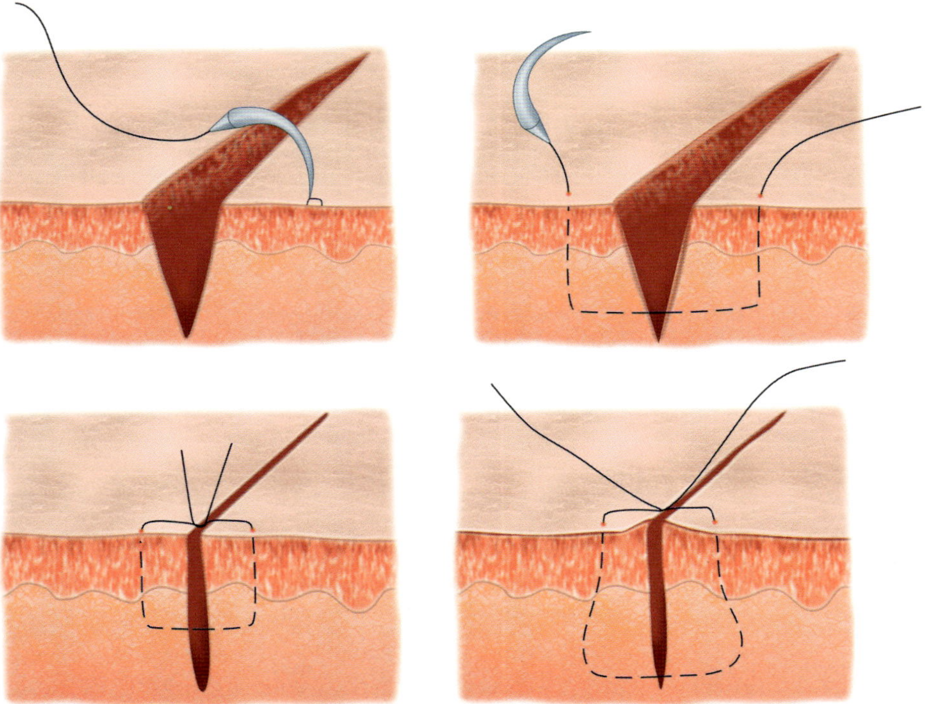

Fig. 22: Simple interrupted suture showing a flask-shaped stitch maximizing wound eversion.

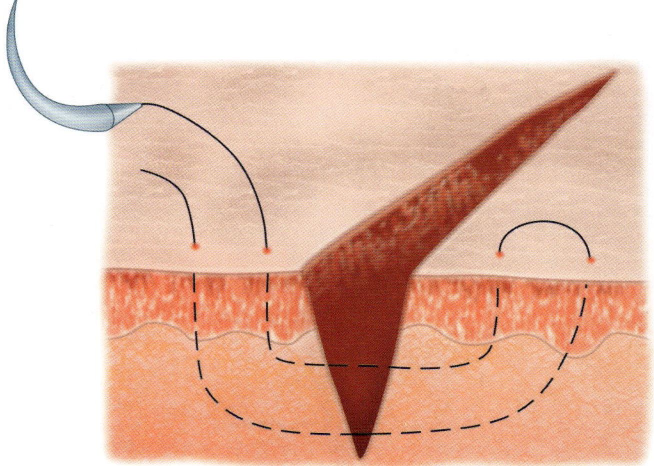

Fig. 23: Vertical mattress suture.

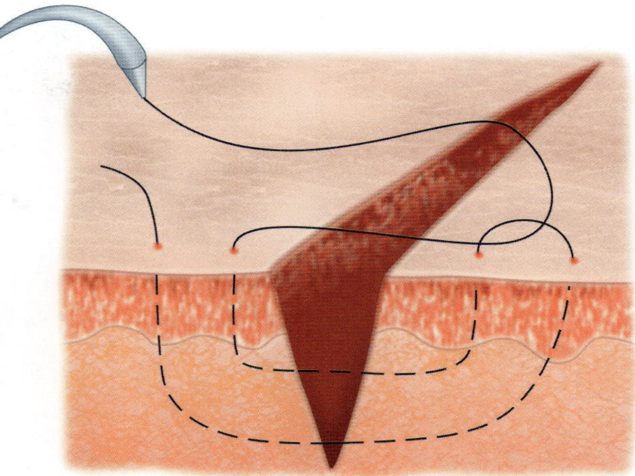

Fig. 24: Pulley stitch.

Advantages

- Interrupted sutures are easy to place and have greater tensile strength.
- They have less potential for causing wound edema and impaired cutaneous circulation when compared to running sutures.
- By altering the depth or angle of the needle, this technique can also be used to approximate the wound edges of uneven thickness.[5] While taking the simple interrupted sutures on the thicker tissue like scalp, the needle is passed deep into the subcutaneous tissue and is curved slightly away from the wound edge so that a large chunk of tissue deep in the wound is encompassed. This helps in controling bleeding too.
- It allows expression of serum or blood from between sutures.

Disadvantage

- The major disadvantage of this technique is that they tend to leave a series of cross-hatched linear scars resembling railroad tracks.[35] The risk of cross-hatching can be minimized by removing sutures early to prevent the development of suture tracks.

ii. Vertical Mattress Sutures

This is an excellent suturing method which provides effective wound support.

Procedure: The vertical mattress suture is a variation of the simple interrupted suture. The needle is introduced 5–10 mm from the wound edge and a deep bite of tissue is taken before exiting the skin in the same position on the opposite wound edge. The needle is then reversed on the needle holder, and the needle is reintroduced 1–3 mm from the second side of the wound and a smaller bite of tissue is taken before exiting on the first side of the wound. A knot can then be secured as shown in Figure 23. The width of the stitch should be increased in proportion to the amount of tension on the wound. That is, the higher the tension, the wider the stitch. Simple interrupted sutures may be placed in between the vertical mattress sutures. Placing each stitch precisely and taking symmetric bites is especially important with this suture.[35-37]

Advantage

- A vertical mattress suture is especially useful in maximizing wound eversion, reducing dead space and minimizing tension across the wound.

Disadvantage

- This suture tends to leave the most obvious and unsightly cross-hatching if not removed early. The risk of cross-hatching is greater because of increased tension across the wound and the four entry and exit points of the stitch in the skin.

Modifications of the Vertical Mattress Suture

a. *Half-buried vertical mattress sutures:* The half-buried vertical mattress suture is a modification of the vertical mattress suture and eliminates two of the four entry points, thereby reducing scarring. The half-buried vertical mattress suture is placed in the same manner as the vertical mattress suture, except that the needle penetrates the skin to the level of the deep part of the dermis on one side of the wound, takes a bite in the deep part of the dermis on the opposite side of the wound without exiting the skin, crosses back to the original side of the wound and exits the skin. Entry and exit points therefore are kept on one side of the wound.[36,37]

   It is used in cosmetically important areas such as the face.

b. *Pulley sutures:* The pulley suture is a modification of the vertical mattress suture. When pulley sutures are used, a vertical mattress suture is placed, the knot is left untied, and the suture is looped through the external loop on the other side of the incision and pulled across. At this point, the knot is tied. This new loop functions as a pulley, directing tension away from the other strands (Fig. 24).[23]

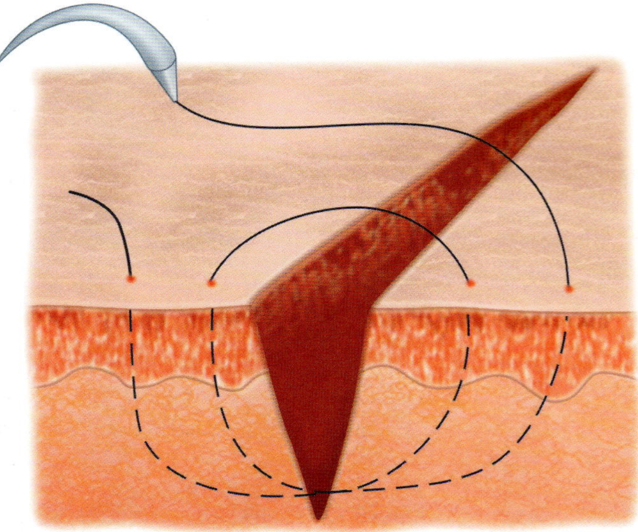

Fig. 25: Far-near near-far pulley stitch.

The pulley suture facilitates greater stretching of the wound edges and is used when additional wound closure strength is desired.

c. *Far-near near-far modified vertical mattress sutures:* Another stitch that serves the same function as the pulley suture is the far-near near-far modification of the vertical mattress suture.

Procedure: The first loop is placed approximately 4–6 mm from the wound edge on the far side and approximately 2 mm from the wound edge on the near side. The suture crosses the suture line and re-enters the skin on the original side at 2 mm from the wound edge on the near side. The loop is completed and the suture exits the skin on the opposite side 4–6 mm away from the wound edge on the far side. This placement creates a pulley effect (Fig. 25).[23]

Advantage: This technique helps to elevate the deeper tissues of the wound and evert the epidermis. It is useful when tissue expansion is desired.[35]

iii. Horizontal Mattress Suture

This is used to reduce the dead space, evert wound edges and helps to reduce high wound tension.[26]

Procedure:[34,35] The horizontal mattress suture is placed by entering the skin 5–10 mm from the wound edge. The suture is passed deep dermally or subcutaneously towards the opposing wound edge at the same level dermally or subcutaneously. The needle should come out on the opposing wound edge equidistant from the insertion. The needle re-enters the skin on the same side of the suture line 5–10 mm laterally. The needle is then passed dermally or subcutaneously to the side of initial penetration and the knot is tied on the surface (Fig. 26).

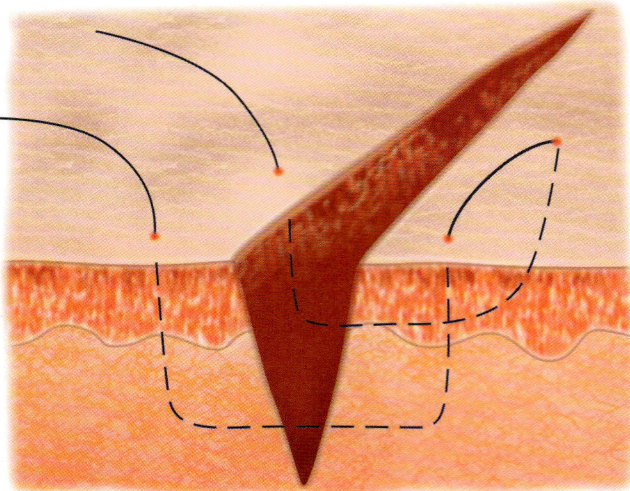

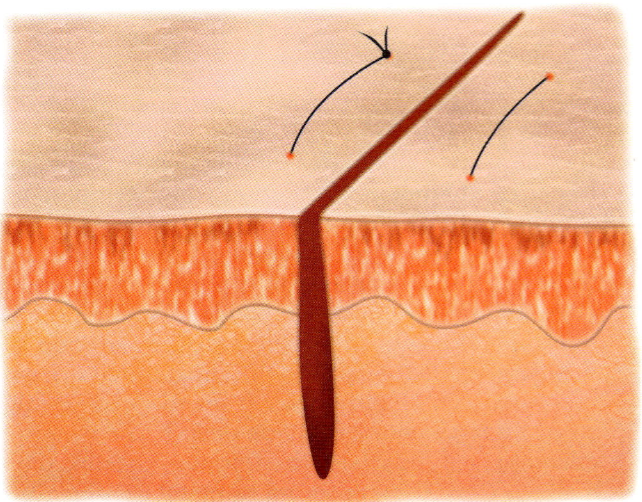

Fig. 26: Horizontal mattress suture.

Advantages

- This is particularly useful in thick glabrous skin (palms and soles).[35]
- This may also be used as a stay stitch to temporarily approximate wound edges allowing placement of simple interrupted or subcuticular stitches. The temporary stitches are removed after the tension is evenly distributed across the wound. However, they have a high-risk of producing suture marks if left in place for longer than 7 days. According to few surgeons, horizontal mattress sutures are superior to their vertical counterparts.[34]

Disadvantage: The risk of strangulation of the dermal blood supply and subsequent edge necrosis if tied too tightly is its chief disadvantage.[34] Taking generous bites, using bolsters, using knot only as tightly as necessary to approximate the wound edges and removing the sutures as early as possible may decrease the risk.

Continuous (Running) Sutures

i. Simple Running Sutures

The simple running suture, otherwise also called as continuous over-and-over suture is an uninterrupted series of simple interrupted sutures (Fig. 27).[26]

Procedure: The suture is started by placing a simple interrupted stitch, which is tied but not cut. A series of simple sutures are placed in succession without tying or cutting the suture material after each pass. Sutures should be evenly spaced, and tension should be evenly distributed along the suture line. The line of stitches is completed by tying a knot after the last pass at the end of the suture line. The knot is tied between the tail end of the suture material where it exits the wound and the loop of the last suture placed (Fig. 28).[34]

Advantages

- Running sutures are useful for long wounds in which wound tension has been minimized with properly placed deep sutures and in which approximation of the wound edges is good.[35]
- Quicker placement and more rapid re-approximation of wound edges, compared with simple interrupted sutures.
- This type of suture may be used to secure a split or full-thickness skin graft. It is also useful over eyelids, ears and the dorsa of hands.[34]
- Less scarring occurs with running sutures compared with interrupted sutures because fewer knots are made with simple running sutures; however, the number of needle insertions remains the same.
- Continuous sutures can also be placed in a locking fashion to provide hemostasis by compression of wound edges especially in scalp wound closures.

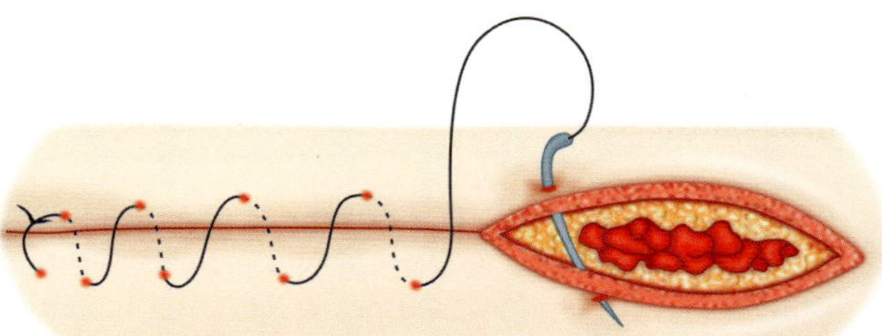

Fig. 27: Simple continuous suture.

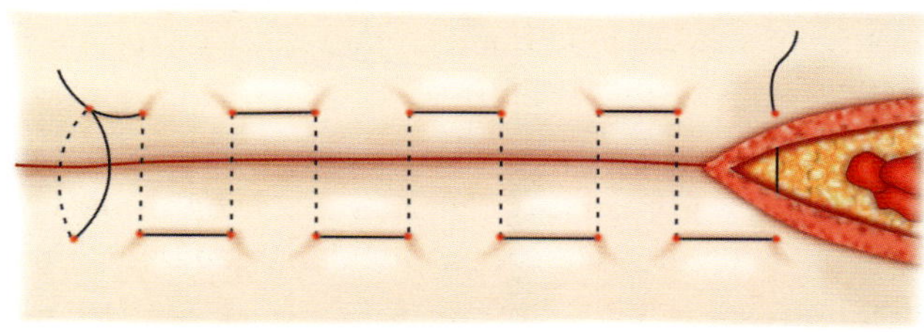

Fig. 29: Running horizontal mattress suture.

Disadvantages

- Possible cross-hatching.
- The risk of dehiscence if the suture material ruptures.
- Difficulty in making fine adjustments along the suture line.
- Can strangulate the blood supply if wounds tension is high.
- It is not as strong as interrupted sutures.

ii. Running Horizontal Mattress Sutures

Procedure: A simple suture is placed, and the knot is tied but not cut. Instead of crossing over the wound prior to re-entering the skin, the running horizontal mattress suture is done by re-entering the skin on the same side through which the suture material is exited (Fig. 29).[35,38] The final loop is tied to the free end of the suture material.

Advantages: The running horizontal mattress suture is used for skin eversion. It is useful in areas with a high tendency for inversion, such as the neck. It can also be useful for reducing the spread of facial scars. Although this technique is slightly more time consuming, it results in smoother and flatter scars as compared to simple running sutures.[38]

iii. Running Locked Sutures

Locked sutures have increased tensile strength.

Procedure: It is a simple running suture where the first knot is tied as in a traditional running suture and may be locked by passing the needle through the loop preceding it as each stitch is placed. This suture is also known as the baseball stitch (Fig. 30) because of the final appearance of the running locked suture line.[23]

Advantage: They are useful in wounds under moderate tension or in those requiring additional hemostasis.

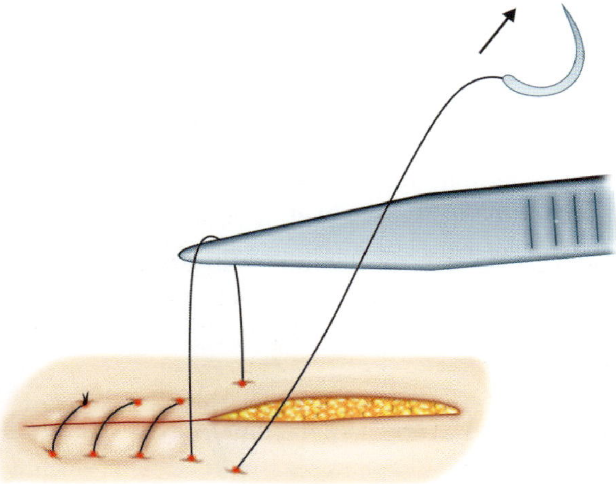

Fig. 28: Control the thread loop with fine forceps as it is tightened to ensure it sits perfectly without snagging on other structures.

Disadvantage: Increases the risk of impairing the microcirculation surrounding the wound and thus can cause tissue strangulation if placed too tightly. Therefore, this type of suture should be used only in areas with good vascularization like scalp.

iv. Dermal-Subdermal Sutures

Procedure: The suture is placed by inserting the needle parallel to the epidermis at the junction of the dermis and the subcutis. The needle curves upward and exits in the papillary dermis, again parallel to the epidermis. The needle is inserted parallel to the epidermis in the papillary dermis on the opposing edge of the wound, curves down through the reticular dermis and exits at the base of the wound at the interface between the dermis and the subcutis and parallel to the epidermis. The knot is tied at the base of the wound to minimize the possibility of tissue reaction and extrusion of the knot. If the suture is placed more superficially in the dermis at 2–4 mm from the wound edge, eversion is increased.[23]

Advantages: It reduces dead space and wound tension. It is used in closing the wound following excision of lipoma or any large epidermal cyst. Absorbable suture material is used.

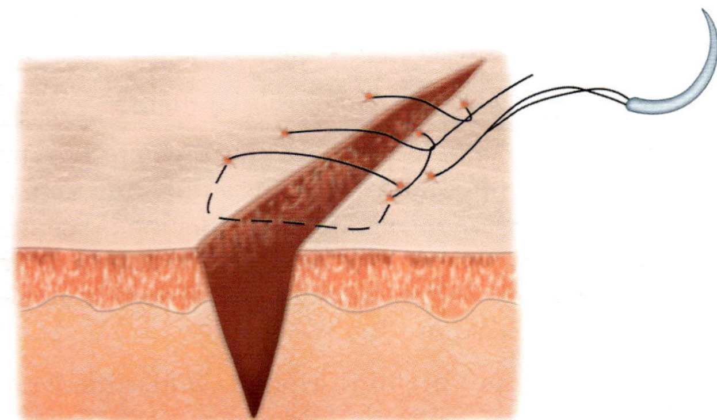

Fig. 30: Running locked suture.

v. Running Subcuticular Sutures

The running subcuticular suture is a buried form of the running horizontal mattress suture.[5] It is valuable in areas in which the best possible cosmetic result is desired. The suture does not provide significant wound strength, although it does precisely approximate the wound edges. Therefore, the running subcuticular suture is best reserved for wounds in which the tension has been eliminated with deep sutures and for closing wounds with equal tissue thickness.[34,35]

Procedure: The needle is introduced 5 mm distal to one wound end and brought out inside the apex of the wound within the dermis. The free end of suture can be tied off on itself, or secured with a bead or crimp. Horizontal bites through the papillary dermis parallel to the skin surface are then taken from alternating sides of the wound working towards the other wound apex. The second epidermal puncture is made when the needle exits 5 mm from the other end of the wound (Fig. 31). Both ends of stitch should be tied off and steristrips may be applied to stabilize the wound surface. This provides close approximation of the skin edges. Care must be taken to ensure that the sutures are placed at the same level. Absorbable or nonabsorbable suture can be used. If absorbable sutures are used, first subcutaneous interrupted sutures should be taken prior to running subcuticular suture. Among nonabsorbable sutures, polypropylene (prolene) which is a monofilament suture with minimal drag is ideal, and it should be removed at 1–2 weeks after suturing.[34]

Advantages

- It results in an excellent cosmetic outcome. Since the epidermis is penetrated only at the beginning and end of the suture line, the subcuticular suture effectively eliminates the risk of cross-hatching and no suture marks are visible.
- It is known to be a useful technique in children when absorbable suture is used so that suture removal is avoided.[35]

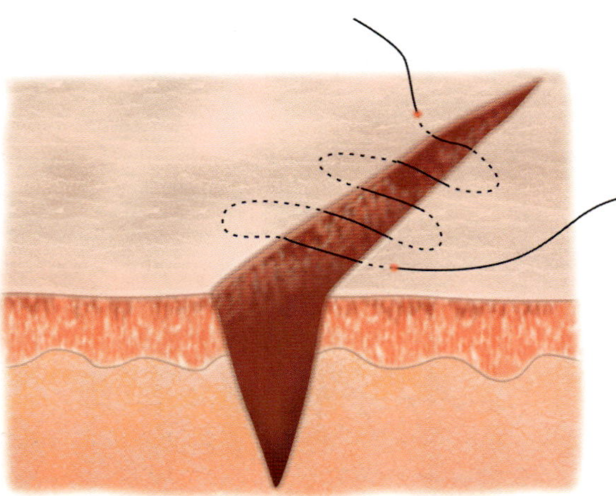

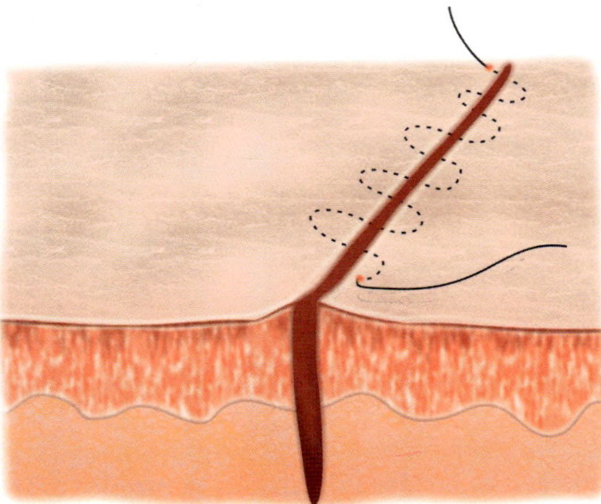

Fig. 31: Subcuticular stitch.

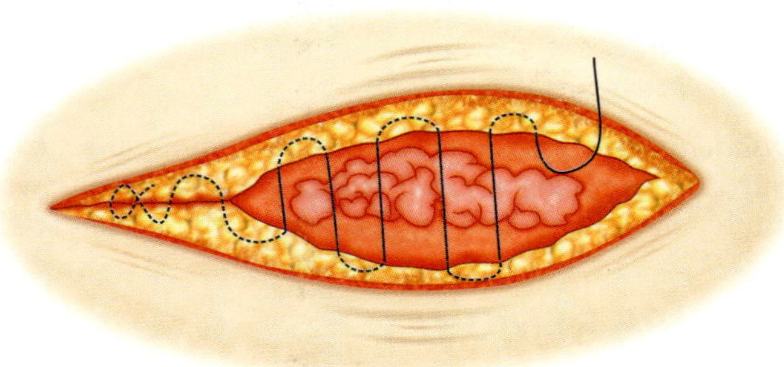

Fig. 32: Running subcutaneous sutures.

Disadvantage: Like any of the running sutures, it is quicker to perform but fails if the suture is cut in just one place.

vi. Running Subcutaneous Sutures

The running subcutaneous suture begins with a simple interrupted subcutaneous suture, which is tied but not cut. The suture is looped through the subcutaneous tissue by successively passing through the opposite sides of the wound. The knot is tied at the opposite end of the wound by knotting the long end of the suture material to the loop of the last pass that was placed (Fig. 32).[36]

Advantage: It is used to close the deep portion of surgical defects under moderate tension.

Disadvantage: It has the risk of suture breakage and the formation of dead space beneath the skin surface.

Special Suturing Techniques

These include tips sutures, purse-string suture and barbed sutures.

Tip Sutures

They are special sutures which have a vital role in flap surgeries as they can keep the flaps in place without causing much damage to flaps.

Commonly used tip sutures are described below:

a. *Half-buried horizontal mattress sutures*
   Procedure: The half-buried horizontal mattress suture or tip stitch begins on the side of the wound on which the flap is to be attached (Fig. 33).[3] The suture is passed through the dermis of the wound edge to the dermis of the flap tip. The needle is passed laterally in the same dermal plane of the flap tip, exits the flap tip, and re-enters the skin to which the flap is to be attached. The needle is directed perpendicularly and exits the skin; then, the knot is tied.[21]

Advantages

- Tip stitch is used primarily to position the corners and tips of flaps and to perform M-plasties and V-Y closures.[34]

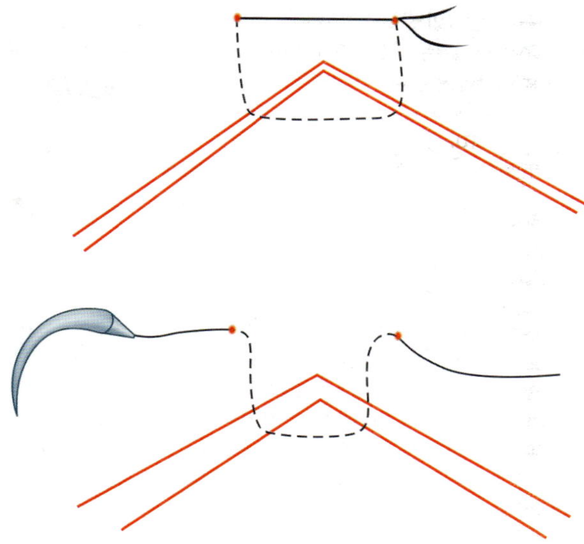

Fig. 33: Tip stitch.

- It helps to have the knots on one side of the suture line with no suture marks on the other side. For example, when insetting the areola in breast reduction, this technique leaves the suture marks on the dark, pebbly areola instead of on the breast skin.

Disadvantage: In larger flaps with greater tension, this technique has been reported to position the flap tip deeper than the surrounding tissue, often resulting in a depressed scar.[34]

b. *Modified half-buried horizontal mattress sutures*
   This stitch places an additional vertical mattress suture superficial to the half-buried horizontal mattress suture.[39] A small skin hook instead of forceps is used to avoid trauma of the flap.
c. *Deep tip stitch*
   The deep tip stitch is essentially a full-buried form of the three corner stitch.[40] The suture is placed into the deep dermis of the wound edge to which the flap is to be attached, passed through the dermis of the flap tip, and inserted into the deep dermis of the opposite wound edge.

Purse-string Suture

It is a buried horizontal mattress suture which is placed in the mid-to-deep part of the dermis to prevent the skin from tearing. This closure provides uniform tension to the wound, enhances hemostasis at the tissue edge, and significantly decreases the size of the defect thus offering excellent long-term cosmetic and functional results.[41]

The purse-string suture may be most appropriate for primary closure for small skin defects or as a partial closure for larger round wounds. It is useful following the local excision of both melanoma and non-melanoma skin cancer. In addition, this technique is especially suitable for patients who insist on maintaining an active lifestyle in the immediate postoperative period, individuals concurrently being treated with anticoagulants, antiplatelet agents or both, and people with extensive postoperative defects that would otherwise require either a skin graft or a large cutaneous flap.

However, if tied too tightly, the suture may strangulate the approximated tissue.[23]

Barbed Sutures

Self-retaining barbed sutures are innovations in non-surgical facial and neck rejuvenation. They can be either absorbable (polydioxanone) or nonabsorbable (polypropylene) variations with microscopic etching that creates the effect of many barb-like as shown in Figure 34. The specialized structure of these stitches enables the repair of tissue that is injured across more than one dermal level without additional tension on the axis point. They are often used for face-lifts (called threadlifts), breast reduction and in tendon repairs in orthopedic surgeries.

The technique to place a barbed suture differs from that of a traditional suture. It has to be carefully measured to match the length of the wound being closed. After being inserted, the end of the suture needs to be pulled to release the barbs and secure the placement of the stitch causing a lifted visual effect. Recovery time and bruising is often much less than traditional face-lift procedures. Polydioxanone barbed configuration allows the suture to be completely subdermal, thus there will be no visible signs of wound closure during and after healing. They are currently available as short APTOS® threads or long WOFFLES® threads. APTOS® threads are useful for malar rounding, facial tightening and firming, and WOFFLES® threads are used as a sling, suspending ptotic facial tissues to the firm, dense tissues of the temporal scalp.[42]

Advantage: The chief advantage is the avoidance of suture knots which facilitates improved blood supply to wound edges, resulting in quicker wound closing time.[43] The knotless configuration greatly reduces the amount of scar tissue that is created during healing in vivo. Although the long-term efficacy of barbed suspension sutures remains unclear, they may allow for a minimally invasive facial lift with few adverse effects.[44]

Disadvantage: Occasionally, there is additional scarring and skin dimpling around the suture placement. The suture may migrate and cause cosmetic abnormality.

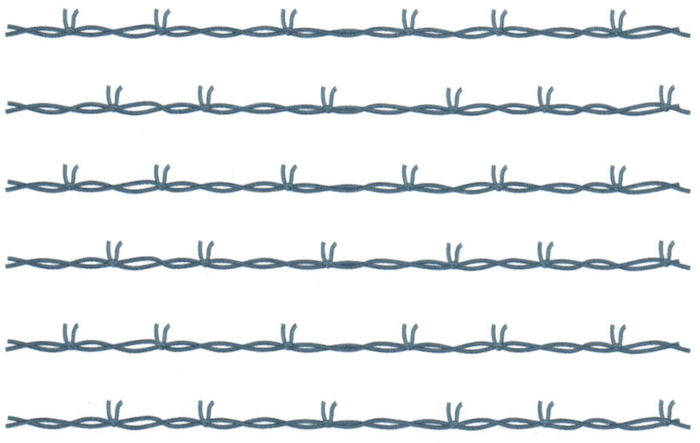

Fig. 34: Barbed suture.

SUTURE REMOVAL

Proper suture removal technique is important to maintain good results after sutures are executed. Prompt removal reduces the risk of suture marks, infection, and tissue reaction.[5,35] To prevent dehiscence and spread of the scar, sutures should not be removed too soon. As a general rule, the greater the tension across a wound, the longer the sutures should remain in place. Sutures should be removed within 1–2 weeks of their placement, depending on the anatomic location as mentioned in Table 8.

Interrupted Suture

After cleansing the interrupted suture with antiseptic lotion, one end of the suture should be grasped with forceps and pulled gently towards one side of the wound, elevating the knot. The opposite side of the suture should then be cut with fine suture scissors immediately under the knot (Fig. 35).[5] Then, the suture is grasped by the knot and gently pulled toward the wound or suture line until the suture material is completely removed. If the suture is pulled away from the suture line, the wound edges may separate. Wound should be examined for any left over sutures. Steristrips may be applied with a tissue adhesive to provide continued supplemental wound support after the sutures are removed.

When multiple sutures are taken, alternate sutures are removed and the wound should be examined for dehiscence. If the wound has healed completely, all sutures can be removed. If dehiscence is seen, remaining sutures are left intact which have to be removed 4–7 days later.

Running Suture

A running suture is removed by cutting its every other loop and grasping the intervening loop with forceps and pulling it out.[5]

Table 8: Removal of suture as per anatomic location.

Anatomic location	Days of suture removal post-implantation
Face and ears	5–7
Eyelids	3–5
Neck	7
Scalp	10
Trunk and upper extremities	10–14
Lower extremities	14–21

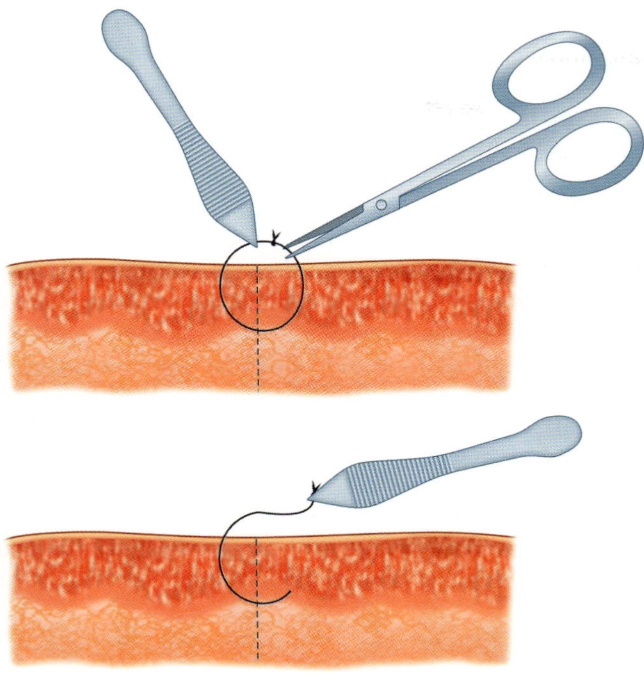

Fig. 35: Suture removal.

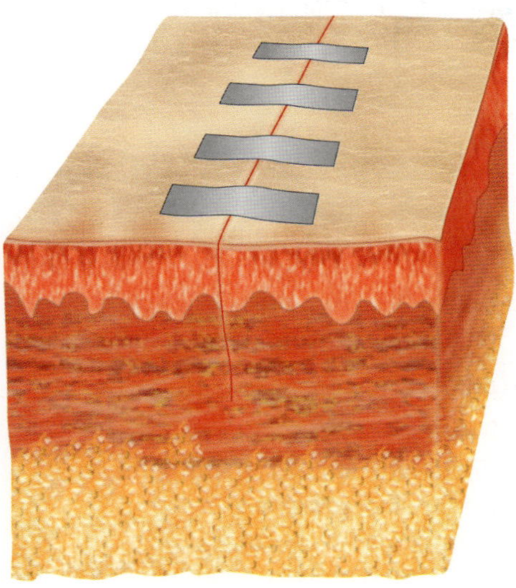

Fig. 36: Skin tapes.

Running subcuticular suture: A running subcuticular suture is removed by cutting the knot at one end and pulling the suture out slowly from the other end to minimize the risk of suture breakage in the wound.[5,35]

ALTERNATIVE WOUND CLOSURE METHODS

While the most common method of closing a wound is with sutures, other materials such as skin tapes, staples or wound adhesives are also useful in certain situations.[34]

Skin Tapes

Wound closure tapes (e.g. Steristrips, Cover-strips) are reinforced microporous nonocclusive material (e.g. paper, plastic, rayon fabric) backed by a thin film of acrylic polymer adhesive (Fig. 36).[7]

Procedure

It is important to first obtain good hemostasis and eversion of the wound edges before using the wound closure tapes. An adhesive solution like tincture of benzoin or mastisol may be applied to the skin before using tapes to enhance its adhesive property.[7,8] Once the adhesive has dried to a tacky feel, strips of tapes should be placed perpendicularly across the wound without overlapping one another. Tapes that are kept dry and clean may remain adherent for up to 1–2 weeks. Tapes have little usefulness in hairy or highly mobile areas. Moisture, soap, and wound exudate decrease the duration of tape adhesion.

Advantages

- They can effectively approximate the low tension wound edges, relieve tension, and prevent inversion of the wound edges.[34]
- They provide extra support to a suture line, when running subcuticular sutures are used or following staples wound closure technique.
- They also provide added strength to the wound when used after suture removal.

Disadvantage

- They are rarely adequate for primary wound closure.

Staples

The principle of mechanical staplers in surgery is exactly the same as paper stapling machines.[3,34] Staples are formed from high-quality stainless steel and are easy to place. They are primarily used in the closure of wounds under high tension on the trunk, extremities and scalp. In dermatological surgery, they are commonly used for closing scalp reductions or to close donor site during hair transplantation.[10] They are also useful to position a skin closure or flap temporarily before suturing and to secure split-thickness skin grafts.[8,10]

Procedure

The central section of the 'U' shaped staple is held while the outer ends are pushed through the skin and then bent

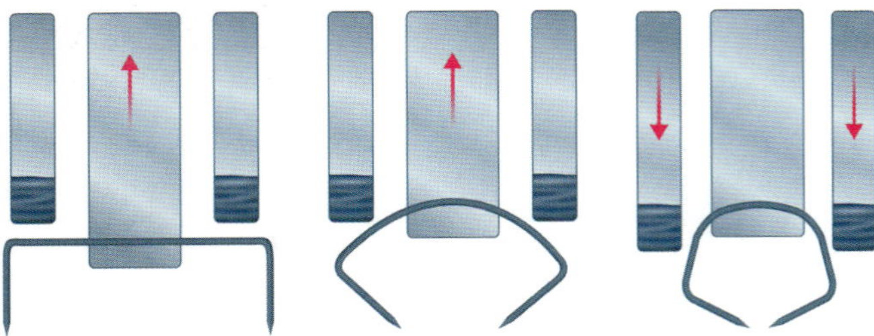

Fig. 37: Skin staples.

so that the ends meet, forming a closed ring (Fig. 37).[34] They are removed by straightening the base of the 'U' to open out the ends so that the staples can be withdrawn.

Advantages

- They are particularly useful for long incisions as they may shorten the wound closure time by 70–80%.
- Decreased risk of infection.
- Improved wound eversion.
- Minimal tissue reactivity.

Disadvantages[10,34]

- Less precise wound approximation and the need for a second operator to evert and reapproximate skin edges during staple placement.
- Staples must be removed early to prevent crosshatch skin marks.
- They are contraindicated in finely contoured areas, over bony prominences, or in highly mobile areas.
- The cost is usually more than that of suture material.

Surgical Adhesives

Skin adhesives have been developed and used widely for more than two decades. They have a role in wound closure, especially in wounds without tension. They do not evert the wound edges by themselves and hence eversion must be provided by deeper sutures.

Most commonly used material is cyanoacrylate adhesives which can be used in combination with, or as an alternative to sutures in wound closure. Two varieties of cyanoacrylates that are available are octyl-2-cyanoacrylate (Dermabond®; Ethicon) and *N*-butyl-2-cyanoacrylate (Indermil®; Syneture).[3,8] The adhesives remains liquid until exposed to water or water-containing tissue, after which it polymerizes within 3 minutes through an exothermic reaction in which a small amount of heat is released forming a flexible film that bonds to the underlying surface.

Procedure

Wound should be completely reapproximated before applying cyanoacrylates as healing may be impaired if the adhesive seeps into the wound bed and may result in foreign body reactions.[34]

Defat the closure site with alcohol or acetone. Octyl-2-cyanoacrylate which is available in prefilled single use vials with various applicator tips is applied in a thin layer over the entire wound and extending 5–10 mm beyond the wound edge. Once the layer is dried (10–30 seconds), another layer is applied. Three to four layers are necessary. *N*-butyl-2-cyanoacrylate requires only a single application by droplet that sets in 30 seconds. No additional bandaging is required, and the patient is advised to not perform wound care at home. By 7–14 days, most of the adhesive sloughs with the epidermis. Topical ointments or creams should not be applied on the wound when adhesives are used as they can weaken the polymerized film and result in wound gaping. Octyl-2-cyanoacrylate is preferred over N-butyl-2 cyanoacrylate as they are three to four times stronger than latter, more flexible and is easier to use.[3] Adhesive is originally sterilized by dry heat and ethylene oxide gas. It is meant for single use only and remaining opened material after each wound closure procedure should be discarded.

Advantages

- They are quick and easy to apply when compared to suturing technique of wound closure. Moreover, it eliminates the trauma to tissues caused by needles and sutures.
- They act as water proof coating and have antibacterial activity against common microbes like staphylococci, *Pseudomonas* and *E. coli*.
- They promote moist wound healing environment which is essential for faster epithelialization.
- They are useful for the closure of simple lacerations in children, uncooperative patients, and for the closure of incisions under casts.
- Needs minimal training.
- Cosmetic outcome is good.
- No postoperative visit is required for removal as it sloughs off naturally over the course of 5–10 days.

Contraindications[3]

- Near the eyes.
- In areas that are highly mobile or subject to friction (e.g. over joints, hands, feet).
- Any wound with evidence of active infection, gangrene or bedsores.
- On patients with known hypersensitivity to cyanoacrylate.
- Patients with peripheral vascular disease.

Laser Wound Closure

Laser welding is an innovative technique which was introduced very recently. The bonding of wounds using laser energy, known as laser welding, has been used on a limited basis as an alternative to traditional wound closure.[8] Compared with previously mentioned closure materials, laser welding is faster, watertight and avoids a

Box 1: Tips for proper wound closure.

- Do not place absorbable sutures superficially as it can lead to permanent suture tracts and result in suture extrusion. Absorbable sutures should always be placed deeper in subcutaneous tissue and lower dermis
- Polyglactin 910 (Vicryl) is an excellent absorbable suture in soft tissue approximation particularly in areas like face, anterior and posterior neck, scalp, superior trunk, nasal and oral mucosa which require sutures with higher tensile strength
- Polypropylene (Prolene), a nonabsorbable suture material is ideal for subcuticular closure in areas like eyelid, periorbital area, nose, pinna, lip, and vermillion which requires less tensile strength
- Monofilament nylon (Ethilon) having its maximal long-term tensile strength property is useful in suturing major musculocutaneous flaps that needs to be closed under significant tension
- Avoid multifilament sutures in contaminated tissues. Monofilament sutures are preferred in infected tissues. However, great care must be taken in handling and tying monofilament suture because crushing or crimping of this suture can weaken the suture leading to premature suture failure
- Smaller suture sizes of 5-0–6-0 is preferred on head and neck surgeries
- Reverse cutting needles with three-eighths inch circle gives best cosmetic outcome, causing minimal trauma
- Grasp the needle with the jaw of the needle holder at its distal portion at the junction of anterior two-third and posterior one-third. This can prevent blunting the cutting point or bending the weaker end of the suture needle
- The jaws of the needle holder must be appropriate to the needle size to hold it securely and prevent rocking, turning, and twisting
- Do not tighten the needle holder excessively. The needle should be held vertically and longitudinally perpendicular to the needle holder
- Tissue bites in simple interrupted suture should be taken at the same level on either side of the wound edges to minimize the possibility of stepping. Simple interrupted sutures lead to cross-hatched linear scars which can be minimized by removing them early
- Use running subcuticular suture for closing wounds with equal tissue thickness. Eliminate the tension with deep sutures before placing running subcuticular suture to achieve the best possible cosmetic result.
- Running subcuticular suture is a useful technique in children when absorbable suture is used so that suture removal is avoided
- Simple running suture may be used to secure a split or full-thickness skin graft. It is also useful over eyelids, ears and the dorsa of hands
- Excellent suturing method to provide effective wound support is vertical mattress suture. Placing each stitch precisely and taking symmetric bites is especially important
- Purse-string sutures should not be tied too tightly as it may strangulate the approximated tissue
- Staples are particularly useful for long incisions as they shorten the wound closure time
- Surgical glues are useful for the closure of simple lacerations in children, uncooperative patients, and for the closure of incisions under casts.

foreign-body reaction. Although collateral thermal injury has prevented its regular clinical use, introduction of laser soldering has shown to minimize this injury. This process involves the application of a biologic "solder" (e.g. bovine serum albumin) prior to temperature-controlled laser welding. Additional studies are necessary to determine its use in dermatologic surgery.

CONCLUSION

Skillful wound closure requires not only knowledge of proper surgical techniques but also knowledge of the physical characteristics and properties of wound closure materials. Today, dermatosurgeon has a significantly increased number of wound closure materials to choose from. While choosing appropriate material, it is important to consider the risk of infection, closure speed, cost, cosmetic results, and wound location. The tips for proper wound closure are mentioned in Box 1.

Wound closure technology has kept its pace of advancement along with the latest techniques in surgery and provides the cosmetic surgical fraternity a wide range of wound closure methods.

REFERENCES

1. Bloom BS, Goldberg DJ. Suture material in cosmetic cutaneous surgery. Journal of Cosmetic and Laser Therapy. 2007;9:41-5.
2. Chang Chu, Howard P, Greisler J, et al. Wound closure biomaterials and devices. Boca Raton, FL: CRC Press; 1997.
3. Doctor HG. Dermabond liquid stitches. Surgeons and Sutures, 3rd edition: Ethicon-Johnson and Johnson; 2005; 27-9.
4. Hiller, Lejaren. Sutures in ancient surgery. Brooklyn, NY: Davis and Geck;1927-38.
5. Kudur MH, Pai SB, Sripathi H, et al. Sutures and suturing techniques in skin closure. Indian J Dermatol Venereol Lerpol. 2009;75(4):425-34.
6. Lai SY, Becker DG, Edlich RF. (2010) Sutures and Needles. [Online] Available from emedicine.medscape.com/article/884838. [Accessed February, 2012].
7. Ammirati CT. Advances in wound closure materials. In: James WD, Cockerell CJ, Maloney ME, et al. (Eds). Advances in Dermatology. Philadelphia: Mosby; 2002; 313-38.
8. Terhune M. Materials for wound closure. [Online] Available from www.emedicine.com/derm/topic825.htm. [Accessed February, 2012].
9. Moy RL, Lee A, Zalka A. Commonly used suture materials in skin surgery. Am Fam Physician. 1991;44:2123-8.
10. Kirk RM. Handling instruments. Basic Surgical Techniques, 6th edition. Churchill, Livingstone; 2010;9-20.
11. Postlethwait RW, Willigan DA, Ulin AW. Human tissue reaction to sutures. Ann Surg. 1975;181:144-50.
12. Bennet RG. Selection of wound closure materials. J Am Acad Dermatol. 1988;18:619-37.
13. Watts GT, Sutures for skin closure. Lancet. 1975;1:581.
14. Lober CW, Fenske NA. Suture materials for closing the skin and subcutaneous tissues. Aesthetic Plast Surg. 1986;10: 245-8.
15. Madsen ET. An experimental and clinical evaluation of surgical suture materials. Surg Gynecol Obstet. 1953;97: 73-80.

16. Conn J, Oyasu R, Welsh M, et al. Vicryl (polyglactin 910) synthetic absorbable sutures. Am J Surg. 1974;128:19-23.
17. Ray JA, Doddi N, Regula D, et al. Polydioxanone (PDS), a novel monofilament synthetic absorbable suture. Surg Gynecol Obstet. 1981;153:497-507.
18. Postlethwait RW, Willigan DA, Ulin AW. Human tissue reaction to sutures. Ann Surg. 1975;181:144-50.
19. Edlich RF, Gubler K, Wallis AG, et al. Wound closure sutures and needles: a new perspective. J Environ Pathol Toxicol Oncol. 2010;29:339-61.
20. Rodeheaver GT, Nesbit WS, Edlich RF. Novafil. A dynamic suture for wound closure. Ann Surg. 1986;204:193-9.
21. Aston SJ. The choice of suture material for skin closure. J Dermatol Surg. 1976;2:57-61.
22. Szarmach RR, Livingston J, Edlich RE. An expanded surgical and needle evaluation and selection program by a healthcare resource management group purchasing organization. J Long Term Eff Med Implants. 2003;13:155-70.
23. Wiggan JM, Elston DM. (2010) Suturing Techniques. [Online] Available from http://emedicine.medscape.com/article/1824895. [Accessed February, 2012]
24. Swanson NA, Tromovitch TA. Suture materials, 1980s: properties, uses, and abuses. Int J Dermatol. 1982;21:373-8.
25. Borges AF. Techniques of wound suture. Elective incisions and Scar Revision. Boston: Little Brown. 1973;65-76.
26. Swanson NA. Basic Techniques. Atlas of Cutaneous Surgery. Boston: Little Brown; 1987;26-49.
27. Edlich RF, Long WB, Gubler KD, et al. Citizen's Petition to Food and Drug Administration to ban cornstarch powder on medical gloves: Maltese cross birefringence. Am J Emerg Med. 2009;27:227-35.
28. Edlich RF, Wind TC, Heather CL, et al. Reliability and performance of innovative surgical double-glove hole puncture indication systems. J Long Term Eff Med Implants. 2003;13:69-83.
29. Edlich RF, Gubler K, Wallis AG, et al. Scientific basis for the selection of skin closure techniques. J Environ Pathol Toxicol Oncol. 2010;29:363-72.
30. Arnold H (Ed). Surgery of the skin and subcutaneous tissue. Farquharson's Textbook of Operative General Surgery, 9th edition: 2005. pp. 1-20.
31. Stegman SJ: Suturing techniques for dermatologic surgery. J Dermatol Surg Oncol. 1978;4:63-8.
32. Richey ML, Roe SC. Assessment of knot security in continuous intradermal wound closures. J Surg Res. 2005; 123:284-8.
33. Adams B, Levy R, Rademaker AE, et al. Frequency of use of suturing and repair techniques preferred by dermatologic surgeons. Dermatol Surg. 2006;32:682-9.
34. Thorne CH. Techniques and principles in plastic surgery. Grabb & Smith's Plastic Surgery, 6th edition. Wolters Kluwer/Lippincott: Williams & Wilkins; 2007;3-14.
35. Popkin GL, Robins P. Closure of skin wounds. Workshop manual for basic dermatological surgery. Kenilworth: NJ. Schering, Inc; 1983;18-36.
36. Zachary CB, Suture techniques. In: Zachary CB, (Ed). Basic Cutaneous Surgery. New York: Churchill Livingstone; 1991; 53-75.
37. Odland PB, Murakuani CS. Simple suturing technique and knot tying. Cutaneous Surgery. In: Wheeland RG (Ed), 1st edition. Philadelphia: WB Saunders Co; 1994;178-88.
38. Stegmen SJ. Suturing techniques for dermatologic surgery. J Dermatol Surg Oncol. 1978;4:63-8.
39. Bechara FG, Al-Muhammadi R, Sand M, et al. A modified corner stitch for fixation of flap tips. Dermatol Surg. 2007; 33:1277-9.
40. Chan JL, Miller EK, Jou RM, et al. Novel surgical technique: placement of a deep tip stitch. Dermatol Surg. 2009;35: 2001-3.
41. Cohen PR, Martinelli PT, Schulze KE, et al. The cuticular purse string suture: a modified purse string suture for the partial closure of round postoperative wounds. Int J Dermatol. 2007;46:746-53.
42. Wu WT. Barbed sutures in facial rejuvenation. Aesthet Surg J. 2004;24:582-7.
43. Kaminer MS, Bogart M, Choi C, et al. Long-term efficacy of anchored barbed sutures in the face and neck. Dermatol Surg. 2008;34:1041-7.
44. Villa MT, White LE, Alam M, et al. Barbed sutures: a review of the literature. Plast Reconstr Surg. 2008;121: 102e-8e.

Chapter 10

Setting Up a Dermatosurgery Unit

HM Omprakash

Key Messages 

- Before designing a dermatosurgery unit, one has to keep in mind the statutory standards and in the end tailor make the facility to meet ones requirement.
- Dermatosurgery unit is viewed as a luxury—but in reality, it is a place of high standard of patient safety with most economical use of manpower and other resources.
- Dermatosurgery unit types could be—Unrestricted type, restricted type or Laser surgery unit.
- Dermatosurgery unit design should look into—location of unit, dimensions, power, water, lighting, instruments and waste disposal.
- Before commissioning a unit one has to look into— trained personnel, sterilization—disinfection services and basic, advanced cardiovascular life support system.

INTRODUCTION

Dermatologists are increasingly performing cutaneous surgery. The surgeries performed range from simple procedures like electrosurgery, biopsies, chemical cauteries, sclerotherapy, soft tissue augmentation, botulinum toxin chemodenervation to more aggressive surgeries such as vitiligo surgery, nail surgeries and more complex labor intensive procedures like hair restoration, liposuction, etc. Since patient's safety is the first concern, it is not only the dermatologist skill which matters but also the infrastructure. A well-equipped, well-designed surgical suite improves the experience for both patients and the dermatologist.[1]

NOMENCLATURE

The units where dermatosurgeries are performed have different nomenclature: the dermatosurgery unit, the operation theater, the ambulatory surgery facility, the office surgery and the free standing outpatient surgery center, outpatient surgical suite. But in this chapter, it shall be known as the dermatosurgery unit.

If the dermatosurgery unit is located in the same premise as the consultation room, patients are already familiar with the surroundings, personnel and prefer this personalized care.

WHY THE NEED FOR SEPARATE DERMATOSURGERY UNIT?

The paucity of financial resources and high cost of leasing or owning separate dermatosurgery unit is forcing many dermatologists to operate on the patient in their consultation rooms. This is putting both the patient and dermatologist at the risk. The risks are infection, anaphylaxis or hemodynamic and airway compromise inherent to the use of topical or infiltration anesthetics, hence the rationale of having a separate dermatosurgery unit with clean if not sterile environment and back up of advanced life support.

Even though it may make sense to use the existing minor or major operation theater of an existing hospital, it has definite drawbacks. Patients attending traditional major operation theater are sick, unlike dermatology patients. To get a slot for surgery at patients or dermatologists convenience is often difficult. Also it would cost more to hire the operation theater on hourly basis.[1]

If the dermatosurgery unit is located in the same premise as the consultation room, patients are already familiar with the surroundings, personnel and prefer this personalized care.

Patients prefer dermatosurgery unit to hospital-based operation theater because the environment is less threatening. If the dermatosurgery unit is located in the same premises as the consultation room, patients are already familiar with the surroundings, personnel and prefer this personalized care.[2]

Thus, the dermatosurgery unit may be housed in a major hospital or private clinic premises or in shared premises with common theater shared by different doctors: plastic surgeons, general surgeons or like minded dermatologist willing to do group practice.[3]

REQUIREMENTS OF A DERMATOSURGERY UNIT

Each dermatologist will have his own likes and dislikes. So before embarking on designing, one has to keep in mind the statutory standards and in the end, tailor make the facility to meet ones requirement.

The Indian standard-basic requirements for hospital planning,[4] the Medical council of India guidelines,[5] the Indian Association of Dermatologist, Venereologist and Leprologist guidelines,[6] have issued guidelines which are of use to a dermatosurgeon.

The International guidelines include American Association for Accreditation of Ambulatory Surgery facilities,[7] Singapore Directives for Private Ambulatory surgical centers providing ambulatory surgery,[8] Netherlands Building Guidelines for a surgical department,[9] WHO guidelines.[10]

However, industry leaders whose publications are opinion makers: Satish S Savant,[11] Walter P Unger[12] should also be referred to before starting a dermatosurgery unit.

THE DERMATOSURGERY UNIT TYPES

There are three types of dermatosurgery zones:
1. Unrestricted zone
2. Restricted zone
3. Laser surgery unit.

Unrestricted Zone

Majority of dermatosurgeries are performed on intact skin, with only resident cutaneous flora. Only the site of surgery requires isolation. Hence, both the patient and dermatologist can enter the operation theater in routine clothes. This is where most procedures such as cryotherapy, electrosurgery, soft tissue augmentation, botulinum toxin chemodenervation, skin biopsies are carried out. Here only topical, infiltration anesthesia is permitted with oral and intramuscular sedation. Spinal, epidural, regional blocks and general anesthesia are not permitted (Fig. 1).[13]

Restricted Zone

But invasive surgeries like vitiligo surgeries, hair transplantation, laser resurfacing require a separate theater. This is the restricted zone (Fig. 2) or the traditional operation theater, wherein the patient, dermatologist must change their dress, don cap, mask and use separate operation theater footwear.[14] General anesthesia, intravenous anesthesia are permitted.[8]

Laser Zone

It is dealt in a separate chapter.

A dermatosurgical theater can include all the zones in the same complex or may include one theater of unrestricted zone.

LOCATION OF THE DERMATOSURGERY UNIT IN THE OFFICE OR HOSPITAL

The Indian standard for hospital planning[4] clearly defines that the traditional operation theater unit be located in Box 1.

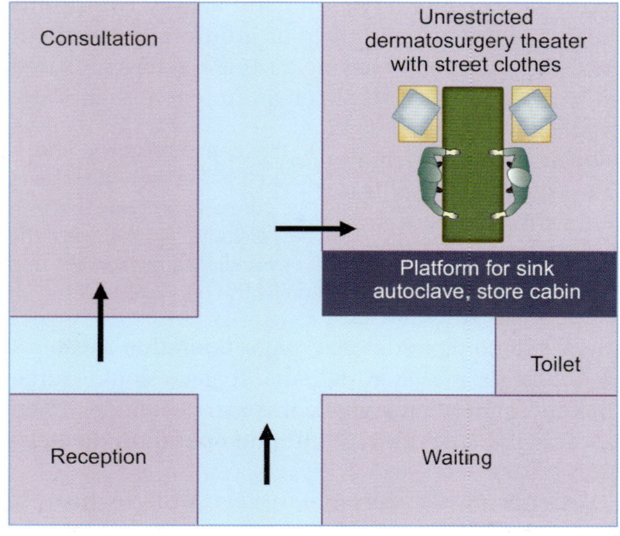

Fig. 1: Unrestricted type of dermatosurgery unit.

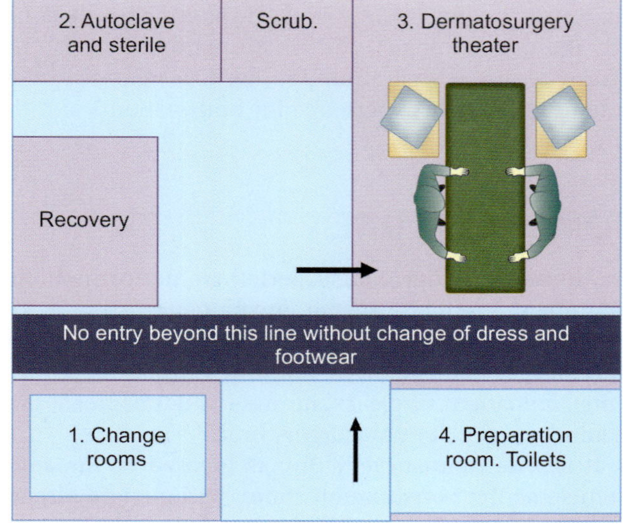

Fig. 2: Restricted type of dermatosurgery unit.

Box 1: Location of the dermatosurgery unit.

- Quiet environment
- Freedom from noise and other disturbance
- Freedom from contamination and possible cross infection
- Maximum protection from solar radiation
- Convenient relationship with surgical ward, intensive care unit, central sterilization, blood bank, radiology, pathology and supply department
- Efficient lift service if located on upper floors
- Lastly the obvious electric supply, ventilation, fire extinguisher and water supply.

What follows is the layouts and requirements of the dermatosurgery unit. These are ideal requirements. Minimal requirements have already been laid out in IADVL taskforce recommendations.[6]

Layout of the Restricted Zone Type of Dermatosurgery Unit

There are four well-defined zones depending upon the degree of cleanliness. Zoning is done to keep the theater free from micro-organisms.

1. *Protective zone*: This includes waiting area, preanesthetic examination room, changing rooms and theater supply rooms.
2. *Clean zone*: This includes theater pack preparation, preoperative room, recovery room.
3. *Aseptic zone or sterile zone:* The sterilization room, operation theater.
4. *Disposal zone or dirty zone*: The soiled instruments and dressings are washed or disposed here.[4]

Guidelines for the Restricted Type of Dermatosurgery Unit Complex

- The door of the complex should be two leaf types with self-closing hinges. The door should be 1 meter wide.
- The floor and side of the passage in the complex should be tiled to withstand repeated washing or else the side walls can be just painted with washable paint and light color.
- The corridor of the complex should be adequate for ease of mobility of trolleys. The required dimensions may be 2 meters.[15]
- Suitable fire alarms and powder type fire extinguishers should be in place (Fig. 3). Carbon dioxide type fire extinguishers are suitable for equipment in the theater, but foam type and water should be not used on lasers and other type equipment in theater.[16]
- Change room should have lockers.
- No window curtains or floor mats are permitted in the premises.
- Scrub zone should have elbow operated or foot operated taps and elbow operated hand disinfectant dispenser. Since water can harbor pseudomonas and other microbes the water should be UV and heat treated.

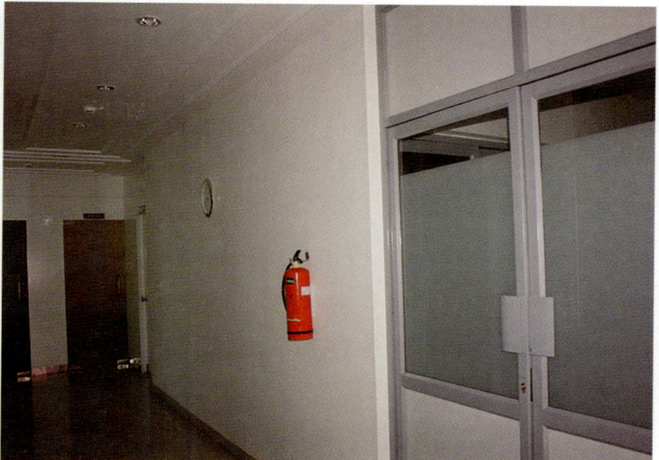

Fig. 3: Note the fire alarms in ceiling, powder type fire extinguishers, tiled floor and washable walls.

Common Features of the Operation Theater of Both Restricted and Unrestricted Type

- The operation theater should be dust proof and moisture proof.
- Corners and junctions of walls, floor and ceiling could be rounded to prevent accumulation of dust and to facilitate cleaning (Fig. 4). The flooring of restricted type theater (Fig. 5) should be seamless and made of epoxy resin. But in the unrestricted type it could be tiled (Fig. 6) or concrete able to withstand repeated washing.
- All doors should be 1.5 meters in width and half leaf type with self-closing devices in place. If laser is in use then the laser usage sign with the wavelength being used should be displayed on the door.
- The dimension of the theater could be 3 × 3 meters[11], 4 × 4 meters[17] or 4 × 5 meters[12] minimum.
- The height of the wall should be 2.6 meters[15] or 3.0 meters.[4]

Lighting of Theater

- Natural light through windows should be provided. But windows should be sealed tight.
- General lighting by ceiling mounted fluorescent tubes at the rate of 1 W per square foot (i.e. for 120 square feet 120 W, 3 tubes of 40 W)[18] is sufficient.
- The artificial light: fluorescent tubes, compact fluorescent lamps (CFL) or light emitting diodes (LED); should match the color of the objects, as they are seen in outdoor natural sunlight. This is called color rendering index (CRI). Sunlight CRI is 100. Tubes and CFL with CRI of 90-98 are available. Also ask for "Daylight" version of the lamps.
- Compact fluorescent lamps and cluster white LED lights can save power and last longer. Tubes have a life

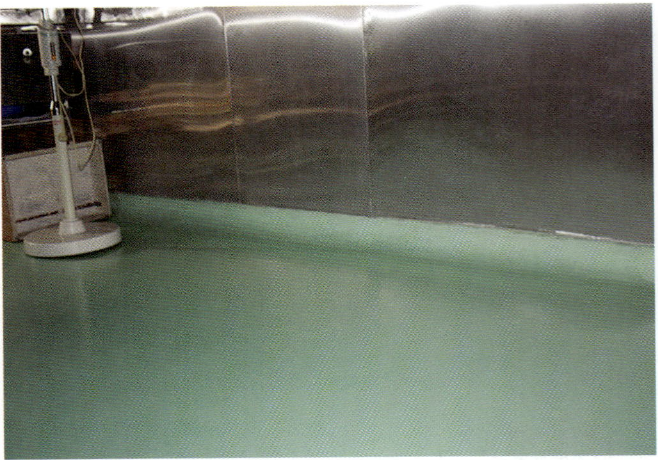

Fig. 4: Restricted theater with rounded corners and epoxy seamless flooring.

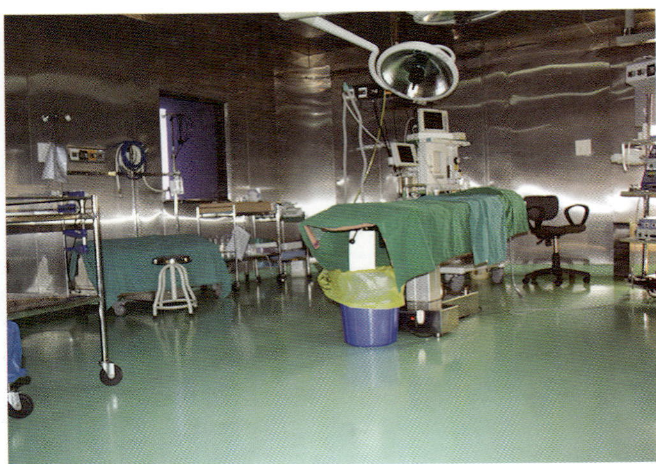

Fig. 5: Restricted theater–seamless epoxy flooring, natural closed window light with washable walls.
Courtesy: Vikram Hospital, Mysore.

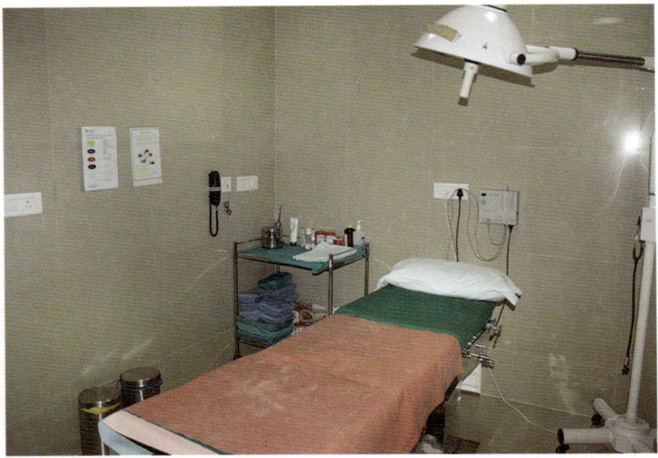

Fig. 6: Unrestricted theater with tiled walls and floors, electrical outlets, phone, OT light, table, trolley, kick bucket for waste.
Courtesy: Vikram Hospital, Mysore.

of 15,000 hours but LED lights last 50,000 hours. But for the long life, low power consumption and being mercury free; LED light requires further standardization as of today.

Operation Theater Light

- Before purchasing a light for the surgical field, check for: (a) intensity of light, (b) size of the illuminated field, (c) production of heat and shadows, (d) ease of changing the position of light and (e) ceiling mounted or floor movable.
- Shadow less lighting delivering 3,000–8,000 foot candles[19] is the basic operation theater light required (i.e. the dental chairs have halogen lamp of 50 W power. Each Watt of power will give 50 foot candle of illumination at the site of surgery. So a 50 W of halogen bulb can roughly give 2,500 foot candles of illumination on the site of surgery).
- For dermatologist looking for precise illumination, single bulb 100 W, 12 V halogen bulb giving 30,000 Lux illumination are available.
- Light-emitting diode operation theater light with long life, low heat are entering the market and may change halogen bulb in future.

Electrical Outlets

- All 3 pin outlet should be located about 1.5 meters above the floor. This is to prevent wires on the floor. There should be good earthing.
- No extension cords or boards are permitted.
- Five ampere and 15 ampere sockets are required. The 5 ampere sockets, on an average 4 should be located on each wall.
- On line UPS are required for lasers and operation theater lights. Preferably, draw the current for costly devices through servo stabilizer which is a one time investment.
- Standby generators should be planned.

Air Conditioning

- Air conditioning minimum requirement is of office type with 10 micron dust filter. In our country, this is basically for operators comfort rather than for clean air supply (applicable only to unrestricted type theater).
- The temperature of theater should be 21° and humidity 50–55%.
- But National Accreditation Board for Hospitals (NABH) does not recommend split and windows AC for restricted type operation theaters.[20]

Operation Table

- Stainless steel operation table, with adjustable head, foot end and arm rest is the heart of the theater. This could be manual or electric power controlled, with foot or fingertip controls.

- The dimension of the table could be a minimum of 1 meter length and 30 cm breadth.[19]
- Dental chairs with the same specification could be used in unrestricted theaters.

Instrument Trolley

- Mayo stand with four wheels is the most preferred instrument trolley. An autoclaved rubber sheet/ mackintosh should be draped on the table over which a sterile pack is placed every time. If simple cloth is placed moisture will percolate down and contaminate the instruments.

Surgeons Stool

- Surgeons stool with wheels and pneumatic height adjustment, controlled by foot in case of dermatologist is already gloved and also with back rest which sometimes could double up as armrest is a good addition (*see* also section on ergonomics).

Waste Containers

- Four main types of wastes are generated in the theater of a dermatologist: (1) blood soaked gauze, (2) latex gloves, (3) glove paper and plastic cover, (4) sharps, needle and syringes. These are segregated at source[21] into: (a) yellow plastic cover, (b) blue plastic cover, (c) white plastic cover, (d) plastic container with disinfectant respectively with the biohazard logo (Fig. 7). Each of the plastic covers is spread out in kick-bucket type steel containers with rubber baskets.

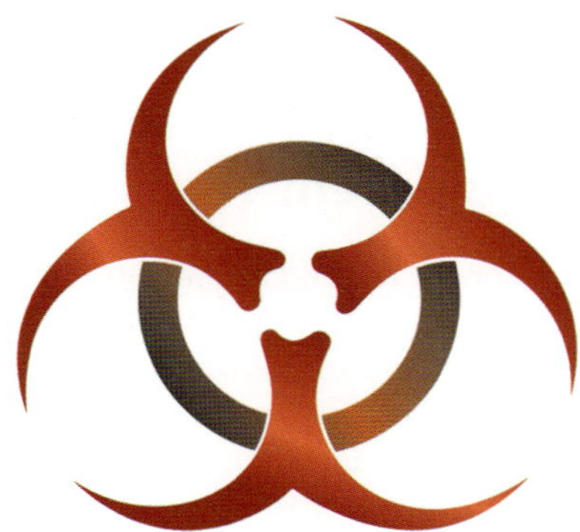

Fig. 7: Biohazard logo.

Surgical Instruments

- The surgical instruments depend upon the type of work and individual surgeon's preference.[11,12] The below Box 2 is not comprehensive and consists of basic requirements for a functional theater.

Specific instruments may be needed according to individual surgeries, for which the reader may consult individual chapters on procedures in respective chapters of this textbook.

ADVANCE CARDIOVASCULAR LIFE SUPPORT

As per government of India and Supreme Court verdict, all personnel in the operation theater should be familiar with basic and advanced life support.[22] Basic life support (BLS) does not require any devices or drugs, but advanced cardiovascular life support (ACLS) does. A standby anesthetist may be necessary for certain procedures. Also it is better to liaison with a local hospital with ICU facility and ambulance service. The reader is referred to the chapter on emergency resuscitation in dermatosurgery for more details.

Advanced cardiovascular life support is taught in batches at various institutes. One should register to these courses, get the precourse material and learn before going to course: (a) BLS and the usage of defibrillator; (b)drugs used in CPR; (c) ECG; (d) understand 10 core cases in ACLS-respiratory arrest case, VF treated with CPR and AED, VF/Pulseless VT case, pulseless electrical activity case, asystole case, acute coronary syndrome case, bradycardia case, unstable tachycardia case, stable tachycardia case and acute stroke case.

The ACLS training involves 3 days: day 1 BLS, day 2 and day 3 ACLS. The training involves-interactive lectures, videos and practice session using mannequin, defibrillator, Ambu bag, ET tubes and drugs. A candidate at the end will have written test and will have to perform BLS and ACLS both in children and adults to pass. Every 2 years, this course has to be repeated.[23]

Advanced life support requires the following drugs and devices (Table 1).[24]

Box 2: Basic requirements for a functional theater.

Forceps	*Sharp instruments*	*Scissors*	Miscellaneous
Cheatles Sponge holding Adson non-toothed Adson toothed Jewellers Mosquito artery Spencer suture removal	Bard parker handle no 3, 4 and 5 Disposable surgical blades no 11, 15 Disposable punch Comedone extractor Curette of 3–4 mm diameter	5 inch blunt and sharp (Lister) Iris scissors Castroviejo	Skin hooks Needle holder-Halsey and box type Nail splitter

Table 1: Drugs and devices for advanced life support.

Devices	Quantity	Drugs	Quantity
Ambu bag	1	Adrenaline 1:1000	10
Laryngoscope with different size blades	1	Atropine 0.6 mg	10
Endo tracheal tube of different size 6–8 no.	1	Sodium bicarbonate (7.5%) ampoules	12
IV cannula adult and pediatric	2	Chlorpheniramine maleate 22.75 mg/ml, 2 cc	10
Drip set	2	Hydrocortisone 100 mg/ml	2
Airway of all size	1	Injection furosemide	10
Stethoscope	1	Aminophylline 250 mg/2 ml ampoules	5
BP apparatus	1	Dopamine 200 mg/5 ml	2
Cardiac monitor with built in defibrillator	1	Normal saline 500 ml	2
Oxygen cylinder with connectors	1	5% Dextrose normal saline 500 ml	2
Suction device	1	Mephentermine 15 mg/ml	5
Disposable syringe	2	Dextrose 25%	2 ampoules

OPERATION ROOM RECORDS

A record containing: (a) patient identity, (b) diagnosis, (c) procedures performed, (d) persons involved in the procedures and (e) complications should be maintained.

This is not only a statutory requirement, but also helping auditing: procedures performed, complications and improvisation of ones' skills.

Surgical Drapes and Attires: Mask, Caps, Suits, Gowns, Gloves, Patient's Suits

Drapes for the operation field are available in different material: cotton and disposable paper or plastic. Cotton is porous and comfortable for the patient. But disposable paper and plastic avoids the need for washing and autoclaving.

Mask definitely protects the dermatologist from splash of blood, injectable anesthetics and most important viral particles during electrosurgery. Surgical wound is protected from operators and assistant secretions in the event of coughing and sneezing; since the aerosol can travel up to 3 meters. Mask should cover both nose and mouth. Cotton, paper and gauze masks should not be used. Paper with synthetic material offer effective barrier.[25] The pore size of the mask should be 1 micron.[26]

Surgical cap should cover the hair on scalp. This prevents contamination of the surgical suit and also the operation site by hair organism.

Surgical suits or theater suits or scrub suits are pants and shirts into which the theater personnel change from street clothes. This has to be cotton and clean but not sterile. These are required for restricted zone of theater.

Gowns are sterile cotton material, full sleeve knee length attires to prevent contamination of the operation site, put on by dermatologist and nurses on surgical suits.

Sterile plastic apron could be donned on surgical suite during dermabrasion to prevent soiling of cotton suite.

Patient suits are required to prevent soiling of the clothes during surgery. They just have to be clean and not sterile.

Gloves can be of latex or non-latex type of various sizes. Double gloving can be practiced when operating on high-risk cases (For hand hygiene, glove donning technique, refer chapters on Sterilization and Disinfection).

Cloth instrument packing is the traditional way of securing the instrument tray. They have to be 270 thread count Pima cotton fabric.The only drawback is the cloth has to laundered every time. Hence nowadays disposable paper crepe type or medical grade plastic paper reels are available (Fig. 8).[27] The storage shelf life varies 1 to 12 months depending upon the material (Fig. 9) (refer the manufacturer guidelines).

Disinfection and Sterilization of Theater Equipment

The reader is referred to the chapter on disinfection and sterilization for detailed description. Specific features are mentioned. Disinfection in the operation theater can be referred to as below:

- Cleaning working surface (category-a).
- Equipment which cannot be autoclaved or need not be autoclaved,e.g. electrosurgery tips, sharps, gloves, linen, OT dresses, stainless steel instruments-comedone expressor, forceps, gallipots (category-b).
- Non-disposable items (category-c).
- Spillages of infectious material.

Cleaning Working Surfaces

Before surgery

- Mop the floor using 0.5 % chlorine solution.
- Using cloth wipe the operation table and trolley with 0.5% chlorine solution (Box 3).

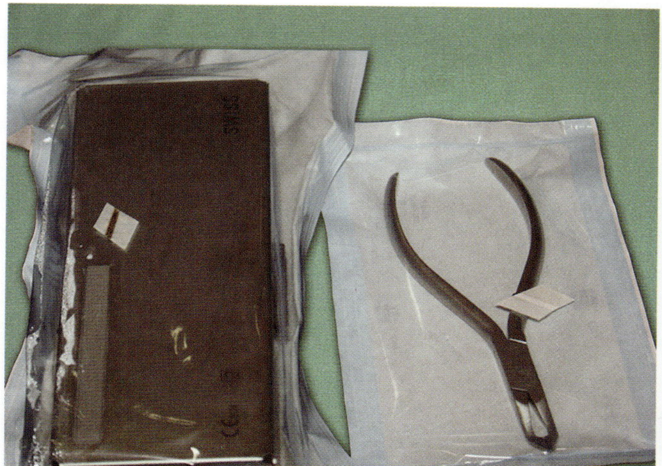

Fig. 8: Medical grade plastic paper pack with one side transparent and autoclave indicator, left autoclaved with black line and right not autoclaved with white line.

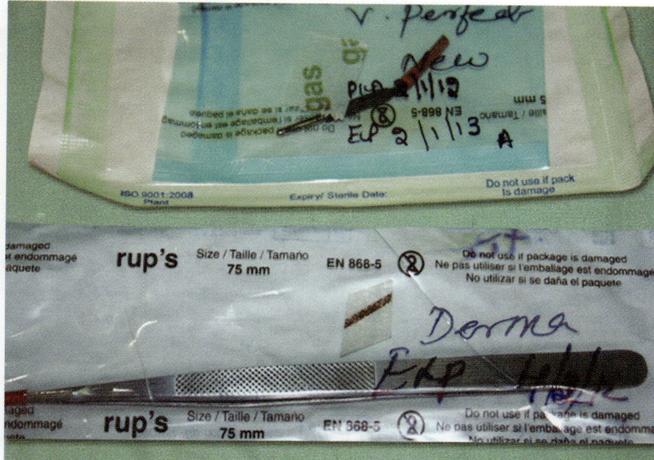

Fig. 9: Top-medical grade plastic reel used to ETO gas sterilize electrosurgery tip expiry date 1 year. Bottom: Forceps autoclaved expiry 1 month.

Box 3: Preparation of 0.5% chlorine solution.

- Procure commercial available bleaching powder
- Add 150 grams in 10 liters of tap water (10 tablespoon or 30 teaspoon)
- First premix the required amount of powder in small quantity of tap water and later add remaining quantity of water
- Use the same day.

After surgery

- Repeat above steps. Keep it ready for next case.

Disinfection of Category "b" and "c" Items

- Items in category "b" and "c" should be collected in separate plastic buckets or basin or waste disposal leak proof plastic container for sharps.
- About 0.5% chlorine solution should be poured and left in contact for minimum of 10 minutes to maximum of 30 minutes. The instruments and linen should be fully immersed in the solution.
- After the "contact" time, wearing mask and thick rubber gloves should be rinsed in tap water or lukewarm water. Do not use very hot water because it coagulates blood and makes it hard to clean.

1. Cleaning removes debris.
2. Disinfection reduces the bacterial and viral load, but does not remove debris or sterilize.
3. Sterilization kills microbes.
4. Sterilization is not a method of cleaning.[10]

- Using a tooth brush to scrub the instruments or brush the clothes.
- Use later, commercial detergents to further clean.
- Do not use soaps as it leaves a precipitate on the steel surface.
- Linen, drapes, suits, gowns, hand towels should be washed with household detergent at 71°C for 25 minutes. Later they can be sterilized or disinfected[10] (Note: drapes, gowns and hand towels require later autoclaving, but not suits).
- After cleansing and disinfecting the instruments and clothes must be dried. Later sent for sterilization as below.

Steam Sterilization (Autoclave)

- Dry the equipment or clothes.
- Wrap the equipment in clothes or paper or medical grade plastic paper pack (Figs. 8 and 9).
- Lay the instruments in the autoclave so that all the surface of the device will come in contact with heat.
- Before packing lay the instruments like scissors in open position.
- Refer the manufacturer's time recommendations for the duration of autoclave.
- Also buy a small autoclave which can be reused many times in a day than large one, once a day. Table top autoclave should be considered.
- Generally, it is 121°C for 15 minutes, pressure of 2.4 bar in porous stainless steel containers.
- The outside of the packs should not be wet, if so the autoclave process has failed.
- Appropriate color indicators should be used on packs to know the adequacy of autoclaving.
- Date of autoclave should be mentioned. The expiry date varies. If polythene bags are used for biopsy trays before autoclaving, sterility is ensured for 8 weeks. If double packed and medical grade plastic paper packs are used the sterility is valid for 1 year.

Chemical Sterilization

- Cleaned, disinfected, dried instruments should be fully soaked in a steel or plastic container having 2% glutaraldehyde for 8-10 hours[10] (Note: For disinfection, the contact time is 20 minutes).

Table 2: Methods of high level disinfection.

Chemical used	Quantity required	Time for disinfection	To be changed	Comment
Formalin in chamber	7 g of formalin for 1 cubic meter area at 20°C (1 g tablet available)	12 hours	Daily	For disinfecting electrosurgery electrodes and cables. For disinfecting sharp instruments Note: It is an irritant and carcinogen
Glutaraldehyde	2.45% concentration	20 minutes	14 days	For disinfecting sharp instruments
Isopropyl alcohol	70%	2 minutes	Daily	Caution: Inflammable near lasers and electrosurgery units

Note: Safer alternatives to formalin chamber and glutaraldehyde should be explored like peracetic acid. Formalin chamber may not be effective in cold areas of the country and cooler nights. Newer agents for high level disinfection and sterilization such as gluteraldehyde + dioxahexane + rust inhibitors at 5% concentration is available for emergency disinfection of equipment within 5 minutes.[28]

- Instruments like scissors should be in open position when soaked.
- After 10 hours, using autoclaved water (100 mL of water autoclaved for 20 minutes and not boiled water) the instruments should be washed, dried and packed, stored in a sterile tray. Note the contact time for high level disinfection (Table 2) is just 20 minutes compared to 10 hours required for sterilization.

OPERATION THEATER FUMIGATION AND/OR SURFACE DISINFECTION

Three agents are currently available for theater fumigation or surface disinfection.

1. *Forty percent formalin solution*: Formalin fumigation overnight either using a fumigator or formalin in a galipot is sufficient.[29] About 500 mL of 40% formalin in 1,000 mL of water, for 1,000 cu feet of operation theater area in an electric boiler/fumigator is the ideal concentration. This requires sealing of windows and doors overnight while fumigating.
2. Glutaraldehyde 5 grams, benzalkonium chloride 5 grams, alkyl urea 3 grams and 1,6-dihydroxy-2, 5-dioxahexane 11.2 grams; all the above in 100 grams packing. Around 0.5% spray or mopping daily may be done. To be left on surface for 20 minutes and later wiped off.
3. Aldehyde free, quick acting-ethanol 10 grams, 2-propanol 9 grams and 1-propanol 6 grams solution in 100 grams to be sprayed before 5 minutes of surgery on the floor, table, light and later wiped.[28] During spraying, no electrical switches to be operated since the sparks can ignite the fumigant.

House Keeping of the Operation Theater

The operation theater needs only be clean of dust and organic matter.

- Daily in the morning the floor, the operation table, chair, light, shelves and sink should be wet mopped free of dust, with water. *Note*: Avoid using broom which could aerosolize the dust. Use of detergent or chemical disinfectant for floor is optional, unless one is planning dermabrasion, skin grafting, hair restoration or liposuction. The wet mop later should be put in a proper place to dry.
- Later, the operation theater trolley should be mopped with a chemical disinfectant or isopropyl alcohol before surgery and between two surgeries.
- The floor and other areas of blood spillage should be mopped with chemical disinfectant or chlorine bleach.
- Cleaning the walls, ceiling on a daily basis is not mandatory but periodic maintenance could be undertaken.
- Use of fan in the operation theater should be avoided as it causes aerosolization of dust.
- If there is an air conditioner, maintenance of the same is necessary. Legionnaires'disease should be a reminder.

But however when invasive surgeries are being carried out: hair restoration, liposuction, complex closures, laser resurfacing; fumigation should be done daily or prior to each surgery.

Operation Theater Etiquettes

- The door of theater should be kept closed always.
- Unnecessary movement in and out of theater should be avoided.
- People with respiratory of skin infection should stay out.
- Staff must respect and maintain the dignity of the patient.
- Patients' privacy and modesty should be respected by all staff at all times.
- Patient must be explained in detail of the diagnosis, anesthesia planned, pain involved, and instrument being used like either laser or electrosurgery, postoperative care including the necessity of dressing, sunscreens or antibiotics, complications expected and their remedy. The next follow-up should be informed prior. If the patient is receiving oral sedation, the necessity of an attendant after surgery should be prior informed. The cost of the therapy should be explained.[30]
- Use of mobile in the operation theater should be restricted. Keep it in silent mode and in case you want to take the call, inform the patient and then proceed.[31]

WASTE DISPOSAL

Each dermatologist clinic and operation theater should be registered with the state health authorities. The waste

Box 4: Ergonomically designed chair.

- The seat height is adjustable with pneumatic pedestal (15–22 inches)
- Good lumbar support
- A seat pan with curved front
- Five pronged base support to prevent the chair from falling
- A good foot rest to prevent the stress of dangling thigh and leg on the hip (Fig. 10).

collected in leak proof plastic bags or plastic cans have to be handed over to the local agents, authorized by health department, for either incineration or land fill on daily basis. No waste should be left overnight in the theater.

Dermatologist in remote area should look into two main options of waste management:

1. *Sharps, plastic syringes, needle*: These should be shred after treatment in chlorine bleach for 12 hours.
2. *Blood soaked gauze*: These should be incinerated after treating in chlorine bleach for 12 hours.[32]

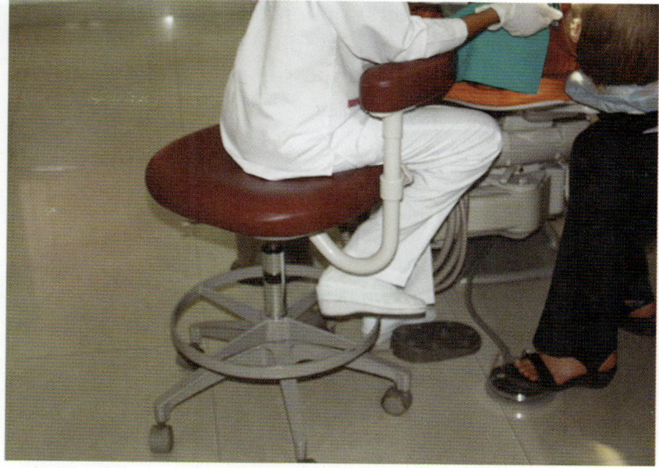

Fig. 10: An ideal chair with good base, foot rest, seat pan, lumbar seat support which can change to hand support and adjustable height.

ERGONOMICS

Ergon (work) + Nomo's (law) is the study focusing on worker's safety and productivity. In a well-designed work atmosphere, the workers should not be able to find any design or architectural deficiency but only concentrate on his/her work at hand.

> Surgeons till now were reluctant to have their work habits analyzed or criticized by others[33]

In the theater during hair transplantation, large area Vitiligo punch grafting and large area electrosurgery, a dermatologist could experience strain in the following four segments: (1) lower limb, (2) back, (3) neck and shoulder and (4) arm, wrist and hand.

But unfortunately surgical training discourages about complaining of stress and fatigue. Surgeons till now were reluctant to have their unique work habits analyzed or criticized by others.[33] However, there is an increasing awareness about these aspects now.

What is the Best Posture during Standing or Sitting?

Standing: During standing the head should be upright on torso, torso upright with the center of gravity over the hips, knees slightly bent and hands by the sides.

Sitting: During sitting one thinks that 90° hip flexion, 90° knee flexion, 90° elbow flexion with back and neck erect is ideal posture which is a myth. The ideal position of hip flexion is 105° with the back supported by the back rest. This puts least pressure on the intervertebral disc.

Which Position is Better—Sitting or Standing?

Both are good depending on the surgery. During standing position, the pressure on the intervertebral disc is 33% lesser than that of sitting. So standing in upright posture is more disc-friendly. But sitting requires 20% less energy than standing. During sitting only a few muscle groups are active and receive oxygenation. The large muscles of lower limbs are inactive and under prolonged tension leading to CO_2 build up and fatigue. The features of ergonomically designed chair have been mentioned in the Box 4.

To reduce the effect of posture on the body, several rules should be kept in mind:

- Change the position frequently.
- All procedures require forward bending putting strain on neck and back so position the operation table in a high visual field range to keep head balanced on spine.
- Arms should be kept next to the body, lifting and moving away from trunk increases strain (this is the neutral position of the arm).
- Precise surgery requires proper visualization and arm support. Ideally the operation table should be at 5-10 cm above elbow height. Elbow height is measured from the floor to the olecranon process of the elbow of the operator.
- Take regular breaks during prolonged surgeries, even before pain or discomfort sets in.
- By this you are preventing injuries.
- A break of 30 seconds is as good as long breaks.[34]

CONCLUSION

A dermatosurgical procedure is deemed successful if there is aseptic wound healing, surgery was painless with minimal blood loss. To achieve this, one has to have a clean, unobstructed work place which is easy to disinfect and in some situations sterilize. This place should have good set of instruments, advanced life support with good lighting. To achieve this, World Health Organization calls for 'sober down to earth planning and design' of theater.

Operation theater should not be viewed as a luxury but in reality, it is a place of high standard of patient safety with most economical use of manpower and other resources.

REFERENCES

1. Geisse JK. The dermatologic surgical suite. Semin Dermatol. 1994;13:2-9.
2. Pamela Phillips, Dirk M Elston, Desiree Ratner, et al. (2009). Outpatient Surgical Suite. 1-6, [online] Available from emedicine.medscape.com/article/1128609. [Accessed February, 2012].
3. Golberg LH, Peterson SR, Silaprint S, et al. The incidence of major complications from mohs micrographic surgery performed in office-based and hospital-based settings. J Am Acad Dermatol. 2005;53:628-34.
4. Indian standard-Basic requirements for hospital planning. IS12433 (part 2), 2001-Reaffirmed 2006;26-39.
5. The minimum standard requirements for the medical college-Amended November 2010. www.mciindia.org. [Accessed Dec 28, 2011].
6. Rajendran SC, Omprakash HM. Standard guidelines for setting up a dermatosurgery theater. Indian J Dermatol Venereal Leprol. 2009;75:76-82.
7. Accreditation for Ambulatory Care. Available from www.jointcommissioninternational.org/ambulatory-care. [Accessed February, 2012].
8. Directives for private ambulatorysurgical centers providing ambulatory surgery, Ministry of health, Singapore. 2007:1-6
9. Building guidelines for a surgical department. Netherlands Board for Hospital Facilities. 2004:1-16
10. Surgical care at the district hospital.WHO. 2003;2-13.
11. Savant SS, Gore D. Instruments, equipment and universal precautions. In: Satish S Savant. Textbook of Dermatosurgery and Cosmetology. Mumbai, India:Association of Scientific Cosmetologists and Dermatosurgeons; 2005;26-34.
12. Unger WP. The surgical suite. In: Unger WP, Shapiro R (Eds). Hair Transplantation. New York: Marcel Dekker; 2004; 833-4.
13. Malkin J. Ambulatory surgical centers. In: Malkin J (Ed). Medical and Dental Space Planning: A Comprehensive Guide to Design, Equipment and Clinical Procedures, 3rd edition. New York: John Wiley and Sons; 2002;334-6.
14. Malkin J. Ambulatory surgical centers. In: Malkin J (Ed). Medical and Dental Space Planning: A Comprehensive Guide to Design, Equipment and Clinical Procedures, 3rd edition. New York: John Wiley and Sons; 2002;352-3.
15. Regulations governing private hospitals and unattached operating theater units. Ministry of Health, Government of South Africa. 1993:8-10.
16. Ridley SA, Parry G. Guidelines for Fire safety in Intensive Care Unit. Intensive Care Society Publication. NHS, UK. 1998:1-16.
17. Lawrence C. Equipment. In: Lawrence C (Ed). An Introduction to Dermatological Surgery, 2nd edition. London: Churchill Livingstone; 2002;9-10.
18. Malkin J. Construction methods and building systems. In: Malkin J (Ed). Medical and DentalSpace planning, A comprehensive guide to design, equipment and clinical procedures.3rd edition. New York: John Wiley and sons; 2002; 556-61.
19. Maritza Perez, Rashmi Lodha, Keyvan Nouri. Surgical equipment and instrumentation. In: Keyvan Nouri, Susana Leal (Eds). Khouri Techniques in Dermatologic Surgery. Missouri: Mosby; 2003;25-31.
20. The revised guidelines for air conditioning system for operation theater. (2010). www.nabh.com. [Accessed February, 2012].
21. Bio-Medical Waste Management and Handling Rules, Second Amendment, 2000.Issued by Ministry of Environment and Forests, Government of India.
22. Female sterilization operation. Ensuring right to safety, dignity and informed choice. Government of India standards. 2005. Order dated 01.03.2005 passed in writ petition {civil} no-209/2003; Ramkant Rai v/s. Union of India and others. Available from www.hrln.org.
23. Field JM, Soderberg ES, Gonzales L, et al. Advanced Cardiovascular Life Support Provider Manual, Professional. Published on behalf of American Heart Association, Texas. 2006:1-142
24. Emergency drugs for both tubectomy and vasectomy camps. In: Standard operating procédures for sterilization services in camps, published by family planning division, Ministry of Health and Family Welfare, Government of India. 2008:30-1.
25. Pratt RJ, Pellowe C, Loveday HP, et al. The epic project: Developing national evidence-based guideline for preventing healthcare based guidelines for preventing healthcare associated infections. Phase I: Guideline for preventing hospital-acquired infections. J Hosp Infect. 2001;47 (supplement): S3-4.
26. Sawchuk WS, Weber PJ, Lowy DR, et al. Infectious papillomavirus in the vapor of warts treated with carbon dioxide laser or electrocoagulation: detection and protection. J Am Acad Dermatol. 1989;21:41-9.
27. Marra DE, Fincher EF, Moy RL. Surgical preparation, facilities and monitoring. In: Roenigk's Dermatologic Surgery. Current Techniques in Procedural Dermatology, 3rd edition. New York: Informa; 2007;1-9.
28. Korsolex, Baccillol agents. Available from www. Bodechemie.de. [Accessed January, 2012].
29. Savant SS, Gore D. Instruments, equipment and universal precautions. In: Savant SS (Ed). Textbook of Dermatosurgery and Cosmetology. Mumbai, India: Association of Scientific Cosmetologists and Dermatosurgeons; 2005;26.
30. Satyanarayana Rao KH. Informed consent: an ethical obligation or legal compulsion? J Cutan Aesthet Surg. 2008; 1:33-5.
31. Operation Theater Standard No-27, Theater Etiquette. Page 75, Royal United Bath Hospital NHS Trust, Theater practice policy, Reference no. 742. 2006.
32. Categories of biomedical waste. Schedule I. Ministry of Environment and Forest, Government of India. Available from envfov.nic.in/legis/hsm/biomed.html.
33. Burguer R. Surgery and Ergonomics. Arch Surg. 1999;134: 1011-6.
34. Jacobs K. Ergonomics for Therapists. Missouri: Mosby; 2008; 1-460.

Chapter

11

Disinfection and Sterilization

Uday Kelkar

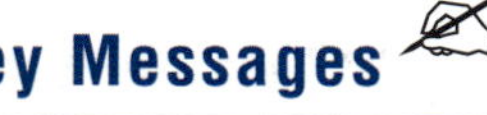

Key Messages

- Dermatosurgeons should be familiar with different processes such as cleaning, disinfection and sterilization.
- Dermatosurgical instruments used in hair transplantation, liposuction, vitiligo surgery, dermabrasion, nail surgery, scar revisions belong to critical device category. Most other instruments are noncritical.
- Handwashing by healthcare personnel is the most important procedure for preventing nosocomial infections and is of two types: (1) Typical surgical scrub and (2) Routine hand scrub.
- Methodical cleaning before high-level disinfection and sterilization removes organic and inorganic materials on the surfaces of instruments and enhances the efficiency of these processes.
- Disinfectants are classified as high-level, intermediate level and low-level disinfectants.
- Sterilization which is an absolute process achieves destruction of all microbes including spores, can be carried out either by physical or chemical methods.

INTRODUCTION

Dermatosurgical practice involves procedures that are performed mostly in outpatient settings and some procedures performed exclusively in operation theater (OT). In dermatological surgery adverse events in the form of infections are not common, but the potential for nosocomial infections does exist. The rates of postoperative infections tend to be low, but have been documented to be ranging from 0.2 to 3.5%.[1-3] Superficial infections occur essentially as a result of breach in the laid down and advocated standard infection control practices. Disinfection and sterilization constitute the foundation and core of standard infection control practices. Maintenance of strict asepsis is essential to minimize postoperative infections and their consequences. Awareness about these practices and principles is of great importance as dermatosurgeons today perform increasing number of procedures. This is particularly so, since many of these procedures are esthetic procedures with possible medicolegal implications. The reader is also suggested to read this chapter in conjunction with Chapter 7 on Universal Precautions.

BASIC PRINCIPLES OF DISINFECTION AND STERILIZATION

Infections can be either of endogenous or exogenous origin. Factors associated with transmission of infective material exogenously in hospitals and clinics include:

- Use of inadequately sterilized equipment.
- Presence of shedders of pathogenic microorganisms amongst the hospital personnel.
- Contaminated environment and contaminated surfaces.[4,5]
- Poor standards in antiseptic precautions.

Appropriate disinfection and sterilization policy is the mainstay of a successful infection control program to ensure that medical and surgical equipment does not transmit infectious pathogens to patients. It is important to appreciate that different practices are needed for different instruments and equipment, and practitioners must identify the right process such as cleaning, disinfection or sterilization, is needed, primarily on the basis of items intended for use.

IMPORTANT DEFINITIONS

- **Sterilization** is defined as a process that destroys or eliminates all forms of microbial life including bacterial endospores. Sterilization is carried out in hospitals and clinics by physical or chemical methods. Sterilization is intended to convey an absolute process.
- **Disinfection** is defined as a physical or chemical procedure performed on inanimate objects such as instruments and environmental surfaces that eliminate many pathogenic microorganisms. High-level disinfection is a procedure that destroys all microorganisms except high numbers of bacterial endospores. Unlike sterilization disinfection is not sporicidal. Few disinfectants will kill spores with prolonged exposure time, and these are called *chemical sterilants*.
- **Decontamination** is defined as removal of pathogenic organisms from objects in order to make them safe to handle.
- **Antisepsis** is defined as a procedure wherein a germicide is used on skin or living tissue with the intention of inhibiting or destroying microorganisms. The term is inappropriately used interchangeably with disinfection. Antiseptics are not designed to be used on medical devices, instruments or environmental surfaces and should not be confused with disinfectants which are too irritating to be used on skin or tissue.
- **Germicide** is a chemical agent that destroys microorganisms on either inanimate objects or living tissue.
- **Cleaning** is a prerequisite for disinfection or sterilization. It is the physical removal of organic material or soil from objects usually done by using water with or without detergents. Generally, cleaning is designed to remove rather than to kill microorganisms.

CLASSIFICATION OF MEDICAL DEVICES

The choice of a sterilization or disinfection procedure depends on the type of items to be processed. A helpful categorization devised by Spaulding stratifies medical equipment into critical, semi-critical and noncritical devices on the basis of the risk of infections implicated with their use.[6]

Critical Devices

Instruments or equipment having a contact with the bloodstream or sterile areas of the body are classified as critical devices. Risk of acquiring infections is significant if these devices are contaminated. Bloodstream catheters, implants, needles, scalpels and surgical instruments are some of the examples of critical devices. Dermatosurgical instruments used in hair transplantation, liposuction, vitiligo surgery, dermabrasion, nail surgery, scar revisions, etc. belong to this category. Critical devices require sterilization prior to use on patients.

Semi-critical Devices

Equipments that come in contact with mucous membrane are considered as semi-critical devices. Although these items come in contact with intact mucous membranes, they do not ordinarily penetrate body surface. Endoscopes, endotracheal tubes, anesthesia breathing circuits, cystoscopes, respiratory care equipment and urinary catheters are examples of semi-critical devices. Sterilization is the preferred method for processing these devices. However, sterilization is not absolutely essential and hence in situations where sterilization is not feasible, high-level disinfection after thorough cleaning is an acceptable alternative.

Noncritical Devices

Devices coming into contact with intact skin of patients are classified as noncritical. The risk of acquiring infections from these devices is minimal. Stethoscopes, cardiac electrodes, crutches, sphygmomanometer cuffs, surfaces of medical equipments and environmental surfaces are grouped under this category. Most instruments used in esthetic procedures such as microdermabrasion, lasers and phototherapy glasses belong to this category. The cleaning and disinfection policy for these depend upon the physical characters of these items or surfaces. It ranges from simple detergent-based cleaning to low-level disinfection methods.

ANTISEPSIS AND NORMAL BACTERIAL SKIN FLORA

Antisepsis is defined as a procedure wherein a germicide is used on skin or living tissue with the intention of inhibiting or destroying microorganisms. It is important to understand the normal skin microorganisms to understand the antiseptics.

Normal human skin is colonized with bacteria; different areas of the body have varied total aerobic bacterial counts. Total bacterial counts on the hands of medical personnel have ranged from 3.9×10^4 to 4.6×10^6. Bacteria recovered from the hands are divided into two categories: transient and resident.[6] The hands of healthcare workers may become persistently colonized with pathogenic flora (e.g. *Staphylococcus aureus*), gram-negative bacilli, or yeast. Investigators have documented that, although the number of transient and resident flora varies considerably from person-to-person, it is often relatively constant for any specific person.[7,8]

Transient flora, which colonizes the superficial layers of the skin, is more common source of the organisms most frequently associated with healthcare-associated infections and are amenable to removal by routine handwashing. They are often acquired by healthcare workers during direct contact with patients or contact with contaminated environmental surfaces within close proximity of the patient. Resident flora (e.g. coagulase-negative staphylococci and diphtheroids, are found in deeper layers of the skin and are more resistant to removal. However, resident flora is less likely to cause infections.

Handwashing

Handwashing by healthcare personnel, the most commonly performed antiseptic procedure, is also the most important procedure for preventing nosocomial infections. When done with plain soap, it results in mechanical removal of microorganisms and if done with detergents containing antimicrobial agents, it results in chemical removal of microorganisms as well. In practice, handwashing is broadly of two types: (1) typical surgical scrub, and (2) routine hand scrub after examining a patient. Surgical hand scrub is an elaborate detailed procedure performed for a minimum 2 minutes; while a casual hand scrub is advocated after patient examination (for details see chapter Universal Precautions). Different handwash antiseptics are discussed below.

Alcohol-Based Hand Scrubs

The majority of alcohol-based hand antiseptics contain isopropanol, ethanol, n-propanol, or a combination of two of these products. Alcohols are usually used as a combination of two alcohols or along with other agents like hexachlorophene, quaternary ammonium compounds, povidone-iodine, triclosan or chlorhexidine gluconate. The antimicrobial activity of alcohols can be attributed to their ability to denature proteins. Alcohol solutions containing 60–95% alcohol are most effective and higher concentrations are less potent because proteins are not denatured easily in the absence of water.

Chlorhexidine: Chlorhexidine gluconate, a cationic biguanide, acts by disruption of cytoplasmic membranes, resulting in precipitation of cellular contents. Chlorhexidine has good activity against gram-positive bacteria, somewhat less activity against gram-negative bacteria and fungi and only minimal activity against tubercle bacilli. The antimicrobial activity of chlorhexidine is only minimally affected by the presence of organic material, including blood. Chlorhexidine has substantial residual activity, addition of low concentrations (0.5–1.0%) of chlorhexidine to alcohol-based preparations results in greater residual activity than alcohol alone.

Iodophors: Iodine molecules rapidly penetrate the cell wall of microorganisms and inactivate cells by forming complexes with amino acids and unsaturated fatty acids, resulting in impaired protein synthesis and alteration of cell membranes. The antimicrobial activity of iodophors can be affected by pH, temperature, exposure time, concentration of total available iodine, and the amount and type of organic and inorganic compounds present (e.g. alcohols and detergents). Iodine and iodophors have bactericidal activity against gram-positive, gram-negative, and certain spore-forming bacteria (e.g. clostridia and *Bacillus* spp.) and are active against mycobacteria, viruses, and fungi. However, in concentrations used in antiseptics, iodophors are not usually sporicidal. Povidone-iodine 5–10% has been classified as a safe and effective agent for use as an antiseptic handwash. The majority of iodophor preparations used for hand hygiene contain 7.5–10% povidone-iodine.

FACTORS AFFECTING THE EFFICACY OF DISINFECTION AND STERILIZATION

The germicidal activity depends on a number of factors, based on intrinsic qualities of the organism and the chemical and external physical environment.[6,9-12]

Number and Location of Microorganisms

All other conditions remaining constant, the larger the number of microbes, the more time a germicide needs to destroy all of them. This emphasizes the need for scrupulous cleaning of medical instruments, before disinfection and sterilization. Meticulous cleaning reduces the number of microorganisms that must be inactivated, increasing the margin of safety when the germicide is used. The location of microorganisms also affects the efficacy of germicides. Medical instruments with multiple pieces need to be disassembled and equipment such as endoscopes that have crevices and channels, need more meticulous disinfection than flat surface equipment, because penetration of the disinfectant into all parts of the equipment is more difficult.

Innate Resistance of Microorganisms

Microorganisms differ greatly in their susceptibility to chemical germicides and sterilization processes. Spores are generally resistant to disinfectants, because the spore coat and cortex act as a barrier. Mycobacteria have a waxy cell wall that prevents disinfectant entry, and gram-negative bacteria possess an outer membrane that acts as a barrier to the uptake of disinfectants.[13,14] The sterilization or disinfection time is dependent upon the time required to destroy the most resistant forms. Prions possess the highest innate resistance to chemical germicides, followed by bacterial spores, coccidia (*Cryptosporidium*), mycobacteria (*M. tuberculosis*), non-lipid or small viruses (poliovirus, and coxsackievirus), fungi (*Aspergillus,* and *Candida*), vegetative bacteria (e.g. *Staphylococcus* and *Pseudomonas*) and lipid or medium size viruses (herpes and human immunodeficiency virus).[15-17]

Concentration and Potency of Disinfectants

With other variables constant and with one exception (iodophors), the more concentrated the disinfectant, the greater its efficacy and the shorter the time necessary to achieve microbial death. However, all disinfectants are not similarly affected by concentration changes. For example, quaternary ammonium compounds and phenol have a concentration exponent of 1 and 6, respectively; thus, halving the concentration of a quaternary ammonium compound requires doubling its disinfecting time, but halving the concentration of a phenol solution requires a sixty-four fold increase in its disinfecting time.[18-20] Length of the contact time with disinfectant thus depends on the potency of the germicide.

Physical and Chemical Factors

Temperature, pH, relative humidity and water hardness affect the disinfection time. The activity of most disinfectants increases as the temperature increases, but some exceptions exist. An increase in pH improves the antimicrobial activity of some disinfectants (e.g. glutaraldehyde, quaternary ammonium compounds) but decreases the antimicrobial activity of others (e.g. phenols, hypochlorites and iodine).[19] Relative humidity is the single most important factor influencing the activity of gaseous disinfectants/sterilants such as ETO, chlorine dioxide and formaldehyde. Water hardness (i.e. high concentration of divalent cations) reduces the rate of kill of certain disinfectants because divalent cations (e.g. magnesium, calcium) in the hard water interact with the disinfectant to form insoluble precipitates.[9,21]

Types of Matter: Organic and Inorganic

Presence of serum, blood, pus, or fecal or lubricant material interferes with the antimicrobial activity of disinfectants. Interference occurs by a chemical reaction between the germicide and the organic matter resulting in a complex that is less germicidal. Chlorine and iodine disinfectants, in particular, are prone to such interaction.[22] Inorganic contaminants like salts have an effect of protecting microorganisms by interfering in the sterilization cycle. Meticulous cleaning of medical devices before any sterilization or disinfection procedure is therefore very important, as organic and inorganic soils can be easily removed by washing.[23]

Duration of Exposure

Items need exposure to the germicide for the appropriate contact time. All lumens and channels of endoscopic instruments must come in contact with the disinfectant. The disinfectant must be introduced reliably into the internal channels of the devices.

Cleaning

As emphasized above, methodical cleaning is necessary before high-level disinfection and sterilization, as the organic and inorganic materials that may persist on the surfaces of instruments interfere with the efficiency of these processes. Cleaning is the process of removing alien material (e.g. soil and organic material) from objects. Cleaning is important for several reasons:

- Instruments and materials used during a procedure are usually covered with blood and remains of tissues; they may have also been in touch with chemicals and fluids, dirt and dust. The tubing of hollow instruments may also be full of these soils. Cleaning plays an immensely important role in this process.
- A major requirement for critical devices is that they should be sterile. However, sterility alone is not sufficient for safe use. An instrument, which is covered with sterile dirt or with remains of chemicals or corrosion, still is a serious health hazard. Thus, all potentially dangerous soil or remains have to be removed by cleaning.
- In case the proteinaceous material dries on the device, the disinfection or sterilization process becomes less effective or ineffective. Surgical instruments should be presoaked or rinsed to prevent drying of blood and to soften or remove blood from the instruments. Ultrasonic cleaners are a useful addition to the available equipments to ensure that the material sticking to the instruments gets dislodged prior to cleaning.
- The process of cleaning reduces the bioburden (the population of microorganisms residing on the materials) considerably (Fig. 1). Reduction of the bioburden ensures that the disinfection or sterilization process will be more effective, as much less organisms have to be killed.
- Cleaning also ensures that the pyrogens and endotoxins are effectively removed.

Methods of Cleaning

Cleaning is normally done using water with detergents or enzymatic products. Cleaning can be either manual

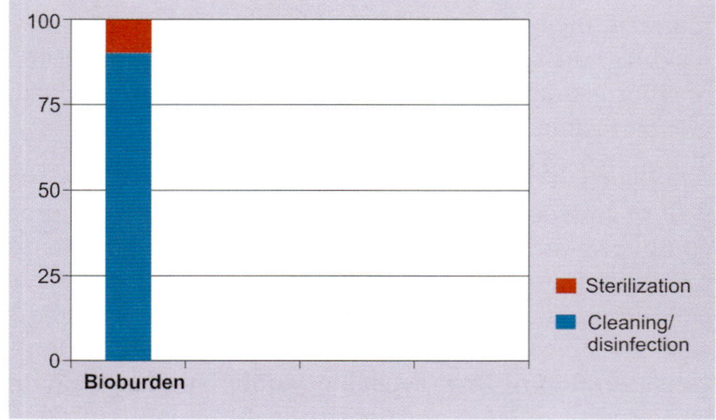

Fig. 1: Graph showing percentage reduction of bioburden.

or automatic. Cleaning is done manually in most of healthcare settings. In manual cleaning, the two essential components are friction and use of fluids. Friction (e.g. rubbing/scrubbing the soiled area with a brush) is an old and dependable method. Fluids usually water under pressure is used to remove soil and debris from internal channels after brushing and when the design does not allow passage of a brush through a channel.[24] It is of vital importance that the instruments should be disassembled as much as possible.

The most common types of automatic cleaners are ultrasonic cleaners (Fig. 2). Ultrasonic cleaning removes soil by cavitation and implosion in which waves of acoustic energy are propagated in aqueous solutions to disrupt the bonds that hold particulate matter to surfaces. The process of sonication can act synergistically to increase the cidal efficacy of a disinfectant.[25]

Washer sterilizers are modified steam sterilizers that clean by filling the chamber with water and detergent through which steam passes to provide agitation. Instruments are subsequently rinsed and subjected to a short steam sterilization cycle.[26] Washer decontaminators act like a dishwasher that uses a combination of water circulation and detergents to remove soil. Washer disinfectors are generally computer controlled units for cleaning, disinfecting and drying solid and hollow surgical and medical equipment. Studies have shown that manual and mechanical cleaning of endoscopes achieves approximately a log 10^4 reduction of contaminating organisms.[27]

Instrument cleaning requires a neutral or near neutral pH detergent solution because such solutions generally provide the best material compatibility profile and good soil removal. Enzymes, usually proteases, sometimes are added to neutral pH solutions to assist in removing organic material. Enzymes in these formulations attack proteins that make up a large portion of common soil (e.g. blood, pus). Cleaning solutions also can contain lipases (enzymes active on fats) and amylases (enzymes active on starches). Enzymatic cleaners are not disinfectants and proteinaceous enzymes can be inactivated by germicides. Enzyme solutions should be used in proper dilution of the enzymatic detergent and contact with equipment for the amount of time specified on the label.[28]

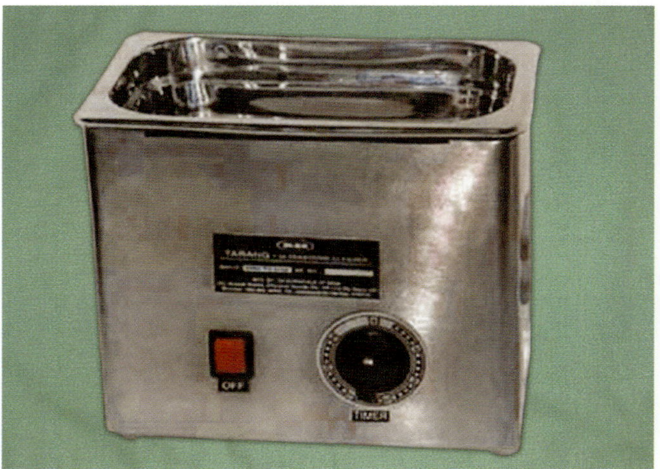

Fig. 2: Ultrasonic cleaner.

Validation of Cleaning Process

Although the effectiveness of high-level disinfection and sterilization mandates effective cleaning, it is rather difficult to validate the cleaning process. The ideal and foolproof method to ensure adequate cleaning is to conduct microbiologic sampling, but this is not practicable and hence not routinely recommended.[29] Visual inspection of the cleaned and dried gadgets is the commonly employed and acceptable method employed in hospitals. Instruments must be individually inspected and be visibly clean (Fig. 3).

DISINFECTION

Disinfection describes a process that eliminates most or all pathogenic microorganisms, except bacterial spores. Since disinfected products are not wrapped, they can be contaminated and do not remain germ-free. Disinfection decreases the population of microorganisms by a limited reduction factor (up to 10^5) in contrast to sterilization, which inactivates all varieties of microorganisms including spores, resulting in a very low probability of persistence. Some disinfectants can kill spores with prolonged exposure time and are called chemical sterilants. The required efficacy of the disinfection process is linked to the intended use and the microorganisms relevant for that use (e.g. bed pans require a lower level of disinfection than a flexible endoscope).

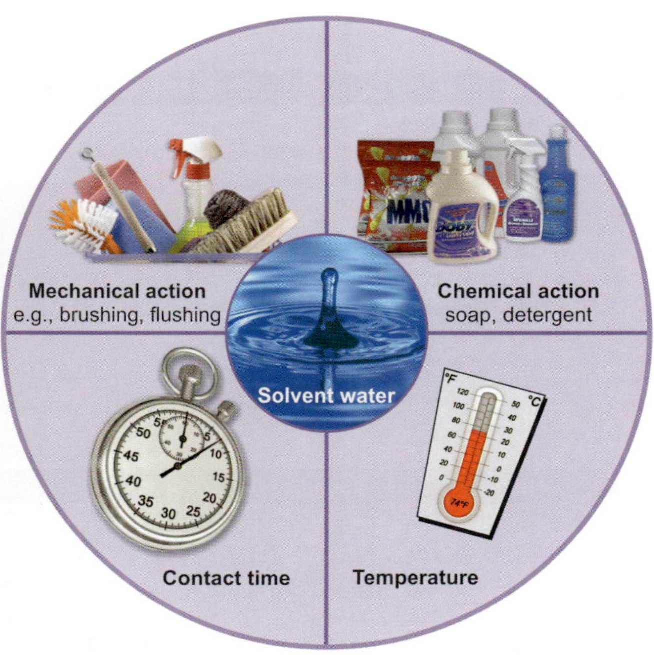

Fig. 3: Cleaning circle—all factors are essential.

For disinfectants, the level and intended spectrum of activity is specified in international standards.

In practice, instruments are usually disinfected by liquid chemicals. The choice of specific cleaning or disinfecting agents is largely a matter of judgment, guided by product label claims and instructions. A single liquid chemical germicide might not satisfy all disinfection requirements in a given practice or facility. Realistic use of liquid chemical germicides depends on consideration of multiple factors, including the degree of microbial killing required; the nature and composition of the surface, item, or device to be treated; and the cost, safety and ease of use of the available agents.

The properties of an ideal antiseptic or disinfectant are shown in Box 1:

Classification of Disinfectants

Disinfectants can be classified in different ways:

- Based on consistency
  - Liquid (e.g. alcohols, phenols)
  - Gaseous (formaldehyde vapor, ethylene oxide)
- Based on spectrum of activity
  - High-level
  - Intermediate
  - Low-level
- Based on mechanism of action
  - Action on membrane (e.g. alcohol, detergent)
  - Denaturation of cellular proteins (e.g. alcohol, phenol)
  - Oxidation of essential sulfhydryl groups of enzymes (e.g. H_2O_2, halogens)
  - Alkylation of amino, carboxyl and hydroxyl group (e.g. ethylene oxide, formaldehyde)
  - Damage to nucleic acids (e.g. ethylene oxide, formaldehyde)

Box 1: Characteristics of an ideal disinfectant.

- Wide spectrum of activity
- Ability to destroy microbes within reasonable period of time
- Activity in the presence of organic matter
- Activity over a wide range of pH
- Stability and shelf life
- Speedy action
- High penetrating power
- Nontoxic, nonallergenic, nonirritative and noncorrosive
- Should not leave nonvolatile residue or stain
- Easily available and reasonable cost

- A commonly used classification which is universally used is as follows (Table 1):
  - *High-level disinfectants*: Chemicals that kill all microorganisms and can act as sterilants if applied for prolonged length of time. However, if spores are present in large numbers, they are not killed.
  - *Intermediate level disinfectants*: They kill all mycobacteria, vegetative bacteria, most viruses and most fungi, but not bacterial spores.
  - *Low-level disinfectants*: Can kill most vegetative bacteria, but only some fungi and some viruses.

Different Agents and Methods

Both chemical and nonchemical methods are available.

Chemical disinfectants: A wide variety of germicides, which differ in their spectrum of activity against various forms of microorganisms, are available (Fig. 4). Chemical composition and structure of the outer cell layers determine the uptake of germicide.

a. *Alcohols:* Alcohols in health care refer to two water-soluble chemical compounds: ethyl alcohol and isopropyl alcohol. These alcohols are rapidly bactericidal against vegetative forms of bacteria; they also are tuberculocidal, fungicidal and virucidal, but do not destroy bacterial spores. Their cidal activity drops sharply when diluted below 50% concentration, and the optimum bactericidal concentration is 60–90% solutions in water (volume/volume).[30] Alcohols act by denaturation of proteins. The mixtures of alcohol and water is more bactericidal because proteins are denatured more quickly in the presence of water than absolute alcohols which have a dehydrating action.[30] Methyl alcohol (methanol) has the weakest bactericidal action of the alcohols. Ethyl alcohol, at concentrations of 60–80%, is a potent virucidal agent inactivating all of the lipophilic viruses (e.g. herpes, vaccinia and influenza virus) and many hydrophilic viruses (e.g. adenovirus, enterovirus, rhinovirus and rotaviruses but not hepatitis A virus (HAV) or poliovirus).[31] Isopropyl alcohol is not active against the nonlipid enteroviruses but is fully active against the lipid viruses. Ethyl and isopropyl alcohol have the ability to inactivate the hepatitis B virus (HBV)[32] and the herpes virus[33] and ethyl alcohol to inactivate human immunodeficiency virus (HIV).[34]

Alcohols have been used effectively to disinfect noncritical devices and to disinfect external surfaces

Table 1: Spectrum of activity of disinfectants.

	Vegetative cells	*Mycobacteria*	*Spores*	*Fungi*	*Viruses*	*Examples*
High-level	+	+	+	+	+	Ethylene oxide gluteraldehyde, formaldehyde
Intermediate level	+	+		+	+	Phenolics, halogens
Low-level	+			+	+/	Alcohols, quaternary ammonium compounds

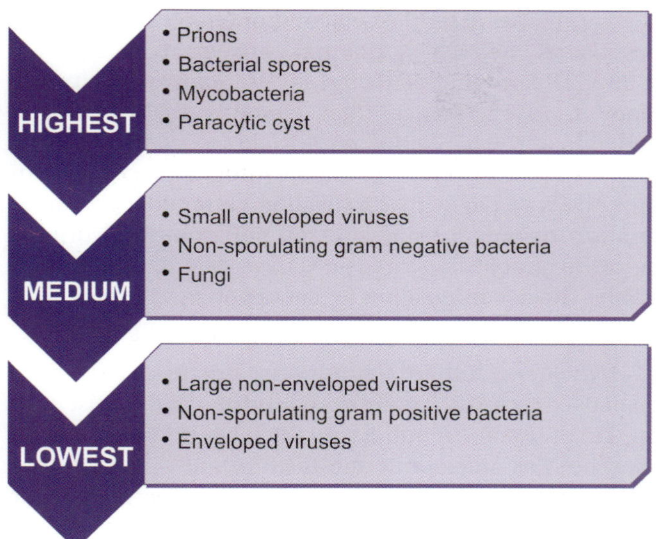

Fig. 4: Resistance of microorganisms to disinfectants in descending order.

of equipment. However, alcohols are not recommended for sterilizing medical and surgical materials as they lack sporicidal action and they cannot penetrate protein-rich materials. Disadvantages of alcohols are:

- They damage the shellac mountings of lensed instruments.
- Tend to swell and harden rubber and certain plastic tubing after prolonged and repeated use.
- Bleach rubber and plastic tiles.[35]
- Alcohols are flammable and consequently must be stored in a cool, well-ventilated area.
- They also evaporate rapidly, making extended exposure time difficult to achieve unless the items are immersed.

b. *Chlorine and chlorine compounds:* Hypochlorites, the most widely used of the chlorine disinfectants, are available as liquid (e.g. sodium hypochlorite) or solid (e.g. calcium hypochlorite). The most prevalent chlorine products is the aqueous solutions of 5–6% sodium hypochlorite, usually called household bleach. They have a broad spectrum of antimicrobial activity, do not leave toxic residues, are unaffected by water hardness, are inexpensive and fast acting,[36] remove dried or fixed organisms and biofilms from surfaces[37] and have a low incidence of serious toxicity.[38] Sodium hypochlorite at the concentration used in household bleach can produce ocular irritation or oropharyngeal, esophageal and gastric burns.[39] Hypochlorites are corrosive in nature specially to metals, are inactivated by organic matter, lead to discoloration of fabrics and release of toxic chlorine gas when mixed with ammonia or acid.[40] The actual microbicidal mechanism of chlorine may be due to a combination of several factors like oxidation of sulfhydryl enzymes and amino acids; ring chlorination of amino acids; loss of intracellular contents; decreased uptake of nutrients; inhibition of protein synthesis; decreased oxygen uptake; breaks in DNA; and depressed DNA synthesis. The microbicidal activity of chlorine is attributed largely to undissociated hypochlorous acid (HOCl). The dissociation of HOCI to the less microbicidal form (hypochlorite ion OCl) depends on the pH. The disinfecting efficacy of chlorine decreases with an increase in pH.[41] Chlorine dioxide, sodium dichloro isocyanurate and chloramine T are the other compounds used as chlorine-releasing agents. The advantage of these compounds over the hypochlorites is that they retain chlorine longer and so exert a more prolonged bactericidal effect.[42] Chlorine solution is used for disinfecting counter tops and floors. It has been recommended for decontaminating blood spills. For small spills of blood on noncritical surfaces, the area can be disinfected with a 1:100 dilution of 5–6% sodium hypochlorite. Hypochlorites and other germicides are substantially inactivated in the presence of blood.[43] Large spills of blood require that the surface be cleaned before a 1:10 (final concentration) solution of household bleach is applied.[44]

c. *Superoxidized water:* Superoxidized water is a relatively new disinfectant with good microbicidal properties.[45] Saline is electrolyzed to create a disinfectant or antiseptics. The solution is nontoxic to biologic tissues. Superoxidized water is generally noncorrosive to equipment. The activity of this disinfectant decreases substantially in the presence of organic material.

d. *Formaldehyde:* Formaldehyde is used as a disinfectant and sterilant in both its liquid and gaseous states. Formaldehyde inactivates microorganisms by alkylating the amino and sulfhydryl groups of proteins and ring nitrogen atoms of purine bases. Formaldehyde alcohol is a chemical sterilant and formaldehyde is a high-level disinfectant. Formaldehyde is sold and used principally as water-based solution called formalin, which is 37% formaldehyde by weight. The aqueous solution is a bactericidal, tuberculocidal, fungicidal, virucidal and sporicidal. Formaldehyde, however, is a potential carcinogen and ingestion of formaldehyde can be fatal. Long-term exposure to low-levels in the air or on the skin can cause asthma like respiratory problems and skin irritation, such as dermatitis and itching. For these reasons, employees should have limited direct contact with formaldehyde and an employee exposure standard for formaldehyde that limits an 8 hours time weighted average exposure concentration of 0.75 ppm.[46] These considerations and its pungent odor and irritating fumes limit its role in sterilization and disinfection processes.

e. *Glutaraldehyde:* Glutaraldehyde is a saturated dialdehyde which is a high-level disinfectant and chemical sterilant. The biocidal activity of glutaraldehyde results from its alkylation of sulfhydryl, hydroxyl, carboxyl, and amino groups of microorganisms, which alters RNA, DNA and protein synthesis. Two percent alkaline glutaraldehyde has excellent cidal action against bacteria, fungi, viruses and a relatively slow action (20 to >30 minutes) against *Mycobacterium tuberculosis.* Aqueous solutions of glutaraldehyde are acidic and generally in this state are not sporicidal. Only when the solution is "activated" (made alkaline) by the use of alkalinating agents to pH 7.5–8.5, does the solution become sporicidal. Once activated, these solutions have a limited shelf life of about 14 days, because of the polymerization of the glutaraldehyde molecules at alkaline pH levels. Newer glutaraldehyde formulations (e.g. glutaraldehyde phenol sodium phenate, potentiated acid glutaraldehyde, stabilized alkaline glutaraldehyde) have a longer shelf life (e.g. use life 2,830 days). The use of glutaraldehyde-based solutions in healthcare facilities is widespread because of their advantages, including excellent biocidal properties; activity in the presence of organic matter (20% bovine serum); and noncorrosive action to endoscopic equipment, thermometers, rubber, or plastic equipment.[47,48] *It is very suitable for most dermatosurgical equipment.*

Acute or chronic exposure to glutaraldehyde can result in skin irritation or dermatitis, mucous membrane irritation (eye, nose, mouth), or pulmonary symptoms.[39] Measures that can be used to resolve these problems include ducted exhaust hoods, air systems that provide 7–15 air exchanges per hour, ductless fume hoods with absorbents for the glutaraldehyde vapor, tight fitting lids on immersion baths, personal protection (e.g. nitrile or butyl rubber gloves but not natural latex gloves, goggles) to minimize skin or mucous membrane contact. Sodium bisulfate can be used to neutralize the glutaraldehyde and make it safe for disposal.

f. *Orthophthalaldehyde:* Orthophthalaldehyde (OPA) is a high-level disinfectant that contains 0.55% 1, 2 benzenedicarboxaldehyde, with a pH of 7.5. OPA, like glutaraldehyde interacts with amino acids, proteins of microorganisms. OPA has excellent microbicidal activity. OPA is effective against a wide range of microorganisms, including glutaraldehyde resistant mycobacteria. OPA kills spores by blocking the spore germination process.

Orthophthalaldehyde has several potential advantages over glutaraldehyde. It has excellent stability over a wide range of pH 3–9, is not a known irritant to the eyes and nasal passages, does not require exposure monitoring, has barely perceptible odor and requires no activation.[49] OPA, like glutaraldehyde has excellent material compatibility.

A potential disadvantage of OPA is that it stains proteins gray including unprotected skin and thus must be handled with caution.[50] Personal protective equipments should be worn when contaminated instruments, equipment and chemicals are handled. In addition equipments must be thoroughly rinsed to prevent discoloration of patient's skin or mucous membrane.

g. *Hydrogen peroxide:* Hydrogen peroxide has excellent bactericidal, virucidal, sporicidal and fungicidal properties. Hydrogen peroxide works by producing destructive hydroxyl free radicals that can attack membrane lipids, DNA and other essential cell components and has shown promise as chemical sterilant in concentrations from 6% to 25%. The product marketed as a sterilant is a premixed, ready to use chemical that contains 7.5% hydrogen peroxide and 0.85% phosphoric acid (to maintain a low pH).[50] The effectiveness of 7.5% hydrogen peroxide at 10 minutes is at par with 2% alkaline glutaraldehyde at 20 minutes in manual disinfection of endoscopes.[51] Hydrogen peroxide should be stored in dark containers to remain stable. The decomposition or loss of potency in small containers is less than 2% per year at ambient temperatures.[52]

h. *Iodophors:* Iodine solutions or tinctures long have been used by health professionals primarily as antiseptics on skin or tissue. Iodophors, on the other hand, have been used both as antiseptics and disinfectants. An iodophor is a combination of iodine and a solubilizing agent or carrier; the resulting complex provides a sustained release reservoir of iodine and releases small amounts of free iodine in aqueous solution. Povidone iodine and other iodophors retain the germicidal efficacy of iodine but unlike iodine generally do not stain and are relatively free of toxicity and irritancy.[53] Free iodine (I_2) contributes to the bactericidal activity of iodophors and dilutions of iodophors demonstrate more rapid bactericidal action than does a full strength povidone iodine solution.

Iodophors are bactericidal, mycobactericidal and virucidal but can require prolonged contact times to kill certain fungi and bacterial spores.[6,54]

i. *Peracetic acid:* Peracetic acid is characterized by rapid action against all microorganisms. Special advantages of peracetic acid are that it lacks harmful decomposition products and enhances removal of organic material and leaves no residue. It remains effective in the presence of organic matter and is sporicidal even at low temperatures. Peracetic acid can corrode copper, brass, bronze, plain steel, and galvanized iron but these effects can be reduced by additives and pH modifications. Peracetic acid is believed to function similarly to other oxidizing agents; that is, it denatures proteins, disrupts the cell wall permeability, and oxidizes sulfhydryl and sulfur bonds in proteins, enzymes and other metabolites.[55]

Peracetic acid inactivates gram-positive and gram-negative bacteria, viruses, fungi, mycobacteria, and bacterial spores.

Peracetic acid is available in combination with hydrogen peroxide (0.23% peracetic acid plus 7.35% hydrogen peroxide) for their synergistic action in inactivating all microorganisms except bacterial spores within 20 minutes.

j. *Phenolic disinfectants:* Phenol has occupied a prominent place in the field of hospital disinfection since its initial use as a germicide by Lister in his pioneering work on antiseptic surgery. Phenol derivatives originate when a functional group (e.g. alkyl, phenyl, benzyl and halogen) replaces one of the hydrogen atoms on the aromatic ring. Two phenol derivatives commonly found as constituents of hospital disinfectants are ortho phenyl phenol and ortho benzyl para chlorophenol. In high concentrations, phenol acts as a gross protoplasmic poison, penetrating and disrupting the cell wall and precipitating the cell proteins. Low concentrations of phenol and higher molecular weight phenol derivatives cause bacterial death by inactivation of essential enzyme systems and leakage of essential metabolites from the cell wall.[56] Commercially available phenolic disinfectants are not sporicidal, but are tuberculocidal, fungicidal, virucidal and bactericidal at their recommended use dilution.

Phenolic germicides are disinfectants for use on environmental surfaces (e.g. bedside tables, bedrails, and laboratory surfaces) and noncritical medical devices. Phenolics are not high-level disinfectants for use with semi-critical items but could be used to preclean or decontaminate critical and semi-critical devices before terminal sterilization or high-level disinfection.

k. *Quaternary ammonium compounds:* The quaternary ammonium compounds are widely used as disinfectants. The quaternaries are good cleaning agents. Each compound exhibits its own antimicrobial characteristics. Some of the chemical names of quaternary ammonium compounds used in health care are alkyl dimethyl benzyl ammonium chloride, alkyl didecyl dimethyl ammonium chloride, and dialkyl dimethyl ammonium chloride. The newer quaternary ammonium compounds (i.e. fourth generation), referred to as twin chain or dialkyl quaternaries (e.g. didecyl dimethyl ammonium bromide and dioctyl dimethyl ammonium bromide), reportedly remain active in hard water and are tolerant of anionic residues.[57]

The bactericidal action of the quaternaries has been attributed to the inactivation of energy producing enzymes, denaturation of essential cell proteins, and disruption of the cell membrane.[57]

Quaternaries available as hospital disinfectants are generally fungicidal, bactericidal, and virucidal against enveloped viruses. They are not sporicidal and generally not tuberculocidal. The quaternaries are commonly used in ordinary environmental sanitation of noncritical surfaces, such as floors, furniture, and walls.

l. *Other germicides:* New disinfectants that require further evaluation include glucoprotamin, tertiary amines and a light activated antimicrobial coating. In preliminary studies, nanoemulsions (composed of detergents and lipids in water) showed activity against vegetative bacteria, enveloped viruses and *Candida*. This product represents a potential agent for use as a topical biocidal agent.[58]

Metals such as silver, iron and copper could be used for environmental control, disinfection of water, or incorporated into medical devices (e.g. intravascular catheters).[59,60] Surfacine is a new persistent antimicrobial agent that may be used on animate or inanimate surfaces. It incorporates a water insoluble antimicrobial compound (silver iodide) in a surface immobilized coating. Surfacine is applied to the animate or inanimate surfaces by spraying or coating without any prior surface treatment.

m. *Ultraviolet radiation:* The wavelength of ultraviolet (UV) radiation ranges from 328 nm to 210 nm (3,280–2,100 A). Its maximum bactericidal effect occurs at 240–280 nm. Mercury vapor lamps emit more than 90% of their radiation at 253.7 nm, which is near the maximum microbicidal activity. Inactivation of microorganisms results from destruction of nucleic acid through induction of thymine dimers. Ultraviolet radiation has been employed in the disinfection of drinking water, air, titanium implants and contact lenses.[61] Bacteria and viruses are more easily killed by UV light than are bacterial spores. Ultraviolet radiation has several potential applications, but unfortunately its germicidal effectiveness and use is influenced by organic matter, wavelength, type of suspension, temperature, type of microorganism and UV intensity, which is affected by distance and dirty tubes. The application of UV radiation in the healthcare environment operating rooms, isolation rooms and biologic safety cabinets is limited to destruction of airborne organisms.

STERILIZATION

Sterilization is defined as a process that destroys or eliminates all forms of microbial life including bacterial endospores. Sterilization is intended to convey an absolute process. Sterilization is carried out in hospitals and clinics by various physical (such as heat) or chemical methods. Recently, a number of newer methods like low temperature sterilization systems (e.g. hydrogen peroxide gas plasma, peracetic acid immersion, ozone) have been developed and are being utilized to sterilize medical devices.[62,63]

Methods of Sterilization

Heat

Heat is considered as the most reliable methods of sterilization for articles that can withstand heat. Heat acts by oxidative effects as well as denaturation and coagulation of proteins. Factors affecting sterilization by heat are:

- Nature of heat: Moist heat is more effective than dry heat.
- Temperature and time: Temperature and time are inversely related. As the temperature increases the time taken for sterilization decreases.
- Number of microorganisms: Direct relation with time.
- Nature of microorganisms: Spores are relatively resistant to heat.
- Type of material and presence of organic matter: In presence of organic matter like proteins, fats, etc. the time taken increases.

Dry heat

Dry heat acts by denaturation of proteins. Articles such as bacteriological loops, tips of forceps, etc. are sterilized by holding them in a Bunsen burner flame till they are red hot.

Incineration: Incineration is a method of terminal destruction of contaminated material. Incineration results in loss of material and hence used only when the article in question like a soiled dressing, bedding, etc. is not to be reused.

Hot air oven: Articles to be sterilized are exposed to high temperature of about 160°C for about 1 hour in an electrically heated oven. Since air is a poor conductor of heat, even distribution of heat inside the oven is achieved by a fan. Heat is transferred to the articles by radiation, conduction and convection.

Glassware, oils, petroleum jelly and powders are materials which are sterilized using hot air oven. Articles to be sterilized must be perfectly dry before placing them in oven. Articles must be placed with sufficient distance between them so that circulation of hot air is uniformly maintained inside the hot air oven. The holding time observed is 60 minutes at 160°C, 40 minutes at 170°C and 20 minutes at 180°C. The hot air oven must not be opened till the temperature inside has not fallen below 60°C to prevent breakage of glassware.

Moist heat

Steam sterilization: Amongst the available methods for sterilization, moist heat in the form of saturated steam under pressure is the most widely used and the most dependable as it is a nontoxic, inexpensive system requiring relatively shorter sterilization time (Fig. 5). It is recommended that all equipments which can withstand the effects of temperature should be sterilized by steam sterilization.[64,65] Moist heat destroys microorganisms by the irreversible coagulation and denaturation of enzymes and structural proteins.

The basic principle of steam sterilization, as accomplished in an autoclave, is to expose each item to direct steam contact at the required temperature and pressure for the specified time. Thus, there are four parameters of steam sterilization: steam, pressure, temperature, and time.[66,67] Pressure serves as a means to obtain the high temperatures necessary to quickly kill microorganisms. Specific temperatures must be obtained to ensure the microbicidal activity. The two common steam sterilizing temperatures are 121°C and 132°C. Recognized minimum exposure periods for sterilization of wrapped healthcare supplies are 30 minutes at 121°C in a gravity displacement sterilizer or 4 minutes at 132°C in a prevacuum sterilizer. Sterilization time further varies depending on the type of item (e.g. metal versus rubber, plastic, items with lumens), whether the item is wrapped or unwrapped, and the kind of sterilizer.

Autoclaves: The different types of steam sterilizers (autoclaves) include:

- Simple "pressure cooker type" laboratory autoclave,
- Steam jacketed downward displacement laboratory autoclave
- High pressure prevacuum autoclave.

In the gravity displacement sterilizer, steam is admitted at the top or the sides of the sterilizing chamber and, because the steam is lighter than air, forces air out from the bottom of the chamber through the drain vent. The gravity displacement autoclaves are primarily used to process laboratory media, water, pharmaceutical products, regulated medical waste and nonporous articles whose surfaces have direct steam contact. The high-speed prevacuum sterilizers are similar to the gravity displacement sterilizers except they are fitted with a vacuum pump (or ejector) to ensure air removal from the sterilizing chamber and load before the steam is introduced. The advantage of using a vacuum pump is that there is nearly instantaneous steam penetration even into porous loads. The different cycle times to be followed are depicted in Table 2.

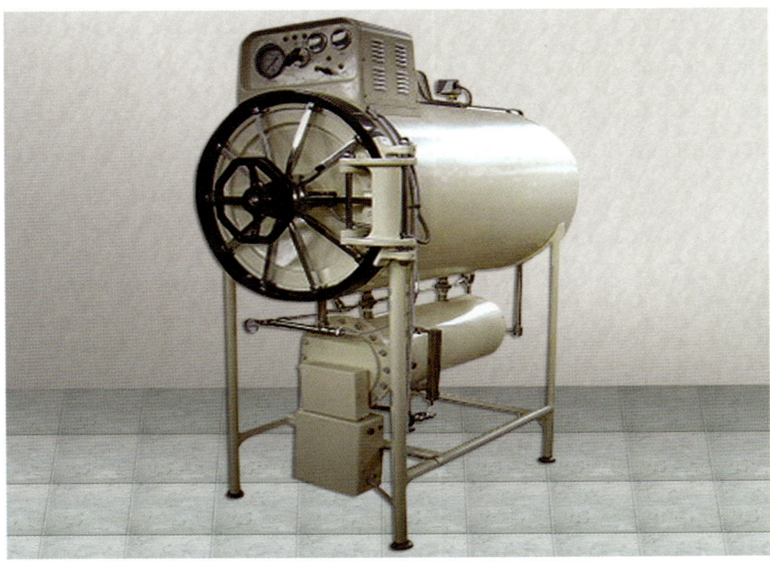

Fig. 5: Horizontal steam sterilizer.

Table 2: Minimum cycle times for steam sterilization cycles.

Type of sterilizer	*Item*	*Exposure time at 121°C*	*Exposure time at 132°C*	*Drying time*
Gravity displacement	Wrapped instruments	30 min	15 min	15–30 min
	Textile packs	30 min	25 min	15 min
	Wrapped utensils	30 min	15 min	15–30 min
Dynamic air removal (e.g. prevacuum)	Wrapped instruments		4 min	20–30 min
	Textile packs		4 min	5–20 min
	Wrapped utensils		4 min	20 min

Source: Modified from Association for the Advancement of Medical Instrumentation[66,67]

Flash sterilization: Flash sterilization is a modification of conventional steam sterilization (either gravity, prevacuum or steam flush pressure pulse) in which the item is placed in an open tray or is placed in a specially designed, covered, rigid container to allow for rapid penetration of steam. Typical sterilization temperatures and times are 132–135°C with 3–4 minutes exposure time for porous loads and instruments.[68,69] Flash sterilization has generally been used as a quick or last resort sterilization method when a unique instrument is urgently needed for a procedure or is dropped on the floor.

The autoclaving process needs periodic monitoring. Chemical indicators are incorporated regularly with autoclaving cycles. Single parameter chemical indicators indicate attainment of a certain temperature by a visible color change. Multiparameter chemical indicators called as integrators indicating temperature, pressure and time are also available. Biological indicators containing spores of *Geobacillus stearothermophilus* (formerly *Bacillus stearothermophilus*) need to be used periodically to substantiate the process of sterilization[10] especially in developing countries like India.[70]

Low Temperature Sterilization Technologies

Ethylene oxide (ETO) has been widely used as a low temperature sterilant since the 1950s. Alternative technologies to ETO with chlorofluorocarbon that are currently available include 100% ETO. ETO with a different stabilizing gas such as carbon dioxide or hydro chlorofluorocarbons (HCFC); immersion in peracetic acid, hydrogen peroxide gas plasma and ozone.

Ethylene oxide: It is a colorless gas that is flammable and explosive. Essential parameters for ETO sterilization are: adequate gas concentration, proper temperature between 37°C and 63°C, relative humidity of 40–80% and correct exposure time.[71] It has been the most commonly used process for sterilizing temperature and moisture sensitive medical devices. Two types of ETO sterilizers are available, mixed gas and 100% ETO. Ethylene oxide cycles are lengthy, costly, and potentially hazardous to patients and staff. The big advantage is that it can sterilize heat or moisture sensitive medical equipment without deleterious effects. ETO is a potential human carcinogen.[72] The mode of action of ETO is considered to be by alkylation of protein, DNA and RNA. ETO inactivates all microorganisms including bacterial spores.

The basic ETO sterilization cycle consists of five stages: preconditioning and humidification, gas introduction, exposure, evacuation, and air washes and takes approximately 2½ hours excluding aeration time. Mechanical aeration for 8–12 hours at 50–60°C allows desorption of the toxic ETO residual contained in exposed absorbent materials. Most modern ETO sterilizers combine sterilization and aeration in the same chamber as a continuous process. ETO is absorbed by many materials. For this reason, following sterilization, the item must undergo aeration to remove residual ETO.

Ethylene oxide is highly useful to sterilize critical items and sometimes semi-critical items which are moisture or heat sensitive and cannot be sterilized by steam sterilization.

Hydrogen peroxide gas plasma: Gas plasmas are generated in an enclosed chamber under deep vacuum using radiofrequency or microwave energy to excite the gas molecules and produce charged particles, many of which are in the form of free radicals. The free radicals interact with essential cell components (e.g. enzymes, nucleic acids) and thereby disrupt the metabolism of microorganisms.

This process has the ability to inactivate a broad range of microorganisms, including resistant bacterial spores. Materials and devices that cannot tolerate high temperatures and humidity, such as some plastics, electrical devices, and corrosion-susceptible metal alloys, can be sterilized by hydrogen peroxide gas plasma.[73,74]

Peracetic acid sterilization: Peracetic acid is a unique cidal agent which has the ability to maintain its efficacy in the presence of organic matter.[75,76] Peracetic acid, a 35% liquid solution is thought to function by denaturing proteins, disrupting cell wall permeability, and oxidizing sulfhydryl and sulfur bonds in proteins.[55]

Other Sterilization Methods

Ionizing radiation: Sterilization by ionizing radiation, primarily by cobalt 60 gamma rays or electron accelerators, is a low temperature sterilization method that has been used for a number of medical products (e.g. tissue for transplantation, pharmaceuticals, medical devices).

The method is suitable for large scale sterilization because of high sterilization costs and is not suitable for healthcare facilities.

Liquid chemical sterilants: Sterilization processes based on liquid chemical sterilants have been used as pointed earlier, but in general, do not convey the same sterility assurance level as sterilization achieved using thermal or physical methods. The use of liquids as sterilants is restricted to reprocessing critical devices that are heat sensitive and incompatible with other sterilization methods.

Filtration: Filtration does not kill microbes, it separates them out. Membrane filters with pore size between 0.2 µm and 0.45 µm are commonly used to remove particles from solutions or liquids which are heat labile like serum, antibiotic solutions, sugar solution or urea solution. Filtration is aided by using vacuum pumps.

Air filters: Air can be filtered using HEPA (high-efficiency particle air) filters. They are usually used in biological safety cabinets, modern operation theaters, positive pressure and negative pressure rooms. High efficiency particle air filters deliver air with a filtering efficacy of 99.97% for particle size of 0.3 µm diameter. The HEPA filters need frequent monitoring by particle counters or similar tests.

Vaporized hydrogen peroxide: Hydrogen peroxide solutions have been in use as chemical sterilants for many years. It is environmentally safe, compatible with all materials and relative ease of operation, installation and monitoring. Few limitations are that cellulose cannot be processed; nylon becomes brittle; and penetration capabilities are less than those of ETO.[77,78]

Ozone: Ozone has been used for years as a drinking water disinfectant. Ozone is produced when O_2 is energized which then split into two monatomic (O_1) molecules. The monatomic oxygen molecules then collide with O_2 molecules to form ozone, which is O_3. Thus, ozone consists of O_2 with a loosely bonded third oxygen atom that is readily available to attach to, and oxidize, other molecules. This additional oxygen atom makes ozone a powerful oxidant that destroys microorganisms but is highly unstable.

Formaldehyde steam: Low temperature steam with formaldehyde is used as a low temperature sterilization method in many European countries. It has certain advantages; the cycle time for formaldehyde gas is faster than that for ETO and the cost per cycle is relatively low. However, ETO is more penetrating and operates at lower temperatures than do steam/formaldehyde sterilizers.

Sterilization Cycle Verification

The efficacy of the sterilization process is measured by the sterility assurance level (SAL) of a product and is defined as the probability of a single viable microorganism persisting on a product after sterilization.[79,80] In short, SAL is an estimate of lethality of the entire sterilization process.

The sterilization procedure should be monitored at different intervals; routinely, on installation, and after repairs by using a combination of mechanical, chemical, and biological indicators to evaluate the sterilizing conditions and indirectly the microbiologic status of the processed items.[66,67,71,81] The mechanical monitors for steam sterilization include the daily assessment of cycle time and temperature by examining the temperature record chart and an assessment of pressure via the pressure gauge. The mechanical monitors for ETO include time, temperature, and pressure records.[71]

Both biological and chemical indicators can be used for verification. Chemical indicators are convenient, are inexpensive. Biological indicator, on the other hand, can measure the microbial killing power of the sterilization process.[82] Chemical indicators are affixed on the outside of each pack to show that the package has been processed through a sterilization cycle, but these indicators do not prove sterilization has been achieved. Chemical indicators usually are either heat- or chemical-sensitive inks that change color when one or more sterilization parameters is achieved. If the internal and/or external indicator suggests inadequate processing, the item should not be used.[83]

Biological indicators are recognized by most authorities as being closest to the ideal monitors of the sterilization process[84,85] because they measure the sterilization process directly by using the most resistant microorganisms (*Bacillus* spores), and not by merely testing the physical and chemical conditions necessary for sterilization. Since the *Bacillus* spores used in biological indicators are more resistant and present in greater numbers than are the common microbial contaminants found on patient care equipment, the demonstration that the biological indicator has been inactivated strongly implies that other potential pathogens in the load have been killed.[86] Steam and low temperature sterilizers (e.g. hydrogen peroxide gas plasma, peracetic acid) should be monitored at least weekly with the appropriate commercial preparation of spores. If a sterilizer is used frequently (e.g. several loads per day), daily use of biological indicators allows earlier discovery of equipment malfunctions or procedural errors and thus minimizes the extent of patient surveillance and product recall needed in the event of a positive biological indicator.[81] Each load should be monitored if it contains implantable objects. If feasible, implantable items should not be used until the results of spore tests are known to be negative.

High-Level Disinfection of Dermatosurgical Operation Theaters

This has been dealt in more detail in the chapter on dermatosurgical theater and only relevant details are mentioned here. A dermatosurgical operation theater should adhere to the definition of a clean room which is defined as; a room in which the concentration of airborne particles is controlled, and which is constructed and used in a manner to minimize the introduction, generation, and retention of particles inside the room and in which other relevant parameters, e.g. temperature, humidity, and pressure, are controlled as necessary. As per available guidelines[87] the ventilation requirements for operating rooms should have an outward air movement in relation to the adjacent area, a minimum of 15 total air changes per hour, a relative humidity of 30–60% and a design temperature of 20–23°C. The use of laminar air flow systems is advised in operation theaters, but their value has not been fully documented for all types of theaters.[88]

Most of the operation theaters continue to use aldehydes for high-level disinfection of the theater environment. It has been observed that there is a general relationship between aerobic bacterial count and risk of infection. There is a significant risk of infection with counts in the range of 700–1,800 bacteria carrying particle (BCP) per cubic meter. However, the risk is slight when the BCP load is less than 180 per cubic meter.[89] Formaldehyde is the commonly used agent either as a gas utilizing potassium permanganate or as dispersed by a sprayer like device. Other agents used as high-level disinfectants essentially through a fogger are hydrogen peroxide, hydrogen peroxide along with silver nitrate, peracetic acid and other chemical compounds of aldehydes. The inanimate surfaces in the operation theater need proper periodic cleaning and disinfection. Grossly contaminated surfaces could be potential source of hospital-acquired infections. The operation theater should be thoroughly washed with water and detergent mixture so as to rid of all spills and proteinaceous materials before a disinfectant is used for mopping the surfaces.

Air Conditioning Units

Opportunistic fungi like *Aspergillus, Rhizopus, Fusarium* and *Penicillium* are capable of proliferating in air conditioning (AC) units. The filters utilized in these units can act as a suitable nidus for growth and proliferation of the pathogenic fungi, the spores of which can be discharged and carried through the theater air. Presence of fungi in AC units and subsequent dispersal of spores could be a potential hazard, especially for the immunocompromised patients. The operating room and clinic AC units should be meticulously maintained and frequently monitored to minimize the chances of growth and proliferation of potentially pathogenic fungi. Split AC units appear to be a safer option than the window mounted AC units.[90]

Staphylococcus aureus and β-hemolytic *Streptococci* are important healthcare associated pathogens and can persist in the environment. They can be shed and infections can occur when healthcare personnel are heavily colonized with these organisms. *S. aureus* and β-hemolytic *Streptococci* have been linked to airborne transmission in operation theaters, burn units, and neonatal units.[91,92] Proper surveillance of the AC units, the disinfectants used, and the personnel working in the operation theater need to be carried out periodically. Periodic and regular screening, and treatment of shedders, and barring them from entering operation theater till the treatment is completed is necessary to minimize the risk of transmission of infections.[5]

The dermatological procedures routinely carried out in clinics and hospitals along with the recommended disinfection/sterilization methods advocated are summarized in Table. 3.[93]

CONCLUSION

Disinfection and sterilization are very important concepts in ensuring safe surgery. World Health Organization has recently commenced a "safe surgery" initiative to help reduce risks involved in surgeries around the world by adhering to proven standards of care. WHO advocates use of a "Surgical Safety Checklist" prior to operative procedure. That the use of checklists significantly reduces the surgical morbidity and mortality has been documented after pilot studies conducted by WHO. The check list (Table 4) is available for downloading at following web address: http://whqlibdoc.who.int/publications/2009/9789241598590_eng_ Checklist.pdf

Table 3: Dermatological equipment requiring disinfection/sterilization.

Name of procedure	*Instruments used*	*Recommended disinfection/sterilization method*
Skin grafting for vitiligo	Stainless punches, disposable punches venesection tray with artery forceps, blades, forceps, scissors	Autoclaving Not to be reused ETO sterilization Autoclaving
Hair transplant	Needles, forceps, cutting boards, blades, plastic blade holders, BP handle artery forceps, Adson's forceps needle holder, plastic bottles for spraying saline	All heat stable material to be autoclaved. Heat labile material ETO sterilization or prolonged exposure to chemical disinfectant like glutaraldehyde, orthophthalaldehyde
Chemical peels	Brushes to apply chemicals on face from the bottle	ETO
Laser	Metal spacers, interchangeable hand pieces of metal or plastic, dedicated goggles	All heat stable material to be autoclaved. Heat labile material ETO sterilization or prolonged exposure to chemical disinfectant like glutaraldehyde, orthophthalaldehyde

Table 4: Surgical safety checklist.

Surgical Safety Checklist

World Health Organization | Patient Safety — A World Alliance for Safer Health Care

Before induction of anaesthesia	Before skin incision	Before patient leaves operating room
(with at least nurse and anaesthetist)	(with nurse, anaesthetist and surgeon)	(with nurse, anaesthetist and surgeon)
Has the patient confirmed his/her identity, site, procedure, and consent? ☐ Yes	☐ **Confirm all team members have introduced themselves by name and role.**	**Nurse Verbally Confirms:** ☐ The name of the procedure ☐ Completion of instrument, sponge and needle counts ☐ Specimen labelling (read specimen labels aloud, including patient name) ☐ Whether there are any equipment problems to be addressed
Is the site marked? ☐ Yes ☐ Not applicable	☐ **Confirm the patient's name, procedure, and where the incision will be made.**	**To Surgeon, Anaesthetist and Nurse:** ☐ What are the key concerns for recovery and management of this patient?
Is the anaesthesia machine and medication check complete? ☐ Yes	**Has antibiotic prophylaxis been given within the last 60 minutes?** ☐ Yes ☐ Not applicable	
Is the pulse oximeter on the patient and functioning? ☐ Yes	**Anticipated Critical Events** **To Surgeon:** ☐ What are the critical or non-routine steps? ☐ How long will the case take? ☐ What is the anticipated blood loss? **To Anaesthetist:** ☐ Are there any patient-specific concerns? **To Nursing Team:** ☐ Has sterility (including indicator results) been confirmed? ☐ Are there equipment issues or any concerns?	
Does the patient have a: **Known allergy?** ☐ No ☐ Yes **Difficult airway or aspiration risk?** ☐ No ☐ Yes, and equipment/assistance available **Risk of >500ml blood loss (7ml/kg in children)?** ☐ No ☐ Yes, and two IVs/central access and fluids planned	**Is essential imaging displayed?** ☐ Yes ☐ Not applicable	

This checklist is not intended to be comprehensive. Additions and modifications to fit local practice are encouraged.

Revised 1 / 2009

Source: http://whqlibdoc.who.int/publications/2009/ 9789241598590_eng_ Checklist.pdf

REFERENCES

1. Amici JM, Roques AM, Lasheras A, et al. A prospective study of the incidence of complications associated with dermatological surgery. Br J Dermatol. 2005;153:967-71.
2. Chan BC, Patel DC. Perioperative management and the associated rate of adverse events in dermatological procedures performed by dermatologists in New Zealand. Australas J Dermatol. 2009;50:23-8.
3. Salanitri S, Gonçalves A, Helene A, et al. Surgical complications in hair transplantation: a series of 533 procedures. Aesthet Surg J. 2009;29:72-6.
4. Ram J, Kaushik S, Brar GS, et al. Prevention of postoperative infections in ophthalmic Surgery. Indian J Ophthalmol. 2001;49:59-69.
5. Kelkar U, Kelkar S, Bal AM, et al. Microbiological evaluation of various parameters in ophthalmic operating rooms. The need to establish guidelines. Indian J Ophthalmol. 2003;51:171-6.
6. Spaulding EH. Chemical disinfection of medical and surgical materials. In: Lawrence C, Block SS (Eds). Disinfection, Sterilization, and Preservation. Philadelphia: Lea & Fibiger; 1968.pp.517-31.
7. Price PB. Bacteriology of normal skin: a new quantitative test applied to a study of the bacterial flora and the disinfectant action of mechanical cleansing. J Infect Dis. 1938;63:301-18.
8. Sprunt K, Redman W, Leidy G. Antibacterial effectiveness of routine hand washing. Pediatrics. 1973;52:264-71.
9. Favero MS, Bond WW. Chemical disinfection of medical and surgical materials. In: Block SS (Ed). Disinfection, Sterilization, and Preservation. Philadelphia: Lippincott Williams & Wilkins; 2001.pp.881-917.
10. Bean HS. Types and characteristics of disinfectants. J Appl Bacteriol. 1967;30:616.
11. Russell AD, Hugo WB, Ayliffe GAJ. Principles and Practice of Disinfection, Preservation and Sterilization. England, Oxford: Blackwell Scientific Publications; 1999.
12. Russell AD. Factors influencing the efficacy of germicides. In: Rutala WA (Ed). Disinfection, Sterilization and Antisepsis: Principles, Practices, Challenges, and New Research. Washington, DC: Association for Professionals in Infection Control and Epidemiology; 2004.pp.162-70.
13. Russell AD, Russell NJ. Biocides: activity, action and resistance. In: Hunter PA, Darby GK, Russell NJ (Eds). Fifty Years of Antimicrobials: Past Perspectives and Future Trends. England: Cambridge University Press; 1995.pp.327-65.

14. Russell AD. Plasmids and bacterial resistance to biocides. J Appl Microbiol. 1997;83:155-65.
15. Gebel J, Sonntag HG, Werner HP, et al. The higher disinfectant resistance of nosocomial isolates of Klebsiella oxytoca: how reliable are indicator organisms in disinfectant testing? J Hosp Infect. 2002;50:309-11.
16. Favero MS, Petersen NJ, Carson LA, et al. Gram-negative water bacteria in hemodialysis systems. Health Lab Sci. 1975;12:321-34.
17. Rutala WA, Cole EC. Ineffectiveness of hospital disinfectants against bacteria: a collaborative study. Infect Control. 1987;8:501-6.
18. Russell AD, McDonnell G. Concentration: a major factor in studying biocidal action. J Hosp Infect. 2000;44(1):1-3.
19. Russell AD. Factors influencing the efficacy of germicides. In: Rutala WA (Ed). Disinfection, Sterilization and Antisepsis: Principles, Practices, Challenges, and New Research. Washington, DC: Association for Professionals in Infection Control and Epidemiology; 2004.pp.162-70.
20. Russell AD. Factors influencing the efficacy of antimicrobial agents. In: Russell AD, Hugo WB, Ayliffe GAJ (Eds). Principles and Practice of Disinfection, Preservation and Sterilization. Oxford: Blackwell Science; 1999.pp.951-1023.
21. Rutala WA. Selection and use of disinfectants in health care. In: Mayhall CG (Ed). Hospital Epidemiology and Infection Control, 2nd edition. Philadelphia: Lippincott Williams &Wilkins; 1999.pp.1161-87.
22. Lewis DL, Arens M. Resistance of micro-organisms to disinfection in dental and medical devices. Nat Med. 1995;1: 956-8.
23. Jacobs P. Cleaning: principles, methods and benefits. In: Rutala WA (Ed). Disinfection, Sterilization, and Antisepsis in Health Care. NewYork, Champlain: Polyscience Publications; 1998.pp.165-81.
24. Reichert M. Preparation of supplies for terminal sterilization. In: Reichert M, Young JH (Eds). Sterilization Technology for the Health Care Facility. Gaithersburg: Aspen Publication; 1997.pp.36-50.
25. Jatzwauk L, Schone H, Pietsch H. How to improve instrument disinfection by ultrasound. J Hosp Infect. 2001;48:S80-3.
26. Schultz JK. Decontamination alternative. Infect Control Hosp Epidemiol. 1990;11:8-9.
27. Roberts CG. Studies on the bioburden on medical devices and the importance of cleaning. In: Rutala WA (Ed). Disinfection, Sterilization and Antisepsis: Principles and Practices in Healthcare Facilities. Washington, DC: Association for professional in infection control and epidemiology; 2001.pp.63-9.
28. Hutchisson B, LeBlanc C. The truth and consequences of enzymatic detergents. Gastroenterol Nurs. 2005;28:372-6.
29. Dancer SJ. How do we assess hospital cleaning? A proposal for microbiological standards for surface hygiene in hospitals. J Hosp Infect. 2004;56:10-5.
30. AliY, Dolan MJ, Fendler EJ, et al. Alcohols. In: Block SS (Ed). Disinfection, Sterilization, and Preservation. Philadelphia: Lippincott Williams & Wilkins; 2001.pp.229-54.
31. Tyler R, Ayliffe GA, Bradley C. Virucidal activity of disinfectants: studies with the poliovirus. J Hosp Infect. 1990; 15:339-45.
32. Bond WW, Favero MS, Petersen NJ, et al. Inactivation of hepatitis B virus by intermediate-to-high-level disinfectant chemicals. J Clin Microbiol. 1983;18:535-8.
33. Tyler R, Ayliffe GA. A surface test for virucidal activity of disinfectants: preliminary study with herpes virus. J Hosp Infect. 1987;9:22-9.
34. Martin LS, McDougal JS, Loskoski SL. Disinfection and inactivation of the human T-lymphotropic virus type III/ Lymphadenopathy-associated virus. J Infect Dis. 1985;152: 400-3.
35. Spaulding EH. Alcohol as a surgical disinfectant. AORNJ. 1964;2:67-71.
36. Rutala WA, Weber DJ. Uses of inorganic hypochlorite (bleach) in healthcare facilities. Clin Microbiol Rev. 1997;10:597-610.
37. Merritt K, Hitchins VM, Brown SA. Safety and cleaning of medical materials and devices. J Biomed Mater Res. 2000;53:131-6.
38. Hoy RH. Accidental systemic exposure to sodium hypochlorite (Clorox) during hemodialysis. Am J Hosp Pharm. 1981;38:1512-4.
39. Weber DJ, Rutala WA. Occupational risks associated with the use of selected disinfectants and sterilants. In: Rutala WA (Ed). Disinfection, Sterilization, and Antisepsis in Health Care. New York, Champlain: Polyscience Publications; 1998. pp.211-26.
40. Reisz GR, Gammon RS. Toxic pneumonitis from mixing household cleaners. Chest. 1986;89:49-52.
41. Hoffman PN, Death JE, Coates D. The stability of sodium hypochlorite solutions. In: Collins CH, Allwood MC, Bloomfield SF, FoxA (Eds). Disinfectants: Their use and Evaluation of Effectiveness. London: Academic Press; 1981. pp.77-83.
42. Griffiths PA, Babb JR, Fraise AP. Mycobactericidal activity of selected disinfectants using a quantitative suspension test. J Hosp Infect. 1999;41:111-21.
43. Bloomfield SF, Miller EA. A comparison of hypochlorite and phenolic disinfectants for disinfection of clean and soiled surfaces and blood spillages. J Hosp Infect. 1989;13:231-9.
44. Chitnis V, Chitnis S, Patil S, et al. Practical limitations of disinfection of body fluid spills with 10,000 ppm sodium hypochlorite (NaOCl). Am J Infect Control. 2004;32:306-8.
45. Selkon JB, Babb JR, Morris R. Evaluation of the antimicrobial activity of a new super-oxidized water, Sterilox®, for the disinfection of endoscopes. J Hosp Infect. 1999;41: 59-70.
46. Occupational Health and Safety Administration. OSHA Fact Sheet: Formaldehyde: Occupational Safety and Health Administration, US Department of Labor; 2002.
47. Scott EM, Gorman SP. Glutaraldehyde. In: Block SS (Ed). Disinfection, Sterilization, and Preservation. Philadelphia: Lippincott Williams & Wilkins; 2001.pp.361-81.
48. Masferrer R, Marquez R. Comparison of two activated glutaraldehyde solutions: Cidex Solution and Sonacide. Respir Care. 1977;22:257-62.
49. Cooke RPD, Goddard SV, Whymant Morris A, Sherwood J, Chatterly R. An evaluation of Cidex OPA (0.55% orthophthalaldehyde) as an alternative to 2% glutaraldehyde for high-level disinfection of endoscopes. J Hosp Infect. 2003; 54:226-31.

50. Rutala WA, Weber DJ. Disinfection of endoscopes: review of new chemical sterilants used for high level disinfection. Infect Control Hosp Epidemiol. 1999;20:69-76.
51. Sattar SA, Taylor YE, Paquette M, et al. In-hospital evaluation of 7.5% hydrogen peroxide as a disinfectant for flexible endoscopes. Can J Infect Control. 1996;11:51-4.
52. Hobson DW, Seal LA. Evaluation of a novel, rapid acting, sterilizing solution at room temperature. Am J Infect Control. 2000;28:370-5.
53. Gottardi W. Iodine and iodine compounds. In: Block SS (Ed). Disinfection, Sterilization, and Preservation. Philadelphia: Lea & Febiger; 1991.pp.152-66.
54. Chang SL. Modern concept of disinfection. J Sanit Eng Div Proc Am Soc Civ Eng. 1971:689-705.
55. Block SS. Peroxygen compounds. In: Block SS (Ed). Disinfection, Sterilization, and Preservation. Philadelphia: Lippincott Williams & Wilkins; 2001.pp.185-204.
56. Prindle RF. Phenolic compounds. In: Block SS (Ed). Disinfection, Sterilization, and Preservation. Philadelphia: Lea & Febiger; 1983.pp.197-224.
57. Merianos JJ. Surface active agents. In: Block SS (Ed). Disinfection, Sterilization, and Preservation. Philadelphia: Lippincott Williams & Wilkins; 2001.pp.283-320.
58. Hamouda T, Hayes MM, Cao ZH, et al. A novel surfactant nanoemulsions with broad spectrum sporicidal activity against Bacillus species. J Infect Dis. 1999;180:1939-49.
59. Weber DJ, Rutala WA. Use of metals and microbicides in the prevention of nosocomial infections. In: Rutala W (Ed). Disinfection, Sterilization, and Antisepsis in Health Care. Champlain, New York: Polyscience Publications; 1995. pp.271-85.
60. Noyce JO, Michels H, Keevil CW. Potential use of copper surfaces to reduce survival of epidemic methicillin resistant. *Staphylococcus aureus* in the healthcare environment. J Hosp Infect. 2006;63:289-97.
61. Russell AD. Ultraviolet radiation. In: Russell AD, Hugo WB, Ayliffe GAJ (Eds). Principles and Practices of Disinfection, Preservation and Sterilization. Oxford: Blackwell Science; 1999.pp.688-702.
62. Garner JS, Favero MS. CDC Guideline for hand washing and hospital environmental control, 1985. Infect Control. 1986; 7:231-43.
63. Rutala WA. Disinfection, sterilization and waste disposal. In: Wenzel RP (Ed). Prevention and Control of Nosocomial Infections. Baltimore: Williams and Wilkins; 1997.pp.539-93.
64. Joslyn L. Sterilization by heat. In: Block SS (Ed). Disinfection, Sterilization, and Preservation. Philadelphia: Lippincott Williams & Wilkins; 2001.pp.695-728.
65. Bucx MJ, Veldman DJ, Beenhakker MM, et al. The effect of steam sterilization at 134 degrees C on light intensity provided by fibre light into laryngoscopes. Anaesthesia. 1999;54: 875-8.
66. Association for the Advancement of Medical Instrumentation. Steam sterilization and sterility assurance in health care facilities. ANSI/AAMI ST46. Arlington, VA, ANSI/AAMIST46, 2002.
67. Association for the Advancement of Medical Instrumentation. Comprehensive guide to steam sterilization and sterility assurance in healthcare facilities, ANSI/AAMIST79, 2006.
68. Joslyn L. Sterilization by heat. In: Block SS (Ed). Disinfection, Sterilization, and Preservation. Philadelphia: Lippincott Williams & Wilkins; 2001.pp.695-728.
69. Crow S. Steam sterilizers: an evolution in design. Infect Control Hosp Epidemiol. 1993;14:488-90.
70. Kelkar U, Bal AM, Kulkarni S. Monitoring of steam sterilization process by biological indicators a necessary surveillance tool for developing countries. Am J Infect Control. 2004;32:512-3.
71. Association for the Advancement of Medical Instrumentation. (1999) Ethylene oxide sterilization in healthcare facilities: Safety and effectiveness. AAMI, Arlington: VA; 1999.
72. National Toxicology Program. http://ntpserver.niehs.nih.gov/.
73. Timm D, Gonzales D. Effect of sterilization on microstructure and function of microsurgical scissors. Surg Serv Management. 1997;3:479.
74. Feldman LA, Hui HK. Compatibility of medical devices and materials with low temperature hydrogen peroxide gas plasma. Med Dev Diag Indust. 1997;19:57-62.
75. Malchesky PS. Medical applications of peracetic acid. In: Block SS (Ed). Disinfection, Sterilization, and Preservation. Philadelphia: Lippincott Williams & Wilkins; 2001.pp.979-96.
76. Bradley CR, Babb JR, Ayliffe GA. Evaluation of the Steris System 1. Peracetic acid endoscope processor. J Hosp Infect. 1995;29:143-51.
77. French GL, Otter JA, Shannon KP, et al. Tackling contamination of the hospital environment by methicillin resistant Staphylococcus aureus (MRSA): a comparison between conventional terminal cleaning and hydrogen peroxide vapour decontamination. J Hosp Infect. 2004;57:31-7.
78. Boyce JM, Havill NL, Otter JA, et al. Impact of hydrogen peroxide vapor room bio decontamination on environmental contamination and nosocomial transmission of Clostridium difficile. The Society of Healthcare Epidemiology of America. 2006;155:109.
79. Favero MS. Sterility assurance: concepts for patient safety. In: Rutala WA (Ed). Disinfection, Sterilization and Antisepsis: Principles and Practices in Healthcare Facilities. Washington, DC: Association for Professional in Infection Control and Epidemiology; 2001.pp.110-9.
80. Oxborrow GS, Berube R. Sterility testing validation of sterilization processes, and sporicide testing. In: Block SS (Ed). Disinfection, Sterilization, and Preservation. Philadelphia: Lea & Febiger; 1991.pp.1047-57.
81. Association for the advancement of medical instrumentation. Good hospital practice: steam sterilization and sterility assurance. AAMI, Arlington: VA; 1993.
82. Rutala WA, Gergen MF, Weber DJ. Evaluation of a rapid readout biological indicator for flash sterilization with three biological indicators and three chemical indicators. Infect Control Hosp Epidemiol. 1993;14:390-4.
83. Association of Operating Room Nurses. Recommended practices for sterilization in perioperative practice settings. Standards, Recommended Practices, and Guidelines. Denver, CO: AORN, 2000.pp.347-58.
84. Schneider PM, Reich RR, Kirckof SS, et al. Performance of various steam sterilization indicators under optimum and suboptimum exposure conditions. In: Rutala WA (Ed).

Disinfection, Sterilization and Antisepsis: Principles, Practices, Challenges, and New Research. Washington, DC: Association for Professionals in Infection Control and Epidemiology; 2004.pp.200-23.

85. Greene VW. Control of sterilization process. In: Russell AD, Hugo WB, Ayliffe GAJ (Eds). Principles and Practice of Disinfection, Preservation and Sterilization. Oxford, England: Blackwell Scientific Publications; 1992.pp.605-24.
86. Maki DG, Hassemer CA. Flash sterilization: carefully measured haste. Infect Control. 1987;8:307-10.
87. Simmons BP. Guideline for hospital environmental control. Atlanta GA: US Department of Health and Human Services, Public Health Service, Centers for Disease Control; 1981.
88. Centers for Disease Control and Prevention, Health care infection control practices advisory committee. Draft guideline for environmental infection control in healthcare facilities, Appendix G; 2001.p.197.
89. World Health Organization. Hospital acquired infections: guidelines to laboratory methods. WHO Regional Publications European Series No.4. Copenhagen; 1978. pp.28-33.
90. Kelkar U, Bal AM, Kulkarni S. Fungal contamination of air conditioning units in operating theaters in India. J Hosp Infect. 2005;60:81-4.
91. Wenzel RP, Veazey JM, Townsend TR. Role of inanimate environment in hospital acquired infections. In: Cundy KR, Ball W (Eds). Infection Control in Healthcare Facilities: Microbiological Surveillance. Baltimore: University Park Press; 1977.pp.71-98.
92. Mortimer EA, Wolinsky E, Gonzaga AJ, et al. Role of airborne transmission in staphylococcal infections. Br Med J. 1966;1:319-22.
93. Patwardhan N, Kelkar U. Disinfection,sterilization and operation theater guidelines for dermatological practitioners in India. Indian J Dermatol Venereol Leprol. 2011;77:83-93.

Chapter

12

Local Anesthesia

KC Nischal

Key Messages

- Most dermatosurgeries are performed under local anesthesia.
- A dermatosurgeon needs to be familiar with various forms of administration of local anesthesia.
- Life-threatening hypersensitivity reactions and systemic toxicity can happen with local anesthetics.
- Topical anesthesia is a useful technique for many minor dermatologic surgeries in adult and pediatric patients as well as pregnant and nursing mothers.

INTRODUCTION

Local anesthesia is analgesia restricted to particular area or field of interest without causing any impairment of consciousness and cognizance. Most of the procedures done by dermatosurgeons are performed on outpatient or day care basis and hence, local anesthesia has been the preferred mode of achieving anesthesia. Though considered safe, the agents used in local anesthesia may rarely cause various systemic side effects with significant morbidity and mortality. The techniques of local anesthesia have expanded to include tumescent anesthesia, which has allowed dermatosurgeons to perform such surgeries as liposuction under local anesthesia. Hence it is important for dermatologists and dermatosurgeons to be aware of these molecules and the different local anesthetic techniques.

HISTORY

Cocaine was the first local anesthetic agent to be isolated by Albert Niemann in 1860. However, it was Carl Köller of Vienna, who pioneered its use in topical anesthesia by introducing it in his ophthalmology practice in 1884. Later on, Halstead innovated its use in infiltrative anesthesia and nerve blocks. Procaine was the first synthetic local anesthetic to be synthesized in 1905 by Alfred Einhorn, a German chemist. Lidocaine, the most popular local anesthetic was synthesized in 1943 by Nils Löfgren, a Swedish chemist. Bupivacaine and prilocaine were introduced later in 1957 and 1959 respectively. As the first local anesthetic cocaine, was a natural alkaloid, all local anesthetic agents were designated with names ending with *caine*.[1-3]

PHARMACOLOGY

Chemical Structure

Local anesthetic agent (LAA) consists of a hydrophobic aromatic ring, an intermediate chain and a hydrophilic tertiary or secondary amine moiety (Fig. 1). Potency, duration of action and thereof, toxicity of local anesthetics is directly proportional to the hydrophobicity of the agent. Local anesthetic agent is classified as an ester (-COO-) or amide (-NH-) based on the intermediate linker. Esters include cocaine, procaine (prototype), chloroprocaine, benzocaine, tetracaine and amides are lidocaine (*prototype*), prilocaine, bupivacaine, mepivacaine, ropivacaine. However, there are local anesthetics which are ketone (dyclonine),[4] amidine, ether (pramoxine) intermediate chain or phenetidine derivatives (phenacaine).

Mechanism of Action

When the nerve is stimulated, the sodium channels open and there is influx of positively charged Na^+ ions changing the negatively charged internal milieu to a positively charged milieu leading to depolarization of membrane.

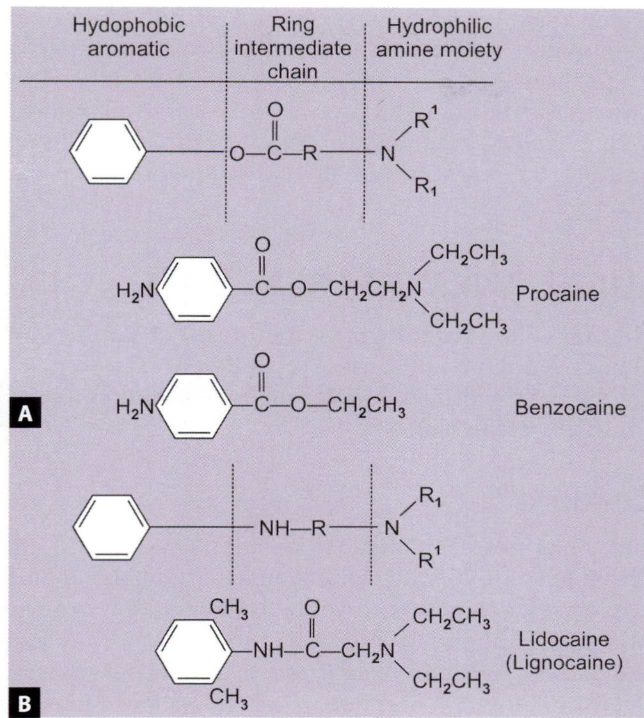

Fig. 1: Structure of ester (A. prototype procaine) and amide (B. prototype lidocaine) local anesthetic agents. Benzocaine is an ester without amine chain.

This generates the action potential which is responsible for nerve impulse generation and conduction. LAA inhibits nerve conduction by blocking these sodium channels. Two theories have been put forth to explain this blockage. Local anesthetic agent either gets incorporated into the nerve membrane thereby compressing the Na^+ channels laterally and blocking the passage of ions or cause conformational changes in the Na^+ channels (*membrane expansion theory*); these LAA may also bind to specific sites in or around Na^+ channels and impede ion flow by plugging the channel (*specific receptor theory*).[3] LAAs have also been observed to bind to potassium channels but at higher concentrations and hence, this action is not of relevance.[5]

Sodium channel is made up of α (contains four homologous domains, I–IV) and β (β1–β4) subunits. The binding site for LAA is located intracellularly and made up of the S6 segments of α, I, III and IV. This site is supposed to be hydrophobic and hence, hydrophobic LAA are more avidly bound to receptor leading to greater potency, longer duration of action and higher toxicity.[5] As the receptor site is intracellular, LAA have to transgress the cell membrane and this is more efficient in its unionized form. However, they bind better with receptor site in ionized form (cationic). Therefore, local anesthetic effects are better in an alkaline pH (less ionized forms, more transcellular migration) than in an acidic pH. Any inflammation makes the local environment more acidic and hence, the potency of LAA decreases locally.[6]

FACTORS INFLUENCING THE POTENCY OF LOCAL ANESTHETIC AGENTS

Chemical Properties of Local Anesthetic Agents

Hydrophobicity has been considered the prime determinant of potency of a LAA. Increasing the size of alkyl substituents increases the hydrophobicity. Receptor site for LAA is intracellular and hence LAA have to transgress cell membrane before it can act. Hence, hydrophobic agents which penetrate better should have better potency. But this is not true always clinically (in vitro, etidocaine is better than bupivacaine. But, in vivo, bupivacaine is more potent than etidocaine). This could be due to other factors influencing the availability of LAA at the action site like vasoconstriction (presence of vasoconstrictor increases local concentration and delayed clearance) or charge of the LAA.

Charge of Local Anesthetic Agents

In solution, LAA exists either as basic uncharged form or charged cationic form. The logarithm of hydrogen ion concentration at which, the concentration of basic form and the ionic form are equal is called as pKa value for that LAA (about 8.0–9.0 for LAA). In an acidic environment like in inflamed tissues, the protonated charged molecules are more than the basic forms. As the cell membrane penetration of charged molecules is poor than the basic forms, the efficacy of LAA decreases. However, there is no consistent increase in the rapidity of onset of action of LAA with increase in concentration of basic form of LAA (alkaline pH of solution increases the basic uncharged form).[7]

Local Vasculature

Vasoconstriction at the site of LAA administration leads to delayed local clearance, thus improving the depth and duration of local anesthesia. Also, higher dosages can be used without significant risk of systemic toxicity. This principle is used in tumescent anesthesia which is discussed later in detail. Cocaine is the only LAA with intrinsic potent vasoconstrictor effect. Hence, other agents need to be combined with vasoconstrictors like adrenaline (1:2,00,000), noradrenaline and phenylephrine to improve the efficacy of LAA. Lidocaine exhibits biphasic dose-dependent action on blood vessels. At lower concentrations as that achieved in plasma on intravenous infusion or nerve block, lidocaine causes vasoconstriction. Whereas at higher concentrations that is achieved during infiltration anesthesia, it causes vasodilatation.[8] On the contrary, in areas with rich vascularity or LAA without vasoconstrictors or intravenous administration of LAA, there is rapid clearance of LAA from the injected site and hence shorter duration of action.

Dosage of LAA

Increasing the dosage of LAA leads to improved anesthesia and reduced latency of action. Increase in the dosage can be either in the form of more quantity (large volume) or quality (higher concentration) of LAA. Larger volumes diffuse over larger areas and hence increase efficacy.[7] Conventionally, higher dosages are associated with higher side effects. However, this does not hold good always because, in tumescent anesthesia, higher dosages are used without risk of adverse effects.

Mixture of LAA

Lidocaine with dimethylsulfoxide produced better cutaneous anesthesia than eutectic mixture of local anesthetics (EMLA) during shock wave lithotripsy.[9] Combination of lidocaine, tetracaine and phenylephrine was better than benzocaine 20%.

Type of Nerve

Sodium channels are more concentrated at myelinated nerve fibers' nodes of Ranvier and evenly distributed throughout the axonal membrane of non-myelinated nerve fiber.[7] Hence, non-myelinated fibers are more susceptible to LAA than myelinated fibers.[1] Smaller fibers have shorter distance over which an electrical impulse can passively propagate and hence, thin nerves get blocked earlier than thick nerves. Hence, on decreasing trend, the order of blockade is autonomic fibers, C fibers, Aδ, Aβ, Aβ and Aα. Therefore after administration of LAA, clinically, pain is lost first, then temperature, touch, deep pressure, finally proprioception and motor functions.

Tachyphylaxis

Local anesthetic agent are usually acidic (pH 4–6) for better aqueous solubility.[2] On infiltration into tissues, due to tissue buffering, an optimal free base concentration is achieved which aids in driving the LAA into the axonal membrane. On repeated injections, the buffering capacity of the tissue reduces thereby causing local acidosis. This reduces the diffusion of LAA across the nerve membrane leading to decreased potency. Tissues with less buffering capacity like cerebrospinal fluid are more prone for this effect.

LOCAL ANESTHETIC AGENTS

Although the mechanism of action of all amide and ester LAA are the same, there are differences in some of their structure, property or function. Following is a brief discussion of the same:[1,5-7]

Cocaine

Cocaine causes sympathetic stimulation (both central and peripheral) by inhibiting norepinephrine reuptake leading to potent vasoconstriction, cardiotoxicity and CNS toxicity. Due to its euphoric actions, it has abuse propensity and hence fallen out from regular use. It has a rapid onset of action and duration of action up to 2 hours. In contrast to other esters, it is metabolized predominantly in liver rather by plasma cholinesterase enzymes.[7]

Procaine

Procaine is the prototype of ester LAA and was the first synthetic LAA. It readily metabolized by plasma pseudocholinesterase (Table 1). It is used for infiltrative anesthesia and nerve blocks. It is safe to be combined with epinephrine. Though it has low toxicity, its potency is also low and hence used only for infiltrative anesthesia.

Benzocaine

Benzocaine differs from other LAA in not having a basic hydrophilic amine side chain (*see* Fig. 1).[6] Benzocaine is a

Table 1: Pharmacological properties of common local anesthetics.

	Procaine	Prilocaine	Lidocaine	Tetracaine	Bupivacaine	Mepivacaine	Ropivacaine
Relative potency (Procaine = 1)	1	1.8	2	8	8	1.5	Same as bupivacaine at high doses, Less than bupivacaine at low doses
Onset of action	2–5 minutes	Longer than lidocaine	<2 minutes	5 minutes	5 minutes	3–5 minutes	–
Duration of action	20–30 minutes	30–90 minutes	30–60 minutes	120–180 minutes	120–240 minutes	45–90 minutes	120–240 minutes
Duration of action with adrenaline	30–45 minutes	120 minutes	120 minutes	–	180–240 minutes	120 minutes	180–240 minutes
Protein binding	60–80%	55%	60–80%	–	82–96%	60–85%	94%
Elimination t½ (in hours)	0.66	1.5	1.6	–	3.5	1.9	4.2

Contd...

Contd...

	Procaine	Prilocaine	Lidocaine	Tetracaine	Bupivacaine	Mepivacaine	Ropivacaine
Metabolism	Hydrolyzed by plasma pseudocholin-esterase	Liver	Liver	Hydrolyzed by plasma pseudocholin-esterase	Liver	Liver	Liver
Excretion	Kidney	Kidney	Kidney	Kidney	Kidney	Kidney	Kidney
Maximum dose*	500 mg (7 mg/kg)	350 mg	300 mg (4.5 mg/kg)	–	175 mg (2 mg/kg)	300 mg	200 mg
Maximum dose with adrenaline	600 mg	550 mg	500 mg (7 mg/kg) Up to 55 mg/kg can be used in Tumescent anesthesia in appropriate setting	–	200 mg	500 mg	250 mg

* This dose increases by about one-third on coadministration with epinephrine.

p-aminobenzoic acid (PABA) derivative and hence cannot be used in patients with PABA hypersensitivity. Due to its poor solubility in water, it stays at site of application for long periods and has low systemic toxicity (poor absorption). Hence it is used for transient pain relief purposes, viz. post insect bite, burns, etc.

Tetracaine

Tetracaine, a PABA derivative is used both for topical as well as spinal anesthesia. It is more potent and toxic than procaine. It can be combined with epinephrine. In view of larger doses required, slow onset of action and greater toxicity, bupivacaine is preferred over tetracaine for nerve blocks.

Chloroprocaine

As the name suggests, chloroprocaine is chlorinated procaine. This leads to increased potency and lesser toxicity. Due to its rapid degradation, there is no risk of toxicity in the neonate and hence it is commonly used in obstetrics. Newer preparations of chloroprocaine contain calcium EDTA as preservative. There are reports of muscle pains due to tetany following its administration due to chelation of calcium by EDTA.

Lidocaine

This is the prototype of amide LAA and also the most commonly used local anesthetic. It is preferred for its fast, longer and potent actions. Concomitant use with epinephrine prolongs the duration of action and enhances the safety when higher doses are used as in tumescent anesthesia. Lidocaine is metabolized in liver and these metabolites (monoethylglycinexylidide and glycinexylidide) also contribute for the cardiovascular and CNS toxicities.[5] Lidocaine causes CNS side effects like anxiety, tinnitus, dysgeusia, tingling and numbness of lips and tongue, dizziness, diplopia, nystagmus, twitching and later, seizures, coma and respiratory distress. Cardiovascular depression may also occur along with these CNS effects. These may occasionally have to be differentiated from signs and symptoms due to epinephrine toxicity.

Bupivacaine

Bupivacaine is more potent and toxic than lidocaine and mepivacaine. As it produces good analgesia at very low doses without affecting the muscular activity, it has been preferred for epidural anesthesia in obstetrics. Due to its extended duration of action, it is an ideal agent for post- operative analgesia. It can be combined with epinephrine. Cardiotoxicity (both central and peripheral) is a major concern with bupivacaine and is aggravated by hypoxemia, hypercarbia and acidosis. It causes ventricular arrhythmias and subsequently myocardial depression. Levobupivacaine is a levo S isomer of bupivacaine and has less cardiotoxicity.

Mepivacaine

Mepivacaine is a potent LAA with rapid onset and intermediate duration of action. The lower pH of fetal blood as well as pKa of mepivacaine leads to ion trapping of this agent. This causes neurobehavioral side effects in neonate and hence less preferred in Obstetrics. Mepivacaine can be combined with epinephrine but cannot be used for topical anesthesia.

Ropivacaine

Ropivacaine has same duration of action as bupivacaine. Though it is less potent, it has better safety profile than bupivacaine. Latter is due to it being an S-stereoisomer.

Motor sparing action of ropivacaine is better than bupivacaine. This is attributable to its low lipophilicity and hence poor penetration of large myelinated motor axons.

Prilocaine

Prilocaine functionally simulates lidocaine except for slightly slower onset of action. Its aromatic ring is metabolized to O-toludine, which can precipitate methemoglobinemia. This effect is seen at doses higher than 8 mg/kg.[10] There is no need for vasoconstrictors with this agent due to its minimal vasodilatation property. CNS toxicity is also less due to greater volume of distribution.

Etidocaine

Etidocaine is more potent and slightly more toxic than lidocaine. It produces more motor inhibition than sensory in contrast to other LAA. Hence, it is not used for epidural analgesia in conduct of normal labor. It can be used with epinephrine.

Dibucaine

Dibucaine is a quinoline derivative with significant toxicities and hence not widely used. It is used in over the counter pain relief products as those used for hemorrhoids, etc.

Articaine

Articaine is an amide LAA with an ester linkage as well. The ester gets hydrolyzed and terminates the action. It has rapid onset of action (1–6 minutes) and short duration of action (about 1 hour).[5]

Pramoxine

Pramoxine is an ether chain containing LAA with antipruritic effect. As it lacks benzoate ester moiety, it can be used in patients with hypersensitivity to other LAA. It is used for topical anesthesia and to alleviate pruritus; but may irritate ocular and nasal mucosa.

Dyclonine

Dyclonine, a ketone LAA has fast and short duration of action like procaine. It has been used for topical anesthesia for relieving the mucositis pain (postradiotherapy or chemotherapy).

Capsaicin

Capsaicin is a natural alkaloid derived from plants of *Solanaceae* family viz. chillies. Capsaicin specific receptors are present only on small diameter sensory neurons, i.e. peripheral unmyelinated C fibers (mediate pain). It causes persistent release of substance P and hence depletes it leading to mitigation of pain. Onset of action is slow (1–2 weeks) and may take 4–6 weeks. Effects last for 3–6 hours. Topical application may cause burning sensation, erythema, pruritus, cough and sneeze.

Diphenhydramine

Diphenhydramine is an antihistamine agent and causes anesthesia by inhibiting sodium channels. On topical application, it is a potent sensitizer and can lead to systemic contact dermatitis. Hence, its use is often restricted for patients sensitive to lidocaine.

As an LAA, diphenhydramine 1% was found to be as efficacious as lidociane 1% but the pain of injection was greater than that of latter.[11] In contrast to lidocaine, buffering does not reduce the pain of injection of diphenhydramine. The onset of anesthesia is usually within 5 mins and lasts for 15 mins to 3 hours.[12,13] It has been safely used both intradermally as well as subcutaneously.[14,15] Recommended dose is 1.5–10 mL. Erythema, irritation, vesiculation, rebound hyperesthesia and skin sloughing (observed only with 5% solution) has been noted with diphenhydramine infiltration. Diphenhydramine has been specially used in the setting of lidocaine sensitivity (level of evidence III, strength of recommendation C).[16]

Doxepin

Doxepin has antipruritic effect on topical application. But, it causes irritation, contact dermatitis, somnolence and hence of doubtful use.

Ambroxol

Ambroxol is a mucolytic commonly used in expectorants. It has a structure similar to local anesthetics and binds to neuronal voltage gated sodium channels more avidly than lidocaine at much lower concentrations. It selectively binds to voltage gated sodium channel 1.8 which is selectively distributed in nociceptive sensory neurons.[17] These receptors tend to express more or redistribute on nociceptive neurons post-nerve injury viz., neuropathies, radiculopathies and neuralgias. It has been used as pastilles to ameliorate pain of pharyngitis. There are reports of high doses being used intravenously as well as orally without any adverse events. Based on these facts, Kern and Weiser effectively treated patients with neuropathic pain with ambroxol 20% cream.[18]

Chlorpheniramine

Chlorpheniramine 1% produces better anesthesia than normal saline; but is more painful than latter. Duration of anesthesia is lesser than lidocaine 1%.[19]

Bacteriostatic saline

Bacteriostatic saline (0.9% Benzyl alcohol with normal saline) has been used as a LAA with level of evidence III and strength of recommendation C in cases of sensitivity to lidocaine.[16,20] Duration of action of bacteriostatic saline is slightly longer than diphenhydramine but lesser than lidocaine.[20] Pain of injection is less than lidocaine.[21]

Metabolism of Local Anesthetic Agents

Drug interactions depend upon how a drug is metabolized and properties of its metabolites. There is a class variation in metabolism of LAA. Ester LAA is metabolized readily by pseudocholinesterase enzyme in blood to aromatic acids and amino alcohols. Pseudocholinesterase enzyme is partially deficient in 4% and totally deficient in 0.1% of population. However, this assumes greater importance when neuromuscular blocker like succinylcholine is being used rather than these agents. Esters like procaine are metabolized to PABA which is further metabolized in liver. However, this PABA can alter the metabolism of sulfur containing medications viz. cotrimoxazole.

Amide LAAs like lidocaine are metabolized in liver by microsomal enzymes. Lidocaine is metabolized predominantly by cytochrome P450 3A4 and to lesser extent by cytochrome P450 1A2 system. Rate of metabolism varies with agent: prilocaine (fastest) greater than etidocaine greater than lidocaine greater than mepivacaine greater than ropivacaine greater than bupivacaine and levobupivacaine (slowest). Various other drugs share this enzyme system for metabolism and hence there is significant interactions of lidocaine with them (Table 2). Therefore, hepatic dysfunction may lead to lidocaine toxicity. Some drugs alter blood supply to liver, thereby affecting metabolism (volatile anesthetics reduce hepatic blood flow leading to reduced amide LAA clearance). Hepatic enzyme systems is immature in infants and may lead to toxicity of lidocaine, bupivacaine and ropivacaine (bupivacaine is often used in obstetrics for epidural analgesia). Amide LAAs are transported to liver by binding to plasma proteins especially alpha 1 acid glycoproteins. Conditions that alter plasma protein levels also alter the delivery of LAA to liver for metabolism and toxicity. Uremia, smoking, surgery increase whereas oral contraceptive pills, neonatal age decrease plasma proteins.

Table 2: Drugs affecting the potency of lidocaine.

Drugs which potentiate lidocaine toxicity	
Antiarrhythmic agents	Amiodarone, disopyramide, quinidine, mexiletine
Antibiotics	Macrolides (clarithromycin, erythromycin), fluoroquinolones (ciprofloxacin, norfloxacin)
Antifungal agents	Ketoconazole, itraconazole, fluconazole
Antidepressants	Nefazodone, fluoxetine, fluvoxamine
Calcium channel blockers	Diltiazem, verapamil, nicardipine
Antiretroviral agents	Protease inhibitors: Ritonavir, indinavir, saquinavir, nelfinavir, atazanavir
Sedatives	Benzodiazepines: Alprazolam, midazolam, triazolam
Others	Danazol, zileuton, tacrine
Nutrients	Grape fruit
Drugs which decrease efficacy of lidocaine	
Antibiotics	Rifamycins: Rifabutin, rifampin, rifapentine
Anticonvulsants	Carbamazepine, phenobarbitone, phenytoin
Antiretroviral agent	Nevirapine

Source: Adopted from Wolverton Comprehensive Dermatologic Drug Therapy, 2nd edition.[1]

Evaluation of Patients for Administration of LAA

Patient should be asked about the history of allergy to any of the LAA or any other medication, presence of systemic illness like hypertension, liver dysfunction, any medications like beta blockers, phenytoin. Informed consent should include specific consent for intradermal test for infiltration local anesthesia.

Method of Administration of Local Anesthesia

Local anesthesia can be topical anesthesia (skin and mucosa), infiltration anesthesia, ring block, field block, regional block, peripheral nerve block and tumescent anesthesia.[1,5,7,22] Nerve blocks and tumescent anesthesia are dealt in separate chapter.

TOPICAL ANESTHESIA

Topical anesthesia involves application of local anesthetic agents over skin or mucosa to cause anesthesia. Pharmacological preparations used are benzocaine, lidocaine 2–10% and tetracaine 2%. Maximal safe dose for topical anesthesia in 70 kg adult is 300 mg for lidocaine and 50 mg for tetracaine. Peak anesthetic effects are seen within 2–5 minutes with lidocaine and 3–8 minutes with tetracaine. Anesthetic action of lidocaine lasts for 30–45 minutes and of tetracaine, 30–60 minutes. Eutectic mixture of local anesthetics (EMLA) is a formulation containing mixture of prilocaine 2.5%/ lidocaine 2.5% or lidocaine 7%/tetracaine 7%. Eutectic mixture of 2.5% lidocaine and 2.5% prilocaine in oil-water emulsion has a melting point (17°C) which is less than either of lidocaine (66–69°C) or prilocaine (36–38°C) and hence exist as liquid at body temperature enhancing its absorption. Depth of analgesia is dependent on the duration of application of EMLA. Maximum depth achieved is 5 mm at the end of 2 hours of application.[23] Eutectic mixture of local anesthetics has been used safely on mucosa.[24-27] It is better than benzocaine or plain lidocaine in producing analgesia on mucosa.[28-30] Dosage of EMLA in adults is 2 g/10 sq.cm. Dose of medication, time of application and maximal area applicable varies in children (Table 3).[22,31,32]

Table 3: Dosage of EMLA in children.

Age and weight	Maximum total dose and time	Maximum application area (cm²)
1–3 months or <5 kg	1 g (1 hour)	10
4–12 months and >5 kg	2 g	20
1–6 years and >10 kg	10 g	100
7–12 years and >20 kg	20 g	200

Eutectic mixture of local anesthetics is FDA-approved only for topical analgesia for intact skin, laser procedures and leg ulcer debridement. It is contraindicated in cases with hypersensitivity, infants below 1 year on methemoglobinemia inducing drugs, those with methemoglobinemia of any cause, glucose-6-phosphate dehydrogenase deficiency, mucosa and pregnancy.[1] Topical anesthetic preparation especially used for abraded or lacerated skin consisting of tetracaine 0.5%, adrenaline 1:2,00,000 and cocaine 11.8% has been used in pediatric emergencies. In view of risk of precipitating seizures, revised formulation with reduced strength of cocaine and adrenaline and more of tetracaine (1%) has been suggested. This preparation cannot anesthetize intact skin and use on mucosa leads to rapid absorption and toxicity. Because of these side effects and the addictive tendency, preparations of lidocaine 4%, epinephrine 1:20,000, tetracaine 0.5% (LET); tetracaine, phenylephrine; prilocaine-phenylephrine and bupivacaine-phenylephrine[33] have been used with varying results.[34] When used in the form of occlusive patch, lidocaine exhibited sustained alleviation of pain for a duration much longer than the actual duration of action of lidocaine.[35] Transdermal diclofenac patch was found to be as effective as EMLA in ameliorating the venous cannulation pain. In comparison to EMLA, it caused less erythema, edema and induration.[36]

Analgesic effects of EMLA was found to be better than 50% nitrous oxide/oxygen gas when used for chronic leg ulcer debridement.[37] EMLA has been safely used not only in open wounds to ameliorate the pain of suturing or dressing[38] but also as primary dressing to reduce pain in leg ulcer.[39] Topical anesthesia is the first line technique for repair of dermal laceration in children (strength of recommendation A, level of evidence I,II).[16]

Application of topical anesthetic agents prior to fractional ablative laser resurfacing (both CO_2 and Erb:Yag) narrowed the ablative width and increased the coagulative depth. However, this was not statistically significant.[40] EMLA causes a 27% reduction in vessel diameter and this is of relevance when pulse dye laser is being contemplated.[41]

Lidoderm: It is 5% lidocaine adhesive patch commonly used for post herpetic neuralgia.[42]

S-caine peel: This is a combination of lidocaine 7% and tetracaine 7% cream and forms a pliable sheet on the skin after application. It is usually applied for 20–30 mins for laser hair reduction and 60 mins for laser tattoo removal. It contains a controlled heating (39°–41°C) system which gets activated by oxygen. This facilitates faster penetration of anesthetics with better anesthesia. Anesthesia was found to be effective till 8.22 mm depth and lasted for 100 mins after its removal.[43,44]

Other topical preparations are Topicaine (lidocaine, both 4% and 5%), Betacaine-LA (lidocaine, prilocaine, dibucaine and phenylepherine), ELA-max cream (liposomal lidocaine at 4% and 5%) and amethocaine (tetracaine 4%).[44] Topical tetracaine 4% with intradermal and subcutaneous infiltration of diphenhydramine provided good anesthesia for wide local excision of nodular BCC followed by flap closure of wound.[15]

INFILTRATION ANESTHESIA

In infiltration anesthesia, local anesthetics are injected directly into the tissue of interest without considering the course of the nerve supplying it. Lidocaine with or without adrenaline is the most commonly used local anesthetic for this indication. Other commonly used agent is bupivacaine. Onset and duration of action are delayed if injected into subcutaneous rather than into dermis. Bupivacaine acts for longer duration than lidocaine even in combination with adrenaline.[45] Adding adrenaline decreases blood loss, reduces the toxicity and increases the duration of action of local anesthetic. Disadvantages of infiltration anesthesia include need for larger volume of LAA for anesthetizing small areas and while performing skin biopsy, there is a risk of distortion of morphologic features of the lesion. When larger surface areas have to be anesthetized, greater volumes with lower concentration (0.3–0.5% lidocaine) can be effectively used.[7]

Ring Block

Ring block is a modification of infiltration anesthesia where LAA is infiltrated all around the area of interest but not into it. This prevents distortion of tissues when histopathology of the tissue is contemplated and also prevents false negative cultures from the interest area. Preservatives in LAA preparations have antibacterial effects and this is avoided by ring block.[1]

Field Block

Here, the LAA is injected subcutaneously to anesthetize area distal to the site of injection. By this technique, larger areas can be anesthetized with lesser quantity of LAA.[5]

Regional Block

Regional blocks can be achieved either by intravenous infusion of LAA (Bier block) or infiltration of LAA around a nerve or nerve plexus (peripheral nerve block). Peripheral nerve blocks are used for hands/foot, fingers/toes and face.[46] Peripheral nerve blocks are classified as minor and major. When a single nerve is anesthetized, it is referred to as minor block. When two or more nerves, nerve plexus or large nerve fiber is blocked more proximally, it becomes a major nerve block. Onset of action is rapid and duration of action can be altered choosing an appropriate LAA or combining LAA with epinephrine.[7] Use of inadequate dose of LAA leads to blockage of peripherally placed and some small, sensitive central nerve fibers. Vasa nervorum is placed in the center; therefore central fibers regain function (sensation) earlier than peripheral nerve fibers.[5] There is a risk of laceration of nerve, transient motor paralysis, intravascular injection and compartment syndrome during peripheral nerve blocks.

Cryoanesthesia

As cooling numbs the skin, it can be used for achieving local analgesia and anesthesia. This technique has been aptly termed as cryoanesthesia. Cryoanesthesia can be employed for both diagnostic as well as therapeutic dermatosurgical procedures. When used for performing skin biopsies, Luck et al. have shown that, it does not interfere with the histological interpretation.[47] Various modalities adopted include, applying ice cubes, vapocoolant sprays and cryosprays. Depending upon the pain sensitivity and tolerance, ice cubes alone can be used for numbing the skin before injecting LAA or used in addition to topical anesthesia. Vapocoolant sprays contain either ethyl chloride or dichlorotetrafluoroethane. Ethyl chloride has to be sprayed from a distance of 3–9 inches taking care so that, there is whitening and not frosting of skin (spray duration 3–7 seconds).[48] Ethyl chloride is inflammable and hence avoided during procedures like cautery or lasers. Liquid nitrogen is used as cryosprays and care should be taken not to cause frosting. Sprays act fast and can be sprayed before injecting LAA or intralesional steroids into keloids or molluscum curettage in children. Forced cold air delivered at a distance of 1 cm for 30 seconds was found to augment the anesthetic effect of topical anesthetic for injecting botulinum toxin for palmar hyperhidrosis.[49] The mean beginning time of anesthesia with forced cold air for non-facial skin was found to be 54.61seconds.[50] Analgesia was much better with ethylchloride spray than EMLA.[51]

LOCAL ANESTHETICS DURING PREGNANCY

The use of local anesthetics during pregnancy is generally acceptable, but after careful consideration. Lidocaine is classified as FDA pregnancy risk category B and epinephrine as category C.[1] Pregnancy has a greater impact on spread and depth of epidural and spinal anesthesia rather than on infiltration or topical anesthesia (latter more commonly practiced by dermatologists and dermatosurgeons). Topical lidocaine is considered safe in comparison to other topical anesthetics during pregnancy; hence other LAAs have not been recommended during pregnancy or lactation.[16]

For the use of topical anesthesia in pregnant and nursing mothers, there is Level of evidence III and strength of recommendation C.[16] Small quantities of lidocaine with epinephrine can be used in pregnant and nursing mothers (level of evidence II, strength of recommendation B).[16] However, following aspects need to be considered when administration of LAA is planned for a pregnant mother.

- Avoiding during organogenesis (15–56 days of gestation) when possible
- Reduce the dose of LAA[7]
- Be alert about vasovagal reactions, which may occur at a higher rate during pregnancy
- Position the patient on her left side to avoid vena caval and aortic compression.

MEASURES TO ALLEVIATE THE PAIN OF LAA INJECTION

Pain of local anesthetic injections can be alleviated by the following measures:[52,53] The reader is also referred to the chapter on analgesics for more details.

- Combining local anesthetic with 8.4% sodium bicarbonate (10:1) to render the pH neutral. Solutions of local anesthetics are acidic (pH 5.0–7.0) and hence cause pain and stinging sensation on infiltration. Solutions of lidocaine with adrenaline is more painful than plain lidocaine as the former is more acidic (pH 3.3–5.5) than latter.[54,55] Reconstituted buffered lidocaine with or without adrenaline can be kept at room temperature for 1 week.[56,57] Buffering the LAA is suggested only for lidocaine. Precipitation happens on buffering bupivacaine and hence it is not recommended.[16]
- Injection of freshly prepared LAA with epinephrine is less painful than a premixed combination. This is because, latter is more acidic to improve stability of epinephrine. Solution can be prepared by mixing 0.3 mL of 1:1000 epinephrine with 30 mL of lidocaine.[58]
- Slow administration of only the required amount of the local anesthetic to prevent tissue distention, which may give rise to pain.
- Precool the concerned area with ice pack for 10 seconds. This gives anesthesia for 2 seconds sufficient for needle prick. Cold air cooling also reduces pain of injection.
- Warming the anesthetic to 40°C[59]: Systematic review and meta-analysis by Hogan et al has revealed that, the pain of injection of LAA can be reduced by warming the injection solution to body temperature.[60]
- Using vibration during injections.

Slow rate of infiltration, precooling, using warm solution and vibrating the skin have level of evidence II and strength of recommendation B.[16] Few other practical tips for making the injections relatively painless are:

- As soon as the needle is introduced into the skin, push some local anesthetic, wait for 1–2 minutes so that the area is anesthetized and then introduce the needle further ahead

- When lesion on the palmar or plantar area is to be anesthetized, it is preferable to introduce the needle through the dorsal thin skin along with the above said technique for infiltration
- Apply topical anesthesia cream if deep infiltration is desired for about 30–60 minutes under occlusion. Application topical anesthesia before infiltrating LAA reduces not only the pain but also the dose of infiltrative LAA.[16]
- Repetitive pinching of skin while injecting local anesthetic.[61]
- Ethyl chloride spray can be used to reduce pain of LAA injection (level of evidence III, strength of recommendation C).[16]

Although it has long been held that finer needles cause less pain, Palmon et al. did not find significant difference in pain when 25-guage and 30-gauge needle were used.[62]

MEASURES TO ACHIEVE RAPID ANESTHESIA AND ANALGESIA

Stratum corneum is a tough barrier which prevents transcutaneous permeation of various molecules. Occlusion of topical anesthetics and local heat application increases the penetration of LAA. Disruption of this barrier definitely enhances the penetration of topically applied agents.

Mechanical methods of disruption include exfoliating the skin like microdermabrasion, degreasing the skin with alcohol or acetone, abrading the skin with lasers (fractional ablative viz., CO_2, Erb:YAG)[63,64] or creating microchannels through dermaroller or fractional microneedling. Jetpeel™ consists of a high velocity spray which contains oxygen and normal saline. This causes gentle exfoliation of skin without dryness.[65] Jetpeel™-3 has been used efficaciously in delivering the local anesthetic but also reduced the dose of botulinum toxin to treat palmar hyperhidrosis.[66] Other methods include inotophoresis, electroporation, sonophoresis and magnetophoresis. The charged molecules are pushed through the skin by low voltage current in iontophoresis and are dependent on the current intensity and duration of treatment. Transient pores are created by short pulses of high voltage current in electroporation. In electroincorporation, there is dielectric breakdown of stratum corneum due to the pulsed electric fields.[67] Depth of anesthesia was more with iontophoresis than electroporation or electroincorporation.[68] Ultrasound waves cause cavitation and steaming which facilitates movement of molecules through skin. Various frequencies are used 20–100 kHz or 0.7–16 MHz for this purpose.[69]

Investigational tool include poly L-lactide microneedle array and biodegradable microneedles which deliver lidocaine.[70,71]

Delivery of drugs through liposomes, niosomes, transferosomes and lipid polymer hybrid nanoparticles have been investigated. Lidocaine loaded lipid polymer hybrid nanoparticles were more efficient in lidocaine delivery than liposomes.[72] Hair follicles are a major route of transcutaneous drug delivery; hence follicular penetration was found to be better with sebum like lipid material of liposomes and with liposomes less or equal to 640 nm diameter.[73] Liposomal tetracaine 5% anesthetized better than EMLA. Niosomes are similar to liposomes but produced from non-ionic surfactants. They are smaller, more stable and penetrate faster than liposomes. Transferosomes are produced from bile salts and they can squeeze through pores of size 5 times lesser than them.[69] EMLA delivered in nanotechnology has shown > 30% reduction in pain within 10 mins of its application.[74]

Hyaluronidase has been used along with LAA as it facilitates the dispersion of the latter leading to faster and better analgesia.[75,76] It also reduced the quantity of LAA by 2.4 folds.[77] Navarre et al. have noted increased pain on injection and reduced duration of action when LAA was combined with hyaluronidase. It may also elicit allergic reactions due to the preservative, thimerosal in it.[78] Due to cross reactivity, individuals sensitive to bee venom should not be administered hyaluronidase. However, there was no evidence of any adverse effect of hyaluronidase on wound healing.[76]

Theoretically, alkalinization of local anesthetics results in reduced ionized to unionized proportion of LAA, thereby reducing the time for onset of action. However, clinical studies have showed inconsistent results and hence routine alkalinization of local anesthetics is not recommended for hastening the effect. Bupivacaine and etidocaine cannot be alkalinized as they tend to precipitate on mixing with sodium bicarbonate.[79] Nerve blocks are done by single, double or multiple injections. Multiple injection technique was found to produce better analgesia than any other method.[80]

Mixtures of LAAs like lidocaine with bupivacaine, bupivacaine with mepivacaine and prilocaine with ropivacaine have been used with intent to achieve faster and long lasting anesthesia. However, there is no sufficient evidence to prove their superiority over the use of single LAA.[16]

MEASURES TO PROLONG THE DURATION OF ACTION OF LAA

Duration of action of local anesthetics is prolonged by addition of adrenaline (1:2,00,000 dilution) or low molecular weight dextran 40 (1:1 dilution) to the local anesthetic. Both the agents delay the clearance of the drug from the site of administration (former by causing vasoconstriction and latter by delaying its systemic absorption) and hence prolong its action.[81] Fentanyl has been used with LAA to enhance the quality as well as the duration of action of LAA. This works on the principle that afferent nerve fibers contain opioid receptors and hence, opioid analgesics placed around the nerve augments the local anesthetic effects.[82]

VASOCONSTRICTORS AND LAA

Vasoconstrictors when used with LAA controls blood loss during procedure and retards local clearance of LAA. This increases efficacy and reduces the risk of systemic toxicity of LAA.[1,2,5,7] Various agents used are as follows:

Epinephrine

Epinephrine is the most common vasoconstrictor used with LAA. It has both alpha (vasoconstriction action) as well beta adrenergic effect (increases blood pressure and pulse rate). Efficacy of lidocaine 1% with epinephrine has been found to be equivalent to lidocaine 2%.[3] Combination of epinephrine with lidocaine is more potent than when former is used with bupivacaine or etidocaine. This is due to high protein binding of latter LAA which itself decreases the clearance of these agents resulting in prolonged action. It takes about 7–15 minutes for achieving optimal hemostatic effect with epinephrine.[1] Dosage of epinephrine in cardiac patients is 40–200 µg (0.04–0.2 mg or 4–20 mL of 1:1,00,000 epinephrine) and in healthy adults is 500 µg (0.5 mg or 50 mL of 1:1,00,000 epinephrine). It has long been held that, use of vasoconstrictors with LAA is contraindicated for areas with end arterial supply like digits/toes, penis, ear lobes and nose tip. Recent evidence suggests that lidocaine with adrenaline is safe for ears, digits, toes and tip of nose.[83-84] Similarly, several studies have demonstrated the safety of lidocaine with adrenaline combination for digits and toes in patients with normal circulatory status.[85-88] Hence, lidocaine with adrenaline may be used with caution, particularly in an otherwise healthy young patient without any vascular insufficieny in injections to fingers and toes, if benefits outweigh the risk of such a combination. However in people with suspected vascular insufficiency, elderly patients, and in patients with unreliable history of previous disease states, such combinations are contraindicated because of the risk of precipitating vascular complications such as gangrene. In such individuals, only plain lidocaine should be used. Based on various studies and reports, the recent guidelines on use of local anesthesia suggest that, LAA with epinephrine can be safely used for regions like ear, nose and digits (Level of Evidence I, II and strength of recommendation A). However, for penis, it is level II with strength of recommendation of B.[16]

Systemic side effects of epinephrine starts after 5–10 mins of injection and lasts for about 10–15 mins.[89] Small quantities of epinephrine with lidocaine can be used in stable cardiovascular patients (level of evidence I,II, strength of recommendation B).[16] Although, there has been debate over the use of vasoconstrictor with LAA for harvesting the split thickness and full thickness graft, there is no consensus on this and hence, it can be used in healthy patients without any vascular insufficiency.

Malignant hypertension can occur with epinephrine-LAA in patients on nonselective beta blockers like propranolol, labetalol, timolol. This is due to unopposed alpha adrenergic activity as protective beta adrenergic effects are blocked by propranolol. However, in view of low doses of epinephrine used, there is no need to discontinue non-selective beta blockers before cutaneous surgeries.[1] Epinephrine also causes CNS side effects like restlessness, tremors, headache, cerebral bleed and cause hypertension in pheochromocytoma and hyperthyroid patients. Being a stress hormone, it increases blood sugars.

Topical epinephrine fails to increase the duration of action of topical anesthetics due to poor penetration of intact skin or mucosa. However, phenylephrine 0.005% can be used for the same purpose.

Levonordefrin

Levonordefrin is an active isomer of nordefrin, which has alpha 1 adrenergic activity and minimal to absent beta adrenergic activity. Because of its latter action, variation in blood pressure and pulse rate is minimal.

Phenylephrine

Phenylephrine has only alpha adrenergic activity and often used in subarachnoid blocks. This is used as an alternative to epinephrine for topical anesthesia.

COMPLICATIONS DURING LOCAL ANESTHESIA

Local Neural Toxicity

Extraneural deposition of LAA as in nerve blocks has been found to be cytotoxic to neuronal cells and Schwann cells through several mechanisms which are less understood. Perez-Castro et al. found that bupivacaine was more toxic than lidocaine, though latter causes more transient neurological symptoms.[90] Damage caused to Schwann cells differ with duration of exposure to LAA and the concentration used. Even at low concentration, bupivacaine caused significant cell death on prolonged exposure. On intermediate duration of exposure, both bupivacaine and ropivacaine were equally toxic. Prolonged extraneural exposure to bupivacaine resulted in significant demyelination and nerve inflammation.[91]

Syncope

Syncope secondary to vasovagal attack (presence of pallor, hyperhidrosis, hyperventilation and hypotension) is common, particularly in anxious patients, and those with unstable autonomic nervous system. It is always advisable to ask about previous syncopal attacks before administration of anesthesia. Vasovagal syncopal attack can be treated by raising the foot end of the bed. For this reason, all procedures needing local anesthesia should be done in supine position. Injection atropine may be helpful in cases that develop bradycardia (Table 4).[46] Hence it is preferable to keep a syringe filled with atropine ready before administration of local anesthesia.

Table 4: Common adverse reactions during administration of LAA and their management.

Signs and symptoms	Cause	Corrective measures
CNS excitation: headache, anxiety, tingling of lips and tongue, twitching, seizures Cardiac depression: Hypotension Respiratory depression	Lidocaine toxicity	Stop further administration of LAA Airway, breathing and circulation management Diazepam for convulsion, ephedrine for hypotension, atropine for bradycardia
Tachycardia, palpitations, apprehension, anxiety, hypertension	Epinephrine	Stop further administration, observe for 10–15 min, reassure patient Esmolol, sotalol may be used for hypertension Phentolamine may be needed
Bradycardia, hypotension, nausea, pallor, dizziness/fainting	Vasovagal syncope	Lower the head end Elevate the leg end monitor vitals and intervene accordingly
Edema, erythema, dyspnea Bronchospasm, tachycardia, hypotension	Anaphylaxis	Intravenous hydrocortisone, adrenaline subcutaneously, bronchodilator (nasal or oral spray) Be prepared for emergency tracheotomy or cricothyroidotomy Lidocaine sensitivity to be performed to prevent such an occurrence

Source: Local and regional anesthetic blocks made simple by Sanchez Jr. et al.

Hypersensitivity Reactions

Hypersensitivity reactions are potentially serious and hence should always be recognized and treated early. However, it must be recognized that true allergic reactions to local anesthetics are rare.[92-94] Vasovagal syncopal attacks are often mistakenly considered as hypersensitivity reactions. Careful evaluation and skin testing is needed for proper diagnosis.[95-97] Sensitivity to local anesthetics may be either due to the anesthetic itself or the preservatives.

Esters are metabolized to PABA which is allergenic. Sensitivity to local anesthetics can be either of type I reaction (anaphylaxis) or type IV (delayed hypersensitivity). Anaphylaxis, though very rare, may be potentially fatal. Ester group anesthetics are more prone to cause anaphylaxis than the amide group anesthetics.[98] Type IV reaction can be either due to amides or ester based local anesthetics. Amides and ester groups of local anesthetics do not cross react. However, within the group, there may be cross-reaction to other agents.[99] Rarely, hypersensitivity can exist in a patient, to both amide and ester group of local anesthetics.[100] Delayed type hypersensitivity reaction may rarely vary with the site of deposition of LAA. Wobser et al. reported 'Compartment Allergy' a case of delayed hypersensitivity to prilocaine which occurred only on patch and superficial subcutaneous application but not on deep subcutaneous injection. He hypothesized that, this could be due to *'lower dendritic cell (DC) density in deeper cutaneous compartments and/or different DC subsets exhibiting distinct functional immunomodulatory properties in the various layers of the skin'*.[101] Hypersensitivity may also be caused by reactions to preservatives (methylparaben) and antioxidants (metabisulphite).[94,96,102]

Skin Testing

Skin testing is an important means of determining possible hypersensitivity. However, both false positives and false negatives may occur.

Skin testing for topical cream anesthesia: Contact hypersensitivity to topically applied anesthetics is infrequent.[94-96] Topical allergic reaction is usually mild, limited to development of dermatitis or contact urticaria. Hence a patch test is not recommended as a routine in all cases. However, where there is a suspicion of hypersensitivity, a patch testing may be performed. Apply about 1–2 mm thick layer of anesthetic preparation over about 1 cm^2 area for 30 minutes and check for history of itching or any erythema or maculopapular rash.

Intradermal testing: All anesthetic injections may be associated with systemic hypersensitivity which may be potentially fatal. Hence intradermal test is mandatory in all such cases. This is performed by injection of lidocaine or bupivacaine with 0.1 mL on flexural forearm about 1–2 inches below the antecubital fossa. If the patient complains of any itching with the development of urticarial rash in the form of erythema, edema and induration at the site of intradermal test, it indicates a positive test, indicating that the patient is hypersensitive to it. In such a situation, it is not safe and ethical to administer/use the same local anesthetic.

Alternatives for Anesthesia in Patients with Lidocaine Hypersensitivity

In cases of hypersensitivity to lidocaine, anesthesia can be achieved by using an anesthetic from the ester group. If there is any allergy to the preservative, then preservative free lidocaine may be used, if such a preparation is available. If there is hypersensitivity to both amide and ester groups, then the alternative would include:[19]

- Diphenhydramine and chlorpheniramine are alternatives though they provided milder anesthesia[11,12,20]
- Benzyl alcohol can also be used for anesthesia[103]
- Intravenous sedation/general anesthesia can be used in a hypersensitive patient, if the circumstances of the case demand
- Cryoanesthesia (discussed earlier).

Prilocaine has caused cross-sensitivity with bupivacaine and pramoxine.[90]

Systemic toxicities with EMLA are usually due to inappropriate technique (large quantities, large surface area of application, and long duration of application), inappropriate local factors (abraded skin, vascular malformations, eczema), inappropriate demographics (prematurity, age less than 3 months) and drug interactions.[104]

Methemoglobinemia

Amide LAA undergoes N-dealkylation and then hydrolysis. However, prilocaine undergoes first hydrolysis which results in formation of orthotoluidine. This product oxidizes ferrous ion (Fe^{2+}) in hemoglobin to ferric (Fe^{3+}) leading to impaired release of oxygen causing hypoxia termed methemoglobinemia. Patients appear cyanotic and their blood is chocolate colored when MetHb level is 3–5 mg%. Doses of prilocaine greater than 10 mg/kg or greater than 600 mg are required for producing this side effect. However, lower doses can cause same side effect in patients with congenital or idiopathic methemoglobinemia, infants less than 6 months (immature NADH reductase enzyme complex),[10,103] glucose-6-phosphate dehydrogenase enzyme deficiency and those on medications which cause methemoglobinemia (viz. dapsone, chloroquine, sulfonamides, primaquine, acetaminophen, phenobarbital, phenytoin, nitroglycerin, nitrofurantoin, nitroprusside, aniline dyes, para-aminosalicylic acid and benzocaine). In mild cases, methemoglobinemia resolves spontaneously or with supportive care like oxygen administration; if severe, intravenous administration of reducing agents like methylene blue, vitamin C may be required. Methylene blue is contraindicated in G6PD deficient individuals and such patients should be treated with ascorbic acid, though latter works much slowly.

Guay in his study of patients of methemoglobinemia secondary to LAA found that maximum cases were due to benzocaine (77 out of 97). Benzoic esters are metabolized similar to anilides and it is hypothesized that, methemoglobinemia could be due to a variation in metabolism and/or elimination of benzocaine. In patients with methemoglobinemia due to benzocaine application on mucosa, there is a high-risk of development of rebound methemoglobinemia after administration of methylene blue for up to 18 hours. Hence, these patients should be carefully monitored after antidote therapy. Methemoglobinemia has also been reported with lidocaine and tetracaine; however, NADH deficiency was not evaluated in them.[10]

Local Anesthetic Systemic Toxicity

Local anesthetic systemic toxicity (LAST) is occurrence of systemic toxicity (cardiovascular and central nervous system) due to administration of local anesthesia. Though not common, it can happen (2–2.8/10,000 peripheral nerve blocks).[105]

Cause, Mechanism and Clinical Features of LAST

Systemic toxicity can occur due to inadvertent intraarterial or intravenous injection as well as systemic absorption. Symptoms due to intra-arterial injections often occur during nerve blocks in head and neck region. Because of proximity to brain, CNS side effects occur very fast and also recover fast due to rapid cerebral circulation. Even low doses may give this side effect. Symptoms due to inadvertent intravenous injection occur within 5 mins and are common with regional blocks when large quantities of LAA (5–10 mL) are used. Symptoms due to systemic absorption are delayed and take about 20–30 min or more. It occurs if large quantities of LAA are used or with continuous LAA infusion or in the presence of risk factors viz., in infants less than 4 months and elderly, severe hepatic dysfunction, advanced cardiac failure, uremia, metabolic acidosis and late pregnancy. Rapid systemic absorption can also occur when LAA is injected in highly vascular areas. The mechanism of toxicity and clinical features are summarized in Table 5. Eventhough there is initial CNS excitation followed by suppression, occasionally, CNS depression can occur directly without preluding excitation phase.[5,7]

All the LAAs are potential cardiovascular depressants, both central and peripheral. CNS side effects precede cardiac side effects and cardiac depression occurs at doses which cause CNS depression. Cardiotoxicity is more

Table 5: Mechanism of toxicity and clinical features of LAST.

System involved	Mechanism of toxicity	Clinical features
CNS system	Initial phase: Inhibition of cerebral cortical inhibitory pathway	Sensory disturbances (perioral paresthesia, dysgeusia), visual disturbances, dysarthria, dizziness, muscle twitching, confusion, convulsions
	Delayed phase: inhibition of excitatory neurons	Mental obtundation, unconsciousness, coma, respiratory arrest
CVS system	Inhibition of Na channels lead to decreased rate of depolarization and propagation of action potentials	Hypertension, tachycardia (due early CNS excitation), dysarrhythmia (bradycardia, tachycardia, ventricular ectopy), reentrant tachyarrhythmia
	Inhibition of calcium channel and sodium-calcium channel leads to reduced myocardial contraction; impairs mitochondrial oxidative phosphorylation; inhibits cAMP production	Myocardial depression, asystole
	Suppress baroreceptor reflex; reduce vascular tone	Hypotension

severe with bupivacaine and etidocaine in comparison to lidocaine. The increased toxicity of bupivacaine is attributed to slower dissociation of bupivacaine from sodium channels during diastole leading to cumulative blockage of channels and a more intense depression of rapid phase of depolarization in Purkinje fibers and ventricular muscles. This leads to ventricular arrhythmias and myocardial depression. Bupivacaine is a racemic mixture of R- and S-stereoisomers and R-isomers are more cardiotoxic. Hence, pure S-stereoisomers of bupivacaine, i.e. ropivacaine (single S-enantiomer) and levobupivacaine (levo-S-bupivacaine) have less cardiotoxicity.[5,7] It is difficult to resuscitate patients with bupivacaine induced cardiac toxicity and hence great caution has to be exercised to prevent inadvertent intravascular injection.

As the symptoms of CNS toxicity are much easier to recognize than cardiovascular collapse, a new ratio encompassing these has been proposed to check potential of LAA to cause these side effects. Cardiovascular collapse/ CNS (CC/CNS) ratio is the ratio of drug dose required to cause catastrophic cardiovascular collapse to drug dose required to cause seizures. Greater the cardiotoxicity, lower is the ratio. Ascending order of this ratio is racemic bupivacaine (lowest), levobupivacaine, ropivaciane and lidocaine (highest). However, CVS toxicity can occur without preceding CNS toxicity irrespective of agent used.[106]

Methods to Mitigate Risk of LAST

The American Society of Regional Anesthesia and Pain Medicine recommends following techniques to reduce the risk of LAST:[107]

1. Minimalistic approach: Use of just adequate dose of LAA is better. Lean body mass is a better index for dose calculation than whole body weight in overweight/ obese individuals. Whenever combination of LAAs is used, lesser doses of each should be used as the side effects can accrue.
2. Choosing right LAA: LAA with higher CC/CNS ratios should be preferred.
3. Safe technique of administration: Aspirate before injecting so as to confirm that needle is not intravascular. Administer LAA as small boluses slowly rather than depositing large doses in a single shot. Maintaining a gap of one circulation time viz., 30–45 seconds between these boluses is a safe practice.
4. Use of marker of intravascular injection: A test dose of epinephrine 5μg/ml of LAA has been used to know the expected response, adverse reaction in case of intravascular injection. An intravascular injection of 3ml of LAA with epinephrine (1:200000) viz., 15 μg of epinephrine causes tachycardia (10 beats/min) and rise in systolic pressure by 15 mm Hg. But this may not be appreciated in elderly patients and those on beta blockers, sedated or under general anesthesia.
5. Ultrasound guided administration of peripheral nerve blocks: this avoids intravascular injection of LAA.

Management of LAST

Most important aspect of management is early recognition of LAST! Monitor the vitals for 30 mins after administration of LAA and keep speaking to patient to recognize any early CNS side effects. Any alteration of mental function or variations of cardiac parameters is LAST. Like in any hypersensitivity or toxicity reactions, maintenance of airway, breathing and circulation is critical for resuscitation of an individual with LAST. Seizures can be effectively treated with benzodiazepines and if refractory may require succinylcholine (*see* Table 4). However, these need anesthetist or an intensivists intervention. CNS or cardiac complications necessitate advanced life support and appropriate timely intervention. Epinephrine <1 mg/kg has been suggested to improve cardiac contractility and maintain blood pressure. Amiodarone is preferred over calcium channel blockers and beta blockers to treat ventricular tachyarrhythmias as latter reduce vascular resistance and also suppress cardiac muscles. Intravenous lipid emulsion therapy, also called as lipid resuscitation has been considered a standard care for resuscitation of LAST.[107] After successful resuscitation, patient should be observed for 12 hours before taking up for intended procedure. Lipid resuscitation is discussed in detail in separate section.

OTHER SIDE EFFECTS

Bruising

Bruising is common in elderly due to thin dermis. Bruise can be localized by immediate application of pressure or ice cubes at the site.

Vasoconstriction

In case of mild ischemia due to lidocaine with adrenaline, apply topical nitroglycerin; for severe cases, start phentolamine 2.5–5.0 mg which is diluted in 4.5–9.0 mL of normal saline.[108]

Myonecrosis

Intramuscular injection of LAA can cause variable muscle necrosis which is also LAA dependent (bupivacaine, chloroprocaine > ropivacaine, procaine, tetracaine).[109]

Drug Fever

Drug fever was noted with EMLA but not plain 2% lidocaine jelly. Drug fever correlated with increase in serum IL-6 levels.[110]

Pseudobullous Dermatosis

Both intraepidermal (subcorneal and suprabasal) as well as subepidermal clefting have been observed with EMLA application. Epidermal necrosis and multifocal clefting was more common with genital lesions secondary to EMLA application.[111,112]

Various adverse reactions noted with EMLA are erythema, edema, pain, allergic contact dermatitis, contact urticaria, purpura, post inflammatory hyperpigmentation and skin necrosis when applied to leg ulcers in patients with disordered microcirculation.[113-116] Loss of vision has been documented during eyelid infiltration secondary to corneal perforation.[117]

Lipid Resuscitation

Intravenous lipids have long been used for parenteral nutrition. It is an emulsion composed of egg phospholipids or soyabean oil in water. It has also been used to treat systemic toxicity of LAA (LAST) and referred as Intravenous lipid emulsion therapy and Lipid rescue. Commonly 20% emulsions are used for this purpose. Among various preparations available, Intralipid™ has maximum studies.

Mechanism of Action of Intravenous Lipids

Various mechanisms have been hypothesized and include,[118,119]

1. Lipid sink: Lipid soluble LAA agents in circulation or tissue binding sites are attracted and absorbed by the intravenous lipids.
2. Influence on cardiac myocyte fatty acid metabolism: LAA inhibit fatty acid metabolism in heart and intravenous lipids counteract this by being an exogenous source of energy.
3. Acts as a positive inotrope
4. Relieves the sodium channel (Nav 1.5) by the drug
5. Regulate carnitine transport, thereby improving fatty acid metabolism in cardiac muscles.

Method of Use

Initially a loading dose of 1.5 mL/kg is administered over 5 mins and subsequently a slow infusion of 0.25 mL/kg/min (i.e., about 18 mL/min if patient is 70 kg) is administered over 30–60 mins. If the hypotension persists, then one or two additional boluses are administered and the dose of continuous infusion is doubled (0.5 mL/kg/min). Continuous infusion is continued for 10 mins after the CVS stability. Maximum recommended dose is 10 mL/kg in initial 30 mins.

Adverse effects of lipid resuscitation include alteration of laboratory tests (renal and liver function test, electrolytes, creatine kinase and total proteins; this tends to persists for 24 hours after administration of intravenous lipids), pancreatitis, pulmonary dysfunction, acute renal failure and deep vein thrombosis.[120]

Positioning of Lipid Resuscitiation for LAST

Even though intravenous lipids have found to reverse CVS and CNS adverse effects of LAAs in some reports, lipid resuscitation cannot be used as first line therapy for LAST. It can be used when all other resuscitative efforts fail. It can be used for treating toxicity due to lipophilic drugs viz., bupivacaine and can be considered for treating toxicity due to other LAAs, amitriptyline and bupropion.[121.122]

Safety Tips When Administering Local Anesthesia

- Ethyl chloride is more inflammable than alcohol; eventhough it vaporizes rapidly, it is safe to avoid it when electrocautery is planned.
- When injecting lidocaine or bupivacaine (especially latter) ensures that the needle is not within a vessel as it can precipitate arrhythmias.
- Avoid using lidocaine with adrenaline, in patients with hypertension, history of Raynaud's phenomenon, peripheral vascular disease, vasospasm, history of thromboembolism, history of thromboangitis obliterans.
- On anesthetizing oral mucosa, ingestion of food has to be avoided for 1 hour as swallowing is impaired and hence can lead to aspiration. Also, there is a risk of tongue bite.
- Whenever mixture of LAA are used, it should be presumed that the toxicities are additive.[7,123,124]

OTHER USES OF LAA

Neuropathic Pain

Intravenous infusion of lidocaine alone or with oral sodium channel blockers has been used successfully in the treatment of neuropathic pain. Interestingly, even though they reduce the neuropathic pain, normal pain and other sensations are unaffected. This could be due to higher doses of anesthetic required to block the normal sensation in comparison to neuropathic pain. Often, the pain relief stays for duration much longer than the elimination t½ of that LAA.

High dose topical capsaicin 8% is better than low dose preparations (0.025%, 0.075%) in the treatment of PHN. However, it is 2nd or 3rd line option for treating PHN.[125]

Premature Ejaculation

As penile hypersensitivity has been hypothesized to be a cause for premature ejaculation, topical anesthesia is used to reduce neuronal excitability thus delaying ejaculation.[96] Lidocaine spray, EMLA, topical eutectic mixture for premature ejaculation (TEMPE) containing lidocaine and prilocaine spray and dyclonine/alprostadil (latter is a vasodilator) cream have been used in its treatment.[126]

Assessment of Polyneuropathy

As small nerves are affected much earlier in diabetic neuropathy, EMLA which effectively inhibit these small fibers has been used to check for early polyneuropathy in diabetes mellitus. Stimulated skin wrinkling test is adopted for the same. Here the area to be tested is exposed to EMLA for 5–30 mins and the wrinkling of skin noted. Wrinkling is due to vasoconstriction mediated by post-ganglionic sympathetic innervation. The advantage of EMLA over water immersion is that, the response is more linear and sustained for 90 mins with former. This test can be used to check the nerve function in leprosy as well.[127]

Antibacterial Property of LAA

It is interesting to know that, some of the topical anesthetic agents have antibacterial properties. Lidocaine 2% showed significant reduction of colonies of *Staph aureus* and *Strept viridians* [90% ($p<0.01$) and 92% ($p<0.001$) respectively]. Clinically, there were no infections after intravitreal injections when subconjunctival lidocaine was infiltrated in comparison to other modalities of anesthesia used for same procedure.[128] Proparacaine, tetracaine also have shown inhibitory action on *Strept viridians* and proparacaine showed the lowest MIC amongst itself, tetracaine and lidocaine.[129]

Others

Continuous infusion of local anesthetic at the site of surgery is required for alleviation of postsurgical pain.[130] Topical anesthesia can be used for tuberculin skin testing without any risk of altered test result.[131] Pramoxine is used for its antipruritic property in many over-the-counter topical antipruritic and antihemorrhoids formulations.[132]

PREPROCEDURE PREPARATION

An anxiolytic administered before any procedure improves patient comfort and avoids occurrence of untoward reactions of patients like restlessness, variations in blood pressure. Midazolam is an ultra-short acting sedative of benzodiazepine group and has anxiolytic, sedative, anticonvulsant and muscle relaxant properties. Hence, it is extensively used in many day care procedures performed on children as well as adults. It is readily absorbed by any route of administration with peak plasma concentration occurring in 20–60 minutes. Midazolam is metabolized in liver and inhibits cytochrome P 250 3A4 enzyme complex potentiating lidocaine toxicity.[1] It has an elimination $t½$ of 2 hours. It is used in a dose of 0.25–0.5 mg/kg in infants less than 6 months and in children between 6 months to 6 years, up to 1 mg/kg stat dose. Toxicity leads to depression of cardiovascular system and CNS. Occasionally, paradoxical muscle excitation may occur. It should be cautiously used in patient with cardiac conditions, open angle glaucoma, myasthenia gravis and elderly individuals.[133]

LOCAL ANESTHETIC FAILURE

Infrequently, there are situations where local anesthesia does not work. This could be due to following factors:[7]

- Increased local blood flow leading to rapid clearance of the LAA.
- Local tissue acidosis (due to conditions like inflammation or infection) leading to enhanced ionization of LAA which retards diffusion of LAA across the axonal membrane.
- Local tissue edema, whereby, LAA has to traverse longer distance to diffuse into nerve membrane.
- Tachyphylaxis (discussed earlier).
- Genetic: some patients with Ehlers-Danlos syndrome show poor response to topical anesthesia.[134]

CONCLUSION

Local anesthesia is an integral part of dermatosurgery and cosmetic surgery. However, LAA can give rise to some life threatening side effects much graver than the risk of procedure itself. Hence, performing surgeons need to be vigilant of the same to render better care to patients and clients.

REFERENCES

1. Huether MJ, Brodland DG. Local anesthetics. In: Wolverton SE (Ed). Comprehensive Dermatologic Drug Therapy, 2nd edition. Philadelphia: Saunders Elsevier; 2007;825-49.
2. Katzung BG, White PF. Local anesthetics. In: Katzung BG, Masters SB, Trevor AJ (Eds). Basic and Clinical Pharmacology, 11th edition. New Delhi: Tata McGraw Hill Education Private Limited; 2009;439-50.
3. Haddox JD, Baumann PL. Local Anesthetics. In: Craig CR, Stitzel RE (Eds). Modern Pharmacology with Clinical Applications, 5th edition. USA: Little, Brown and Company (Inc.); 1997;347-53.
4. Wheeler DE. Bronchography using dyclonine hydrochloride anesthesia (4 N-butoxy-beta-piperidino-propiophenone-hydrochloride). Dis Chest. 1960;37:193-5.
5. Caterall WA, Mackie K. Local anesthetics. In: Brunton LL, Chabner BA, Knollman BC (Eds). Goodman & Gilman's The Pharmacological Basis of Therapeutics, 12th edition. USA: McGraw-Hill; 2011;565-82.
6. Local anesthetics and other drugs affecting sodium channels. In: Rang HP, Dale MM, Ritter JM, Flower RJ (Eds). Rang and Dale's Pharmacology, 6th edition. Philadelphia: Churchill Livingstone Elsevier; 2007;638-44.
7. Berde CB, Strichartz GR. Local anesthetics. In: Miller RD, Eriksson LI, Fleisher LA, Wiener-Kronish JP, Young WL (Eds). Miller's Anesthesia, 7th edition. Philadelphia: Churchill Livingstone Elsevier; 2010;913-39.
8. Johns RA, DiFazio CA, Longnecker DE. Lidocaine constricts or dilates rat arterioles in a dose-dependent manner. Anesthesiol. 1985;62:141-4.
9. Kumar S, Kumar S, Ganesamoni R, et al. Dimethyl sulfoxide prospective randomized study to compare the efficacy of cutaneous anesthesia in shock wave lithotripsy. Urol Res. 2011;39:181-3.
10. Guay J. Methemoglobinemia related to local anesthetics: a summary of 242 episodes. Anesth Analg. 2009;108:837-45.
11. Green SM, Rothrock SG, Gorchynski J. Validation of diphenhydramine as a dermal local anesthetic. Ann Emerg Med. 1994;23(6):1284-9.

12. Xia Y, Chen E, Tibbits DL, et al. Comparison of effects of lidocaine hydrochloride, buffered lidocaine, diphenhydramine, and normal saline after intradermal injection. J Clin Anesth. 2002;14(5):339-43.
13. Pavlidakey PG, Brodell EE, Helms SE. Diphenhydramine as an alternative local anesthetic agent. J Clin Aesthet Dermatol. 2009;2(10):37-40.
14. Chen A, Loquias EJ, Roshan R, et al. Safe Use of Subcutaneous Diphenhydramine in the Inpatient Hospice Unit. Am J Hosp Palliat Care. 2016 Sep 13. pii: 1049909116668160. [Epub ahead of print]
15. Pickett LE, Macdonald J. Injectable diphenhydramine used as anaesthetic for wide local excision with flap closure. J Cutan Med Surg. 2016 Dec 5. pii: 1203475416681760. [Epub ahead of print]
16. Kouba DJ, LoPiccolo MC, Alam M, et al. Guidelines for the use of local anesthesia in office-based dermatologic surgery. J Am Acad Dermatol. 2016;74(6):1201-19.
17. Leffler A, Reckzeh J, Nau C. Block of sensory neuronal Na+ channels by the secreolytic ambroxol is associated with an interaction with local anesthetic binding sites. Eur J Pharmacol. 2010;630(1-3):19-28.
18. Kern KU, Weiser T. Topical ambroxol for the treatment of neuropathic pain. An initial clinical observation. Schmerz. 2015;29 (Suppl 3):S89-96.
19. Orhan ME, Yüksel U, Bilgin F, Doğrul A. Comparison of the local anesthetic effects of chlorpheniramine, midazolam, lidocaine, and normal saline after intradermal injection. Med Sci Monit. 2007;13(4):PI7-11.
20. Bartfield JM, Jandreau SW, Raccio-Robak N. Randomized trial of diphenhydramine versus benzyl alcohol with epinephrine as an alternative to lidocaine local anesthesia. Ann Emerg Med. 1998;32(6):650-4.
21. Wilson L, Martin S. Benzyl alcohol as an alternative local anesthetic. Ann Emerg Med. 1999 May;33(5):495-9.
22. Mysore V, Nischal KC. Guidelines for administration of local anesthesia for dermatosurgery and cosmetic dermatology procedures. Indian J Dermatol Venereol Leprol [serial online]. 2009 [cited 2012 Jan 18];75:68-75.
23. Bjerring P, Arendt-Nielsen L. Depth and duration of skin analgesia to needle insertion after topical application of EMLA. Br J Anaesth. 1990;64:173-7.
24. Vickers ER, Marzbani N, Gerzina TM, et al. Pharmacokinetics of EMLA cream 5% application to oral mucosa. Anesth Prog. 1997;44:32-7.
25. Sohmer B, Bryson GL, Bencze S, et al. EMLA cream is an effective topical anesthetic for bronchoscopy. Can Respir J. 2004;11:587-8.
26. Barcohana N, Duperon DF, Yashar M. The relationship of application time to EMLA efficacy. J Dent Child (Chic.). 2003;70:51-4.
27. Bernardi M, Secco F, Benech A. Anesthetic efficacy of an eutectic mixture of lidocaine and prilocaine (EMLA) on the oral mucosa: prospective double-blind study with a placebo. Minerva Stomatol. 1999;48:39-43.
28. Al-Melh MA, Andersson L. Comparison of topical anesthetics (EMLA/Oraqix vs. benzocaine) on pain experienced during palatal needle injection. Oral Surg Oral Med Oral Pathol Oral Radiol Endod. 2007;103:e16-20.
29. McMillan AS, Walshaw D, Meechan JG. The efficacy of EMLA and 5% lignocaine gel for anaesthesia of human gingival mucosa. Br J Oral Maxillofac Surg. 2000;38:58-61.
30. Rylander E, Sjöberg I, Lillieborg S, et al. Local anesthesia of the genital mucosa with a lidocaine/prilocaine cream (EMLA) for laser treatment of condylomata acuminata: a placebo-controlled study. Obstet Gynecol. 1990;75:302-6.
31. Brodland DG, Huether MJ. Local anesthetics. In: Wolverton SE (Ed). Comprehensive Dermatologic Drug Therapy. Philadelphia: WB Saunders Company; 2001;736-66.
32. Package insert Prilox™. Neon Labs, India.
33. Smith GA, Strausbaugh SD, Harbeck-Weber C, et al. Prilocaine-phenylephrine and bupivacaine-phenylephrine topical anesthetics compared with tetracaine-adrenaline-cocaine during repair of lacerations. Am J Emerg Med. 1998;16:121-4.
34. Smith GA, Strausbaugh SD, Harbeck-Weber C, et al. New non-cocaine-containing topical anesthetics compared with tetracaine-adrenaline-cocaine during repair of lacerations. Pediatrics. 1997;100:825-30.
35. Zink KA, Mayberry JC, Peck EG, et al. Lidocaine patches reduce pain in trauma patients with rib fractures. Am Surg. 2011;77:438-42.
36. Agarwal A, Gautam S, Gupta D, et al. Transdermal diclofenac patch vs eutectic mixture of local anesthetics for venous cannulation pain. Can J Anaesth. 2007;54:196-200.
37. Traber J, Held U, Signer M, et al. Analgesic efficacy of equimolar 50% nitrous oxide/oxygen gas premix (Kalinox®) as compared with a 5% eutectic mixture of lidocaine/prilocaine (EMLA®) in chronic leg ulcer debridement. Int Wound J. 2016 Aug 8. doi: 10.1111/iwj.12652. [Epub ahead of print]
38. Park SW, Oh TS, Choi JW. Topical EMLA Cream as a Pretreatment for Facial Lacerations. Arch Plast Surg. 2015;42(1):28-33.
39. Purcell A, Marshall A, King J, et al. Eutectic mixture of local anaesthetics (EMLA) 5% cream as a primary dressing on a painful lower leg ulcer. J Wound Care. 2012;21(7):309-10, 312, 314.
40. Punyaratabandhu P, Wanitphakdeedecha R, Pattanaprichakul P, et al. The effect of pre-operative topical anaesthetic cream on the ablative width and coagulative depth of ablative fractional resurfacing laser. Lasers Med Sci. 2016 Nov 24. [Epub ahead of print]
41. Tollan CJ, MacLaren W, Mackay IR. Topical anaesthetic effects on skin vasculature with potential implications for laser treatment. Lasers Med Sci. 2016;31(4):611-7.
42. Baron R, Allegri M, Correa-Illanes G, et al. The 5% lidocaine-medicated plaster: its inclusion in international treatment guidelines for treating localized neuropathic pain, and clinical evidence Pain Ther. 2016;5(2):149-69. Epub 2016 Nov 7. Supporting its Use.
43. Wallace MS, Ridgeway B, Jun E, et al. Topical delivery of lidocaine in healthy volunteers by electroporation, electroincorporation, or iontophoresis: an evaluation of skin anesthesia. Reg Anesth Pain Med. 2001;26(3):229-38.
44. Friedman PM, Mafong EA, Friedman ES, Geronemus RG. Topical anesthetics update: EMLA and beyond. Dermatol Surg. 2001;27(12):1019-26.
45. Thomson CJ, Lalonde DH. Randomized double-blind comparison of duration of anesthesia among three commonly with lignocaineversuseutecticmixtureoflocal anesthetics: used agents in digital nerve block. Plast Reconstr Surg. 2006;118:429-32.

46. Sanchez JP, Balingit JS, McCutcheon R, et al (Eds). Local and Regional Anesthetic Blocks Made Simple. Philippines: Nazarene Printers; 2002.
47. Luck L, Longley BJ. Cutaneous cryoanesthesia does not affect histopathology of biopsy specimens. Cutis. 1999;64:225-6.
48. Campbell JR, Maestrello CL, Campbell RL. Allergic response to metabisulfite in lidocaine anesthetic solution. Anesth Prog. 2001;48:21-6.
49. Patel R, Halem M, Zaiac M. The combined use of forced cold air and topical anesthetic cream for analgesia during the treatment of palmar hyperhydrosis with botulinum toxin injections. J Drugs Dermatol. 2009;8:948-51.
50. Sari E, Sandikci MM, Bakar B, et al. Estimated beginning time of local anesthesia effectiveness in forced cold air application: A preliminary study. J Cosmet Laser Ther. 2016;18(1):22-4.
51. Irkoren S1, Ozkan HS, Karaca H. A clinical comparison of EMLA cream and ethyl chloride spray application for pain relief of forehead botulinum toxin injection. Ann Plast Surg. 2015 Sep;75(3):272-4.
52. Mutalik S. How to make local anesthesia less painful? J Cut Aesth Surg. 2008;1:37-8.
53. Radha Atal-Shah. Anaesthesia in dermatosurgery. In: Satish S. Textbook of Dermatosurgery and Cosmetology, 2nd edition. Mumbai: ASCAD; 2005;53-64.
54. Christoph RA, Buchanan L, Begalla K, et al. Pain reduction in local anesthetic administration through pH buffering. Ann Emerg Med. 1988;17:117-20.
55. Hruza GJ. Anesthesia. In: Bolognia JL, Jorizzo FL, Rapini RP (Eds). Dermatology. New York: Elsevier Science; 2003; 2233-42.
56. Stewart JH, Cole GW, Klein JA. Neutralized lidocaine with epinephrine for local anesthesia. J Dermatol Surg Oncol. 1989;66:572-4.
57. Stewart JH, Chinn SE, Cole GW, et al. Neutralized lidocaine with epinephrine for local anesthesia. J Dermatol Surg Oncol. 1990;16:842-5.
58. Grekin RC, Auletta MJ. Local anesthesia in dermatologic surgery. J Am Acad Dermatol. 1988;19:599-614.
59. Dinehart SM. Topical, local, regional anesthesia. In: Wheeland R (Ed). Cutaneous Surgery. Philadelphia: WB Saunders; 1994;102-12.
60. Hogan ME, vanderVaart S, Perampaladas K, et al. Systematic review and meta-analysis of the effect of warming local anesthetics on injection pain. Ann Emerg Med. 2011;58(1):86-98.e1
61. Fosko SW, Gibney MD, Harrison B. Repetitive pinching of the skin during lidocaine infiltration reduces patient discomfort. J Am Acad Dermatol. 1998;39:74-8.
62. Palmon SC, Lloyd AT, Kirsch JR. The effect of needle gauge and lidocaine pH on pain during intradermal injection. Anesth Analg. 1998;86:379-81.
63. Tian T, Luo Y, Jiang T, et al. Clinical effect of ablative fractional laser-assisted topical anesthesia on human skin: A randomized pilot study. J Cosmet Laser Ther. 2016;18(7):409-12.
64. Meesters AA, Bakker MM, de Rie MA, et al. Fractional CO_2 laser assisted delivery of topical anesthetics: A randomized controlled pilot study. Lasers Surg Med. 2016;48(2):208-11.
65. Golan J, Hai N. JetPeel: a new technology for facial rejuvenation. Ann Plast Surg. 2005;54(4):369-74.
66. Iannitti T, Palmieri B, Aspiro A, et al. A preliminary study of painless and effective transdermal botulinum toxin A delivery by jet nebulization for treatment of primary hyperhidrosis. Drug Des Devel Ther. 2014;8:931-5.
67. Hofmann GA, Rustrum WV, Suder KS. Electro-incorporation of microcarriers as a method for the transdermal delivery of large molecules. Bioelectrochemistry and Bioenergetics. 1995;38:209-22.
68. Wallace MS, Ridgeway B, Jun E, et al. Topical delivery of lidocaine in healthy volunteers by electroporation, electroincorporation, or iontophoresis: an evaluation of skin anesthesia. Reg Anesth Pain Med. 2001;26(3):229-38.
69. Kumar M, Chawla R, Goyal M. Topical anesthesia. J Anaesthesiol Clin Pharmacol. 2015;31(4):450-6.
70. Nayak A, Das DB. Potential of biodegradable microneedles as a transdermal delivery vehicle for lidocaine. Biotechnol Lett. 2013;35(9):1351-63.
71. Baek SH, Shin JH, Kim YC. Drug-coated microneedles for rapid and painless local anesthesia. Biomed Microdevices. 2017;19(1):2.
72. Wang J, Zhang L, Chi H, et al. An alternative choice of lidocaine-loaded liposomes: lidocaine-loaded lipid-polymer hybrid nanoparticles for local anesthetic therapy. Drug Deliv. 2016;23(4):1254-60.
73. Lauterbach A, Müller-Goymann CC. Applications and limitations of lipid nanoparticles in dermal and transdermal drug delivery via the follicular route. Eur J Pharm Biopharm. 2015;97(Pt A):152-63.
74. Gagliano-Jucá T, Castelli MR, Mendes GD, et al. Pharmacokinetic and pharmacodynamic evaluation of a nanotechnological topical formulation of lidocaine/prilocaine (nanorap) in healthy volunteers. Ther Drug Monit. 2015;37(3):362-8.
75. Remy M, Pinter F, Nentwich MM, et al. Efficacy and safety of hyaluronidase 75 IU as an adjuvant to mepivacaine for retrobulbar anesthesia in cataract surgery. J Cataract Refract Surg. 2008;34:1966-9.
76. Wohlrab J, Finke R, Franke WG, et al. Clinical trial for safety evaluation of hyaluronidase as diffusion enhancing adjuvant for infiltration analgesia of skin with lidocaine. Dermatol Surg. 2012;38:91-6.
77. Schulenburg HE, Sri-Chandana C, Lyons G, et al. Hyaluronidase reduces local anaesthetic volumes for sub-Tenon's anaesthesia. Br J Anaesth. 2007;99:717-20.
78. Nevarre DR, Tzarnas CD. The effects of hyaluronidase on the efficacy and on the pain of administration of 1% lidocaine. Plast Reconstr Surg. 1998;101:365-9.
79. Chassard D, Berrada K, Boulétreau P. Alkalinization of local anesthetics: theoretically justified but clinically useless. Can J Anaesth. 1996;43:384-93.
80. Chin KJ, Handoll HH. Single, double or multiple-injection techniques for axillary brachial plexus block for hand, wrist or forearm surgery in adults. Cochrane Database Syst Rev. 2011;6:CD003842.
81. Kaplan JA, Miller ED, Gallagher EG. Postoperative analgesia for thoracotomy patients. Anaesth Analg. 1975;54:773-7.
82. Sindjelic RP, Vlajkovic GP, Davidovic LB, et al. The addition of fentanyl to local anesthetics affects the quality and duration of cervical plexus block: a randomized, controlled trial. Anesth Analg. 2010;111:234-7.
83. Häfner HM, Röcken M, Breuninger H. Epinephrine-supplemented local anesthetics for ear and nose surgery: clinical use without complications in more than 10,000 surgical procedures. J Dtsch Dermatol Ges. 2005;3:195-9.

84. Häfner HM, Schmid U, Moehrle M, et al. Changes in acral blood flux under local application of ropivacaine and lidocaine with and without an adrenaline additive: a double-blind, randomized, placebo-controlled study. Clin Hemorheol Microcirc. 2008;38:279-88.
85. Lalonde D, Bell M, Benoit P, et al. A multicenter prospective study of 3,110 consecutive cases of elective epinephrine use in the fingers and hand: the Dalhousie Project clinical phase. J Hand Surg Am. 2005;30:1061-7.
86. Thomson CJ, Lalonde DH, Denkler KA, et al. A critical look at the evidence for and against elective epinephrine use in the finger. Plast Reconstr Surg. 2007;119:260-6.
87. Krunic AL, Wang LC, Soltani K, et al. Digital anesthesia with epinephrine: an old myth revisited. J Am Acad Dermatol. 2004;51:755-9.
88. Wilhelmi BJ, Blackwell SJ, Miller JH, et al. Do not use epinephrine in digital blocks: myth or truth? Plast Reconstr Surg. 2001;107:393-7.
89. Son HW, Park SH, Cho HO, et al. Epinephrine-induced lactic acidosis in orthognathic surgery: a report of two cases. J Korean Assoc Oral Maxillofac Surg. 2016;42(5):295-300.
90. Perez-Castro R, Patel S, Garavito-Aguilar ZV, et al. Cytotoxicity of local anesthetics in human neuronal cells. Anesth Analg. 2009;108:997-1007.
91. Yang S, Abrahams MS, Hurn PD, et al. Local anesthetic Schwann cell toxicity is time and concentration dependent. Reg Anesth Pain Med. 2011;36:444-51.
92. Gall H, Kaufmann R, Kalveram CM. Adverse reactions to local anesthetics: Analysis of 197 cases. J Allergy Clin Immunol. 1996;97:933-7.
93. Swanson JG. Assessment of allergy to local anesthetic. Ann Emerg Med. 1983;12:316-8.
94. Phillips JF, Yates AB, Deshazo RD. Approach to patients with suspected hypersensitivity to local anesthetics. Am J Med Sci. 2007;334:190-6.
95. Eggleston ST, Lush LW. Understanding allergic reactions to local anesthetics. Ann Pharmacother. 1996;30:851-7.
96. Boren E, Teuber SS, Naguwa SM, et al. A critical review of local anesthetic sensitivity. Clin Rev Allergy Immunol. 2007;32:119-28.
97. Berkun Y, Ben-Zvi A, Levy Y, et al. Evaluation of adverse reactions to local anesthetics: experience with 236 patients. Ann Allergy Asthma Immunol. 2003;91:342-5.
98. Macy E. Local anesthetic adverse reaction evaluations: The role of the allergist. Annals Allergy Clin Immunol. 2003;91:319-20.
99. González-Delgado P, Antón R, Soriano V, et al. Cross-Reactivity among local anesthetics in a case of allergy amide-type to mepivacaine. J Investig Allergol Clin Immunol. 2006;16:311-3.
100. Caron AB. Allergy to multiple local anesthetics. Allergy Asthma Proc. 2007;28:600-1.
101. Wobser M, Gaigl Z, Trautmann A. The concept of "compartment allergy": prilocaine injected into different skin layers. Allergy Asthma Clin Immunol. 2011;7:7.
102. Huang W, Vidimos A. Topical anesthetics in dermatology. J Am Acad Dermatol. 2000;43:286-98.
103. García F, Iparraguirre A, Blanco J, et al. Contact dermatitis from prilocaine with cross-sensitivity to pramocaine and bupivacaine. Contact Dermatitis. 2007;56:120-1.
104. Tran AN, Koo JY. Risk of systemic toxicity with topical lidocaine/prilocaine: a review. J Drugs Dermatol. 2014;13(9):1118-22.
105. El-Boghdadly K, Chin KJ. Local anesthetic systemic toxicity: Continuing Professional Development. Can J Anaesth. 2016;63(3):330-49.
106. Di Gregorio G, Neal JM, Rosenquist RW, et al. Clinical presentation of local anesthetic systemic toxicity: a review of published cases, 1979 to 2009. Reg Anesth Pain Med. 2010;35(2):181-7.
107. Checklist for Treatment of Local Anesthetic Systemic Toxicity. Available on https://www.asra.com/content/documents/asra_last_checklist.2011.pdf
108. Krunic AL, Wang LC, Soltani K, et al. Digital anesthesia with epinephrine: an old myth revisited. J Am Acad Dermatol. 2004;51:755-9.
109. Tasch MD, Butterworth JF. Adverse reactions to local anesthetics. In: Lobata EB, Gravenstein N, Kirby RR (Eds). Complications in Anesthesiology. Philadelphia: Lippincott Williams & Wilkins; 2008;865-78.
110. Kamata M, Tada Y, Yazawa N, et al. Drug fever caused by eutectic mixture of local anesthetic cream. J Investig Allergol Clin Immunol. 2011;21(5):421.
111. Kieliszak CR, Griffin JR, Pollinger TH, et al. Pseudo-bullous dermatosis induced by topical anesthetic agent-clues to this localized toxic reaction. Am J Dermatopathol. 2017;39(2):e19-e22.
112. Lewis FM, Agarwal A, Neill SM, et al. The spectrum of histopathologic patterns secondary to the topical application of EMLA® on vulvar epithelium: clinicopathological correlation in three cases. J Cutan Pathol. 2013;40(8):708-13.
113. Pérez-Pérez LC, Fernández-Redondo V, Ginarte-Val M, et al. Allergic contact dermatitis from EMLA cream in a hemodialyzed patient. Dermatitis. 2006;17:85-7.
114. Waton J, Boulanger A, Trechot PH, et al. Contact urticaria from Emla cream. Contact Dermatitis. 2004;51:284-7.
115. Cervigón I, Torres-Iglesias LM, Palomo A. Purpura after application of a eutectic mixture of local anesthetic. Actas Dermosifiliogr. 2008;99:499-500.
116. Stahl M, Meyer C, Haas E, et al. Leg ulcer progression caused by topical anesthesia with EMLA cream. J Dtsch Dermatol Ges. 2008;6:566-8.
117. Parikh M, Kwon YH. Vision loss after inadvertent corneal perforation during lid anesthesia. Ophthal Plast Reconstr Surg. 2011;27:e141-2.
118. Bartlett D. Intravenous lipids: antidotal therapy for drug overdose and toxic effects of local anesthetics. Crit Care Nurse. 2014;34(5):62-6; quiz 67.
119. Nadrowitz F, Stoetzer C, Foadi N, et al. Leffler A. The distinct effects of lipid emulsions used for "lipid resuscitation" on gating and bupivacaine-induced inhibition of the cardiac sodium channel Nav1.5. Anesth Analg. 2013;117(5):1101-8.
120. Cao D, Heard K, Foran M, et al. Intravenous lipid emulsion in the emergency department: a systematic review of recent literature. J Emerg Med. 2015;48(3):387-97.
121. Gosselin S, Hoegberg LC, Hoffman RS, et al. Evidence-based recommendations on the use of intravenous lipid emulsion therapy in poisoning. Clin Toxicol (Phila). 2016;54(10):899-923.
122. Levine M, Hoffman RS, Lavergne V, et al. Systematic review of the effect of intravenous lipid emulsion therapy for non-local anesthetics toxicity. Clin Toxicol (Phila). 2016;54(3):194-221.
123. Kyttä J, Heavner JE, Badgwell JM, et al. Cardiovascular and central nervous system effects of co-administered lidocaine and bupivacaine in piglets. Reg Anesth. 1991;16:89-94.

124. Munson ES, Paul WL, Embro WJ. Central nervous-system toxicity of local anesthetic mixtures in monkeys. Anesthesiol. 1977;46:179-83.
125. Laklouk M, Baranidharan G. Profile of the capsaicin 8% patch for the management of neuropathic pain associated with postherpetic neuralgia: safety, efficacy, and patient acceptability. Patient Prefer Adherence. 2016;10:1913-8.
126. Linton KD, Wylie KR. Recent advances in the treatment of premature ejaculation. Drug Des Devel Ther. 2010;18:1-6.
127. Ping Ng KW, Ong JJ, Nyein Nyein TD, et al. EMLA-induced skin wrinkling for the detection of diabetic neuropathy. Front Neurol. 2013;4:126.
128. Tustin A, Kim SJ, Chomsky A, et al. Antibacterial properties of 2% lidocaine and reduced rate of endophthalmitis after intravitreal injection. Retina. 2014;34(5):935-42.
129. Reynolds MM, Greenwood-Quaintance KE, Patel R, et al. Selected antimicrobial activity of topical ophthalmic anesthetics. Transl Vis Sci Technol. 2016;5(4):2.
130. Fustran Guerrero N, Dalmau Llitjós A, Sabaté Pes A. Continuous infusion of local anesthetic at the site of the abdominal surgical wound for postoperative analgesia: a systematic review. Rev Esp Anestesiol Reanim. 2011;58: 337-44.
131. Beydon N, Lebras MN, de Lauzanne A, et al. Randomized study of the effect of topical anesthesia on tuberculin skin test reaction size in children. Pediatr Infect Dis J. 2010;29:180-2.
132. Pramoxine. (online). Last updated on 08 March 2017. Available from https://medlineplus.gov/druginfo/meds/a682429.html [Last accessed on 24 March 2017]
133. Midazolam information from DrugsUpdate. Available from http://www.drugsupdate.com/generic/view/312. [Last accessed 24 March 2017].
134. Arendt-Nielsen L, Kaalund S, Bjerring P, et al. Insufficient effect of local analgesics in Ehlers Danlos type III patients (connective tissue disorder). Acta Anaesthesiol Scand. 1990;34:358-61.

Chapter 13

Tips and Tricks for Using Local Anesthesia for Dermatosurgical Procedures

Dhepe Niteen V

Key Messages

- Local anesthesia is widely used in dermatosurgery and esthetic surgery
- Injection of local anesthetic agents can be painful for the patient and with a few tips and tricks, this discomfort can be decreased
- Local anesthesia techniques such as tumescent anesthesia and nerve block anesthesia have various newer indications nowadays, that help in carrying out even painful invasive dermatosurgery procedures without any discomfort

INTRODUCTION

Most dermatosurgical procedures are amenable to various depths of local anesthesia. This is not only comfortable but have extraordinary safety profile making most dermatosurgical procedure an office-based, walk-in-walk-out procedures. Here are some tips and tricks on how local anesthesia can be made safer and more effective (Box 1).

Box 1: Types of local anesthesia for cosmetic procedures.

- Non-pharmacological anesthesia
  - Vocal anesthesia
  - Tactile or vibration anesthesia
- Topical anesthesia: Needleless anesthesia techniques
  - Creams
  - Iontophoresis, sonophoresis, microporation
- Cold anesthesia
  - Cryogens
- Fractional drug delivery
- Infiltration anesthesia
  - Tips to make infiltration less painful
  - Nerve blocks
- Tumescent local anesthesia
  - Tips for liposuction
  - Non-liposuction indications of tumescence
- Tips and tricks in special situation
  - Hair transplantation
  - Laser hair reduction
  - Tattoo removal
  - Full-face resurfacing
  - Hyperhidrosis
  - Lips surgery
  - Extensive area vitiligo surgery

NON-PHARMACOLOGICAL ANESTHESIA

Vocal Anesthesia

Make the patient comfortable. Do not rush to the procedure immediately. Start a friendly talk to distract his attention. Hold the patient hands gently. Ask them to focus on breath, count while inspiration and expiration.[1]

Tactile or Vibration Anesthesia[2]

Application of a vibrator will reduce the pain sensitivity. Higher the amplitude, lesser the pain perception. Apply the vibrator on site of treatment before starting and in adjacent proximal area during treatment. You can use a handheld neck or back massager as a handy tool.

TOPICAL ANESTHESIA: NEEDLELESS ANESTHESIA TECHNIQUES

Topical Creams of Anesthesia

- An eutectic mixture of local anesthetics (EMLA) (lidocaine and/or prilocaine), has to be applied for a minimum of 45 minutes to 2 hours according to the composition of the EMLA. It has to be applied under occlusion for its optimum effect.

- Effect of EMLA lasts for 10–15 minutes maximum after cream removal. So aim at starting procedure immediately after occlusion removal. It is a wise practice to shave, paint and sterilize the area before applying the cream. Also remove the cream from only half the part applied to start the procedure and remaining whenever required.
- *Cling film occlusion*: Cling film is used to wrap food items which can very conveniently be used as occlusion method. Entire face is covered with apertures made for nose and mouth.
- The area can be treated with microdermabrasion or a very light dose of fractional lasers to enhance penetration. This will enhance the penetration and occlusion time which will be reduced to as early as 5–10 minutes.[3]

Iontophoresis[4]/Sonophoresis[5]/ Microporation

Electricity in iontophoresis and sound waves in sonophoresis are used to enhance penetration of ions through the skin via sweat glands, hair follicles and sebaceous glands.

Various solutions preferably in ionic form can be used with iontophoresis and sonophoresis. Vitamin C infusion with this technique after microdermabrasion is the most popular cosmetic indication.[6,7]

Cold Anesthesia

Cryogens

- Anesthetic sprays, such as fluoroethyl or eythlene chloride, provide effective topical anesthesia for small lesions that are completely intraepidermal, for example, molluscum contagiosum.[8]
- These sprays produce a skin frost. Approximately for 10–12 seconds, anesthesia is applied at the procedure area after which the ambient skin temperature returns back to normal and anesthesia disappears.
- Periocular zone area and inhalation should be avoided.[8]

FRACTIONAL DRUG DELIVERY

- It was observed during a research in 2003 that one light pass of the erbium: Yttrium aluminum garnet (Er:YAG) laser works by altering integrity of the stratum corneum and increases transcutaneous permeation of lidocaine.[9]
- Fractional CO_2 laser created deep vertical still narrow channels of ablation into skin which delivered a drug, methyl 5-aminolevulinate (MAL) with full thickness uniform distribution.[8]
- A very light dose of fractional laser is applied before application of topical creams. This may enhance penetration and reduce application time to 5–10 minutes.[3]
- Full-face CO_2 laser resurfacing is a quiet painful procedure. Applying 2% lignocaine diluted in water to 1:4 and is used to sprinkle after each pass of fractional laser will subsequently pass less painful (author's technique).
- Use of *ultrasound pull and push waves*. A novel device "Legato II" by Alma used ultrasound waves to push the solution forms through fractional channels to have enhanced and deeper penetration.
- Penetration enhancement techniques to be used within 15–30 minutes of fractional laser.
- Recent studies have shown that these channels remain patent only for couple of minutes and they are filled with fibrin clot thereafter.

INFILTRATION ANESTHESIA[10]

- With intradermal injections, the anesthesia is almost immediate, stays longer but it is usually painful, while with injection into the subcutaneous tissue, the anesthesia is usually delayed but has a shorter duration.
- The pain during a local anesthetic (LA) injection is due to the acidic pH of the solution. It can be minimized by addition of a 1:10 dilution of sodium bicarbonate (8.4%) solution to the anesthesia solution.
- Speed of injection is another factor determining pain through compression of nerve endings. So slow and steady infiltration is recommended to avoid pain.
- *A field or ring block* is a variation of infiltration anesthesia. The anesthetic injections are given all around the lesion. Both superficial and deep planes are to be infiltrated. Author advised deep plane infiltration first then superficial one to make it comfortable. This will limit volume of anesthesia fluid infiltrated into operative field avoiding distortion of anatomy.

Nerve Blocks[10]

- If the local anesthetic solution is infiltrated around the main nerve trunk, achieving loss of sensation in the entire area of sensory distribution of that particular nerve.
- The commonly employed nerve blocks are for the digits and for the central face, because both areas are painful to anesthetize using local infiltration.
- To prevent intravascular injection of neighboring veins and arteries, frequent aspirations are recommended.
- Author's technique: Locate nerve by palpation, infiltrate a little in dermis first, wait for few minutes to start numbing effect. Then inject deep till the nerve right on periosteum slowly.

Digital Nerve Block[10]

Two methods exist for achieving a digital block

1. Ring block (more common)
2. Metacarpal or metatarsal head technique

Ring Block

- Enter the dorsolateral margin of the finger or the toe, at the level of webspace. Use 26 gauge short needle and preferably plain lignocaine.
- Enter at 3 o'clock and 9 o'clock position on digit infiltrate deep, then move the needle dorsally towards 12 o'clock to inject and then withdraw the needle and reroute to palmar surface, i.e. toward 6 o'clock.
- Avoid injecting too much of the fluid as not adrenaline but the pressure due to excess volume is more frequent cause of ischemia and digital necrosis.

Metacarpal or Metatarsal Head Technique

- Palpate the heads of the metacarpals or metatarsals, inject from dorsal side right there perpendicular to the skin, till you reach the subcutaneous level just below plantar surface.
- This blocks the digital nerves right before entering the digits.
- Slow infiltration, plain lignocaine and frequent aspiration will ensure safety preventing ischemia.

Reducing the Pain of Local Anesthesia[10]

- Reducing the needle prick pain[11]
  - Talk to patient, explain what to expect
  - Sometimes mild sedation could be used
  - Use EMLA cream on site of needle pricks
  - Use as small gauge needle as possible
  - Long-acting LA agent for longer procedure
  - Insert needle slowly, inject slowly a little quantity, reinject from already injected area
- Reducing the pain associated with tissue distension
  - Inject slowly
  - Injecting into subcutaneous fat
  - Inject deep layer first then superficial
- Reducing the pain due to tissue irritation
  - Acidic pH of LA irritates the nerve endings causing pain
  - Buffer the LA solution with sodium bicarbonate to elevate the pH of LA fluid to tissue fluid.[12]

TUMESCENT LOCAL ANESTHESIA[13,14]

This technique of local anesthesia is most popularly used during liposuction. It is also used during various dermatosurgical procedures. It involves the injection of LA diluted in very high volumes of normal saline (NS) or RL in combination with adrenaline and other agents. The plasma levels of LA usually peak 8–12 hours after infiltration. It is interesting to note that maximum safe dose of lignocaine in LA is 3–5 mg/kg but in tumescent technique the safe dose is 55 mg/kg, according to the American Academy of Dermatology (AAD) guidelines on liposuction.

Tumescence Infiltration Technique

- Small infiltration at sites of needle or cannula entry
- Infiltrate with needle or cannula
- Deep infiltration first then superficial
- Pallor and turgor of tissue is desired end-point.

Discomfort during the infusion may be due to the following:
- High infusion rate
- Rapidly advancing an infusing cannula which can be avoided by initiating infusion with needle prior to using infusion cannula.

Tips for Liposuction

- Tumescent technique is *gold standard*
- Tumescent anesthesia should not be combined with other forms of anesthesia such as intravenous or general anesthesia
- Concentrations of lignocaine and adrenaline varies from body region to region.

Non-liposuction Indications of Tumescence

- It can be used in all types of dermatological surgery involving larger operating area.
- Excision of large melanocytic nevus.
- In extensive keloid treatment, tumescence will help in avoiding complications of general anesthesia and make a painful procedure like SCAAR FX laser treatment painless.
- In laser sweat ablation (LSA), tumescence technique not only makes it a painless procedure but also separates the deeper layer of vascular bundle from the operative field in axillary area.

TIPS AND TRICKS IN SPECIAL SITUATIONS

Hair Transplantation[15]

- Local anesthetic during strip removal: Inject 1 cm below lower margin of the strip. The occipital scalp is innervated by cervical nerves traveling from below.
- Zigzag technique (Dr Vasa technique, author's personal communication). Inject at one point perpendicular to skin, inject 0.5–1 mL. Withdraw the needle till dermis then reroutes at 45° again, inject 1 mL. Wait for 2 minutes. Inject 1 cm lateral vertically through already numb area, reroute at 45° laterally. This will give virtually painless picks if sufficient time is invested before each prick.

Tumescent anesthesia and nerve blocks are used in recipient area.

Body Hair Transplant[16]

- Compared with scalp donor, body donor areas are larger and hence diluted lignociane solutions are used.
- Dosage of lignociane used should be monitored to avoid toxicity.

Laser Hair Reduction[17]

- *Cooling:* Ice cooling before starting the procedures
- During the procedure using forced cooled air (Zimmer Cryo) helps in minimizing the pain
- *Postprocedure ice cooling:* For very apprehensive patients, topical anesthetic cream may be used.

Tattoo Removal

Tumescent technique can be considered in tattoo removal of large area.

Three-tier Anesthesia for Full-face Resurfacing (Author's Technique)[18]

- Topical EMLA at points of nerve blocks and sites of needle pricks of tumescent anesthesia
- Small quantity infiltration of tumescent fluid at EMLA applied sites and wait for couple of minutes
- Inject large volume of tumescent fluid on nerves and then on entire face
- 100–200 mL of tumescent fluid may be used over entire face slowly over 40–60 minutes.
- Typical composition of tumescent fluid on face: RL 500 mL, 1 mL adrenaline, 5 cc soda bicarbonate, lignocaine 40 mL, 10 mg of triamcinolone acetonide

Hyperhidrosis[19]

- Palmoplantar hyperhidrosis is treated with injection of botulinum toxin type A. The injection is often very painful.
- Mark the points of injections. Topical ice application for 10–30 seconds right on the points will reduce pain.
- Topical EMLA is useful. Wrist block or foot block is effective but needs experience.
- Axillary hyperhidrosis is treated with 1470 nm optical fiber laser and procedure is called laser sweat ablation. Tumescent anesthesia makes this procedure painless and outpatient. 100–200 mL of tumescent fluid infiltrated into each axilla will separate skin from underlying neurovascular structures.

Lip Surgery[20]

- Bilateral infraorbital block is used for numbing upper lips while bilateral mental blocks for lower lips. Topical EMLA is also used
- "Kiss the ice": Kissing ice cubes for 10–20 seconds just before injecting will reduce pain.

Extensive Area Vitiligo Surgery

In extensive area of vitiligo surgery, tumescent technique is used to eliminate the risk of general anesthesia.

PEARLS

- Local anesthesia makes cosmetic procedures safe, day care and more acceptable to the patients.
- Topical EMLA cream is the most common form of LA.
- Vocal anesthesia in form of reassurance to patient, talking with them will reduce dose of LA.
- Field blocks and nerve blocks are useful in selected areas on a smaller area.
- Tumescent local anesthesia is an interesting modification of local infiltration that numbs a large area of tissue for longer period with great safety.
- Local anesthesia is an art as well as science that need to be mastered for making cosmetic procedures painless and safe.

REFERENCES

1. Spiegel H, Spiegel D. Trance and Treatment Clinical Use of Hypnosis. New York: Basic Books; 1978.
2. Smith KC, Comite SL, Balasubramanian S, et al. Vibration anesthesia: A noninvasive method of reducing discomfort prior to dermatologic procedures. Dermatol Online J. 2004;10(2):1.
3. Baron ED, Harris L, Redpath WS, et al. Laser-assisted penetration of topical anesthetic in adults. Arch Dermatol. 2003;139(10):1288-90.
4. Green SS. Iontophoresis as a tool for anesthesia in dermatology surgery: an overview. Dermatol Surg. 2001;27: 1027-30.
5. Nassar A, Ghomey S, El Gohary Y, et al. Treatment of striae distensae with needling therapy versus microdermabrasion with sonophoresis. J Cosmet Laser Ther. 2016;18(6):330-4.
6. Lee GS. Intravenous vitamin C in the treatment of post-laser hyperpigmentation for melasma: A short report. J Cosmet Laser Ther. 2008;10(4):234-6.
7. Banga AK, Bose S, Ghosh TK. Iontophoresis and electroporation: comparisons and contrasts. Int J Pharm. 1999;179(1):1-19.
8. Scarborough D, Bisaccia E, Schwen W, et al. Anesthesia for the dermatologic surgeon. International Journal of Dermatology. 1989;2:629-37.
9. Baron ED, Harris L, Redpath WS, et al. Laser assisted penetration of topical anesthetics in adults. Arch Dermatol. 2003;139:1288-90.
10. Auletta MJ, Grekin RC. Clinical application of local anesthesia. In: Local Anesthesia for Dermatologic Surgery, 1st edition. New York: Churchill Livingstone; 1991. pp. 41-78

11. Auletta MJ, Grekin RC. Tricks to make the delivery of local anesthesia less painful. In: Local Anesthesia for Dermatologic Surgery, 1st edition. New York: Churchill Livingstone; 1991. pp. 79-84.
12. Skidmore RA, Patterson JD, Tomsick RS. Local anesthetics. Dermatol Surg. 1996;22:511-22.
13. Klein JA. Anesthesia for liposuction in dermatologic surgery. J Dermatol Surg Oncol. 1988;14:1124-32.
14. William Hanke C, Sattler G (Eds). Liposuction. New Delhi: Elsevier; 2007.pp. 21-32.
15. Seager DJ, Simmons C. Local anesthesia in hair transplantation. Dermatol Surg. 2002;28:320-28.
16. Umar S. Use of body hair and beard hair in hair restoration. Facial Plast Surg Clin N Am. 2013; 21(3):469-77.
17. Stephanie DG, Graber EM. Laser hair removal: a review. Dermatol Surg. 2013;39(6):823-38.
18. Hanke CW. The tumescent facial block: tumescent local anesthesia and nerve block anesthesia for full-face laser resurfacing. Dermatol Surg. 2001;27(12):1003-5.
19. Smith KC, Comite SL, Storwick GS. Ice minimizes discomfort associated with injection of botulinum toxin type A for the treatment of palmar and plantar hyperhidrosis. Dermatol Surg. 2007;33(1 Spec No.):S88-91.
20. Carruthers J, Carruthers A (Eds). Soft Tissue Augmentation. New Delhi: Elsevier; 2006, pp.155-9.

Chapter 14

Tumescent Local Anesthesia

Jayashree Venkataram, Venkataram Mysore,
Aniketh Venkataram

Key Messages

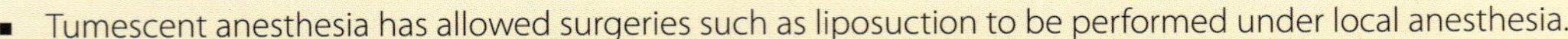

- Tumescent anesthesia has allowed surgeries such as liposuction to be performed under local anesthesia.
- Proper knowledge of pharmacology of lignocaine is necessary for administration.
- It should not be combined with other types of anesthesia such as intravenous anesthesia.

INTRODUCTION

Tumescent local anesthesia (TLA) is a form of local anesthesia, which has been used for several dermatosurgical procedures, particularly liposuction. It uses very dilute solution of anesthetic agent such as lignocaine in large quantities. The word tumescent means tumid—firm and swollen (Figs. 1 and 2). It has revolutionized the administration of anesthesia for cutaneous procedures, particularly liposuction and has made it possible for performing surgeries under local anesthesia, which were other wise being done under general anesthesia.

PRINCIPLE

The procedure consists of using a local anesthetic-epinephrine-saline mixture (also called Klein's solution), over a wide area to provide anesthesia and analgesia, using sufficient quantity of lidocaine far in excess of the conventional dosage. The underlying principle here is that contrary to conventional thinking, larger doses of lidocaine, even up to 45–55 mg/kg body weight can be administered safely with this modification called tumescent technique. Conventional teaching has widely regarded, without adequate pharmacological proof, that the safe upper limit for lidocaine administration is 6 mg/kg body weight. In a radical departure from this hitherto accepted fact, Klein showed that, in tumescent anesthesia, much higher doses can safely be administered, because, in tumescent anesthesia, rate of absorption of lidocaine is slow, leading to smaller peak values and hence lesser toxicity.[1]

Subcutaneous infiltration of large volumes of this solution causes the targeted tissue to become temporarily swollen and firm. The resulting increased subcutaneous interstitial pressure spreads the solution through adjacent tissues by bulk flow. Lidocaine the toxicity is a function of serum lidocaine concentration and since concentration is low, the toxicity is less. Diluted epinephrine produces intense local vasoconstriction, slows systemic absorption of lidocaine, and thus reduces peak serum lidocaine concentrations, which reduces the risk of systemic lidocaine toxicity (Box 1).[2,3]

CONCENTRATIONS

The usual tumescent solution concentration used by dermatologic surgeons is 0.05–0.1% lidocaine. The concentration of adrenaline or epinephrine is at 1:1,000,000–1.5:1,000,000. About 10 mEq of sodium bicarbonate is added to 1 liter of tumescent solution to raise pH and to prevent stinging (due to acidic pH of lidocaine). The recommended usual dose is 35 mg/kg body weight and maximum dose of lidocaine is 55 mg/kg body weight for most patients.[4,5] The recommended concentration of epinephrine in tumescent solutions is 0.5–1.5 mg/L. The total dosage of epinephrine should be minimized, within these limits and usually should not exceed 50 μg/kg.[6,7]

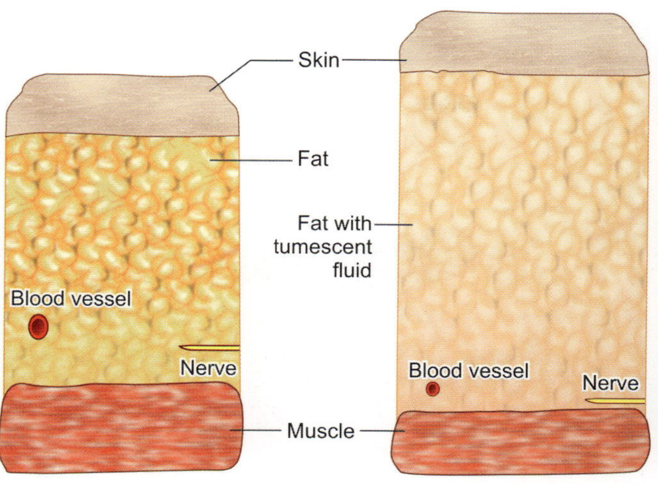

Fig. 1: Tissue before and after tumescent anesthesia—schematic diagram.

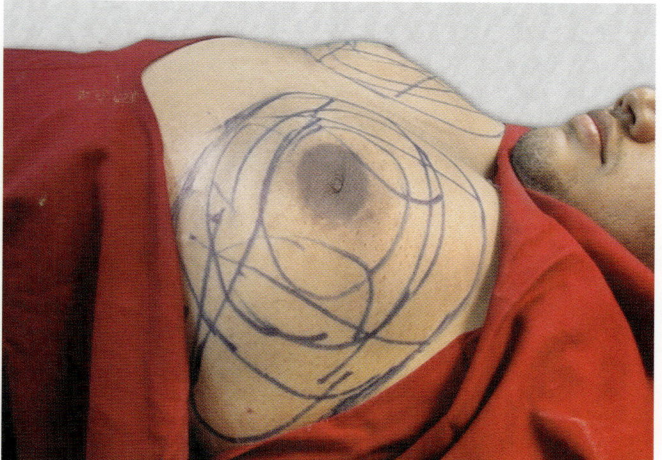

Fig. 2: Male breast after tumescence—swollen and firm.

Box 1: The reasons for the slow absorption of lidocaine.[3]

- Subcutaneous fat has a low volume of blood flow
- Lidocaine is lipophilic and is easily sequestered in fat
- Diluted epinephrine in saline solution ensures vasoconstriction, thus minimizing systemic absorption and bleeding
- The large volume of tumescent solution itself compresses blood vessels by hydrostatic pressure
- The very low dilution of lidocaine in Klein's solution does not achieve the gradient required for systemic absorption
- Most of the solution is removed during aspiration, minimizing the quantity and duration available for absorption.

Thus tumescent anesthesia is like a suggestion: slow sustained release tablet.

Table 1: Tumescent anesthetic solution for liposuction: concentrations.

Lidocaine	*Epinephrine*
500 mg (0.05%)	with 0.5 mg (1:2 million) or
750 mg (0.75%)	with 0.75 mg (1:1.5 million) or
1000 mg (0.1%)	with 1 mg (1:1.5 million)
Sodium bicarbonate	10 mEq (10 mL of 8.4% NaHCO3)
Triamcinolone	10 mg (an optional ingredient)
Physiologic saline	1000 mL of 0.9% NaCl

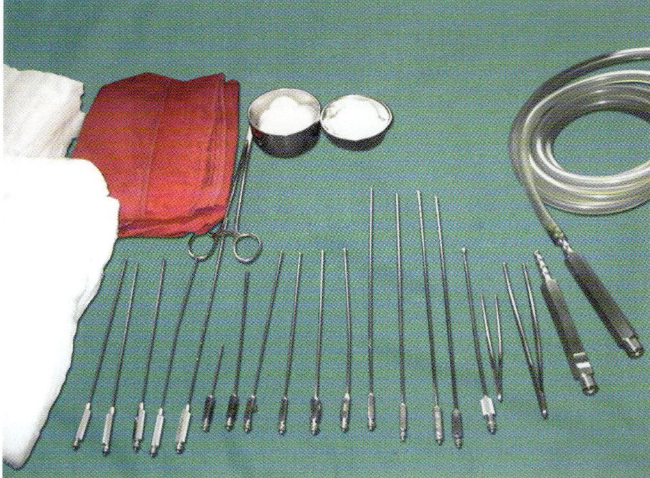

Fig. 3: Cannulae used for infiltration.

PROCEDURE

Tumescent anesthesia is classically used in liposuction and it has made liposuction a safe and gold-standard method of surgery and hence is described in detail:

1. Adits are small holes made for insertion of infiltration cannulae. These are done with 1.5–2 mm dermal punches at different locations of the area under infiltration anesthesia with 1 mL of 2% lignocaine.
2. Tumescent fluid is prepared as discussed above (Table 1). The required lidocaine dosages are dependent on appropriate epinephrine concentration in the tumescent solution. The concentration of lignocaine and epinephrine should be carefully calculated for each area, in relation to weight of the patient.[8,9]
3. Infiltration of tumescent fluid: The delivery system for tumescent solution consists of fluid, infiltration cannulae of size 0.5–1 mm (Fig. 3) infusion bags, infiltration pressure cuffs (Fig. 4), an infiltration pump (Fig. 5) to hasten delivery of the fluid. About 2–3 liters of fluid is infiltrated gradually, in different directions, first into deeper layers of fat and then into the superficial layers. The end point is a firm feel of the skin which makes the skin swollen and difficult to grasp. It is important to be slow and to avoid jerky, sudden movements to avoid pain. Normally it takes about 1–2 hours for proper anesthesia.

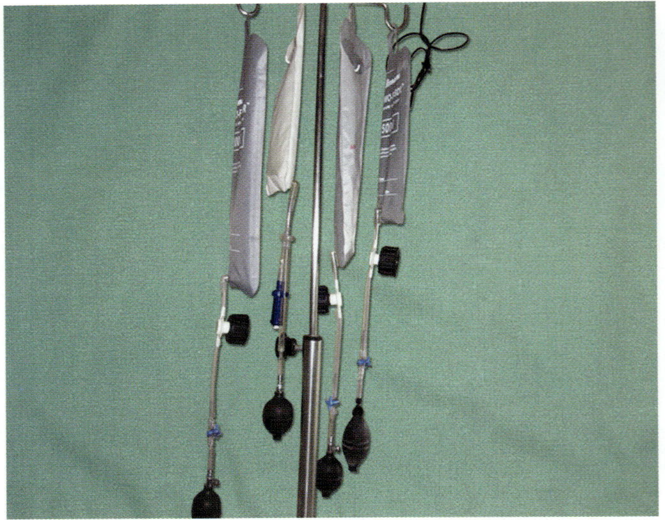

Fig. 4: Infiltration cuffs.

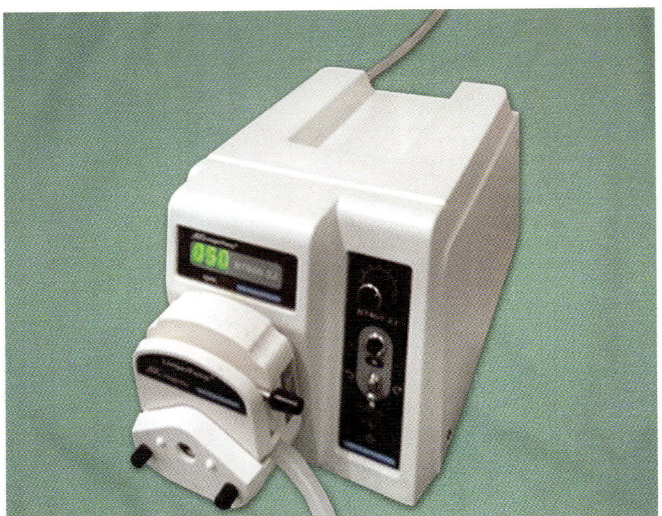

Fig. 5: Infiltration pump.

Table 2: Recommended area wise dosages of lidocaine.

Area	Lidocaine dosage per liter	Lidocaine dosage in volume
Abdomen, upper and lower	750–1000mg/L	800–2000 mL
Hip (flank, or love handle)each side	750–1000mg/L	400–1000 mL
Lateral thigh, each side	600–750mg/L	500–1200 mL
Anterior thigh each side	600–750mg/L	600–1200 mL
Proximal medial thigh, each side	750–1000mg/L	250–700 mL
Knee	750–1000mg/L	200–500 mL
Male breast, each side	1000–1500mg/L	300–800 mL
Sub mental area-chin	750–1000mg/L	100–200 mL

Table 2 shows formulation of tumescent solution for different areas.[10]

4. *Detumescence*: It is important to wait for about 30 minutes after tumescence, for the infiltration fluid to percolate properly in all layers of fat and its full pharmacological effects to take effect. This is indicated by the slight decrease in firmness and the ability to grasp the skin.

Advantages of tumescent anesthesia in liposuction:[11,12]

1. Profound local anesthesia
2. Reduced surgical blood loss due to vasoconstriction
3. The reduction of IV fluid requirements
4. Enhanced aesthetic results—as tumescence reduces contours by swelling the tissue
5. Enhanced postoperative pain relief caused by persistent fluid in the fat
6. Enhanced overall safety—while deaths have been reported after liposuction in general anesthesia, tumescent liposuction has been remarkably safe

OTHER INDICATIONS FOR TUMESCENT ANESTHESIA

Fat Transfer

Fat transfer involves liposuction first and hence always needs tumescent anesthesia. It has been suggested that lignocaine may induce stem cell apoptosis and hence may have a negative impact on adipose derived stem cells.[14] Goldman et al. have suggested that tumescent liposuction without lignocaine may be used when fat transfer is planned and ropivacaine be used instead.

Hair Transplantation

Tumescent anesthesia has been routinely used in hair transplantation, in both strip and follicular unit extraction (FUE) methods.[15] In donor area, tumescence helps in the following ways:

- Tumescence lifts the skin from galea and hence avoids injury to larger vessels and nerves
- It controls bleeding by producing vasoconstriction
- Prolongs anesthesia
- Makes the skin tumid and aids dissection and extraction of hairs
- It is also useful in body hair extraction where a larger area has to be anesthetized.

In the recipient area, it is useful in the following ways:

- It controls bleeding by producing vasoconstriction—prevents popping and allows dense packing
- Prolongs anesthesia.

Tumescence over recipient area has one disadvantage—it contributes to postoperative swelling.

Other Surgeries

Tumescent anesthesia has been used for a number of other surgeries such as vitiligo surgery, venous surgeries

Table 3: Plasma lidocaine concentration and toxicity.

3–6 μg/mL	Subjective pharmacologic effects
5–9 μg/mL	Objective toxicity
8–12 μg/mL	Seizures, cardiac depression
12 μg/mL	Coma
20 μg/mL	Respiratory arrest
26 μg/mL	Cardiac arrest

(striping, endovenous laser ablation, stab ligation),[16-20] acne scarring (subscission, resurfacing, microneedle radiofrequency),[21] Hand surgery,[22] lipomas,[23] breast augmentation,[24] axillary hyperhidrosis,[25] burn scar surgeries and other procedures.[26-30]

Other Anesthetics

Apart from lignocaine, other anesthetic agents such as prilocaine and ropivacaine have been used, though infrequently.[37]

ADVERSE EVENTS WITH TUMESCENT ANESTHESIA

Over the last three decades, tumescent anesthesia has proved to be remarkably safe. The technique has stood its test of time and has established itself as a gold-standard method in liposuction and also useful in several other surgeries. Side effects have been few and nonserious. Several safety studies are available in liposuction[38,39] and these are dealt in detail in the chapters on liposuction.

Adverse events associated with TLA may be due to[40]:

- Lack of pharmacological awareness of this form of anesthesia
- Casual attitude and lack of protocols in calculation of dosage
- Clinician's error in calculation of dosages and fluids, such as inadvertent IV delivery of tumescent solution, miscommunication leading to excessive lidocaine in the tumescent lidocaine solution
- Drug interactions that reduce lidocaine metabolism by impairing cytochrome P450 1A2 and 3A4. The reader is referred to the chapter 12 on local anesthesia for the list of drugs which can affect lignocaine metabolism
- Combination formulations of tumescent solutions using bupivacaine, mepivacaine, or triamcinolone
- Pre-existing medical conditions.

Mild side effects include nausea, vomiting, drowsiness, lightheadedness, paresthesias, tinnitus, blurred vision, nystagmus, ataxia, slurred speech, confusion, etc. The threshold serum concentration for these signs of mild lidocaine toxicity is 6 μg/mL.[40] Respiratory depression vasodilatation, hypotension, suggest serious toxicity. Table 3 shows plasma lignocaine concentration and toxicitiy. These side effects can be avoided by due diligence and adherence to standard dosages.[41]

USE OF OTHER FORMS OF ANESTHESIA WITH TUMESCENT ANESTHESIA

Oral anxiolytics, sedatives, or narcotic analgesics may be used with tumescent liposuction at dosages that are not associated with respiratory depression. Oral clonidine has been shown to have beneficial effects in reducing pulse rate, hypertension due to its sympatholytic effects and reducing postoperative syncope due to its atropine like effect.[9] Lorazepam or diazepam and paracetamol are recommended. Intramuscular anxiolytics, sedatives, or narcotic analgesics should be used with great caution with tumescent liposuction and only after full consultation with the anesthetist as the dose-response relationships can vary widely and may be associated with respiratory depression. Intravascular anxiolytics, sedatives, or narcotic analgesics should be avoided as they may, be associated with increased risk of mortality and morbidity if not used properly. They may however, be used only if the procedure is performed by an experienced dermatosurgeon in a hospital setting with full intensive care unit (ICU) facilities and only if an anesthetist is present during the procedure and for postoperative care. The use of inhalational (general) anesthesia for tumescent liposuction is not recommended.

SUMMARY

Tumescent anesthesia introduced by Jeffrey Klien is one of the most significant inventions in cutaneous surgeries particularly liposuction. However, this needs proper pharmacological knowledge and appreciation of anatomy of the region.

PEARLS

- Tumescent anesthesia should be administed carefully, slowly, and gradually
- Other forms of anesthesia such as intravenous and general anesthesia should not be combined with tumescent anesthesia
- Maximum dose of lignocaine should not exceed 55 mg/kg body weight.

REFERENCES

1. Klein JA. Anesthesia for liposuction in dermatologic surgery. J Dematol Surg Oncol. 1988;14:1124.
2. Lillis PJ. Liposuction surgery under local anesthesia: Limited blood loss and minimal lidocaine absorption. J Dermatol Surg Oncol. 1988;14:1145.
3. Klein JA. The tumescent technique for liposuction. Am J Cosmetic Surg. 1987;4:263.
4. Klein JA. Tumescent technique for regional anaethesia permits lidocaine doses of 35 mg/kg for liposuction. J Dermatol Surg Oncol. 1990;16:248.
5. Klein JA. The tumescent technique: Anesthesia and modified liposuction technique. Dermatol Clin. 1990;8:425.
6. Lillis PJ. The tumescent technique for liposuction surgery. Dermatol Clin. 1990;8:439.

7. Lillis PJ. Liposuction surgery under local anaesthesia: limited blood loss and minimal lidocaine absorption. J Dermatol Surg Oncol. 1988;14:1145-8.
8. Klein JA. The tumescent technique for liposuction surgery. J Am Acad Cosmetic Surg. 1987;4:263-7.
9. Klein JA. Tumescent technique for local anesthesia improves safety in large-volume liposuction. Plast Reconstr Surg. 1993;92:1085-98.
10. Klein JA. Anesthetic formulation of tumescent solutions. Dermatol Clin. 1999;17:751-9.
11. Ostad A, Kageyama N, Moy RL. Tumescent anesthesia with a lidocaine dose of 55 mg/kg is safe for liposuction. Dermatol Surg. 1996;22:921-7. [PubMed]
12. Habbema L. Safety of liposuction using exclusively tumescent local anesthesia in 3,240 consecutive cases. Dermatol Surg. 2009;35:1728-35.
13. Wang WZ, Fang XH, Williams SJ, et al. Lidocaine-induced ASC apoptosis (tumescent vs. local anesthesia). Aesthetic Plast Surg. 2014;38(5):1017-23. doi: 10.1007/s00266-014-0387-2. Epub 2014 Aug 7.
14. Goldman JJ, Wang WZ, Fang XH, et al. Tumescent Liposuction without Lidocaine. Plast Reconstr Surg Glob Open. 2016;4(8):e829. doi: 10.1097 GOX.0000000000000830. eCollection 2016.
15. Sattur S. Anesthesia for hair Transplantation. In: Venkataram Mysore (Ed). Hair Transplantation, Jaypee Brothers Medical Publishers, New Delhi; Ch 22 .pp.138-45.
16. Cavallini A, Marcer D, Bernardini G, Ferrari Ruffino S. Endovenous laser ablation of great saphenous veins performed using tumescent cold saline solution without local anesthesia. Ann Vasc Surg. 2014;28(4):951-6.
17. Jibiki M, Miyata T, Futatsugi S, et al. Effect of the wide-spread use of endovenous laser ablation on the treatment of varicose veins in Japan: a large-scale, single institute stu dy. Laser Ther. 2016;25(3):171-177.
18. Cohn MS, Seiger E, Goldman S. Ambulatory phlebectomy using the tumescent technique for local anesthesia. Dermatol Surg. 1995;21:315-8.
19. Vuylsteke ME, Mordon SR. Endovenous laser ablation: a review of mechanisms of action. Ann Vasc Surg. 2012;26: 424-33.
20. Bush RG, Hammond KA. Tumescent anesthetic technique for long saphenous stripping. J Am Coll Surg. 1999;189:626-8.
21. Taylor MB, Zaleski-Larsen L, McGraw TA. Single session treatment of rolling acne scars using tumescent anesthesia, 20% trichloracetic acid extensive subcision, and fractional CO_2 laser. Dermatol Surg. 2017;43;70-4.
22. Prasetyono TO, Lestari PA.The onset and duration of action of 0.2% lidocaine in a one-per-mil tumescent solution for hand surgery. Arch Plast Surg. 2016;43(3):272-7. doi: 10.5999/aps.2016.43.3.272.
23. Morioka D, Sato N, Ohkubo F. Excision of large lipomas using tumescent local anesthesia. J Cutan Med Surg. 2016; 20(3):263-5.
24. Rusciani A, Pietramaggiori G, Troccola A, et al. The outcome of primary subglandular breast augmentation using tum-escent local anesthesia. Ann Plast Surg. 2016;76(1):13-7.
25. Feldmeyer L, Bogdan I, Moser A, et al. Short- and long-term efficacy and mechanism of action of tumescent suction curettage for axillary hyperhidrosis. J Eur Acad Dermatol Venereol. 2015;29(10):1933-7.
26. Bussolin L, Busoni P, Giorgi L, et al. Tumescent local anesthesia for the surgical treatment of burns and postburn sequelae in pediatric patients. Anesthesiology. 2003;99: 1371-5. [PubMed]
27. Gümüs N. Tumescent infiltration of lidocaine and adrenaline for burn surgery. Ann Burns Fire Disasters. 2011;24:144-8. [PMC free article] [PubMed].
28. Blome-Eberwein S, Abboud M, Lozano DD, et al. Effect of subcutaneous epinephrine/saline/local anesthetic versus saline-only injection on split-thickness skin graft donor site perfusion, healing, and pain. J Burn Care Res. 2013;34:e80-6. [PubMed]
29. Behroozan DS, Goldberg LH. Dermal tumescent local anesthesia in cutaneous surgery. J Am Acad Dermatol. 2005;53:828-30. [PubMed]
30. Girard C, Debu A, Bessis D, et al. Treatment of Gorlin syndrome (nevoid basal cell carcinoma syndrome) with methylaminolevulinate photodynamic therapy in seven patients, including two children: interest of tumescent anesthesia for pain control in children. J Eur Acad Dermatol Venereol. 2013;27:e171-5. [PubMed]
31. Kendler M, Micheluzzi M, Wetzig T, Simon JC. Electro-chemotherapy under tumescent local anesthesia for treat-ment of cutaneous metastases. Dermatolog Surg. 2013;39: 1023-32. [PubMed]
32. Stoffels I, Dissemond J, Schulz A, et al. Reliability and cost-effectiveness of complete lymph node dissection under tumescent local anaesthesia vs. general anaesthesia: a retrospective analysis in patients with malignant melanoma AJCC stage III. J Eur Acad Dermatol Venereol. 2012;26:200-6. [PubMed]
33. Ramon Y, Barak Y, Ullmann Y, et al. Pharmacokinetics of high-dose diluted lidocaine in local anesthesia for facelift procedures. Ther Drug Monit. 2007;29:644-7. [PubMed]
34. Abramson DL. Tumescent abdominoplasty: an ambulatory office procedure. Aesthetic Plast Surg. 1998;22:404-7. [PubMed]
35. Kayaalp C, Olmez A, Aydin C, Piskin T. Tumescent local anesthesia for excision and flap procedures in treatment of pilonidal disease. Dis Colon Rectum. 2009;52:1780-3. [PubMed]
36. Kendler M, Simon JC, Wetzig T. Local anesthesia with lidocaine and prilocaine, using the tumescent technique, for the radiofrequency ablation of lower extremity varicose veins. Int J Dermatol. 2013;52(6):739-44. doi: 10.1111/ijd.12025. Epub 2013 Apr 28.
37. Breuninger H, Hobbach PS, Schimek F. Ropivacaine: an important anesthetic agent for slow infusion and other forms of tumescent anesthesia. Dermatol Surg. 1999;25(10):799-802.
38. Coldiron BM, Healy C, Bene NI. Office surgery incidents: what seven years of Florida data show us. Dermatol Surg. 2008;34:285-91. [PubMed]
39. Hanke W. Cox SE, Kuznets N, Coleman WP 3rd. Tumescent liposuction report performance measurement initiative: National survey results. Dermatol Surg. 2004;30:967-78.
40. Klein JA, Kassarjdian N. Lidocaine toxicity with tumescent liposuction. A case report of probable drug interactions. Dermatol Surg. 1997;23:1169-74.
41. Venkataram M. Tumescent liposuction: Standard guidelines of care. Indian J Dermatol Venereol Leprol. 2008;74:S54- S60.

Chapter

15

Nerve Blocks in Dermatosurgery

Savitha AS, Venkataram Mysore

Key Messages

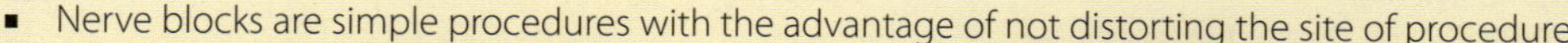

- Nerve blocks are simple procedures with the advantage of not distorting the site of procedure
- Large areas can be anesthetized with single injections and minimum quantity of anesthesia
- Complications are vascular puncture and bleeding, nerve damage.

INTRODUCTION

As dermatologists are venturing to perform more procedures both aesthetic and surgical, patient comfort and pain avoidance during these procedures should also be given prime importance.

Nerve block is an important mode of anesthesia involving injection of anesthetic agent directly to the nerve or in its vicinity, and has several advantages. These blocks can be useful in procedures like full face dermabrasion, botulinum toxin injections to palms and soles, vitiligo surgery, nail surgery, hair transplantation, and fillers. Nerve blocks are ideal when a single nerve innervates the region of anesthesia.

ADVANTAGES OF NERVE BLOCKS

- Simple procedure carried out in day care or outpatient setting
- Small quantities of drugs will anesthetize large areas, thus minimizing the risk of systemic toxicity
- There is no local distortion of tissues, thus preserving appearance
- Preferred option for areas like digits, face and ears
- Nerve blocks are better tolerated by the patient as the number of injection pricks are less, this further reduces the risk of needlestick injury to the surgeon.
- Acts longer
- Avoids multiple pricks and hence causes less pain.

DISADVANTAGES OF NERVE BLOCKS

- The surgeon should be well versed with anatomy of the nerve and needs training
- To cover large areas sometimes multiple blocks have to be given
- Takes longer time to act
- Failure rate is high
- Local hemostasis due to adrenalin is not there
- Vascular puncture, bleeding, nerve damage, and local anesthetic systemic toxicity are general risks in peripheral nerve block regardless of technique or block location.

CONTRAINDICATIONS TO NERVE BLOCKS IN GENERAL

- Known allergy or sensitivity to the anesthetic agent
- Infection at the injection site
- If anatomical landmarks are distorted
- Uncooperative patient
- Physician's lack of familiarity with nerve block.

INDICATIONS

Nerve blocks can be used in most places instead of local infiltration to the lesion. Few special dermatological indications will be mentioned along with the respective blocks.

ANESTHETIC AGENTS[1]

Lignocaine is the commonly used anesthetic agent. Other drugs which are used as long-acting agents are ropivacaine, bupivacaine and mepivacaine. For routine dermatologic procedures lignocaine is sufficient.

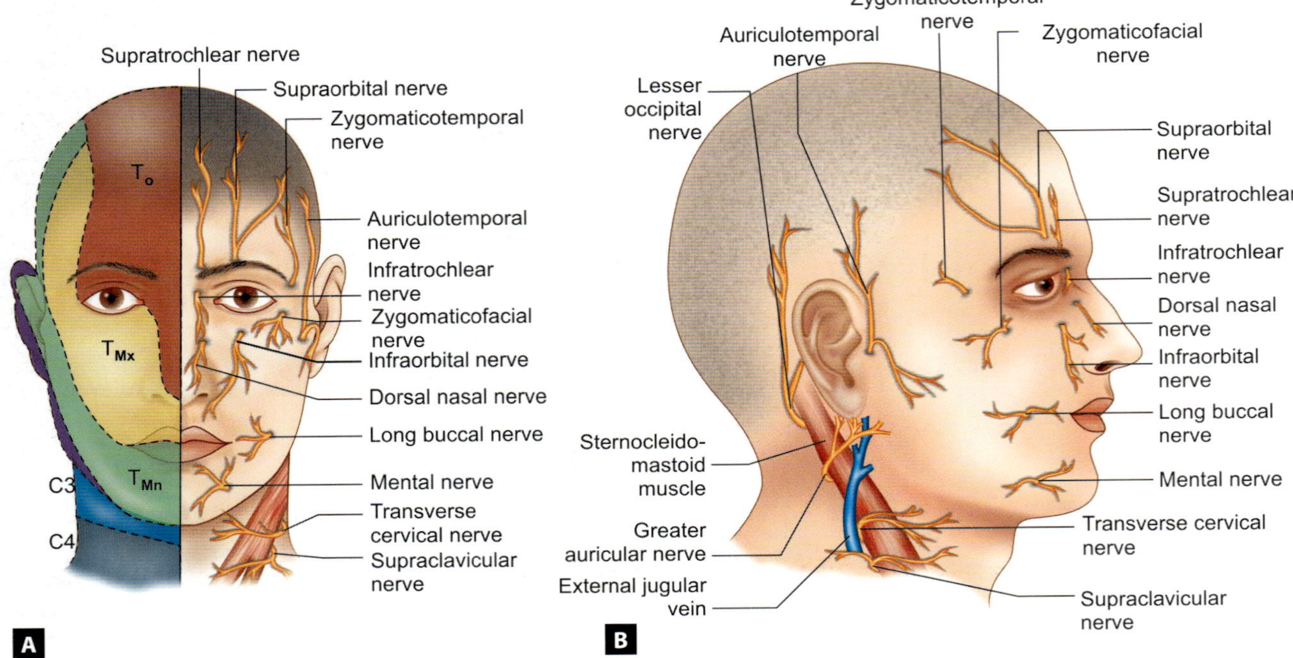

Figs. 1A and B: Sensory innervations of face.

The long-acting agents can be used in procedures which take a long time and also those which have some postoperative discomfort like hair transplantation. Though epinephrine certainly has analgesic benefit when used with short- and intermediate-acting local anesthetics, studies with long-acting local anesthetics (e.g. ropivacaine) failed to show an increased duration of analgesia with coadministration of epinephrine. With increased use of ultrasound and potential concerns about neurotoxicity, its use with long-acting agents in nerve blocks is debated. Epinephrine is a valuable marker for intravascular injection. Recent recommendations are to use epinephrine for nerve blocks done without ultrasound guidance, or blocks in which the needle tip and local anesthetic spread is not adequately visualized, as a safety measure to detect intravascular injection.

PREPARATION

Before nerve block is given, the procedure, risks, and potential complications have to be explained to the patient, and consent obtained. A review of regional anatomy and the location of nerves and other important structures also are essential before the injection.

The area to be anesthetized is surgically prepared by cleaning with povidone-iodine prior to injection.

FACIAL NERVE BLOCKS

Dermatological Indications

Hair transplantation, fat fillers, dermal grafts, dermabrasion, subcision, laser resurfacing, and blepharoplasty.

All the sensory innervation of the face is by the trigeminal nerve and the superficial cervical plexus (Fig. 1).

Supraorbital Nerve Block

The supraorbital nerve block is simple and easy with a very high success rate.

Anatomical Landmark[2]

Supraorbital nerve exits the supraorbital foramen, and divides into medial and lateral branches, each branch accompanied by its artery (Fig. 2).

Position

The patient can be positioned either supine or seated in a semi-recline position with head resting, (to avoid the patient from falling due to vasovagal syncope if any), facing the person performing the block.

Procedure

- The supraorbital foramen is located with the pulp of the index finger of nondominant hand and marked with the pen. To locate the supraorbital foramen, the patient is asked to look straight ahead and imagine a line drawn vertically from the pupil up toward the inferior border of the supraorbital ridge. Then palpate along the supraorbital ridge until a subtle notch is felt; this is the supraorbital foramen
- Another method is to place three fingers centered vertically over glabella, the major branches of supraorbital nerve emerge just lateral to the fingers (Fig. 3).[3]

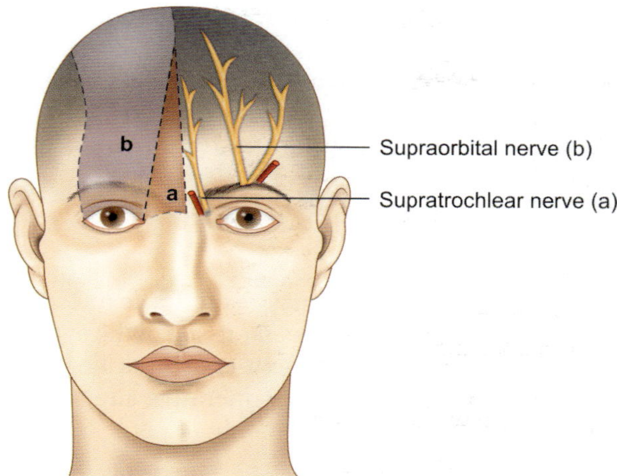

Fig. 2: Supraorbital and supratrochlear nerve and areas supplied by them.

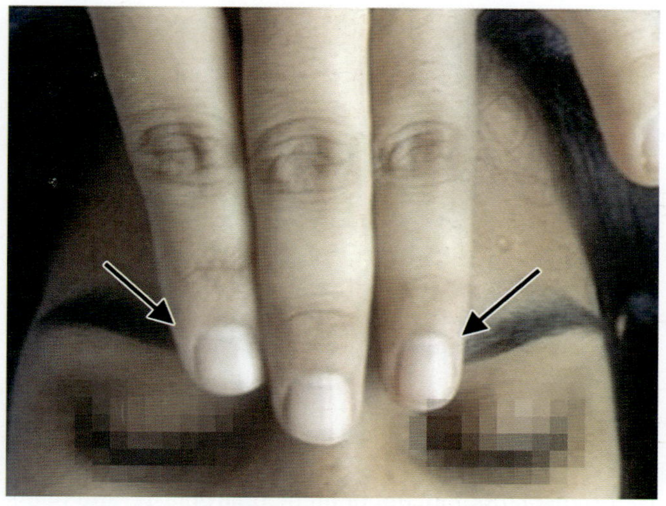

Fig. 3: Surface marking of supraorbital notch.

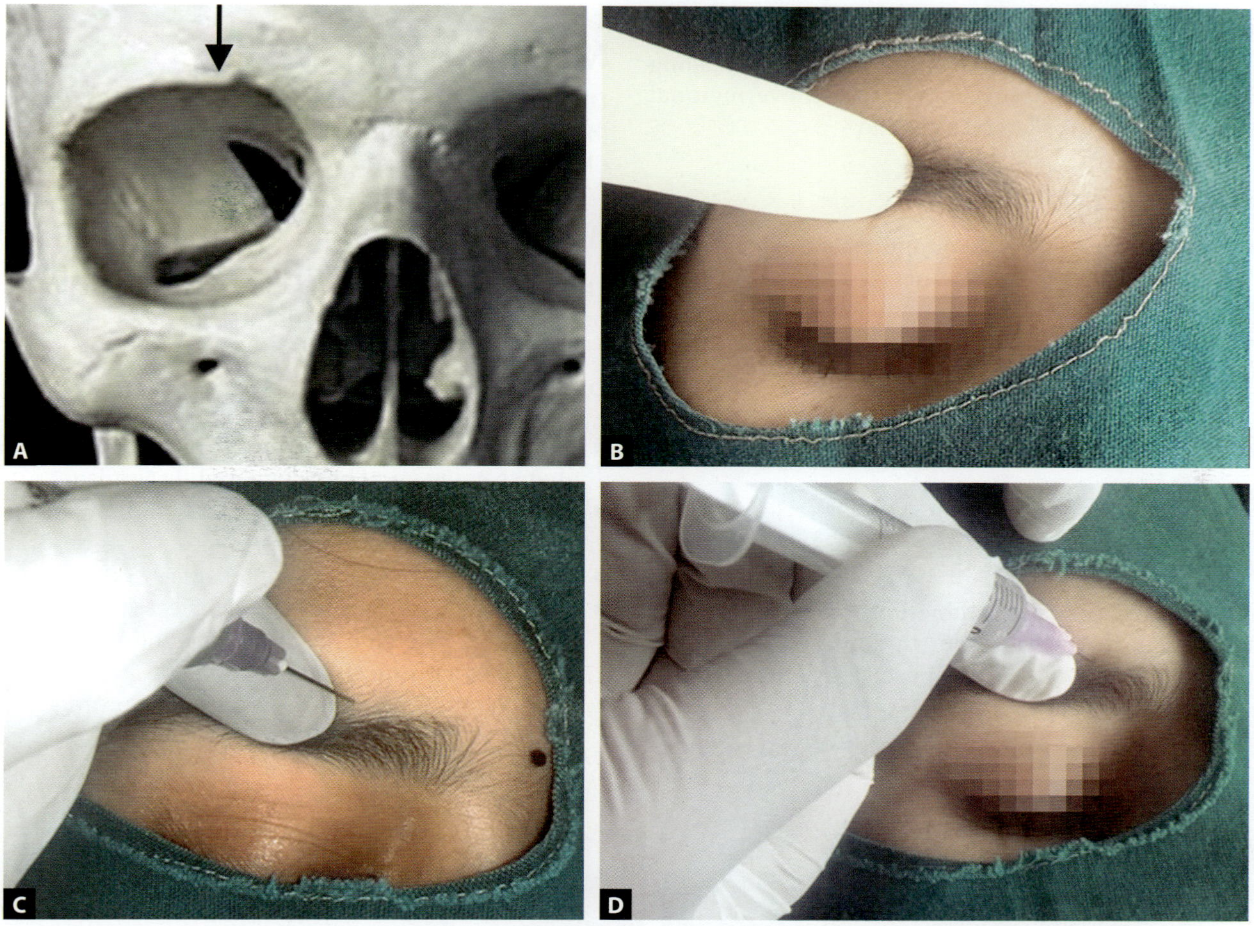

Figs. 4A to D: (A) Supraorbital notch; (B) Palpate the supraorbital notch with index finger of nondominant hand; (C) Insert the needle at the lateral margin of the notch; and (D) Deposit 1.5–2 mL of anesthetic with needle slowly advancing medially.

- Insert the needle just lateral to the foramen, the needle will seek bone contact at the edge of the foramen within 1 cm (Figs. 4A to D)
- Inject very slowly 1.5–2 mL of anesthetic solution with the needle facing medially
- A discrete massage supports the diffusion of the anesthetic
- To prevent swelling of the anesthetic into the upper eyelid, it is recommended to firmly place either a finger or a roll of gauze under the orbital rim.[4]

Caution

Advance the needle medially to avoid penetration of the foramen.

Complications

- The puncture of the supraorbital artery
- A transitory palpebral ptosis can be seen, by diffusion of the product towards the elevator muscle of the eyelid
- Paresthesias sequels in the territory of the nerve may occur, because of an edema of the nerve, strangled in its foramen.[4]

Special Indications

Hair transplantation, upper lid blepharoplasty, and fillers in forehead.

Supratrochlear Nerve Block

The supratrochlear nerve block is often performed along with the supraorbital nerve block to achieve regional anesthesia over the ipsilateral forehead.

Anatomical Landmark

Supratrochlear nerve is smaller and exits the orbit 1 cm more medially than supraorbital nerve, above the trochlea (pulley) of the superior oblique muscle (Fig. 2). Some patients may have either a supratrochlear foramen or an absent supratrochlear notch instead.

Position

Same as that of supraorbital block.

Procedure

- As the supratrochlear foramen or notch can be hard to palpate (or even absent in some patients), the supraorbital foramen is often used as a landmark
- The target area for insertion is on the supraorbital ridge approximately 1 cm medial to the supraorbital notch, between the notch and the bridge of the nose (Figs. 5A and B)
- A discrete massage supports the diffusion of the product.

Complications

- Swelling or ecchymosis may result if the anesthetics infiltrates into the loose areolar tissue of the eyelid
- Puncture of the angular vein causing a hematoma (potentially obstructing the operative site) has also been described.[4]

Special Indications

Hair transplantation, upper lid blepharoplasty, and filler injections.

Nasal Nerve Block

Dorsal nasal nerve is branch of anterior ethmoidal nerve; provides sensory innervation to the skin of the lower half of the nose (Figs. 6 and 7).[5]

Anatomical Landmark

The nasal nerve emerges at the lower border of the nasal bone 6–10 mm from the midline (Fig. 6).

Procedure (Figs. 8A to C)

- With the nondominant hand palpate the junction between the nasal bone and mobile cartilage
- Insert the needle 5 mm lateral to midline and inject 1 mL of the anesthetic agent
- Repeat the procedure on other side
- Alternately both nerves can be accesses with a single injection, insert the needle in the midline and advance inferolaterally on either side.

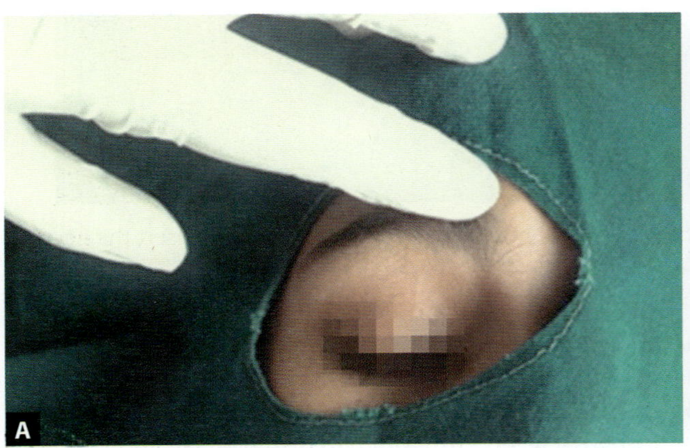

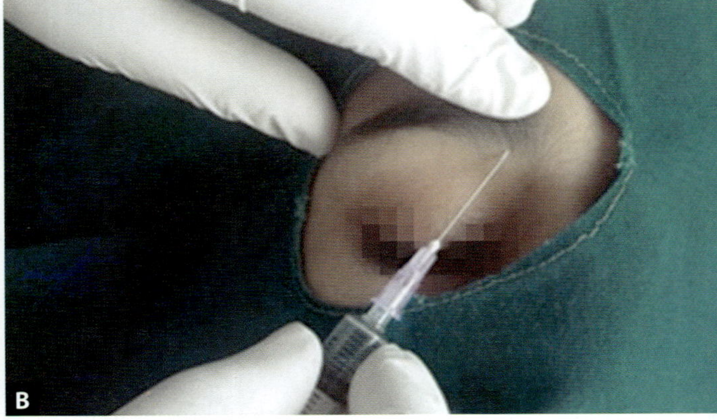

Figs. 5A and B: Supratrochlear nerve block: insertion is on the supraorbital ridge approximately 1 cm medial to the supraorbital notch.

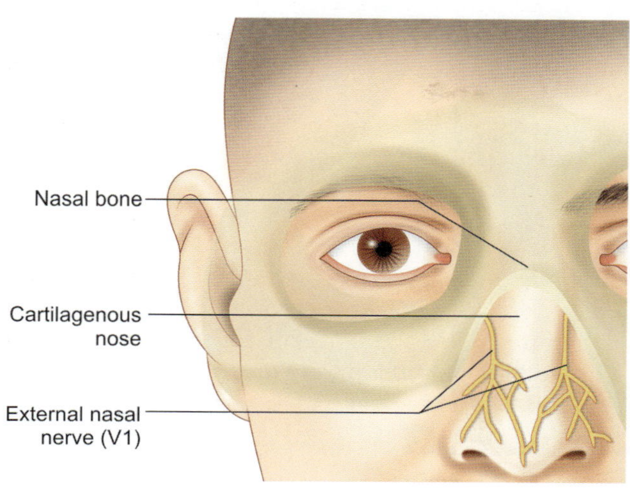

Fig. 6: Nasal nerves.

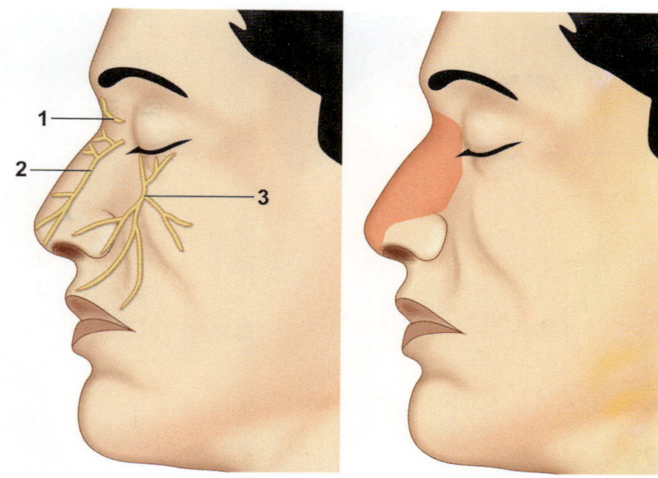

Fig. 7: Nerve supply to the nose (1: Infratrochlear, 2: Dorsal nasal, and 3: Infraorbital, area in red is supplied by dorsal nasal nerve).

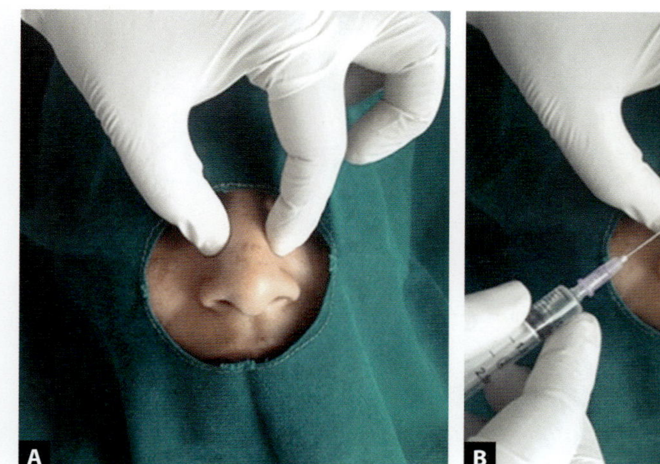

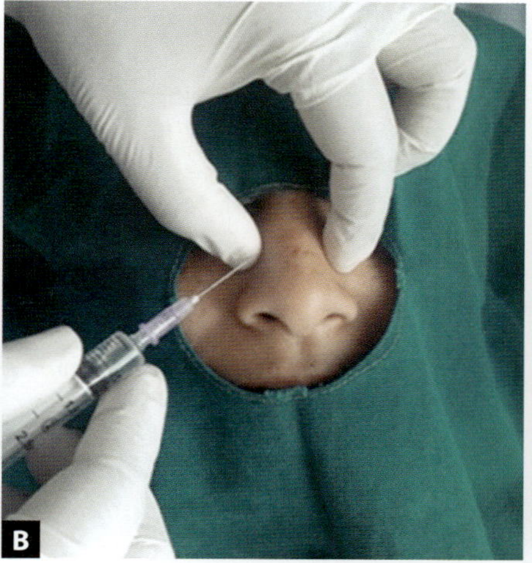

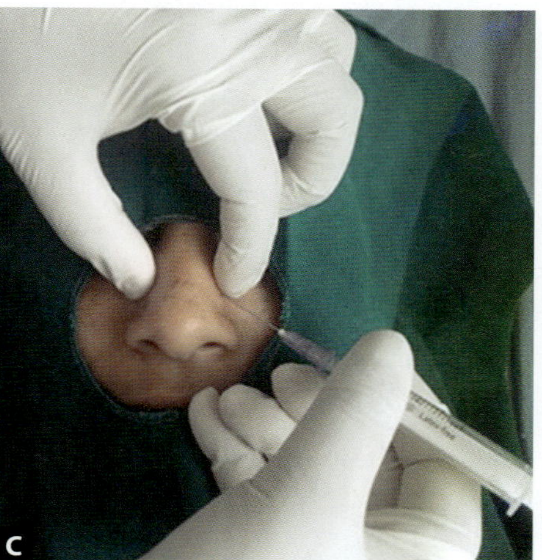

Figs 8A to C: (A) With your nondominant hand, palpate the junction between the firm nasal bone and mobile nasal cartilage; (B) Insert the needle 5–10 mm lateral to midline and inject 1 cc of anesthetic; and (C) Repeat the procedure on the other side.

Regional Anesthesia to the Nose (Figs. 9A to C)

- Two injections will be necessary to block the area completely
- First is at the root of the nose, at the level of the interior angle of the eye, an infiltration, with more close to the nasal bone, with a direction towards the nasal base—blocks the infratrochlear and nasal nerve
- Second, in the axis of nasal alar; towards its base and alar joint—blocks the area of infraorbital nerve
- The injection must be particularly slow because the area is very sensitive: 1 mL on the first site and 1.5 mL of anesthetic solution, on the second site.[4]

Special Indications

Rhinoplasty, and nose shaping with fillers.

Infraorbital Nerve Block

Anatomical Landmark (Fig. 10)

The infraorbital nerve leaves by the infraorbital foramen located at 4–7 mm below the infraorbital bone edge.

Procedure

Extraoral technique (Figs. 11A to D):

- To locate the infraorbital foramen, the patient is asked to look straight ahead and imagine a line drawn vertically from the pupil down to the superior border of the infraorbital ridge. Then palpate along the ridge until a subtle notch is felt; this is the infraorbital notch. The infraorbital foramen is located about 4–7 mm below this notch
- The point of puncture is done on the level of the lateral edge of the foramen

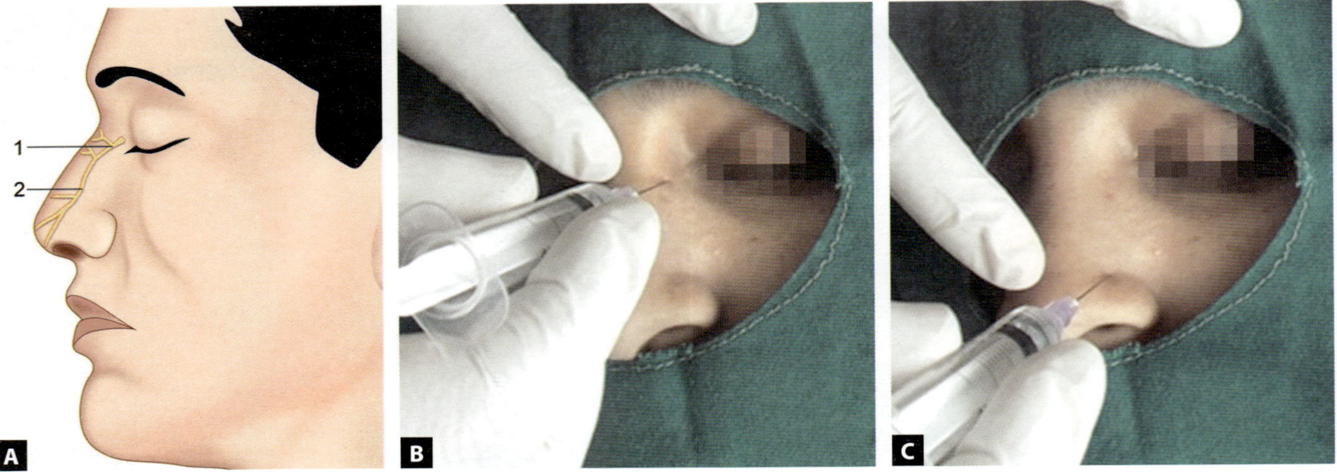

Figs. 9A to C: Regional block to nose. (A) 1: Infratrochlear nerve, 2: Nasal nerve; (B) Infiltration at root of nose 1 mL; and (C) Infiltration at the ala, 1.5 mL.

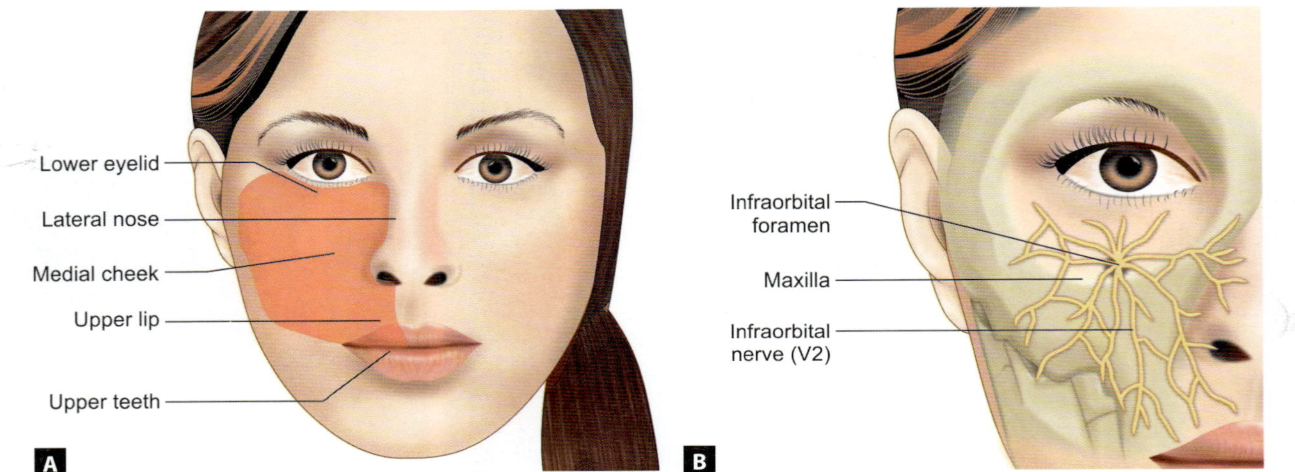

Figs. 10A and B: Infraorbital nerve sensory supply.

- The needle will seek the bone contact (with less than 10 mm) at the edge of the foramen
- The needle should be directed cephalic and medially and inject 1.5–2 mL of anesthetic after withdrawing
- The axis of the infraorbital foramen look towards the ala of the nose, it is better to prick with a needle directed towards the root of the nose (Figs. 11A to D).[6]

Caution: During the extraoral technique, the needle is in very close proximity to the facial artery. Because of this proximity, avoid adding vasoconstrictors to the anesthetic agent.

Complications

- The puncture of the infraorbital artery
- Paresthesias due to an edema of the nerve strangled in its foramen
- Transitory paralysis of the extrinsic muscles of the ocular sphere by orbital passage of the anesthetic solution.

Endo-oral Method and Three and Half Method (Figs. 12A to C)[7]

- Palpate the infraorbital foramen with the middle finger of nondominant hand
- Hold the lip with the thumb and index finger
- Insert the needle at the upper canine tooth into the buccal recess directed towards the foramen. As the needle is inserted between the canine and first premolar, it is called three and a half method
- Inject 2–3 mL of anesthetic after aspiration to rule out intravascular placement.

Caution: Difficult and more sensitive with risks of dysesthesias with injection in the infraorbital foramen.

Special Indications

Acne scar surgeries, dermal fillers, fat transplants, dimple creation procedures, and upper lip surgeries.

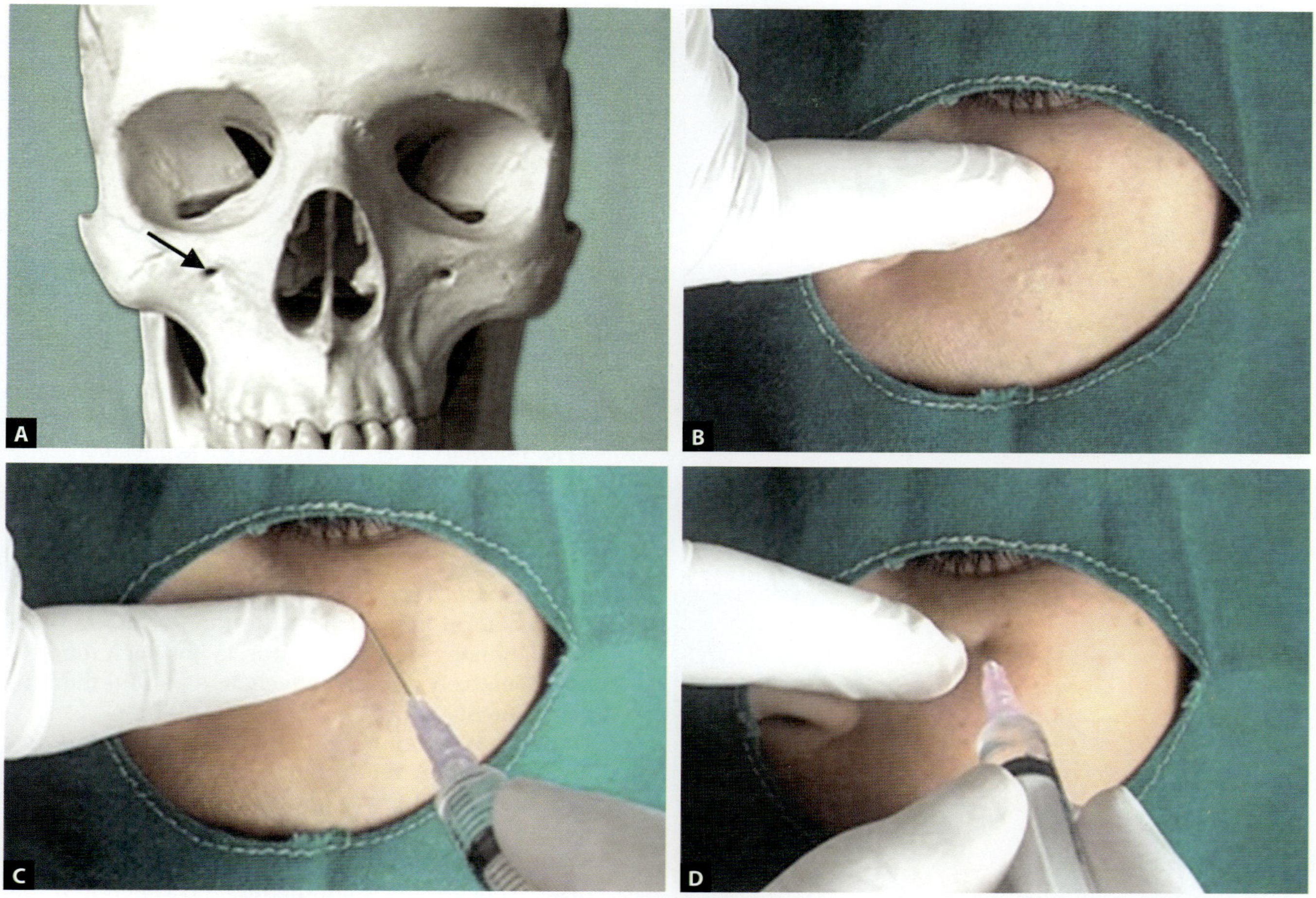

Figs. 11A to D: Extraoral method for infraorbital block. (A) Infraorbital foramen; (B) Palpate the foramen 5–7 mm below the infraorbital notch; and (C and D) Insert needle medially.

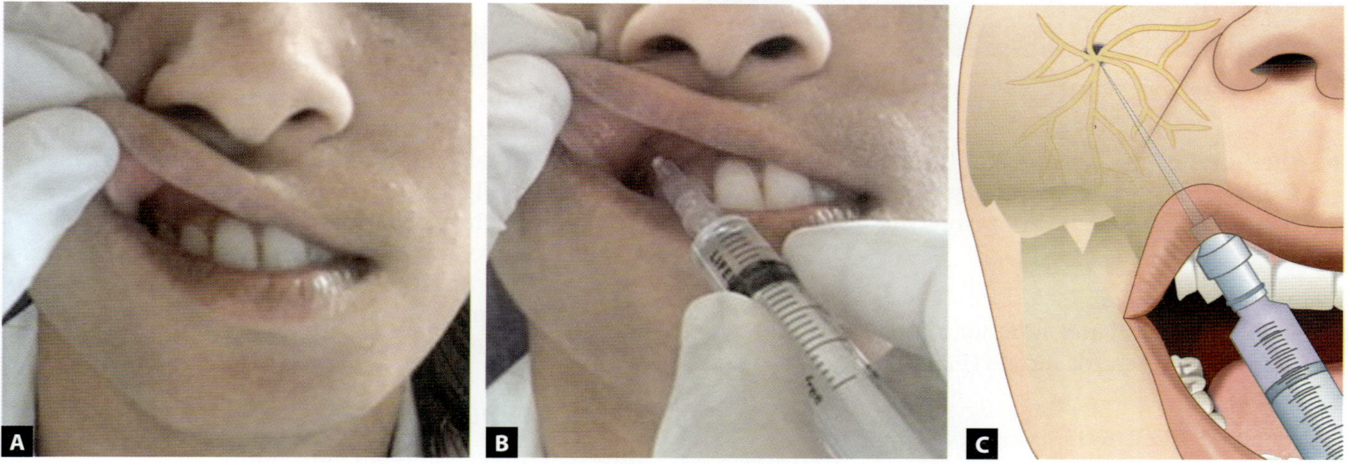

Figs. 12A to C: Intraoral method for infraorbital block. (A) Palpate infraorbital foramen; (B) Insert needle between incisor and first premolar into buccal recess; and (C) Schematic diagram of the block.

Long Buccal Nerve

The buccal nerve is situated just beneath the soft tissue and not within bone, so the success rate is very high. It is a pure sensory nerve and supplies the upper lip at the angle of the mouth (Fig. 13).

Procedure

Intraoral method (Fig. 14):[8,9]

- Injection site is located on the buccal mucosa distal to the third molar

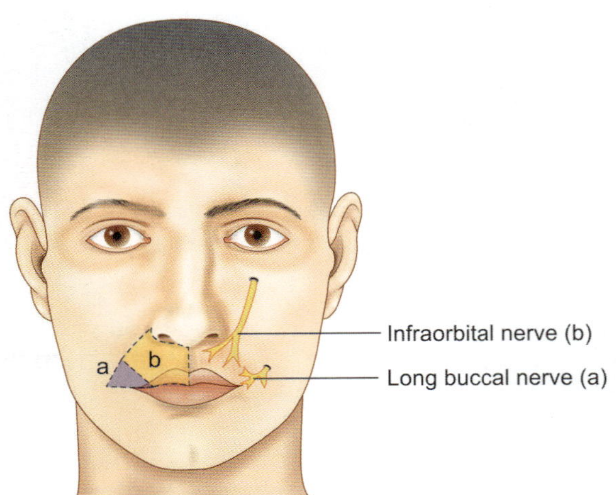

Fig. 13: Long buccal nerve and area supplied by it.

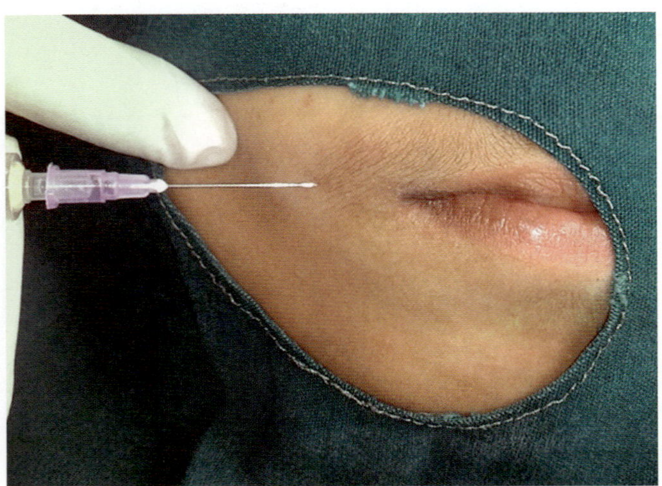

Fig. 15: Transcutaneous long buccal nerve block.

- The bevel of the needle should be toward the bone and inserted at a depth of 1–3 mm with the buccal soft tissue lateral and taut. The syringe should be parallel to the occlusal plane.

Transcutaneous method:
Inject 2–3 cm lateral and superior to angle of mouth with needle pointing towards mouth (Fig. 15).

Special Indications

Procedures at the angle of the mouth, and lip augmentation.

Mental Nerve

Anatomical Landmark

The mental nerve is the terminal branch of the inferior alveolar nerve. It enters the face through the mental foramen and supplies the inferior lip and the chin (Fig. 16).

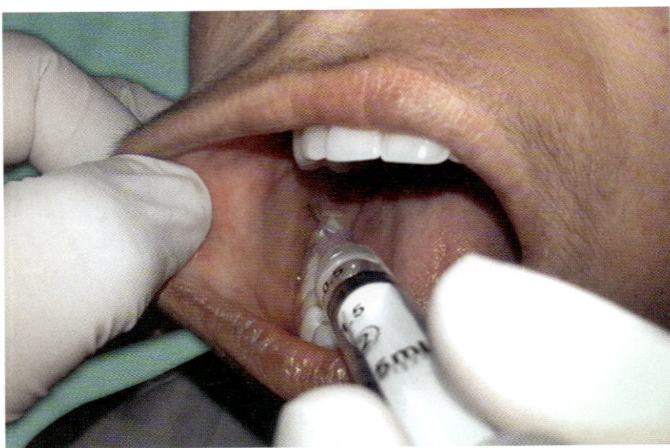

Fig. 14: Long buccal nerve block—intraoral method.

Procedure

Intraoral approach (Fig. 17):
- The intraoral approach to the mental nerve block with adjunctive topical anesthesia has been reported as subjectively and objectively less painful than the percutaneous approach.[10]
- The mental foramen is palpable between the two lower premolar teeth. Locate the mental foramen with the nondominant hand, insert the needle along the lower gum line into the buccal fold between the premolar teeth near the foramen. As the needle is inserted between two premolars it is called four and half method
- Do not place the needle directly into the foramen. Aspirate and inject 2–3 mL of anesthetic.

Transcutaneous route
- Mental foramen is located 1 cm inferior and slightly anterior to the second premolar. It is in line with the mid-pupil on forward gaze. Line drawn through supraorbital, and infraorbital foramen passes mental foramen (Fig. 18).[11]
- Insert needle at a point overlying mental foramen
- Advance needle perpendicular to bone until periosteum is reached, withdraw the needle and inject 2–3 mL of anesthetic near but not in the mental foramen, redirect needle if paresthesias or sharp pain occurs.

Special Indications

Lower lip surgery, and filler injections.

NERVE BLOCKS FOR HAIR TRANSPLANTATION

Sensory Supply of Scalp[12]

The following six sensory nerve branches of either the trigeminal nerve or the cervical nerve supply the scalp as shown in Figure 19.

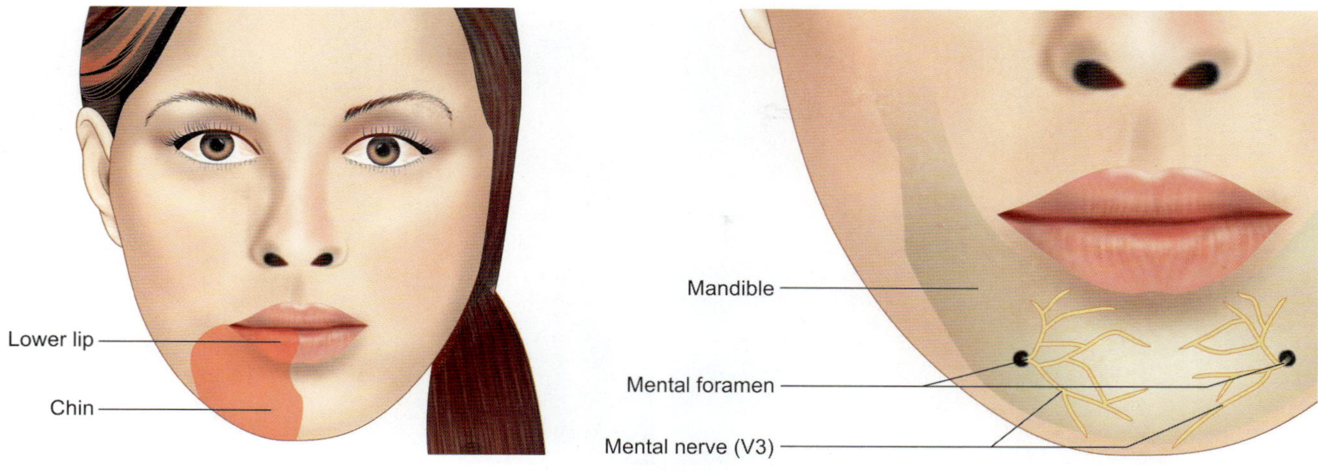

Fig. 16: Mental nerve and area supplied by it.

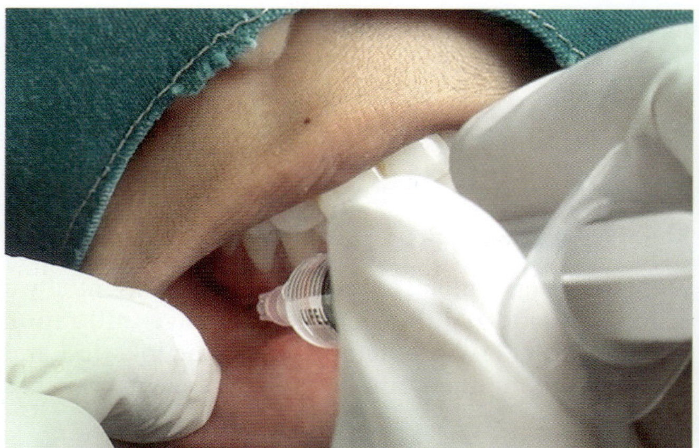
Fig. 17: Transoral mental nerve block—four and half method.

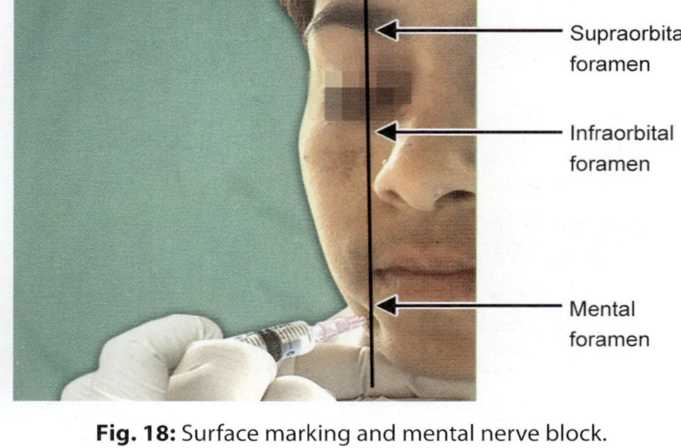

Fig. 18: Surface marking and mental nerve block.

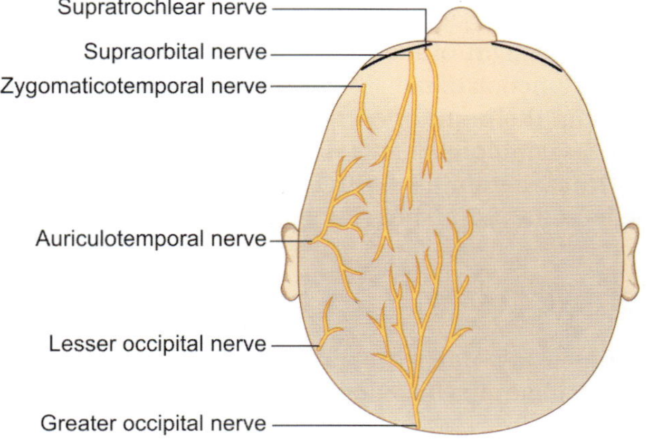

Fig. 19: Sensory supply of scalp.

The common blocks used in hair transplantation are:[3]

- Greater occipital nerve block
- Supraorbital and supratrochlear nerve block
- Auriculotemporal block
- Zygomaticotemporal block.
  With these blocks most of the scalp can be anesthetized.

Greater Occipital Nerve Block

Anatomical Landmark

The greater occipital nerve runs on the lateral aspect of external occipital protuberance along with the occipital artery which lies medial to it.

Procedure

- The patient is in prone or lateral position
- Place three fingers on superior nuchal line with middle finger on the external occipital protuberance, point on injection is just lateral to the lateral fingers on either side (Fig. 20). Inject about 1 mL of anesthetic lotion on either side.

Zygomaticotemporal Nerve Block

Anatomical Landmark

The nerve lies 1.5 cm lateral to the outer canthus on the zygomatic arch. It emerges through a foramen located on the anterior wall of temporal fossa (Fig. 21).

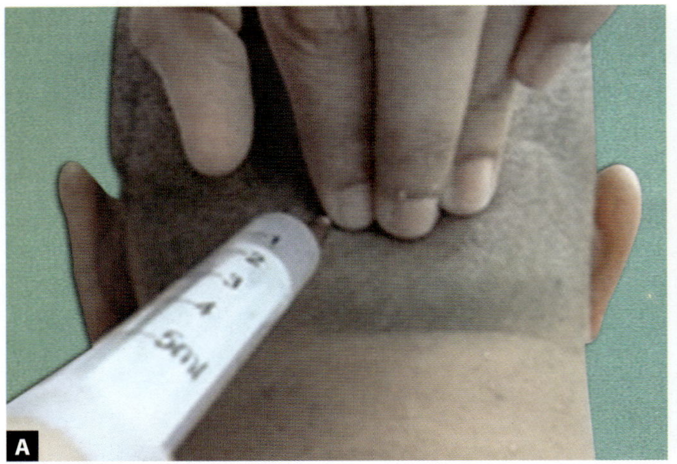

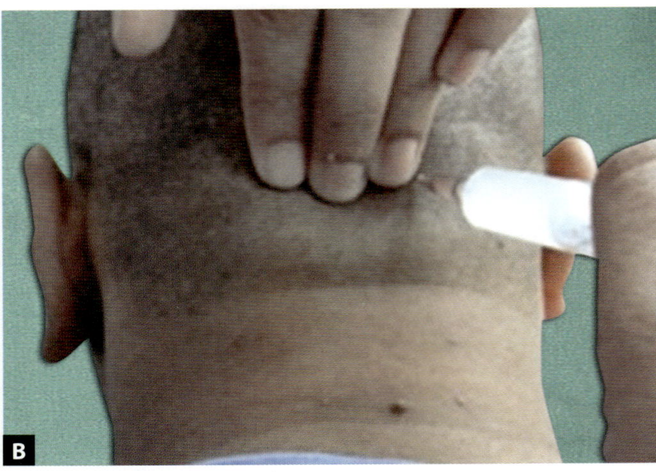

Fig. 20: Greater occipital nerve block.

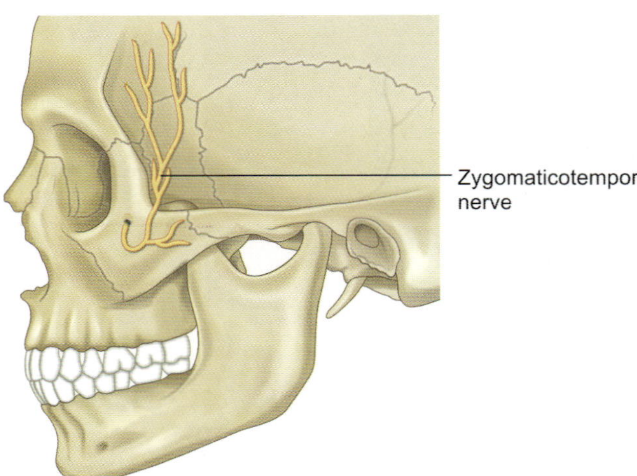

Fig. 21: Zygomaticotemporal nerve.

Procedure

- Palpate the lateral orbital rim at the level of frontozygomatic suture which is usually palpable
- Place the index finger in the depression posterior to lateral orbital rim, insert the needle just behind the finger
- The needle is slowly advanced down along the posterior border of the lateral orbital rim. Aspirate and inject 1.5–2 mL of anesthetic agent (Fig. 22).

Auriculotemporal Nerve Block

Anatomical Landmark

This nerve originates from the posterior trunk of mandibular nerve and passes in front of the tragus in close proximity to superficial temporal artery. It supplies part of the auricle, temporal and temporoparietal area of scalp.

Procedure

Palpate the temporal artery as it crosses the zygomatic arch near the root of the zygoma. This gives an approximate location of the nerve. Infiltrate about 2 mL of anesthetic in the area to block the nerve and terminal branches (Fig. 23).

UPPER LIMB BLOCKS

Radial Nerve Block[13]

The radial nerve block at the wrist level is essentially a field block and requires a more extensive infiltration because of its less predictable anatomic location and division into multiple, smaller, and cutaneous branches (Fig. 24).

Procedure (Figs. 25A to D)

- Palpate the radial styloid and radial artery to establish landmarks
- Inject 2–3 mL of anesthetic lateral to the radial artery, at the junction of radial styloid and palmar crease
- From the point of entry continue the field block till dorsal midpoint of the wrist.

Other method is to direct the needle from lateral to medial side of snuff box (Fig. 26).

Complications

- Residual paresthesia due to an inadvertent intraneuronal injection.

Median Nerve Block (Same as Wrist Block)

Anatomical Landmark

At the wrist, the median nerve lies within the carpal tunnel, deep and radial to the palmaris longus (PL) tendon and medial to the flexor carpi radialis (FCR) tendon (Fig. 27).

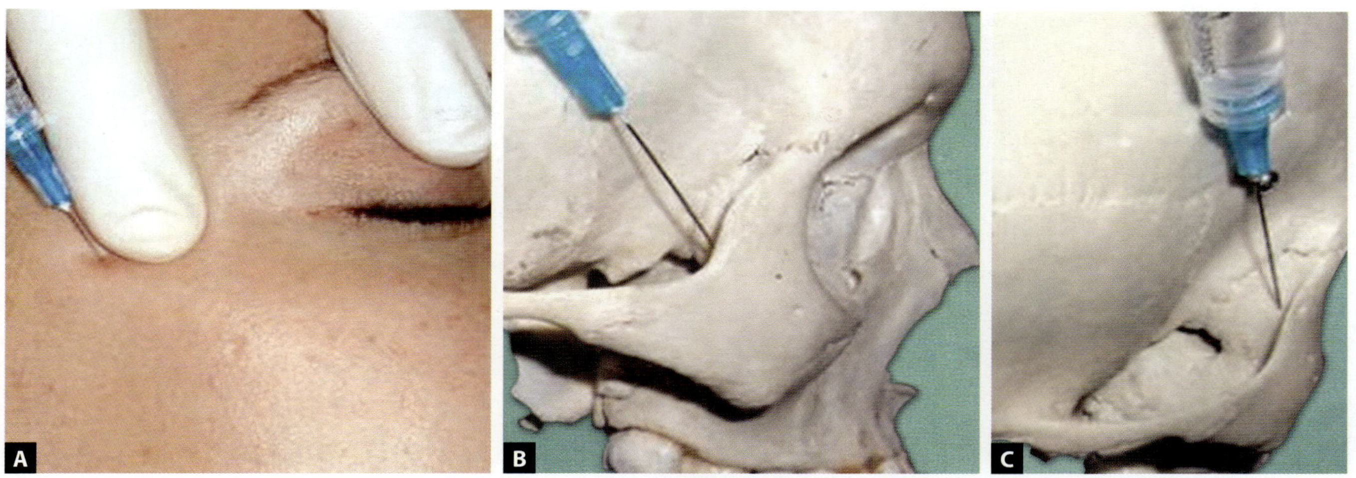

Figs. 22A to C: Zygomaticotemporal nerve block.

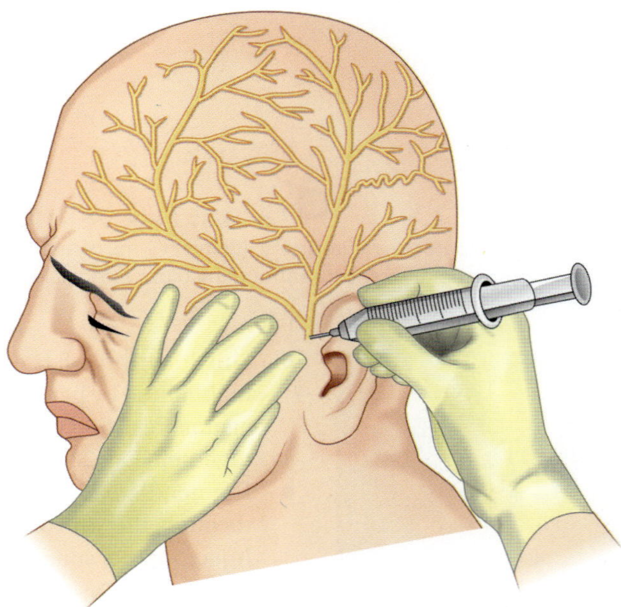

Fig. 23: Auriculotemporal nerve block.

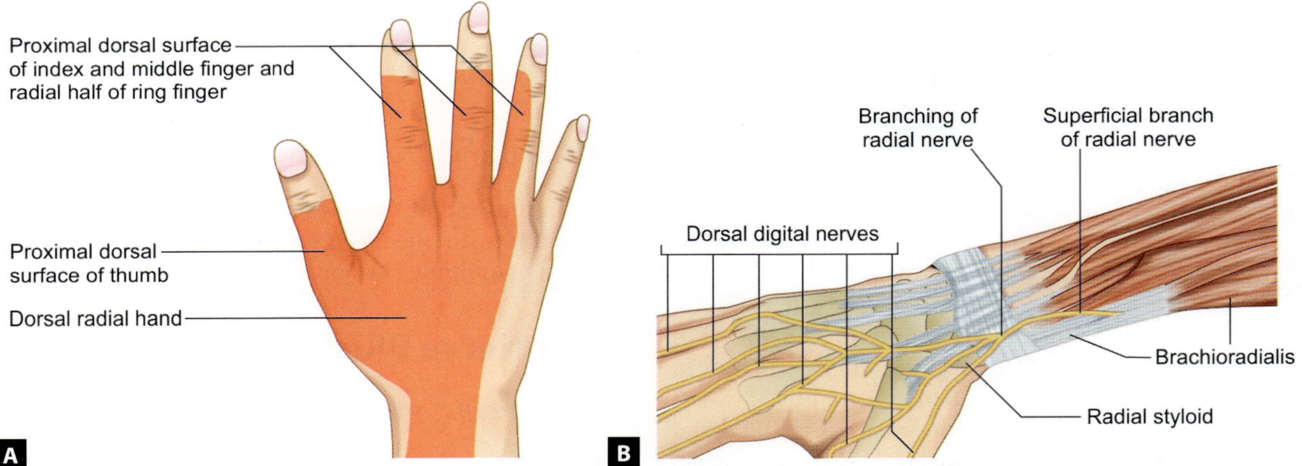

Figs. 24A and B: Branches of radial nerve and sensory supply.

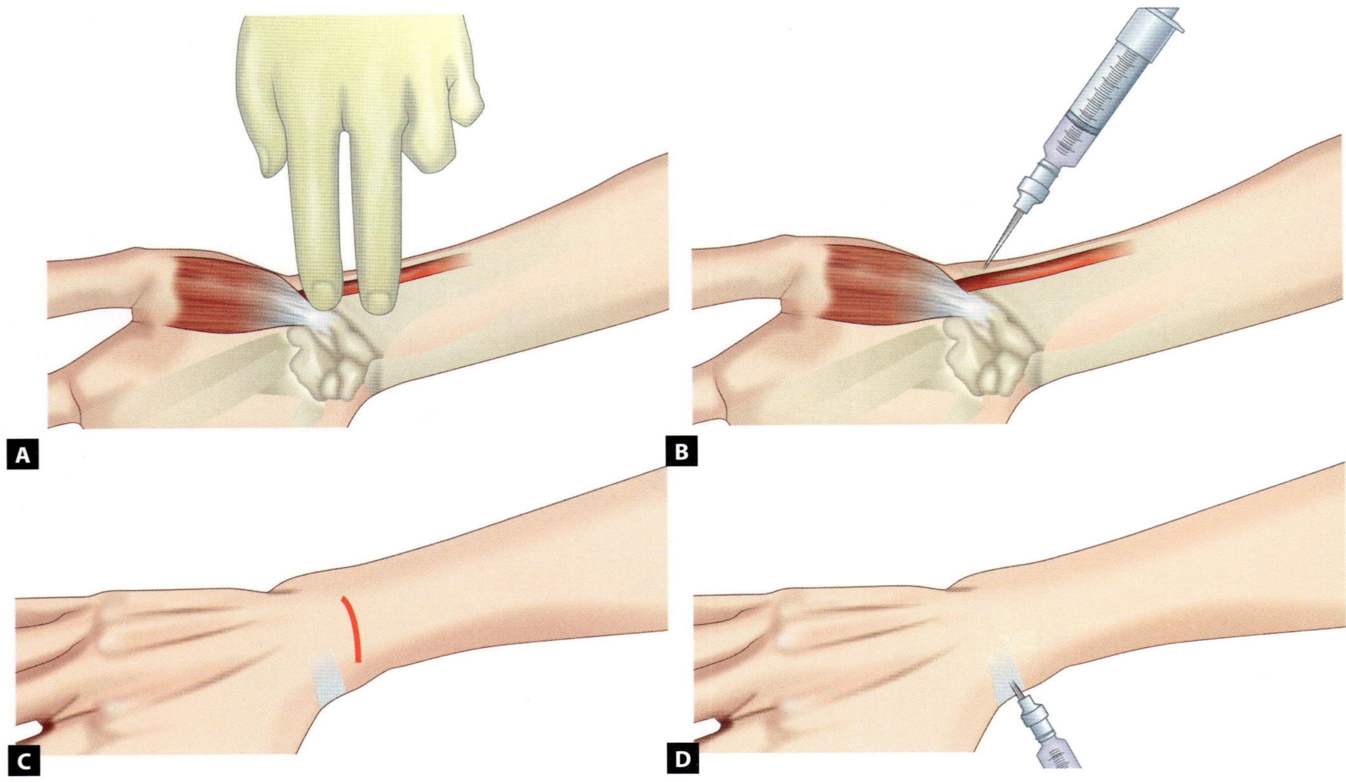

Figs. 25A to D: Radial nerve block. (A) Palpate the radial artery; (B) Inject 2 mL of anesthetic lateral to radial artery; and (C and D) From point of entry continue the block to dorsal aspect.

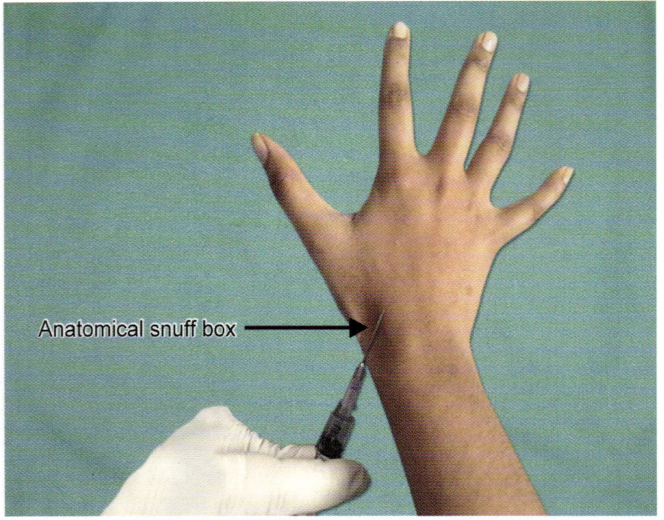

Fig. 26: Radial nerve block by injecting across anatomical snuff box.

Procedure (Figs. 28A and B)

- The needle is inserted perpendicular to the skin between the PL and FCR tendons, angled such as to place the needle tip directly beneath the PL
- The injection is made 2–3 cm proximal to the distal crease of the wrist to avoid injecting within the carpal tunnel
- The location of the PL and FCR tendons can be highlighted by having the patient flex the middle finger against resistance or pinch the thumb and little finger together (Fig. 28)
- The needle is inserted to a depth of 1–2 cm. Passage through the fibrous flexor retinaculum may be felt. Injecting in a space too deep is better than in a space too shallow, as the retinaculum prevents anesthetic from reaching the nerve if injected too superficially. An anesthetic volume of 3–5 mL is appropriate
- To include the peripheral (palmar) branches, a small wheal of anesthetic is placed subcutaneously as the needle is withdrawn and massaged gently over the volar wrist.

Special Indications

Median and radial nerve blocks can be utilized during botulinum toxin injections for palmar hyperhidrosis, and removal of multiple corn or warts.

Ulnar Nerve Block

Anatomical Landmark

At the wrist the ulnar nerve lies lateral to flexor carpi ulnaris tendon (Fig. 29).

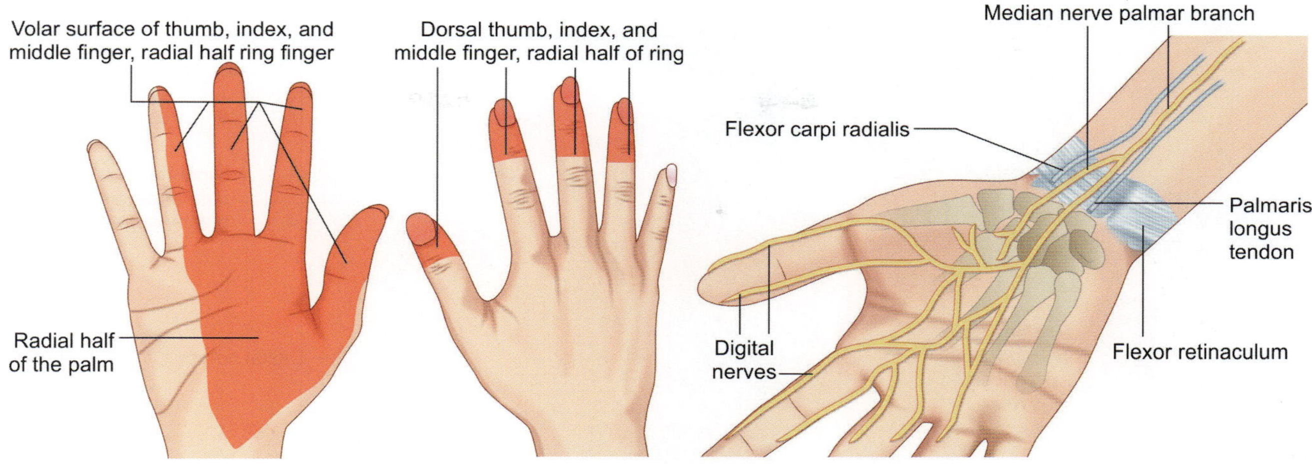

Fig. 27: Branches of median nerve and sensory supply.

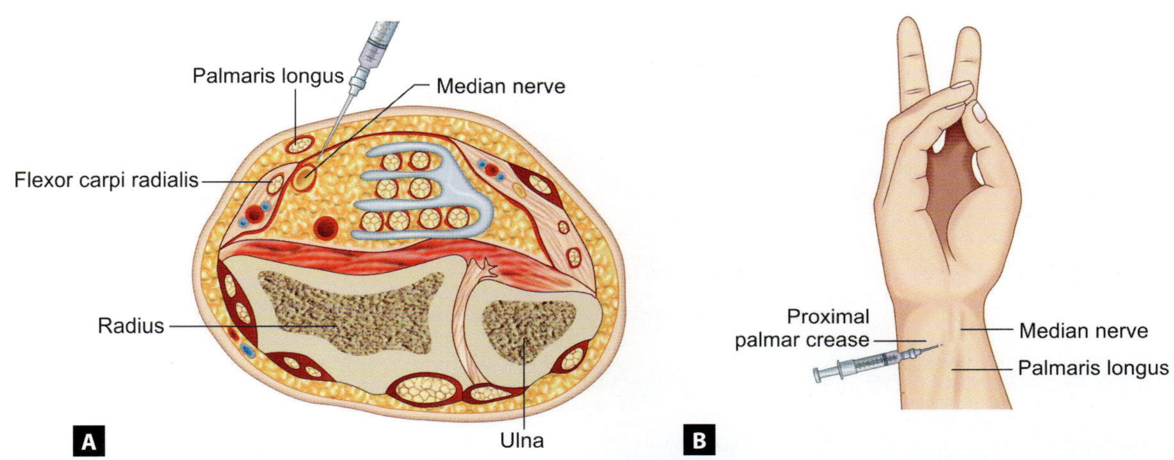

Figs. 28A and B: Median nerve block. (A) Anatomical location of nerve; and (B) Schematic representation of median nerve block.

Procedure (Figs. 30A to D)

- Dorsiflexion at the wrist joint is the position for injection of anesthesia, this makes the flexor carpi ulnaris tendon prominent (Fig. 30A)
- Insert the needle beneath the tendon or just lateral to it, to a depth of 2–3 cm, (Fig. 30B), eliciting paresthesia indicates proper placement. Withdraw the needle several cms, before infiltrating the nerve. About 2 mL of anesthetic agent needs to be deposited
- To infiltrate the dorsal branches, insert the needle medial to the tendon and proceed medially for about 2 cm (Fig. 30C)
- The pisiform bone also can be used as a landmark, infiltrating the agent lateral to it (Fig. 30D).

Digital Nerve Blocks

Anatomy[14]

Each digit is innervated by four digital nerves. The two palmar digital nerves innervate the palmar aspect of the digit and the nail bed, whereas the dorsal nerves innervate the dorsum of the digit (Fig. 31).

Proximal Digital Nerve Block (Fig. 32)

- Patient's hand should be placed flat on the table with palm down
- The syringe is inserted perpendicularly into the web space, just distal to the metacarpal-phalangeal (MP) joint, lateral to extensor tendon
- The anesthetic is injected slowly through the dorsal aspect of the web space, slowly advance the needle straight down toward the volar aspect of the web space, and slowly infiltrating the surrounding tissues of the web space
- The needle should not pierce the volar aspect of the web space
- Withdraw the needle and repeat the procedure on the other web space of the involved digit
- The toes (except the great toe) can be effectively anesthetized in the same manner.

Caution: Direct the needle inwards and downwards.

Transthecal Block (Fig. 33)[15]

- Place the patient's hand on the sterile field with the palm up

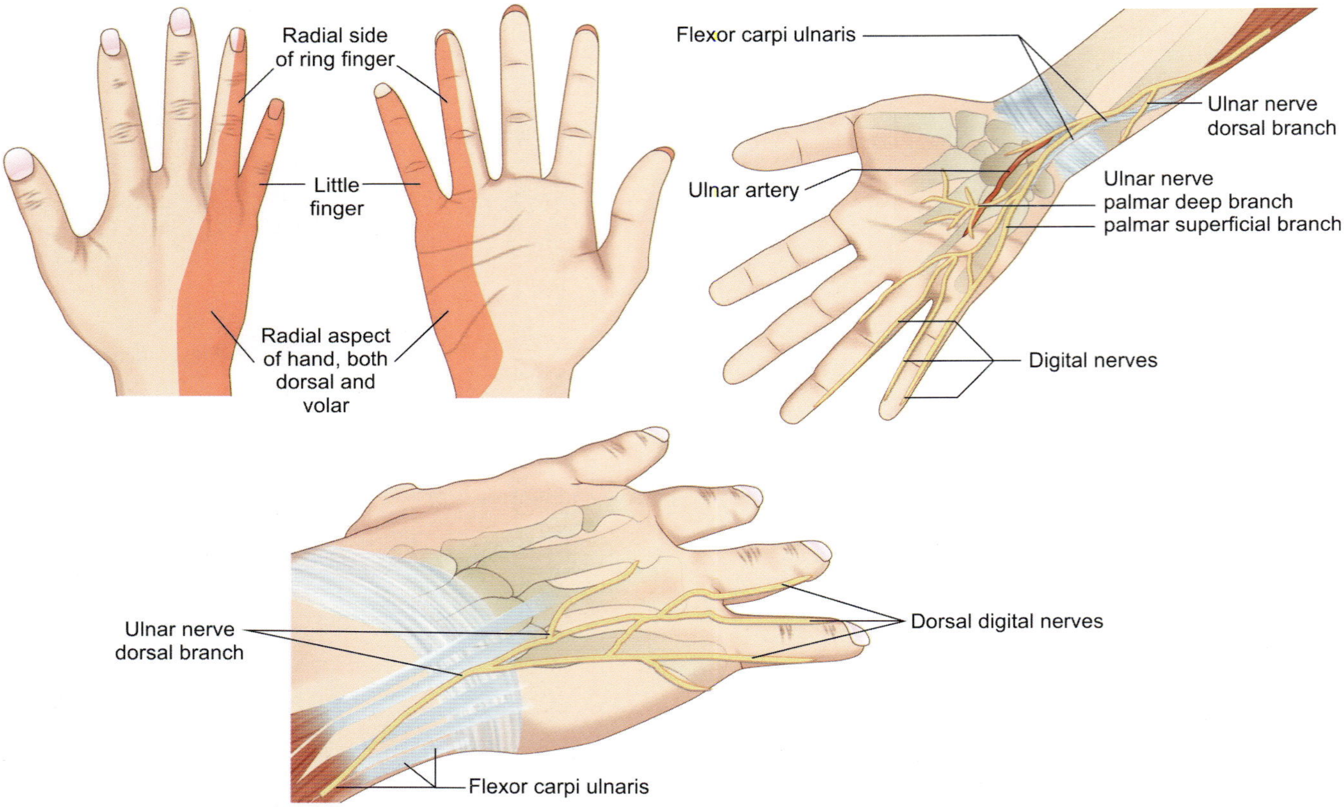

Fig. 29: Branches and sensory supply of ulnar nerve.

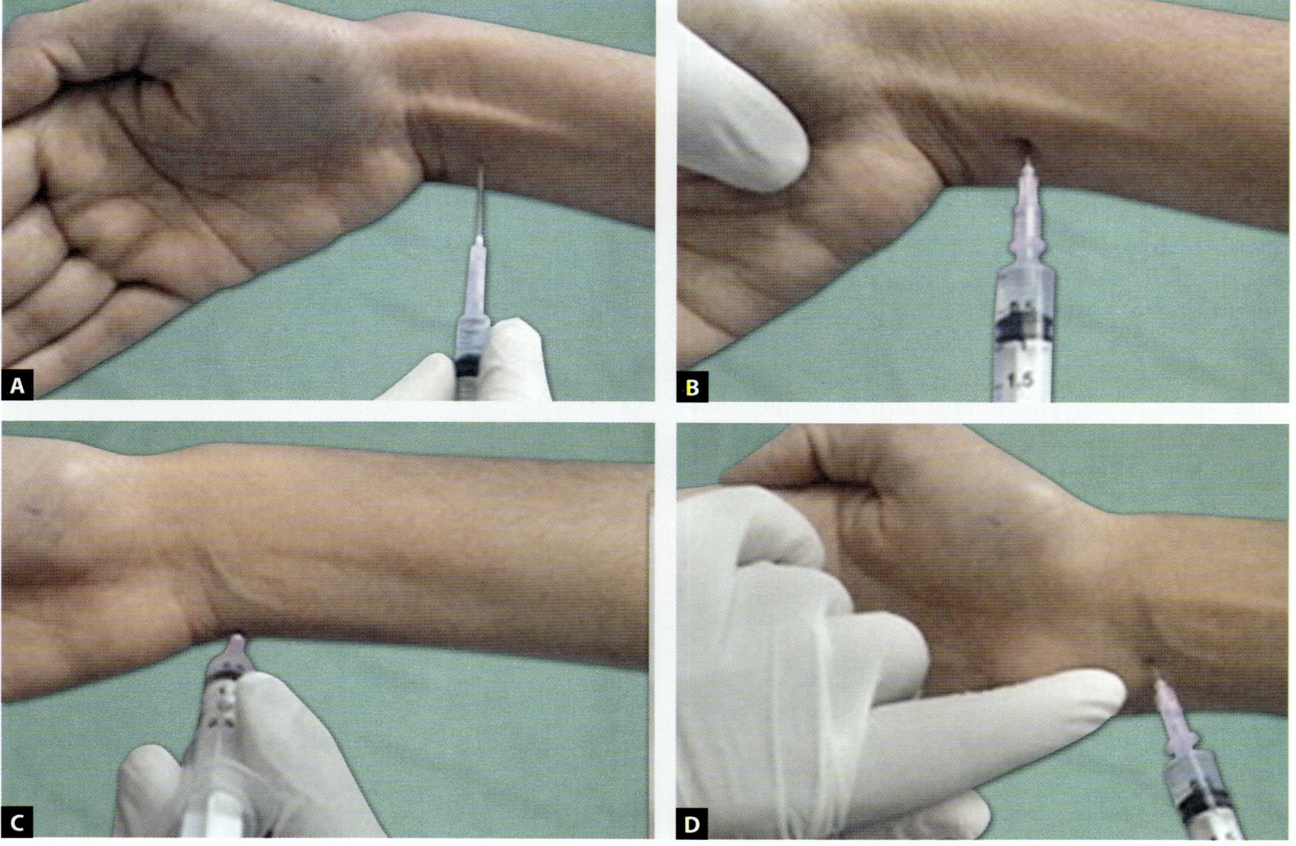

Figs. 30A to D: Ulnar nerve block.

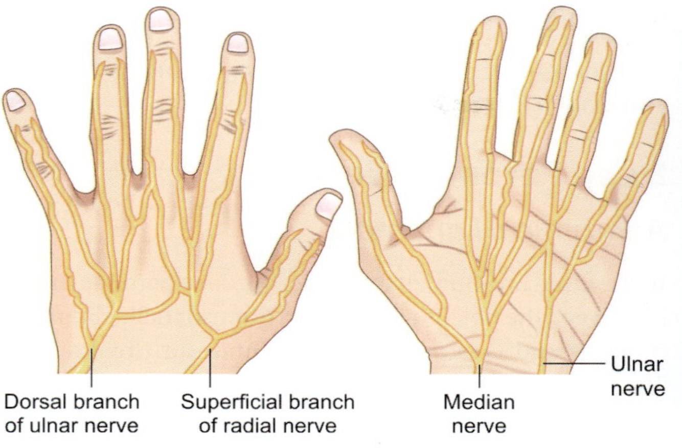

Fig. 31: Palmar and dorsal digital nerves.

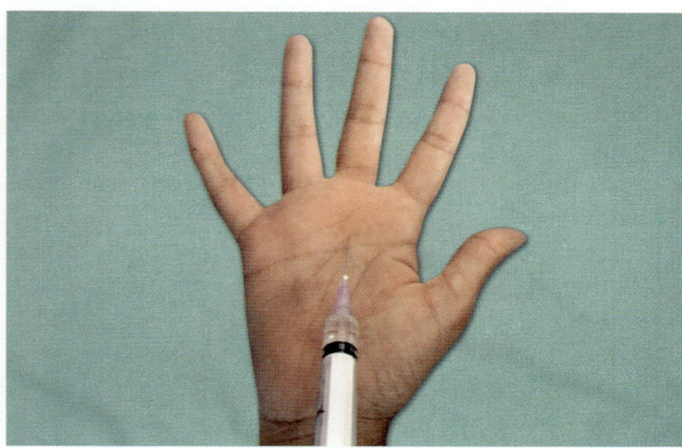

Fig. 33: Transthecal block.

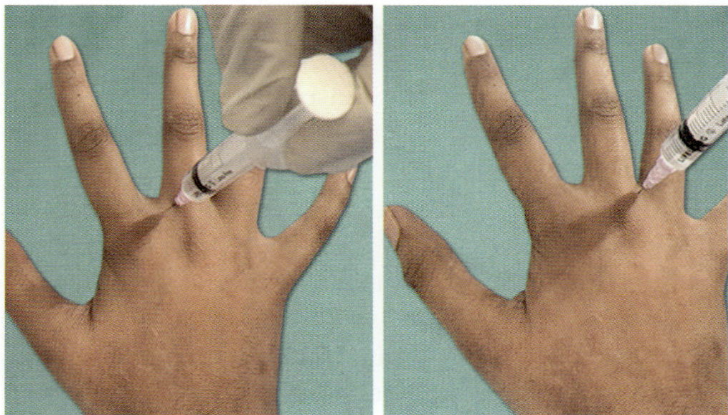

Fig. 32: Proximal digital nerve block.

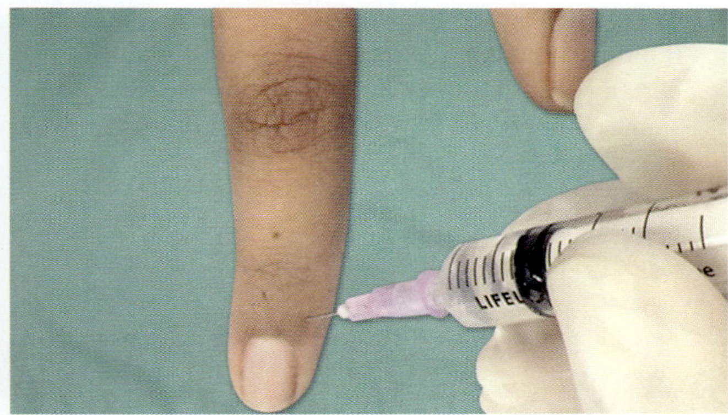

Fig. 34: Distal digital block.

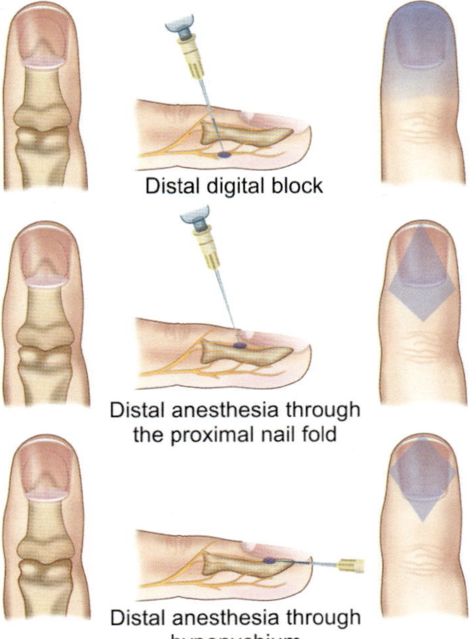

Fig. 35: Three types of distal digital blocks with areas covered.

- Locate the flexor tendon sheath by palpating it at the distal palmar crease
- Insert the needle at a 45° angle just distal to the distal palmar crease
- Inject the anesthetic, it should flow freely. If resistance is met, reposition the needle by slowly withdrawing it
- Studies have shown that transthecal blocks to be as effective as ring blocks for digital analgesia.

Distal Digital Block (Wing Block)[16]

Distal digital block offers total nail unit anesthesia. Here the needle is inserted 2–3 mm proximal to the junction of proximal and lateral nail fold. Insert the needle vertically and advance towards ventral aspect injection about 0.5–1 mL of anesthetic agent (Fig. 34). Three types of distal digital blocks with areas covered are illustrated in Figure 35.

LOWER LIMB BLOCKS

The sensory supply of lower limbs is depicted in Figure 36.

Posterior Tibial Nerve Block

Anatomical Landmark

At the level of ankle, the posterior tibial nerve can be found midway between the medial malleolus and the heel. The nerve lies beneath the flexor retinaculum (Fig. 37).

Procedure (Figs. 38A to D)[17]

- Start by palpating the medial malleolus and advance posteroinferiorly toward the Achilles tendon, until the pulsation of the posterior tibial artery is felt
- Mark the point 0.5–1 cm superior to the posterior tibial artery
- If the artery is not palpable, mark a point 1 cm superior to the medial malleolus and slightly anterior to the Achilles tendon
- Advance the needle through the skin towards the tibia at a 45° angle in a mediolateral plane, just posterior to the artery
- Wiggle the needle slightly to induce paresthesia. If elicited, aspirate to make sure the needle is not in a vessel, wait for the paresthesia to resolve, and inject 3–5 mL
- If paresthesia is not elicited, advance the needle at a 45° angle until it meets the posterior tibia. Withdraw 1 cm and inject 5–7 mL of anesthetic while withdrawing needle another 1 cm.

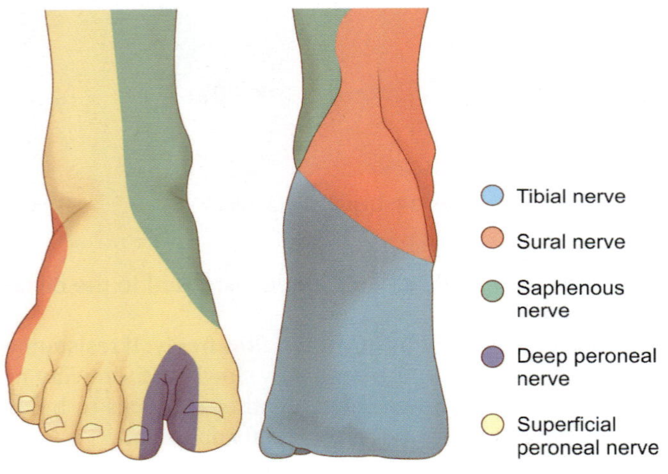

Fig. 36: Sensory supply of lower limb.

Special Indications

Excision of multiple corn, or ablation of multiple warts, and plantar hyperhidrosis

Deep Peroneal Nerve

Anatomical Landmark

In the distal one third of the ankle, the deep peroneal nerve is between the tibialis anterior and extensor hallucis longus muscles and is superficial to the anterior tibial artery. The nerve crosses the ankle deep to the extensor hallucis longus tendon about 12.5 mm proximal to the ankle, and courses between the extensor hallucis longus and extensor digitorum longus tendons (Fig. 39).

Procedure (Figs. 40A and B)[18]

- Identify the tendon of extensor hallucis longus by big toe dorsiflexion against resistance. A groove is felt just lateral to the tendon
- The deep peroneal nerve lies lateral to the tendon and the dorsalis pedis artery. The needle entry site is about 2 cm distal to the intermalleolar line, just lateral to the dorsalis pedis artery pulse
- Advance the needle through the skin in a perpendicular manner until bone is encountered, usually within 2–3 cm
- Withdraw the needle slightly to prevent periosteal injection
- Patients may experience paresthesia in the first web space. If paresthesia occurs, withdraw the needle slightly until the paresthesia disappears and inject 2 mL of the local anesthetic
- To increase the block success, the needle may be redirected 30º medially and laterally and an additional 2 mL of the anesthetic injected.

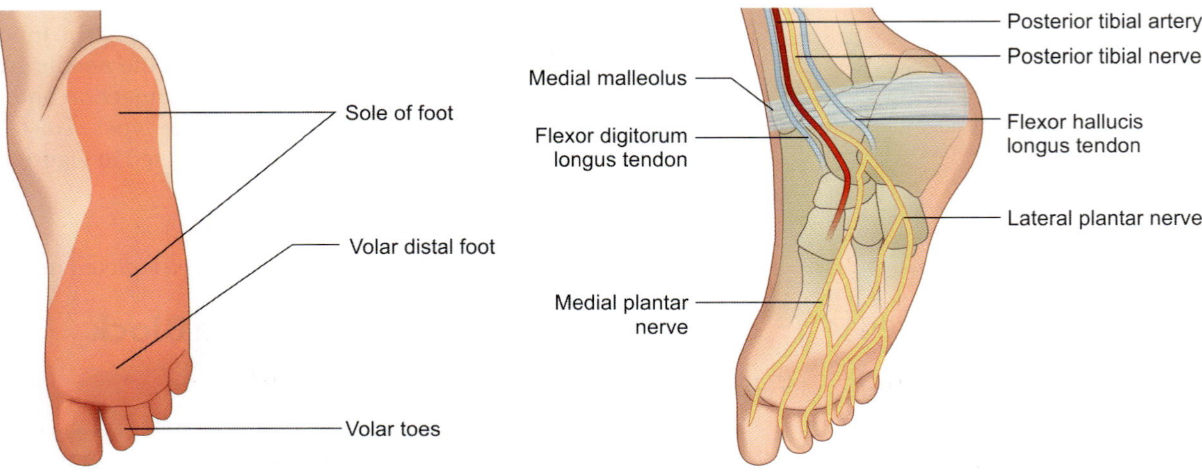

Fig. 37: Posterior tibial nerve and area supplied by it.

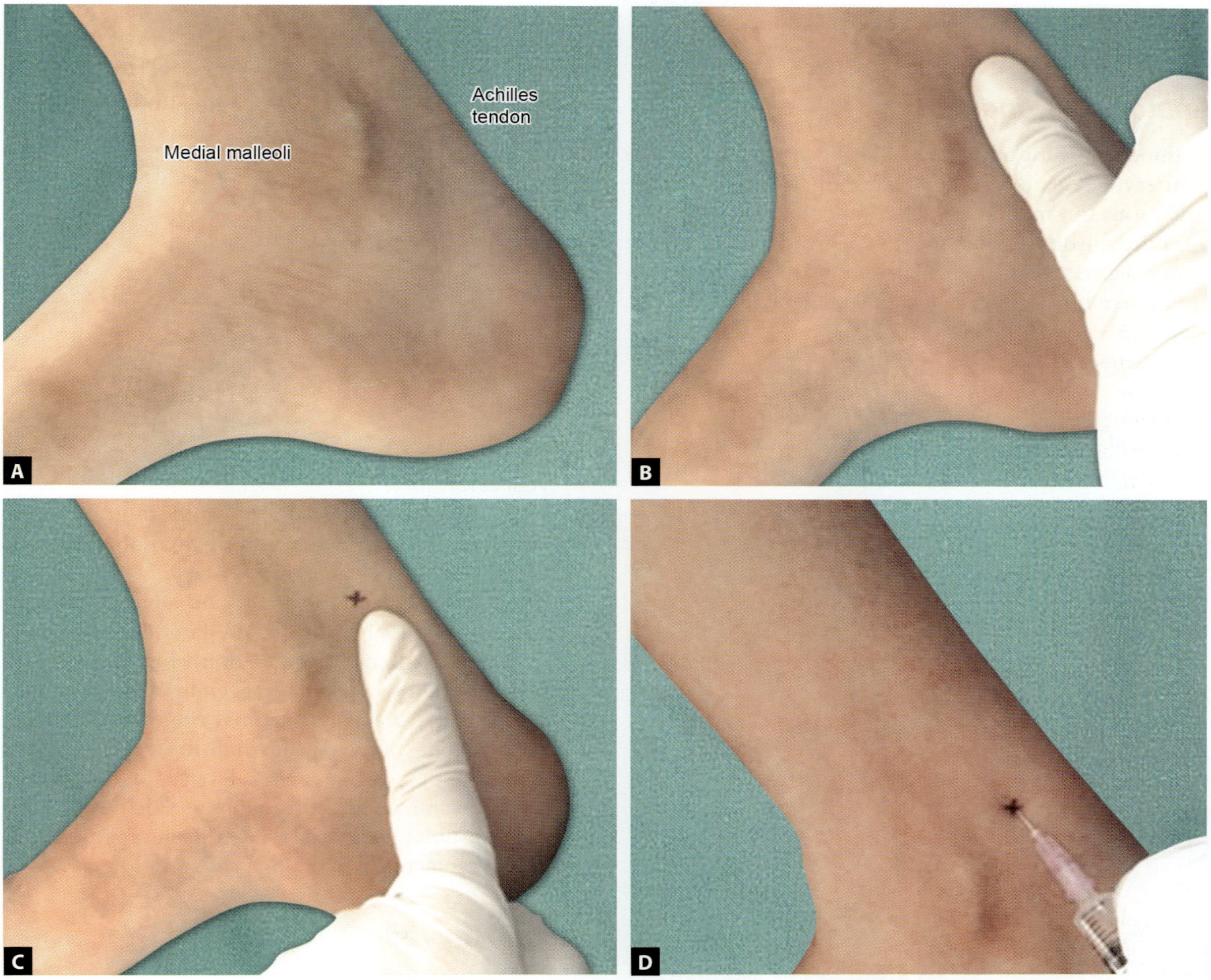

Figs. 38A to D: (A and B) Palpate posterior tibial artery between medial malleoli and Achilles tendon; (C) Mark a point 1 cm superior to artery; and (D) Advance the needle towards tibia and inject 3 mL of anesthetic agent.

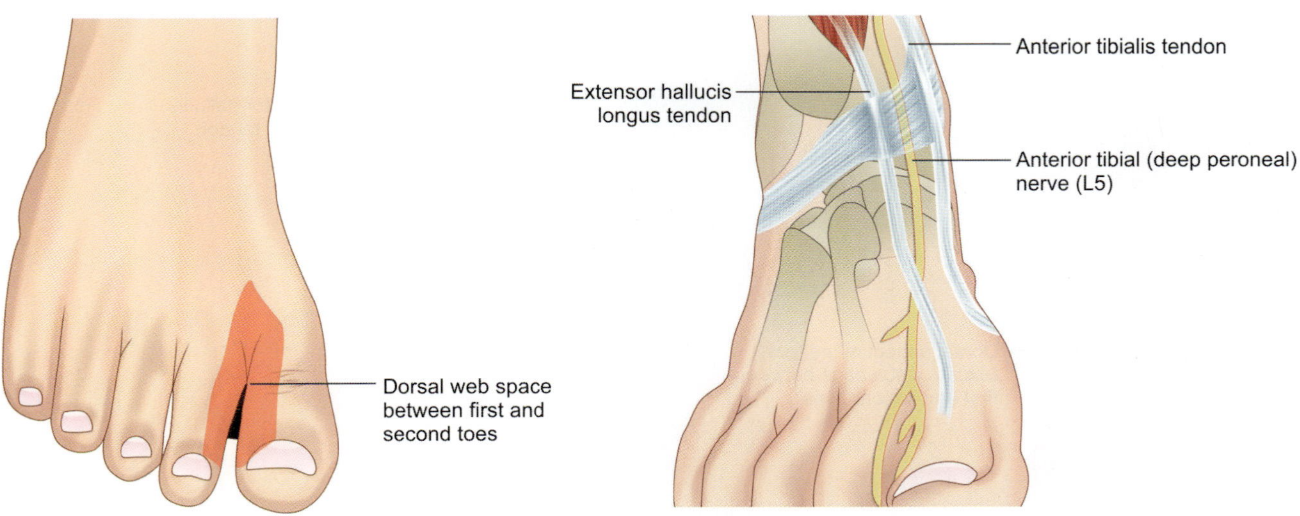

Fig. 39: Deep peroneal nerve and area supplied by it.

Superficial Peroneal Nerve Ankle Block

Anatomical Landmark

In the distal third of the leg, superficial peroneal nerve pierces the deep fascia to become superficial. The nerve splits into the medial dorsal cutaneous nerve and the intermediate dorsal cutaneous nerve, which give rise to the dorsal digital nerves. It lies lateral to extensor digitorum longus tendon at the level of lateral malleoli (Fig. 41).

Procedure (Figs. 42A and B)

- Draw a line from the distal anterior aspect of the lateral malleolus to the anterior border of the medial malleolus (Fig. 42A)

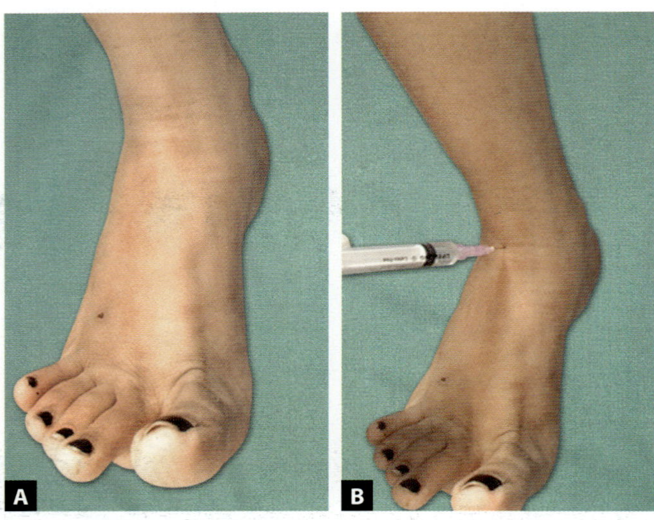

Figs. 40A and B: Deep peroneal nerve block. (A) Tendon of extensor hallucis longus made prominent by big toe dorsiflexion; and (B) Inject lateral to the tendon.

- Place an initial skin wheal of lidocaine anterior to the distal medial malleolus
- Insert the needle through the skin wheal and infiltrate 6–10 mL in a transverse fashion until the lateral malleolus is reached (Fig. 42B).

Saphenous Nerve Block[19]

Anatomical Landmark

At the level of ankle, the saphenous nerve is found between the medial malleolus and the anterior tibial tendon, just lateral to the saphenous vein (Fig. 43).

Procedure

- Palpate the medial malleolus and the great saphenous vein at the ankle
- Mark the site 1.5 cm superior and anterior to the anterosuperior border of the medial malleolus (Fig. 44)
- Insert the needle at this point and advance laterally in a transverse line toward the lateral malleolus to identify the anterior tibial tendon while the foot is in dorsiflexion (dorsiflexion exaggerates the tendon)
- Also identify the anterior tibial ridge by advancing further in the transverse line while the foot is in plantar flexion
- Advance the needle through the skin toward the anterior tibial tendon in a superficial transverse line, without injecting the tendon itself.

Sural Nerve[20]

Anatomical Landmark

Sural nerve enters the foot posterior to the lateral malleolus (Fig. 45).

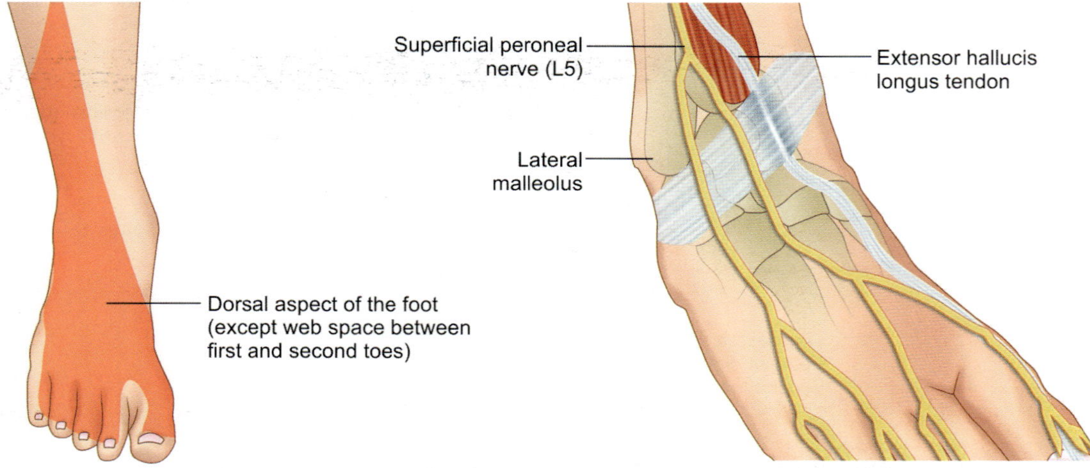

Fig. 41: Superficial peroneal nerve and area supplied by it.

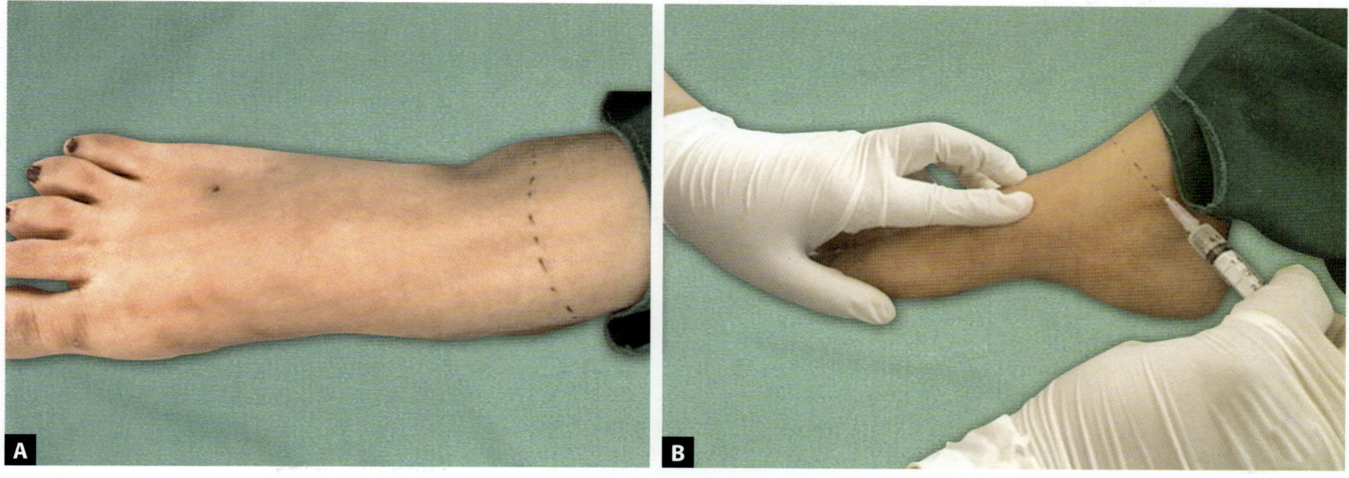

Figs. 42A and B: Superficial peroneal block.

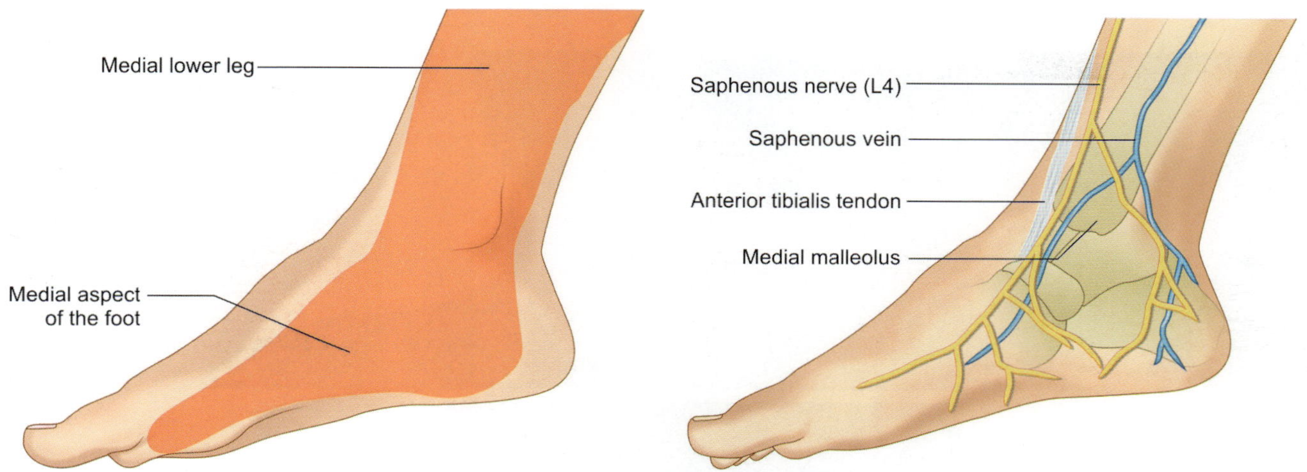

Fig. 43: Saphenous nerve and area supplied by it.

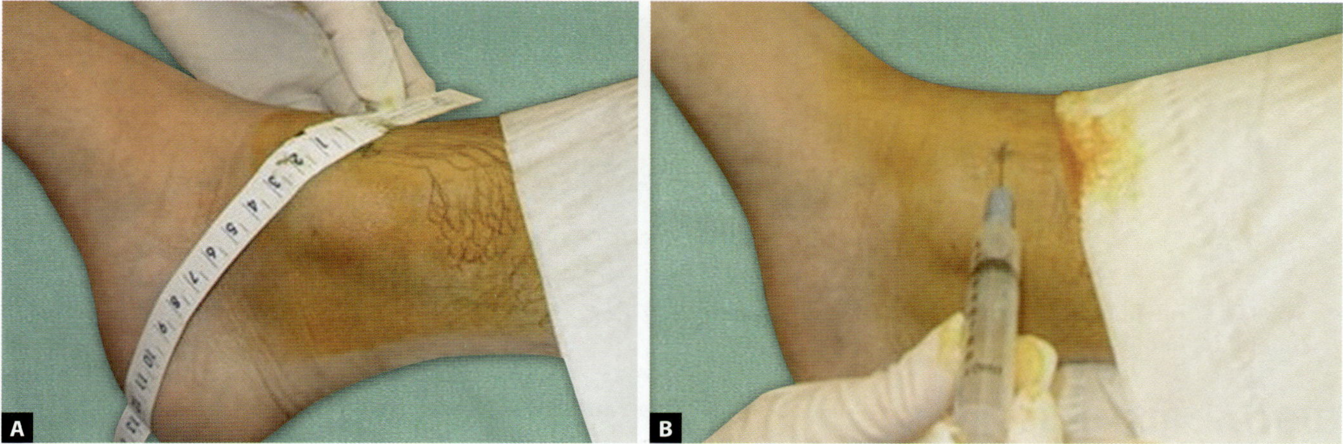

Figs. 44A and B: Saphenous nerve block.

Procedure (Figs. 46A to C)

- Locate the posterior border of the lateral malleolus and the Achilles tendon (Fig. 46A)
- Mark the site just lateral to the Achilles tendon, between the two landmarks (Fig. 46B)
- Insert the needle and move the needle angling toward the lateral malleolus (Fig. 46C)

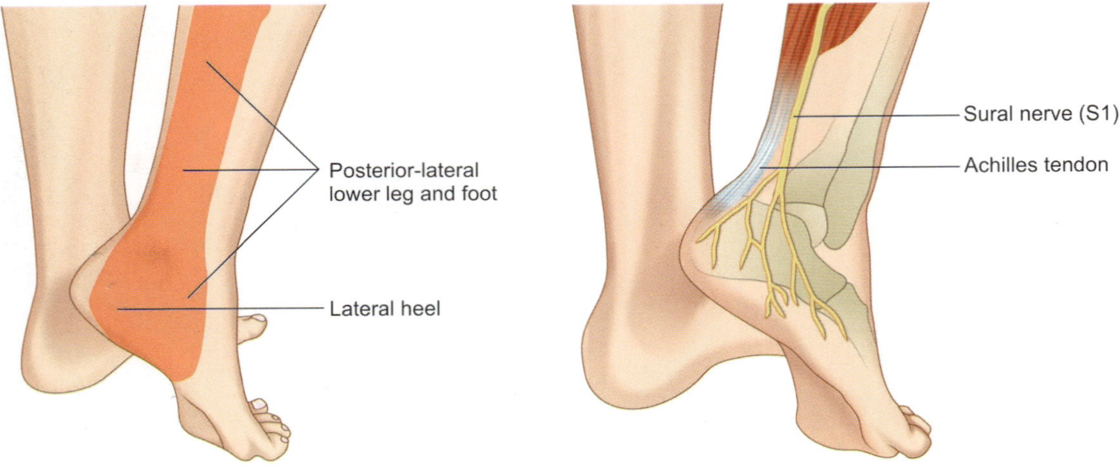

Fig. 45: Sural nerve and area supplied by it.

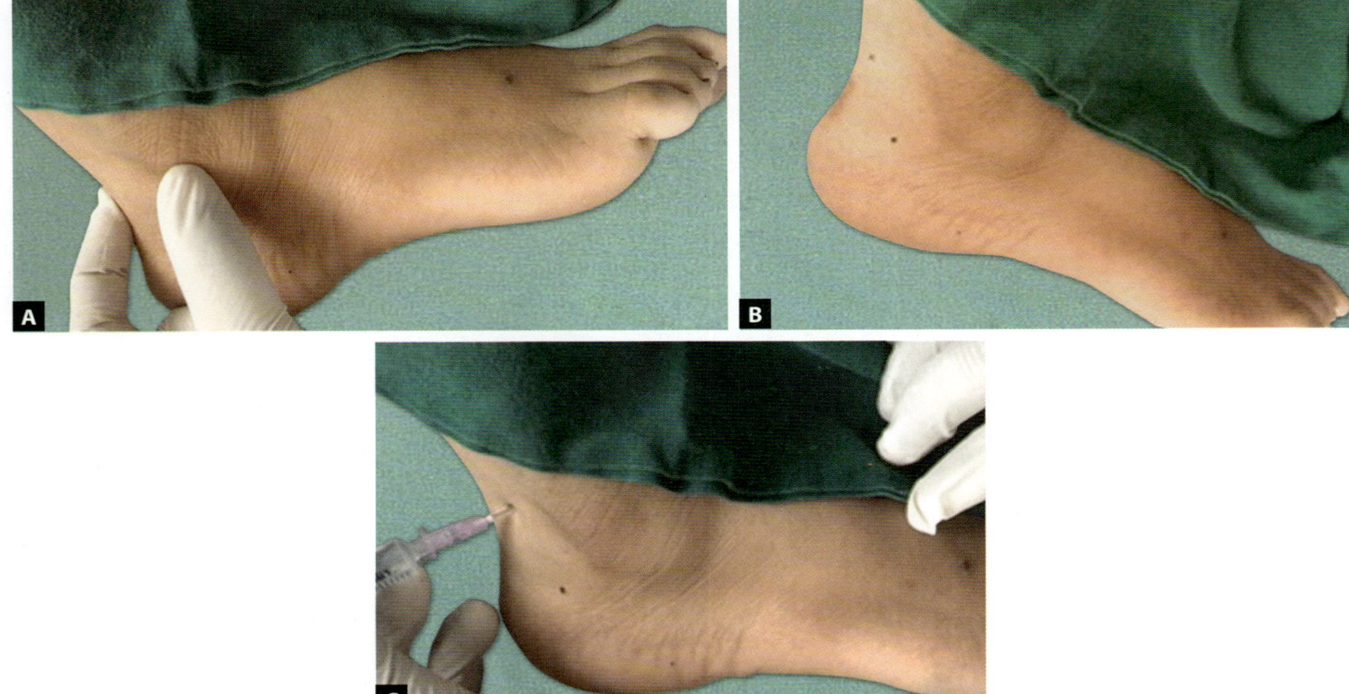

Figs. 46A to C: Sural nerve block.

- Inject 5–7 mL of lidocaine in a transverse line until the lateral malleolus is reached.

DIGITAL BLOCKS (FIG. 47)

Web space block is similar to that in upper limb.

Three-sided Digital Block[21]

This type of digital block is effective in anesthetizing the great toe, but it can be used for any digit.

Procedure (Figs. 48A to C)

- Place the extremity with plantar side down
- Insert the needle at a 90° angle at the medial aspect of the digit, just distal to the metatarsal-phalangeal joint (Fig. 48A)
- Slowly inject the anesthetic as the needle is advanced toward the volar or plantar side, without piercing the volar skin (Fig. 48B)
- Slowly withdraw the needle and redirect it medially

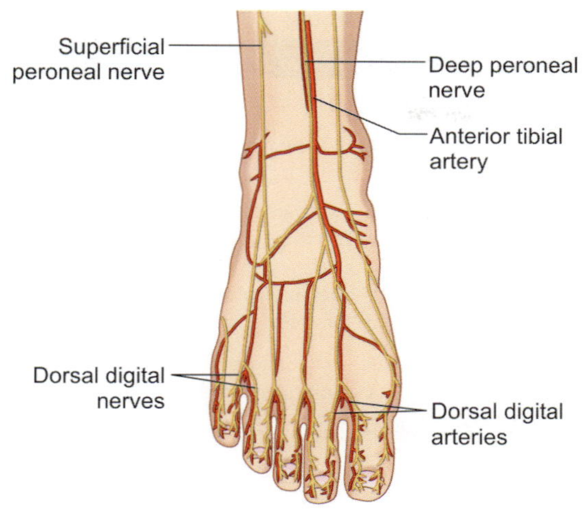

Fig. 47: Nerve supply to the digits of lower limbs.

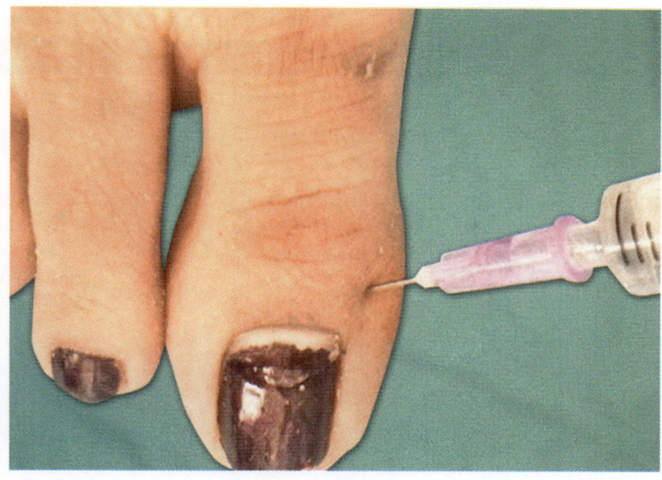

Fig. 49: Wing block for great toe.

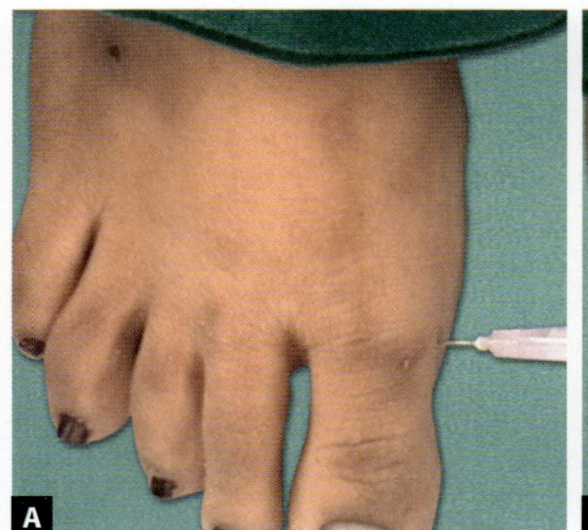
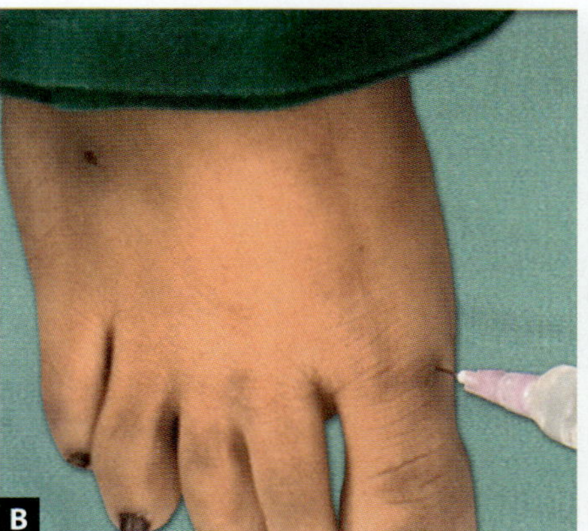
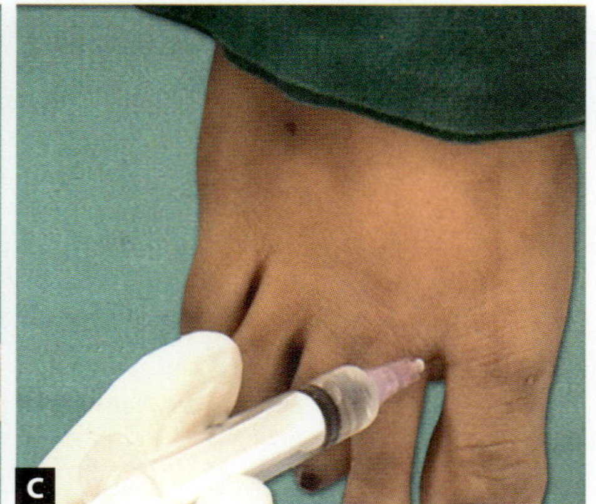

Figs. 48A to C: Three-sided digital block.

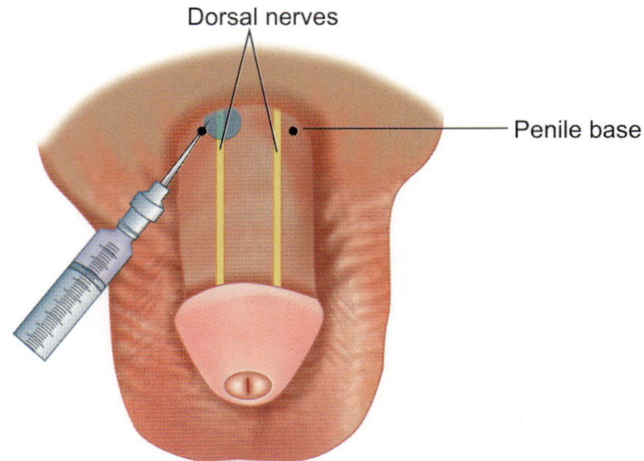

Fig. 50: Dorsal penile nerve block.

- Advance the needle slowly from medial to lateral side while the anesthetic is injected
- Withdraw the needle
- Make another injection over the already anesthetized skin at the lateral aspect of the digit, with the needle at 90°, advancing it from the dorsal to ventral aspect, as was done medially (Fig. 48C).

Distal Digital Block (Wing Block)

Distal digital block offers total nail unit anesthesia. Here the needle is inserted 2–3 mm proximal to the junction of proximal and lateral nail fold. Insert the needle vertically and advance towards ventral aspect injection about 0.5–1 mL of anesthetic agent (Fig. 49).

PENILE BLOCK

- The right and left dorsal penile nerves should be blocked as proximally to the base of the penis as possible
- The point of injection is 2- and 10-O'clock positions at the base of penis (Fig. 50)
- The needle should be directed toward the center of the shaft, to a depth of about 0.5 cm or until loss of resistance is felt to suggest that the tip of the needle is within the Buck fascia
- Aspirate to ensure that the needle is not in a blood vessel, and slowly inject about 2 mL of local anesthetic on each side

Table 1: Common peripheral nerve blocks practiced in dermatosurgery.

Nerve	*Anatomical landmark*	*Technique*
Supraorbital nerve	Exits through supraorbital notch	Insert needle just below the eyebrow along midpupillary line
Supratrochlear nerve	Present beneath the medial end of eyebrow	Insert needle 1 cm below and lateral to the medial tip of eyebrow
Infraorbital nerve	Exits from infraorbital foramen present about 7 mm below the infraorbital margin in midline	Intraoral route: Insert the needle vertically upwards with tip pointing towards the foramen in the gingivolabial sulcus between the 3rd and 4th teeth from midline (3½ method) Extraoral route: Insert needle at midpoint between alar groove and upper nasolabial fold with tip directed towards foramen
Long buccal nerve	Emerges 2–3 cm upper and lateral to the angle of mouth	Insert needle 2–3 cm lateral and superior to the angle of mouth with needle pointing towards mouth and inject in a fanning technique
Mental nerve	Emerges from the mental foramen	Insert needle in the gingivolabial sulcus in between the 4th and 5th teeth from the midline (4½ method)
Median nerve	Situated deep to palmaris longus and medial to flexor carpi radialis	Ask the patient to slightly flex at wrist and appose thumb and little finger tightly. Now insert the needle beneath the plamaris longus with needle pointing laterally and inferiorly
Ulnar nerve	Present beneath and lateral to flexor carpi ulnaris. It is also, proximal and lateral to pisiform	Insert needle proximal and lateral to pisiform bone. Alternatively, needle can be introduced between flexor carpi ulnaris and ulnar artery at the level of proximal wrist crease. Direct the needle below and outwards (lateral)
Radial nerve	Anatomical snuff box at the radial side of wrist	Mark the anatomical snuff box by asking the patient to abduct and hyperextend the thumb and all 4 fingers. Insert the needle just proximal and radial to the anatomic snuff box with the needle directed across the snuff box from lateral to medial
Dorsal digital nerve	Dorsolateral to extensor digital tendon and just beneath the superficial vein	At the level of webspace, insert the needle at 20° angle or just into subcutis lateral to extensor tendon. Needle should be directed inwards and downwards
Palmar digital nerve	Lateral to flexor tendon	Insert the needle at 30° into subcutis lateral to flexor tendon. Needle should be directed medially and inferiorly
Posterior tibial nerve	Situated between Achilles tendon and medial malleolus, close to bone	Insert the needle anterior to Achilles tendon at the level of medial malleolus with needle directed towards posterior border of malleolus Hit the bone and slightly withdraw and inject
Deep peroneal nerve	Medial to extensor digitorum longus at the level of lateral malleolus	Ask the patient to dorsiflex the foot with slight eversion. Insert the needle just medial to extensor digitorum longus at the level of lateral malleolus. Needle should be inserted perpendicular to skin
Superficial peroneal nerve	Lateral to extensor digitorum longus tendon at the level of lateral malleolus	Ask the patient to dorsiflex the foot with slight eversion. Insert the needle just lateral to extensor digitorum longus at the level of lateral malleolus. Needle should be directed towards the lateral malleolus
Saphenous nerve	Situated anterior to medial malleolus and posteromedial to tibialis anterior tendon	Palpate the tibialis anterior tendon by asking the patient to dorsiflex and invert the foot. Introduce the needle slightly posteromedial to tibialis anterior tendon at the level of superior border of medial malleolus
Sural nerve	Anterior to Achilles tendon at the level of lateral malleolus	Insert the needle just anterior to Achilles tendon at the level of lateral malleolus with the needle directed towards the posterior border of lateral malleolus
Dorsal digital nerve of toes	Dorsolateral to extensor digital tendon	At the level of webspace, insert the needle at 45° angle. Needle should be directed inwards and downwards towards the webspace
Palmar digital nerve of toes	Lateral to flexor tendon	Insert the needle at 30° into subcutis lateral to flexor tendon. Needle should be directed medially and inferiorly
Penile nerve (at Pubic Symphysis)	Lower border of pubis symphysis	Place index and middle finger tips over the lower border of symphysis pubis at the base of penis on dorsal aspect in midline. Introduce the needle between the slightly spread index and middle finger. Needle should be directed perpendicular to skin and push it inferior to the lower margin of pubic symphysis
Dorsal penile nerves	They are paired and present 1 cm lateral to midline alongside dorsal penile artery or posterolateral to visible cutaneous dorsal vein in postpubertals	Hold the penis with thumb in midline just distal to penile base and introduce the needle perpendicular to skin and progress anterolaterally
Ventral ramus of penile nerve	Situated at the base of penis in midline on ventral side	Hold and lift the skin of ventral side with thumb and index finger at the base of penis. Insert the needle close to base of penis, lateral and just below the tip of the thumb

Source: Adopted from Local and Regional Anesthetic Blocks Made Simple by Sanchez et al.

- An alternative method is to inject 2 mL of local anesthetic on either side of the midline, avoiding injecting into the superficial dorsal penile vein.

CONCLUSION

Table 1 summarizes the different nerve blocks used in dermatosurgery.

Tips and Pearls

- The key to successful regional anesthesia is familiarity with the local anatomy of the nerve and its associated landmarks
- To help avoid injecting anesthetic into the nerve, the patient is told to signal if any paresthesia is felt in the region of needle insertion. If paresthesia is elicited, the needle must be withdrawn 1–2 mm before the anesthetic is injected to avoid intraneural injection
- To decrease the risk of directly injecting into an artery or vein, aspirate prior to injection
- A few blocks are of easy and durable acquisition: supraorbital, infraorbital, mental, and nasal very safe from serious complications
- On the other hand the blocks carried out in the "plexus" beginning, like the maxillary nerve and the mandibular nerve, are more delicate, with a rate of less raised success, even for accustomed, and with risks of complications raised in the literature. These are out of purview of dermatologists.

REFERENCES

1. Brummett CM, Williams BA. Additives to Local Anesthetics for Peripheral Nerve Blockade. Int Anesthesiol Clin. 2011;49(4):104-16.
2. Shin KJ, Shin HJ, Lee SH, et al. Emerging Points of the Supraorbital and Supratrochlear Nerves in the Supraorbital Margin With Reference to the Lacrimal Caruncle: Implications for Regional Nerve Block in Upper Eyelid and Dermatologic Surgery. Dermatol Surg. 2016;42(8):992-8.
3. Sattur S. Donor area strip harvesting. In: Mysore V (Ed). Hair transplantation. New Delhi: Jaypee Brothers Medical Publishers (P) Ltd; 2015. pp. 141-4.
4. A Pulcini, JP Gueri, European Society of Regional Anesthesia (ESRA). (2007). Regional blocks. [online] Available from http://nesra.co.uk/files/training/education/Handbook%20of%20Regional%20Anesthesia%20ESRA.pdf. [Accessed February, 2017].
5. Hornung DE. Nasal anatomy and the sense of smell. Adv Otorhinolaryngol. 2006;63:1-22.
6. Taleghani K, Sternbach G. Infraorbital nerve block. In: Rosen P, Chan TC, Vilke GM, Sternbach G (Eds). Atlas of Emergency Procedures. St Louis: Mosby Press; 2001. pp. 160-1.
7. Byrne KM, Hedges JR. Infraorbital nerve block: intraoral approach. In: Roberts JR, Hedges JR, Custalow C (Eds). Clinical Procedures in Emergency Medicine, 4th edition. Philadelphia: Elsevier; 2004.
8. Khoury JN, Mihailidis S, Ghabriel M, et al. Applied anatomy of the pterygomandibular space: improving the success of inferior alveolar nerve blocks. Aust Dent J. 2011;56(2):112-21.
9. Dental Hygiene. (2017). Review of long buccal nerve block. [online] Available from www.dentalhygiene411.com/administration-of-local-anesthetics/long-buccal-nerve-block. [Accessed February, 2017].
10. Syverud SA, Jenkins JM, Schwab RA, et al. A comparative study of the percutaneous versus intraoral technique for mental nerve block. Acad Emerg Med. 1994;1(6):509-13.
11. Ling Tan FF, Schiere S, Reidinga AC, et al. Blockade of the mental nerve for lower lip surgery as a safe alternative to general anesthesia in two very old patients. Local Reg Anesth. 2015;8:11-4.
12. McMinn NH, Hutchings RT, Logan BM. Color Atlas of Head and Neck Anatomy, 2nd edition. Baltimore: Mosby-Wolfe; 1995. pp. 161-3.
13. The New York School of Regional Anesthesia (NYSORA). (2017). Wrist block. [online] Available from www.nysora.com/posts/view/94. [Accessed February, 2017].
14. Agur A, Ming L. Grant's Atlas of Anatomy, 10th edition. Lippincott: Williams & Wilkins; 2003. pp 78-84.
15. Low CK, Wong HP, Low YP. Comparison between single injection transthecal and subcutaneous digital blocks. J Hand Surg Br. 1997;22(5):582-4.
16. Tahiliani S. Surgery of nails. In: Mysore V (Ed). ACSI Textbook on Cutaneous and Aesthetic Surgery. New Delhi: Jaypee Brothers Medical Publishers (P) Ltd; 2012. pp. 484-97.
17. Brown DL. Ankle block. In: Gray AT (Ed). Atlas of Ultrasound-Guided Regional Anesthesia, 2nd edition. Philadelphia: Elsevier Saunders; 2013. pp. 129-33.
18. Kelly JJ, Spektor M. Nerve blocks of the thorax and extremities. In: Roberts JR, Hedges JR, Custalow C (Eds). Clinical Procedures in Emergency Medicine, 4th edition. Philadelphia: Elsevier Saunders; 2004. pp. 584-9.
19. Myerson MS, Ruland CM, Allon SM. Regional anesthesia for foot and ankle surgery. Foot Ankle. 1992;13(5):282-8.
20. Russell DF, Pillai A, Kumar CS. Safety and efficacy of forefoot surgery under ankle block anaesthesia. Scott Med J. 2014;59(2):103-7.
21. Flarity-Reed K. Methods of digital block. J Emerg Nurs. 2002;28(4):351-4.

Chapter

16

Hemostasis in Dermatologic Surgery

T Salim

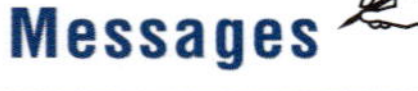

- Proper hemostasis is vital for ensuring proper postoperative results and prevent complications.
- Detailed history, particularly with reference to drug intake should be sought in all cases posted for surgery.
- Electrocautery and suture techniques should be appropriately used to control intraoperative bleeding.

INTRODUCTION

Bleeding has always been a concern in all surgeries including dermatologic surgery. Control of the bleeding process is essential for achieving an optimal surgical outcome. Methods to control bleeding and repair wounds have existed for many years. Dermatologic surgery is usually a mild form of surgery and hence serious problems of hemostasis are rare. However, problems can be encountered in surgeries such as hair transplantation and other excisions on scalp, liposuction, flap surgeries on face, etc. Hence dermatosurgeons should be familiar with all aspects of hemostasis.

HISTORY

Efforts have ranged from the use of raw meat by the ancient Egyptians[1] to the use of dried plasma in World War I to achieve hemostasis.[2] The Egyptians used a mixture of wax, grease and barley in an effort to stop bleeding.[3] In ancient Greece, hemostatic herbs were applied to wounds suffered in combat.[4] Native Americans are thought to have used scrapings of the inside of animal hides mixed with hot sand and eagle down as topical hemostatic agent.[5] More traditional techniques have included applying pressure, electrocautery and suturing. In the last decade, however, advances in biotechnology have resulted in an explosive growth of topical hemostatic agents which are available to the modern dermatologic surgeon.

DEFINITION

Hemostasis can be defined as a tightly regulated process that maintains the blood flow through the vasculature simultaneously as a thrombotic response to tissue damage occurs.[6] Hemostasis is blood clot formation at the site of vessel injury. It is a complex interaction between platelets, plasma proteins, and coagulation and fibrinolytic pathways. Hemostasis aims at reducing the amount of blood loss, as well as preventing rebleeding, hematoma formation and need for repeated surgery.

MECHANISMS OF HEMOSTASIS

Understanding the mechanisms of hemostasis and thrombosis is critical to the management and stabilization of a patient undergoing any dermatologic surgical procedure. Maintaining hemostasis requires a complex interaction of the vessel wall, platelets, and the coagulation and fibrinolytic systems (Fig. 1).[7,8] There are two main phases of hemostasis: primary (i.e. the cellular phase) and secondary (i.e. the humoral phase). The clotting

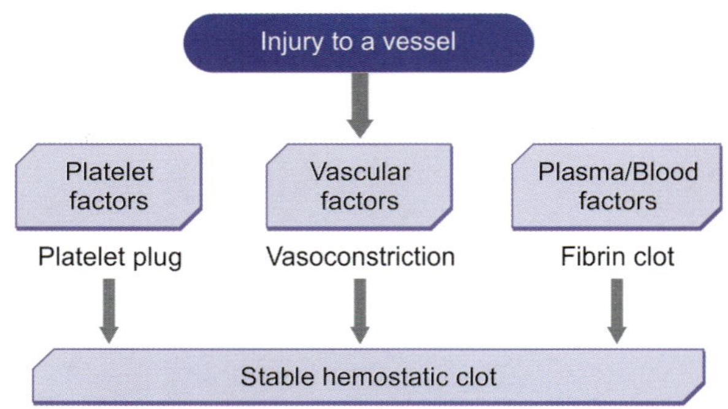

Fig. 1: Factors that contribute to normal hemostasis.

cascade involves the sequential activation of proenzymes in a stepwise response, which ultimately provides local generation of fibrin lattices that reinforce the platelet plug (Fig. 2).

Primary Hemostasis

Primary hemostasis begins immediately after endothelial disruption and is characterized by vasoconstriction, platelet adhesion and formation of a soft aggregate plug.[9] The first phase of hemostasis involves vasoconstriction at the site of injury and is elicited by the release of serotonin and thromboxane A2 (TXA2). The immediate vasoconstrictive period reduces blood flow through the injured tissue and provides some initial protection to the loss of circulating volume in the vascular compartment.

Circulating Von Willebrand factor attaches to the subendothelium at the site of injury within few seconds after the injury and adheres to the glycoproteins on the surface of platelets. As platelets adhere to the injured surface, they are activated by contact with collagen-exposing receptors that bind circulating fibrinogen. A soft plug of aggregated platelets and fibrinogen is formed.[6,9] This phase of hemostasis is short-lived and the soft plug can easily be sheared from the injured surface.[9]

Secondary Hemostasis

The soft platelet plug is stabilized during secondary hemostasis to form a clot. Vasoconstriction and the resultant reduction in blood flow are maintained by platelet secretion of serotonin, prostaglandin and thromboxane while the coagulation cascade is initiated. The coagulation cascade is a series of dependent reactions involving several plasma proteins, calcium ions and blood platelets that lead to the conversion of fibrinogen to fibrin[9,10] (Fig. 2). Coagulation factors are produced by the liver and circulate in an inactive form until the coagulation cascade is initiated. Then each step of the cascade is initiated and completed via a series of sequential and dependent coagulation factor activation reactions. In the final steps, thrombin converts the soluble plasma protein fibrinogen to the insoluble protein fibrin, while simultaneously converting factor XIII to factor XIIIa. This factor conversion stabilizes the fibrin and results in cross-linking of the fibrin monomers, producing a stable clot.[9,10]

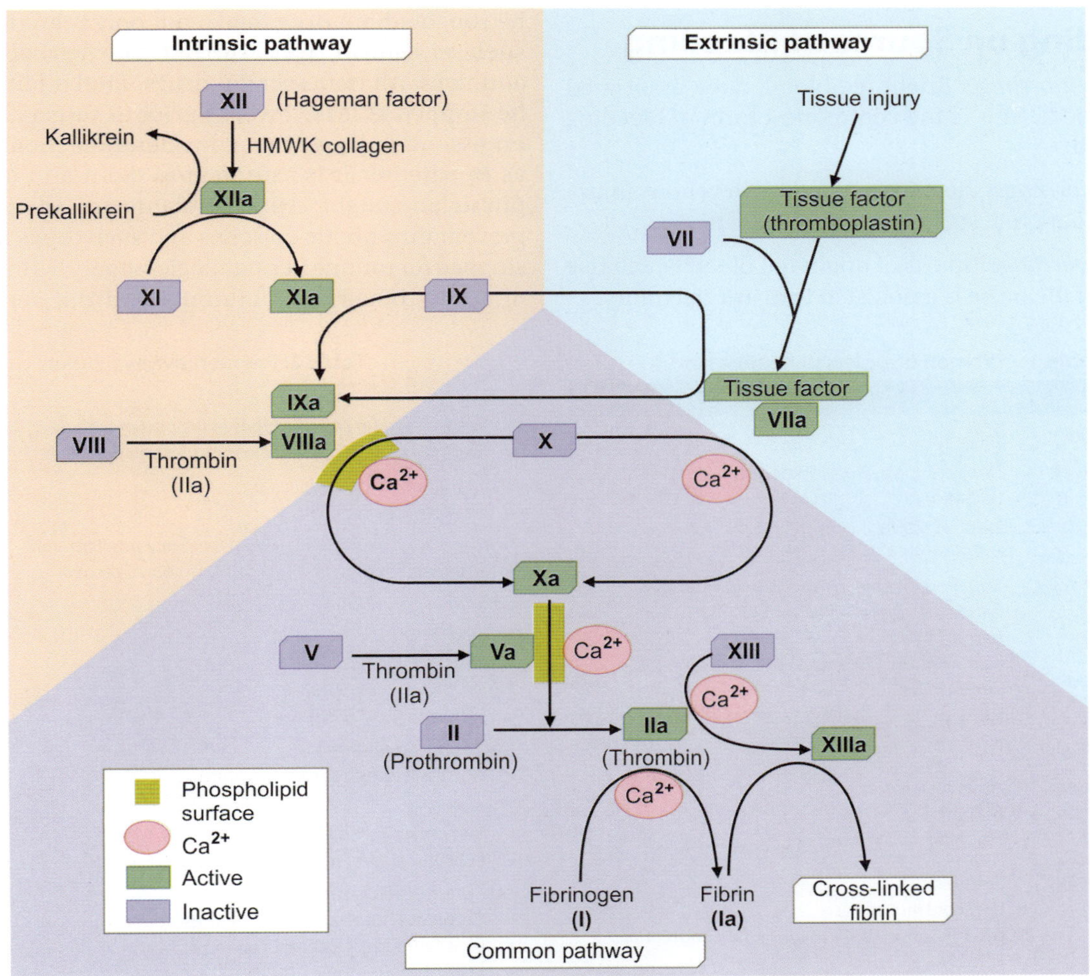

Fig. 2: The clotting cascade.

TYPES OF BLEEDING IN DERMATOLOGIC SURGERY

Hemorrhage can be classified depending on the source of bleeding and time of bleeding.[9]

Depending on Time of Bleeding

Primary hemorrhage: This is the commonest form of bleeding occurring intraoperatively.

Reactionary hemorrhage: This type of bleeding usually follows primary hemorrhage within 24 hours of surgery. Common causes for reactive hemorrhage in dermatologic surgery are slipping of ligature, clot dislodgement, cessation of reflex vasospasm and weaning of tumescence in tumescent anesthesia. This can result in hematoma formation with secondary infection and wound dehiscence.

Secondary hemorrhage: This is a form of bleeding which occurs between 7 days and 14 days after surgery. Sloughing of a part of the vessels or infection of a surgical wound can lead to this type of bleeding. This is rarely encountered in dermatologic surgery.

Depending on Source of Bleeding

Capillary hemorrhage: Bright red blood, often associated with rapid ooze. This is the commonest form of bleeding encountered.

Venous hemorrhage: Bleeding secondary to venous injury presents as dark red, steady copious flow of blood.

Arterial hemorrhage: Spurts of bright red blood which rise and fall with the pulse is associated with arterial injury.

Table 1: Common disorders of hemostasis.

Class	*Example*
Hypocoagulability	
Impaired platelet function	Drugs (e.g. aspirin, clopidogrel) Radiation Splenomegaly Autoimmune
Impaired clotting activity	Impaired protein synthesis (e.g. vitamin K) Classic hemophilia (Factor VIII; ~80% of all hemophilias) Hemophilia B (Factor IX; ~ 15% of all hemophilias) Hemophilia C (Factor XI; ~5% of all hemophilias)
Hypercoagulability	
Increased platelet function	Atherosclerosis Diabetes Smoking
Increased clotting	Pregnancy Oral contraceptives DIC (disseminated intravascular coagulation) activity

Source: Table adapted from: http://www.pathoplus.com/ blood.htm

APPROACH TO EFFECTIVE HEMOSTASIS IN DERMATOLOGIC SURGERY

The approach should include the following steps:

- Preoperative evaluation:
  - History and examination
  - Lab investigations
- Intraoperative techniques
- Postoperative techniques.

Preoperative Evaluation

Evaluation of a patient preoperatively will identify patients at risk and effective hemostatic measures can be implemented. Several factors can contribute to the occurrence of intraoperative bleeding related to either the surgical procedure itself or the individual patient.[10,11]

A careful history will identify patients at risk for bleeding disorders (Table 1). History should include detailed questions about factors surgery (Table 2). This will prove more beneficial than any test. Patients on medications for other ailments should be evaluated to identify drugs affecting hemostasis. Particularly, information should be sought about drug intake not only prescription drugs such as aspirin, warfarin but also herbals and food additives. All nonessential drugs, food additives should be stopped at least 2 weeks prior to surgery. If patent is on essential drugs, due consideration should be given as to whether it is safe to stop them and advice from physician sought. Anticoagulants are administered to prevent thrombotic episodes and such drugs need not be stopped for routine dermatologic surgery, as the likelihood of severe bleeding is minimal and the consequences

Table 2: Preoperative evaluation.

History:

History of bleeding complications in the past procedures:

- Dental extraction, teeth cleaning, invasive surgery

History of spontaneous bleeding:

- GI bleeding, Epistaxis

History of large hematoma after a relatively small trauma:

- Profuse bleeding after minor cuts and scratches

Conditions contributing to bleeding:

- Alcoholism
- Liver diseases

Inheritable coagulopathies:

- Hemophilia, VW disease

Use of anticoagulants:

- NSAIDs, Vitamin E, Ginkgo Biloba

Examination:

- Site of the lesion to be operated
- Ecchymosis, Petechiae, etc.

Laboratory investigations:

- Complete blood count with platelet count
- Bleeding time, clotting time
- Prothrombin time along with INR
- Partial thromboplastin time

Table 3: Factors contributing to intraoperative bleeding.

- Surgical incisions
- Tissues not amenable to suturing
- Low-pressure suture lines
- Anticoagulant medications
- Diffuse capillaries (e.g. large surfaces)
- Unseen sources of bleeding
- Coagulopathies and platelet dysfunction

of stopping the anticoagulant potentially serious and life threatening. Questions about any previous bleeding episodes, particularly during injury or dental extractions should be asked. Proper physical examination should be done to detect any evidence of bleeding tendency such as ecchymoses and petechiae. The type of bleed and hemostatic techniques vary with site. Preoperative examination thus helps the surgeon to plan most effective method of hemostasis according to the site. If any bleeding tendencies are suspected or detected during examination, they can be further evaluated and confirmed by proper laboratory screening. The laboratory screening should include bleeding time, platelet counts, prothrombin time (PT), International Normalized Ratio (INR) and partial thromboplastin time.

The **bleeding time** is a study of platelet function and will be prolonged in patients on aspirin, nonsteroidal anti-inflammatory drugs (NSAIDs), those with defective platelets and decreased platelet number. In contrast, **platelet count** is more specific and will only be abnormal if there is a quantitative deficiency of platelets.[12]

The **PT** detects abnormalities in extrinsic and common pathways of coagulation and will be increased by the use of warfarin and dicoumarin, but not heparin. Routine preoperative INR, bleeding time and PT may not always be helpful in predicting operative and postoperative bleeding. A normal PNR does not rule out the possibility of bleeding, but a high supratherapeutic INR (> 5), indicates a significant risk of postoperative bleeding.[13] The **partial thromboplastin time** (PTT) reveals defect in intrinsic and common pathways and will be prolonged with both heparin and warfarin.

Hence, the coagulation of profile has to be studied in its entirety and in relation to history and circumstances of each patient.

Intraoperative Measures

There are several factors which may lead to intraoperative bleeding (Table 3). Dermatologic surgeons have an array of options to control bleeding, including mechanical and thermal techniques and devices as well as pharmacotherapies and topical agents (Tables 4 and 5).

Rapid and effective hemostasis allows the surgeon to retain visualization of the surgical field. This can both reduce the procedure time and the risk of accidental injury.[7] Adequate lighting and wound retraction is essential to detect the source of bleed. Suction can be used to increase visibility in case of increased intraoperative bleeding.[12]

Table 4: Techniques for maintaining hemostasis in surgery.[14]

Mechanical techniques
- Direct pressure
- Sutures
- Staples
- Ligating clips
- Fabric pads
- Gauzes
- Sponges
- Blood component/replacement therapy

Thermal techniques
- Electrocautery
- Hemostatic scalpel
- Laser

Chemical techniques
- Pharmacotherapy
- Hypotensive anesthesia
- Epinephrine
- Vitamin K
- Protamine
- Desmopressin
- Aminocaproic acid
- Tranexamic acid

Topical hemostats
- Collagen
- Cellulose
- Gelatins
- Thrombins

Topical sealants and adhesives
- Fibrin sealants
- Synthetic glues

An anxious patient is more likely to bleed more, due to increased sympathetic activity. It is therefore important to allay the anxiety of the patient, if necessary by administering a tranquillizer. Likewise preoperative hypertension too may lead to bleeding.

Role of Anesthesia in Preventing Intraoperative Bleeding

Adrenaline in concentration of 1:100,000, when given along with lignocaine has significant vasoconstrictive effect and thereby prevent bleeding. However, it takes 30 minutes after infiltration for this effect to set in. Tumescent anesthesia is the use of large quantity of saline mixed with adrenaline and lignocaine. It has the twin effects producing anesthesia and also decreasing intraoperative bleeding due to the vasoconstrictive effect of adrenaline. A detailed discussion on this technique can be found in chapters on hair transplantation and liposuction.

Measures to Reduce Blood Flow to the Site of Operation

Intraoperative measures to reduce the blood flow to the surgical field are of great use in routine dermatologic surgical procedures.

Table 5: Mechanism of action, advantages/recommended use, and disadvantages/caution against use for topical hemostatic agents.

Hemostatic agent	Products	Mechanism of action	Advantages/ Recommended use	Disadvantages/Caution against use
Gelatin	Gelfoam, Gelfilm, Surgifoam, Abgel	Provides physical matrix for clotting initiation	Effectively controls small vessel bleeding May be used to control bleeding from bone Recommended as hemostatic plug wrapped in oxidized cellulose Absorbed by the body within 4–6 weeks Nonantigenic Neutral pH allows use with biologic agents	Should not be used in closed spaces as significant swelling may compress nerves Use around brisk arterial bleeding can dislodge sponge. May embolize if in an intravascular compartment
Oxidized cellulose	Surgical	Provides physical matrix for clotting initiation, low pH contributes to coagulative necrosis	Low pH has antimicrobial effect Very good handling characteristics (cotton-like consistency, best when applied dry) Does not stick to instruments Typically dissolves in 2–6 weeks	Must not be used with other biologic hemostatic agents (e.g. thrombin) because of low pH Low pH may increase inflammation of surrounding tissue
Microfibrillar collagen (MFC)	Avitene Ultrafoam, Avitene Ultrawrap, Helistat, Helitene, Instant, Endo Avitene	Platelet adherance and activation	No significant swelling Absorbed in less than 8 weeks Can control wide areas of parenchymal bleeding Effective despite profound heparinization because of its mechanism of action	Less effective in patients with thrombocytopenia Sticks to operator's gloves
Thrombin	Thrombin-JMI (bovine), Evithrom (human plasma-derived), rh Thrombin/Recothrom (recombinant human)	Converts fibrinogen to fibrin to form clots, activation of clotting factors	Effectively controls minor bleeding from capillaries and small venules when pressure or ligature is insufficient Easy application Fast acting	May bind to neural structures immunologic response, and possible increase in coagulopathy and thrombosis
Fibrin sealants	Tisseel, Evicel, Crosseal	Thrombin and fibrinogen mixed at site of application; thrombin cleaves fibrinogen to fibrin that forms clots	Effective in heparinized patients Can be used for skin grafting, Tisseel and Evicel good for venous oozing from raw surface	Before application, wounds must be cleaned of antiseptics containing alcohol, iodine, or heavy metal ions that can denature applied thrombin and fibrinogen
Platelet sealants	Vitagel	Microfibrillar collagen and thrombin combined with patient's plasma-derived fibrinogen and platelets	Platelets from patients strengthen clot while proteins in gel facilitate tissue regeneration	Need for centrifugation and preuse processing
Polyethylene glycol hydrogels	Coseal	Two synthetic polyethylene glycol polymers that mix and cross-link in wound site	Good mechanical sealant for vascular reconstructions Is not exothermic, does not cause inflammation, and does not potentiate bacterial infection	Swelling up to 4 times initial volume after 1 day, and can continue swelling
Cyanoacrylates	Dermabond	Liquid monomers form polymers in the presence of water, and glue surfaces together	Use as a replacement for sutures (5–0) for wounds on the face, extremities and torso Full binding strength within 2.5 minutes, attains strength of healed tissue after 7 days Forms waterproof barrier	Difficult to use in jagged lacerations Must not use for bites, puncture or crush wounds Not recommended on mucosal surfaces, axilla or perineum
Fibrin dressings	Dry fibrin sealant dressings	Freeze-dried (lyophilized) fibrinogen and thrombin on gauze dressing	Initial success with US forces with Iraq and Afghanistan under FDA investigational drug protocol Effectively stops bleeding from large surface abrasions Longer shelf-life than fibrin sealants and does not need mixing at site of application	Not FDA approved Needs strong packaging due to brittleness

Contd...

Contd...

Hemostatic agent	***Products***	***Mechanism of action***	***Advantages/ Recommended use***	***Disadvantages/Caution against use***
Chitin dressings	Rapid deployment hemostat (RDH)	Vasoconstriction, mechanical sealing, mobilization of RBCs, clotting factors, platelets	Intended for emergency field use by first responders Effective for minor wounds	Varied results for severe wounds like splenic lacerations in animal model
Chitosan dressings	HemCon	Deacylated form of chitin, similar mechanism	Intended for emergency field use by first responders Initial success with US forces with Iraq and Afghanistan Has antimicrobial properties	Animal testing yields inconsistent results Contains chitosan from shellfish, so do not use in patients with shellfish allergies
Mineral zeolite dressings	QuikClot	Molecular sieves absorb water at site of wound to increase concentration of clotting factors, platelets, RBCs	Intended for emergency field use by first responders Powdered form effective for low-pressure bleeding, Zeolite embedded in mesh for high pressure bleeding	Caution with high pressure bleeds as they can force powdered form out of wound

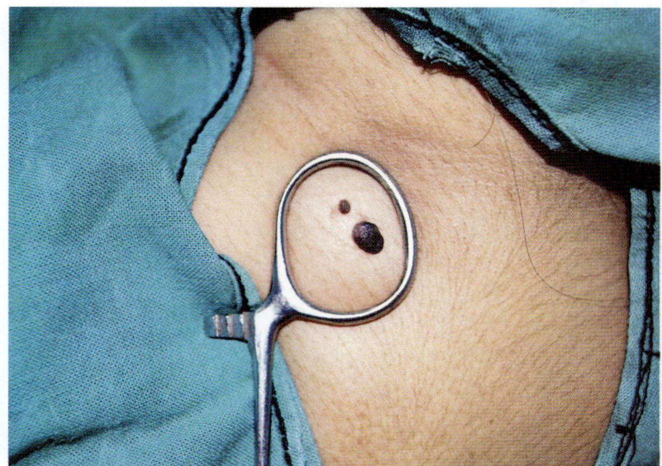

Fig. 3: Circumferential pressure hemostasis using ring of artery forceps.

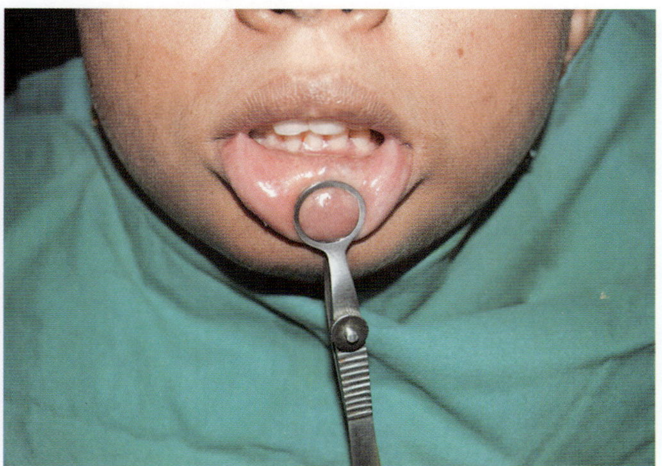

Fig. 4: Circumferential pressure hemostasis using chalazion ring forceps.

Direct pressure: Application of direct pressure or compression at a bleeding site is often the surgeon's first choice to assist in the control of bleeding. It is often an underutilized tool for hemostasis. Constant pressure with surgical pad or mop for 10–20 minutes is effective in reducing capillary oozing and small venous hemorrhage.[12] Other mechanical methods, including sutures, staples, and ligating clips, are useful if the source of bleeding is easily identifiable and able to be sealed.

Tourniquet: Use of Tourniquet and pressure cuffs with intermittent release is of great value in surgeries of extremities. Tourniquet used in nail surgeries allows the surgeon to retain visualization of the surgical field.

Circumferential pressure hemostasis: Tourniquets and pressure cuffs cannot be used on area like trunk, scalp, tongue, lips, etc.

Circumferential pressure is a simple hemostatic method useful in these situations. Finger ring of an artery forceps or a needle holder pressed firmly around the lesion to be excised, exerts uniform circumferential pressure (Fig. 3). This achieves effective hemostasis attaining a bloodless field in situations like scalp biopsy.[14]

For minor procedures on lips and tongue; circumferential pressure hemostasis can be achieved by the help of a simple device called chalazion ring forceps. Chalazion ring forceps is used in ophthalmologic surgery for incision and curettage of meibomian cyst. It has a flat plate on one of the handle and a ringed rim on other handle which can be clamped over the plate. The plate of the forceps can be pushed under lip or tongue in base position so that the ring is placed around the lesion to be excised. The screw is then tightened until the ring fits snugly so as to immobilize the lesion. This stabilizes the lesion as well as provides hemostasis (Fig. 4). Circumferential pressure hemostasis using chalazion ring forceps is useful in procedures on lips, toungue, such as biopsy, excision of mucocele, pyogenic granuloma, etc.[15]

Sutures: Larger vessels may need to be identified clamped and ligated. After ligation, vessel can be tied with suture or electrosurgical device can be used. An absorbable suture is used to tie off the vessel using a figure-of-eight suture or a simple suture.[12,16]

Presuturing technique: This technique can be utilized in excision surgeries in order to prevent excessive blood loss during the surgery. Sutures are passed under the lesion to be excised. These are tied immediately after excising the lesion (Figs. 5A to D). This technique is useful in treating vascular lesions like pyogenic granuloma and in biopsies on scalp (Figs. 6A and B).

Figure of eight suture: This is a suture technique to achieve effective hemostasis in area where there is diffuse bleeding and difficulty to pinpoint the source of bleeding. This suture technique is different from figure of eight suture used for ligating vessels. Suture is made as shown in Figures 7A and B. The circumferential pressure compresses the bleeding vessels so as to attain hemostasis (Figs. 8A and B).

Thermal techniques: Thermal techniques, such as hemostatic scalpels and lasers, also have become viable surgical options to reduce bleeding in dermatologic surgery. Much of the bleeding caused by cutaneous surgery can be controlled by electrocautery, electrocoagulation or electrodessication. Bipolar electrocautery systems are simple devices useful in dermatologic surgical settings. However, care should be taken to minimize damage to surrounding tissue.[12] Too liberal use of electrocautery can contribute to a wider postoperative scar.

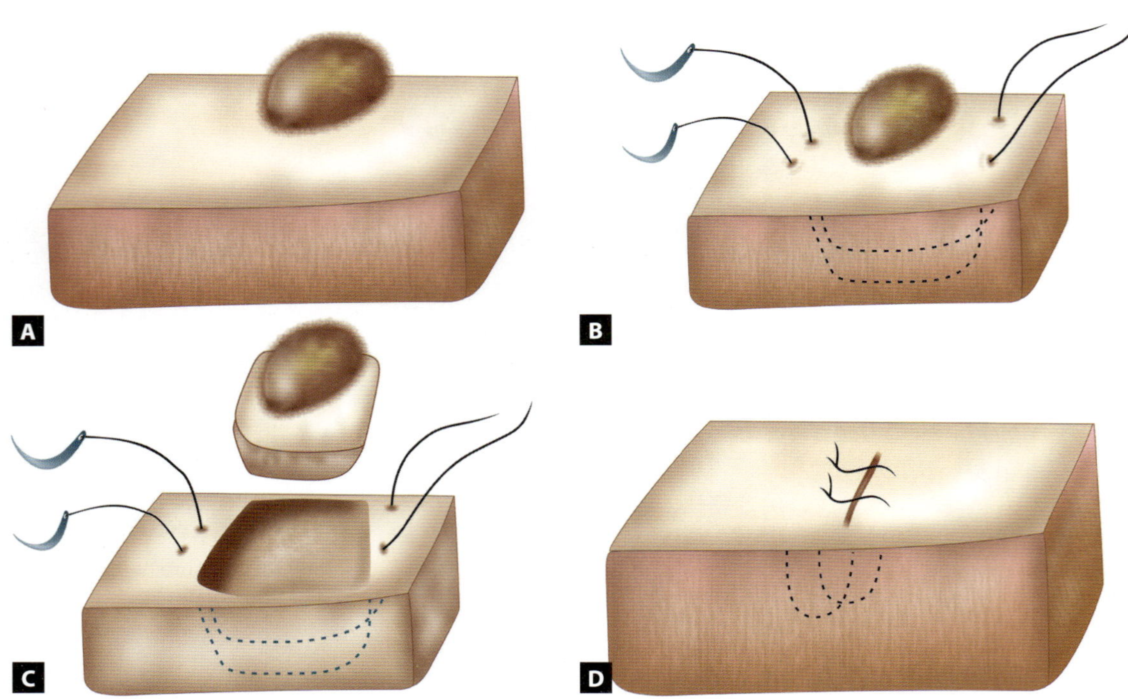

Figs. 5A to D: Presuturing technique.

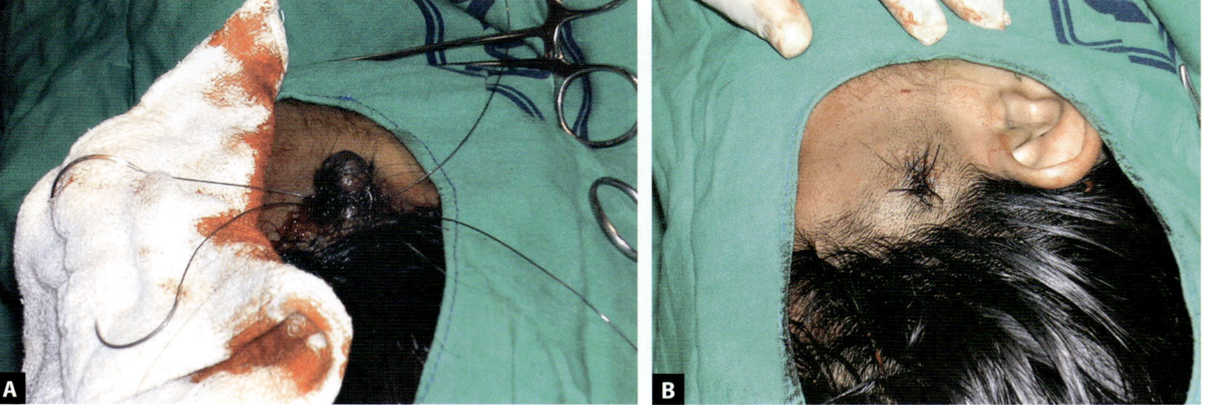

Figs. 6A and B: Presuturing technique for granuloma pyogenicum on face.

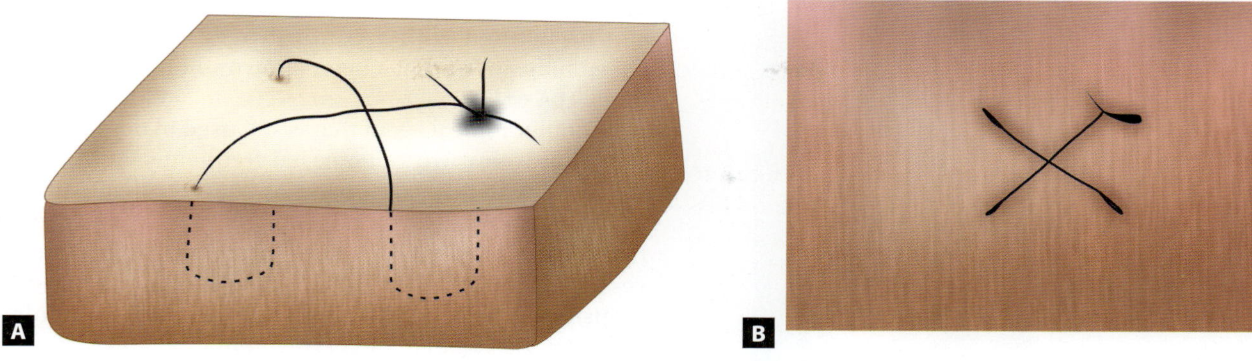

Figs. 7A and B: Figure-of-eight suturing.

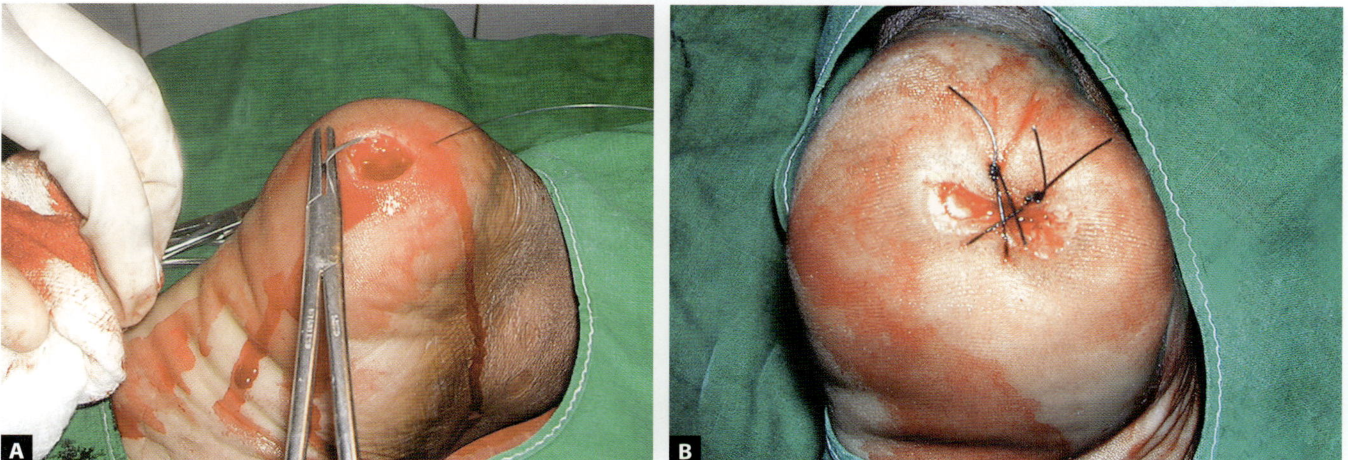

Figs. 8A and B: Figure-of-eight suturing.

Bipolar radiofrequency paired with conductive saline is a new wound sealing method effective in dermatologic surgery.[17] Bipolar radiofrequency paired with conductive saline effectively achieved hemostasis in patients undergoing dermatologic surgery and reduced problems associated with traditional bipolar electrosurgery. It is helpful in the setting of larger flaps and when patients are taking blood thinners. Better visualization of the field and less surgical time; creating a clean wound bed. This employs a bipolar mono terminal configuration and can be safely used in patients with implanted electronic devices, such as permanent pacemakers, automatic implantable cardioverter defibrillators (AICDs), and cochlear implants. All actively bleeding vessels, even actively pulsatile arterial bleeds, were controlled and sealed without the use of hemostats or other instruments. The investigators observed no char, burning, or collateral tissue destruction with saline-coupled bipolar electrosurgery.

Continuous wave CO_2 laser at 10,600 nm wavelength targets water as a chromophore and blocks small blood vessels. This is useful in laser blepharoplasty.

Hemostatic agents: Topical hemostatic agents can be applied directly to the bleeding site and may prevent continuous unrelenting bleeding throughout the entire procedure and into the postoperative recovery period. Hemostasis using topical agents also can avoid the adverse effects of systemic hemostatic medications, such as "unwanted" blood clots. Table 5 summarizes the currently available topical hemostatic agents useful in dermatologic surgery.[18] In surgical procedures where the amount of blood loss is unpredictable, topical hemostats can be used sparingly when blood loss is minimal and more liberally during severe bleeding. Furthermore, as hemostasis is attained and maintained at the bleeding site, there may be prolonged benefit with respect to postoperative blood loss.

Caustic Hemostatic Agents

Topical caustic agents commonly used in dermatosurgical procedures include, aluminum chloride, ferric subsulfate (Monsel's solution) silver nitrate, and zinc chloride paste (Figs. 9A and B). These agents are effective, easy to use and have made many surgeries cost-effective. They work by coagulating proteins leading to tissue necrosis and eschar formation enhancing thrombus formation and hemostasis.[19] Properties of caustic hemostatic agents are given in Table 6.

Aluminum chloride is the most widely used topical agent in dermatologic surgery as it is effective and

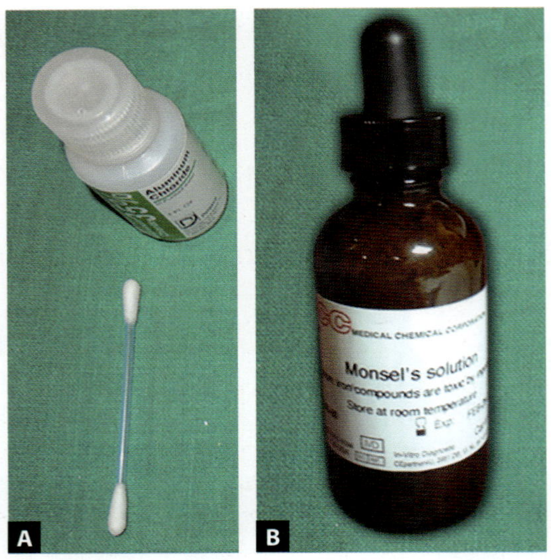

Figs. 9A and B: (A) Silver chloride solution with cotton tipped applicator; (B) Monsel's solution.

does not lead to pigmentation of the skin. This solution can be applied with a cotton-tipped applicator after shave biopsies and has been shown to be very effective (Figs. 10A to C).

Another topical agent that is still used in dermatologic procedures, but with decreased frequency, is Monsel's solution, which is composed of 20% ferric subsulfate. It has an acidic pH which is thought to contribute to its hemostatic properties eliciting protein precipitation in vessels and oxidization.[19] It is effective after punch or shave biopsies but is used less frequently due to its tattooing effect on the skin. Less hyperpigmentation and tattooing of the skin occur with a 10% ferrous sulfate solution when applied to the skin for 1-2 hours postoperatively.

Silver nitrate is commonly used in the treatment of small wounds and is particularly effective in the cauterization of pyogenic granulomas of the hand. Application of the silver nitrate creates a thin eschar, which sloughs off within several days and may cause permanent

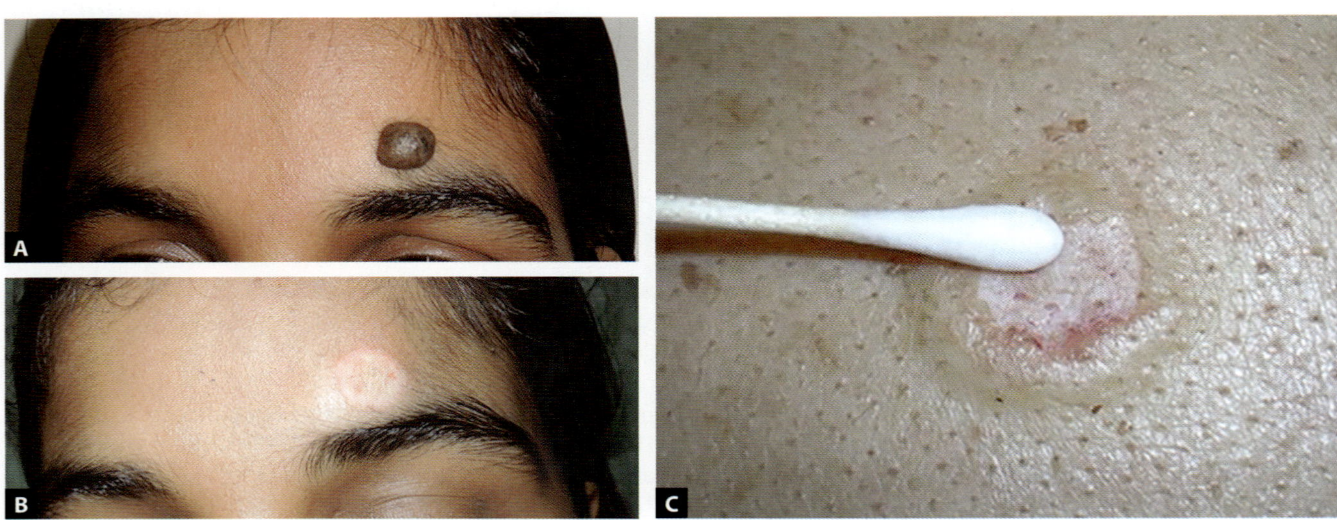

Figs. 10A to C: (A) Compound nevus before shave excision; (B) Application of silver chloride to achieve hemostasis; (C) After excision effective hemostasis achieved.

Table 6: Properties of caustic hemostatic agents.

Hemostatic agent	*Application*	*Mechanism of action*	*Advantages*	*Disadvantages*
Aluminum chloride 20-70% solution	Solution can be applied with a cotton tipped applicator after shave excision.	Precipitates proteins causing coagulation of vessels.	Inexpensive. Less likely to cause pigmentation.	Can be used only on superficial wounds
	Aluminum chloride sticks are also available.		Easily accessible and easy to apply	
Ferric subsulfate 20% solution (Monsel's solution)	Solution can be applied with a cotton tipped applicator or gauze pad.	Precipitates proteins intravascularly and oxidizes tissues.	Inexpensive. Excellent hemostasis. Easy to apply	Intradermal ferruginous deposits causes tattooing of the skin after use
Zinc chloride (Moh's paste)	Paste that can be applied topically. Left on for up to 48 hours.	Precipitates proteins causing coagulation of small vessels	Effective in providing hemostasis to metastatic cutaneous wounds.	Can be very painful and irritating to the patient
Silver nitrate	Solution can be applied with a cotton tipped applicator	Precipitates proteins	Used in the treatment of small wounds. Effective in the cauterization of pyogenic granulomas	May cause permanent skin pigmentation

skin pigmentation.[20] One of the oldest topical hemostatic agents known as "Moh's paste" was created by Frederic Mohs in 1941.[21] Zinc chloride is the main component of the paste, and it can be applied with a tongue depressor, cotton tipped applicator, or incorporated into gauze. It is effective in providing hemostasis to metastatic cutaneous wounds.[22]

Postoperative Care and Instructions

Pressure dressings are recommended for first 24 hours postoperatively in almost all cases. A nonadherent dressing covering the wound or suture line followed by layers of gauze and then elastic dressing will provide adequate compression. Patients should be advised to limit activity after surgery. Leg end elevation should be advised to patients with surgical wound over the legs in order to minimize the oozing.

Postoperative Bleeding

The most common time for the bleeding to occur is during the first few hours of surgery, when the clots are quite fragile and vasodilatation can occur. If the bleeding is not controlled with direct pressure, it needs to be explored with attention for its cause which is tackled accordingly. Usually wound needs to be opened either partially or fully for exploration. Lidocaine without adrenaline can be used to avoid missing bleeding vessels with vasoconstriction. Cautery or suture can be used for ligation of bleeding vessels. Wound can be resutured after a period of observation.[12]

Ecchymoses are a result of blood lying within the tissue plains. Periorbital, perioral and genital areas are more prone for ecchymoses. They usually resolve with time, ice packs and elevation. Hematoma formation has to be ruled out.

Hematoma occurs when blood collects under closed wound. There is no visible bleeding but only swelling and tenderness of sudden onset. This can lead to wound dehiscence or necrosis. Early hematoma is a gelatinous mass that can be expressed partially opening the wound and applying gentle pressure. In case of larger hematoma, complete evacuation has to be done followed by suturing the source of bleed. In case of doubt of further bleed; a drain should be placed for next 24 hours.[12]

Seroma is a collection of transudative serum in a closed space. These can cause increased pressure and wound compromise. This is well managed by inserting a large bore 18-gauge needle. Fenestrations are made on skin grafts to prevent seroma.

Postoperative bleeding can be highly daunting and threatening to patients and hence, it is important to provide a checklist to patients in whom such bleeding is anticipated (Box 1).

Box 1: Postoperative instructions to patients.

- If there is any bleeding noted, do not be anxious
- Lie down, elevating the area of bleeding
- Apply firm pressure for 15 minutes with cotton pad
- If bleeding continues, call the telephone number provided.

Anticoagulants and Blood Thinners during Cutaneous Surgery[13]

The risk of life-threatening thromboembolism associated with even brief cessation of blood thinners is significant. Unfortunately, primary care providers may be unaware of the bleeding risks associated with cutaneous procedures such as Mohs excision and wound repair. The cutaneous surgeon should be aware of the various techniques and tools to reduce the risk of intraoperative and postoperative bleeding in patients taking blood thinners. Notwithstanding, bleeding complications carry far less morbidity and mortality than that of thromboembolism. Evidence continues to mount favoring blood thinner maintenance during cutaneous surgery and hence, anticoagulants should be continued during the dermatosurgical procedures.

CONCLUSION

Control of the bleeding process is essential for achieving an optimal surgical outcome. Effective hemostasis simplifies many techniques in dermatologic surgery. Electrosurgical devices and newer topical agents and gels effectively tackle surgical bleeding. Anticoagulants and blood thinners should be continued during cutaneous surgery.

REFERENCES

1. Shekarriz B, Stoller ML. The use of fibrin sealant in urology. J Urol. 2002;167:1218-25.
2. Radosevich M, Goubran HI, Burnouf T. Fibrin sealant: scientific rationale, production methods, properties, and current clinical use. Vox Sang. 1997;72:133-43.
3. Sigerist H. A history of medicine. New York, NY: Oxford University Press; 1951.
4. Aris A. Hemostatic herbs. Ann Thorac Surg. 2002;74:1291.
5. Stone E. Medicine among the American Indians. New York, NY: PB Hoeber; 1932.
6. Lundblad RL, Bradshaw RA, Gabriel D, et al. A review of the therapeutic uses of thrombin. Thromb Haemost. 2004; 91:851-60.
7. Gabay M. Absorbable hemostatic agents. Am J Health Syst Pharm. 2006;63:1244-53.
8. Adams GL, Manson RJ, Turner I, et al. The balance of thrombosis and hemorrhage in surgery. Hematol Oncol Clin North Am. 2007;21:13-24.
9. Hemostasis. In: Porter RS, Ed. (2005). The Merck Manuals Online Medical Library. [online] Available from http://www.merck.com/mmpe/sec11/ch134/ch134a.html. [Accessed February, 2012].

10. Oz MC, Rondinone JF, Shargill NS. FloSeal Matrix: new generation topical hemostatic sealant. J Card Surg. 2003; 18:486-93.
11. Morikawa T. Tissue sealing. Am J Surg. 2001;182(2 Suppl): 29S-35S.
12. Nouri K, Khouri SL. Techniques in dermatologic surgery; Elsevier; 2003;85-91.
13. Schanbacher CF. Anticoagulants and blood thinners during cutaneous surgery: always, sometimes or never? Skin Therapy Lett. 2004;9:5-7.
14. Harahap M. Excision of small lesions on the scalp. Surgical gems in dermatology 1st edition. New York: Journal Publishing Group; 1988;73-4.
15. Ceiley R, Bodian E. Biopsy of oral lesions. Surgical gems in dermatology, 1st edition. New York: Journal publishing group; 1988;15-7.
16. Samudrala S. Topical hemostatic agents in surgery: a surgeon's perspective. AORN J. 2008;88:S2-11.
17. Nelson A, Schanbacher C. New wound-sealing method effective in dermatologic surgery. American Society for Dermatologic Surgery (ASDS). 2011. Annual meeting. November 5, 2011.
18. Achneck HE, Sileshi B, Jamiolkowski RM, et al. A Comprehensive review of topical hemostatic agents efficacy and recommendations for use. Ann Surg. 2010; 251:217-28.
19. Palm MD, Altman JS. Topical hemostatic agents: a review, Dermatol Surg. 2008;34(4):431-45.
20. Quitkin HM, Rosenwasser MP, Strauch RJ. The efficacy of silver nitrate cauterization for pyogenic granuloma of the hand. J Hand Surg Am. 2003;28(3):435-8.
21. Mohs F. Chemosurgery: A microscopically controlled method of cancer excision. Arch Surg. 1941;42(2):279-96.
22. Kakimoto M, Tokita H, Okamura T, et al. A chemical hemostatic technique for bleeding from malignant wounds. J Palliat Med. 2010;13(1):11-3.

Chapter 17

Antithrombotic Therapy and Dermatosurgery

Vaishalee Kirane, Aniketh Venkataram

Key Messages

- Risk assessment is needed to decide whether to discontinue the Antithrombotics or not before dermatosurgery like Hair Transplant.
- In low risk cases, Antiplatelet drugs like Aspirin can be continued.
- For stopping Warfarin or to start LMWH, prescribing physician needs to be consulted.

INTRODUCTION

As the number of patients seeking dermatosurgery is rising, so is the number of patients on antithrombotic drugs for cardiac comorbidities. There is a significant area of overlap in these two groups, particularly in middle-aged males, who are increasingly seeking dermatosurgery. Hence, the dermatosurgeon needs to be aware of the protocols and precautions of these patients, particularly when he is planning for surgeries associated with some bleeding such as hair transplantation, liposuction, flaps and grafts, dermabrasion, etc. In simple terms, the questions to be answered are:

Should antithrombotics be stopped for a dermatosurgery?

- If yes:
  - What are the protocols to be followed?
  - Is the risk of thrombosis justifiable for a cosmetic procedure?
- If no:
  - Can dermatosurgery still be performed safely and successfully?
  - What additional precautions are needed during surgery?

As a baseline recommendation, in order to decrease the risk of excessive bleeding, it would be prudent to advise avoidance or discontinuation of different agents which inhibit platelet function and clotting.[1] Box 1 contains a list of prescription medications that can increase the risk of bleeding. This list can also be given to the patients in the preoperative instruction package.[2] *However, the issue is more complex and needs a thorough understanding of the need for potentially life-saving drugs and at the same time, safe performance and fulfillment of a patient's emotional need for a cosmetic surgery.*

BRIEF OVERVIEW OF ANTITHROMBOTICS

There are two main classes of drugs which are shown here.

1. Antiplatelets:
   - Inhibit platelet aggregation and function
   - Affect bleeding time
   - Prevention of thrombosis in patients after coronary stent implantation/stroke/myocardial infarction
   - For example, aspirin, ticlopidine, clopidogrel, abciximab, eptifibatide.
2. Anticoagulants:
   - Inhibit the coagulation pathway
   - Affect clotting time. Normally target international normalized ratio (INR) 2.0–3.0/2.5–3.5
   - Atrial fibrillation, mechanical heart valves, venous thromboembolism
   - For example, warfarin, rivaroxaban, dabigatran.

Aspirin

Platelet activation and the production of platelet products are enhanced by thromboxane, the synthesis of which is inhibited by cyclooxygenase enzyme. Aspirin inhibits cyclooxygenase enzyme and thus interferes with platelet function.[3] A study by Lawrence C showed that

Box 1: Medications that can increase bleeding

• Aceclofenac	• Indomethacin
• Acetylsalicylic acid	• Ketoprofen
• Clopidogrel	• Naproxen
• Danazol	• Pentoxifylline
• Diclofenac	• Piroxicam
• Dicoumarol	• Sertraline
• Dipyridamole	• Sulindac
• Escitalopram	• Ticlopidine
• Enoxaparin	• Tranexamic acid
• Fluoxetine	• Warfarin
• Ibuprofen	

intraoperative bleeding complications occurred only in patients receiving aspirin who had a prolonged bleeding time. Patients with a normal bleeding time can continue aspirin or nonsteroidal anti-inflammatory drug (NSAID) therapy before dermatologic surgery.[3] Another study showed the use of anticoagulants and platelet inhibitors can increase the risk of intraoperative and postoperative hemorrhagic complications in cutaneous surgery.[4] NSAIDs action of inhibiting cyclooxygenase is reversible and dependent on the presence of the circulating drug and therefore its half-life. For example, Ibuprofen has a short half-life and further, is a nonessential drug unlike aspirin.

Warfarin

Warfarin depletes the reduced form of vitamin K and thus interferes with the production of vitamin K-dependent clotting factors II, VII, IX, and X. It is a life-saving medication and stoppage of the drug can lead to serious medical episode. Its stoppage for a cosmetic procedure raises ethical questions. However, a number of practitioners have carried out hair transplants on patients who did not discontinue their warfarin and have reported acceptable levels of intraoperative and postoperative bleeding.[4] If warfarin is discontinued, then long-acting heparin is to be started 6 days prior to the date of surgery. The last dose of heparin is given on the morning of the day before surgery and restarted soon after surgery as is deemed fit by the managing physician—usually 36 hours. Warfarin is restarted at the same time as the heparin is discontinued.

Clopidogrel

Clopidogrel bisulfate is an inhibitor of adenosine diphosphate-induced platelet aggregation. It is frequently prescribed in order to reduce atherothrombotic events for patients with cardiac stents, recent myocardial infarction, or stroke as well as for those with established peripheral arterial disease.

Platelets exposed to clopidogrel are affected for the remainder of their lifespan (approximately 7–10 days). Thus, it will need to be stopped 7–10 days before surgery and only with the agreement of the prescribing physician.

Manchikanti et al. showed that the recommendations derived from the comprehensive assessment of the literature and guidelines are to continue NSAIDs and low-dose aspirin during interventional techniques. However, the recommendations for discontinuation of antiplatelet therapy with platelet aggregation inhibitors like clopidogrel, ticlopidine is variable with clinical judgment to continue or discontinue based on the patient's condition and the risk factors. Low-molecular-weight heparin (LMWH) may be discontinued 12 hours prior. Warfarin should be discontinued or INR be normalized to 1.4–2 or less based on risk factors.[5]

RECOMMENDATIONS FOR PERIOPERATIVE MANAGEMENT OF ANTITHROMBOTICS

There are two main factors which guide the perioperative management:

1. Risk of bleeding if antithrombotics continued—dermatosurgery is classified low-risk for serious bleeding as far as morbidity/mortality concerned. However, any undue bleeding might affect the cosmetic outcome even though it may not harm the patient.
2. Risk of thrombosis if antithrombotics are stopped—normally classified into low-risk and high-risk (Table 1). Such a risk is not acceptable for a cosmetic surgery.

This risk assessment has to be taken into consideration and cardiologist seeing the patient should also be consulted to decide on a plan of action jointly. A proposed plan is shown here.

Management of Anticoagulants[6,7]

- Warfarin stopped or reduced for 5 days prior to surgery
- International normalized ratio lowered to 1.5, checked day before surgery
- If high-risk of thromboembolism
  - Bridging anticoagulation with LMWH from 4 days prior to 3 days postsurgery.
- Low-risk of thromboembolism
  - No need for bridging anticoagulation
- Warfarin resumed evening of surgery.

Table 1: Classifications of risk antithrombosis

High-risk	*Low-risk*
▪ Any mechanical heart valve ▪ Atrial fibrillation with $CHADS_2$ score >2 or history of stroke or transient ischemic attack or rheumatic valvular heart disease ▪ Recent venous thromboembolism (within 3 months) ▪ Recurrent venous thromboembolism receiving long-term anticoagulation	▪ Atrial fibrillation with $CHADS_2$ score of ≤ 2 and no history of stroke or transient ischemic attack ▪ Single venous thromboembolism occurring >3 months ago and with no other risk factors

Table 2: Summary of recommendations for perioperative management

Day	Anticoagulant	Antiplatelet
–5	Stop warfarin in all	Stop clopidogrel
–4	Start LMWH in high-risk cases	Aspirin continued throughout
–3		
–2		
–1	Measure INR. Last dose of LMWH 24 hours prior to surgery	
Surgery	Restart warfarin in evening	
+1	LMWH dose 24 hours after surgery	Restart clopidogrel
+2		
+3	Last dose of LMWH	
+4	Measure INR, continue regular warfarin dose	

Abbreviations: LMWH, low-molecular-weight heparin; INR, international normalized ratio

Management of Antiplatelets

- Aspirin is continued throughout the perioperative period. It need not be stopped
- Clopidogrel stopped 5–7 days prior to surgery, restarted within 24 hours of surgery.

If the patient has undergone a stent placement recently, then antiplatelet drugs are critical and cannot be stopped. Hence, the surgery should be postponed for the following durations:

- 6 weeks for bare metal stents
- 12 months for drug-eluting stent.

Intraoperative Precautions[6,7]

Patients on antithrombotics are at increased risk of bleeding, both in the donor as well as the recipient area. This can interfere with surgery cause and postoperative hematoma affecting the cosmetic outcome.

Bleeding can be reduced by adequate amount of tumescent fluid during surgeries such as hair transplantation. However, this may raise the blood pressure and pulse rate, and hence should be discussed with the cardiologist. Any bleeding can also be controlled with adequate and patient gauze compression.

CONCLUSION

With proper knowledge and precautions, dermatosurgery can be safely performed in patients on antithrombotics. The perioperative management of the commonly used antithrombotics is summed up in Table 2.

REFERENCES

1. Langtry JA, Maddin WS, Carruthers JA, et al. Is there a rationale for the drugs used in hair transplantation surgery? Dermatol Surg. 1998;24:967-71.
2. World Federation of Hemophilia. (2017). Drugs that can cause bleeding. [online] Available from http://www.wfh.org/en/page.aspx?pid=639. [Accessed February, 2017].
3. Lawrence C, Sakuntabhai A, Tiling-Grosse S. Effect of aspirin and nonsteroidal anti-inflammatory drug therapy on bleeding complications in dermatologic surgical patients. J Am Acad Dermatol. 1994;31:988-92.
4. Goldsmith SM, Leshin B, Owen J. Management of patients taking anticoagulants and platelet inhibitors prior to dermatologic surgery. J Dermatol Surg Oncol. 1993;19:578-81.
5. Manchikanti L, Falco FJ, Benyamin RM, et al. Assessment of bleeding risk of interventional techniques: a best evidence synthesis of practice patterns and perioperative management of anticoagulant and antithrombotic therapy. Pain Physician. 2013;16(2 Suppl):SE261-318.
6. Douketis JD, Spyropoulos AC, Spencer FA, et al. Perioperative management of antithrombotic therapy: antithrombotic therapy and prevention of thrombosis, 9th ed: American College of Chest Physicians Evidence-Based Clinical Practice Guidelines. Chest. 2012;141(2 Suppl):e326S-50S.
7. Yagyu K. Guidelines for perioperative antithrombotic therapy in hair restoration surgery: management of patients with coronary heart disease, mechanical heart valve, and atrial fibrillation. Hair Transplant Forum Int. 2012;22(2):1-5.

Chapter 18

Management of Dermatosurgical Emergencies

Murali Chakravarthy

Key Messages

- Though dermatosurgeries are office procedures, surgical emergencies may occur, though they are rare.
- Dermatological surgeons should be fully aware of procedures for resuscitation in such eventualities.
- Syncope, bleeding and issues concerning lignocaine use are the common events that might occur.
- Monitoring devices, basic resuscitation equipments, adequate trained staff are needed to manage an emergency.
- The adage "If you are prepared for an emergency, it ceases to exist" appears to be apt under these situations.

INTRODUCTION

Office-based dermatologic procedures and cosmetic surgeries performed on a day care basis have become the trend of the day. Such procedures are supported by anesthesiologists at certain centers and by resident doctors or nurses at others. The support provided by the anesthesiologists in these situations is referred to as "Monitored Anesthesia Care".[1] Complications, though uncommon, have been reported in 6% of such procedures: bleeding or hematoma in 3%, infections in 2% and vasovagal reactions in 1%. Bleeding occurred more frequently in menor in patients taking anticoagulation, antiplatelet or immunosuppressive agents or in; in prolonged procedures. Vasovagal reactions were associated with age younger than 50 years.[2,3]

The preparedness of the dermatologists in dealing with such crises affects the outcome of the situation. With the society getting more and more litingant, it is time that dermatologists attend to quality and safety issues while dealing with these "patients", who do not usually suffer from disease. The emphasis is on the patient safety and adequate infrastructure to deal with the complications that may arise during the procedure. Availability of the monitoring devices, basic resuscitation equipments, adequate trained staff and the ability to manage an emergency should be always borne in mind of the dermatologic surgeons prior to starting the scheduled procedure at the office.[4,5] It may be misconceived by a few dermatologic surgeons that complications are rare and therefore the therapeutic agents and knowledge to deal with the crises at their office may not be required. Providing infrastructural support to deal with crises in day care surgery not only makes the day care procedures safer for the patient, but also avoids potential medicolegal complications. This chapter discusses the spectrum of emergencies that are commonly encountered by the dermatosurgeon and the basic guidelines to manage these emergency situations. Dermatologic surgery is mostly cosmetic; therefore, the potential for medicolegal issues is high in the event of adverse outcome. In the author's view, the entire team in the dermatologic surgeon's procedure room should be trained to provide at least basic life support (BLS), if not advanced cardiac life support (ACLS). Dermatologic surgeons need to practice and adopt "Safe surgery saves lives" campaign as proposed by World Health Organization.[6] A few of the points for safe surgery are mentioned in Box 1.

Several emergency issues may be encountered in the practice of surgical dermatology.[7] These are illustrated in Box 2.

ANAPHYLAXIS

Anaphylaxis is a sudden violent manifestation of an acute immunological reaction, which might become life threatening at times. It is produced by a complex mechanism involving the immune system. The manifestation may vary from pruritus, urticarial in milder cases and inspiratory stridor, laryngeal edema, bronchospasm,

Box 1: Patient safety issues that have to be practiced in dermatosurgical patients.

- Identify all the patients by name, check if the patient has consented to the procedure. All adult patients should consent themselves
- Ask the patient to show the site and side of the procedure
- Take history of allergies, if any
- Instruct the patient to continue all the medications that he has been prescribed
- Insert an intravenous cannula and maintain a running drip of ringer lactate. Other fluids such as dextrose and saline may be infused depending on the requirement
- In diabetic patients check the blood sugar by 'glucostrip' method
- Connect electrocardiogram and pulse oximetry in all the patients. If access to chest is difficult to obtain, loose fitting clothes allowing access to chest may be worn
- Prepare the local anesthetic infiltration yourself. If you have a well-organized team, all medications should be loaded while a witness confirms the name of the medication
- It is author's practice to load 1:200,000 adrenaline in a 20-mL syringe for all cases (It is prepared by diluting 1 mg or 1 mL of adrenaline to 10 mL; discard 9 mL of this and dilute the remaining 1–20 mL). This solution may be used to treat several problems such as hypotension, bradycardia, bronchospasm, anaphylaxis, allergy among others

Box 3: Management of anaphylaxis.[9]

- Place the patient supine on the examination table, preferably Trendelenburg position (head down)
- Loosen the clothing
- Assess the vital signs: Heart rate, blood pressure and oxygen saturation
- Maintain airway, breathing and circulation
- Start oxygen by face mask
- Efforts to minimize further antigen exposure should be made. Call for help. It is prudent to have a mechanism to call for help without having to leave the patient such as a call bell or "code blue"
- Secure an intravenous access if not already in place
- Adrenaline is the drug of choice. About 0.3–0.5 mL of adrenaline, 1:1,000 is administered intravenously or subcutaneously or intramuscularly. Repeat dose at 5–10 minute interval. It is the author's practice to inject 4–5 mL of 1:200,000 adrenalines intravenously when bronchospasm, severe hypotension and bradycardia are encountered
- If the patient has severe hypotension, start intravenous fluids, preferably colloid if not improving, start inotropes such as dopamine
- Nebulized beta agonists such as albuterol with or without intravenous aminophylline may be considered in patients with severe bronchoconstriction. Simultaneously ranitidine 1 mg/kg IV, while a steroid may prevent a delayed reaction. Give hydrocortisone, 5 mg per kg, or approximately 250 mg intravenously (prednisone, 20 mg orally, can be given in mild cases)
- Monitor patients for 2–4 hours for a minor attack and in case of severe anaphylaxis, preferably admit the patient and monitor for 24 hours

hypotension, cardiac arrhythmias in more severe ones. Classic anaphylaxis manifests with a massive cardiovascular collapse within minutes of exposure to the offending antigen. The outcome in such events depends mainly on the preparedness of the team. It is a good practice to start the monitoring devices prior to any interventions. It has been shown that presence of a professional watching the patient's vitals improves the detection of anaphylaxis and its treatment.[8]

Common causes of such anaphylaxis in a dermatologic practice are adverse reactions to intravenous antibiotic

Box 2: Various emergency issues.

- Anaphylaxis
- Syncope
- Lignocaine-related issues
- Breathlessness
- Chest pain
- Bleeding
- Acute stroke
- Status epilepticus
- Hypotension
- Hypoxia
- Cardiac arrest

Box 4: Tips for avoiding syncopal attacks.

- Explaining the patient about the procedure and allaying anxiety often helps in reducing the incidence of syncope as also performing the procedures in a supine position
- Shielding the eyes and placing a surgical sheet to block the patient view from the operated area may help prevent the occurrence of syncope. A distracting conversation may be beneficial
- Following the procedure, the patient should slowly sit up and be observed for several minutes while postoperative instructions are being discussed. Sitting up suddenly and standing immediately after the procedure could also result in syncope after the completion of the procedure.[11]

agents, local anesthetic agents and other allergens such as latex rubber. Box 3 shows management of anaphylaxis.

Anaphylactoid reactions are similar but are not immunologically mediated. They may be prevented by prior administration of corticosteroids and antihistaminic agents. These are common subsequent to administration of radiological ionic dyes and a few anesthetic agents such as atracurium and suxamethonium which are likely to release histamine.[10] However, these are not common in dermatosurgical practice.

SYNCOPE

Syncope is a vagal-mediated unconsciousness, commonly associated with extreme bradycardia and at times pulseless states. It is commonly encountered in anxious patients. It is often confused with anaphylaxis, if it occurs after an injection. Starting of an intravenous cannulation, surgical incision in inadequately anesthetized areas and even sight of blood might trigger it. An early sign of syncope, prior to loss of consciousness, is profuse sweating and cold skin. Vagal-induced bradycardia in the setting of decreased systemic vascular resistance can initiate collapse. Pseudoseizure activity may occur, characterized by brief clonic activity. Blood pressure may initially decrease but is restored with supine position. The tips for avoiding syncopal attacks are mentioned in Box 4.

Management of Syncope

Place the patient in supine and preferably in a head down (Trendelenburg) position. Monitor vital parameters such as heart rate, blood pressure and pulse oximetry. Reassure the patient; that may all be necessary in addition to the recumbent posture. Start intravenous access. Administer injection atropine 1 mg if heart rate is less than 40 per minute and intravenous fluids if blood pressure continues to be low. If alone, one should call for help and step up the monitoring only after minimal monitoring has been started to begin with.

LIGNOCAINE-RELATED ISSUES

Patients with multiple allergies and atopy are more likely to develop lignocaine allergy.[12] Most of the adverse reactions that are clinically seen are in fact manifestation of the over dosage of the local anesthetic by inadvertent intravascular injection in extremely vascular areas such as the scalp and face. It can also occur in cases of tumescent liposuction when dosages over 55 mg/kg are used. In such cases, signs of over dosage are often delayed. A case of lignocaine over dosage leading to death late at mid night, after liposuction has recently been reported.[13] Toxic reactions to lignocaine resulting from over dosage cause central nervous system or myocardial depression or excitation, perioral numbness, nausea, seizures or coma. Vasovagal syncope may be misdiagnosed as an allergic reaction and should be distinguished properly.

Methylparaben and propylparaben are the preservatives added to lignocaine and various cosmetics to increase their shelf life. Some of the adverse reactions seen during administration of lignocaine may indeed be due to these preservatives.[14] Patients who are allergic to sulfa drugs may develop adverse reactions to 'sulfites' which are added as preservatives to lignocaine. Anxiety regarding the use of needles, and/or the effects of epinephrine in lignocaine can lead to palpitations, panic attacks and vasovagal events that the patient may remember as an allergic reaction. Patients admitting to having had previous incorrectly allergic reactions should be properly investigated prior to submitting for dermatologic surgery. The dermatologic surgical procedure in patients with allergic manifestations may be electively performed under general anesthesia and management of such cases in a hospital with a full back up should be planned.[15] More information on local anesthetics and their allergic reactions is provided in the chapter on Local Anesthesia in Dermatosurgery.

BREATHLESSNESS

The etiologies of breathlessness may be cardiac, respiratory or anxiety related. Patients with asthma and obstructive airway disease should be well investigated by a pulmonologist and rendered 'dry' before scheduling for dermatologic surgery. Such patients should be advised to use the routine inhalers before arriving for surgery.[16] Dermatologic surgeons should also check the preoperative 'basal' values of oxygen and carbon dioxide. In the absence of this knowledge one may treat in vain to achieve magic numbers of partial pressures of more than 100 mm Hg and carbon dioxide of less than 40. Patients with 'cardiac asthma' should be well prepared with diuretic and peripheral vasodilator therapy. At times cardiac patients manifest with dyspnea when subjected to myocardial ischemia. Even young obese individuals might present with dyspnea of cardiac origin. Patients with respiratory compromise should not be operated without the guidance of pulse oximetry. If the oxygen saturation decreases during surgery, methods to administer the bronchodilator nebulization must be kept handy. Dyspnea which does not abate with treatment, whether of cardiac or pulmonary origin is a reason to stop the scheduled procedure and to reschedule at a later convenient time. Dyspnea due to anxiety will respond well to a small intravenous dose (0.5–1 mg) of anxiolytic such as midazolam. Appropriate preoperative counseling is sufficient in most patients to avoid anxiety related problems.

CHEST PAIN

Chest pain may be a manifestation of not only coronary arterial ischemia but also anxiety. However, fear, stress of pain and procedure can also precipitate an acute myocardial infarction in any patient prone for ischemia. Although most dermatologic surgical procedures are day care and performed in young healthy individuals, at times, if a high-risk patient is being subjected to esthetic surgery, thorough evaluation would be mandatory.

If a patient complains of chest pain during the procedure, place the patient supine and check the vitals. Activate physician/emergency medical services. Record an electrocardiogram, which may be compared against the basal. If you are suspecting coronary ischemia, a tablet of nitroglycerine 5 mg should be placed immediately under the tongue. One must be aware of possible headache and hypotension following this measure. An intravenous (IV) cannula should be inserted immediately (if not already done) and a patent IV line is important for further management. If with these measures the chest pain settles and the patient is hemodynamically stable, one can proceed with the surgery. If the pain is unabated and electrocardiographic changes persist or worsen, the scheduled procedure should be deferred with. Patient may undergo the scheduled procedure after a consult with a cardiologist.

Patients at risk for myocardial ischemia should be thoroughly evaluated and medically optimized prior to the procedure. In the author's opinion, it may be wise to have 'monitored anesthesia care' for all patients.

BLEEDING

A major surgical bleeder is rare in cutaneous surgeries. A patient receiving antiplatelet medications for concomitant comorbidities may pose special issues. Such patients may be better prepared by stopping the antiplatelet medication at least for 2 weeks prior to the planned procedure. Although the hemorrhage associated with cutaneous surgery may not be life threatening, its other effects such as causing a menacing hematoma and lifting of flaps compromising their viability may be of nuisance value.[17,18] For more information on hemostasis reader is referred to the chapter on Hemostasis.

ACUTE STROKE

Patients on antiplatelet or antithrombotic therapy[19] and their sudden discontinuation, patients with carotid bruit, patients with prior history of stroke, patients with cardiovascular disease are all at potential risk for stroke.[18] Pre-procedural evaluation by a physician or a neurologist has to be considered in such patients. During the procedure, the dermatologist's role chiefly concerns the detection phase of a sudden neurologic deficit. This may include an alteration in consciousness (confusion, coma and seizures), aphasia, dysarthria, facial weakness or asymmetry, extremity weakness, paralysis, sensory loss, ataxia, visual loss or vertigo. Immediately activate the physician or emergency medical services. A definitive hospital-based intervention must occur within 3 hours of the onset of the stroke symptoms to be beneficial. Meanwhile attend to the ABCs (airway, breathing, circulation) of resuscitation and monitor vitals and manage accordingly till the physician arrives.

STATUS EPILEPTICUS

Dermatologists do encounter disease with potential epileptic manifestations in conditions such as tuberous sclerosis, systemic lupus erythematosus (Box 5). It is wise to obtain any past history of seizures and antiseizure medications.[20] If the patients are epileptic on treatment, one should advise them to continue the treatment until the day of surgery.

Box 5: Management of status epilepticus.

- Stop the ongoing procedure. First priority is always the maintenance of airway. Use an oral or nasopharyngeal airway as and when required (inserting these airways are out of the routine for dermatological surgeons, it is advisable for them to learn the insertion of these airways from their anesthesia or critical care colleagues)
- If available, oxygen can be delivered by face mask
- Monitor the vital signs
- Place the patient on a soft, flat surface away from sharp objects
- Look for and prevent tongue bite
- If seizures has stopped and the patient is breathing and has a pulse, place the patient in a recovery position (modified lateral position).It will allow the clearance of any pooled secretions
- Secure a peripheral intravenous line and send blood sample for blood glucose, serum electrolytes
- The benzodiazepine midazolam or lorazepam 1–2 mg or diazepam 5–10 mg intravenously will stop the seizures
- Call for physician and evaluate for seizures etiology and further management options

COLLAPSE

Most commonly syncope, anaphylaxis, hypoglycemia and cardiac arrest are reasons for collapse of a patient. These issues may be addressed as discussed in the chapter. However, associated with a vasomotor collapse are some of the key issues mentioned below which need attention.

HYPOTENSION

Low blood pressure may result from bleeding, syncope, anaphylaxis, acute myocardial infarction, and secondary to medications such as sedatives/anesthetic agents. Patient may complain of giddiness (or orthostatic hypotension).

Management

Place the patient in supine position and check vital signs such as, pulse rate and blood pressure. Treat the underlying cause. Tachycardia with low blood pressure indicates blood loss, start the patient on intravenous fluid crystalloids. Ringer's lactate 5–10 mL/kg bolus over 15 minutes can be administered and the blood pressure checked. If good response continues, intravenous fluid (Ringer's lactate) at the rate of 2–4 mL/kg/hour may be continued. If there is no response to the fluids, check for continued blood loss; send a sample of blood for checking the hemoglobin level. In the absence of matched donor blood, it is vital to maintain the circulating blood volume by administration of colloids such as starch solutions. More damage might be caused by allowing hypovolemia than anemia.[21,22] If hypotension persists, one should seek a physician's opinion and have a provision for starting an inotropic infusion such as injection dopamine 5 μg/kg/min should be commenced.

HYPERTENSION

Known hypertensives, elderly, female, anxious patients are prone for increased blood pressure during the procedure. Accelerated hypertensive patients can also present with giddiness, severe headache. Optimization of blood pressure for known hypertensives, reassuring the patients, premedicant such as alprazolam, sedatives such as midazolam, lorazepam would help in the control of blood pressure. Involvement of a physician would be helpful if basic interventions do not reduce the blood pressure.

Dermatological Procedures and Infection Control

Infections after dermatological procedures are not only rare but usually insignificant. These procedures are majorly aesthetic ones and these 'patients' do not suffer from any major systemic illnesses; the expectation about outcomes are usually high. Absence of infection after the procedure is one such expectation. The dermatologic surgeon must attend to the infection control measures in providing clean ambience while conducting the procedure, using standard precautions, preoperative decolonization of methicillin-resistant *Staphylococcus aureus* (MRSA) and surgical prophylaxis. Postprocedure, the patients may be advised about care of the wound and reporting early if signs of infection come up.

Preoperative preparation: It is a common knowledge that *Staphylococcus aureus* is a common cutaneous commensal; it is impossible to eradicate it. While conducting surgical operations requiring skin incision, the colony count of these organisms have to be reduced.

The methods to achieve this are:

a. *Preoperative chlorhexidine 2% v/v wash:* The patients have to bathe twice daily for 3 preoperative days. This solution cannot be applied over the scalp and face. Those wishing to operate on the scalp and the face may use triclosan solution.
b. *Intranasal mupirocin ointment:* All the surgical patients must be requested to use mupirocin ointment twice daily for 5 days preoperatively. This decolonizes the nasal mucosa of MRSA.
c. *Surgical preparation:* It is recommended that we must use chlorhexidine tincture 2% w/v to prepare the skin. This solution has been found to be superior to using povidone iodine; its residual action is longer than that of povidone iodine. Whether chlorhexidine or povidone iodine is used, one must wait for at least 3 minutes prior to incision. The commonly found practice of 'rubbing off' excess solution using a gauze should be shunned and instead, the solution must be allowed to dry by itself; only then the antibacterial effect is maximized.
d. *Preoperative surgical prophylaxis:* It is recommended by Center for Disease Control and Prevention that a single dose of first or second generation cephalosporin be administered intravenously 15–60 minutes prior to incision. Administering 1.5 g of cefuroxime suffices in most adults. If the surgery continues beyond 4 hours, a similar dose must be administered.
e. *Normoglycemia and normothermia*: It has been shown that intraoperative blood sugar and temperature maintenance is absolutely essential. Cutaneous surgeries are no exception to these recommendations.

HYPOXEMIA

Patient developing desaturation during the procedure requires attention. Hypoxemia may be secondary to pain induced hypoventilation, pulmonary embolism (during liposuction), cardiac failure, bronchospasm due to anaphylaxis.

Management

The management steps of hypoxemia are mentioned below:

- Stop the procedure and start oxygen by face mask, 4 L/minute.
- Talk to the patient and encourage them to breathe deeply.
- Assess the vitals, talk to the patient. Reassure him.
- Determine the underlying cause.
- Notify the physician.
- Treat the underlying cause.

CARDIAC ARREST[7,23]

The most common cause of cardiac arrest is ventricular fibrillation, other arrhythmias like pulseless ventricular tachycardia, pulseless electrical activity also lead to cardiac arrest.

Cardiac arrest is confirmed when the patient is not responding, pulse is not felt, blood pressure is not recordable. Immediate measures to be taken are:

- Activate the emergency department/notify the physician or an anesthesiologist.
- Start cardiopulmonary resuscitation as per American Heart Association (AHA) guidelines 2010.[23]
- Start chest compression at the rate of 100/minute.
- Get an automated external defibrillator device. Diagnose ventricular fibrillation and defibrillate.
- Continue chest compressions.
- Begin ventilation.
- Administer oxygen.
- Obtain intravenous access.
- Administer epinephrine or vasopressin.
- Assess adequacy of Clinical Practice Redesign efforts.
- Intubate trachea.
- Additional drug therapy.
- Post-resuscitation care and shift of the patient to a higher medical center for further management.

NERVE INJURY

Inadvertent nerve damage is one of the most dreaded complications of dermatologic surgery. Effects of local anesthesia, inadvertent pressure or tension due to positioning are the common cause. Nerve injuries may result in transient either reversible or permanent. Patients should always be warned of the possibility of nerve injury during the discussion of the informed consent. Patient should be frequently asked about any discomfort induced by prolonged positioning.

GENERAL RESUSCITATION PLAN AT THE DERMATOLOGIC OFFICE

Training of each and every staff member at the dermatologic office with clearly defined roles for each staff is a must in managing an emergency scenario (Box 6).

Preferably, an anesthetist should be available on the premises, particularly when surgeries such as liposuction

Box 6: General resuscitation plan.

- Dermatologist or a physician should play role of team leader
- Patient is assessed by the team leader, and he assigns tasks to his team members
- Assigned staff member activates the emergency medical services or a physician or an anesthesiologist
- One staff member gets the automated external defibrillator and attaches it to the patient to analyze the rhythm and shock accordingly
- One staff member plays the role of chest compressor and other staff member takes care of airway
- Another staff member can serve as the recorder of the event times, serial vital signs measurements, securing intravenous access; administer medications and communication with the family members

are being performed. In his absence, a person trained in ACLS should be available.

Various roles played by the staff members can be practiced several times so that they can act accordingly in an emergency situation. Cardiopulmonary resuscitation (CPR) training which includes BLS and ACLS are conducted by various health organizations in accordance with AHA. All the staff members should undergo the BLS course whereas the dermatosurgeon/team leader or the nursing staff should undergo both BLS and ACLS course.

LIST OF RESUSCITATION EQUIPMENT

The basic resuscitation equipments in the form of crash cart should be made available in each dermatologist's office (Fig. 1):

Telephone remains the most important piece of emergency equipment in the dermatosurgeon's office; it provides the first link in the chain of initiating the emergency medical services process.

Crash cart should comprise of:

- Portable oxygen cylinder with face mask or nasal prongs, oral or nasopharyngeal airways, intravenous cannulas, tubings, fluids and suction apparatus.
- Medications: Epinephrine 1:1,000, lorazepam, diazepam, diphenhydramine, dextrose 50%, nitroglycerine tablets, baby aspirin.
- Automated external defibrillators (AED) are computerized devices consisting of adhesive electrodes which recognize cardiac rhythms and deliver an electrical shock across the chest wall to terminate the ventricular fibrillation. They are portable and user friendly. Adhesive electrodes are placed over the patient's cardiac apex and upper right chest to detect the cardiac rhythm. With audible and visual prompting, the device advises the operator to press the button and deliver a defibrillating shock.
- Laryngoscope, endotracheal tubes, AMBU bag.
- The crash cart inventory should be periodically reviewed and renewed as necessary.
- Cardiopulmonary resuscitation is a life-saving measure which supports pumping of blood by the heart thus allowing oxygen to reach the brain. It is more effective when done as early as possible. The conduct of CPR is guided by AHA guidelines recently updated in 2010.[23]
- Cardiopulmonary resuscitation includes recognition of cardiac arrest, activating emergency medical services (EMS), and to get an AED, performing BLS and ACLS.
- Components of BLS: The primary survey "circulation airway breathing".
- Circulation: Chest compression keeps the blood pumping to the vital organs. It is done at the rate of 100 compressions per minute, at an adequate depth of 2–2.5 inches, and allowing complete chest recoil.
- Airway and breathing: Opening the patient's airway by performing the head tilt chin lift, and give breath by mask-mouth. Chest compression to ventilation ratio is 30:2.
- Defibrillation: Once the AED arrives, switch on the defibrillator; attach the adhesive electrodes to the patient's chest. Clear the patient and once the defibrillator analyzes the rhythm, follow the defibrillators instructions.

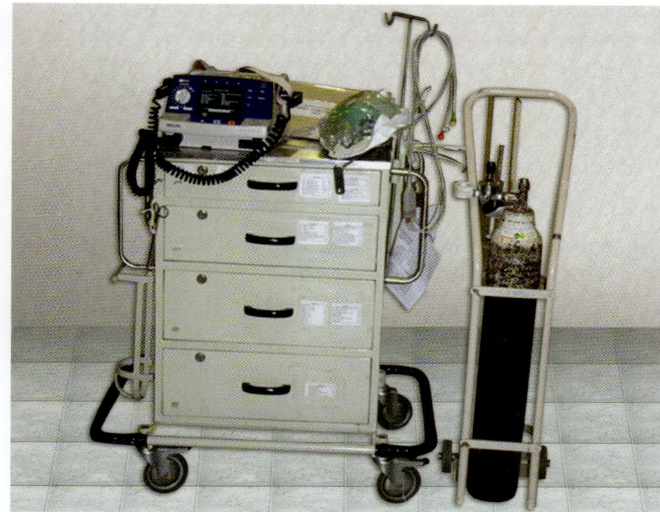

Fig. 1: Crash cart used by the author.

All the medic and paramedic staff members in the dermatology setup should be trained in performing the BLS, performing the chest compressions, maintaining the airway, handling the AED.

Components of ACLS: The Secondary Survey

- Circulation: Obtain intravenous access, attach ECG leads and monitor for arrhythmias or cardiac arrest. Use of drugs/IV fluids to manage rhythm and blood pressure.
- Airway: Maintain the airway patency—use of airways, advanced airway management if needed using a laryngeal masks airway/endotracheal tube.
- Breathing: Give supplemental oxygen; assess the adequacy of ventilation by noting the chest rise, oxygen saturation, capnography (expired carbon dioxide measurement).

Box 7: Tips for avoidance of complications.

- Thorough preoperative evaluation, optimal management of the coexisting medical illness[24]
- Preprocedural counseling, premedication to allay anxiety. Explanation in detail the procedure, postprocedural care
- Basic monitoring facilities: Pulse oximetry, noninvasive blood pressure, electrocardiogram should be made available
- Avoidance of drugs which has previously caused reactions
- Involvement of anesthesiologist (Standby anesthesiologists to provide monitored anesthesia care) as and when required, at the earliest and discussion of various anesthetic options available in the conduct of safe procedure
- Establishment of clear postprocedural instructions

- Differential diagnosis: Find and treat the reversible causes for cardiac arrest, which is easily remembered in a mnemonic form as 5 Hs and 5 Ts.
  - Hs: Hypovolemia, **h**ydrogen ion (acidosis), **h**yper/**h**ypokalemia, **h**ypoglycemia, **h**ypothermia.
  - Ts: Toxins, **t**amponade, **t**ension **p**neumothorax, **t**hrombosis (coronary and pulmonary), **t**rauma.
- General supportive care of the patient and specific pharmacologic therapy aimed at underlying event causing cardiac arrest should be initiated once the patient is successfully resuscitated.

DOCUMENTATION OF THE EVENTS

All adverse events and the measures taken are to be documented, discussed with the patient, and a discharge summary of the event to be issued to the patient. The exact time of the event may not be relevant but the flow of events and their management may be important. Such documentations are important from the medicolegal view point too.

There are certain tips given for the avoidance of complications in Box 7.

CONCLUSION

Complications in dermatosurgery office based-procedures although rare, do occur, and the outcomes of such events are related to the initial diagnosis and early management. Thorough preprocedural evaluation and identification of high-risk patients,[24] optimization of coexisting medical illness with medications will go a long way in preventing adverse events during the procedure. Good communication and patient rapport are important. High-risk cases, technologically advanced procedures should be scheduled under monitored anesthesia care and in a hospital with full-fledged emergency backup facility. A well-planned and organized office setup under the leadership of a dermatologist proves to be beneficial to the patients and reduce the medicolegal complications too.

REFERENCES

1. Bing J, McAuliffe MS, Lupton JR. Regional anesthesia with monitored anesthesia care for dermatologic laser surgery. Dermatol Clin. 2002;20;123-34.
2. Amici JM, Rogues AM, Lasheras A, et al. A prospective study of the incidence of complications associated with dermatological surgery. Br J Dermatol. 2005;153:967-71.
3. Fader DJ, Johnson TM. Medical issues and emergencies in the dermatology office. J Am Acad Dermatol. 1997;36:1-16.
4. Chan BC, Patel DC. Perioperative management and associated rate of adverse events in dermatological procedures performed by dermatologists in New Zealand. Australas J Dermatol. 2009;50:23-8.
5. Natalie LS. Dermatologic surgical complications. Medscape; 2009.
6. World Alliance for Patient Safety. Guideline 15. WHO guidelines for safe surgery. Geneva: World Health Organization; 2008.
7. Gloster HM. Acute emergencies in the dermatology office. In: Fader D (Ed). Complications in Cutaneous Surgery. United Kingdom,: Springer Science Publications; 2008.
8. Tang AW. A practical guide to anaphylaxis. Am Fam Physician. 2003;68:1325-33.
9. The diagnosis and management of anaphylaxis. Joint Task Force on Practice Parameters, American Academy of Allergy, Asthma and Immunology, American College of Allergy, Asthma and Immunology, and the Joint Council of Allergy, Asthma and Immunology. J Allergy Clin Immunol. 1998;101:S465-528.
10. Lieberman P. Anaphylaxis and anaphylactoid reactions. In: Middleton E (Ed). Allergy: principles and practice. 5th edition. St. Louis: Mosby; 1998. pp. 1079-89.
11. Parry SW, Kenny RA. The management of vasovagal syncope: a review. Q J Med. 1999;92:697-705.
12. Gmyrek R. Local and regional anesthesia. Medscape reference; 2011.
13. Araujo LM, Amaral JL. Allergy to lidocaine: case report. Rev Bras Anestesiol (online). 2004;54:672-6.
14. Grzanka A, Misiolek H, Filipowska A, et al. Adverse effects of local anaesthetics—allergy, toxic reactions or hypersensitivity. Anestezjol Intens Ter 2010;42:175-8.
15. Venkataram M, Nischal KC. Guidelines for administration of local anesthesia for dermatosurgery and cosmetic dermatology procedures. Ind J Dermatol Venereol Leprol. 2009;75:68-75.
16. Licker M, Schweizer A, Ellenberger C, et al. Perioperative medical management of patients with COPD. Int J Chron Obstruct Pulmon Dis. 2007;2:493-515.
17. Alcalay J, Alkalay R. Controversies in perioperative management of blood thinners in dermatologic surgery: continue or discontinue? Dermatol Surg. 2004;30:1091-4.
18. Rausher EG. Overview preoperative evaluation and management: Medscape; 2011.
19. Kovich O, Otley CC. Thrombotic complications related to discontinuation of warfarin and aspirin therapy perioperatively for cutaneous operations. J Am Acad Dermatol. 2003;48:233-7.
20. Gloster HM. Acute emergencies in dermatology office. Complications in cutaneous surgery. United Kingdom: Springer Publications; 2007;15.
21. Bacter CR, Canizaro PC, Shires GT, et al. Fluid resuscitation of hemorrhagic shock. Postgrad Med. 1970;48:95-9.
22. Krausz MM. Initial resuscitation of hemorrhagic shock. World J Emerg Surg. 2006;1:14.
23. American Heart Association, Cardiopulmonary resuscitation 2010 guidelines.
24. Leshin B, McCalmont TH. Preoperative evaluation of the surgical patient. Dermatol Clin. 1990;8:787-94.

Chapter

19

Pharmacology of Analgesic and Anxiolytic Drugs used in Dermatosurgery

Shyamanta Barua, Umashankar Nagaraju

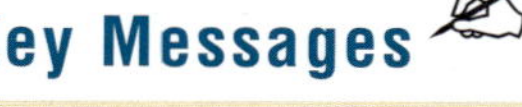

- Prevention and treatment of pain is important aspect of esthetic surgery.
- Pain in dermatosurgical procedures is usually mild.
- Clonidine and midazolam are useful preoperative medications in dermatosurgery.
- Tramadol is a useful analgesic in dermatosurgery.
- Many analgesics have drug interactions which should be considered prior to surgery.

INTRODUCTION

Pain relief during and after surgery is an important aspect of intra- and postoperative management. This is particularly relevant in esthetic surgeries, which are desired by the patient, where fear of pain is an important factor which often dissuades prospective clients from undergoing the procedure. Proper pain management, therefore, contributes to greater patient satisfaction. Hence, proper understanding of analgesia is essential for dermatosurgeons.

This chapter presents a brief description of pharmacology of analgesics and anxiolytics used in dermatosurgery. The reader is referred to pharmacology books[1-6] for detailed description of drugs; what is outlined here is an approach to the management of pain.

PATHOPHYSIOLOGY OF PAIN

Algesia or pain is an ill-defined, unpleasant sensation, usually evoked by an external or internal noxious stimulus. Analgesics are the drugs that relieve pain by acting on the central nervous system (CNS) or on the peripheral pain mechanisms, without significantly altering consciousness. There are two components in pathophysiology of pain:

1. The central component through which afferent inputs generate a pain sensation.
2. The peripheral component in which nociceptive afferent neurons are activated by noxious stimuli.

There are two main categories of pain:

1. Integumental pain: superficial, related to skin, muscle and joints.
2. Visceral pain: deep seated, related to heart, stomach, kidney and gallbladder.

Integumental pain is easier to manage and most dermatosurgeries do not involve the muscles, joints and bones. The skin and the subcutaneous structures are relatively immobile, making the analgesic plan a fairly simple one. In contrast, the movement of the painful structure in thorax and upper abdomen renders the analgesic plan complex. Thus, the issue of pain relief in dermatosurgical practice is not as complex as in other dynamic areas of the body such as thorax and upper abdomen. Integumental pain can be managed therefore with milder drugs.

ANALGESICS

Classification

Analgesics are divided into two broad groups, viz:

1. *Opioid/narcotic/morphine-like analgesics*: These act primarily at the level of the spinal cord and brain.
2. *Nonopioid/non-narcotic/nonsteroidal anti-inflammatory antipyretic analgesics*: These act primarily at peripheral sites to inhibit the synthesis or activity of pain-sensitizing substances like prostaglandins (PGs).

Opioid Analgesics

Morphine is the prototype opioid analgesic. The sites of opioid analgesia include peripheral nervous system and both spinal and supraspinal brain areas, particularly the limbic system. They reduce both the sensory as well as the affective (emotional) components of pain. They are generally more effective against dull, continuous pain such as deep seated visceral pain than a sharp intermittent integumentary pain. Different opioid drugs and their dosages are shown in Table 1.

Adverse Effects

These appear at parenteral doses of morphine higher than 15 mg and include respiratory depression, constipation, bronchospasm, postural hypotension, urinary retention, nausea and vomiting, and urticaria and itching. Tolerance and dependence frequently develop on prolonged and repeated use. Serious toxicity is produced by 50 mg of morphine and the lethal dose in humans is estimated to be 250 mg.

Contraindications

- Bronchial asthma
- Hypotension
- Hepatic damage
- Hypertrophy of prostate
- Head injury
- Hypothyroidism
- Biliary colic
- Extremes of age
- Undiagnosed acute abdominal pain.

Drug Interactions

Phenothiazines, tricyclic antidepressants, monoamine oxidase (MAO) inhibitors, amphetamine and neostigmine potentiate morphine and other opioids, either by retarding its metabolism or by a pharmacodynamic interaction at the level of central neurotransmitters. On the other hand, morphine retards absorption of many orally administered drugs by delaying gastric emptying.

Table 1: Distinctive features of opioid analgesics.

Drug	Receptor activity			Parenteral dose (mg)
	μ	κ	δ	
Morphine	+++	+	+	10–15
Codeine	++	+	+	60
Dextropropoxyphene	++	+	+	60–100
Etorphine	+++	+++	+++	0.01
Fentanyl	+++	–	+	0.05–0.1
Heroin	+++	+	+	3–5
Methadone	+++	–	–	5–10
Meperidine	+++	+	+	50–100
Tramadol	+	–	–	50–100

Drugs Used in Dermatosurgery

As stated earlier, pain in dermatosurgical procedures is not very intense and hence drugs such as morphine or pethidine are rarely needed. Commonly used drugs include tramadol and dextropropoxyphene.

a. *Tramadol:* It is a commonly used drug in dermatosurgery. It is a centrally acting analgesic that relieves pain by opioid effects (mediated almost exclusively through μ receptors) as well as additional mechanisms such as its serotonergic and noradrenergic effects. It is indicated for mild-to-moderate short-lasting pain and can also be used to allay anxiety. Dose: 50–100 mg oral/intramuscular (IM)/slow intravenous (IV) infusion (children 1–2 mg/kg) 4–6 hourly. Maximum dosage is 400 mg/day orally and 600 mg/day parenterally.
   Side effects include nausea, vomiting, sweating, itching and constipation. Hence, it is often prescribed with domperidone to offset the onset of nausea and vomiting. Drowsiness has been reported. Seizures, though rare, may occur as a complication. It undergoes metabolism via cytochrome P 450 system and hence dosage may need to be reduced in patients with liver and renal function alterations.
   The efficacy and relative safety make tramadol a commonly used drug to relieve severe pain in dermatosurgery, after procedures such as hair transplantation.
b. *Dextropropoxyphene:* This is an opioid analgesic with mild to moderate pain relief effect. Propoxyphene is a synthetic derivative of methadone and its analgesic properties reside in the dextro-isomer dextropropoxyphene. It is a μ opioid receptor agonist, similar to codeine. It is used to treat mild pain; additionally it has antitussive and local anesthetic effects. Dextropropoxyphene (30–100 mg) is sometimes combined with acetaminophen, paracetamol (325–600 mg) or acetylsalicylic acid. It exhibits local anesthetic property by virtue of depressing the compound action potential in a reversible dose dependent way. The drug has been withdrawn in US and UK due to risk of dependency.

Nonsteroidal Anti-inflammatory Drugs

All drugs in this class have analgesic, antipyretic and anti-inflammatory actions in different measures (Box 1). In contrast to the opioid analgesics, they do not depress CNS, do not produce physical dependence, have no abuse liability and are weaker analgesics. They act primarily on peripheral pain mechanisms, but also in the CNS to raise pain threshold.

Mechanism of Action

Nonsteroidal anti-inflammatory drugs (NSAIDs) inhibit the cyclooxygenase (COX) enzyme in the arachidonic acid cascade to prevent the synthesis of prostanoids

Box 1: Classification of nonsteroidal anti-inflammatory drugs.

- Nonselective cyclooxygenase (COX) inhibitors
  - Salicylates: Aspirin
  - Propionic acid derivatives: Ibuprofen, naproxen, ketoprofen
  - Anthranilic acid derivatives: Mefenamic acid
  - Arylacetic acid derivatives: Diclofenac, aceclofenac
  - Oxicam derivatives: Piroxicam
  - Pyrrolo-pyrrole derivative: Ketorolac
  - Indole derivative: Indomethacin
  - Pyrazolone derivatives: Phenylbutazone, oxyphenbutazone
- Preferential COX-2 inhibitors
  - Nimesulide, Meloxicam, Nabumetone
- Selective COX-2 inhibitors
  - Rofecoxib, Celecoxib, Valdecoxib, Etoricoxib, Parecoxib
- Analgesics-antipyretics with poor anti-inflammatory action
  - p-aminophenol derivative: Paracetamol (acetaminophen)
  - Pyrazolone derivatives: Metamizol, Propyphenazone
  - Benzoxazocine derivative: Nefopam

Table 2: Features of nonselective COX inhibitors and selective COX-2 inhibitors.

Action	*COX-1/COX-2 inhibitors*	*COX-2 inhibitors*
Analgesic	+	+
Antipyretic	+	+
Anti-inflammatory	+	+
Antiplatelet aggregatory	+	-
Gastric mucosal damage	+	-
Renal salt/water depletion	+	+
Delay/prolongation of labor	+	+
Ductus arteriosus closure	+	?
Asthma precipitation	+	-

[PGs, prostacyclin (PGI_2), and thromboxane (TXA)] (Fig. 1). There are two types of cyclooxygenase enzymes, namely COX-1 and COX-2. A third form, COX-3, has also been recently identified. The majority of traditional NSAIDs are nonselective inhibitors of both COX-1 and COX-2, although they vary in the degree of COX inhibition (Table 2).

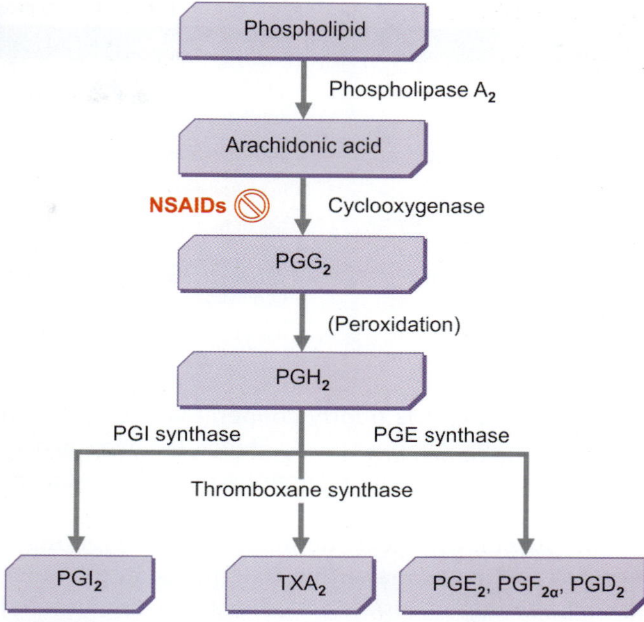

Fig. 1: Schematic representation of site of action of NSAIDs.

Dosage

Aspirin is effective in low doses (0.3–0.6 g, 6–8 hourly). Analgesic effect is maximal at around 1,000 mg (single dose). The doses of the other commonly used NSAIDs are as follows:

- Ibuprofen 400 mg BD
- Mefenamic acid 250–500 mg TDS
- Diclofenac sodium 50 mg TDS oral, 75 mg deep IM
- Aceclofenac 100 mg BD
- Piroxicam 20 mg BD for 2 days followed by 20 mg OD
- Ketorolac 15–30 mg IM or IV every 4–6 hours, 10–20 mg 6 hourly oral
- Metamizole 0.5–1.5 g oral/IM/IV
- Nimesulide 100 mg BD
- Meloxicam 7.5–15 mg OD
- Nabumetone 500 mg OD
- Celecoxib 100–200 mg BD
- Etoricoxib 60–120 mg OD
- Parecoxib 40 mg oral/IM/IV every 6–12 hours
- Nefopam 30–60 mg TDS oral, 20 mg IM 6 hourly.

Adverse Effects

Nonsteroidal anti-inflammatory drugs have several side effects as below:

- Gastrointestinal: gastric irritation, erosions, peptic ulceration, gastric bleeding/perforation, esophagitis
- Renal: sodium and water retention, chronic renal failure, interstitial nephritis, papillary necrosis
- Hepatic: raised transaminases, hepatic failure
- CNS: headache, mental confusion, behavioral disturbances, seizure precipitation
- Hematological: bleeding, thrombocytopenia, hemolytic anemia, agranulocytosis
- Others: asthma exacerbation, nasal polyposis, skin rashes, pruritus, angioedema.

Drug Interactions

Drug interactions are frequent and may be potentially serious (Table 3). Since patients often consume these drugs, without prescription or on long-term basis, proper history is important.

ANXIOLYTICS

Most dermatosurgeries are performed under local anesthesia and hence patient cooperation is vital.

Table 3: Drug interactions with NSAIDs.

	Pharmacodynamic	Pharmacokinetic	
Diuretics	↓ diuresis	Oral anticoagulants	Metabolism inhibited;
β-blocker	↓ antihypertensive effect	Sulfonylureas	competes for plasma
ACE inhibitors	↓ antihypertensive effect	Phenytoin	protein binding
Anticoagulants	↑ risk of *gastrointestinal* bleed	Valproate	
Sulfonylureas	↑ risk of hypoglycemia	Digoxin	↓ renal excretion of
Alcohol	↑ risk of bleed	Lithium	interacting drug
Cyclosporine	↑ nephrotoxicity	Aminoglycosides	
Corticosteroids	↑ risk of *gastrointestinal* bleed	Methotrexate	

An anxious patient is poorly cooperative; anxiety also leads to bleeding intraoperatively. Hence, relieving anxiety through pharmacological and nonpharmacological means is important.

Nonpharmacological methods include creating a pleasant ambience, reassuring staff, music in the background, reading materials and above all calm, assured presence of the dermatosurgeon. These are particularly important in children and in dermatosurgeries such as vitiligo surgeries, tumor excisions and hair transplantation.

Commonly used anxiolytics are diazepam, lorazepam and midazolam.

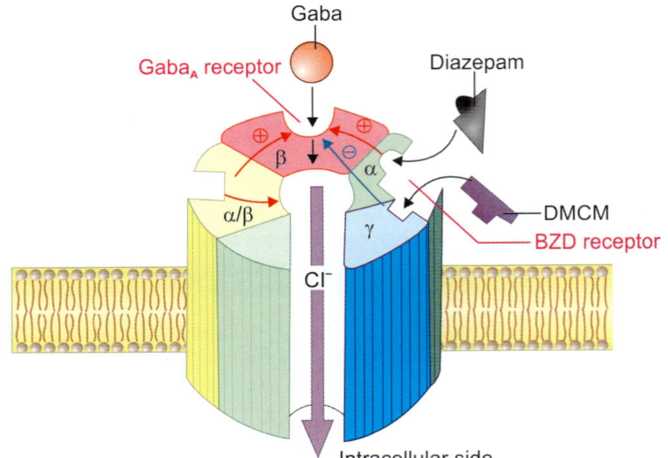

Fig. 2: Schematic depiction of $GABA_A$-benzodiazepine receptor-chloride channel complex. The chloride channel is gated by the primary ligand GABA. The benzodiazepine (BZD) receptor modulates $GABA_A$ receptor in either direction: agonists like diazepam facilitates, while inverse agonists like DMCM hinder GABA mediated Cl^- channel opening.
Source: Textbook of Pharmacology (6th Edn). Jaypee Brothers Medical Publishers, New Delhi, 2006).

Diazepam

Diazepam is a long-acting benzodiazepine. It acts by binding to a specific subunit on the gamma amino butyric acid A ($GABA_A$) receptor (Fig. 2) at a site that is distinct from the binding site of the endogenous GABA molecule. The $GABA_A$ receptor is an inhibitory channel which, when activated, decreases neuronal activity. Peak blood levels after the IV and IM administration of diazepam injection are reached within 15–30 minutes respectively whereas it takes 1 hour after a single oral dosing. The acute half-life is 2–3 hours with a slower decline thereafter.

Required dose is 2–10 mg IM or IV. In children dosage is 1 mg/4.5 kg.

Special precautions:

- Intramuscular: Diazepam injection should be injected deeply into the muscle.
- Rapid injection or the use of veins with too small a lumen carries the risk of thrombophlebitis. Intravenous injection should be directed into a large lumen vessel, such as an antecubital vein, and the ampule solution should be administered slowly (e.g. 5 mg/minute).
- Resuscitative facilities should be available as respiratory arrest is a possible complication.
- After parenteral administration, ambulation should be delayed at least 1 or 2 hours or until complete alertness is restored.
- Pregnancy: Being considered under FDA pregnancy category D, its usage in pregnancy and lactation should be limited only to emergencies.
- Elderly: The benefits of benzodiazepines are least and the risks are greatest in the elderly. The elderly are at an increased risk of dependence and are more sensitive to the adverse effects such as memory problems, daytime sedation, impaired motor coordination, and increased risk of motor vehicle accidents and falls.

Lorazepam

Lorazepam is a high-potency short-to-intermediate-acting 3-hydroxy benzodiazepine drug that has all five intrinsic benzodiazepine effects: anxiolytic, amnesic, sedative/hypnotic, anticonvulsant, antiemetic and muscle relaxant. Its mechanism of action is similar to that of diazepam, i.e. interaction at benzodiazepine binding sites, which are located on $GABA_A$ receptors in the CNS.

It is fast acting. Its relatively potent amnesic effect, with its anxiolytic and sedative effects, makes lorazepam a useful drug for premedication. Oral lorazepam is given 90–120 minutes before procedures and intravenous lorazepam as late as 10 minutes before procedures. It is given in the dosage as 1 mg tablet orally or 2 mg/ml intravenously. It has a relatively high addictive and abuse potential, a fact of importance, but not relevant in dermatosurgery.

Midazolam

Midazolam is an ultra-short-acting benzodiazepine derivative, with a rapid onset of action, high effectiveness and low toxicity level. The drug is commonly used as a preanesthetic medication for inducing sedation and amnesia before dermatosurgical procedures. It has potent anxiolytic, skeletal muscle relaxant, and sedative properties.

As with other benzodiazepines, almost all of the properties of midazolam can be explained by the actions of benzodiazepines on $GABA_A$ receptors. It enhances the effect of the neurotransmitter GABA on the $GABA_A$ receptors (↑ frequency of chloride channel opening) resulting in neural inhibition. Midazolam is water-soluble and fat-soluble in physiologic pH. It is freely soluble in alcohol and acetone.

Recommended Dosage

Oral

- Child: ≥ 6 months: Single dose of 250–500 µg/kg, up to a maximum of 20 mg.
- Younger patients (6 months to <6 years) may require up to 1 mg/kg.

Intramuscular

- Adult: 70–100 µg/kg (usual dose: 5 mg) given 20–60 minutes before surgery by deep IM injection.
- Child: ≥ 1 year: 80–200 µg/kg given 20–60 minutes before surgery by deep IM injection.
- Elderly: 20–50 mcg/kg given 20–60 minutes before surgery by deep IM injection.

Intravenous

- Adult: Initially, upto 2.5 mg given over at least 2–5 minutes, 5–10 minutes before procedure. Repeat after at least 2 minutes, if necessary. Usual total: 3.5–5 mg. Maximum total: 7.5 mg.
- Child: 6 months–5 years: Initial: 50–100 µg/kg given over 2 minutes, increase slowly at 2 minutes interval upto a total of 600 µg/kg, maximum total dose: 6 mg.
- Child: 6–12 years: 25–50 µg/kg given over 2 minutes and increase slowly at 2 minutes interval up to a total of 400 µg/kg; maximum total dose: 10 mg.
- Elderly: Initially 1–1.5 mg given over 2 minutes, increased by increments of 0.5–1 mg at 2 minutes intervals as needed.

Special precautions:

- Avoid midazolam in conjunction with opioids or other sedatives, as there is increased potential risk for respiratory depression, airway obstruction, or hypoventilation.
- Intravenous administration should be done only in the presence of adequate measures and trained staff for resuscitation.
- Concomitant use of grapefruit juice should be avoided as bioavailability of oral midazolam will be increased.
- It is in category D in pregnancy safety and hence, is better avoided in pregnancy and lactation.

Clonidine

It is an α_2 adrenergic agonist primarily used as an antihypertensive drug. As premedication, oral clonidine 5 µg/kg given 30 minutes prior to surgery reduces the requirement of lignocaine acid and prolongs the duration of analgesia without significant side effects and hence has found use in dermatosurgery, dental surgery and other surgeries.[7-10] Clonidine is routinely administered by most liposuction surgeons as a preoperative medication, along with anxiolytics.[11] Clonidine has recently been used in several other surgical procedures such as arthroscopy and in obstetric analgesia as an adjuvant both preoperatively and postoperatively.

Clonidine[12] has been used as a preoperative medication for its antisympathetic, antihypertensive, anxiolytic, sedative, anesthetic, analgesic effects. Effects of clonidine which can be beneficial in dermatosurgery patients include:

- Antihypertensive effects because of its central hypotensive effect as an alpha 2 adrenergic agent. Clonidine lowers intraoperative and postoperative responses to anesthetics and surgical stress.
- Sedative effects: Clonidine induces sedation because of its alpha 2 adrenergic effect. It also synergistically increases the potency of benzodiazepines such as lorazepam.
- Anxiolytics: Clonidine has anxiolytic effect independent of its sedative effect.
- Narcotic analgesic effects: Clonidine both supplements and minimizes the need for narcotic analgesics and therefore prevents respiratory depression.
- Clonidine prolongs the action of lignocaine in peripheral blocks.
- Clonidine induces bradycardia and hypotension and also has antiarrhythmic effect. Thus, it effectively counteracts tachycardia induced by epinephrine in tumescent fluid.

USE OF ANALGESICS AND ANXIOLYTICS IN DERMATOSURGERY PATIENTS

Dermatosurgeries are generally mild and severe pain is not a feature in most surgeries. However, pain can occur after hair transplantation (strip excision), surgeries on scalp, scar revisions, flaps and grafts, etc. (Box 2). Proper

Box 2: Dermatosurgeries which are associated with significant pain.

- Hair transplantation by strip method (e.g. FUT)
- Vitiligo surgery (split skin grafting) of large areas
- Some scar revisions and flaps
- Full face resurfacing by dermabrasion
- Ablative lasers
- Phenol peels

counseling about pain and its management should form an integral part of preprocedure consultation.

Pain and Patient Counseling

Pain perception is an extremely variable function and patients vary greatly in the amount of pain felt. In many, this is the main fear before surgery and "how much pain will I have" is a frequently asked question during counseling. Hence, enough time should be spent on explaining to patients about this aspect; their anxiety should be allayed that pain, while it may occur, will be prevented/treated by appropriate drugs. Patient can be asked a direct question "are you a nervous person?", "how was the pain in your previous surgery?", "would you prefer an anxiolytic before surgery?". Previous history of dental extractions serves as a useful guide and indicator.

Anxiolytics are preferred preoperatively, whereas analgesics are normally recommended postoperatively to relieve pain and inflammation.

Analgesics and Hemostasis

Some of the NSAIDs can adversely affect surgical outcome by interfering with the hemostasis, wound healing and hence, necessitate discontinuation for an adequate duration prior to surgery or require constant patient monitoring.[10,11] This is definitely so for NSAIDs administered for nonlife-saving indications, which may need to be stopped before surgery.[13-14] Aspirin is commonly used by patients with ischemic heart disease and irreversibly inhibits the COX activity of platelets resulting in anticoagulant effect.[13] Platelet recovery occurs in 2 weeks after stopping aspirin. However, in such instances, stopping the drug for better hemostasis, needs to be assessed in the light of possible cardiovascular risk that the stoppage of drug may bring about. It is also well known, that serious bleeding is rare in dermatosurgical procedures. Hence, it is generally not necessary to stop aspirin prior to surgery. Careful assessment should be done of the given situation and opinion of a physician sought before stopping the drug.

Choice of Analgesic

While choosing the analgesics in dermatosurgical patients, one should check the following pre-existing comorbidities and the medications that the patient is consuming; as mentioned in the text above, drug interactions are quite common among analgesics and other medications. Most commonly used oral analgesic medications include diclofenac and tramadol. In addition to oral analgesics, the other modalities such as suppositories of diclofenac sodium, transdermal patches of opioids and nonopioids could be tried. One should keep in mind that the multimodal analgesic plan is not only contemporary but will decrease the side effect of any one drug. The drugs commonly used in multimodal therapy are:

- Intravenous paracetamol at a dose of 1 g administered once in 8 hours
- Transcutaneous diclofenac (NuPatch®) or fentanyl
- Rectal suppositories of paracetamol or diclofenac
- Oral analgesics such as tramadol, paracetamol, diclofenac sodium, ketorolac, piroxicam or nimesulide.

Additional Modalities for Pain Relief

As mentioned above, use of drugs such as midazolam and clonidine preoperatively can help in better management of pain. Infiltrating the incision with long acting local anesthetic agents such as bupivacaine (0.06%) not only provides instant analgesia but continues to provide it for about 5–6 hours. At a few centers, in hair transplant surgery, continuous infiltration of local anesthetic agents using elastomeric pump has been used with good analgesic outcomes. Injection of triamcinolone acetate at the site of suture and recipient area in hair transplantation may reduce postoperative edema and hence reduce pain.

It is wise to practice a combination of one or more of the groups of medications/techniques mentioned above to get the maximum benefit of the components of the combinations.

Tips

- No single drug is superior to all others for every patient. Choice of drug is thus largely empirical. The nature of the surgical procedure along with consideration of risk-factors in the given patient governs selection of the analgesic. Past experience of the patient, acceptability and individual preference are also to be considered.
- For dermatological procedures and surgery, tramadol, ketorolac, diclofenac, nimesulide or aspirin may be suitable.
- For pediatric patients, only paracetamol, ibuprofen and naproxen are to be used.
- Paracetamol is the safest analgesic in pregnancy while low-dose aspirin is probably the second best drug.
- Midazolam is the preferred anxiolytic used before dermatosurgeries.
- Clonidine is a useful preoperative drug.
- Avoid anxiolytics in pregnancy and lactation.
- Postoperative infiltration of bupivacaine and triamcinolone at the site of surgery can help reduce pain.

ACKNOWLEDGMENTS

The contribution of Drs Murali Chakravarty, Pradip Kumar S, Manoj Krishnamachar and Venkataram Mysore is gratefully acknowledged.

REFERENCES

1. Yaksh TL, Wallace MS. Opioids, Analgesia, and Pain Management. In: Brunton LL, Chabner BA, Knollmann BC (Eds). Goodman and Gilman's: The pharmacological basis of therapeutics (12th edn). New York: McGraw-Hill Medical Publishing Division; 2011;481-526.
2. Tripathi KD. Nonsteroidal anti-inflammatory drugs and antipyretic-analgesics. In: Essentials of Medical Pharmacology (6th edn). New Delhi: Jaypee Brothers Medical Publishers (P) Ltd; 2006;184-201.
3. Sharma HL, Sharma KK. Nonsteroidal anti-inflammatory agents, drugs for gout and antirheumatic drugs. In: Principles of Pharmacology (2nd edn). Hyderabad: Paras Medical Publishers; 2011;363-81.
4. Trevor AJ, Way WL. Sedative-Hypnotic drugs. In: Katzung BG, Masters SB, Trevor AJ (Eds). Basic and Clinical pharmacology (11th edn). New York: The McGraw- Hill Medical Publishing Division; 2009;371-86.
5. Satoskar RS, Rege NN, Bhandarkar SD. Analgesics-antipyretics and nonsteroidal anti-inflammatory drugs. In: Pharmacology and Pharmacotherapeutics (22nd edn). Mumbai: Popular Prakashan Pvt. Ltd; 2009;161-81.
6. Das MM, Dutta SK. Narcotic analgesics. In: Ghosh R (Ed). Modern Concepts on Pharmacology and Therapeutics (24th edn). Kolkata: SK Ghosh and Others; 1989;250-69.
7. Pratap JN, Shankar RK, Goroszeniuk T. Co-injection of clonidine prolongs the anesthetic effect of lidocaine skin infiltration by a peripheral action. Anesth Analg. 2007;104:982-3.
8. YaDeau JT, LaSala VR, Paroli, et al. Clonidine and analgesic duration after popliteal fossa nerve blockade: randomized, double-blind, placebo-controlled study. Anesth Analg. 2008;106:1916-20.
9. Madan R, Bharti N, Shende D, et al. A dose response study of clonidine with local anesthetic mixture for peribulbar block: a comparison of three doses. Anesthesia and analgesia, World Congress of Anaesthesiologists No. 12, Montreal; 2001;1593-7.
10. Mishunin YuV, Ostreikov IF, Nazarov NA, et al. Combined use of local anesthetic with clonidine in cases of tooth extraction. Stomatologiâ. 2005;33-5.
11. Klein J. Tumescent anesthesia and microcannular liposuction: Mosby Publications; 2000;201-4.
12. Venkataram M, Shivashankar, Venkataram J. Use of clonidine as a preoperative drug in hair transplantation. ISHRS meeting at Montreal; 2009.
13. Patrono C. Aspirin as an antiplatelet drug. N Engl J Med. 1994;330:1287-8.
14. Proper SA, Fenske NA, Burnett SM, et al. Compromised wound repair caused by perioperative use of Ibuprofen. J Am Acad Dermatol. 1998;18:1173-4.

Chapter

20

Pain Management in Dermatosurgery

Manoj GK, Venkataram Mysore

Key Messages

- Modern-day dermatosurgeries are office-based, and performed under local anesthesia with little or no sedation
- A thorough preoperative patient assessment, counseling with relevant investigations is compulsory
- Peri-operative multimodal analgesic approach enhances better surgical outcome
- Well-structured postoperative instructions will have a positive outcome on the patient's recovery.

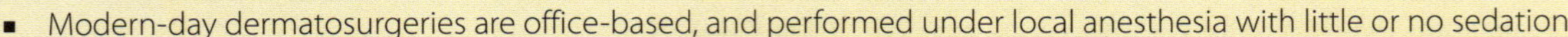

INTRODUCTION

With increasing types and number of dermatosurgeries being performed by the dermatologist, perioperative pain relief has now assumed importance. Pain at sites like scalp, face, etc. may be severe and stressful. While large majority of procedures are performed under local anesthesia (LA), demand for sedation, anxiolysis and analgesia has increased. The request profile is for a rapid onset as well as a long lasting action. The intravenous route and the usage of fast-acting sedatives and analgesics has assumed greater interest. A complete understanding of pain, its pathways and various modes of pain relief and anxiolysis goes a long way in enhancing prevention as well as treating pain, restoring confidence and satisfaction of the patient. This is particularly important as aesthetic patients are internet savvy, fully aware patients and demand a higher degree of care. This chapter highlights the importance of sedation, monitoring and appropriate use of analgesics for dermatological procedures. Details of drugs used as sedatives and analgesics are described elsewhere in the textbook.

DEFINITIONS

Analgesia: It is a state of absent perception of pain. This state can be achieved using Local, Oral, Topical, Intravenous (IV), Intramuscular, Regional anesthesia etc.

Anxiolysis: It is a drug-induced state during which patients respond normally to verbal commands. Although cognitive function and coordination may be impaired, ventilation and cardiovascular functions are unaffected. This can be achieved using short-acting benzodiazepine-midazolam or selective partial alpha-2 agonist clonidine.

Sedation: It is a technique of administering drugs to induce a state that allows patients to tolerate unpleasant procedures while maintaining cardiopulmonary function. A degree of lowering of consciousness is a characteristic of the procedure. While administering drugs for sedation the following scale has to be kept in mind (Table 1).

The objective of sedation and or analgesia in dermatosurgery is to achieve a level of sedation comparable to 'level 1-3' using appropriate pharmacological techniques.

Requirement of sedation in dermatosurgeries is subjective and variable. While some patients may not require any intervention, others may require anxiolysis or conscious sedation. Increasing sedation and analgesia influences physiological parameters of the patient as highlighted in the following table. Large majority require only monitoring and anxiolysis. Table 2 provides details of levels of sedation.[1]

Anesthesia: It may be local or general anesthesia or regional anesthesia. Local anesthesia is most commonly

Table 1: Levels of sedation.

Level 1	Fully awake
Level 2	Drowsy
Level 3	Apparently asleep but arousable by normal speech
Level 4	Apparently asleep responding to a standardized physical stimulus like Glabellar tap
Level 5	Asleep, but not responding to, physical stimuli

Table 2: Continuum of depth of sedation: Definition of general anesthesia and levels of sedation/analgesia.

	Minimal sedation (anxiolysis)	*Moderate sedation/ analgesia (conscious sedation)*	*Deep sedation/analgesia*	*General anesthesia*
Responsiveness	Normal response to verbal stimulation	Purposeful response to verbal stimulation	Purposeful response following repeated or painful stimulation	Unarousable even with painful stimuli
Airway	Unaffected	No intervention required	Intervention may be required	Intervention often required
Spontaneous ventilation	Unaffected	Adequate	May be inadequate	Frequently inadequate
Cardiovacular function	Unaffected	Usually maintained	Usually maintained	May be impaired

Reflex withdrawal from painful stimulus is not considered a purposeful response. Minimal sedation (anxiolysis) is used for dermatosurgery
Courtesy: "Practice guidelines for sedation and analgesia by non-anesthesiologists "Anesthesiology. 1996:84;459-71.

used in dermatosurgery and has been covered extensively in other chapters. General anesthesia is rarely used in dermatosurgery. Some instances where it is useful include extensive vitiligo surgery (megasessions), dermabrasion, removal of large number of warts in an uncooperative child. General anesthesia is a drug -induced loss of consciousness during which patients are not arousable even to painful stimuli. This is achieved by a combination of drugs like opioids, induction agents like propofol and muscle relaxants. Patients often require assistance in maintaining a patent airway and positive pressure ventilation because of depressed spontaneous ventilation. A qualified practitioner should be present to provide anesthesia during the procedure. Regional anesthesia is less frequently used in dermatosurgery and include spinal, epidural, or nerve blocks.

Concept of Monitored Anesthesia Care (MAC)[2]

Modern-day dermatosurgeons employ the assistance of anesthesiologist/nurse-assistance for sedation/ analgesia during various procedures. Conscious sedation is used to provide anxiolysis in patients undergoing local anesthetic procedures like hair transplantation, etc. It enables prolonged procedures to be performed and provide a degree of amnesia, a safe sedation, anxiolysis and pain relief. MAC implies the potential for a deeper level of sedation than provided by sedation/analgesia and is always administered by an anesthesiologist provider[3] Appropriate equipment for care and resuscitation should be available. Sedation does not compensate for inadequate local anesthesia. For conscious sedation, the College of Anesthetist Guidelines[4] states that pulse oximetry and blood pressure monitoring are the minimum requirement.

PATIENT SELECTION FOR DERMATOSURGERY

Usually, the majority of patients undergoing dermatosurgery are healthy. However, elderly patients and those with concurrent diseases are increasingly being included. The physiological effects of pain in these patients pose a challenge for perioperative management. Concurrent use of drugs for various comorbidities and their interaction with LA, intraoperative bleeding should be monitored. Box 1 shows details of conditions which need to be carefully assessed while planning dermatosurgery.[5]

Box 1: Preoperative evaluation.

It is necessary for the patient to discuss with the doctor prior to surgery, if drugs are used routinely for the following conditions:
- Hypertension
- Asthma/COPD
- Cardiac dysrhythmias
- Angina
- Epilepsy
- Neurological diseases like parkinsons

Source: Choudhary S, Begani MM, Mulchandani D. Choice of anesthesia for day care surgery. Bombay Hospital Journal. 2015;57:2.

American Society of Anesthesiologists (ASA)[6] physical status classification system is used to assess the fitness of patients before surgery. ASA has adopted six categories for the evaluation of the patient. Although debatable, this classification helps to predict risk vs benefit of surgery as depicted in Table 3.

ANALGESIA

In 1996, the International Association for the Study of Pain (IASP) defined pain as 'an unpleasant, sensory and emotional experience associated with actual or potential tissue damage, or described in terms of such damage'.

Nociception is the neural process involving the transduction and transmission of a noxious stimulus to the brain via a pain pathway. Pain is the result of a complex interplay between signaling systems, modulation from higher centers and the unique perception of the individual. Nociceptors are receptors in tissues which are activated specifically by painful stimuli. Nociceptors are, therefore, the free nerve endings of nerve fibers. There are two main fiber types: A-delta and C fibers. The transduction of noxious stimuli begins with peripheral nociceptors,

Table 3: ASA* classification.

ASA PS Classification	Definition	Examples, including, but not limited to
ASA I	A normal healthy patient	Healthy, nonsmoking, no or minimal alcohol use
ASA II	A patient with mild systemic disease	Mild diseases only without substantive functional limitations. Examples include (but not limited to): Current smoker, social alcohol drinker, pregnancy, obesity (30 < BMI < 40), well-controlled DM/HTN, mild lung disease
ASA III	A patient with severe systemic disease	Substantive functional limitations; one or more moderate-to-severe diseases. Examples include (but not limited to): Poorly controlled DM or HTN, COPD, morbid obesity (BMI ≥ 40), active hepatitis, alcohol dependence or abuse, implanted pacemaker, moderate reduction of ejection fraction, ESRD undergoing regularly scheduled dialysis, premature infant PCA < 60 weeks, history (> 3 months) of MI, CVA, TIA, or CAD/stents.
ASA IV	A patient with severe systemic disease that is a constant threat to life	Examples include (but not limited to): Recent (< 3 months) MI, CVA, TIA, or CAD/stents, ongoing cardiac ischemia or severe valve dysfunction, severe reduction of ejection fraction, sepsis, DIC, ARD or ESRD not undergoing regularly scheduled dialysis
ASA V	A moribund patient who is not expected to survive without the operation	Examples include (but not limited to): Ruptured abdominal/thoracic aneurysm, massive trauma, intracranial bleed with mass effect, ischemic bowel in the face of significant cardiac pathology or multiple organ/system dysfunction
ASA VI	A declared brain-dead patient whose organs are being removed for donor purposes	

*American Society of Anesthesiologists (ASA). Last approved by the ASA House of Delegates on October 15th, 2014.
ASA I and II are appropriate for dermatosurgery.

travelling along the A-delta and C fibers to dorsal root ganglion.[7] Their axons synapse in the dorsal horn, ascend along spinothalamic tract to thalamus and the cortex as shown in Figure 1. Dermatosurgeons rely mainly on anti inflammatory drugs and only infrequently use centrally acting drugs like opioids.

General Principles of Pain Relief

Optimal perioperative pain control for dermatosurgeries should be effective and safe, produce minimal side effects, facilitate recovery, and be easily managed by patients after discharge. It should follow the principle of providing a general background level of analgesia sufficient to permit normal activity, together with the use of additional analgesic supplements to cover any painful activity. An approach to breakthrough medications in addition to regular round-the-clock medication leads to an improved pain relief, mobility, and sleep.[8]

Multimodal Analgesia

The mainstay of perioperative analgesia is LA with oral, intramuscular, intravenous, and transdermal patch as supplementary sedation/analgesia. Although the most effective analgesic, opioids are associated with nausea, vomiting, and sedation that may delay discharge.[9] Non-opioid approach such as additional infiltration of LA at the wound site at the end of surgery, surgeon's reassurance and relaxation, and proper counseling are effective multimodal methods for an uneventful perioperative period.

Preventive multimodal analgesia has become the gold standard. This includes opioid as well as nonopioid analgesics. Nonopioid analgesics are increasingly used as adjuvants before, during, and after surgery to facilitate smooth recovery after the procedure. Combination of drugs help reduce the dose of individual drug and therefore prevent the side effects. Administering Paracetamol/NSAIDs along with alpha-2 agonist (clonidine when indicated) prior to start of surgery decreases the noxious influx by the LA infiltration in surgical field prior to incision. They also act on different levels of the pain pathway and have synergistic action.

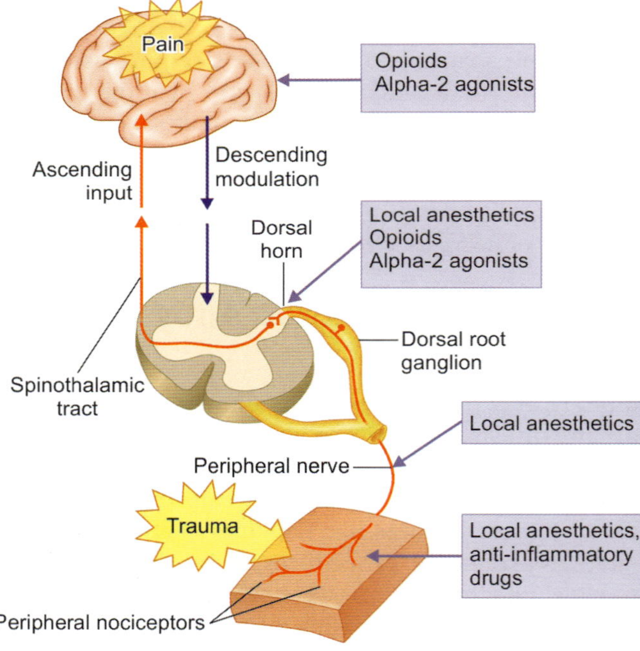

Fig. 1: The pain pathway and interventions that can modulate activity at each point.

Courtesy: Kehlet. H, Dahl JB, The value of "multimodal" or "balanced analgesia" in postoperative pain treatment. AnesthAnalg. 1993; 77:1049

Routes of Drug Administration

The intravenous route is preferred for conscious sedation because it has a faster onset of action and is more predictable as well as easier to titrate the doses. A reliable IV access should be maintained throughout the procedure. Intravenous sedation is employed only under the supervision of an anesthesiologist and nurse-anesthetist.

Optimal conscious sedation/analgesia is achieved when the patient:

- Maintains consciousness
- Independently maintains airway
- Retains protective reflexes (swallow and gag)
- Responds to physical and verbal command
- Is calm and not anxious
- Experiences acceptable pain relief
- Has minimal changes in vital signs
- Is cooperative during the procedure
- Has mild amnesia for the procedure
- Recovers to preoperative status safely and promptly

Equipment

Procedures for which sedation is used often occur in unfamiliar and isolated places and by nonanesthetists. following equipment are necessary during the procedure:

- Fully equipped crash cart, with emergency and resuscitative drugs, airway and ventilatory equipment and defibrillator
- Electrocardiogram (ECG) monitor and display
- Noninvasive blood pressure (BP) monitor
- Oximeter monitor
- Stethoscope
- 100% oxygen source with administration supplies
- Suction source and supplies
- IV supplies

Table 4: Advantages of LA with conscious sedation and analgesia in dermatosurgery.

Advantages to the patient:
• Avoidance of GA with its related complications
• Minimal postoperative nausea and vomiting
• Improved postoperative pain relief
• Ability to communicate with staff during surgery
• Ability to observe the procedure
• Early ambulation and discharge
Advantages to the surgeon:
• Enables accurate assessment of function before the end of surgery
• Allows discussion of operative technique and treatment option
• Enables modification of technique
Advantages to the hospital:
• Shortened patient's time in recovery room
• Reduced postoperative nursing time

Courtesy: Modified from analgesia for day-case surgery, N Rawal; British Journal of Anesthesia. 87(1):73-87.

- Capnography for end-tidal carbon dioxide ($EtCO_2$) measuring side-stream capnograph using face masks.
- Sedative, analgesic and reversing agents

LA with sedation offers the anesthesia personnel and the surgeon great flexibility in tailoring the degree of anesthesia to the needs of the patient. It helps the patient undergo lengthy and complex dermatosurgeries as office-based procedures and is then promptly and safely discharged home. Table 4 highlights the various advantages of LA with sedation.

Complications of conscious sedation: Serious complications are rare, but all sedatives and narcotics can cause adverse effects even in recommended doses (Box 2). Precautions are to be exercised in patients with comorbidities, and on various drugs.

Strategies for Perioperative Pain Management

Optimal perioperative pain control for dermatosurgeries should be effective and safe, produce minimal side effects, facilitate recovery and be easily managed by patients at home. Analgesic/sedation techniques should allow the patient to communicate with the Staff, allow for oral intake of liquids and a "rest room" break. Allowing time or the LA to act before incision and constantly checking for pain through communication with the patient allows for a smooth conduct of the procedure.

Recovery

Post-procedure patients are monitored for giddiness, vasovagal attacks, bleeding, nausea and pain. An area for observation by nursing staff until the patient has returned to pre-procedure state should be earmarked.

Instructions to all sedated patients:

- should be accompanied by a responsible person
- should not drive, operate machinery, and make important decisions for at least next 24 hours

Factors affecting speed of recovery:[10]
1 Length and type of procedure
2 Type of sedation employed
3 Pre existing co morbidities
4 Procedure done under LA vs Sedation

Box 2: Complications of conscious sedation.

- Dose-dependent respiratory depression hypoventilation are treated with supplemental oxygen.
- Transient hypotension and bradycardia and treated by stopping the procedure, change of posture, fluids, atropine and sympathomimetics.
- Vasovagal attacks are related to prolonged position. During the procedure, patient should be encouraged to sit up gradually and then assume the standing posture.

Choice of Analgesia after Discharge

Oral analgesics are the mainstay of continuing pain control at home, and it is important to ask patients to take them preemptively and regularly, starting before the effect of the LA has worn off. For mild pain, weak analgesic like paracetamol is sufficient; for moderate pain a combination of NSAIDs with a weak opioid like oral Tramazac is effective. A combination of paracetamol, weak opioid and NSAIDs, as a part of balanced analgesic approach will effectively take care of postoperative pain.

SUMMARY

The administration of sedation/analgesia for dermatosurgeries is a highly specialized skill. Clinicians must be trained to recognize the fine line between a tranquil amnestic patient and an unconscious, unresponsive patient. Preoperative education's audiovisual material and an information pamphlet are helpful tools, giving the patient time to be psychologically prepared for the procedure. Pre-emptive analgesia and balanced sedation help in smooth conduct of dermatosurgeries and its recovery. Long-acting local anesthetic like bupivacaine should be chosen for prolonged analgesic effect. All surgeons should be encouraged to use bupivacaine for wound infiltration. However, patients should be warned that the effects will wear off and that they should take another analgesic before it happens, particularly before going to bed night after surgery. Since most dermatosurgeries are office based, combination of LA with minimal sedation is sufficient and lasts the entire duration of procedure. If upon discharge the patient is alert, has minimal pain, and no nausea and vomiting, then the surgical experience was a positive one.

REFERENCES

1. Malamed SF. Sedation: A Guide to Patient Management, Elsevier Health Sciences, Introduction to Sedation. 2009, 5th edition. pp. 10-3.
2. Ghisi D, Fanelli A, Tosi M, Nuzzi M, Fanelli G. Monitored anesthesia care. Minerva Anesthesiol. 2005;71(9)533-8.
3. Barash P. Clinical Anesthesia, Lippincott Williams & Wilkins, Monitored Anesthesia Care. 2013, 7th edition 824.
4. Newton M, Blightman K. Guidance on the provision of sedation services. Royal College of Anesthetists' Guidelines for the Provision of Anesthesia Services, 2016, chapter 19.
5. Choudhary S, Begani MM, Mulchandani D. Choice of anaesthesia for day care surgery. J Bombay Hospital. 2015;57:2.
6. Mohamed Daabiss American Society of Anaesthesiologists physical status classification, Indian J Anaesth. 2011; 55(2):111-5.
7. Kehlet H, Dahl JB. The value of "multimodal" or "balanced analgesia" in postoperative pain treatment. Anesth Analg. 1993;77:1049.
8. Pain Management in Ambulatory Surgery; Jan G Jakobsson Pharmaceuticals (Basel). 2014; 7(8):850-65.
9. Marquardt HM, Razis PA. Prepacked take-home analgesia for day care surgery. Br J Nurs. 1996;5:1114-8
10. N Rawal. Analgesia for day case surgery: Br J Anaesth. 2001; 87:73-87.

Chapter 21

Antibacterial Agents in Dermatosurgery

Pradyumna Vaidya, Ragunatha S

Key Messages

- Infectious complications, either local or remote, following dermatosurgical procedures are an important concern.
- Overall infection rate following dermatosurgical procedures is very low.
- Most infections are acquired during surgery by contamination of endogenous bacterial flora at the site of surgery. Droplet infection, fomites are the other routes.
- Antibiotic prophylaxis is recommended based on the class of surgical wound.
- Majority of wounds following dermatosurgical procedures belong to clean and clean-contaminated wound which do not require antibiotic prophylaxis.
- As there are no uniform guidelines, inappropriate use of antibiotics in dermatosurgery may lead to increased drug resistance and adverse drug reactions.
- Sterile surgical technique, proper postoperative wound care, close monitoring of wound healing and adequate treatment of post-operative wound infection as and when it occurs, is a sound strategy.

INTRODUCTION

The main objective of any dermatosurgical procedure is to achieve a good cosmetic outcome. Infection at the site of surgery is one of the important factors that determine the outcome of surgery. All dermatosurgical procedures result in damage to the skin barrier to a lesser or greater extent, thereby predisposing the patient to the risk of infection. Though prophylactic administration of antibacterial agents minimizes the risk of infection, lack of data on their role in dermatosurgery is leading to inappropriate use and development of bacterial resistance. Furthermore, antibacterials can cause adverse reactions and rarely serious anaphylactic reactions. There are also known interactions between antibacterials and several medications administered for underlying health problems. Therefore, there is a need to understand the factors responsible for infection and the role of antibacterial agents in dermatosurgery, and to follow appropriate guidelines for the use of anitibiotics, both for prophylaxis and treatment of infections.

The purpose of this chapter is to review the literature regarding the use of topical and systemic antibiotics prophylactically, intraoperatively and postoperatively in various dermatosurgical procedures. Although the primary focus will be on traditional excisional or cold steel surgery, the use of these medications for more specialized procedures in the field of dermatology such as facial resurfacing, chemical peeling, liposuction and other cosmetic surgical procedures, will also be briefly addressed. The reader is also referred to the chapter on disinfection and sterilization, dermatosurgical operation theater and also universal precautions for additional information on related topics.

FACTORS RESPONSIBLE FOR INCREASED RISK OF INFECTION

Several factors related to patient, disease and dermatosurgical procedure determine the risk of infection (Table 1). All these factors should be carefully evaluated as a part of preoperative preparation through clinical history, examination and investigations.

Factors Related to Patient

Gram-positive cocci, in particular staphylococci are the most common organisms causing infection at the site of

Table 1: Factors responsible for increased risk of infection.[1,2]

Factors related to patient ▪ Staphylococcal colonization and carrier state ▪ Preexisting inflammatory cutaneous disorders, e.g. atopic dermatitis, psoriasis ▪ Underlying debilitating systemic diseases ▪ Chronic smoking
Factors related to disease ▪ Site of involvement ▪ Type and extent of disease
Factors related to dermatosurgical procedure ▪ Failure of aseptic precaution ▪ Improper sterilization of instruments ▪ Improper preparation of surgical site ▪ Type of dermatosurgical procedure ▪ Extensive destruction of tissue ▪ Prolonged duration of procedure ▪ Inadequate wound care

Box 1: Patient and environmental risk factors in the development of surgical site infections.

Patient risk factors	*Environmental risk factors*
• Malnutrition • Obesity • Advancing age • Diabetes mellitus • Chronic renal sufficiency • Peripheral vascular disease • Immunosuppression • Corticosteroid use • Concurrent remote infection • Bacterial colonization	• Length of the operation • Surgical technique • Preoperative preparation

surgery. History of recurrent staphylococcal infections (furunculosis), recent bacterial skin infection or active infection elsewhere indicates possibility of staphylococcal colonization or carrier state. Similarly, certain inflammatory cutaneous disorders like atopic dermatitis and psoriasis also increase the risk of infection with staphylococci. Patients with chronic and debilitating systemic diseases like diabetes mellitus, renal failure, liver failure, chronic obstructive pulmonary diseases, severe malnutrition and immunodeficiency disorders are susceptible to infection secondary to immunosuppression caused either by disease or immunosuppressive drugs used to treat these disorders. Smoking also increases the risk of surgical site infection.[1,2] Accompanying Box 1 shows the host and environmental factors leading to infections after surgery.

Factors Related to Disease

Based on the site of involvement and type of lesion, surgical wound is categorized into four types. The necessity of antibiotic prophylaxis depends on the type of wound (Table 2).[3,4] Dermatological procedures performed at certain sites are associated with increased infection rate. These include procedures below waist, and around the lip and ear.[5-7] The surgical excisions on

Table 2: Recommendation of antibiotic prophylaxis based on type of surgical wounds.[3,4]

Wound status	*Skin condition, site and surgical techniques*	*Antibiotic prophylaxis*
Clean	Noninflamed, non contaminated skin using sterile surgical technique	No
Clean, contaminated	Contaminated areas such as the axilla, perineum, or mucosal areas without gross spillage and minor breaks in sterile technique	Yes
Contaminated	Major deviations in sterile technique, community-acquired traumatic wounds, obviously inflamed skin, or gross spillage across a mucosal surface	Yes
Infected	Grossly contamination with foreign bodies, devitalized tissue or purulence	Yes

extremities, excision of squamous cell carcinoma and basal cell carcinoma, length of excision and patient status as an ex-smoker (ceased smoking in past 10 years) have been reported as independent risk factors for surgical site infections after dermatological surgeries.[8]

Factors Related to Dermatosurgical Procedure

Most pathogens causing surgical site infection arise from adjacent cutaneous or mucosal flora. Hence, appropriate use of antiseptic agents for preparation of surgical site and scrubbing of hands is essential for prevention of contamination. The type of procedure, extent of tissue destruction, duration of procedure and postoperative care also play an important role in the occurrence of infection at the site of surgery. Dermatosurgical procedures involving flaps and grafts especially around the lip and ear are associated with increased infection rate.[5-7] Hematoma at the site of wound acts as a good medium for growth of bacteria and a barrier to immune response.[6] Expanding hematoma and extensive tissue destruction form a nidus for infection. In general surgical procedures, it has been demonstrated that the infection is higher in procedures that extend beyond 3 hours.[9] However, majority of dermatosurgical procedures do not last more than an hour except hair transplantation, vitiligo surgery and liposuction.[10] Preparation of the site by shaving of hairs prior to surgery also increases the risk of infection.[2] Initial 24–48 hours of postoperative period is critical after which the wound is more resistant to contamination. However, dressing change, manipulation or exposure of wound during this period can increase the chance of contamination and subsequent infection.[11] A good sterile surgical technique and patient education regarding proper wound care minimizes all the factors responsible for surgical site infection. Accompanying Box 2 shows the common sites and procedures associated with increased risk of infection.

Box 2: Procedure locations and surgical techniques at increased risk for surgical site infection.

- Lower extremity, especially leg
- Groin
- Wedge excision of lip or ear
- Skin flaps on nose
- Skin grafting

ORGANISMS CAUSING INFECTIONS IN DERMATOSURGERY

Skin has both resident flora and transient flora. Resident flora consists of organisms on the skin that are relatively stable in number and composition. These bacteria vary among locations on the body and among individuals. Resident bacteria live on the stratum corneum and in the outermost layers of the epidermis. Transient florae which lie on the surface of the skin are derived from exogenous sources and vary widely. Skin flora is usually nonpathogenic and are either commensals (which are not harmful to their host, but offer no benefit) or mutualistic (which offer a benefit). However, resident microbes may occasionally cause skin diseases and enter the blood stream causing life-threatening diseases particularly in immunosuppressed patients.[12] The most frequent source of microbial contamination of surgical skin wounds is from endogenous cutaneous or mucosal flora present at the site (Table 3).[1,12,13]

ROLE OF ANTIBACTERIAL AGENTS IN DERMATOSURGERY

Prophylaxis for Prevention of Bacterial Endocarditis and Noncardiac Prosthesis Infection

The two main prerequisites or events that should occur to cause infective endocarditis are formation of noninfective thrombotic endocarditis and bacteremia leading to deposition of bacteria on noninfective thrombus resulting in subsequent proliferation.[2] A few studies which investigated bacteremia associated with dermatosurgical procedures have demonstrated low incidence of bacteremia, and in positive cases it lasted for first 15 minutes of procedure.[3] Highest risk of bacteremia in dermatology is associated with manipulation of infected skin lesion or abscess.[14]

Therefore, American Heart Association recommends prophylactic antibiotic in high-risk patients undergoing Mohs' surgery and any dermatological procedure with inflamed or infected skin. Patients belonging to high-risk category include those with the history of infective endocarditis; *prosthetic valve or prosthetic material used for valve repair; cardiac vulvopathy in a patient with previous cardiac transplantation; unrepaired congenital heart disease; repaired congenital heart disease within 6 months of procedure; or repaired congenital heart disease with residual defect at or adjacent to the site of prosthetic device or patch.* Irrespective of type of dermatosurgical

Table 3: Normal bacterial flora and common causative organisms responsible for infection and their antibacterial sensitivity depending upon the various sites of involvement.[1,11,12]

Site of procedure/ infection	*Normal bacterial flora*	*Infective organism*	*Antibiotics for prophylaxis and overt infection*
Glabrous skin	*Staphylococcus epidermidis, Micrococci, corynebacteria*	*S. aureus, Streptococcus pyogenes*	Cephalexin, Cloxacillin
Perineum/groin	*S. epidermidis, Corynebacteria, Micrococci, Acinetobacter,* Gram-negative organisms from intestine, anerobes	*S. aureus, Enterococcus, Escherichia coli*	Ciprofloxacin, Ofloxacin
Axilla	*S. epidermidis, corynebacteria, Micrococci, Acinetobacter, Propionobacterium acnes*	*S. aureus, Enterococcus, E. coli*	Ciprofloxacin
Nasal vestibule	*S. epidermidis, Micrococci, corynebacteria, S. aureus*	*S. aureus*	Cephalexin, Cloxacillin
External auditory canal	*S. epidermidis, corynebacteria, Proteus, E. coli, Neisseria catarrhalis, N. flora*	*S. aureus, E. coli, Pseudomonas*	Ciprofloxacin, Levofloxacin
Vulva	*S. epidermidis, corynebacteria, Enterococcus, E. coli*	*S. aureus, Enterococcus, E. coli*	Ciprofloxacin, Levofloxacin
Oral mucosa	*Streptococcus viridans, Peptostrepatococcus*	*Streptococcus viridans*	Amoxicillin
Infective endocarditis	——	*S. aureus, S. pyogenes*	Cephalexin, Amoxicillin
Prosthetic valve endocarditis	——	Early: *S. epidermidis, Gram-negative bacilli*	Cephalexin, Amoxicillin

Flowchart 1: Guidelines for prophylaxis in dermatosurgical procedures.

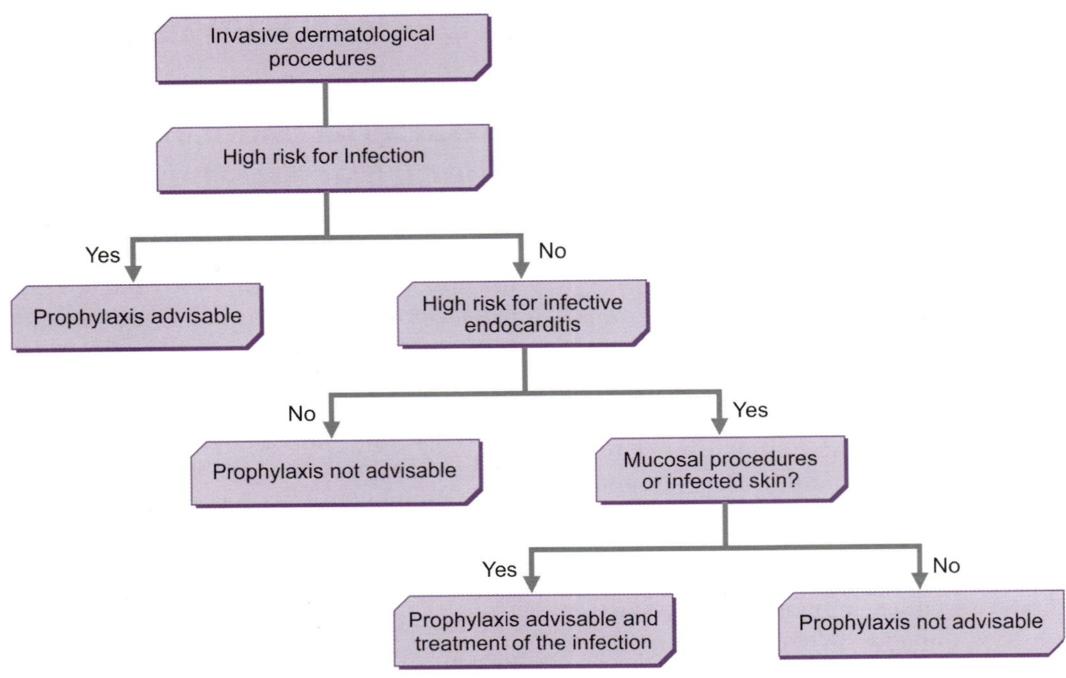

(Flowchart modified from Antibiotic prophylaxis in dermatologic surgery: Advisory statement 2008. Wright TI, Baddour LM, Elie FB, Roenigk RK. J Am Acad Dermatol Volume 59, Number 3, 464-473.)

procedure to be performed, except in cases posted for Mohs' surgery, antibiotic prophylaxis is not recommended to prevent endocarditis if the skin is intact, noninflamed and noninfected.[1]

Similarly, in patients with a prosthesis, as high level of bacteremia is required for infection of joint and vascular prosthesis, prophylactic antibiotic is not recommended for dermatosurgical procedures involving uninfected skin. If the skin is infected and the implantation is recent, the infection should be treated adequately before procedure.[4]

Antibiotic prophylaxis would not be indicated for noninvasive procedures, including botulinum toxin, nonablative laser procedures or percutaneous intravascular procedures, such as sclerotherapy.

Flowchart 1 shows the guidelines for prophylaxis in dermatosurgery. Box 3 shows recommended antibiotics and their dosages for prophylaxis in dermatosurgery.

Box 3: Recommendations for prophylactic antibiotics.

1. Surgical site infection prophylaxis
   a. Area—lips, ears, skin grafts, lower limbs, groins—cephalexin 2 gm orally
   If allergic—clindamycin 600 mg, azithromycin/clarithromycin 500 mg orally
2. Infective endocarditis
   a. Nonoral sites—cephalexin 2 gm orally
   If allergic—clindamycin 600 mg, azithromycin/clarithromycin 500 mg orally
   b. Oral sites—amoxicillin 2 gm orally
   If allergic—clindamycin 600 mg, azithromycin/clarithromycin 500 mg orally

Prevention of Surgical Wound Infection

Any measures taken to prevent surgical wound infection should decrease the risk of contamination of wound from existing skin flora. Sterile surgical technique and antibiotic prophylaxis are considered as good preventive measures. In general practice, non-sterile clean boxed gloves can be used for minor skin excisions.[15] The infection rate following dermatological procedures is very low and it has been reported to be around 1.3%.[16-19] In Mohs' micrographic surgery, the incidence of infection is 2.5%. Hence, most of the wounds following dermatosurgical procedures (skin biopsy, elliptical excision, electrosurgery, cryotherapy) belong to clean and clean-contaminated wounds. Considering the risk and benefit ratio, prophylactic antibiotics are recommended only for contaminated and infected (dirty) wounds.[1] However, due to lack of enough evidence, it is important to individualize the need for antibiotic prophylaxis based on various factors responsible for infection (Table 1). The use of prophylaxis is justified only when the cost of treating and morbidity of infection is significantly more than the cost and morbidity associated with prophylaxis.[20]

To be effective, the antibiotic should be active against the organisms most likely to cause infection in the area treated and should be present at the site during the procedure or shortly thereafter as all wound infections occur due to contamination of surgical site in this period. Therefore, route and timing of administration of prophylactic antibiotics is crucial. Antibiotics administered postoperatively do not get incorporated into the wound and are therefore less effective.

Hence, preoperative or intraincisional administration of antibiotics is preferred.[4] As majority of the dermatosurgical procedures are performed in an outpatient office setting, parenteral administration of antibiotic is impractical. So, effective oral antibiotic administered 60 minutes before the procedure is advised (Table 3). Oral cephalexin 2 g 30–60 min before lower limb excisions, though not statistically significant, has reduced the absolute risk of infection by 23.2% and relative risk by 65%. But, potential benefit offered by this prophylaxis need to be analyzed further.[21]

To overcome the disadvantages associated with preoperative antibiotics such as inconvenience of administration, drug resistance and possible adverse effects, intraincisional injection of small dose of antibiotic is considered as a good alternative for prevention of surgical site infection. Intraincisional injection of 0.5 mg/ml of nafcillin[18] or 40 µg/ml of clindamycin[19] in 1% buffered lidocaine and 1:100,000 epinephrine given at the site of surgery approximately 15 minutes before Mohs' surgery showed significantly less wound infection rate compared to placebo (local anesthetic). This method has the advantages of convenience of administration, decreased cost, less systemic effects and thus minimal side effects, drug interactions and drug resistance.[4]

For similar reasons, postoperative application of topical antibiotics has been a common method of antibiotic prophylaxis among dermatologists. However, this practice is contrary to the scientific basis that the wound contamination occurs before the wound closure and postoperative application of antibiotic is ineffective.[4] Moreover, topical antibiotics like neomycin and bacitracin have resulted in increased incidence of allergic contact dermatitis.

Studies comparing efficacy of petrolatum or paraffin and topical antibiotics (bacitracin or mupirocin) in prevention of infection have demonstrated statistically insignificant difference in infection rate at surgical site.[22,23] Therefore, simple wound dressing with non-antibiotic topical agents that provides a moist wound environment is recommended for prevention of surgical site infection.[10]

Treatment of Infected Wound

Postoperative wound infection acquired during the procedure usually manifests between 4 and 10 postoperative days as swelling, erythema and tenderness at the site of surgery. There may be associated malodorous purulent discharge. Immediate intervention is to remove the suture or any foreign body, drain the abscess and send the pus for culture and sensitivity. Empirical antibiotic is started which covers presumed organisms known to cause infection at the site (Table 3). The wound may be covered with sterile gauze or left open to heal by secondary intention.[2] The occlusive postoperative dressing also predisposes to infection with dermatophytes or candida. The presence of vesicles, pustules or scales with erythema on the skin surrounding the wound indicates fungal infection. If any of these signs are present only at the site of application of antibiotic or adhesive plaster, allergic contact dermatitis is suspected.[11]

Any dermatosurgical procedures involving deeper penetration of tissue like liposuction have the risk of invasive infections. The organisms are inoculated into deeper tissues through contaminated instruments (e.g. cannulae). Fatal necrotizing fasciitis caused by *Streptococcus pyogenes* and infection by *Rapidly Growing Atypical Mycobacteria* (RGM) have been reported following liposuction. The latter, commonly caused by *Mycobacterium fortuitum, M. chelonae* complex and *M.abscessus* presents between 1 week and 8 weeks postoperatively as local erythema, induration, microabscesses and serous discharge. Dehiscence of previously closed wound, delayed wound healing, absence of clinical response to conventional antibiotics or sterile routine culture should alert the possibility of infection with RGM. Clarithromycin taken continuously for more than 3 months is considered as drug of choice for infection with RGM.[24]

SPECIAL SITUATIONS IN DERMATOSURGERY

Majority of dermatosurgical procedures are conducted in an office-based setup usually lasting less than 1 hour. These procedures are simple, resulting in minor wounds with low infection rate. However, some dermatosurgical procedures such as hair transplantation, vitiligo surgery, facial resurfacing and liposuction require special consideration regarding antibiotic prophylaxis because these procedures last longer than 1 hour with relatively large, deep and multiple wounds predisposing to infection. Unlike routine dermatosurgical procedures, these surgeries are conducted in an operation theater with strict aseptic precautions. The resulting wounds are clean with less infection rate and therefore, antibiotic prophylaxis is generally not recommended.[11] However, considering the site of surgery, the extent and depth of injury associated with these procedures and more importantly the cosmetic nature of these procedures, in practice, most surgeons routinely administer prophylactic antibiotics. In patients with history of herpes labialis undergoing facial resurfacing either with laser or deep chemical peels, prophylactic antiviral therapy (acyclovir) is recommended.

SYSTEMIC AND TOPICAL ANTIBIOTICS

Topical antibiotics are used by dermatologist routinely postoperatively. Many topical agents are available to make

Table 4: Commonly used topical antibiotics and antimicrobials.

Silver sulfadiazine	Silver sulfadiazine has an excellent antimicrobial activity against gram-positive and gram-negative bacteria, as well as yeast. It is majorly used in burn cases. Dermatologists use this molecule very sparingly because of reports of contact sensitivity, bone marrow suppression and few cases of argyria
Mupirocin	Topical antibiotic produced by fermented *Pseudomonas fluorescens*. Spectrum of activity against gram-positive aerobic bacteria (*Staphylococcus aureus* and MRSA) and *Streptococcus*. It is bacteriostatic at low concentrations and bactericidal at high concentration. It does not interfere with wound healing. Prolonged use may increase the risk of resistant organisms. Less risk of cross resistance development. It rarely causes allergic sensitization. It is one of the most widely topical antibiotic used in postdermatosurgical procedures.
Fusidic acid	Sodium sulfate 2% is a salt of fusidic acid derived from *Fusidium coccineum*. It is bacteriostatic. It is only effective against gram-positive bacteria such as *Staphylococcus* and *Corynebactrium* species. There is less incidence of allergic sensitization and no cross sensitization observed.
Retapamulin	Retapamulin is a derivative of the naturally occurring pleuromutilin, produced by *Pleurotus mutilus* (now called *Clitopilus scyphoides*), an edible mushroom. Retapamulin is effective against gram-positive and some gram-negative organisms. It includes *Streptococcus pyogenes, Streptococcus agalactiae*, β-hemolytic streptococci, *Streptococcus viridans, Staphylococcus aureus*, Coagulase-negative staphylococci, *Propionibacterium* spp (including *P. acnes*), *Prevotella* spp, *Porphyromonas* spp, *Fusobacterium* spp, *Bacteroides and Clostridium*. It is a bacteriostatic drug, but may be bactericidal at high concentration
Nadifloxacin	It is a fluoroquinolone antibiotic. It is effective against infection caused by gram-positive and gram-negative organisms. No cross sensitization reported
Bacitracin	Polypeptide antibiotic derived from culture of *B. subtilis*. Mainly effective against gram-positive cocci and bacilli. Also effective against few gram-negative organisms. It does not penetrate the intact skin. Allergic contact dermatitis may occur
Polymyxin B	It is bactericidal, cationic polypeptide antibiotic effective against gram-negative bacilli except *Proteus*
Neomycin	It is obtained from the species of *Actinomycete streptomyces* and is an aminoglycoside antibiotic. It is more effective against most of the aerobic gram-negative organisms. It is one of the most common allergic contact sensitizer. Rarely anaphylaxis may occur. Though widely used in the initial period due to its common sensitizer property its use is declining
Metronidazole	It is a synthetic, nitroimidazole antibacterial effective against anaerobic organisms. It also has an anti-inflammatory effect

a choice as stated earlier. But the use of topical antibiotics is again controversial.[22,23] There have been increased report of contact sensitivity after topical use of antibiotics. In view of this, use of topical antibiotics in dermatologic surgery should be considered only in contaminated or infected class III or IV wounds. The high incidence of contact dermatitis, the insignificant decrease in infection rates and the relatively high cost compared with white petrolatum may warrant a reduction in the use of such agents in class I or II wounds. Commonly used antibiotics include silver sulphadiazine, mupirocin, fucidic acid, nadifloxacin, neomycin, retapamulin. Table 4 provides information about the commonly used topical antimicrobial drugs, and Table 5 summarizes the spectrum of activity of commonly used antibiotics.

Table 5: Systemic antibiotics and their spectrum of activity.

Antibiotic	*Spectrum of activity*
Cloxacillin	Excellent gram-positive coverage, including *Staphylococcus* aureus. Minimal gram-negative or anaerobic coverage except *Peptostreptococcus*
Amoxicillin	Aminopenicillin, which expands its gram-negative coverage but not *Pseudomonas*. Good anaerobic activity. Limited *S. aureus* coverage
Cephalexin/ cefadroxil	Excellent gram-positive coverage, including *S. aureus*. Limited gram-negative coverage. No anaerobic coverage except peptostreptococci.
Clindamycin	Excellent gram-positive and anaerobic activity, including *S. aureus*. No gram-negative coverage
Erythromycin	Good gram-positive and anaerobic activity. Variable *S. aureus* activity. Limited gram-negative coverage
Azithromycin	Similar to erythromycin but thought to have better *S. aureus* activity
Ciprofloxacin	Broad-spectrum antibiotic with excellent gram-negative coverage, including *Pseudomonas*. Has variable activity against gram-positives and anaerobes
Levofloxacin	Similar to ciprofloxacin but better gram-positive activity, including *S. aureus*. Variable *Pseudomonas* coverage

CONCLUSION

- Surgical site infection, infective endocarditis and infection of noncardiac prostheses following a dermatosurgical procedure is an important concern.
- Careful preoperative evaluation of patient for potential risk factors; good surgical technique with standard aseptic precaution; and proper postoperative wound care are essential for prevention of infectious complications of dermatosurgical procedures.
- Current literature reveals very low infection rate following dermatosurgical procedures and there are only a few indications where antibiotic prophylaxis is recommended for prevention of infectious complications.
- Till further evidences accumulate regarding role of antibiotic prophylaxis in dermatosurgical procedures, sterile surgical technique, proper postoperative wound care, close monitoring of wound healing and adequate treatment of postoperative wound infection as and when it occurs is a better strategy than inappropriate use of prophylactic antibiotics.

REFERENCES

1. Maragh SL, Otley CC, Roenigk RK, et al. Antibiotic prophylaxis in dermatosurgery: updated guidelines. Dermatol Surg. 2005;31(1):83-91.
2. Hass AF. Antibiotics. In: Robinson JK, Hanke CW, Siegel DM, Fratila A (Eds). Surgery of the Skin, 2nd edition. Philadelphia: Mosby-Elsevier; 2010;85-93.
3. Hass AF, Grekin RC. Antibiotic prophylaxis in dermatologic surgery. J Am Acad Dermatol. 1995;32(2):155-79.
4. Hirschmann JV. When antibiotics are unnecessary. Dermatol Clin. 2009;27(1):75-83.
5. Dixon AJ, Dixon MP, Askew DA, et al. Prospective study of wound infections in dermatosurgery in the absence of prophylactic antibiotics. Dermatol Surg. 2006;32(6):819-26.
6. Rogues AM, Lasheras A, Amici JM, et al. Infection control practices and infectious complications in dermatological surgery. J Hospital Infect. 2007;65(3):258-63.
7. Wahie S, Lawrence CM. Wound complications following diagnostic skin biopsies in dermatology inpatients. Arch Dermatol. 2007;143(10):1267-71.
8. Heal CF, Buttner PG, Drobetz H. Risk factors for surgical site infection after dermatological surgery. Int J Dermatol 2012; 51: 796-803
9. Schweinberger MH, Roukis TS. Wound complications. Clin Podiatr Med Surg. 2009;26(1):1-10.
10. Del Rosso JQ. Wound care in dermatology office: where are we in 2011? J Am Acad Dermatol. 2011;64(3):S1-7.
11. Stasko T. Complications of cutaneous procedures. In: Roenigk RK, Roenigk Jr HH (Eds). Roenigk and Roenigk's Dermatologic Surgery: Principles and Practice, 2nd edition. New York: Marcel Dekker; 1996;149-75.
12. Hay RJ, Adriaans BM. Bacterial Infections. In: Burns T, Breathnach S, Cox N, Griffiths C (Eds). Rook's Textbook of Dermatology, 8th edition. Oxford: Wiley-Blackwell; 2010; 30.2-30.5.
13. Messingham MJ, Arpey CJ. Update on the use of antibiotics in cutaneous surgery. Dermatol Surg. 2005;31(8):1068-78.
14. Wright TI, Baddour LM, Berbari EF, et al. Antibiotic prophylaxis in dermatologic surgery: advisory statement 2008. J Am Acad Dermatol. 2008;59(3):464-73.
15. Heal CF, Sriharan S, Buttner PG, Kimber D. Comparing nonsterile to sterile gloves for minor surgery: a prospective randomised controlled noninferiority trial. Med J Aust 2015;202:27-31.
16. Futoryan T, Grande D. Postoperative wound infection rates in dermatologic surgery. Dermatol Surg. 1995;21(6):509-14.
17. Whitaker DC, Grande DJ, Johnson SS. Wound infection rate in dermatologic surgery. J Dermatol Surg Oncol. 1988;14(5):525-8.
18. Griego RD, Zitelli JA. Intra-incisional prophylactic antibiotics for dermatologic surgery. Arch Dermatol. 1998;134(6): 688-92.
19. Huether MJ, Griego RD, Brodland DG, et al. Clindamycin for intraincisional antibiotic prophylaxis for dermatologic surgery. Arch Dermatol. 2002;138(9):1145-8.
20. Rafati M, Shiva A, Ahmadi A, Habibi O. Adherence to American society of health-system pharmacists surgical antibiotic prophylaxis guidelines in a teaching hospital. J Res Pharm Pract. 2014;3(2):62-6
21. Smith SC, Heal CF, Buettner PG. Prevention of surgical site infection in lower limb skin lesion excisions with single dose oral antibiotic prophylaxis: a prospective randomised placebocontrolled double-blind trial. BMJ Open 2014;4:e005270
22. Smack DP, Harrington AC, Dunn C, et al. Infection and allergy incidence in ambulatory surgery patients using white petrolatum vs bacitracin ointment. A randomized controlled trial. JAMA. 1996;276(12):972-7.
23. Dixon AJ, Dixon MP, Dixon JB. Randomized clinical trial of the effect of applying ointment to surgical wounds before occlusive dressing. Br J Surg. 2006;93(8):937-43.
24. Murillo J, Torres J, Bofill L, et al. Skin and wound infection by rapidly growing mycobacteria; an unexpected complication of liposuction and liposculpture. Arch Dermatol. 2000; 136(11):1347-52.

Section 2

Standard Cutaneous Surgical Techniques

Section Outline

- Simple Dermatosurgical Procedures: Biopsy, Curettage and Chemical Cautery
- Simple Excisions
- Electrosurgery
- Radiofrequency in Dermatology
- Cryotherapy
- Surgical Management of Cutaneous Cysts and Lipomas
- Flaps for Facial Reconstruction
- Flap Surgeries: A Dermatologist's Perspective
- Scar Revision
- Dermabrasion
- Keloids and Hypertrophic Scars

Chapter 22

Simple Dermatosurgical Procedures: Biopsy, Curettage and Chemical Cautery

Dhanashree Bhide

Key Messages
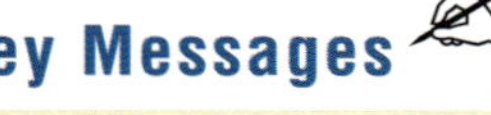

- A dermatosurgeon should be familiar with different biopsy techniques, such as punch, excision, incision, shave biopsies, as well as special requirements in difficult areas such as scalp, mucosa and nail.
- Curettage is a simple and useful procedure to treat superficial lesions.
- Chemical cautery with trichloroacetic acid, phenol and other caustics yield satisfactory results in several skin conditions, but should be done carefully to avoid postinflammatory pigmentation in Indian skin.

INTRODUCTION

This chapter describes easy-to-perform but common and useful procedures, like skin biopsy, cauterization and curettage in day-to-day dermatosurgery practice. There is stepwise description of different biopsy techniques, the various chemical cauterizing agents used along with their recommended concentrations and techniques of curettage with their indications. The correct and scientific methods for practicing these effective, but comparatively simple and inexpensive procedures are explained with appropriate diagrams and photographs.

SKIN BIOPSY

Skin biopsy is a very important and commonly performed office procedure in dermatology practice. This is an era of net savvy patients, evidence-based medicine, litigations and demand for the proof of clinical judgment. Hence, biopsy becomes an important documentary evidence for supporting the diagnosis made and also the basis for starting the treatment.

In biopsy, cells or tissues are removed by using different techniques for examination. Biopsy "Bio" means life and "Opsia" means to view. Biopsy means to view life. It can be excisional, incisional or a needle aspiration biopsy (Box 1).

It is an art to choose correct site for perfect dermatological diagnosis. Everyone should master different techniques and apply the correct technique appropriate for that condition.

History

One of the earliest diagnostic biopsies was developed as early as 1013–1107 AD by the Arab physician Abulcasim. A needle was used to puncture a goiter and the material was examined.[1] Skin biopsy technique in modern times was introduced over 100 years ago. Before this, the histological diagnosis was done in connection with autopsies or necropsies. The term "biopsy" was coined by a dermatologist Ernest Besnier in 1879. As local anesthesia facilities were not available that time, it was not a commonly performed procedure. Local anesthesia was brought in use by an ophthalmologist Karl Koller in late1800[2] when he instilled cocaine solution to perform pain-free cataract surgery. A year after this cocaine was injected in skin by William Halsted an American surgeon. Around end of 19th century, the infiltration anesthesia practice began and then the biopsy was performed on routine basis. Heinrich Auspitz and Hans von Hebra introduced sharp spoon in 1876. Punch instrument was originally used to trephine cut through skull bone. Its use was documented in abscess removal from tibia in 1852. A discotome was created by Watson in 1877 to remove traumatic tattoos.[3] In 1878, Watson described punch use in correction of accidental gunpowder disfigurement,[4] Edward L Keyes in 1887 described punch for dermatology use.[3] He used the

Box 1: Different types of biopsy.
- In excisional biopsy, entire lump or suspicious area is removed
- In incisional biopsy, only small sample from the affected area is removed by preserving the histological architecture of the cells
- In fine needle aspiration biopsy, tissue sample is removed with the needle. In attempting this, the histological architecture of cells may not be preserved

punch initially to remove powder crystals in the face of a youth due to firecracker injury. He deviced serial sized punches. There was a difference in the diameter of half a millimeter between the two consecutive sizes.[3]

Various modifications in the design as well as the uses were considered.

Rotary drill by Urbach, disposable punch, punch for autograft experiments,[5] use in hair transplant by Norman Orentreich[6] and Samuel Agres[6] were some of the modifications. The use of punch in acne scar surgery was suggested by Orentreich and Waine Johnson.[3]

Basic Anatomy

It is important to have the knowledge of relaxed skin tension lines (RSTL) to determine the incision.[7] Properly taken incision, which is parallel to RSTL lines, gives a better and cosmetically acceptable scar especially on the face. The RSTL lines can be made prominent by giving gentle lateral pressure in the area to be treated or by asking the patient to perform specific action (Figs. 1A and B).

Indications for Skin Biopsy[8,9]

Indications for skin biopsy are described in Table 1.

Contraindications

There are no absolute contraindications for diagnostic biopsies. However, the procedure should be performed with caution in following situations:
- Active infection at local site.
- Bleeding tendencies or patients on anticoagulants (aspirin, warfarin).
- Allergies to local antiseptics or to local anesthetics.
- Keloidal tendency.
- Systemic conditions such as uncontrolled diabetes mellitus.

Site Selection[8]

According to the Pathogenesis of the Lesion

1. *For inflammatory lesions:* When the disease is in the process of evolution choose a lesion with most advanced inflammatory change or from an active border. It is always good to include adjacent normal tissue for comparison.
2. *For bullous diseases:* Early lesions should be biopsied to get more specific results. Lesions within 48 hours of their appearance give the best results.

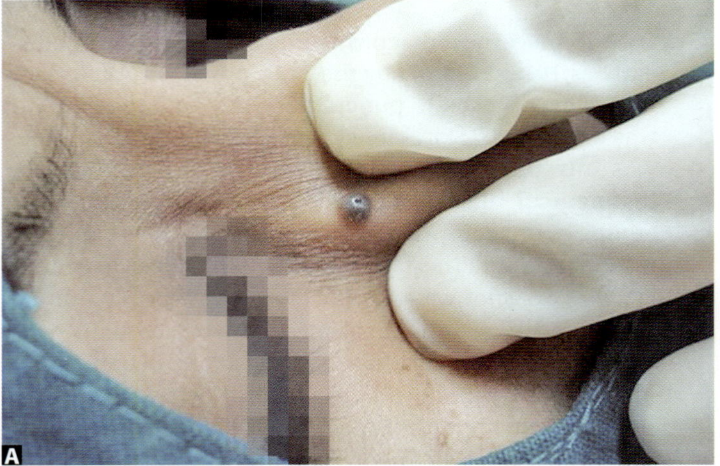

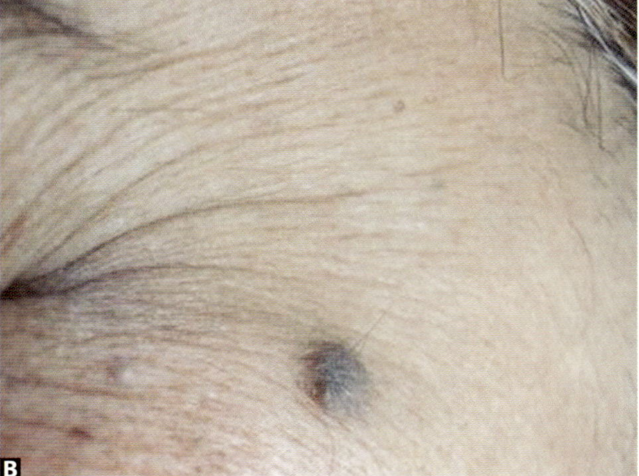

Figs. 1A and B: (A) RSTL lines made prominent by gentle lateral pressure; (B) RSTL lines made prominent by tightly closing the eyes.

Table 1: Skin biopsy indications.

Diagnostic	*Prognostic*	*Therapeutic*	*Special tests*	*To evaluate effect of treatment*
▪ When clinical diagnosis not possible or doubtful ▪ In all bullous and suspected neoplastic conditions ▪ To confirm the clinical diagnosis	In lupus erythematosus to do lupus band test (clinically uninvolved skin sent for direct immunofluorescence study)	Excisional biopsy in conditions like nevi, granuloma annulare, basal cell carcinoma, etc.	▪ Immunofluorescence ▪ Special stains ▪ Electron microscopy	For example, in leprosy before and after starting the treatment

3. *Suspected malignancy*: If it is small lesion, excise it completely with adequate clearance on all sides.

According to the Size of the Lesion

- Small lesions may be removed entirely.
- Large lesions, central part may be biopsied. Avoid crusted excoriated areas.

For Special Procedures

- Direct immunofluorescence in vesiculobullous disorders: Perilesional skin.
- Lupus band test in collagen vascular disease: Clinically uninvolved skin.

Points to Remember while Choosing the Site for Biopsy[10]

- Avoid friction areas as there may be secondary changes.
- In case of polymorphic eruptions, more than one biopsy may be required.
- Normally, a well-formed lesion should be chosen for biopsy except in Henoch Schnölein purpura, dermatitis herpetiformis and suspected subepidermal blisters when very early lesions should be biopsied.
- In urticaria pigmentosa, instead of infiltration anesthesia, use of a field block to avoid mast cell degranulation is advised.

Tips for Getting Better Results[8,11,12]

- Try to remove the vesicle intact.
- Bulla can be biopsied at the edge trying to keep the roof attached if it cannot be removed entirely.
- Try to avoid important cosmetic areas like face, deltoid area, chest (chances of hypertrophic scarring), tibia (delayed healing), groins and axillae (high incidence of secondary infection) as far as possible.
- Avoid biopsy in burnt out lesions, lesions altered by trauma or prior treatment.

Diagnostic accuracy of biopsy specimen can be increased if correct site, correct technique and appropriate transport medium is chosen (Tables 2 and 3).

Types of Skin Biopsy Techniques

1. Shave biopsy
2. Punch biopsy
3. Incisional biopsy
4. Excisional biopsy
5. Other procedures

Table 2: Site, type of biopsy and lesion selection.[11,12]

Disease	*Type of biopsy*	*Site and type of lesion*
Autoimmune bullous diseases	Small vesicles and perilesional skin-punch biopsy Large bulla: 1. Scooped shave biopsy extending up to reticular dermis 2. Incision biopsy from the edge involving the perilesional skin	▪ Preferred site trunk ▪ Extremities to be avoided
Epidermolysis bullosa	Saucerised removal of intact bulla preferred	▪ Blisters less than 12 hours duration ▪ Induce blister at a site where patient normally blisters can use pencil eraser, gloved finger or cotton swab ▪ Gentle traction given in downward direction ▪ And twist given in each direction by 180° till erythema produces ▪ Give lag period of 5 minutes before biopsy ▪ Avoid topical anesthesia which may induce artificial blisters
Vasculitis	Punch or deep shave biopsy	▪ For H and E well established purpuric lesion >72 hours ▪ For DIF fresh lesion less than 24 hours except in IgA vasculitis for which established lesion may be chosen
Panniculitis	▪ Deep incision biopsy ▪ Avoid punch biopsy as it is likely to leave behind inflamed or necrotic fat ▪ If at all punch is to be used electric rotary power punch may be used	▪ Apply alcohol to skin surface and allow to evaporate ▪ Take about 6 mm size biopsy ▪ Divide and send for culture and special stains ▪ The edge of necrotic focus ideal for this
Lupus and dermatomyositis	Punch biopsy	▪ Established but still active lesion ▪ For long-standing disease specimen from active lesion >6 months duration
SJS/TEN vs SSSS	Shave biopsy including entire epidermal thickness	Sheets of desquamating skin adequate sample
Scarring alopecia	Punch biopsy 4 mm and above	Avoid active edge Prefer established lesion
Nonscarring alopecia	Punch biopsy 4 mm and above	▪ Alopecia areata or syphilis-active lesion of recent onset is preferred ▪ Patterned alopecia and TE-established area more than 6 months

(SJS: Stevens-Johnson syndrome; TEN: Toxic epidermal necrosis; SSSS: Staphylococcal scalded skin syndrome; TE: Telogen effluvium; DIF: Direct immunofluorescence).

Choice of Procedure

Shave Biopsy

This is suitable for lesions confined to epidermis or raised above the skin, e.g. skin tags, seborrheic keratoses. However, it cannot be used when malignancy is suspected.

Punch Biopsy

This is the most commonly used biopsies.

Excisional Biopsy

Excisional biopsy is suitable for lesions which cannot be removed with punch because of their large size or due to their location or due to their depth.

Incisional Biopsy

Incisional biopsy can be used in large lesions to excise small portion of the tissue.

Pre-procedure Counseling

Obtain informed consent and counsel about possibility of a small scar, particularly when biopsy is planned on face or other cosmetically important area.

Instruments necessary for different types of biospies are shown in Table 4.

Chemical Hemostatic Agents

Chemicals which can be used to achieve hemostasis, such as 20% aluminum chloride in absolute alcohol, Monsels solution (ferric sulfate), trichloroacetic acid, silver nitrate are useful, particularly for shave biopsy. A solution called BotroClot (sterile hemocoagulase solution) can also be used. The active ingredient is purified hemocoagulase enzyme complex isolated from *Bothrops atrox* or *Bothrops jararaca*, species of South American snakes. It is atoxic and arrests the capillary bleeding by accelerating the physiological process of hemostasis. 5–10 drops of the solution can be used depending upon the severity of bleeding. It should be consumed within one month after opening the container. It is available as 10 mL solution in plastic container.

Table 3: Transport medium according to type of study.

Type of study	*Transport medium*
Light microscopy H and E	Formalin
Direct immunofluorescence	▪ Normal saline, liquid nitrogen, Michel medium, or Zeus medium ▪ N saline gives highest yield and send without freezing ▪ Samples sent in liquid nitrogen require thawing
Immunohistochemistry	Formalin fixed paraffin embedded blocks
Electron microscopy	2.5% glutaraldehyde solution
Microorganism culture	Nonbacteriostatic saline

Transport Medium[11,12]

For hematoxylin and eosin staining, 10% buffered formalin is adequate. Commercially available formalin is 40% which should be diluted 1 in 4 before use.

For immunofluorescence—Michaels solution if laboratory is located at a distance. Phosphate buffered saline in a cold pack can be used if laboratory is located within 4 hours (Table 3).

Steps Common to All Minor Procedures

1. Correct documentation with clinical photograph.
2. Informed written consent.
3. Universal precautions.
4. Proper sterilization of instruments.
5. Cleaning with betadine and spirit.
6. Marking the area before infiltration.
7. Infiltration of local anesthesia—1% xylocaine with or without adrenaline, depending upon the site. While infiltrating, try to elevate the lesion by raising a wheal which allows the lesion to prop up.
8. Postprocedure dressing, topical and oral antibiotic and suture removal when indicated.
9. Carefully label the specimen including patient and physicians name, date and location of the lesion.

Procedure of Biopsy

Shave Biopsy

Shave biopsy has the advantages of being quick, needs little training, does not require suturing for closure, faster healing and good cosmetic result. However, its disadvantage is that deeper dermis and subcutaneous fat are not available for examination and hence, the method is unsuitable for deeper pathologies.

Table 4: Instruments for biopsy.

For shave excision	*For punch biopsy*	*For incision and excision biopsy*
▪ Blades No. 15 or 11, razor blade or cutting scissors straight or curved ▪ BP handle No. 3 ▪ Chemical hemostatic agents or electrocautery for fulguration	▪ Biopsy punches 1–10 mm ▪ Optimum size 4 mm ▪ Cutting scissors ▪ Forceps atraumatic ▪ Skin hook	▪ Blades No. 15 or 11 ▪ BP handle No. 3 ▪ Atraumatic forceps—Adson's forceps ▪ Cutting scissors ▪ Suture material—needle holder ▪ Skin hook

Steps (Figs. 2A to H)

Steps involved in shave biopsy are as follows:

1. Stabilize the lesion between the thumb and forefinger in a direction perpendicular to RSTL lines.
2. A vertical cut is put at the periphery of the lesion using 11 or 15 No. scalpel blade attached to No. 3 BP handle.
3. Blade is held parallel to the skin surface and then passed through the lesion through the cut that is already made at the periphery.

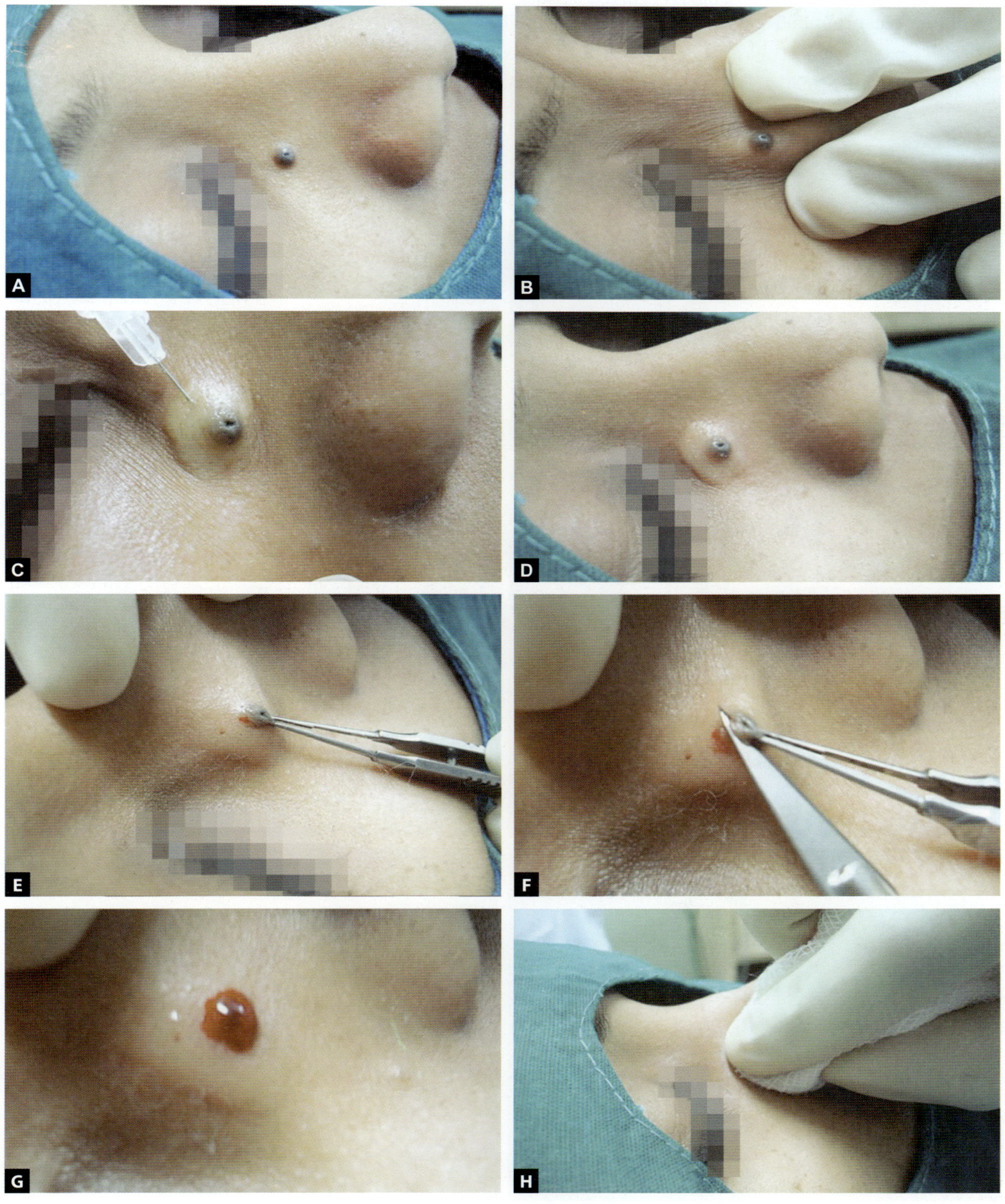

Figs. 2A to H: Steps of shave biopsy: (A) Mole on the nose; (B) RSTL lines made prominent; (C) Local anesthesia infiltration; (D) Lesion gets elevated; (E) Vertical cut at periphery; (F) Biopsy with blade parallel to surface; (G) Bleeding at site; (H) Hemostasis by firm pressure.

4. The blade is advanced through the lesion by a smooth sweeping stroke rather than a sawing motion while grasping the lesion with forceps.
5. Hemostasis is achieved by firm pressure or with the chemicals mentioned before the procedure can also be performed by using halved razor blade or curved scissors.
6. Antibiotic cream applied and a gauze dressing is given.

Alternative Methods

Scissor technique (Figs.3A to E)

For pedunculated lesions, biopsy with scissors is simple and effective option. Operator's clinical judgment is important while sending the sample for histopathological examination.

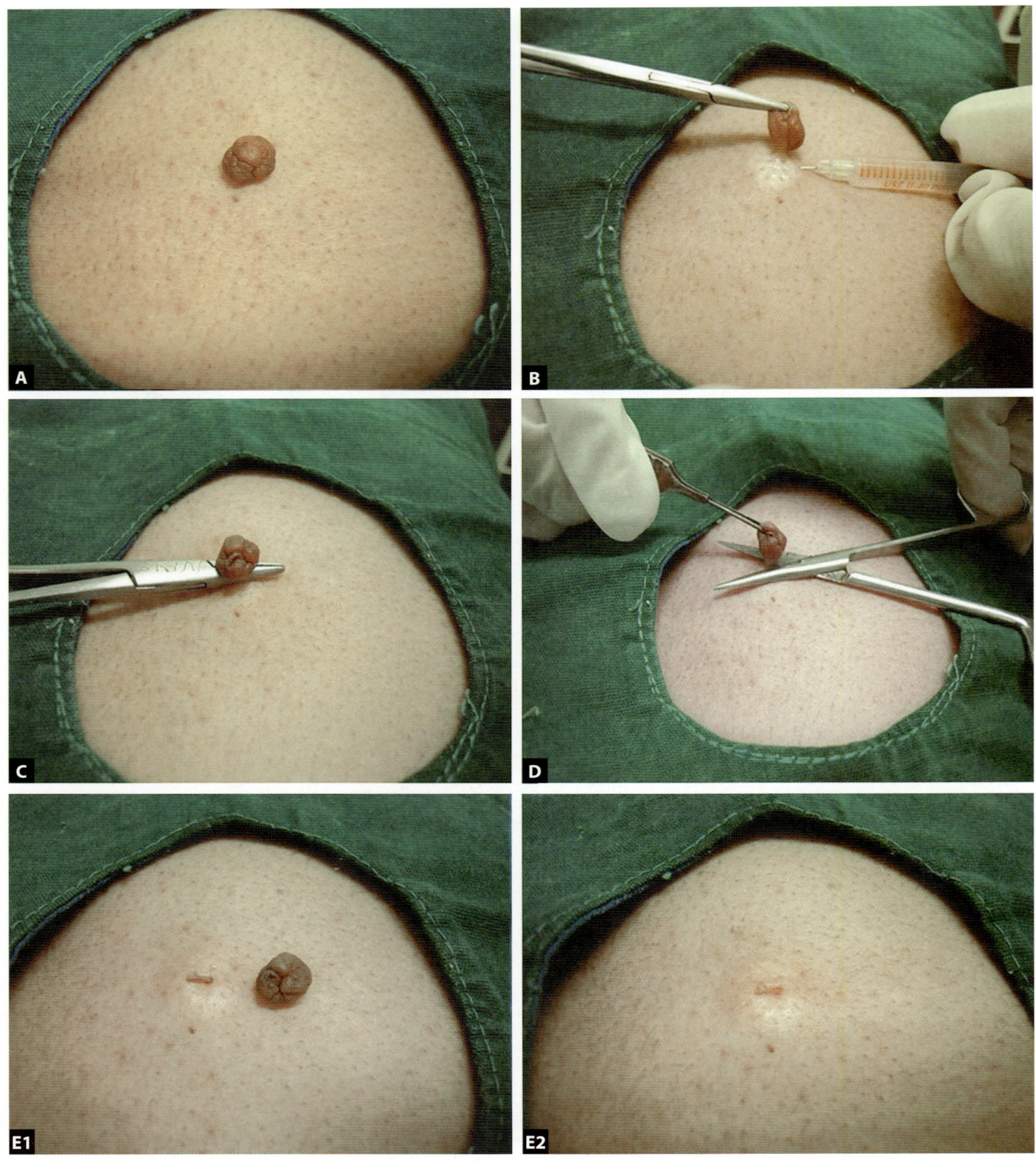

Figs. 3A to E: Shave biopsy (scissor technique). (A) Skin tag; (B) Local infiltration; (C) Base crushed with straight artery forceps; (D) Lesion excised with scissors; (E1 and E2) Immediately after procedure.

Shave Biopsy Using a Razor Blade (Fig. 4)

A razor blade can be broken into half and bent along its longitudinal axis. It is then held between the thumb and other fingers. Holding the blade without handle gives great flexibility. Horizontal sawing motion is used to the desired depth in the dermis. Superficial lesions can be easily removed by this technique. This blade has an advantage of being flexible and extremely sharp.[13,14]

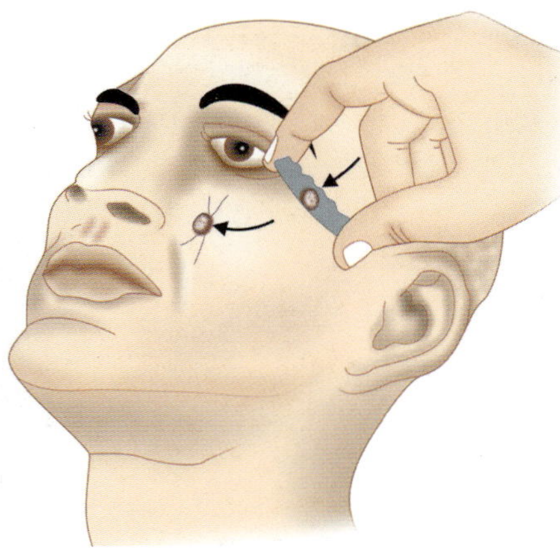

Fig. 4: Shave biopsy using a razor blade.

Punch Biopsy

Punch biopsy is indicated for routine histopathological examination as a therapy to remove small lesions like nevi. If lesion is totally removed, it is excisional punch biopsy. If the lesion is partially removed, it is incisional punch biopsy.

Its advantages are that it is simple, heals with minimal scar. However, it is unsuitable for lesions having pathologies deeper to subcutaneous tissue, such as leiomyoma, dermatomyositis and in difficult anatomical location, e.g. nasal cartilage.

Procedure of punch biopsy

Steps (Figs. 5A to J) of punch biopsy are as follows:

1. Common steps as mentioned above.
2. Routinely a 4 mm punch is chosen.
3. Traction given in a direction perpendicular to long axis of resting skin tension lines.
   While performing scalp biopsies, rim of the ring of a large artery forceps is pressed against the scalp surface.
4. Punch is held vertically and a steady pressure is applied.
5. Punch is rotated in a clockwise manner till tissue cast is completely separated from collagen fibers of reticular dermis and the punch reaches the subcutis. At this stage there is feeling of give away.
6. Punch is withdrawn.

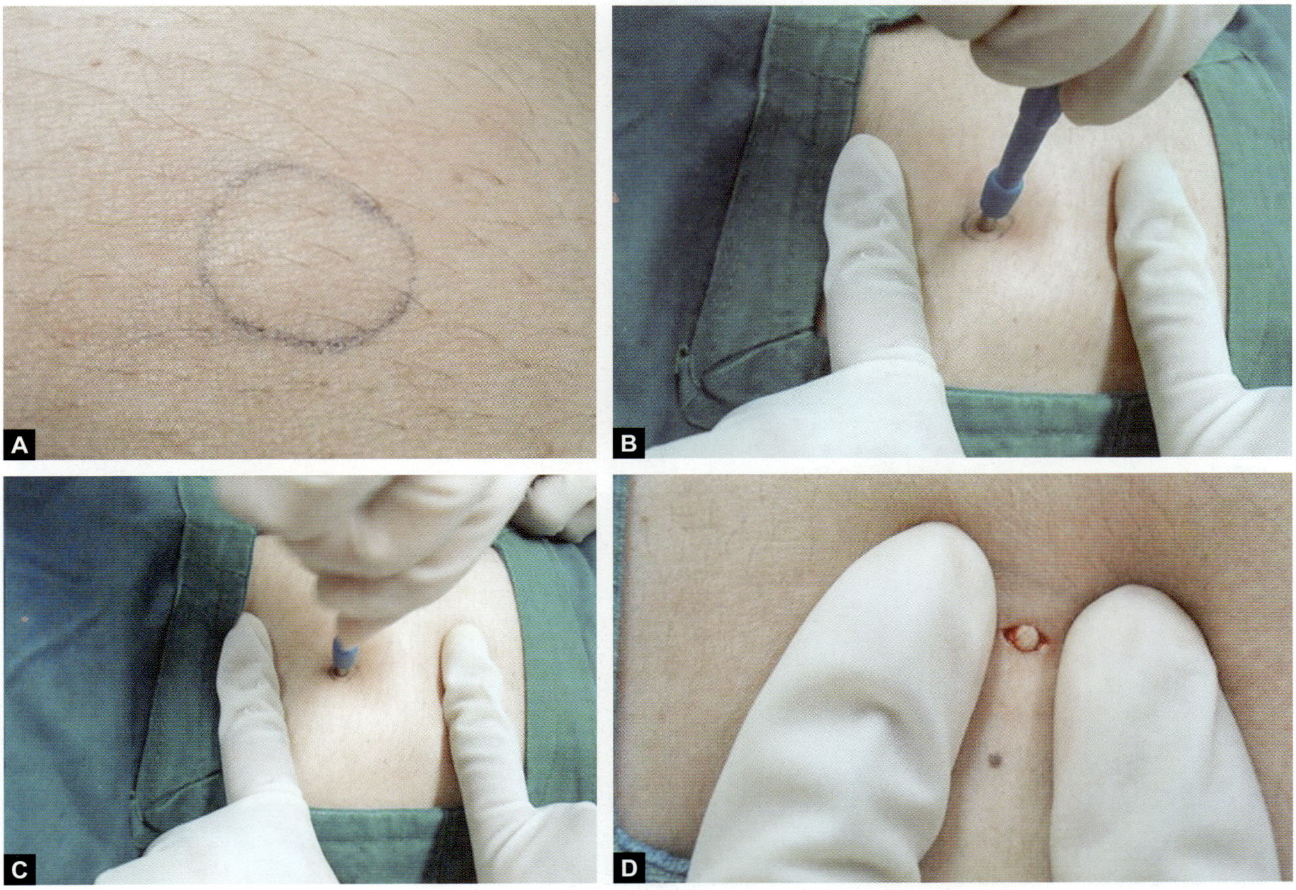

Figs. 5A to D: Steps in punch biopsy. (A) Site marked; (B) Punch held in vertical direction. Traction is given perpendicular to RSTL lines; (C) Punch rotated in clockwise manner; (D) Circular defect relaxes into an ellipse.

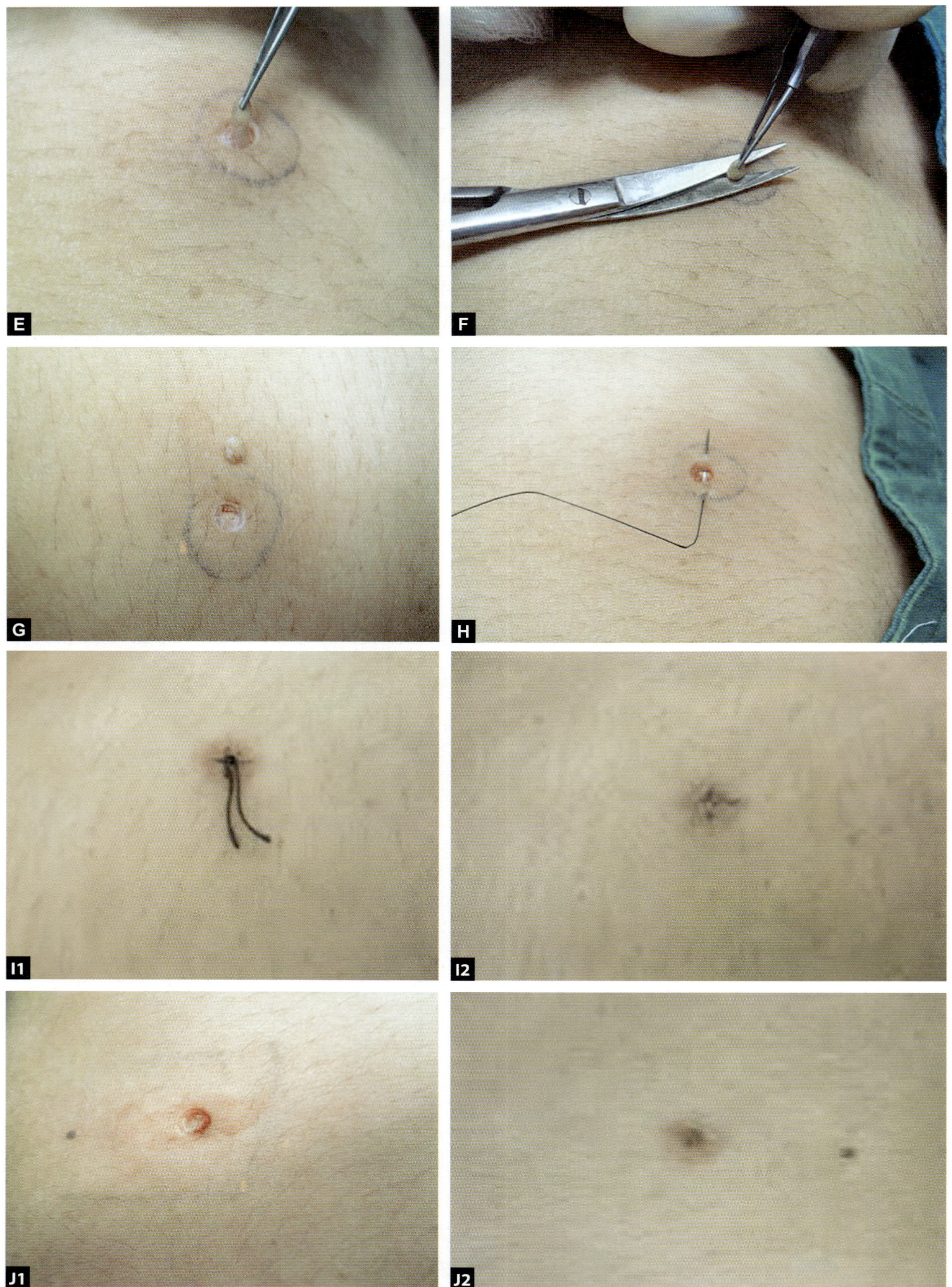

Figs. 5E to J: Procedure of punch biopsy. (E) Column of tissue grasped with forceps; (F) Tissue cut with scissors; (G) Biopsy specimen; (H) Suture taken; (I1 and I2) Healing after 1 week with suture; (J1 and J2) Healing after 1 week without suture.

7. Tissue cast is lifted with fine forceps or a needle to avoid crushing and damage. It is then cut at the base with scissors.
8. On releasing the tension, the circular biopsy defect relaxes into ellipse.
9. The wound is sutured for better healing with interrupted sutures by using 5/0 prolene and dressing is given. For defects up to 3 mm suture may not be taken in areas that are not important cosmetically.
10. Sutures removed after 7–10 days.

Excisional Biopsy

Excisional biopsy is indicated for removing benign or malignant lesions, which can be removed and closed by primary closure. As entire lesion is removed, it is both diagnostic and therapeutic modality. Its advantages are that entire specimen available for histology and since the wound is sutured, it heals with good cosmetic result. However, training is needed for performing the procedure and skill needs to be acquired. If excision is incomplete, chances of recurrence are high.

Steps (Fig. 6)

1. Basic steps as mentioned.
2. While infiltration, give a field block.
3. Draw an ellipse using a surgical marker, methylene blue or gentian violet. Apex of ellipse should have 30° angle on each side. The length should be 3 times the width. Two to five millimeters margin of normal skin, around the margin, should be included.
4. Area is kept taught and scalpel with No. 15 blade is held like a pencil.
5. Begin the incision at the apex holding the blade perpendicular to the skin.
6. As the incision progresses blade is angled to 45° to cut the tissue with the belly of the blade.
7. At the end of the incision again the scalpel is lifted vertically to prevent the excision from extending beyond the end point.
8. Same steps repeated on other side.

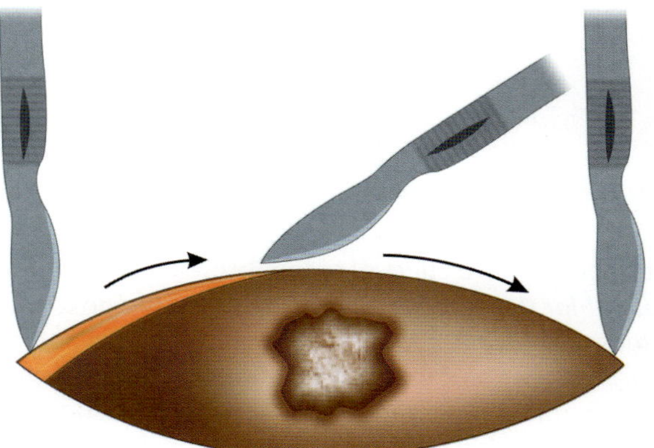

Fig. 6: Scalpel movement.

9. Ellipse of tissue separated from underlying tissue with scalpel or dissecting forceps.
10. Interrupted suture taken for larger and deeper defects suturing is done in two layers.
11. Dressing done after applying antibiotic cream.
12. Sutures removed after 5–10 days depending on the area.

Incision Biopsy (Wedge Biopsy)

Incisional biopsy is performed when tissue sample is required to perform special tests like culture, microscopy, e.g. deep fungal infections, cutaneous tuberculosis, mycosis fungoides, and for diseases that can spread beyond the clinically visible margin, e.g. malignancies. By including the normal looking skin, exact extent of spread of malignancy can be determined.

Steps (Figs. 7A to D)

1. Basic steps as mentioned before.
2. In this type, biopsy is performed from active edge of the lesion in a wedge shape including the normal skin. Alternatively it can be performed by using biopsy punches of size 5 mm and above.
3. Other steps are similar to excision biopsy. The only difference is in incision biopsy only part of the lesion is removed rather than the entire lesion (Fig. 8).

Other Techniques[9]

Curette biopsy

This biopsy can be performed without local anesthesia using a sharp curette. Friable part of the lesion can be scraped off with the curette and sent for histological examination. This sample may be adequate for the diagnosis but fails to determine the depth and lateral spread of the lesion and hence is not commonly performed.

Skin surface biopsy

This biopsy is done to inspect the stratum corneum. It is useful in detection of mites in scabies, dermatophytes and other microorganisms. It can be useful for research purpose, e.g. sampling of follicular casts (microcomedones) to determine the density of sebaceous follicles in different areas of face.

Procedure

1. Cyanoacrylate gel is applied on the skin surface.
2. A glass slide is pressed on top for 1 minute.
3. Slide is then rolled off from the skin surface and examined under low power after staining.
4. As the glue is costly and not easily available, this procedure is not performed routinely.

Oral biopsy[11]

Oral mucosal biopsy can be performed by the same technique as skin biopsy. However, there may be difficulties in performing the biopsy at this site due to various reasons:

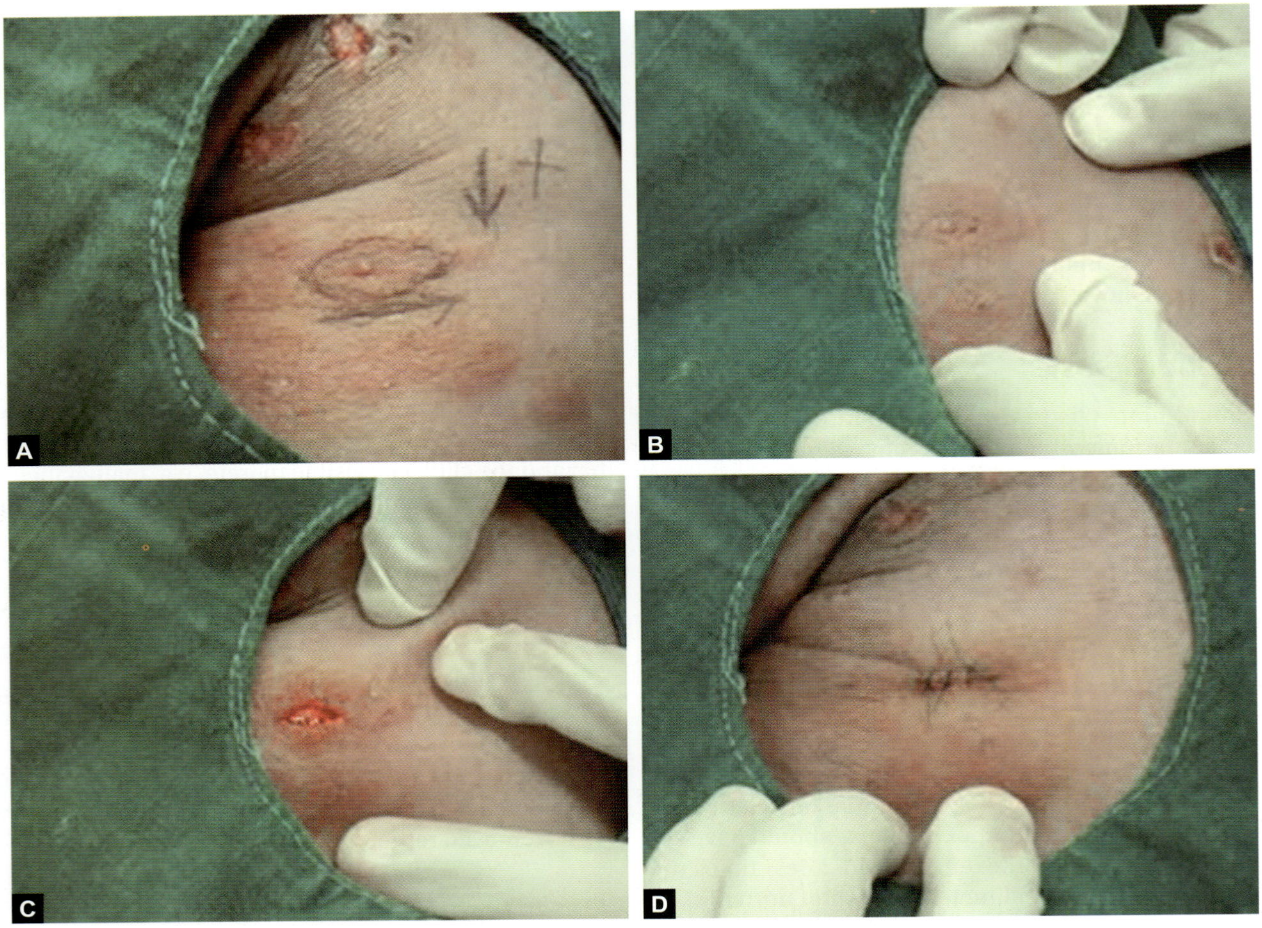

Figs. 7A to D: Incision biopsy. (A) Ellipse marked parallel to RSTL lines; (B) Skin is made taut; (C) Elliptical incision is taken and tissue is removed; (D) Closure with interrupted sutures.

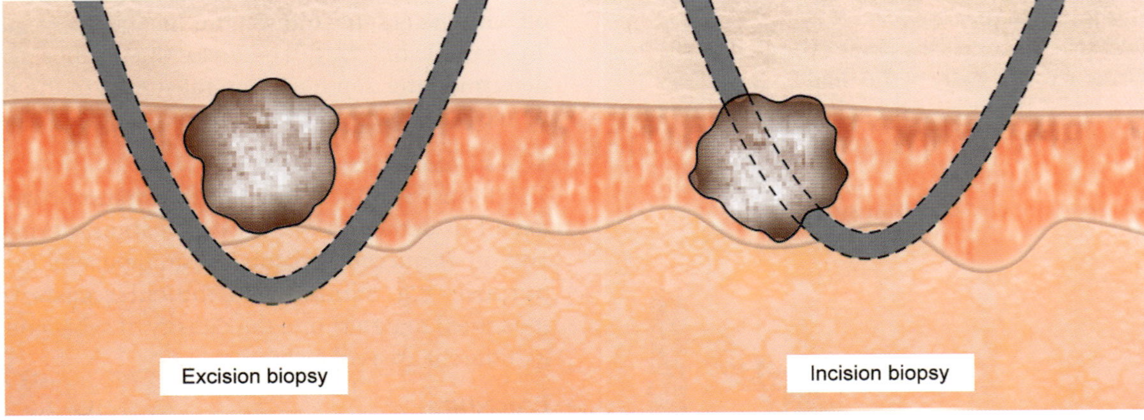

Fig. 8: Difference between incision and excision biopsy.

1. Area is vascular; hence achieving hemostasis may be difficult.
2. Access is difficult due to enclosed cavity.
3. To achieve adequate light in the oral cavity can be difficult.

The moist conditions due to saliva and extensive microflora make antiseptic scrub pointless. To achieve good hemostasis, wait for 10 minutes after infiltrating the anesthetic to have effect of epinephrine. *A chalesion clamp is useful for the biopsies on the lips, anterior buccal mucosa or tongue to achieve hemostasis and to prevent slipping of tissue.* Another tool that can help to have better access is a plastic or metal cheek retractor. Grasping the tissues with dry cotton gauze allows firm grip. A punch biopsy can be easily performed for getting full thickness specimen. For dome-shaped lesions, incisional or shave excision technique are useful. The area opposite to the second upper molar should be avoided as the duct of parotid gland opens there. While performing biopsies on the floor, area of sublingual salivary gland should be carefully approached. Suturing with silk is useful as this type of suture is easy to work with in a cramped space. This suture is nonirritating and remains soft. Wounds heal rapidly and with few complications.

Scalp biopsy[9]

As scalp is very vascular, achieving hemostasis is crucial. Xylocaine with adrenaline about 2–3 mL to tumescence the area is useful. The ring of the artery forceps can be used to give circumferential pressure to achieve bloodless field during surgery (Fig. 9). A cotton tipped applicator is also very useful to control bleeding. Surrounding hairs need to be properly taped to prevent interference. KY jelly is useful to keep the hairs away from the biopsy field.

It is also important to do the biopsy in a direction parallel to hair growth to avoid transecting the follicles. This will prevent development of a patch of alopecia. Also the biopsy should reach the subcutis, so that bulbs of terminal follicles are included. Always use at least 4 mm punch for biopsy. Two biopsies are preferred, one each for vertical and horizontal sectioning.

Nail biopsy[13]

It is performed for the diagnosis of tumors of nail apparatus and to diagnose a particular condition when the nails are dystrophic. Caution should be exercised in patients with diabetes, scleroderma and peripheral vascular disease. It is performed by giving digital block at the base of the digit. The anesthetic used is xylocaine, preferably without adrenaline.

For nail bed biopsy, either a punch technique or a longitudinal elliptical biopsy technique is used. For punch biopsy, prior soaking in water helps to soften the nail plate. For elliptical biopsy, nail plate is separated from nail bed and cut away to expose the lesion.

For matrix biopsy nail is avulsed and nail fold is reflected to expose the matrix. Then a transverse elliptical biopsy is performed. A longitudinal biopsy can be performed in nail dystrophies to obtain a specimen containing nail matrix, nail bed and nail plate. More details can be found in the chapter on Nail Surgery.

Biopsy on palms and soles[14]

The skin in these areas is thick and inelastic. Hence, it is difficult to approximate the wound of biopsy. The incision should be taken parallel to the flexion creases or it should cross high tension areas at 45° angle. This prevents wound dehiscence. This area would require proper undermining and correct suture placement.

Complications of Biopsy

Though rare, the following complications may occur:

- Secondary infection
- Scarring
- Bleeding and hematoma formation
- Damage to underlying nerves and blood vessels in deep excisions
- Allergy to adhesive tape
- Rarely allergy to local anesthetic agent causing anaphylaxis

Tips for Better Procedural Outcome

Refer Figures 22.10 to 22.12.

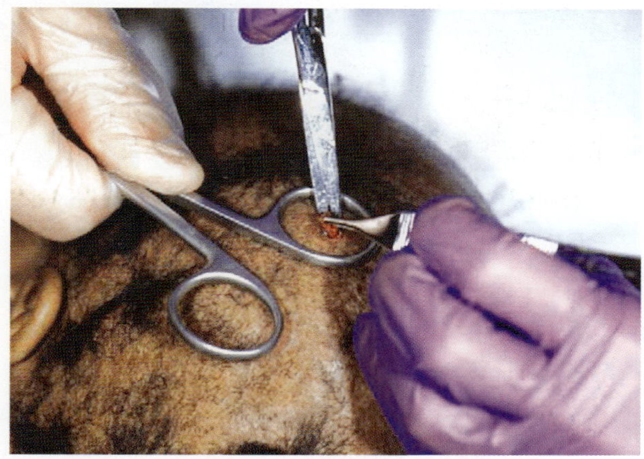

Fig. 9: Using the ring of the artery forceps for hemostasis.

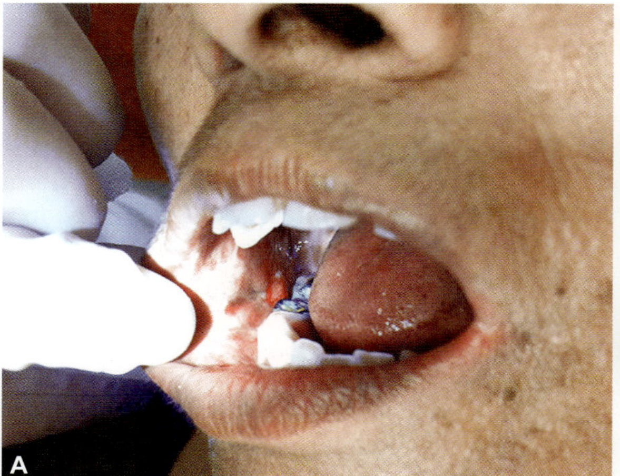

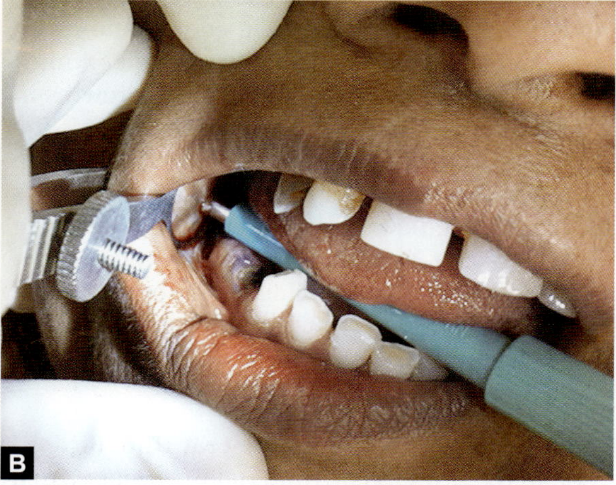

Figs. 10A and B: Taking sample from oral mucosa. (A) Use of chalasion clamp; (B) Use of long spinal needle for infiltration of anesthesia.

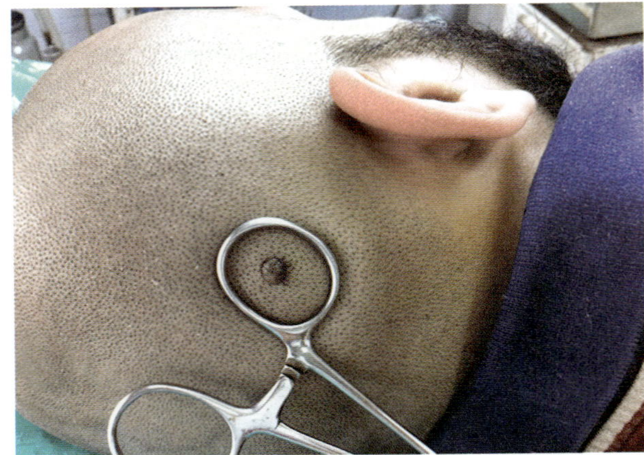

Fig. 11: Taking sample from scalp or from a vascular skin lesion. Use of eye of an artery forceps to give firm pressure.

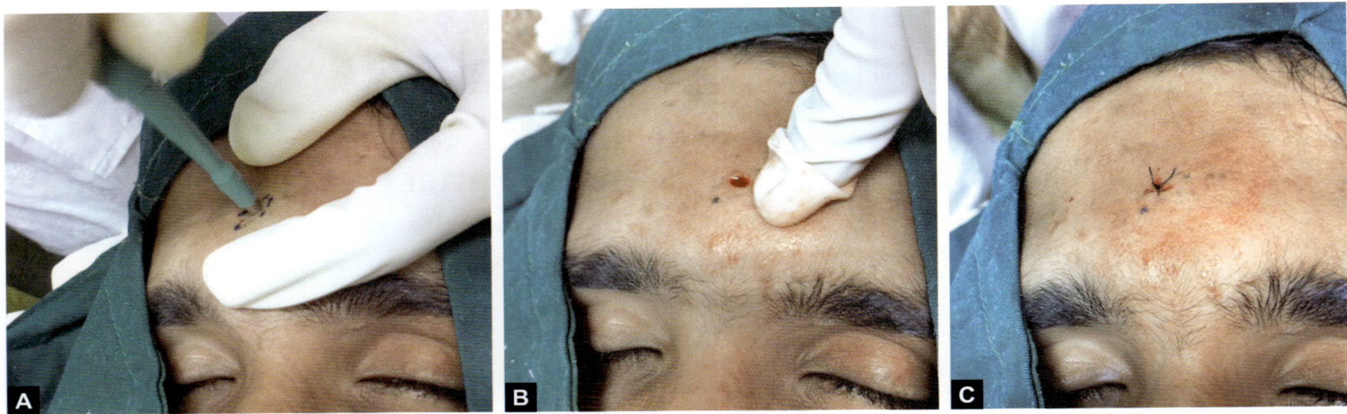

Figs. 12A to C: Taking sample from face. Even after punch biopsy single stay suture can be taken to give cosmetically acceptable scar.

CURETTAGE

Introduction

It is a scraping or scooping technique used to remove soft tumors or tissues by using a simple instrument called curette.

The word *curet* is derived from old French word *Curet (Kyuret)*. The meaning of curet is to cure and cura means care. The tip of curette can have scoop, hook or gauge. The treatment can be used alone or in combination with cryosurgery, chemical cautery or electrodessication. It is a very useful technique for removing small growths in locations with firm base like ears, nose and forehead. The aim of curettage is to remove the skin lesion completely with minimum destruction of normal tissue. It has the advantages of being a quick procedure, simple, inexpensive and even can be done without any local anesthesia. However, it cannot be used for deeper lesions and healing is done by secondary intention, hence can lead to infection and scarring.

Historical Aspect[3]

The use of curette was adapted around year 1870. Richard Vokman (1830–1889), a surgeon from Halle Germany, used scraping spoon in skin practice.[3] It was then called Scharfer Loflel (sharp spoon) or Volkman instrument. In gynecology procedures, a curette created by JCA Recamier, a French surgeon was used. A dermatologist from Philadelphia Louis A Duhring (1845–1913) regarded it as the most valuable remedial measure. It was later modified by different cutaneous surgeons. The changes were suggested by Henry Pifford and George Henry Fox (1846–1937) of New York and also by Henrick Auspitz (1835–1886) and Hans von Hebra (1847–1902). Initially the changes in curette for acne use were recommended by L Duncan Bulkley. A roller for compressing acne papules and pustules was deviced by Piffard. The modifications suggested in acne curette by Jay Frank Schamberg (1870–1913) of Philadelphia and Paul Gerson Unna (1850–1929) of Hamburg Germany are still popular in practitioners. Volkmann's spoon was also used for scar treatment. The scars were scraped in order to stimulate new tissue formation.

- Solar keratosis
- Keratoacanthoma
- Viral warts
- Molluscum contagiosum
- Pyogenic granuloma
- Skin tags
- Milia

- For taking sample for fungal scraping (blunt end)
- For obtaining shave biopsy in difficult areas like outer ear canal, umbilicus and medial canthus.

Contraindication

- Malignant tumors

Instruments

Surgical curette of desired shape and size **(*Fig. 13*)**: Spoon and ring curettes are commonly used. The most popular is 4 mm or 6 mm ring curette.[15]

Procedure[18,19]

The procedure can be done either under surface cream anesthesia using Eutectic mixture of lignocaine and prilocaine (EMLA), lignocaine infiltration, or rarely with any anesthesia as in case of molluscum contagiosum.

Techniques of Curettage[17,18]

Fountain Pen Technique (Fig. 14A)

In this technique curette is held between the thumb, index and middle finger. The base of the palm of the curettage hand, and the tips of ring and little fingers rest upon the skin to give stability. The skin should be stretched with the other hand. This helps to precisely guide the curette, so as to remove the lesion in a single incision.

Common indications

- Seborrheic keratosis.

Potato Peeler Technique (Fig. 14B)

In this technique, handle of the curette is held in the distal interdigital fold of index finger and supported by the other

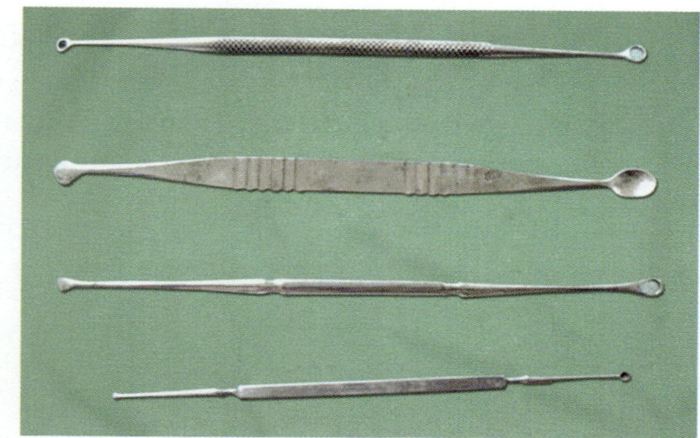

Fig. 13: Curettes of different types.

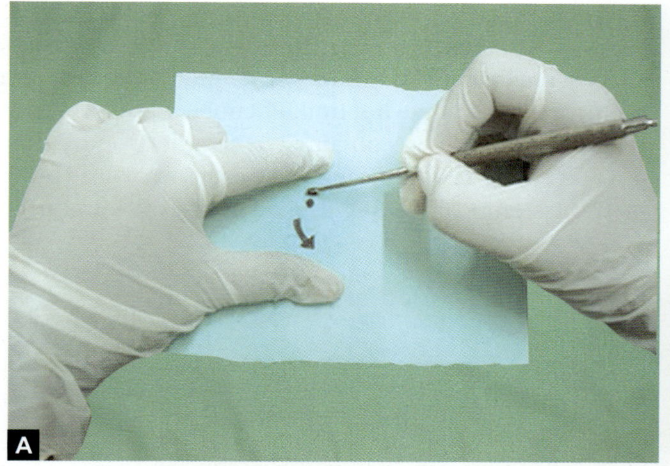

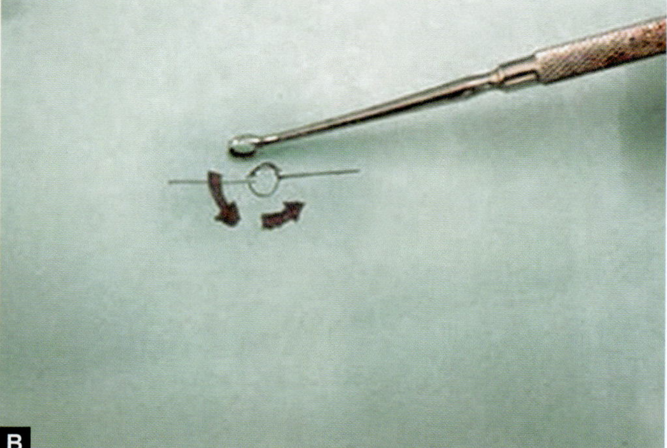

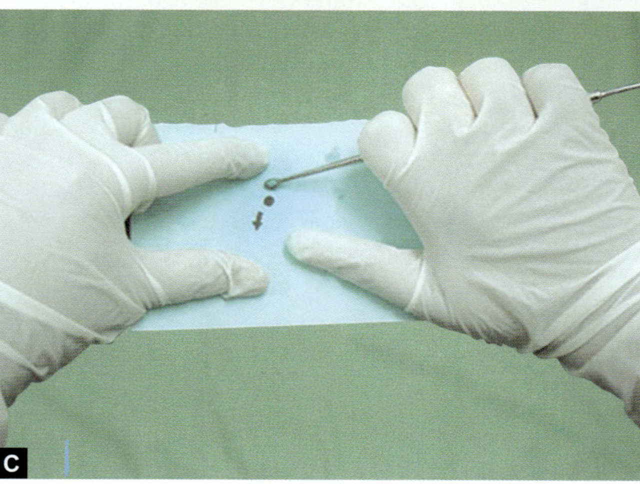

Figs. 14A to C: Different curettage techniques. (A) Fountain pen grip; (B) Direction of curettage; (C) Potato peeler grip.

three fingers. The thumb provides a stable base. This technique is preferable for hard or tough skin growths. Post-procedure hemostasis can be achieved by pressure, topical hemostatic agents or by electrodessication.

Curettage for different indications such as scrappings for fingus, filiform wart and menucleation of molluscum contagiosum are shown in Figures 15 to 17 respectively.

Tips

For extraction of milia back side of a curette can be used with 18 gauge needle. A defect is created in epidermis and lateral pressure is applied with the back side of curette to enucleate the milia.[18]

Postoperative Care

Minimal care is needed which includes keeping the wound dry and applying an antibiotic ointment and a simple daily dressing.

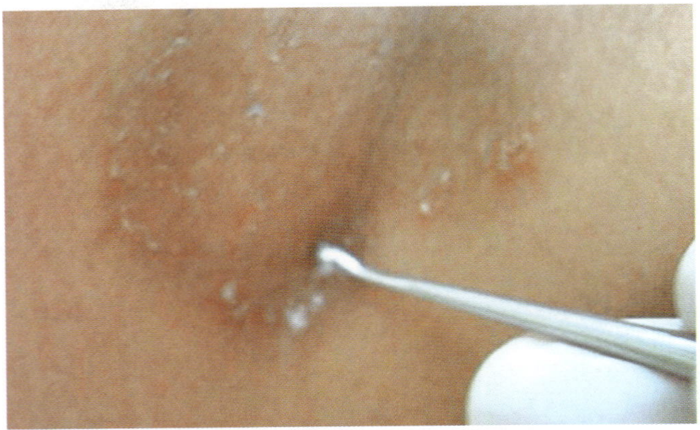

Fig. 15: Fungal scraping with blunt end of curette.

Complications

Uncommon-bleeding may occur, but can easily be controlled by using hemostatic agents as discussed earlier.

Summary

Thus curettage is a simple alternative to excision and can give very good results with comparatively less costly instruments. It is safe and economical option in small clinics.

CHEMICAL CAUTERY

Introduction

In cauterization process, a tissue is either destroyed or it is used for clotting the blood. The process of cauterization is carried out by using heat, cold or chemicals. When chemical agents are used to carry out this process it is called chemical cautery or chemocautery. It is very simple, easy to perform procedure, not requiring any specialized training or equipments and can give excellent results in appropriate settings and has good patient compliance.

Historical Aspects

Chemocautery was used in early 20th century in the treatment of sinus. In pre-antibiotic era, cauterization was also used as means to minimize the infection. The term cautery refers to white hot iron. Phenol was discovered in 1834 by Rounge. It was obtained in chemically pure state by Lauret in 1840. Its antiseptic properties were used by Sir Joseph Lister in 1827–1912. The caustics were introduced

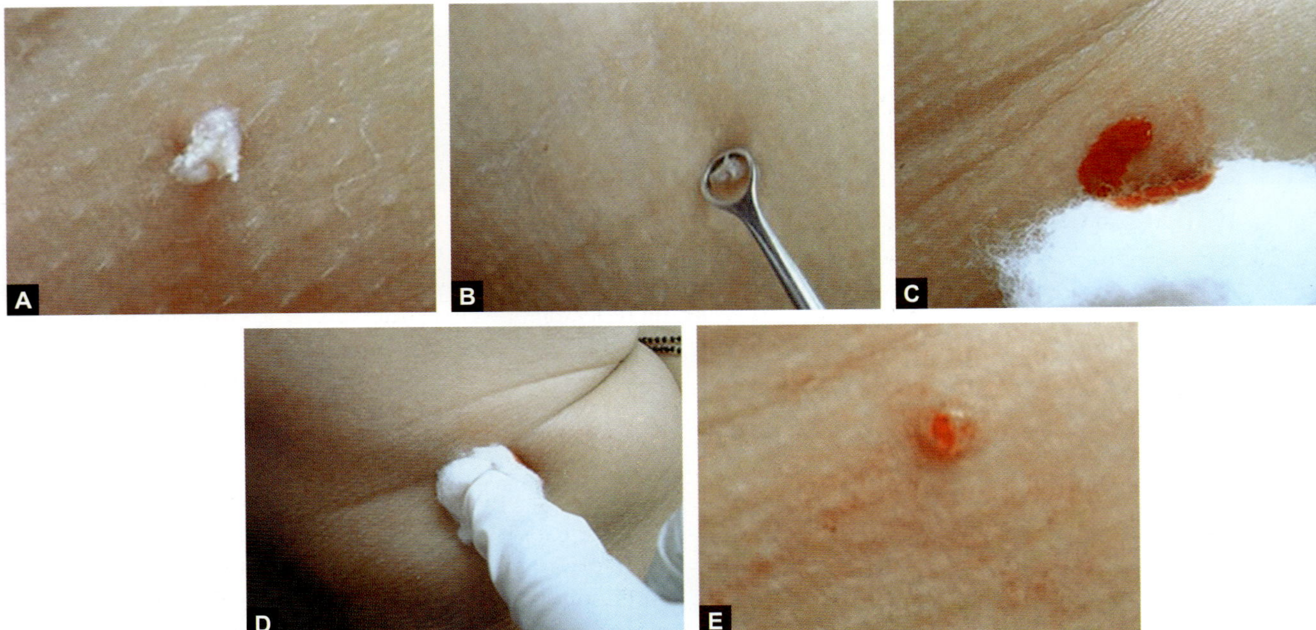

Figs. 16A to E: (A) Filiform wart; (B) Curettage; (C) Post-treatment bleeding; (D) Firm pressure; (E) Hemostasis achieved.

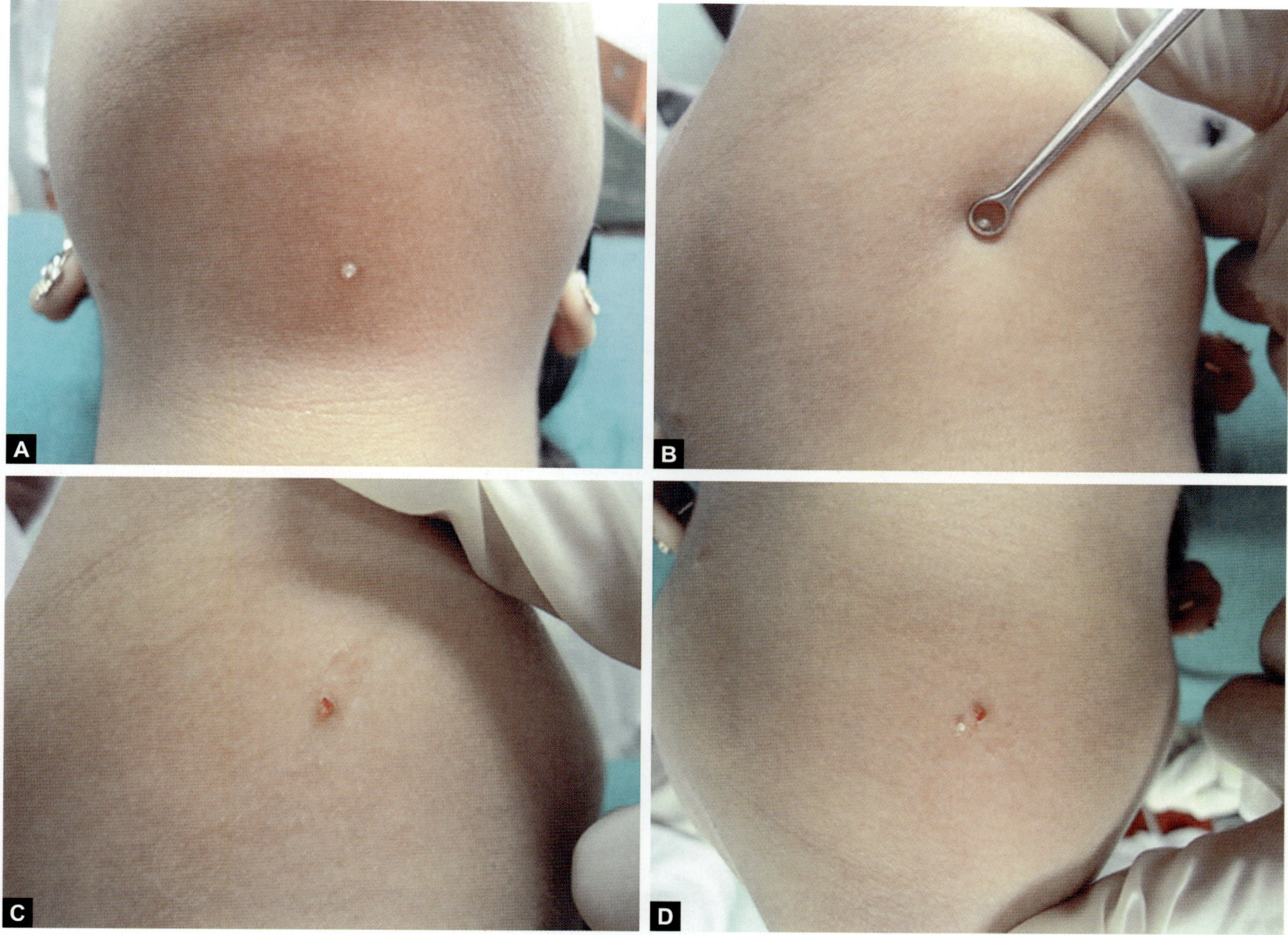

Figs. 17A to D: (A) Molluscum contagiosum; (B) Ring curette used for enucleation; (C) Immediately after curettage; (D) Enucleated molluscum body.

in dermatotherapy in 1880s. The word caustic means to burn. To reduce hypertrophic lesions, use of nitric acid, acetic acid and sulfuric acid was recommended by Pifford. Use of salicylic acid for treating callosities, corns and warts was suggested by Carl Heitzmann (1836–1894).[3] Use of trichloroacetic acid was noted by Charles N Davis (1861–1939) of Philadelphia. Various concentrations of salicylic acid were studied by Samuel Monarch of New York (around 1934). He reported that the useful concentration is in the range of 15–50%.[3]

Commonly used agents in dermatology office are:

- Trichloroacetic acid
- Phenol
- Podophyllin
- KOH
- Salicylic acid
- $AgNO_3$
- Formalin

Different caustic agents, their concentrations, indications and complications are shown in Tables 5 and 6.

Trichloroacetic Acid

This is very commonly used acid because of its safety and easy availability; it is available as crystals. To prepare the desired concentration, it is diluted with distilled water. To make 30% solution, 30 g is to be dissolved in 100 mL distilled water. It is applied with wooden stick (Figs. 18A to D). There is an immediate erythema and frosting. The scab forms which falls after 5–8 days (Figs. 19A to D). It can be repeated at weekly intervals. Once frosting takes place neutralization is not possible. In case of accidental spillage, the acid can be washed away by water or alcohol.

Phenol[19,20]

Full strength phenol consists of 88% phenol solution with water. It causes tissue necrosis at any concentration and therefore needs to be used with caution. It also acts on cutaneous nerve endings causing local anesthesia. It is particularly useful for nail matricectomy after avulsing the required strip of nail plate (Fig. 20).

Table 5: Different caustic agents, their concentrations and indications.[23-31]

Chemical	*Concentration*	*Mechanism of action*	*Indications*
TCA	30–70%	▪ Caustic, hemostatic, styptic agent ▪ Causes precipitation and coagulation of skin proteins	▪ Warts, molluscum contagiosum, xanthelasma, pyogenic granuloma (50–70%) ▪ Acrochordons, seborrheic keratoses, actinic keratoses (30–50%) ▪ Freckles, Lentigines (20–30%)
Phenol	50–88%	▪ Bactericidal (>1%) ▪ Fungicidal (>1.3%) ▪ Local anesthetics ▪ 50%—deep peelant ▪ >80%—coagulation of proteins ▪ <80%—keratolytic	Warts, molluscum contagiosum, xanthelasma, nail matricectomy, pyogenic granuloma, prurigo nodularis
Podophyllin	▪ 25% to be freshly prepared in tincture benzene or alcohol or flexible collodion—most commonly used ▪ Can use from 10–40%	▪ Cytotoxic ▪ Binds to intracellular microtubules and causes mitotic arrest in metaphase ▪ Inhibits RNA synthesis	▪ Warts on mucosal surfaces—condyloma accuminata ▪ Plantar warts ▪ Superficial epitheliomas and keratoses
KOH	10–20%	Dissolves keratin	Molluscum contagiosum
Salicylic acid	▪ 5–20% with equal amount of lactic acid and flexible collodion ▪ 60% ointment ▪ 40% plaster	Tissue destruction	Warts
$AgNO_3$	In solid form or solution >5%	▪ Germicidal ▪ Astringent ▪ Caustic	▪ Aphthous ulcer ▪ Fissures ▪ Excessive granulation tissue
Formalin	5–20%	▪ Hardening and drying of skin ▪ Psychotherapeutic response	Multiple plantar warts

Table 6: Complications of different caustic agents.

Chemical	*Source*	*Contraindications if any*	*Side effects*
TCA	▪ As crystals ▪ Analog of acetic acid		Post-inflammatory hypo- or hyperpigmentation, ulceration and scarring
Phenol	▪ As crystals or liquid ▪ Aromatic substance derived from benzene	Keloidal tendency, active infection, if needs to be used in large areas rule out renal, hepatic or cardiac dysfunction	▪ If >3 mL used cardiac arrhythmias ▪ Also hepatotoxic and nephrotoxic
Podophyllin	Roots of plants	▪ Pregnancy-suspected teratogenicity ▪ Very large lesions (not to exceed 0.5 mL) or 10 cm^2 per sitting	▪ Erosive changes in adjacent skin, peripheral neuropathy, psychotoxic confusional states, adynamic ileus, renal damage, leucopenia, thrombocytopenia ▪ Abortion
KOH			Irritation and stinging
Salicylic acid			▪ Systemic toxicity in large quantities ▪ Salicylism—tinitus, headache
Silver nitrate ($AgNO_3$)	▪ Sticks and solution ▪ Sticks prepared by fusing silver salt with sodium chloride		Burning sensation, dark brown pigmentation on repeated application, chemical burns
Formalin			Excessive irritation, sensitization

Podophyllin

It is a chemically complex extract obtained from roots of plants, *Podophyllum peltatum* (American) or *P. emodi* (Indian). It is also known as Mandrake or Mayapple. The cytotoxic agent is podofilox—the active ingredient in the resin. The procedure is simple. Podophyllin is applied with a cotton stick applicator or with a swab over the lesion (Figs. 21A and B). Care should be taken to prevent leakage to surrounding areas by covering with Vaseline. It is allowed to dry and patient is asked to wash it after 2–4 hours. Repeated application can be done after a week as necessary.

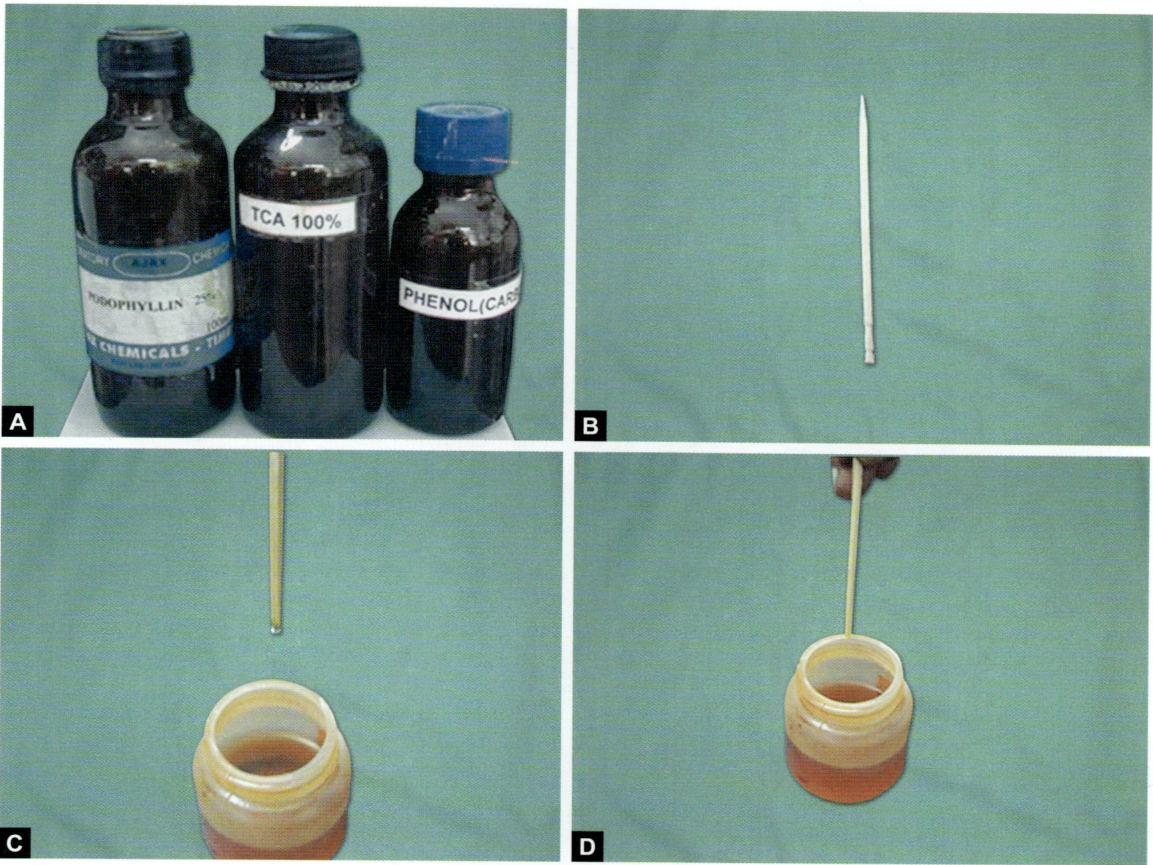

Figs. 18A to D: (A) Chemical cauterizing agents; (B) Wooden stick and not a plastic coated stick chosen; (C) Hanging drop should not be used; (D) Excess chemical is removed.

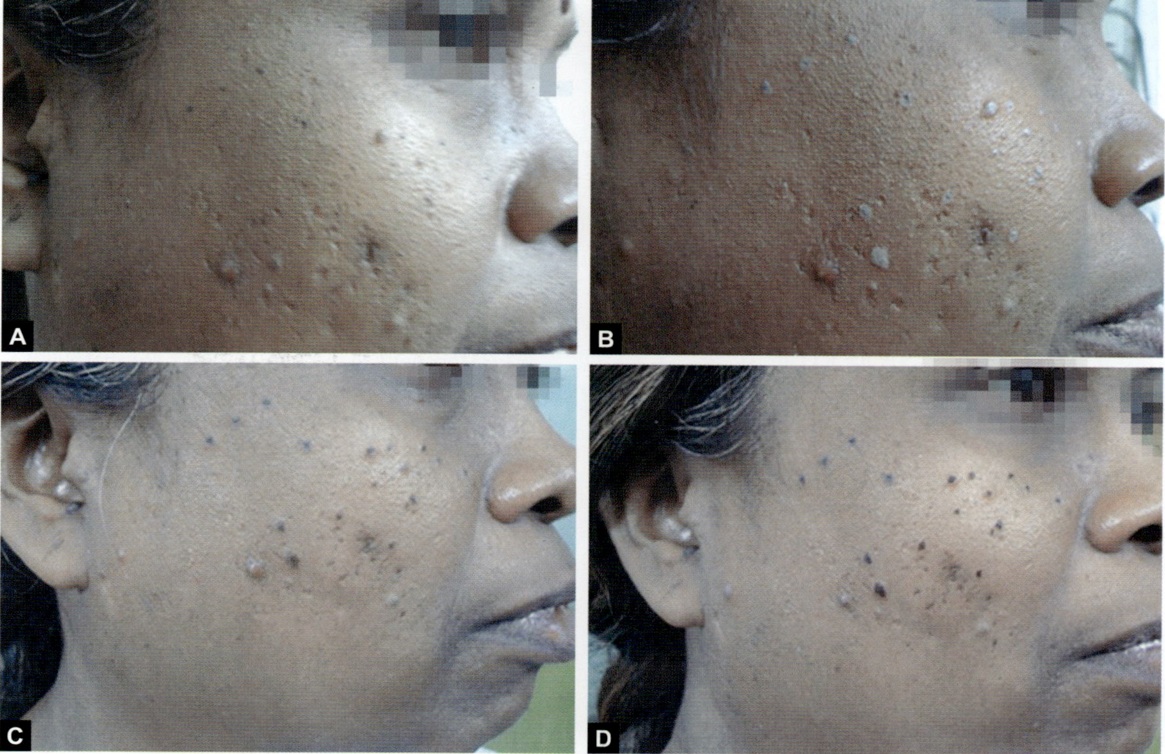

Figs. 19A to D: Sequential changes after chemical cautery. (A) Pretreatment; (B) Immediate frosting; (C) Day 1 post-treatment; (D) Day 3 post-treatment.

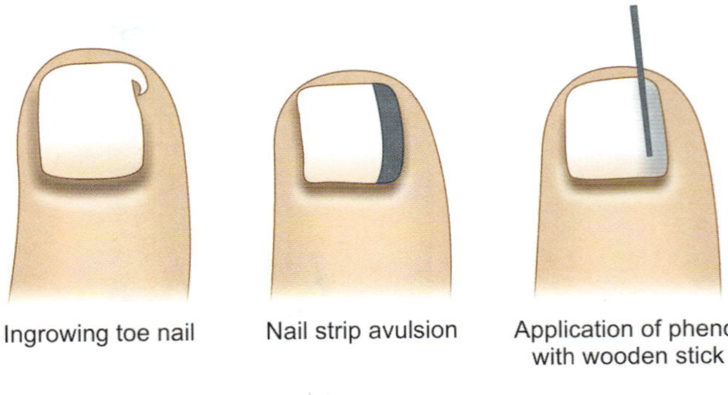

Fig. 20: Nail matricectomy and phenol cauterization.

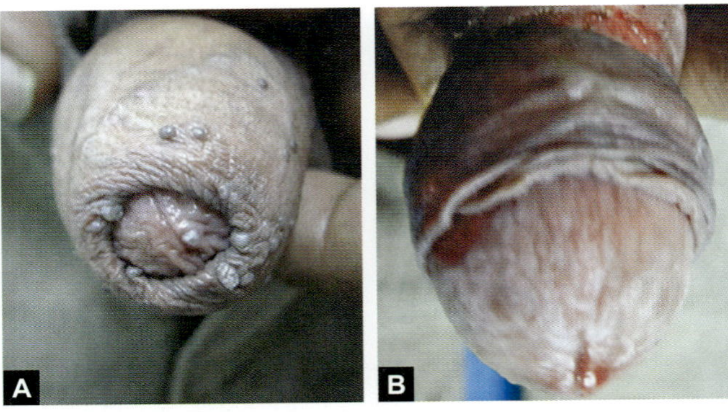

Figs. 21A and B: Chemical cautery with podophyllin. (A) Condyloma accuminata—before treatment; (B) Condyloma accuminata—after treatment.

CONCLUSION

Thus, this simple and inexpensive technique can be immensely useful if proper precautions are taken. We can achieve excellent results for most of the commonly seen dermatological problems in day-to-day OPD practice by chemocautery.

REFERENCES

1. Anderson JB, Webb AJ. Fine needle aspiration biopsy and the diagnosis of thyroid cancer. British Journal of Surgery. 1987;74:292-6.
2. Bobrow JC, Belcher MH. Surgery for cataract in lens and cataract section II. 2010-2011:91-162.
3. Parish LC. Historical aspects of cutaneous surgery. Wheeland Cutaneous Surgery, 1st edition; 1994. pp. 3-11.
4. Lahiri K. Evolution and evaluation of autologous mini punch grafts in vitiligo. Ind J Dermatol. 2009;54(20):159-67.
5. Lowenthal LJA. Punch biopsy with autograft. AMA Arch Dermatol Syphilol. 1953;67:629.
6. Orentreich N. Autografts in alopecias and other selected dermatological conditions. Ann NY Acad Sci. 1959;83: 463-79.
7. Wilhelmi BJ, Blackwell SJ, Phillips LG. Langers lines: to use or not to use. Plast Reconstr Surg. 1999;104(1):208-14.
8. Algure PC, Mathes BM. Skin biopsy techniques for the internist. J Gen Intern Med. 1998;13(1):46-54.
9. Savant Satish S. Skin biopsy techniques. Textbook of Dermatosurgery and Cosmetology, 2nd edition; 2005. pp. 72-80.
10. Nischal U, Nischal KC, Uday K. Techniques of skin biopsy and practical consideration. Journal of Cutaneous and Aesthetic Surgery. 2008;1(2):107-11.
11. Dirk M Elston, Erik J Stratman, Stanley J Miller, et al. Skin biopsy: Biopsy issues in specific diseases. J Am Acad Dermatol. January 2016:1-14.
12. Erik J Stratman, Dirk M Elston, Stanley J Miller, et al. Skin biopsy: Identifying and overcoming errors in the skin biopsy pathway. J Am Acad Dermatol. January 2016:19-24.
13. Huerter CJ. Simple Biopsy Techniques in Wheeland Cutaneous Surgery, 1st edition; 1994. pp. 159-70.
14. Shelley WB. The razor blade in dermatologic practice. Cutis. 1975;16:843-5.
15. Saraf V. Nail Biopsy in Manual of Dermatologic Surgery; 1999. pp. 108-12.
16. Savant Satish S, Gore D. Applied anatomy for the derma-to-surgeon. Textbook of Dermatosurgery and Cosmetology, 2nd edition; 2005. pp. 3-11.
17. Adam JE. The technique of curettage surgery. J Am Acad Dermatol. 1986;15;697-702.
18. Savant SS. Curettage. Textbook of Dermatosurgery and Cosmetology, 2nd edition; 2005. pp. 92-9.
19. Saraf V. Curettage. Manual of Dermatologic Surgery; 1999. pp. 134-41.
20. Chan CY, Creed RD, Browning JC, et al. Alternative use of a curette. Dermatology Online Journal. 2007;13(3):7.
21. Rubin AI, La Natra Nicole, Stiller MJ. Other topical medications. Fitzpatricks Dermatology in General Medicine, Vol. 2, 6th edition; 2003. pp. 2362-9.
22. Franklin A. Phenol cauterization of nail matrix remnants. J Dermatol Surg Oncol. 1987;13:1324-5.
23. Savant SS. Chemical cauterization. Textbook of Dermatosurgery and Cosmetology, 2nd edition; 2005. pp. 107-16.
24. Robinson JK, Hruza GJ. Dermatologic surgery: introduction and approach. Fitzpatricks Dermatology in General Medicine, Vol 2, 6th edition; 2003. pp. 2517-29.
25. Ghalla MP. Skin biopsy. Manual of Dermatologic Surgery; 1999. pp. 95-107.
26. Burnett JW, Crutcher WA. Viral and rickettsial infections. In: Moschella SL, Hurley HJ (Eds). Dermatology, Vol. 2, 2nd edition; 1987. pp. 694-5.
27. Maddin S. Dermatologic therapy. In: Moschella SL, Hurley HJ (Eds). Dermatology, Vol. 2, 2nd edition; 1987. pp. 1946-77.
28. Chi SG, Song CH, Lee WJ. TCA matricectomy and aluminium splint fixation for the treatment of pincer nails. Dermatol Surg. 2010;36(9):1493-5.
29. Cannon PS, Ajit R. Efficacy of TCA (95%) in the management of xanthelesma palpebrum. Clinical Exp Dermatol. 2010;35(8):845-8.
30. Ramsay G, Caldwell D. Phenol cauterization for ingrown toenails. Archives of Emergency Medicine. 1986;3:243-6.
31. Pascher F. Systemic reactions to topically applied drugs. Int J Dermato1. 1978;7:768.

Chapter

23

Simple Excisions

Vinay Saraf, Ragunatha S

Key Messages

- Important steps in simple elliptical excision of lesion include planning the ellipse, incision, dissection of lesion, undermining of defect and hemostasis.
- Undermining is essential to reduce the tension on wound margins. Undermining facilitates wound closure; avoids unnecessary vascular compromise; everts the wound margins; enhances the cosmetic outcome after scar contraction and prevents spread of scar at high wound tension areas.
- A good suture technique should ensure closure of dead space in subcutaneous tissue, decreased wound tension, and good approximation and eversion of wound margins.

HISTORY OF CUTANEOUS SURGERY

Surgery is a Greek word meaning 'hand work'. Excision means cutting out an organ, tumor or other tissue. In 6th century BC, Sushrutha, father of surgery in ancient India, wrote *Sushrut Samhita*, wherein he described hundred and twenty instruments, three hundred surgical procedures and eight categories of surgeries including plastic surgery. He used herbal juice which was similar to modern day anesthesia. His descriptions included excision surgery. In Egypt, China and Arab countries, in 3500 years ago, the surgeries being practiced were mainly excision and reconstructive surgery. The first description of Skin Tension Lines (STL) was made by Dupuytren in 1834. He demonstrated that circular incisions produced linear wounds. Langer is credited with major work on this subject. In 1973, Borges published drawings of Resting STLs (RSTLs). He demonstrated that RSTLs were of more importance than wrinkle lines and indicated that they were identical for all individuals. He constructed detailed line maps which have been referred to as the correct direction for placement of incisions.[1-4]

INTRODUCTION

The elliptical (fusiform) excision is the mainstay and workhorse of cutaneous excisional and reconstructive surgery.[5] Majority of simple cutaneous excisions are done by performing the elliptical or fusiform excision. Proper planning and execution of this procedure needs good understanding of anatomy of skin, wound healing, tumor biology, RSTLs, and functional considerations of head, neck and face.[6] Thorough understanding of these basic principles will help the surgeon to execute the procedure meticulously, giving excellent cosmetic outcome.

INDICATIONS

The following are the indications for simple excisions:

- Simple excision without suture (small benign lesions):
  - Mucoceles
  - Hamartomas
  - Small epidermal inclusion cyst
- Elliptical excision (moderate to large lesions):
  - Benign:
    - Sebaceous cyst
    - Lipoma
    - Fibroma
    - Epidermoid cyst
    - Nevi
  - Malignant:
    - Basal cell carcinoma
    - Noninvasive squamous cell carcinoma
    - Bowen's disease

- Modifications in simple excision:
  - Excision with full thickness graft or rotation flap:
    - Large malignant lesions
  - Punch incision:
    - Sebaceous cyst
    - Lipoma.

CONTRAINDICATIONS

- Infected lesions
- Patients with history of keloidal tendency and bleeding tendency
- Patients on anticoagulants
- Recent isotretinoin use
- Uncontrolled diabetes and debilitating conditions
- Unreliable patients

REQUIREMENTS: EQUIPMENTS AND MATERIALS

Equipments and materials required during each step of excisional surgery should be kept ready for smooth conduction of procedure. The following is the checklist of requirements for cutaneous excisional surgery:

- Counseling
  - Consent form
  - Patient instruction slip
- Surgical preparation of the site
  - Antiseptic solutions: Surgical spirit, povidone-iodine
  - Surgical drapes: Hole cloth towel
- Local anesthesia
  - Injection lignocaine (1 or 2%) with or without epinephrine (1:100000)
  - Insulin syringe, or syringe with 0.5 inch 30-guage needle
- Excision of the lesion
  - Sterile steel tray
  - Skin marking pen (to mark the lesion and ellipse)
  - Scalpel handle
  - Scalpel blade number 15
  - Cutting scissors straight and curved
  - Adson's serrated forceps, toothed and plane
  - Skin hooks
  - Small mosquito artery forceps
- Wound closure
  - Suture materials (absorbable/nonabsorbable sutures)
  - Cutting needles
  - Needle holder
- Wound dressing
  - Spirit swabs
  - Guaze pieces
  - Dressing pads
  - Adhesive plaster or micropore
  - Antibiotic cream
- Suture removal
  - Suture cutting scissor
- Skin biopsy
  - Ten percent formalin
  - Histopathology requisition form
  - Empty clean vials with label to provide details of patient.

PREOPERATIVE PREPARATIONS

Patient education and counseling, assessment of risk factors for complications and prophylactic antibiotics administration are important aspects of preoperative preparation.[3,7,8]

Counseling

As is true with all cosmetic dermatosurgery procedures, informed consent is a must. Information about the procedure, complications, postoperative care and outcome of the surgery must be provided to the patient. All queries about the procedures should be duly addressed, and expected results should be explained. Avoid patient with unrealistic expectation and suspicion about surgeon's credibility and charges.

Preoperative Evaluation of Patients

Thorough systemic examination and specific inquiries must be made to identify risk factors which may affect the surgical outcome (Box 1).[2,3,9]

Prophylactic Antibiotics

The antibiotic prophylaxis is recommended only for patients with a high-risk of endocarditis (e.g. prosthetic heart valves or systemic pulmonary shunts). Role of routine antibiotic prophylaxis in cutaneous surgery is not established. The prophylactic antibiotic therapy should cover both staphylococci and streptococci.

Universal Precautions

The surgeon must prepare himself with universal precaution for patient's safety and for his own safety, never forgetting that we are practicing in HIV era. Universal precautions are strictly followed whenever there is potential risk of contact with blood or other body fluids. Masks and protective eyewear or face shield are worn if splatter of blood is anticipated.

SURGICAL PREPARATION OF SITE

The affected area, e.g. face, is washed with soap and water 2–3 times, and all make-up, contact lenses and ornaments are removed, and handed over to a patient's relative. As far as possible see that one responsible person, preferably a relative, accompanies the patient. The operative area must be thoroughly cleansed with surgical scrub (Fig. 1), preferably with povidone-iodine followed by methylated spirit, and then painted with povidone-iodine. The area must be isolated by sterile drapings (Fig. 2). Hole towels are a better choice for draping.

Box 1: Preoperative evaluation of the patient.

Medical history and examination
- Bleeding disorders
  - Bleeding tendencies
  - Any current drug history, e.g. anticoagulants, antiplatelet agents
- Hypersensitivity reactions
  - Drug hypersensitivity, including anesthetics
  - Allergic contact dermatitis to topical applications or adhesive tapes
- Abnormal wound healing
  - Keloid formation
  - Delayed wound healing
- Transmission of infections
  - Human immunodeficiency virus infection
  - Hepatitis B and hepatitis C infections
- Postoperative infections
  - Damaged, infected skin
  - Diabetes
  - Debilitation
  - Hypogammaglobulinemia
  - Anemia
  - Severe malnutrition
  - Long-term antibiotic therapy
  - Corticosteroids therapy
  - Immunocompromised states
  - Emotional stress
  - Poor hygiene

Investigations
- Complete blood count
- Bleeding time, clotting time, prothrombin time
- Fasting blood sugar
- Blood VDRL
- ELISA for HIV
- Serology for hepatitis B and hepatitis C

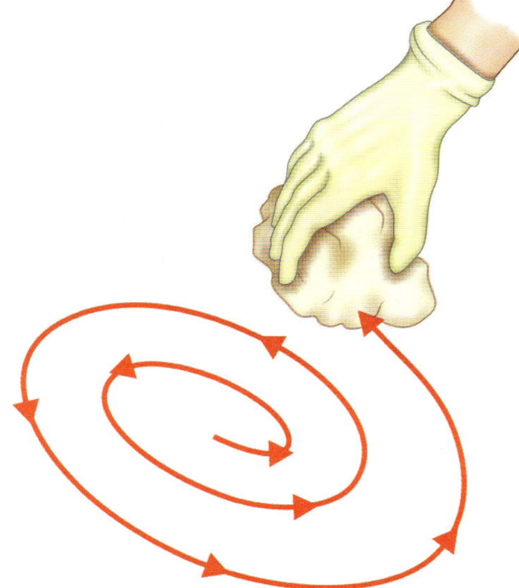

Fig. 1: Cleaning, surgical preparation should be started in the center going peripherally.

LOCAL ANESTHESIA

Always use xylocaine with adrenaline unless contra-indicated. Addition of adrenaline provides bloodless surgical field; allows the use of greater volume of anesthetic agent; longer duration of anesthetic effect and avoids reinjection if the procedure lasts for longer time. The recommended maximum safe dose of lignocaine in a 70 kg man with adrenaline is 7 mg/kg body weight (500 mg) and without adrenaline is 3 mg/kg body weight (200 mg).

TECHNIQUE OF ELLIPTICAL EXCISION

Small benign lesions, such as mucoceles, hamartomas and small epidermal inclusion cysts, can be removed without suture under local infiltration anesthesia using a scalpel blade or small scissor. The lesion is held with small toothed forceps for precise removal of the lesion at the base. The hemostasis is maintained by pressure or Monsel's solution (ferric chloride) or electrodessication. The resulting wound, usually small, is left to heal by secondary intention under surgical dressing.[2,4,7] However, for larger lesions, elliptical excision is preferred. Important steps in elliptical excision of lesion include planning the ellipse, incision, dissection of lesion, undermining of defect and hemostasis.

Planning the Ellipse

This is a very important step as it determines the outcome of procedure. Proper planning results in least noticeable scar without compromising the function. Figures 3 show some of the instruments used. Figure 6 demonstrates administration of local anesthesia. Well-planned incision line should run parallel to the favorable lines of closure, i.e. RSTLs or MSTLs. The incision line so planned not only makes the scar inconspicuous but it also heals faster, and gives a higher tensile strength. Maximum STL are usually, but not always, congruent with relaxed STL. These lines can be made obvious by pinching

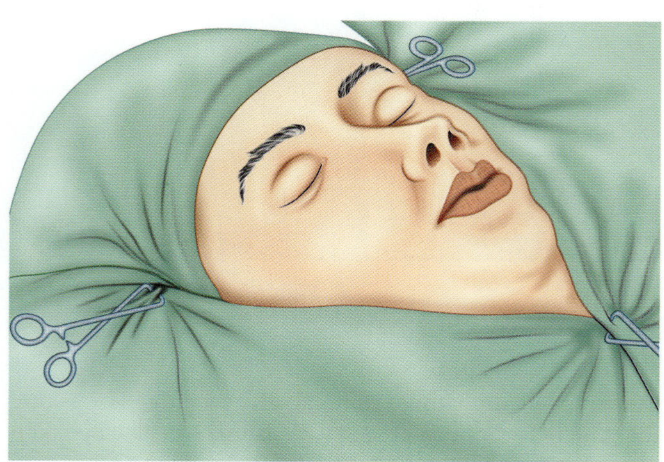

Fig. 2: Draping the surgical area is necessary for asepsis.

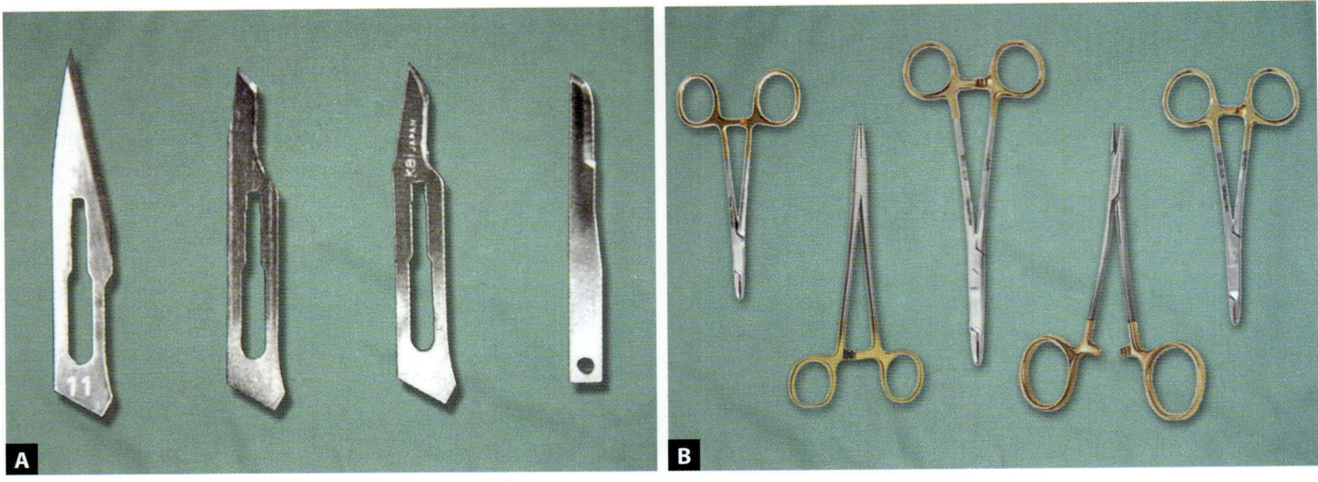

Figs. 3A and B: Scissors, needle holder and scalpel blades.

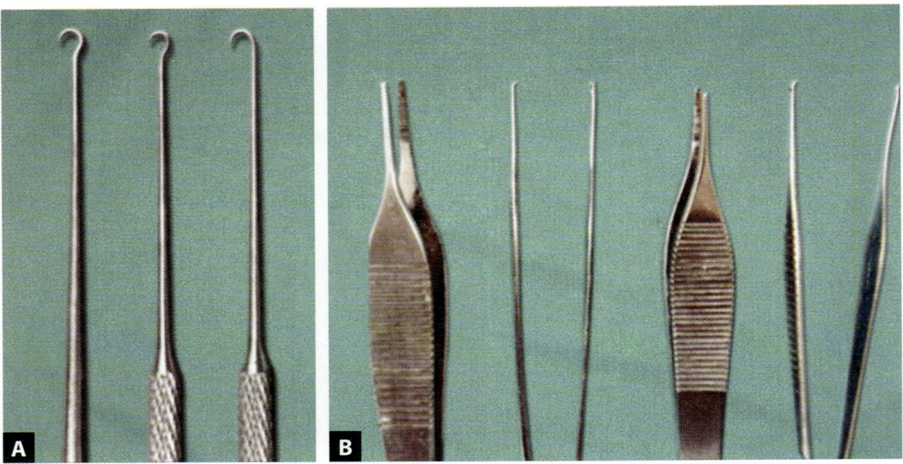

Figs. 4A and B: Skin hooks (A), and forceps (B).

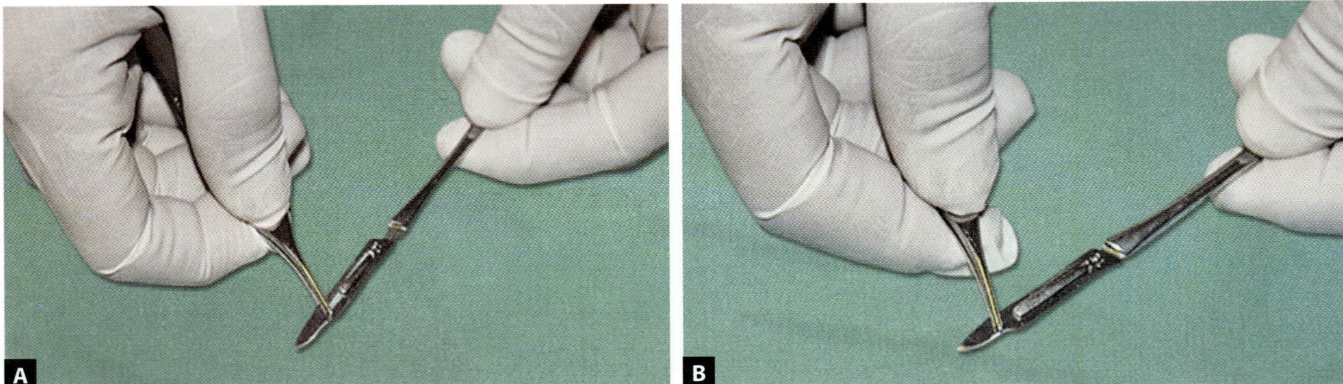

Figs. 5A and B: Mounting the 15 number blade on scalpel handle.

the skin in all directions. They can also be judged by asking the patient to smile or grimace. Incisions can also be taken along the wrinkle lines, or skin folds. Another option is to make a circular incision and wait for some time to allow it to turn into an oval shape after undermining the edges. Before final closure the oval shape can be converted into an ellipse. The length to width ratio of the ellipse or fusiform excision should be 3:1 or 4:1. The tips of the ellipse should meet at 30º angle (Figs. 7 and 8).[2,3,7] For malignant lesions include 3–4 mm normal appearing margins (Box 2).

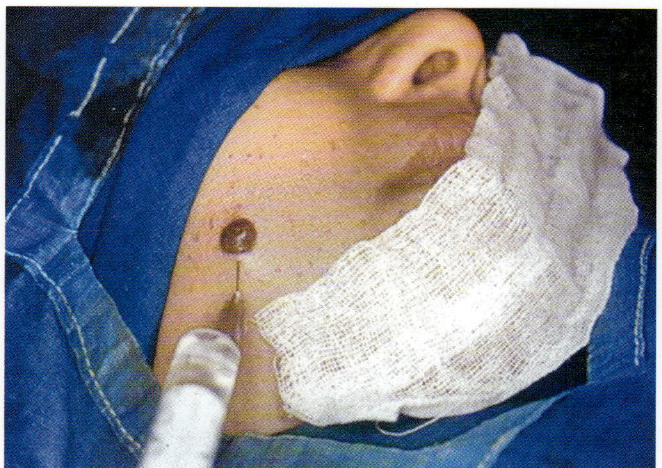

Fig. 6: Local field block is being given.

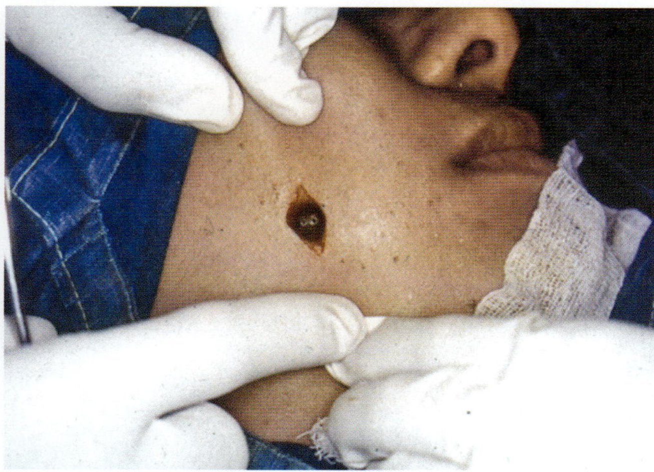

Fig. 7: The tips of the ellipse meet at 30° angle.

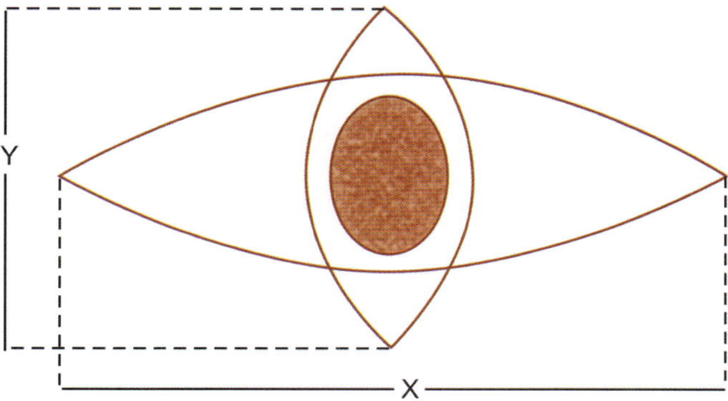

Fig. 8: Length to width ratio of the ellipse should be 3:1 or 4:1.

Box 2: Planning the ellipse.

- Favorable lines of closure (MSTLs)
- Cosmetic units (Face)
- Nature of lesion removed
- Functional consideration (Lower eyelid)
- Dimensions
- Margins
- Fusiform excision variation
- Skin preparation and marking the ellipse

Always consider the cosmetic units of the face because scars restricted to single cosmetic unit hide well as compared to the scars crossing multiple units. The cosmetic units of the face are chin, perioral region, cheek, periorbital region, nose, forehead, glabella and temple. For further details, refer to the chapter on facial anatomy.

Nature of the lesion removed is also an important factor. For benign lesions, the surrounding normal skin excised is minimal, and on the other hand for malignant lesions, sufficient surrounding normal looking tissue is included in the excision to prevent recurrences.[5,10,11]

The shape of the lesion also plays an important role in deciding the excision line. For oval-shaped lesion, the long axis of the incision line must run parallel to the long axis of the lesion. This will shorten the length of the scar.[2,3] When taking incisions near lips or eyes, functional considerations are very important to prevent lip retraction and ectropion, respectively.[2,5,12]

Variations in fusiform excision are required especially when operating on curved surfaces, e.g. cheeks and arms. Lazy S, also called as S plasty, is the preferred incision (Figs. 9A to D). Aim of the S plasty is to lengthen the ultimate length of the scar between two endpoints of the wound. This is particularly useful on the convex surfaces of cheeks and extremities where the tendency of horizontal contraction of the scar is high. The horizontal and vertical dimensions of the ellipse should be in 3:1 or 4:1 proportion. The long axis of the ellipse should run parallel to the long axis of the lesion otherwise it can result into depressed scar. By lengthening the scar, the horizontal forces of contraction will pull and straighten the 's', rather than resulting in depressed scar.[2,7] Marking the incision line of the ellipse before injecting local anesthesia is essential as the anesthetic will distort the tissue, and vasoconstriction may obscure the margins.[2,4] Alternately, a punch can be used to perform an elliptical excision (Fig. 10).

Incision

Figures 11 to 19 show different steps of incision. To get the best cosmetic results, several aspects of incision need to be addressed. To avoid cross-hatching, the tips of the ellipse must meet at a fine point which prevents unnecessary injury and extension of the incision beyond that point (Figs. 11 and 12). The scalpel handle must be held perpendicular to the skin at the initiation of the incision. Then tilt the scalpel at 45° angle (Fig. 13A) and incise through the margin till the other end is reached. Then turn the blade again perpendicular to the skin surface. For smaller incisions 15c or 11 number blade is used.[2,3] Incise perpendicularly (Fig. 13B) through the dermis

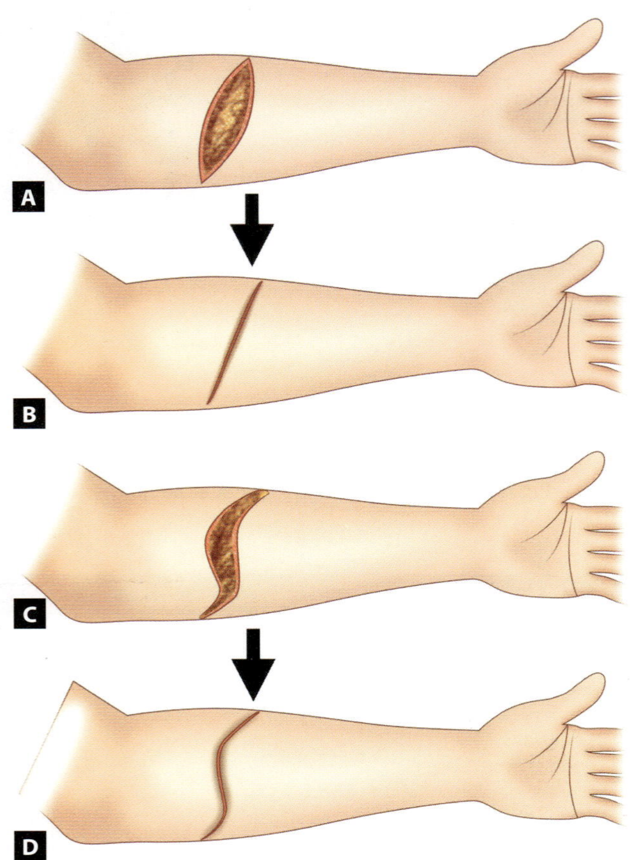

Figs. 9A to D: S-shaped incision. (A) Circumferential closure of a wound on a convex surface; (B) Will create tissue protusions at the ends; (C) An S-plasty design; (D) Allows the terminal ends to remain in the same horizontal plane.

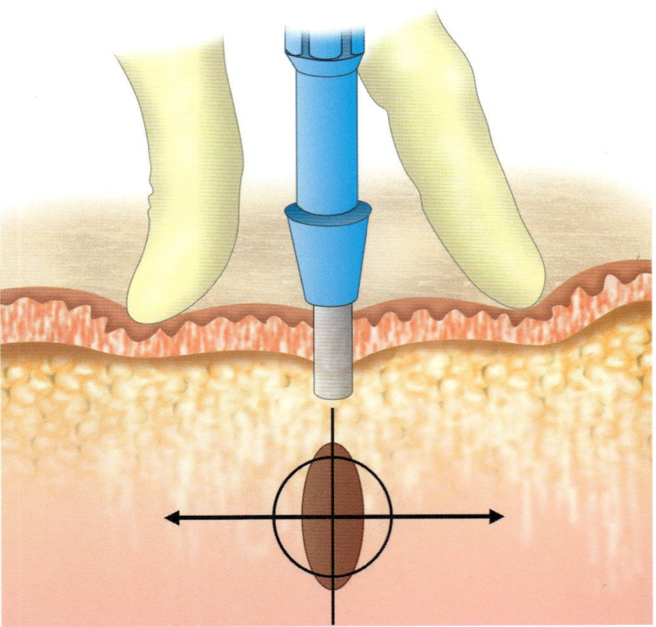

Fig. 10: Alternatively a punch excision can be done which can be converted to ellipse for final closure by stretching the punch wound.

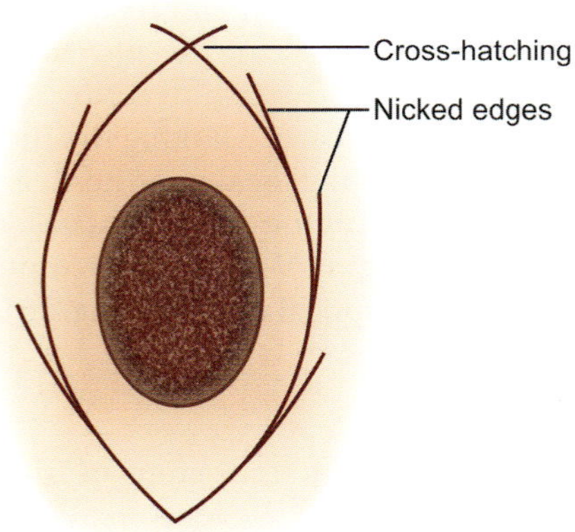

Fig. 12: Avoiding cross-hatching.

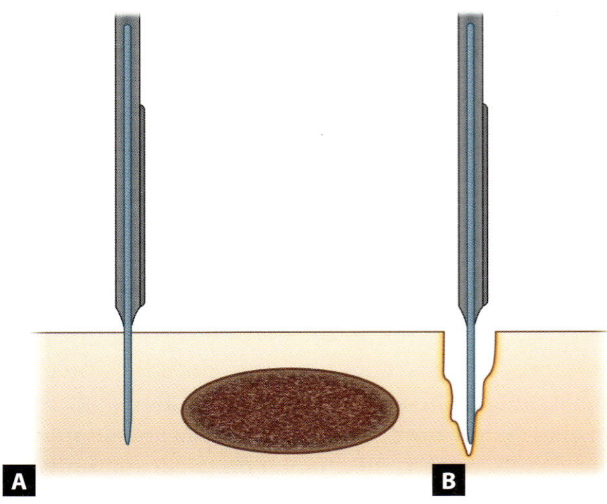

Figs. 11A and B: Scalpel handle must be held perpendicular to the skin (A); avoid staircasing (B).

up to the subcutaneous fat which everts the skin margins for cosmetically acceptable wound closure. In hairy areas, pass the scalpel blade parallel to the hair follicle to avoid follicle transection and subsequent bald area around the scar (Fig. 13C).[2,7] Perfect movement of the scalpel in straight line is important (Fig. 13D) Number of passes through the dermis should be minimum to avoid "staircasing" effect (Fig. 11) and compromise of approximation of the wound margins.[2,4] Right angled incision helps in better wound closure (Fig. 13E).

Dissection of Lesion

Avoid boat-shaped excision by removing desired depth of tissue up to the depth of the incision at the two ends (Figs. 15A and B). Removal of less amount of tissue at both ends causes protrusions at both ends resulting in pseudo-dog-ears (Figs. 16A and B).[2,3,7]

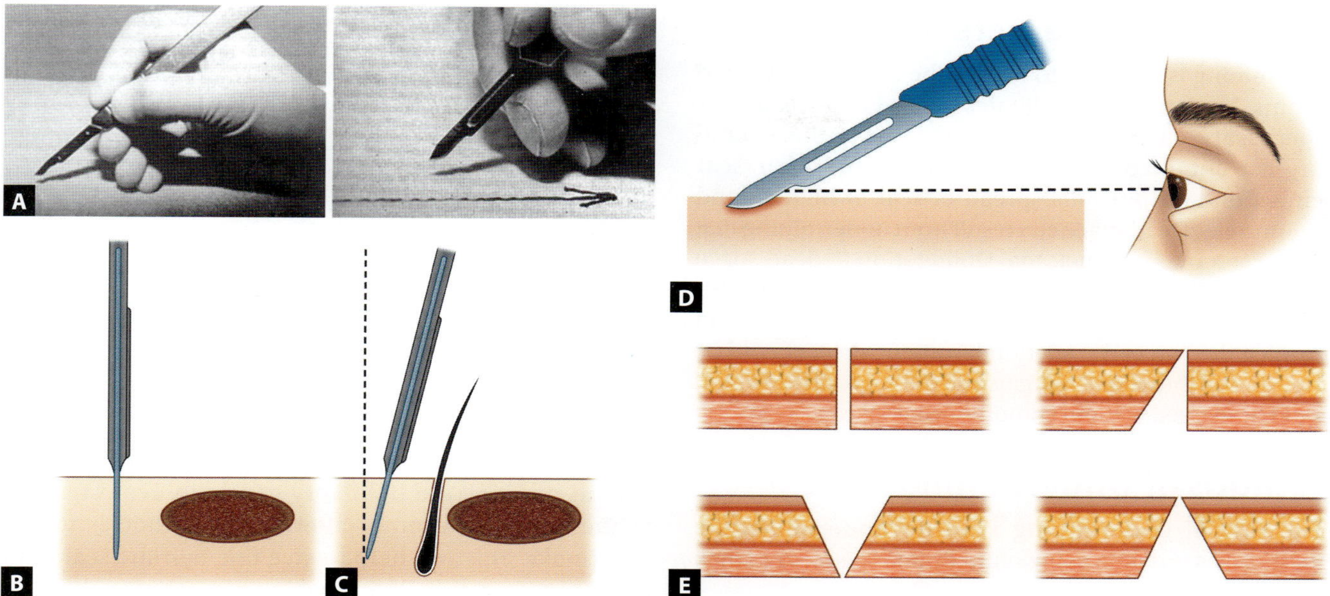

Figs. 13A to E: (A) Scalpel should always move toward the surgeon; (B) Incise perpendicularly through the dermis up to the subcutaneous fat; (C) In hairy areas, pass the scalpel blade parallel to the hair follicle to avoid follicle transection; (D) Perfect movement of the scalpel in straight line is important; (E) Right angle incision is must to get good alignment of the suture line.

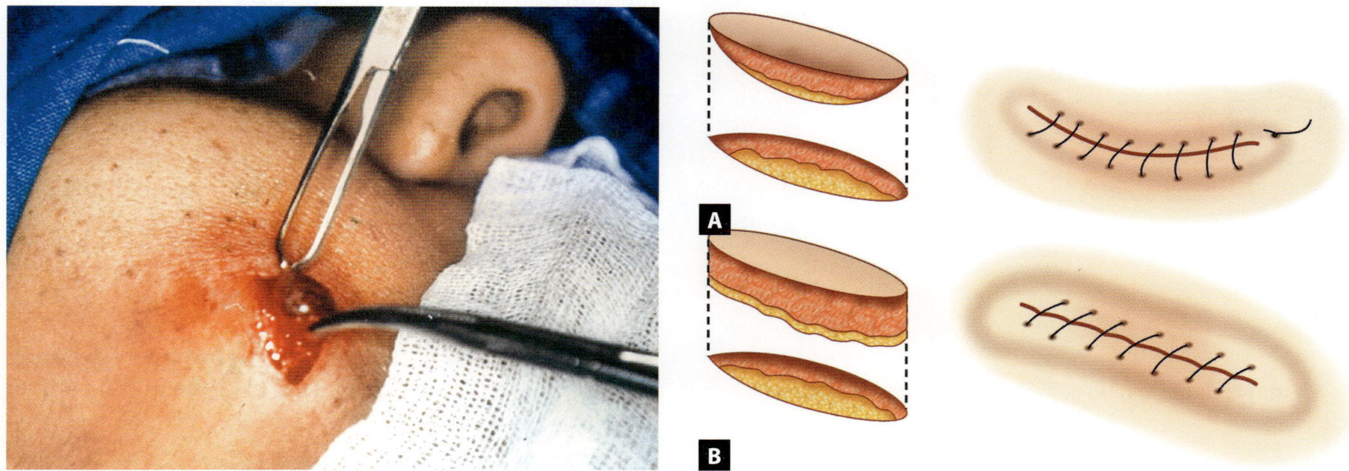

Fig. 14: Dissecting the lesion.

Figs. 15A and B: Avoid boat-shaped incisions.

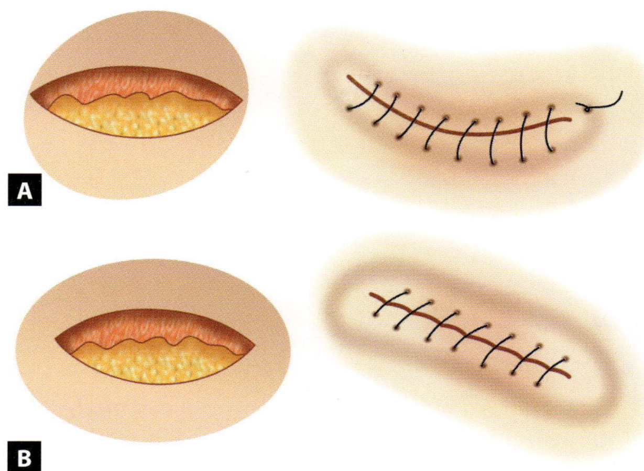

Figs. 16A and B: Depth of tissue removal should be uniform to avoid pseudo-dog ears.

Undermining the Defect

Undermining is essential to reduce the tension on wound margins. Undermining facilitates wound closure; avoids unnecessary vascular compromise; everts the wound margins; enhances the cosmetic outcome after scar contraction and prevents spread of scar at high wound tension areas. Dead space can result from undermining that leads to seroma or hematoma. Obliteration of dead space can be done although this is not imperative (Figs. 17 to 19).

Undermining must be done all around the wound including the two ends. After undermining there should be no tension on the wound margins and the edges of the wound should be everted without compromising vascularity.[2,3,7]

Methods of Undermining

Basic rule of undermining is to do undermining as superficial as possible using blunt tipped scissors or small artery forceps. Author's choice is mosquito forceps; it is a smallest artery forceps. On scalp, it is carried out below the galea aponeurotica which avoids cutting the hair follicles, and supports the suture tension required for closure of the scalp wounds. It is also a bloodless plane thus results in minimal or no bleeding. However, forehead is not undermined at deep subcutaneous tissue level because deeper undermining might result in sensory denervation of the scalp. Undermining on cheeks, chin and temple should be carried out at superficial subcutaneous tissue level to avoid injury to superficial motor nerves. On trunk and extremities undermining is done above muscle fascia at deep subcutaneous tissue level. On hands and feet with minimal subcutaneous tissue undermining is done just below the dermis. During undermining the wound margins are held very gently to avoid trauma to the margins. Another alternative method is to use skin hooks. This will help to give fine hairline scar with excellent cosmetic outcome which is the goal of elliptical excision.[2,3,7]

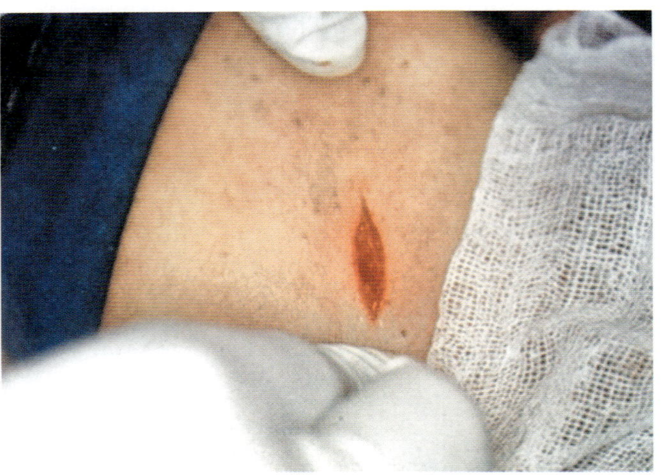

Fig. 17: Undermining completed after smooth incisions.

Hemostasis

Incision and undermining invariably lead to transection and nicking of blood vessels resulting in hematoma. It can be avoided by achieving hemostasis with clamping, ligation, electrocauterization or simple pressure. In case of cautery, ensure that it is used minimally. Otherwise it results in a lot of dead tissue in the wound which can act as a nidus for infection and hamper wound healing. Suturing is also a good option to stop bleeding.[2,3]

CLOSURE OF THE WOUND

This is a very important aspect of excision surgery. By using correct suture material, suture technique and timing of

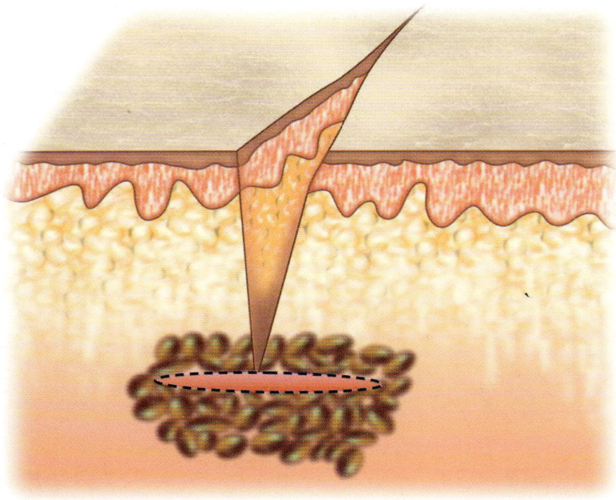

Fig. 18: Dead space can result from undermining.

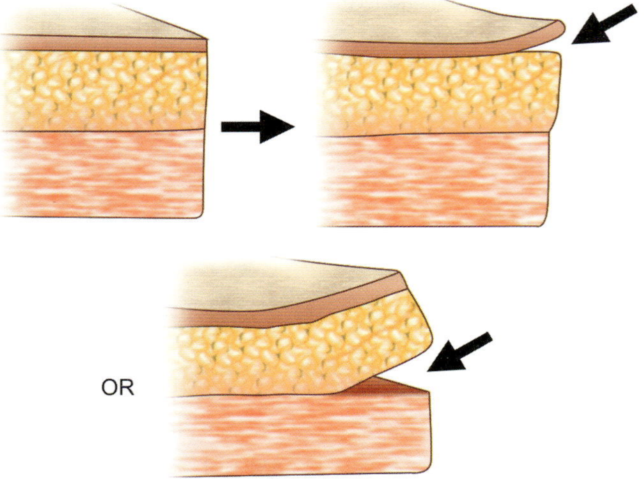

Fig. 19: Different depths of undermining.

suture removal, excellent cosmetic results can be obtained. A well-approximated, everted wound with minimal suture tracking is ideal outcome of simple excision surgery. Various modifications of suture techniques can be used in cutaneous surgery with each technique having its advantages and disadvantages to achieve best possible cosmetic results.[13]

OTHER SIMPLE EXCISION METHODS

The standard elliptical excision may not be suitable for excision of skin lesions in certain age groups and anatomical sites. In such situation, different excision techniques are utilized to give good cosmetic result with minimal scarring.

Circular Excision and Purse-String Closure

It is an effective technique used for excision of circular facial skin lesions in children. Apart from infantile hemangioma (at any stage of evolution), other skin lesions treated successfully with this technique include Spitz nevus, pyogenic granuloma, pilomatricoma, vascular malformations and pigmented nevus.[14] In infantile hemangioma, circular excision and purse-string closure converts large circular lesion into a small ellipsoid scar by significantly reducing the transverse and longitudinal dimensions of the lesion. If required, the ellipsoid scar can be revised subsequently to a linear scar of same length. Hence, the smallest possible scar with minimal distortion of surrounding tissue can be achieved by this method.[15] However, to avoid pleat formation, this method is not indicated for lesions on the free margins such as periorbital region, or on the upper or lower lip.[16]

Intralesional Excision and Primary Closure

The long scar and dog ear formation of elliptical excision and pleat formation of circular excision can be overcome by intralesional excision and primary closure. Infantile hemangiomas, involuting or involuted, are suitable for intralesional excision because of expanded dome-shaped tissue, and excess and redundant skin which permit easy scooping of fibrofatty tissue and closure of wound edge without tension, respectively. In this method, intralesional elliptical resection with dull apical angles and primary closure is performed without extending the incision into the normal skin. A small outermost portion of the lesion is preserved intentionally. If the residual lesion is large, then the same procedure can be repeated 2–3 times at the interval of 3 months each. Intralesional excision is not indicated for hemangiomas in proliferative phase because of excessive intraoperative bleeding and brittle residual tissue.[16]

POSTOPERATIVE CARE AND WOUND DRESSING

Postoperatively the wound is cleaned to remove blood and residual antiseptic. Dressing is applied in four layers comprising of occlusive ointment, a nonadherent gauze material, an absorbent cushion made of cotton covered with gauze material on both sides and adhesive tape to secure the dressing (Fig. 20). Dressing must kept dry all the time and the patient is instructed accordingly. If the dressing gets soiled it has to be replaced immediately. First redressing is to be done after 24 hours. The patient is trained to do subsequent dressings on his own till suture removal.

COMPLICATIONS AND THEIR MANAGEMENT[3]

With good planning technique and aseptic precautions, complications in cutaneous surgery are very rare. Patients should be warned and informed about them preoperatively. The surgeon should be able to recognize and manage them whenever they occur.

Hematoma

Hematomas are seen within 24–48 hours after surgery and they manifest as swelling, erythema and tenderness at wound site. Hematomas are evacuated promptly by partially or completely opening the wound. Resuturing can be done if hematoma develops within early 24 hours provided the wound is not infected. Otherwise the wound is kept open and allowed to heal by second intention. Scar revision can be done at later date. Very small hematomas need not be opened; they can be managed with warm compresses till resolution.

Infection

Infection is a rare event in cutaneous surgery. The recorded incidence is less than one percent. If the wound is frankly

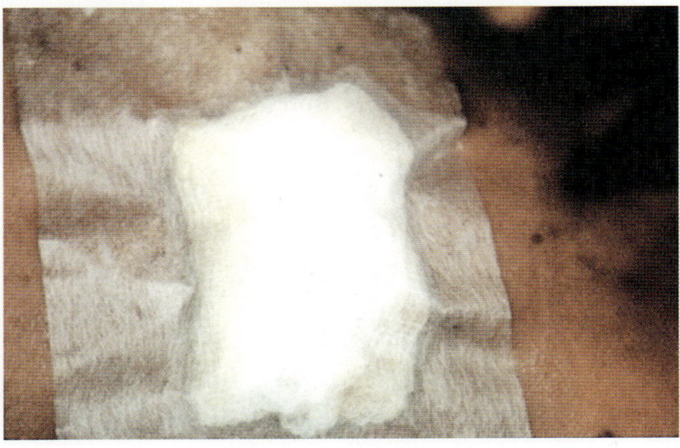

Fig. 20: Three layered dressing.

infected, it is imperative that all the sutures be removed and patient is started on antibiotics. Author prefers to give tetanus toxoid injection and intravenous antibiotic preoperatively and to start the patient on an antibiotic course postoperatively for one week.

Dehiscence

The wound pulls apart in dehiscence usually as a result of underlying infection and/or hematoma. These causes should be promptly managed allowing the wound to heal by second intention. Delayed scar revision can be done at a later date.

Necrosis

Necrosis is a rare complication of simple excision surgery. It occurs only if the wound is closed under high tension thereby compromising the vascularity of the wound margins. The course of action should be suture removal, debridement of the necrotic tissue and allowing the wound to heal by second intention. Corrective scar revision is undertaken at a later date.

Dog-ear

A skin protrusion present at the end of excision is commonly referred to as a dog-ear. These protrusions are caused by the presence of redundant skin at the ends or dressing sites of an excision. The amount of tissue protrusion formed in a given wound is fundamentally determined by the amount of rotation, advancement and intrinsic tissue elasticity of the surrounding skin. The local surface contours also contribute to the final degree of tissue protrusion. Circumferential closures performed on highly convex surfaces, such as the arm, will result in tissue protrusions at the end of the closure. If excess subcutaneous fat is present at the apex of an excision, the resultant elevation of the angle of closure may mimic a tissue protrusion. Removal of excess fat with adequate undermining of the apex will invariably result in the dissolution of the pseudo-dog-ear.[3]

Methods of Dog-ear Correction

Before planning the removal of dog-ear, it is often beneficial to partially close the wound edges to determine whether a tissue protrusion will form.

Linear Repair

This is simple, easy to perform and useful when it is desirable to extend the excision in a straight line. The apex of tissue protrusion is elevated with a skin-hook to define the geometry of tissue protrusion in the shape of a standing cone. The apex of the cone is drawn to one side so that the base of the tissue protrusion is in line with the long axis of the anticipated wound closure. The base is incised and undermined to free up a triangular wedge of tissue. The triangular section is then draped over the underlying wound edge with gentle tension and the base is incised over the line of closure. The wound is then repaired in a straight line.

Other methods of dog-ear repair are curved repair, hockey stick repair, l-shaped repair, T-shaped repair and N-plasty repair.[3]

Summary of Dog-ear Repair

Closure of even the most carefully planned and executed excision may result in the development of tissue pro-trusions. Understanding the dynamics of tissue movement and elasticity allows anticipation and subsequent correction of dog-ears. An attempt should always be made to place the final incision lines parallel to the RSTLs. Proper design and execution of these techniques provides critical difference between an average and an excellent cosmetic outcome. Figures 21 to 23 show the different steps of excision in different situations-scar excision, scrofuloderma and neurofibroma, respectively.

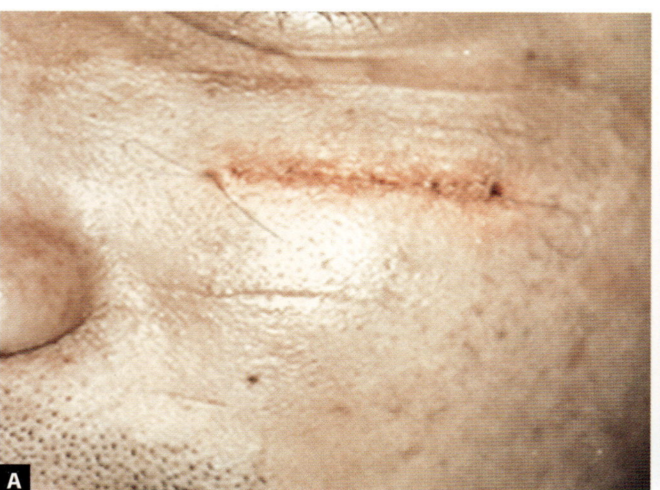

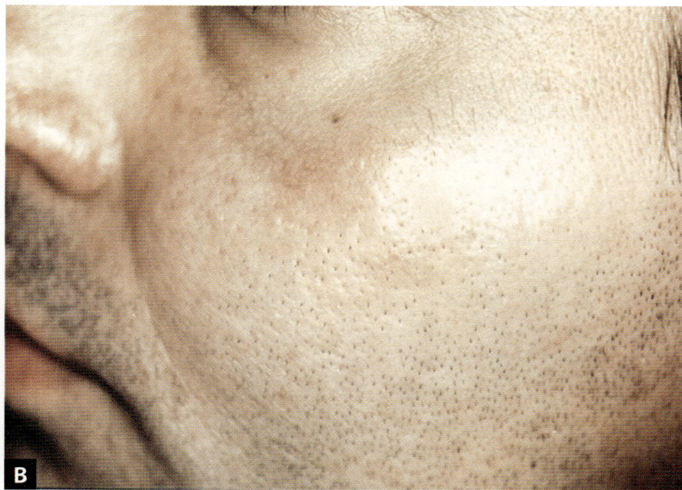

Figs. 21A and B: (A) Scar excision (before); (B) Scar excision (after).

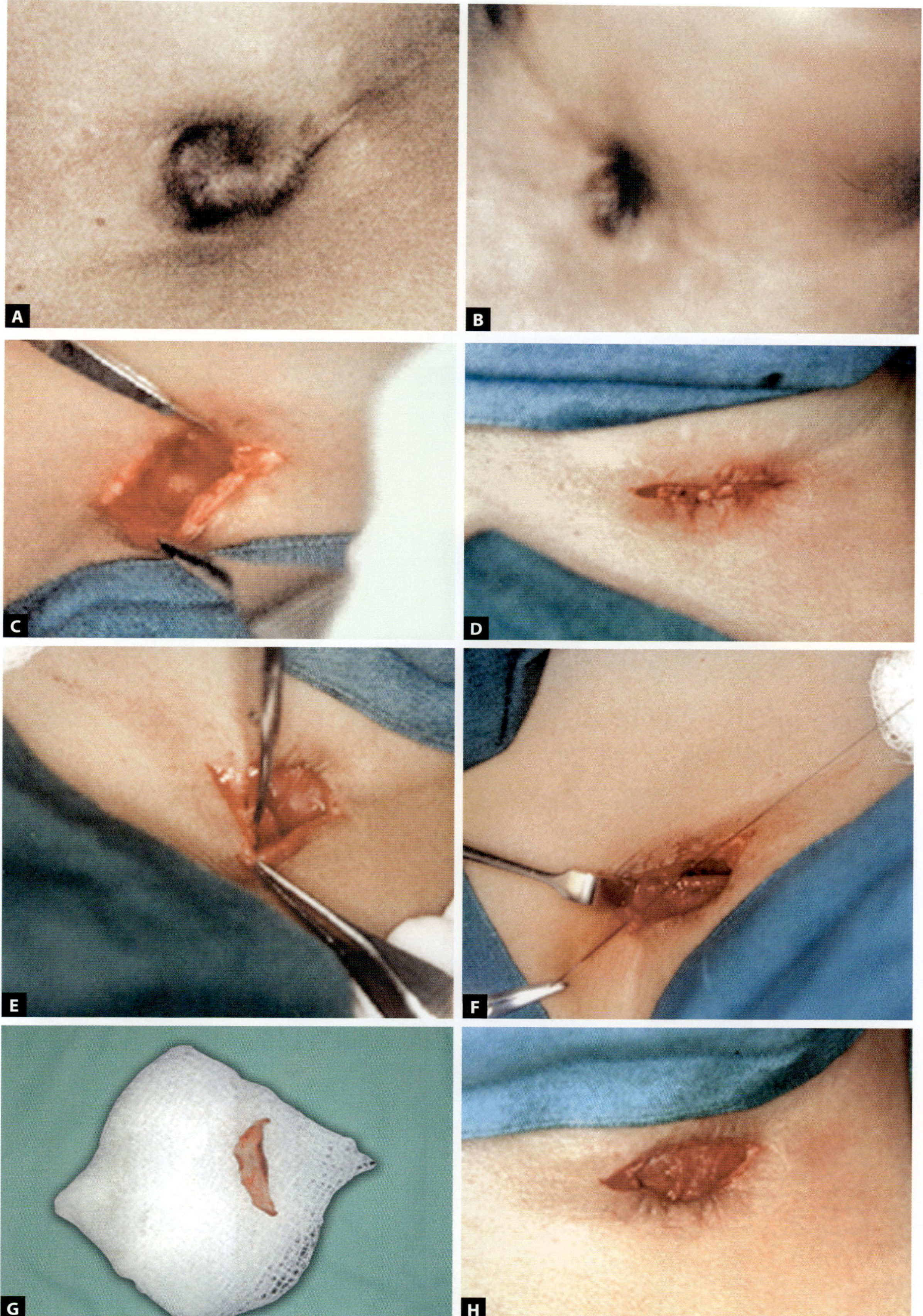

Figs. 22A to H: Deep scar following scrofuloderma, with complete atrophy of subcutaneous tissue. Undermining the defect: Scrofuloderma.

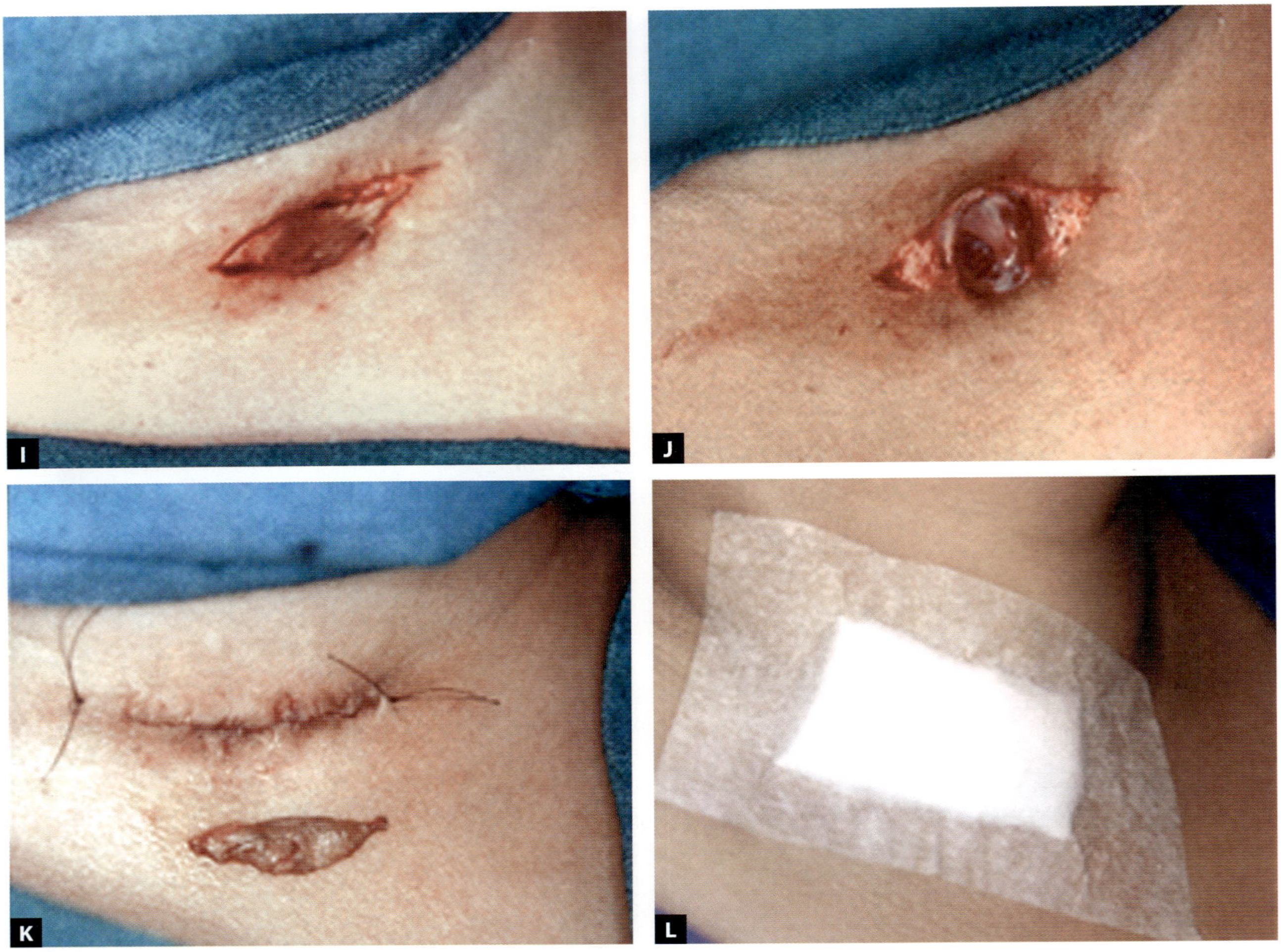

Figs. 22I to L: Excision and suturing done with occlusive dressing.

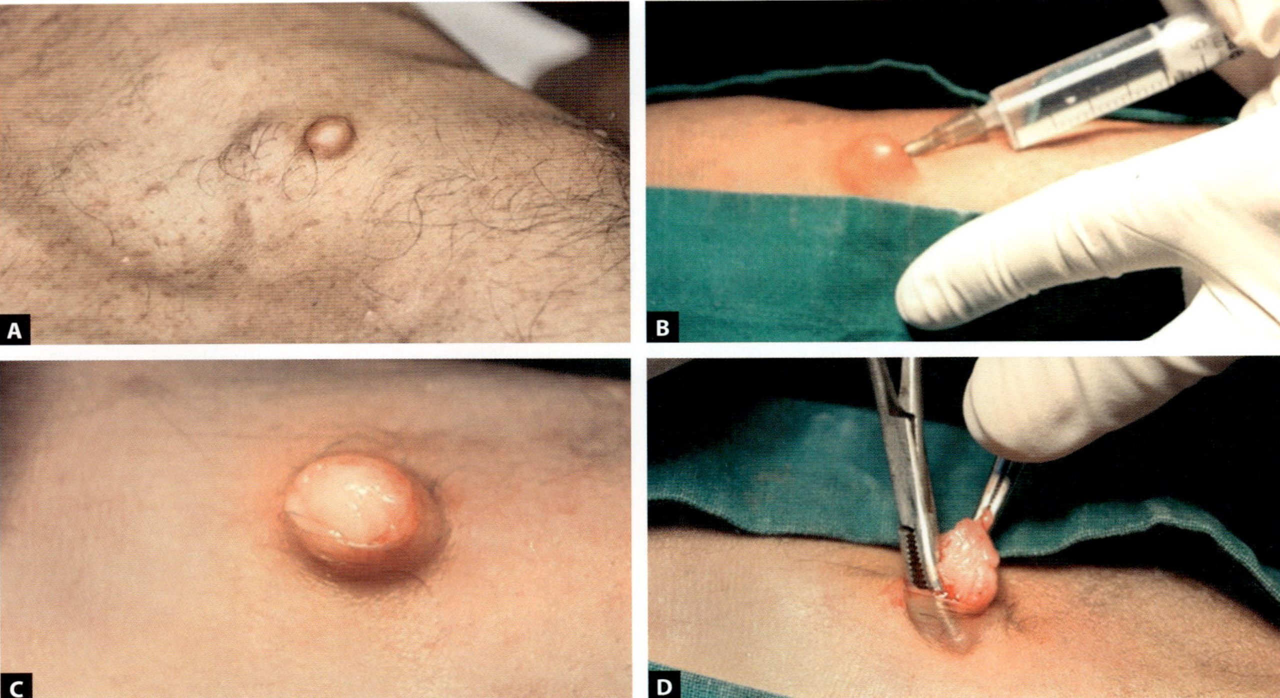

Figs. 23A to D: Excision of neurofibroma. (A) Neurofibroma; (B) Field block for neurofibroma; (C) After blunt dissection; (D) Blunt dissection in progress.

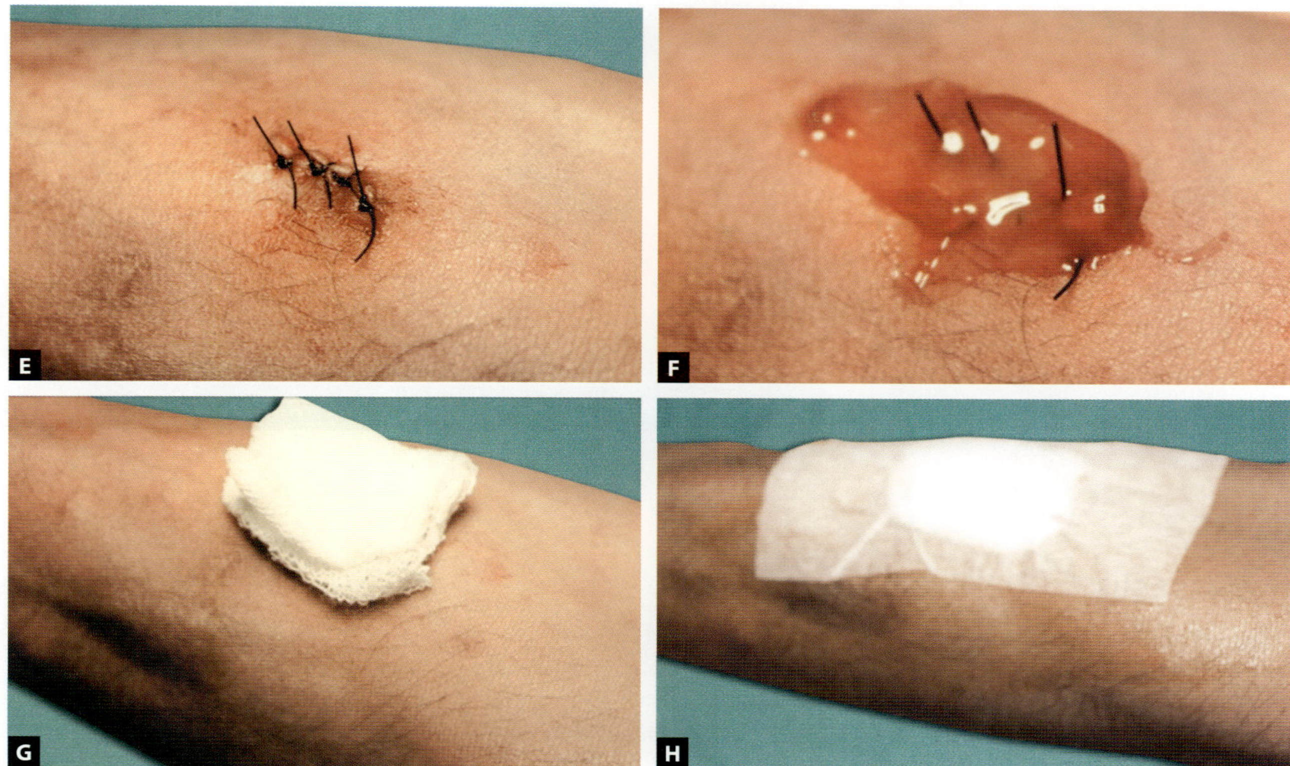

Figs. 23E to H: (E) After suturing; (F) Povidone-iodine applied; (G) Nonocclusive gauze piece applied; (H) Dressing completed in three layers with micropore tape.

Box 3: Advantages of elliptical excision.

- Inexpensive
- Costly equipments are not required
- Excellent cosmetic results
- No tissue destruction
- Not a blind procedure
- Good specimen can be obtained for histopathology

CONCLUSION

Elliptical excision is a cornerstone of cutaneous excisional surgeries because of several advantages (Box 3). Understanding the basic principles of anatomy, wound healing, anesthesia, lines of closure, STL, tumor biology, surgical techniques of incision, suturing and wound care are the prerequisites for cutaneous simple excision surgery. Mastery over these principles gives an excellent cosmetic result satisfying both the patient and the operating surgeon.

REFERENCES

1. Stegman SJ, et al. Basics of Dermatologic Surgery. Chicago, Year Book; 1982.
2. Leshin B. Proper planning and execution of surgical excisions. In: Ronald D (Ed). Cutaneous Surgery, Wheeland. 1994;15:171-7.
3. Goldberg LH. Cold steel surgery. In: Lask GP, Moy RL (Eds). The Ellipse, Principles and Techniques of Cutaneous Surgery. 1996;15:165-70.
4. Perez M. Skin Biopsy Techniques. In: Nouri K, Leal-Khouri S (Eds). Techniques in Dermatologic Surgery.
5. Webster RC, Smith RC. Cosmetic principles in surgery on the face. J Dermatol Surg Oncol. 1978;4:397-402.
6. Bennett RG. Fundamentals of Cutaneous Surgery. CV Mosby, St. Louis; 1988. pp.353-444.
7. Leal-Khouri S, et al. Suturing techniques. In: Nouri K, Leal-Khouri S (Eds). No Techniques in Dermatologic Surgery. 2003;11:71-3.
8. Hruza GJ. Suturing techniques. In: Lask GP, Moy RL (Eds). Principles and Techniques of Cutaneous surgery. 1996; 16:171-85.
9. Chernosky ME. Scalpel and scissors as seen by the dermatologist. In: Epstein E, Epstein E Jr. (Eds). Skin Surgery, 6th edition, Philadelphia, Saunders; 1987. p. 88.
10. Stegman SJ. Planning closure of a surgical wound. J Dermatol Surg Oncol. 1978;4:390-3.
11. Zitelli JA. Tips for a better ellipse. J Am Acad Dermatol. 1990;22:101-3.
12. Spicer TE. Techniques of facial lesion excision and closure. J Dermatol Surg Oncol. 1982;8:551-6.
13. Stegman SJ. Suturing techniques for dermatologi surgery. J Dermatol Surg Oncol. 1978;4:63-8.
14. Hassanein AH, Couto JA, Greene AK. Circular excision and purse-string closure for pediatric facial skin lesions. J Craniofac Surg. 2015;26:1611-2.
15. Mulliken JB, Rogers GF, Marler JJ. Circular excision of hemangioma and purse-string closure: the smallest possible scar. Plast Reconstr Surg. 2002;109:1544-54. discussion 1555.
16. Nomura T, Osaki T, Ishinagi H, Ejiri H, Terashi H. Simple and easy surgical technique for infantile hemangiomas: intralesional excision and primary closure. Eplasty 2015;15:15:e3.

Chapter 24

Electrosurgery

Rashmi Sarkar, Vivek Nair

Key Messages

- Electrosurgery is an effective modality for the treatment of a variety of skin lesions.
- A good understanding of the different waveforms that are generated and their purpose is essential to using it effectively.
- Four types of procedures can be done: electrodessication, electrofulguration, electrocoagulation and electrosection.
- Electrode tips should be sterilized with an appropriate method before use. Disposable tips are another option.
- The electrosurgical plume can transmit infection and hence it is essential for the operating physician to wear a mask and gloves. A smoke evacuator is helpful in further decreasing this risk.

INTRODUCTION

Electrosurgery remains an indispensable tool for the modern dermatologist. It is one of the first things one learns during dermatology postgraduation training and has kept its place despite the increasing use of ablative lasers. Though offering certain advantages these lasers remain out of reach for many practitioners and institutions. The humble electrosurgical machine remains important because of its portability and inexpensiveness.

HISTORY

The first true use of electrosurgery dates back to the last decade of the 19th century when Joseph River, a Parisian physician, used an arcing current to treat a cutaneous carcinoma. Franz Nagelschmidt had used electrical current for treating patients with articular and circulatory problems before this, but he utilized the deep heating effect of current (*diathermy*), as opposed to the superficial destructive changes typical of electrosurgery.[1]

During the early 1900's another physician named Simon Pozzi coined the term *fulguration* to describe the use of high frequency, high voltage, low amperage current to treat skin cancers. Doyen furthered the technique by introducing a grounding plate in the circuit, which allowed deeper penetration of the current - a technique he termed *electrocoagulation*.

A decade later William Clark coined the term *dessication* to describe the effect when tissues were destroyed by dehydration. This required a current with a higher amperage and lower voltage than that used for fulguration and coagulation.

William T. Bovie developed the modern electrosurgical device in the 1920s and it was used for the first time by Dr Harvey Cushing at Peter Bent Brigham Hospital in Boston on October 1, 1926, to successfully remove an enlarging, vascular myeloma from the head of a 64-year-old patient. The low powered Hyfrecator, meant for regular office use, was introduced in 1940.[2]

FUNDAMENTALS

At the outset it is important to differentiate Electrosurgery from Electrocautery. The earliest forms of Electrosurgery used direct current to generate heat in a metal tip which was then used for burning tissue and coagulating blood vessels through the passive transfer of heat. The patient was not a part of the electric circuit. This is the strict definition of the term 'Electrocautery'. As will be explained later this is different from modern Electrosurgery where the patient is a part of the electrical circuit.

It is also important to understand how an electrosurgical machine works to be able to use it most effectively. To do this we must also refamiliarize ourselves with certain electrical terms.

ELECTROSURGICAL TERMS

Ampere: An ampere is a unit of measure of the rate of electron flow or current in an electrical conductor. It is measured as the flow of electrons during a given period of time. A higher value denotes faster current flow.

Voltage: Also known as electromotive force, voltage is a quantitative expression of the potential difference between two points in an electrical field. It is the force driving a current against the resistance of the circuit. Thus the greater the voltage, the higher is the flow of electric current in a circuit.

Damping: There are basically two types of waves generated by an electrosurgical circuit - damped and undamped (Fig. 1).

A *damped wave* is one whose amplitude of oscillation decreases with time eventually going to zero. This is the natural state of an electrical wave generated by a spark gap circuit for example. The more rapidly the waves return to zero the more damped is the wave and vice versa. By increasing the resistance in the oscillating circuit, longer rest periods are generated between subsequent wave trains, and greater damping is produced.

An *undamped wave* is one that has constant equal waves of unchanging amplitude. There is no tendency to zero and this requires special circuitry whereby each oscillation receives an increase in energy by a feedback mechanism and equal amplitude oscillations are produced. A triode vacuum circuit is capable of producing a fully undamped wave.[3]

The term rectified as applied to current dynamics refers to the conversion of alternating current (AC) into direct current (DC) as occurs in most everyday electrical appliances since they need DC to work. However many authors seem to use it as a synonym for damping, with undamped sine waves considered rectified, and damped sine waves considered unrectified. This forms a continuous spectrum with relatively undamped waves considered partially rectified.

ELECTROSURGICAL UNITS

Electrosurgical units (ESU) are appliances which produce oscillating (sine) electromagnetic (EM) radiation. Since the frequency of the EM radiation used for Electrosurgery is in the same bandwidth as that used for radio transmission these waves are often called radio waves and the ESUs themselves radiofrequency (RF) machines.

There are various types of electrosurgical generators, each operating in a particular bandwidth and having different power outputs. Traditional ESU's like the Hyfrecator and newer RF machines differ only in the frequency of radiation emitted - the former emit EM radiation around 500 kHz while the latter generate higher frequency radiation, around the 2.5 to 4 MHz mark.

The electrosurgical circuit consists of a coil wire, condensers, and an air gap. The air gap may be a spark gap, a vacuum tube (diode, triode) or a solid-state transistor.[3] The properties of these three types of circuits are summarized in Table 1.

MONOPOLAR ELECTROSURGERY

Monopolar electrosurgery is the most commonly used electrosurgical modality. It utilizes two electrodes. The *active electrode* is used at the surgical site whereas the *patient return electrode* (PRE or dispersive electrode) is somewhere else on the patient's body. This latter is sometimes also incorrectly called the ground plate; however its purpose is not to carry the current to ground but back to the ESU to complete the circuit, and hence the term is inappropriate. This usage dates back to the 1960's when electrosurgical generators were "ground referenced," i.e. the flow of electrons was in relation to earth ground. This created a potentially hazardous situation because the current would seek the path of least resistance to ground and in certain instances this was not the ground plate of the electrosurgical unit. Several cases of electrical burns resulted at the sites of current exit in these inadvertent

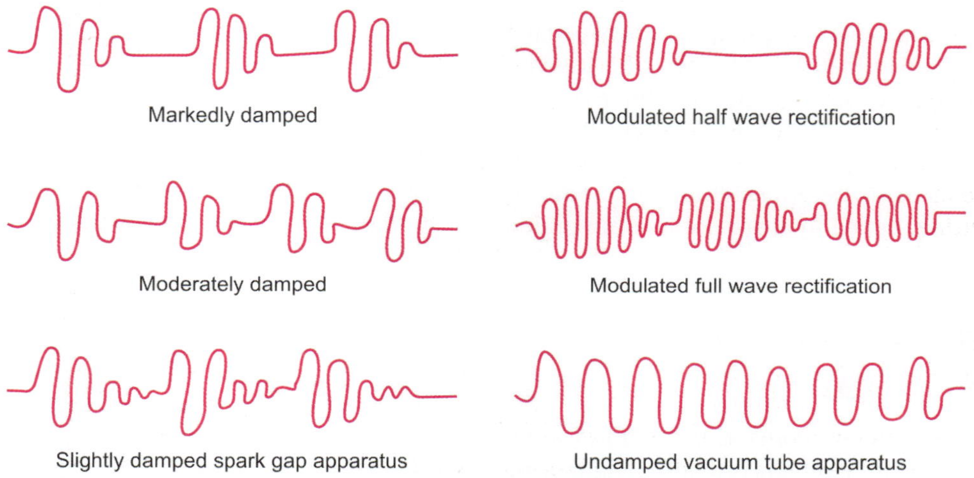

Markedly damped

Modulated half wave rectification

Moderately damped

Modulated full wave rectification

Slightly damped spark gap apparatus

Undamped vacuum tube apparatus

Fig. 1: Waveforms used in electrosurgery.

Table 1: Electrosurgical circuits.[3]

Circuit	Features
Spark gap circuit	Produces markedly damped current, suitable for electro-dessication (ED) and electrofulguration (EF). Seen in low cost ESUs. EF is a unique property of the spark gap current.
Vacuum tube circuit	Partially undamped current is produced, which besides ED provides a coagulative effect and is thus suitable for electrocoagulation (EC). EF is not possible.
Solid state circuit	More uniform undamped waves are produced and these are capable of the electrosection (ES) in addition to EC and ED. EF is not possible. These units are quite expensive.

Note: High end ESUs have all three circuits within the same machine and are thus capable of the full range of ES, EC, ED and EF.

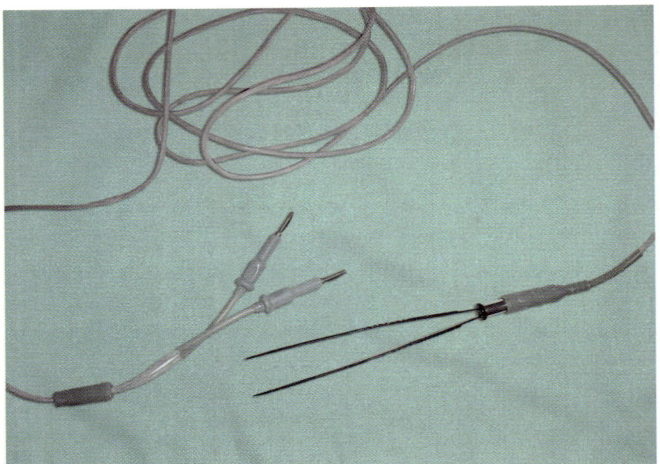

Fig. 2: Bipolar Electrodes.

return circuits (e.g. electrocardiogram pads, metal parts of the operating table, etc.). This potential hazard was eliminated with the introduction of generators that were isolated from ground, confining the current flow to the circuit between the electrode and the patient return electrode, which offered a low-resistance pathway for current to return to the generator from the patient.[4]

As is obvious from the preceding discussion, the patient is a part of the electrical circuit in Monopolar Electrosurgery and current actually flows through the body. Certain ESUs like the Hyfrecator do not use a PRE and rely on the patients self capacitance providing a current sink, a phenomenon known as displacement current,[5] as well as the current seeking its own ground through the operating table, across the floor, into the ground and then back to the ESU through the wall outlet. So even in monoterminal electrosurgery the patient is a part of the electric circuit. In such circuits patient safety is maintained since the ESUs are typically of low power.

BIPOLAR ELECTROSURGERY

In Bipolar Electrosurgery both the active and return electrode functions are performed at the site of surgery by the two limbs of a forcep type electrode (Fig. 2). Here the patient is not part of the electric circuit as no current passes through the body apart from the tissue between the limbs of the forceps. In dermatology this method is used for obtaining hemostasis in surgeries such as cancer resections and donor strip dissection in hair transplantation. It is very difficult to obtain a cutting effect with bipolar electrodes as there is tissue charring before reaching temperatures sufficient for cutting, hence they are not recommended for this purpose.

ELECTRICAL CURRENT AND THE HUMAN BODY

Electrons orbit the nuclei of atoms. Current flows when electrons of one atom jump into the orbit of a neighboring atom thereby displacing resident electrons due to their negative charge. This process is repeated resulting in the flow of electrons. Electrons only flow in closed circuits, hence the importance of grounding electrical appliances. If electrons encounter resistance, heat is produced. This resistance is known as impedance.

A free flow of charge carriers is called an electric current. When the charge carriers are electrons, as in metals and semiconductors, the current is '*Electronic*' and when the charge carriers are ions, as in liquids, the current is '*Ionic*'. Electrical conduction in the body is primarily due to conductivity of the interstitial fluid, and hence mostly ionic in nature.[1]

When electric current encounters tissue impedance, electrical energy is converted to thermal energy (heat). Tissue effects depend on the speed of this process, which in turn is dependent on the type of current applied, current density and its power. Current density is a measure of the concentration of electric current. A higher current density results in a higher concentration of joule heating and the rate of temperature rise in the tissue is directly proportional to it. Higher rates result in instant vaporization of tissue water (intracellular as well as extracellular) resulting in an explosive cutting effect, while slower rates result in less dramatic changes leading to tissue dehydration, denaturation of proteins and coagulum formation. This latter provides excellent hemostasis.

Practically current density is directly proportional to the strength of the applied current and inversely proportional to the surface area of the active electrode. Hence thin wire type electrodes are preferred for electrosection and larger ball type electrodes for electrocoagulation.

The type of current also has a major role in the tissue effects produced. Completely undamped waves have very little rest periods between subsequent waves, and thus the heat energy generated in the tissue is so intense that cells vaporize - thereby producing a cutting effect. In damped or partially damped current longer rest periods between subsequent wave trains decelerate the tissue destruction to a slow dehydration of cellular water and proteins.

Neural and muscle cells are electrically excitable due to the voltage gated ion channels present in their cell membranes. Such stimulation can cause acute pain, muscle spasm and even cardiac arrest. This sensitivity is inversely proportional to the frequency of the applied current. Alternating current frequency refers to the number of cycles the current sine wave goes through in one second and is measured in Hertz (Hz). Commercially available current cycles at 60 cycles per second and this can be fatal. However when the frequency is increased into the kilo hertz range, muscle and nerve sensitivity keeps decreasing and is virtually nil above 100,000 cycles per second (i.e. 100 kHz).[6] This increase in frequency is accomplished by the oscillating circuit of the ESU. A voltage of several thousand volts is also required for electrosurgery and this is done by the step up transformers in the power circuit of the ESU. In this way the low voltage (220V), low frequency (60 Hz) commercial current is converted to the high voltage, high frequency current required for electrosurgery.[3]

ELECTROSURGICAL METHODS

Electrodessication

"*Desiccate*" is a Latin word, meaning to dry. This is a monoterminal method utilizing a high frequency, very high voltage, low amperage damped current as typically generated by a spark gap circuit. Current from solid-state circuits and vacuum tube circuits can be used for electrodessication by reducing the power. The electrode is placed in contact with skin resulting in tissue destruction. The destruction extends for some distance below the epidermis and is characterized by denaturation of proteins, dehydration of tissue and thrombosed blood vessels.

Electrofulguration

"*Fulgur*" is a Latin word, meaning an act of lightening. Again a monoterminal method electrofulguration is identical to electrodessication apart from the fact that the electrode is held away from the skin to produce a spark that arcs across the air gap to reach the skin.The current needs to be of very high voltage to be able to do this and electrofulguration is a hallmark of the spark gap circuit. Solid state and vacuum tube circuits cannot produce this current. Tissue effects are identical to those seen in electrodessication but damage is very superficial and therefore electrofulguration is best suited for treating purely epidermal lesions like flat warts.

Electrocoagulation

"*Coagulate*" is a Latin word, meaning to clot. Electrocoagulation is a biterminal method utilizing a high frequency damped current that has a lower voltage and higher amperage as compared to an electrodessicating current. All three electrosurgical circuits can produce this current. Tissue effects are similar but more pronounced leading to hyalinization of tissue and excellent hemostasis (electrodessication or electrofulguration may be considered as mild electrocoagulation). The field of destruction is large, as is lateral heat spread from the operative site, and more scarring is an inevitable consequence. Hence this current is only used where cosmesis is of secondary concern, as in while treating the base of a curetted basal cell carcinoma. When used to seal bleeders in an operative field a thin electrode should be used and current only passed for a very short duration of time to avoid scarring.

Electrosection

"*Section*" when used as a verb means to cut or divide into parts. Electrosection is again a biterminal method and the current employed has the lowest voltage and the highest amperage of all electrosurgical currents. The waveforms are either slightly damped or undamped. A completely undamped current produces a purely cutting effect whereas a slightly damped current produces cutting with some coagulation (hemostasis), and therefore a more bloodless incision. The latter is preferred for skin surgery. A vacuum tube or solid-state circuit produces the ideal current for electrosection, however biterminal application of a spark gap current can also produce cutting.

Electroepilation

Electroepilation refers to the destruction of the hair follicle using an electric current. Traditionally direct current has been used for this but now most electroepilation is done using high frequency alternating current, partly due to the machines available in the market and partly due to the shortened procedure time with alternating current. Electroepilation remains the only permanent method of hair removal. On an average 3-4 three-monthly cycles are required to convert the hair follicle into a fibrotic band incapable of producing hair.

Direct current (low voltage, low amperage) removal is safer (less likely to scar) and less painful than alternating current epilation, but it takes longer. Current flows from the active electrode (negative pole) to the indifferent electrode (positive pole). The strong polarity around the electrodes produces chemical ionization by electrolysis (hydroxide ions at the negative pole and metallic ions at the positive pole). The hydroxide ions liquefy tissue with minimal pain and thus produce concentrated destruction of the hair follicle around the extremely thin treatment electrode (needle electrode). The larger indifferent electrode harmlessly disperses the metallic ions. A 0.5 to 1.0 milliamp current is applied for 15-60 seconds for electrolysis.[3]

High frequency alternate current epilation does not work through electrolysis but through thermal destruction of the hair follicle. The needle electrode is connected to the active electrode input of the ESU and slipped into the hair follicle opening, parallel to the hair shaft, till the bottom

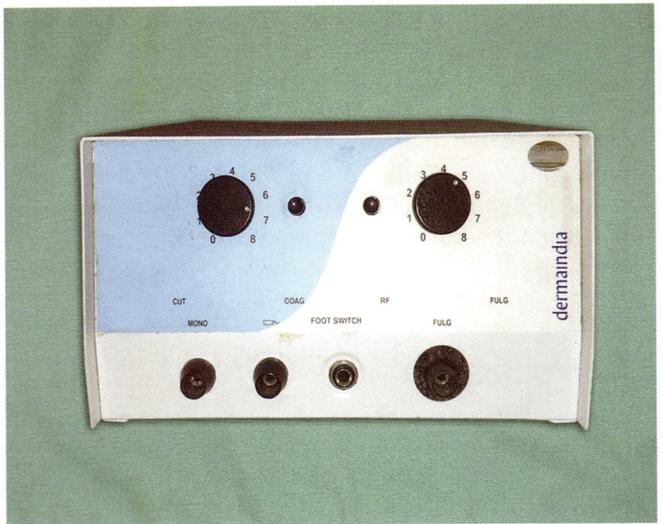

Fig. 3: DermaIndia RF machine with Fulguration mode.

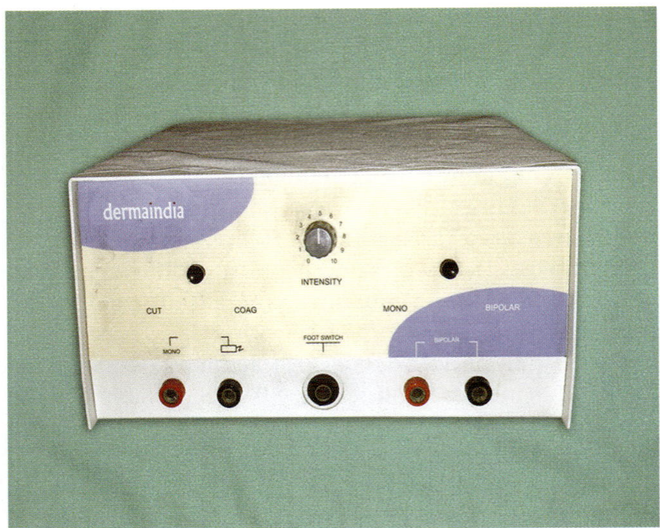

Fig. 4: DermaIndia RF Machine without Fulguration mode.

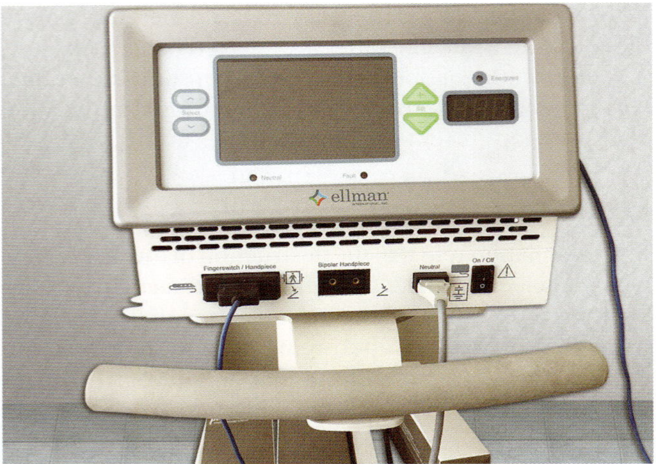

Fig. 5: Ellman RF Machine.

of the hair follicle. It is good practice to ask the patient to shave 4-5 days prior to the procedure since this enables targeting only the hair in anagen phase.[3] The procedure utilizes a very low power setting and thus a patient return or dispersive electrode is not required. 3-6 bursts of current, of less than one second duration, are given either manually or automatically. When done correctly the hair can then be very easily removed from the hair follicle. If too much power is used scarring can result. Using insulated needles prevents scarring. Hair being treated in one session must be 3-4 mm apart.[3] Intervening hair can be treated at a later date, usually after 2-4 weeks. Multiple sittings may be required to permanently destroy a hair follicle and when a large number of hairs are being treated the whole process can take many months, even years. Therefore laser hair removal is the preferred modality for hair reduction unless the hairs are non-pigmented, very fine or resistant to the laser, in which case electroepilation of hair is a very useful adjunct.

BLENDED CURRENTS

As can be seen from the discussion so far, various types of currents are used in electrosurgery, ranging from pure cutting to pure coagulation. Most electrosurgical use in dermatology requires the cutting function. However a purely cutting current would be very hard to work with, as there would be no hemostasis and therefore considerable bleeding. Hence some coagulation current is always mixed with the cutting current even in ESUs which have the 'Cut' mode selected in a two mode system (Cut or Coag). Similarly a purely coagulation current would produce too much tissue destruction and hence is mixed with some cutting current.

Typically, an office unit has one or two blend modes, and an operating room unit has between two and four blend modes. For example the DermaIndia MegaSurg (Figs. 3 and 4) is a two-mode system producing a 70% cut and 30% coag current in the 'Cut' mode and a 40% cut and 60% coag current in the 'Coag' mode. Higher end instrument like the Ellman Surgitron EMC (Fig. 5) has four modes – 'Cut' (90% cut, 10% coag), 'Cut & Coag' (50% cut, 50% coag), 'Coag' (10% cut, 90% coag) and 'Fulgurate' (markedly damped coag). Operating room units like the Aaron 2100 may offer up to nine modes.

PROCEDURE

Indications

As summarized in Table 2, electrosurgery has a wide variety of indications. Levels of evidence for its use have also been provided wherever possible.

Contraindications

There are no absolute contraindications for electrosurgery. Relative contraindications include active infection in the area to be treated, bleeding diathesis, debilitated patients,

Table 2: Lesions treatable with electrosurgery (ES).[7-42]

Lesion	Es as choice of treatment
Verruca plana [7]	Third line
Verruca vulgaris [7]	Third line
Acrochordons [8]	First line
Seborrheic keratosis [9]	First line
Dermatosis papulosa nigra [9]	First line
Molluscum contagiosum [10]	Third line
Melanocytic nevus [11]	Third line
Actinic keratoses [12-14]	Third line
Telangiectasia [15-16]	Second line
Freckles	Third line
Syringomas [17, 21]	First line
Sebaceous cyst	Second line
Pyogenic granuloma [18-20]	First line
Trichoepithelioma [21]	Second line
Basal cell carcinoma [22-24]	First line
Squamous cell carcinoma [25]	First line
Bowens disease [26-27]	First line
Bowenoid papulosis [28]	Second line
Keratoacanthoma [29]	First line
Angiokeratomas [30-31]	Second line
Rhinophyma [32-33]	Second line
Fox fordyce disease [34]	Second line
Lymphangioma circumscriptum [35]	Second line
Sebaceous gland hyperplasia [36]	First line
Spitz nevus [37]	Second line
Anogenital warts [38]	Second line
Mycobacterium marinum infection [39]	Third line
Resurfacing	Third line
Epilation [40]	Second line
Xanthelasma [41]	Second line
Mucous cysts [42]	Third line

Note: Levels of evidence: A – Double blind RCT, B – Clinical trial with ≥20 subjects lacking adequate controls, C – Clinical trial with < 20 subjects, D - ≥ 5 case reports in the literature, E - < 5 case reports in the literature

keloidal tendency, diagnostic confusion with melanoma, and infections transmissible by the electrosurgical plume, viz. HIV, Hepatitis B and C. Precautions required in patients with Implantable Electronic Devices like cardiac pacemakers will be dealt with later.

PREOPERATIVE PREPARATION

The patient must be counseled as to the healing time following the procedure. This simple practice will save a lot of patient anxiety later. Most patients will recover within 2-4 weeks but when post inflammatory hyperpigmentation occurs recovery can take 3-6 months. Sometimes it is not possible to remove a lesion without scarring and this must also be clearly explained to the patient beforehand. It is useful to ask the patient whether he or she has ever had local anesthesia in the past, to rule out hypersensitivity to lignocaine. When large lesions are being treated electrosurgically, it is important to get a complete hemogram and bleeding parameters done preoperatively. In an ideal scenario all patients should also be checked for HIV, HBsAg and Anti-HCV beforehand but this is mostly impractical. It is therefore essential to practice universal precautions while doing electrosurgery, or at the very least wear gloves and a mask.

All patients must sign an informed consent form prior to the procedure.

Preoperative photographs of all patients is a good habit to cultivate. Again, however, due to the commonplace and benign nature of many of the conditions treated with electrosurgery, it is more practical to take preoperative photographs of those patients being treated exclusively for cosmetic indications (e.g. facial melanocytic nevi). Photographs in natural light are best. When this is not available it is better to use a camera stand, long exposure time and bright room illumination rather than a flash, so as to get an accurate representation of the area to be treated.

The hand piece of the electrosurgical electrode as well as the patient return plate must be cleaned before the procedure for every patient. This can be done with either spirit or betadine. Allow the spirit to dry completely before use.

ANESTHESIA

Local anesthesia (topical or injectable) is sufficient in most cases. EMLA cream (Eutectic mixture of local anesthetics) is suitable for many superficial lesions such as plane warts and acrochordons; it needs to be applied under occlusion 30–120 min prior to the procedure, depending on the topical agent being used. Local infiltration with 2% Xylocaine with 1:100,000 adrenaline is better for bigger or deeper lesions. In body areas supplied by terminal arteries (e.g. tip of the nose, ear lobes, fingertips, glans penis) 2% Xylocaine without adrenaline should be used. For warts and skin cancers do not inject directly below the lesions since this can create tracts for the migration of infected/ malignant cells. Instead infiltrate around the periphery or give a ring, nerve or field block.

Procedure

Make sure the patient is sitting or lying comfortably. The procedure room should be well ventilated and well lit. An exhaust fan or smoke evacuator should be used in rooms with inadequate ventilation. Ask the patient to remove all metal jewelry in the vicinity of the treatment area and in the path of the current to the patient return electrode.

Clean the area to be treated with betadine and then drape it. Do not use spirit for cleansing. For very dirty areas savlon can be used before the betadine – please note that savlon contains chlorhexidine and this is toxic to the eyes and middle ear, hence savlon (or any other chlorhexidine containing antiseptic) is contraindicated on the face and scalp.[50] Ensure that there are no explosive materials like oxygen cylinders near the operative field and that the electrosurgical wall outlet is properly grounded.

When the dispersive plate or patient return electrode is used it should make good contact with the bare skin of a well-vascularized part of the patient's body. Not doing so can result in increased current density at the site of the current leaving the body and cause secondary burns or shocks. The patient must maintain firm contact with the electrode throughout the procedure. Loose contact can result in current concentration and skin burns.

The dispersive electrode is usually 3 × 5 inches in size and should be insulated at the clip connection of the metal plate. The plate itself should not be rusted and free of points, angles or bends. It should also not be in contact with any metal part of the operating table.

Electrosurgery in Different Situations

The first step while assessing which type of electrosurgical technique to use for a dermatological condition is to estimate its depth and vascularity. The more vascular a lesion is, the more coagulating current will be required while treating it. Very large or deep lesions like giant condylomas may be better treated with surgery. Pedunculated lesions like acrochordons can be removed by electrosection of the pedicle. Electrosection is also used in place of scalpel incision to remove lesions like compound melanocytic nevi. The most common electrosurgical mode used in day-to-day practice is electrodessication. Sessile lesions like verruca vulgaris, verruca plana, molluscum contagiosum, syringomas, seborrheic keratosis, dermatosis papulosa nigra, trichoepithelioma and actinic keratosis can be treated successfully with this modality. Electrofulguration offers the best cosmesis and is appropriate for small intraepidermal lesions like milia and verruca plana. The authors like to use electrofulguration as the first step for many types of lesions traditionally treated with electrodessication. The subsequent crust is removed gently using a saline soaked gauze resulting in removal of the top layer of the epidermis. This allows better appreciation of the depth of a lesion, and can then be followed by electrodessication for deep lesions. This technique allows excellent cosmesis. For superficial lesions the crust can be left on, allowing it to drop off spontaneously in 3-5 days. This has the advantage of lesser pain during the recovery period and possibly faster healing as the crust acts as a natural cover to the skin healing underneath. However leaving the crust on prevents examination of the base which is very important in lesions like warts, molluscum and melanocytic nevi where recurrences often occur from residual infection or melanocytes. Electrocoagulation is best suited for vascular lesions like cherry and spider angiomas, telangiectasias and pyogenic granulomas. Since it causes tissue destruction well removed from the site of electrode application, both vertically and horizontally, it is also very useful for treating the base of basal cell carcinomas after curettage and for lesions like sebaceous hyperplasia where the lesion extends well into the dermis.

While removing a mucosal cyst, use the cut mode to excise the cyst in a circumferential manner working at the junction of the cyst wall and the normal mucosa. The base should be then electrofulgurated. For a cutanes cyst, the electrosurgical probe is used as a scalpel and the cut mode is selected. A small electrosurgical incision is given across the length of the cyst after which blunt dissection and careful current application is used to dissect the cyst from the surrounding tissue. With proper technique the entire cyst can be removed without rupture.

The lesions of lymphangioma need to be dessicated at the base. Just cauterizing the vesicles is not enough. There is always some degree of scarring with effective electrodessication in this indication. Even after this the recurrence rate is quite high, because of the presence of deeper cisterns.

Choice of Electrodes: Choice of electrode is important in determining final result. In general straight wire electrodes are used for cutting and fine tissue removal, loop/diamond/triangular planning electrodes are used for removing heavier tissue, tissue planning and contouring, and ball electrodes are useful for coagulation. Increased power settings are required for an electrode in motion and less power for a stationary electrode. As a rule of thumb the power used should be the minimum required to accomplish the given task. Excess power will cause sparking and charring while too little power will cause electrode drag. Correct power setting only comes with experience and for new practitioners practicing on moist lean meat at room temperature can be valuable.

With electrodessication and electrocoagulation the electrode should be in contact with the tissue before the current is applied and current flow should cease before the electrode is removed.[3] This prevents arcing of the current and inadvertent electrofulguration of vital structures like the cornea while operating on periorbital syringomas for example. For electrosection the electrode should be activated and held very close to the tissue (actual contact can be made but is not essential). This results in current concentration in the tip and a rapid cutting effect. The electrode should be moved with a feathery touch and deliberate slow speed followed by removal of the electrode and lastly deactivation of the current. There is no danger of current arcing here, as the spark gap circuit is not the current source.

As mentioned earlier electrosurgery should not be used in patients with cardiac pacemakers since malfunction of the pacemaker can occur. Electrocautery is the procedure of choice in such patients.

POSTOPERATIVE INSTRUCTIONS

Post-procedure application of an antibiotic ointment is good practice. This or petrolatum jelly should be continued for 5–7 days since wounds heal best in a moist environment. Sunscreen use is a must for photo-exposed areas like the face and arms, to minimize post-inflammatory erythema and hyperpigmentation. Erythema generally lasts 2–4 weeks but hyperpigmentation, if it occurs, can last many months without treatment. Some practitioners prefer priming the skin with tretinoin or hydroquinone for 2 weeks prior to procedure to minimize this side effect. Oral antibiotics and painkillers are only required when large lesions like a basal cell carcinoma, squamous cell carcinoma or certain pyogenic granulomas are treated.

COMPLICATIONS

Most complications are related to poor operative technique and include gouging of tissue, deep cuts and burns. Bleeding can be minimized with appropriate current setting but small arterioles can sometimes be nicked and this requires pressure packing for 10 minutes to stop the bleeding. Alternatively, if the bleeder can be located a short burst of a coagulating current can stop the bleeding. As with all invasive procedures secondary infection can occur as a result of infection either during the procedure or after. Some pain is common for 1-2 days after electrosurgery but this is usually mild and can be managed with NSAIDs.

PRECAUTIONS

Recent research has shown that the electrosurgical plume can contain live viruses (e.g. HPV) and is possibly infective.[45,46] Hence a facemask and goggles are an absolute must while treating infective lesions like warts and mollusca. If possible patients should be screened for HIV, Hepatitis B and Hepatitis C but this Smoke evacuator ' (Fig. 6)' is not always possible in busy practices. A smoke evacuator can thus be a valuable investment. If this is not available, the procedure room should have an exhaust fan. In addition, a small hand held fan should be used to blow the electrosurgical plume away from the operator's face.

Spirit or other flammable cleansers like acetone should never be used in an electrosurgical field since they can catch fire when a current is applied. The bright lights of an operating theater may make this blue flame nearly invisible resulting in extensive burns before the problem is detected. Electrosurgical machines also should not be placed near oxygen cylinders due to the risk of an explosion.

STERILIZATION OF ELECTROSURGICAL PROBES

Contrary to what was previously believed electrosurgical electrodes are not self-sterilizing, and herpes and hepatitis virus transfer has been proven to occur through contaminated electrodes.[47,48] Recent recommendations are thus for the use of disposable electrodes. This is quite expensive, so a more economical alternative is to sterilize the electrodes with glutaraldehyde or another suitable method of sterilization like ethylene oxide gas before use. Glutaraldehyde is non-corrosive to metal and does not damage rubber or plastic. The minimum exposure time with glutaraldehyde is 20 min (kills most bacteria, viruses, mycobacteria, and fungi at concentrations > 2%) but electrodes should preferably be immersed for at least 3 hours to make sure Bacillus and Clostridial spores are inactivated as well.[51]

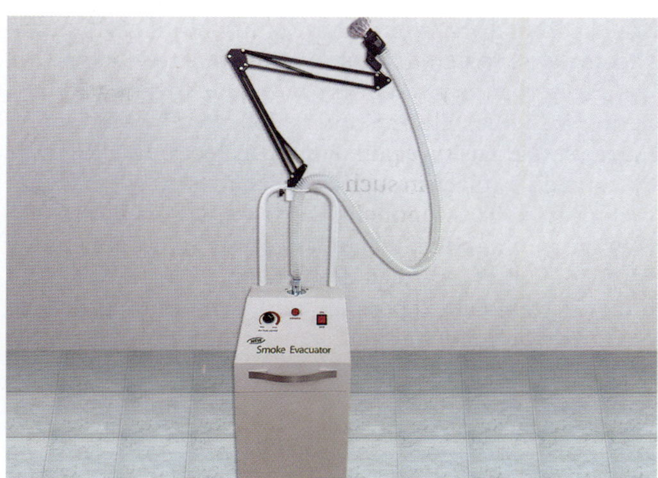

Fig. 6: Smoke Evacuator.

Though most ESUs are hardy machines requiring little maintenance they should be inspected by the vendor if there is any sign of malfunction such as excess heating or sparking. The unit must always be properly grounded when in use and the wire connections should be in good repair.

ELECTROSURGERY IN PATIENTS WITH AN IMPLANTABLE ELECTRONIC DEVICES

Implantable electronic devices (IED) are now being used for a number of conditions, the most common being cardiac IEDs (pacemakers and defibrillators) and cochlear implants. Other IEDs include vagal nerve stimulators, sacral nerve stimulators, spinal cord stimulators, and gastric pacemakers. Electromagnetic waves from an ESU can theoretically cause temporary IED device malfunction. However modern IEDs have numerous safety mechanisms to prevent this from happening. Furthermore most complications have been observed only with high-powered surgical ESUs and office based ESUs are much safer. However because of the theoretical risk, certain precautions are prudent. Turn off the IEDs when this can be done safely for the length of the procedure (e.g. deep brain stimulators, spinal cord stimulators and gastric pacemakers). When this can not be done (cardiac IEDs), use Electrocautery whenever possible. The second best option is Bipolar Electrosurgery, followed by Monopolar Electrosurgery using a patient return electrode (PRE). The PRE should be place in such a fashion that the current path excludes the IED. Monopolar Electrosurgery without a PRE is not recommended. Electrosurgery should not be done within 15 cm of a cardiac device without prior clearance from a cardiologist. If possible cardiac monitoring should be done when any method apart from Electrocautery is used.[43, 44, 49]

Tips

- Pedunculated lesions like acrochordons can be removed by electrosection of the pedicle. Electrosection is also used in place of scalpel incision to remove lesions like compound melanocytic nevi.
- Electrofulguration offers the best cosmesis and is appropriate for small intraepidermal lesions like milia and verruca plana.
- Electrocoagulation is best suited for vascular lesions like cherry and spider angiomas, telangiectasia and pyogenic granulomas.
- The power used should be the minimum required to accomplish the procedure.
- Avoid Monopolar devices that do not use a Patient Return Electrode (e.g. Hyfrecator) in patients with Implantable Electrical Devices.

SUMMARY

- Electrosurgery is an effective modality for the treatment of a variety of skin lesions.
- A good understanding of the different waveforms that are generated and their purpose is essential to using it effectively. The most frequently used current serves a cutting function but also has coagulative effects thereby providing a bloodless incision.
- Four types of procedures can be done: electrodessication, electrofulguration, electrocoagulation and electrosection. Of these electrodessication and electrofulguration only require one electrode whereas electrocoagulation and electrosection require two. That is they are bipolar in nature.
- Contrary to popular belief the active electrode of an electrosurgical unit is not self-sterilizing and transmission of infection, particularly viral infection, can occur. Therefore the electrode tips should be sterilized with an appropriate method before use. Disposable tips are another option.
- The electrosurgical plume can also transmit infection and hence it is essential for the operating physician to wear a mask and gloves. A smoke evacuator is helpful in further decreasing the risk.

REFERENCES

1. Massarweh NN, Cosgriff N, Slakey DP. Electrosurgery: History, principles, and current and future uses. J Am Col Surgeons. 2006;202(3);520-30.
2. Goldwyn RM. Bovie: The man and the machine. Ann Plast Surg. 1979;2:135-53.
3. Blankenship ML. Electrosurgery, electrocautery and electrolysis. Int J Dermatol. 1979;18:443-52.
4. Moak E. Electrosurgical unit safety: the role of the perioperative nurse. AORN J. 1991;53:744-52.
5. Jackson JD. Classical Electrodynamics, 3rd edition. Wiley. 1999; p. 238.
6. Kelly HA, Ward GE. Electrosurgery. Philadelphia: WB Saunder Company; 1932:1-9.
7. Gibbs RC, Scheiner AM. Long-term follow-up evaluation of patients with electrosurgically treated warts. Cutis. 1978;21:383-4.
8. Choudhary ST. Treatment of an unusually large acrochordons by shave excision and electrodessication. J Cutan Aesthet Surg. 2008;1(1):21-2
9. Motley R. Skin tumours: seborrheic warts. Dermatol Pract. 1997;5:6-7.
10. Smith KJ, Skelton H. Molluscum contagiosum. Recent advances in pathogenetic mechanisms and new therapies. Am J Clin Dermatol. 2002;3:536-45.
11. Walton RG, Cox AJ. Electrodessication of pigmented nevi. Arch Dermatol. 1963;87:342-9.
12. Drake LA, Ceilley RL, Cornelison RL, et al. Guidelines of care of actinic keratoses. Committee on Guidelines of Care. J Am Acad Dermatol. 1995;32:95-8.
13. Schwartz RA. The actinic keratosis: A perspective and update. Dermatol Surg. 1997;23(11):1009-19.
14. Jeffes EW, Tang EH. Actinic keratosis: Current treatment options. Am J Clin Dermatol. 2000;1(3):167-79.
15. Goldman MP, Weiss RA, Brody HJ, et al. Treatment of facial telangiectasias with sclerotherapy, laser surgery, and/or electrodessication: a review. J Dermatol Surg Oncol. 1980;6 (10):794-5.
16. Rowland Payne CM, Somaiah N, Neal AJ, Glees JP. The Hyfrecator: a treatment for radiation induced telangiectasia in breast cancer patients. Br J Radiol 2005;78(926):143-6.
17. Karma P, Benedetto AV. Intralesional electrodessication of syringomas. Dermatol Surg. 1997;23:921-4
18. Bunse T, Kuhn A, Groth W, Mahrie G. Therapeutic problem. Angiolymphoid hyperplasia with eosinophilia. Hautartz. 1993;44:225-8.
19. Malakar S, Malakar RS. Crushing assisted shave excision and electrodessication: A novel approach to treat granuloma pyogenicum. Indian J Dermatol Venereol Leprol. 2000;66(1):29-31.
20. Ghodsi SZ, Raziel M, Taheri A, et al. Comparison of cryotherapy and curettage for the treatment of pyogenic granuloma: a randomized trial. Br J Dermatol. 2006;154 (4):671-5.
21. Gim YC. Office surgery: electrodessication in syringomas and trichoepithelioma. Singapore Med J. 1987;28(4):336-7.
22. Silverman MK, Kopf AW. Grin CM, et al. Recurrence rates of treated basal cell carcinomas. Part 2: curettage-electrodessication. J Dermatol Surg Oncol 1991;17:720-6.

Sheridan AT, Dawber RPR. Curettage, electrosurgery and skin cancer. Australas J Dermatol. 2000;41:19-30.

24. Werlinger KD, Upton G, Moore AY. Recurrence rates of primary nonmelanoma skin cancers treated by surgical excision compared to electrodessication-curettage in a private dermatological practice. Dermatol Surg. 2002; 28(12): 1138-42.

25. Reschly MJ, Shenefelt PD. Controversies in skin surgery: electrodessication and curettage versus excision for low risk, small, well-differentiated squamous cell carcinomas. J Drugs Dermatol. 2010;9(7):773-6.
26. Ahmed I, Berth-Jones J, Charles-Homes S, et al. Comparison of cryotherapy with curettage in the treatment of Bowen's disease: a prospective study. Br J Dermatol. 2000;143: 759-66.
27. Cox NH, Eedy DJ, Morton CA. Guidelines for management of Bowen's disease. Br J Dermatol. 1999;141:633-41.
28. Schwartz RA, Janniger CK. Bowenoid papulosis. J Am Acad Dermatol. 1991;24(2 Pt 1):261-4.
29. Nedwich JA. Evaluation of curettage and electrodessication in the treatment of keratoacanthomas. Australas J Dermatol. 1991;32:137-41.
30. Buljan M, Poduje S, Situm M, et al. Multiple angiokeratomas of the vulva: Case report and literature review. Acta Dermatovenereol Croat. 2010;18(4):271-5.
31. Novick NL. Angiokeratoma vulvae. J Am Acad Dermatol. 1985;12(3):561-3.
32. Greenbaum SS, Krull EA, Watnick K. Comparison of CO_2 laser and electrosurgery in the treatment of Rhinophyma. J Am Acad Dermatol. 1988;18:363-8.
33. Clark DP, Hanke CW. Electrosurgical treatment of Rhinophyma. J Am Acad Dermatol. 1990;22:831-7.
34. Pasricha JS, Nayyar KC. Fox-Fordyce disease in the postmenopausal period treated successfully with electrocoagulation. Dermatologica. 1973;147:271-3.
35. Noyes AWF. A case of lymphangioma circumscriptum. Br Med J. 1993;1:1159.
36. Bader RS, Scarborough DA. Surgical pearl: intralesional electrodessication of sebaceous hyperplasia. J Am Acad Dermatol. 2000;42(1 Pt 1):127-8.
37. Gambini C, Rongioletti F. Recurrent Spitz nevus. Case report and review of the literature. Am J Dermatopathol. 1994; 16(4):409-13.
38. Stone KM, Becker TM, Hadgu A, Kraus SJ. Treatment of external genital warts: a randomized clinical trial comparing podophyllin, cryotherapy, and electrodessication. Genitourin Med. 1990;66:16-19.
39. Jolly WH Jr, Seabury JH. Infections with Mycobacterium marinum. Arch Dermatol. 1972;106:32-6.
40. Richards RN, McKenzie MA, Meharg GE. Electroepilation (electrolysis) in hirsutism. 35,000 hours' experience on the face and neck. J Am Acad Dermatol. 1986;15(4 Pt 1):693-7.
41. Dincer D, Koc E, Erbil AH, Kose O. Effectiveness of low-voltage radiofrequency in the treatment of Xanthelasma palpebrarum: a pilot study of 15 cases. Dermatol Surg. 2010; 36(12):1973-8.
42. Ozlugedik S, Titiz A, Yilmas YF, et al. Radiofrequency excision of a larger postcricoid mucous cyst. B-ENT. 2007: 3(2):79-81.
43. Riordan AT, Gamache C, Fosko SW. Electrosurgery and cardiac devices. J Am Acad Dermatol. 1997;37(2 Pt 1):250-5.
44. Yu SS, Tope WD, Grekin RC. Cardiac devices and electromagnetic interference revisited: new radiofrequency technologies and implications for dermatologic surgery. Dermatol Surg. 2005;31(8 Pt 1):932-40.
45. Bigony L. Risks associated with exposure to surgical smoke plume: a review of the literature. AORN J. 2007;86(6):1021-4
46. Ulmer BC. The hazards of surgical smoke. AORN J. 2008; 87(4):735-8.
47. Clover GB, Peutherer JF. Herpes simplex virus dissemination by Hyfrecator electrodes. Br J Dermatol. 1987;177:627.
48. Sheretz EF et al. Transfer of Hepatitis B virus by contaminated needle electrodes after electrodessication in simulated use. J Am Acad Dermatol. 1986;15(6):1246.
49. Voutsalath MA, Bichakjian CK, Pelosi F, et al. Electrosurgery and implantable electronic devices: Review and implications for office based procedures. Dermatol Surg. 2011;37 (7):889-99.
50. Steinsapir KD, Woodward JA. Chlorhexidine keratitis: Safety of chlorhexidine as a facial antiseptic. Dermatol Surg. 2016.
51. Centers for Disease Control and Prevention (CDC). Guideline for Disinfection and Sterilization in Healthcare Facilities, 2008.

Chapter

25

Radiofrequency in Dermatology

Yashwant Tawade, Ekta Romi

Key Messages 

- Radiofrequency uses radio waves at a frequency of 3.8 MHz.
- It is superior to electrosurgery as it has a coagulation mode, causes less heating and therefore less scarring.
- Radiofrequency can be used to treat a number of benign growths and some malignant growths.
- It has also been used in esthetic indications such as blepharoplasty and resurfacing.
- It should be used in caution in patients who are using implanted electrical devices such as pacemakers.

INTRODUCTION

Electrosurgery has been in practice for many years and has been an important asset to a Dermatologist. In electrosurgical units, household electric supply is modified by passing through oscillating circuit which increases its frequency.[1] Radiofrequency refers to high frequency alternating electrical current at the frequency range which is usually used for radio wave communications. The radiosurgical unit is recent addition which operates at a frequency of 3.8 MHz (Fig. 1). It is much more superior to electrocautery and has an advantage of coagulation mode. The minimal collateral damage with this instrument results in esthetically pleasant scars.

HISTORY[2]

In medical science, the use of electric current has been documented since the discovery of electricity. Initially, low voltage direct current was used in electrocauterization and similarly, it was also used to pass chemicals through skin. At the beginning of this century, very high frequency electrical current and voltage were used for fulguration and desiccation. Low frequency alternating currents were used in physiotherapy to cause contractures of muscle fibers. Major breakthrough was invention of electric transformer with the help of which it was possible to produce current of varying frequencies and voltages. Similarly, equipments with very high voltages and frequencies were developed. At the same time, it was found that alternating currents above certain frequency do not produce muscle contraction. This was the principal used in diathermy equipment. In these instruments, the electric current was passed through the patient and heat generated was used for both cutting and coagulation. Later operating room type devices were developed which operate from 500 to 2000 kHz. The instruments having this range make the electrode hot which contracts the tissue.[1] The recent development is the development of instruments having frequency above 3000 kHz (3 MHz), which does not heat the electrode. These instruments are called radiosurgery instruments as they operate at a frequency of 3.8 MHz, which is within the marine radio band.

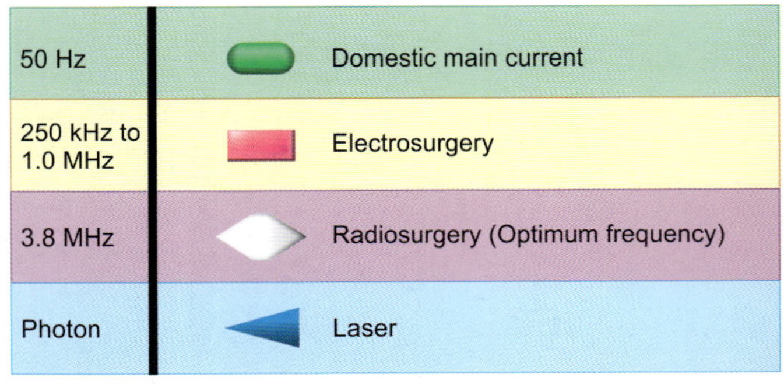

Fig. 1: Different frequencies with applications.

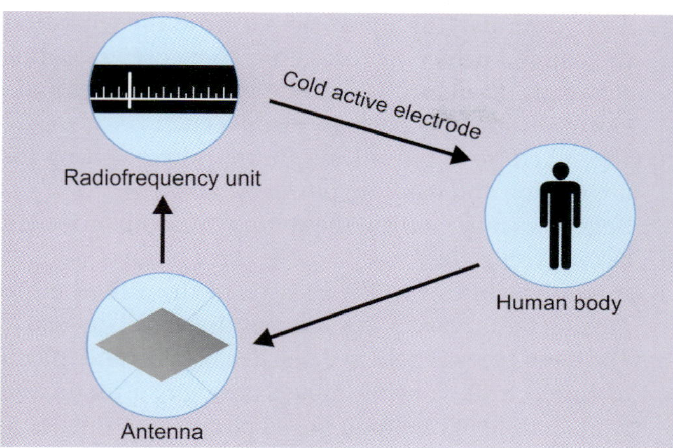

Fig. 2: Electrosurgery with radiofrequency current.

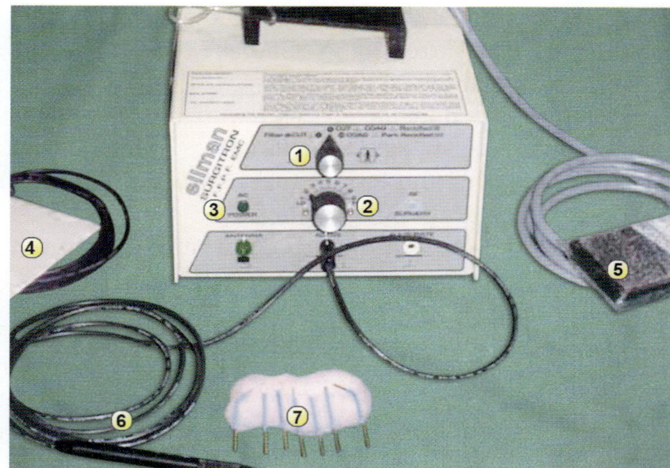

Fig. 4: Components of RF unit.

DIFFERENCES BETWEEN ELECTROSURGICAL CIRCUIT (RF) AND ELECTROCAUTERY CIRCUIT[3]

Radiofrequency

The electric current flows through patient's body and then to the return electrode and back to the Radiofrequency unit. The treatment electrode acts as a conductor that only passes current and therefore remains cool (Fig. 2).

Electric Cautery

The treatment electrode heats the metallic probe that is then applied to the tissue. In electrocautery no current flows through the patient's body (Fig. 3).

MECHANISM OF ACTION OF RADIOFREQUENCY WAVES

The radiofrequency unit consists of a transformer which changes the main voltage to a high voltage and high frequency. Resistance to the passage of the radio waves through tissue generates heat and that boils the water, resulting in steam ultimately causing cutting or coagulation of the tissue. The high frequency 3.8 MHz waveform is modified by filtering which results in continuous nonpulsation flow of current that produces cutting flow with minimum coagulation. Maness et al.[4] found that 3.8 MHz is the optimal frequency for cutting soft tissues. This high frequency current is then further modified by filtering and rectification to produce one of the four waveforms.

1. Fully-filtered rectified—90% cutting, 10% coagulation.
2. Fully-rectified waveforms—50% cutting, 50% coagulation.
3. Partially rectified waveforms for hemostasis, epilation and telangiectasia
4. Fulgurating current.[4]

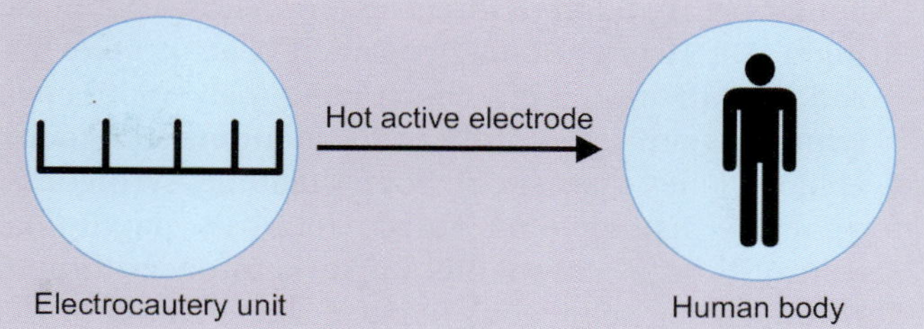

Fig. 3: Electrosurgery device.

RADIOSURGICAL UNIT (FIG. 4)

Basic Parts of Radiosurgical Unit

1. Power source
2. Oscillating circuit
3. Patient circuit-ground plate and hand piece.

Components of Radiofrequency Device

1. Switch to select waveform
2. Dial to select power setting
3. On Off indicator light
4. Antenna/Ground plate
5. Foot switch
6. Hand piece
7. Electrodes set—
    i. very thin wire loop of different shapes (round, triangular and diamond)
    ii. thin wire tip—needle electrode
    iii. ball electrode.

In all radiosurgery machines smoke is produced which has got an unpleasant smell of burning.

INDICATIONS OF RADIOFREQUENCY[5-16]

1. Infections: Verrucae and molluscum contagiosum.
2. Metabolic: Xanthelasma, xanthomas.

3. Benign skin conditions: Freckles, dermatoses papulosa nigra (DPN), granuloma pyogenicum, acne, acrochorodon (skin tags), milia, cherry angiomas, spider nevi, lymphangioma circumscriptum, adenoma sebaceum, Hailey-Hailey disease, trichoepithelioma, syringoma, apocrine histiocytoma, stucco keratosis, papilloma, neurofibroma, cutaneous horn, keratoacanthoma, rhinophyma, sebaceous hyperplasia, steatocystoma multiplex.
4. Senile skin conditions: Actinic keratosis, seborrheic keratosis and senile lentigines.
5. Nail procedures: Nail matrixectomies, surgical hemostasis of ingrown toe nail and onychogryphosis.
6. Cosmetic indications: Mole removal, telangiectasia, unwanted hair removal, scar revision and resurfacing, earlobe repair, development of flaps, oculoplastic procedures and blepharoplasty.
7. Malignant skin tumors: Squamous cell carcinoma, basal cell carcinoma, dermatofibroma protuberans and carcinoma in situ lesions of skin and orogenital mucosa.

RADIOFREQUENCY IN COMBINATION WITH OTHER MODALITIES[6,17]

1. With cryotherapy for warts, small skin tags, seborrheic keratosis and cherry angiomas.
2. With diode laser for wrinkles, improvement of texture and treatment of facial venous malformations.
3. With sclerotherapy for acquired lymphangiectasis.

Patient Selection

1. Detailed history should be taken, e.g.
   i. Keloidal tendency, H/o blood thinning agents/ Antiplatelet drugs,
   ii. H/o herpes simplex (prophylactic acyclovir is needed),
   iii. H/o pace maker,
   iv. H/o previous local anesthesia
2. Counseling regarding limitations and complications
3. Tendency to hyperpigment.

Anesthesia

Most superficial lesions need only EMLA or injection Xylocaine 2% with or without adrenaline. For full face resurfacing sedation or general anesthesia is required.

Procedure

1. Consent
2. Preparation of site as per surgical technique. Avoid spirit.
3. Desired electrode is fixed to the hand piece.
4. The electrode is placed on the saline soaked gauze and RF machine is activated and deactivated.
5. After each use the tip of the electrode is wiped on the rough surface of the saline soaked gauze, thus removing all debris and dirt. This helps to clean the electrode and only partially disinfect it.
6. The machine is put on minimum power setting for fulguration and medium power for ablation.
7. Beginners may confirm the setting by trying on a soap cake or wet gauze.
8. It is advisable to wet the tissue with saline before passing radio waves. This reduces tissue resistance.
9. The hand piece is held in a pen like fashion and the tip of the electrode is swiftly moved through the tissue. The contact time of the tip of the electrode with the tissue should be very brief.
10. It is advisable to remove the lesions in parts for better cosmetic results.
11. After removing the lesion, finishing touches of flushing the area with surrounding skin has to be done using different electrodes.
12. Holding the pedunculated lesion with forceps helps to minimize the tissue damage (Fig. 5).
13. After removing the lesion, the area is cleaned and dressed with antiseptic dressing.
14. Most of the time, prophylactic antibiotics are not needed except in case of infected lesions.
15. Analgesics may be given if needed.
16. Normal healing time is 8 to 15 days depending on type, size and site of lesion (Figs. 6A to C).
17. Post-procedure care instructed.

FACTORS AFFECTING THE RESULTS OF RADIOFREQUENCY[18]

1. Electrode size—When a small electrode is used, lower power is required. The finest possible should be used to cut thin eyelid skin.

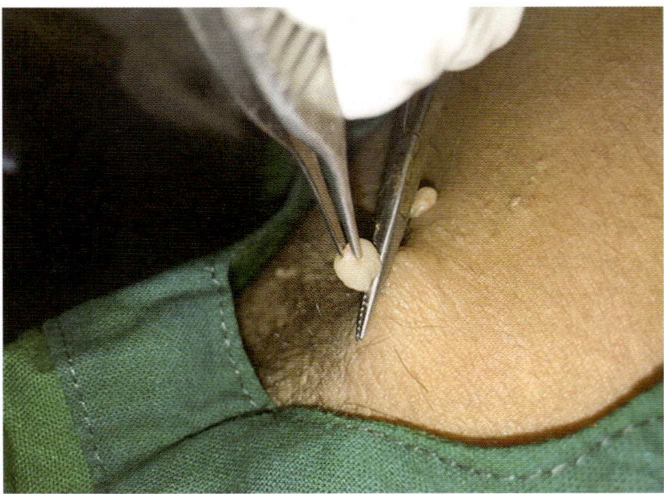

Fig. 5: Crushing the base of the lesions with an artery forceps.

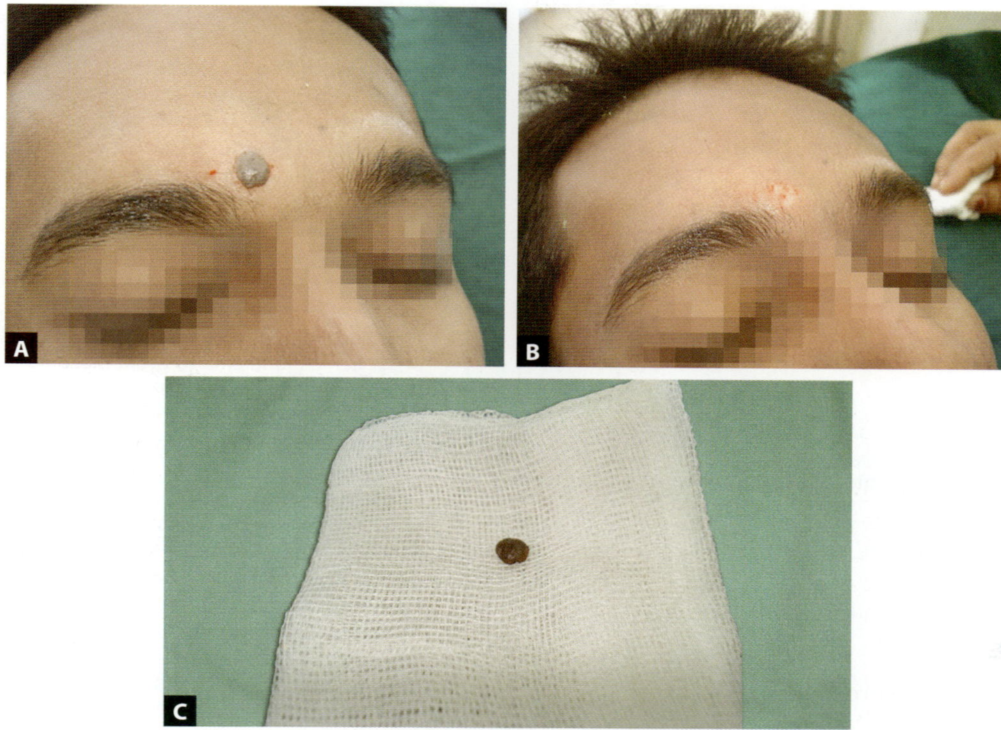

Figs. 6A to C: (A) Intradermal mole before radiofrequency excision; (B) Intradermal mole after radiofrequency excision; (C) Lesion after removal.

2. Electrode type—needle electrodes are good for incisions, loop electrodes to excise small skin lesions or to shave superficial lesions and diamond electrodes for elliptical excisions. For epilation of eye lashes or to treat facial telangiectasia use of insulated needles with active tip is better.
3. Power setting—When the power setting is correct, the electrode flows smoothly through the tissue with no charring or resistance. Insufficient power causes tissue adherence. Charring results from excessive power.
4. Waveform selection—as per Table 1.
5. Position of the electrode—Keeping the electrode tip perpendicular to the skin prevents excessive contact of the electrode. Care should be taken that uninsulated part of the probe should not touch the normal tissue.
6. Moistening of the lesion—It is advisable to moisten the lesion using cold saline soaks for easy movement of electrode through the tissue.
7. While using the cutting mode no pressure should be applied. Excessive pressure causes more damage to the tissue.
8. Electrode contact time—It should be minimized to prevent heat damage.

METHOD OF STERILIZATION OF ELECTRODES[7]

It has been recommended by CDC that, where facilities are available, hand piece and electrodes can be sterilized by ETO. However, where such facilities are not available 2% glutaraldehyde can be used. Even soaking the electrodes for more than 5 minutes is adequate for disinfection. Devices soaked in Glutaraldehyde must also be soaked in sterile water in order to remove residual amount of the germicide which can be harmful to tissue.

Precautions[6,19-23]

1. Radiofrequency is a relative contraindication in patients with pace makers. The return electrode should be placed between the device and the surgical site to reduce the chances of complications in patients with pacemakers or any other metal device. Alternate methods such as scalpel surgery, electrocautery or CO_2 laser should be preferred in patients with pacemakers.
2. Avoid spirit like inflammable antiseptics
3. Avoid the procedure in presence of oxygen cylinders due to risk of explosion.

Table 1: Properties of radio waves.

Sl. No.	Waveform	Function	Lateral spread
1.	Fully filtered, fully rectified	Pure cutting	Least
2.	Fully rectified	Cutting with coagulation	More
3.	Partially rectified	Coagulation	Most
4.	Fulguration	Superficial destruction and coagulation	More

4. Use smoke evacuator
5. Use disposable electrodes or properly sterilized electrodes.
6. Use foot switch intermittently with rest period gap. Continuous pressure damages the instrument and it is harmful to the patient.
7. Wear surgical masks and eye protection while treating lesions with HPV.

Complications

1. Laceration, deep wounds, hemorrhage
2. Sepsis
3. Scarring (Fig. 7)
4. Pigmentary changes
5. Transmission of infection from one patient to another through electrodes.
6. Burns
7. Cardiac arrhythmias.

Advantages

1. Simple and safe office procedure
2. Easy to operate
3. Wide range of application
4. Minimal bleeding
5. Insulated probes prevent excessive damage
6. Low maintenance cost.

Tips and Pearls

- Use radiofrequency on a wet lesion.
- Do not keep the foot handle pressed for a long time.
- Use the right energy and the right mode for optimum results.
- Always take history of pacemakers before performing radiofrequency.
- Use a smoke evacuator.
- For syringoma surface anesthesia is inadequate especially in the upper eyelid and hence infiltration anesthesia is required. This makes the lesions less prominent and therefore marking the lesions with a marker is necessary before infiltrating. Use the ball electrode as the lesion is roundish (Fig. 8)
- In Pyogenic granuloma to avoid bleeding, first coagulate the lesion from above so the lesions becomes hard, easy to remove with less bleeding.
- For moles, demarcation may be done with a straight probe before excision (Fig. 9).
- In case of mole with a few hair, after removal of the mole, the roots of the few hair may be destroyed with a straight probe without damaging the surrounding skin. A smooth finishing touch may be given using the straight probe on the borders.
- Bloodless field helps to precisely destroy the tissue without destroying the normal tissue. This can be achieved by using a rubber band, tourniquet or eye of the artery forceps (Figs. 10 and 11).
- For small size superficial lesions fine tip electrode and contact method in cutting mode with low power gives better results with less collateral damage.
- For large size superficial lesions large tip electrode with fulguration mode with medium power is preferred.
- For medium depth lesions medium to large tip electrode, contact method is preferable.
- For deep infiltrated lesions large tip electrode with contact method and cutting mode is recommended (Figs. 12A and B).

OTHER USES OF RADIOFREQUENCY TECHNOLOGY[23-25]

Radiofrequency technology has now been used in esthetic medicine for treatment of skin rejuvenation and acne scars. It is different from lasers as it uses electric current rather than light. It is independent of specific chromophore, therefore, it is safe for all types of skin. Radiofrequency induces an electrothermal reaction in targeted tissue, the pattern of which depends on resistance of tissue. There are various devices like unipolar, bipolar, multipolar, microneedling fractional RF for various treatments in esthetic medicine. (Details of nonablative radiofrequency was discussed in another chapter in the previous edition Chapter 56).

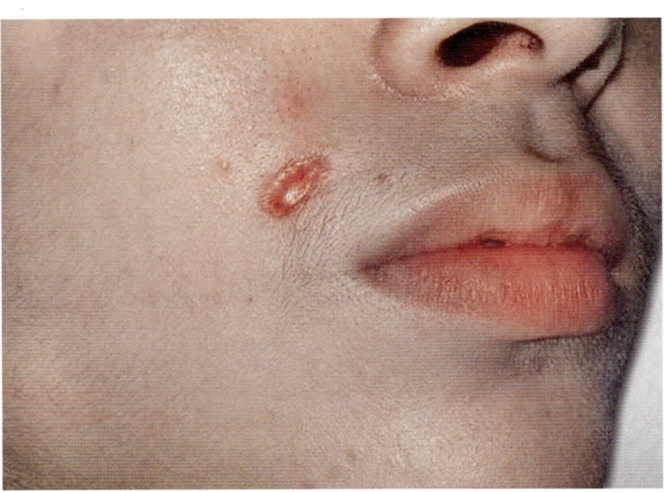

Fig. 7: Scarring produced by radiofrequency.

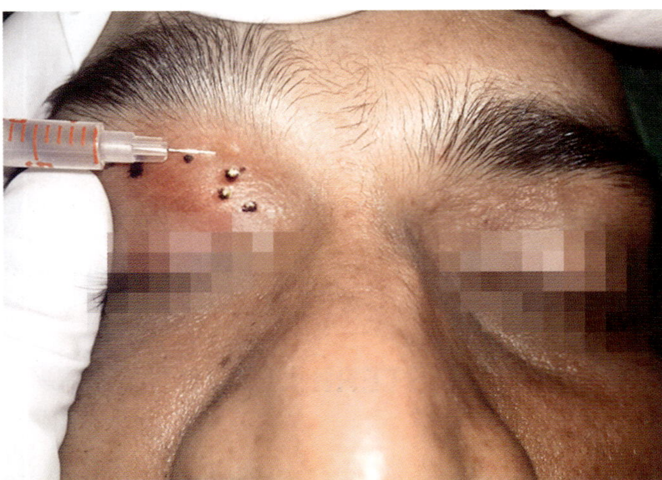

Fig. 8: Syringomas marked before infiltration.

Appendix 1 provides details of parameters for different skin conditions.

Appendix 2 shows a model consent form for radiofrequency procedure.

CONCLUSION

Radiofrequency is a better tool as compared to electrocautery and has advantages like less bleeding, cutting as well as coagulation ability, minimal tissue trauma, faster healing and good esthetic results (Figs. 12A and B).

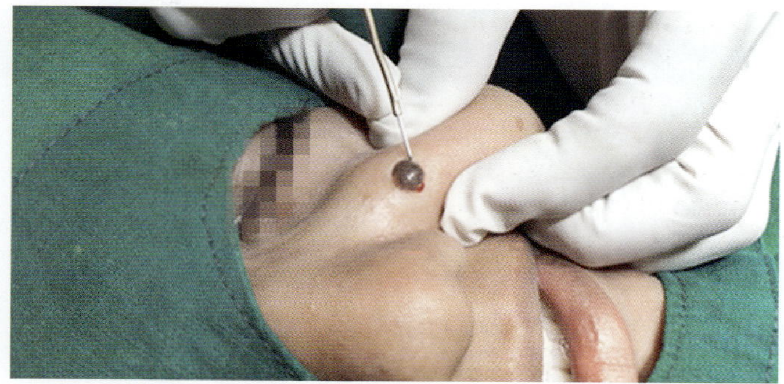

Fig. 9: Demarcation of the mole with a straight probe.

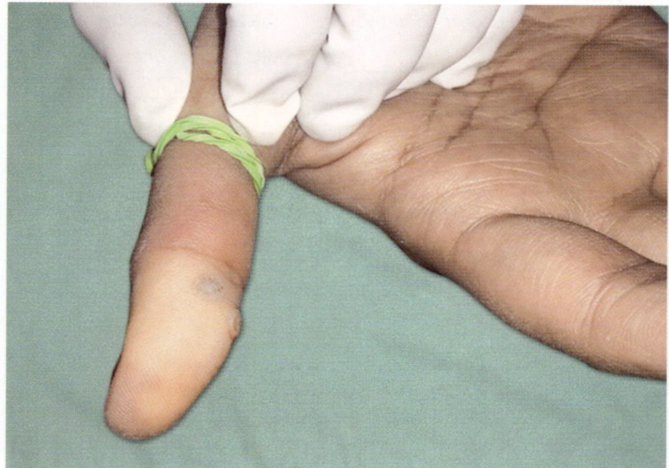

Fig. 10: Use of rubber band to achieve bloodless field.

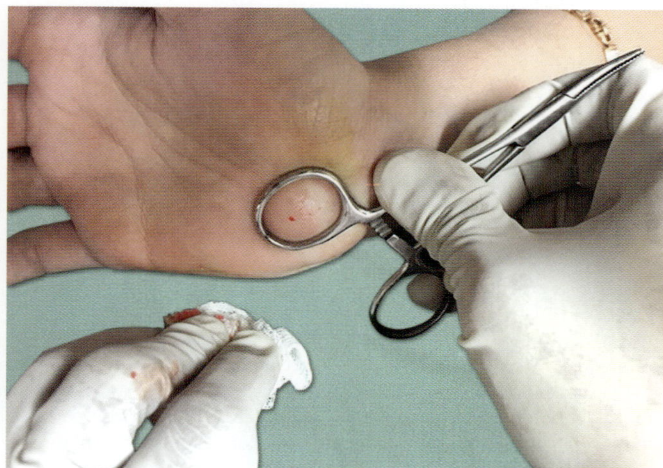

Fig. 11: Use of artery forceps for bloodless field.

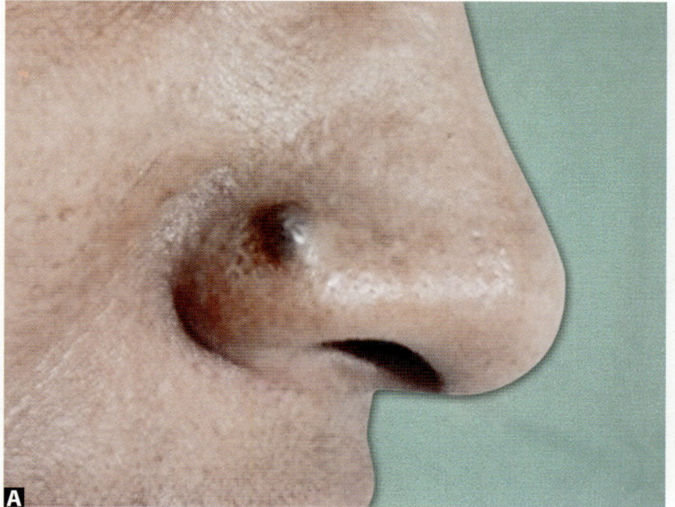

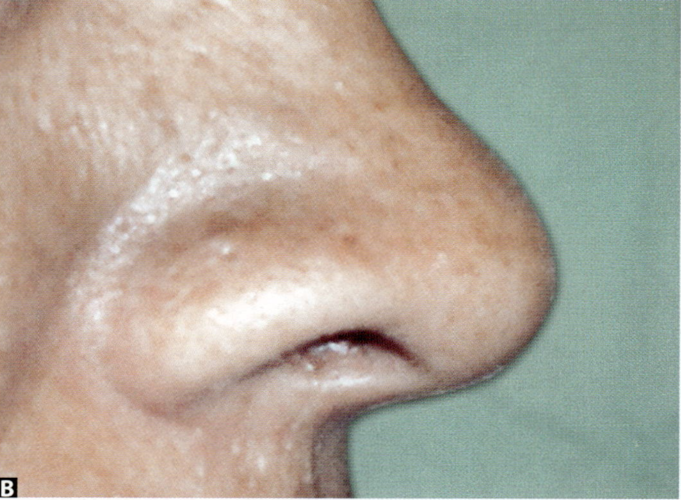

Figs. 12A and B: (A) Intradermal mole before removal; (B) Intradermal mole on nose after excision. Note the excellent esthetic results.

Appendix 1: Indications, anesthesia, power settings and type of electrode while doing radiofrequency surgery.[7]

Indications	*Anesthesia*	*Power settings*	*Type of electrode*
DPN V Plana Molluscum	Xylocaine 2%	Between 1.5 and 2.5 Cut +coagulate in fulguration	Narrow, sharp tipped
Verrucae			Angled with a sharp tip
Epidermal nevi Mole Seborrheic keratosis Skin tags	Xylocaine 2%	Between 2.5 and 3 Cut + Coagulate Coagulation of the base for hemostasis	Wire loop Small ball tip
Granuloma pyogenicum	Xylocaine 2%	Between 3.0 and 3.5 Coagulate	Small ball tip
Rhinophyma/ Resurfacing	Xylocaine 2% Ice packs	Between 2.5 and 3 Cut + Coagulate Coagulation of the base for hemostasis	Wire loop Small ball tip
Epilation	EMLA and Ice pack	Between 1.5 and 2	Epilation microneedle

Appendix 2: Consent form for radiofrequency surgery.[7]

I ______________________________Age __________Sex______,

here by authorize Dr.________________ to operate on myself or on

______________________________, who is my__________ (relation),

with radiofrequency surgery for the treatment of ____________________ ____________________, Dr ______________ has explained the procedure(s), technique and I understand the same. I consent to the administration of any anesthesia considered necessary or indicated in the judgment of the surgeon and/or anesthetist. My Physician / Surgeon / Anesthetist has/ have adequately explained to me about the alternative available treatments for this condition, possible outcome, risk involved and possible consequences associated with this procedure / surgery, and also about the prognosis if this procedure / surgery is not done. I have understood that fully.

It has been also explained to me by Dr____________ that during the course of the procedure / surgery, unforeseen condition may be revealed, that may necessitate intervention or an extension of the procedure(s). I therefore, authorize my surgeon, his/her assistants, anesthetist, or his/her designees to perform such procedure(s) if the need arises. I authorize the examination by an authorized pathologist, of the tissue excised during the surgery and/or disposal of such tissue in accordance with the clinic / hospital policies. I also give full consent to take pre and post operative clinical photographs / video shooting before, during and after the procedure, for the purpose of continuing medical education, publication and presentation in medical conferences. I understand that, this will remain confidential. All my questions have been fully answered to my fullest satisfaction.

I certify that I have read and fully understood the above consent. All the blanks or statements requiring insertion or completion were duly filled in before I signed.

Signature of patient/ Guardian — Signature of Doctor

Name & Address:

Tel number:

Signature & Name of Witness

REFERENCES

1. Bridestine JB. Use of ultra-high frequency Electrosurgery (Radiofrequency) for cosmetic surgical procedures. Dermatol Surg. 1998;24:397-400.
2. Brown JS, Ost J. Radiosurgery for minor operations in general practice. Cosmetic Dermatology. 2000;33-6.
3. Taheri A, Mansoori P, Sandoval LF, et al. Electrosurgery: part I. Basics and Principles. J Am Acad Dermatol. 2014;70 (4):591.e1-14.
4. Mane5s WL, Roeber FW, Clark RE, et al. Histological evaluation of electrosurgery with varying frequency and wave forms. J Prosthetic Dent. 1978;40:304-8.
5. Pollack SV. Clinical applications. Electrosurgery of the skin. 1st edn. New York: Churchill Livingstone; 1991;27-9.
6. Sachdeva S, Dogra A. Radiofrequency ablation in Dermatology. Indian J Dermatol. 2007;5293:134-7.
7. Mutalik S. Standard guidelines for electrosurgery with radiofrequency waves. Indian J Dermatol, Venereal Leprol. 2009;75(suppl 2):83-9.
8. Valinsky MS. Treatment of verrucae via radiowaves surgery. J Am Pediatric Med Assoc. 1990;80:482-8.
9. Wyre HW. Extirpation of warts by a loop cautery and cutting current. J Dermatol Surg Oncol. 1977;3:520-22.
10. Swaroop MR, Nischal KC, Gowda CMR, et al. Radiofrequency ablation of adenoma sebaceum. J Cutan Aesthet Surg. 2008;1(2):2:89-91.
11. Nandini AS, Mysore V. Hailey-Hailey disease: a novel method of management by radiofrequency surgery. J Cutan Aesthet Surg. 2008;1(2):92-3.
12. Hanumanthiah HC. Radiosurgical ablation of solitary trichoepithelioma. J Cutan Aesthet Surg. 2008;1(1):27-8.
13. Clarke DP, Hanke CW. Electrosurgical treatment of rhinophyma. J Am Acad Drematol. 1990:22;831-7.
14. Choudhary S, Koley S, Salodkar A. A modified technique for Steatocystoma multiplex. J Cutan Aesthet Surg. 2010;3(1): 25-28.
15. Grekin RC, Tope WD, Yarbororough JM, et al. Electrosurgical facial resurfacing. Arch Dermatol. 2000;136:1309-16.
16. Patidar S. Excision of basal cell carcinoma with radiofrequency ablation. J Cutan Aesthet Surg. 2008;1(1):29-30.
17. Khunger Niti. Combination technique of radiofrequency ablation with sclerotherapy in acquired lymphangiectasis of the vulva. J Cutan Aesthet Surg. 2009;2(1):33-5.
18. Raus P, Mestens E. Evaluation of radiosurgery as a cosmetic surgery technique. Int J Aesthet Restorative Surg. 1997;5(2): 96-100.
19. Pollack SV. Potential hazards of electrosurgery. Electrosurgery of the skin. 1st edition, New York: Churchill Livingstone; 1991;71-2.
20. Sebben JE. The hazards of electrosurgery. J Am Acad Dermatol. 1987;16:869.
21. Sebben JE. Electrosurgery and cardiac pacemakers. J Am Acad Dermatol. 1983;9:457.
22. Mutalik S. Radiofrequency in Dermatosurgery. J Cutan Aesthet Surg. 2008;1(2):94.
23. Taheri A. Mansoori P, Sandoval LF, et al. Electrosurgery: part II. Technology, applications and safety of electrosurgical devices. J Am Acad Dermatol. 2014;70(4):607.e1-12.
24. Gold M, Biron J. Treatment of acne scars by fractional bipolar radiofrequency energy. J Cosmet Laser Ther. 2012;14:172-8.
25. Chandrashekar BS, Sriram R, Mysore R. Evaluation of Microneedling Fractional radiofrequency for treatment of Acne Scars. J Cutan Aesthet Surg. 2014; 2(7):93-7.

Chapter 26

Cryotherapy

Sujay Khandpur

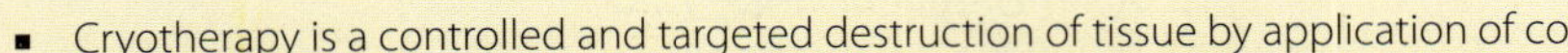

Key Messages

- Cryotherapy is a controlled and targeted destruction of tissue by application of cold.
- It is a simple, cost-effective, efficacious and esthetically acceptable modality for treatment of various dermatoses.
- It can be used safely in elderly patients and in pregnant women.
- It is indicated in the treatment of a wide variety of skin conditions including benign tumors, acne, pigmented lesions, viral infections, inflammatory dermatoses, infectious disorders and various premalignant and malignant tumors.
- Cryotherapy is an OPD procedure with limited complications.

INTRODUCTION

Cryotherapy is a controlled and targeted destruction of diseased tissue by application of a cold substance. It is used for the treatment of diverse benign lesions and well-circumscribed premalignant and malignant tumors.

In the present age, despite the advent of several ablative procedures like radiofrequency or laser therapy, cryosurgery continues to occupy a very important position in the therapeutic armamentarium of a dermatologist. It is a very safe, inexpensive, reproducible, repeatable and simple office procedure. It requires short preparation time, is a sutureless procedure with minimal risk of infection and no anesthesia is usually required. It can be performed at any age including elderly patients with pacemakers in whom electrocautery is contraindicated, those on anti-coagulants, patients allergic to anesthetic agents, patients with transmissible conditions such as HIV and hepatitis, during pregnancy and over most of the body sites. It provides high healing rates even in difficult areas with excellent cosmetic results if performed appropriately. In view of all these advantages, it is regarded as a treatment of choice by many dermatologists for various benign and malignant dermatoses.

HISTORY OF CRYOTHERAPY

The Egyptians used cold to treat injuries and inflammation as early as 2500 BC. In 1840s, Arnott used salt solutions containing crushed ice at –18° to –24°C to freeze breast, cervical, and skin cancers. In 1892, James Dewar of Great Britain designed the first vacuum flask, which facilitated storage and handling of liquefied gases. The first clinical application of liquid air (–190°C) was in 1889 by Campbell White of New York, who used either a swab, spray, or a brass roller device to treat diverse skin conditions, including lupus erythematosus, herpes zoster, chancroid, warts, and epitheliomas. Solidified carbon dioxide (–78.5°C), which was commonly used as a refrigerant and easily obtained where soda-fountain supplies were sold, was introduced into clinical use by Dr William Pusey of Chicago. He treated warts, vascular nevi, lupus erythematosus, lupus vulgaris, and epitheliomas. In the 1920s, Irving and Turnacliff described good results of liquid oxygen (–182.9°C) in warts lichen planus, but it was hazardous as it was combustible. Following World War II, liquid nitrogen (–196°C) became commercially available. In 1950, this cryogen was introduced into clinical practice by Dr Ray Allington, who described the technique of using cotton swabs dipped in liquid nitrogen for treatment of a variety of non-neoplastic skin diseases. Modern cryo-surgery began through the collaborative work of Irving Cooper and Arnold Lee who built a cryosurgical probe that became the prototype. In 1967, Setrag Zacarian introduced a handheld self-pressurized device, which after some modifications became the first commercially available handheld cryosurgical device.

MECHANISM OF CRYOABLATION

Tissue destruction occurs as a result of rapid heat transfer from the tissue causing tissue injury, vascular stasis and occlusion and inflammation.

On spraying the cryogen, there is rapid transfer of heat from the tissue to the cryogen with ice formation in the extracellular compartment. The extracellular solutes are concentrated, setting up an osmotic gradient with movement of fluid extracellularly and concentration of solutes within the cell leading to cell damage. The ice crystals also damage the cell membrane mechanically. Moreover, intracellular ice formation occurs damaging the organelles like mitochondria and endoplasmic reticulum. There is severe vasoconstriction and endothelial damage due to cold temperature leading to platelet aggregation and microthrombi formation producing ischemic necrosis of the tissue. There is inflammation in response to cell death causing further destruction.

Necrosis occurs at the center of the treated area, when temperature reaches around 40°C. However, away from the center, where temperature is higher, only partial destruction but sufficient to cause cell death by apoptosis, occurs. These temperatures can be measured by using a thermocouple and thereby achieve precision in management.

There is differential sensitivity of each cell or tissue to cryodamage, with melanocytes and deeper epidermal cell layers being very sensitive and dermal collagen being cryoresistant. The extent of damage is determined by duration of spray, technique, and the cryogen used. While rapid freezing leads to quick cell death, slow thawing causes the prolongation of the freezing time, leading to improved results (called rapid freeze-slow thaw cycle). While a single freeze-thaw cycle may be adequate for small benign lesions, repeated cycles are needed for larger and malignant lesions.

CRYOTHERAPY FACILITY

Cryotherapy can be undertaken in a physician's office procedure room or minor theater with high degree of aseptic precautions. A fully equipped minor OT with good lighting, appropriate minimal sterilization and storage facilities is desirable.

The commonly used cryogens include:

Cryogen	*Boiling point*
Liquid nitrogen (most commonly used)	–196°C
Nitrous oxide	–89°C
Solidified CO_2 (Dry ice, CO_2 snow)	–78°C
Chlorodifluoromethane	–41°C
Dimethyl ether and propane	–24°C, –42°C

The cryogens, especially liquid nitrogen can be obtained from liquid nitrogen gas plants set up in various institutes or through various gas companies.

CRYOSURGERY EQUIPMENTS (FIG. 1)

1. *Cryogun/cryogen spray canister*: It is a portable, lightweight, handheld device with a controllable trigger to begin and end cooling.
   Portable tabletop devices are also available.
2. *Cryospray nozzle, cryoprobes, spray tips, neoprene or polystyrene cones.*

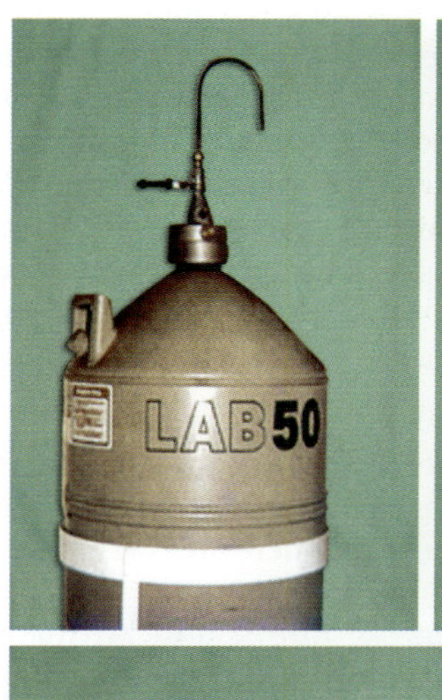

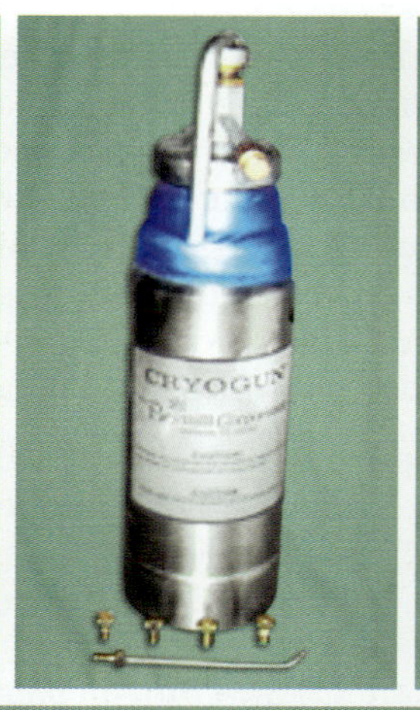

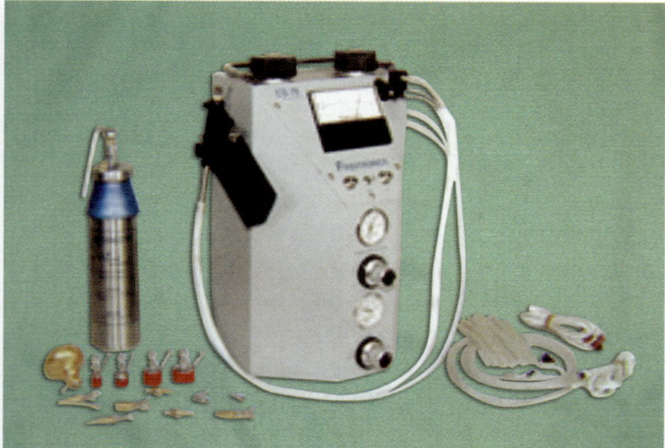
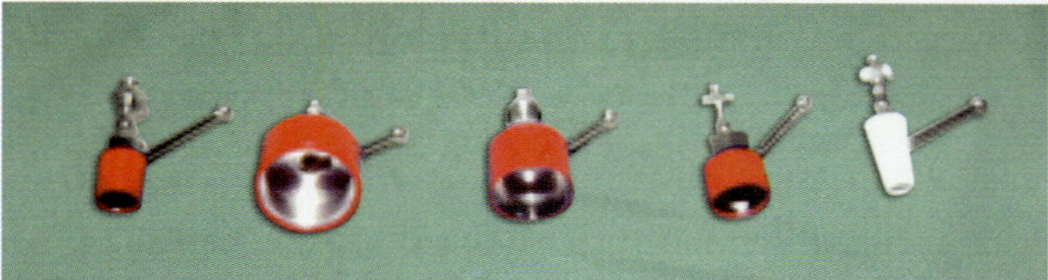
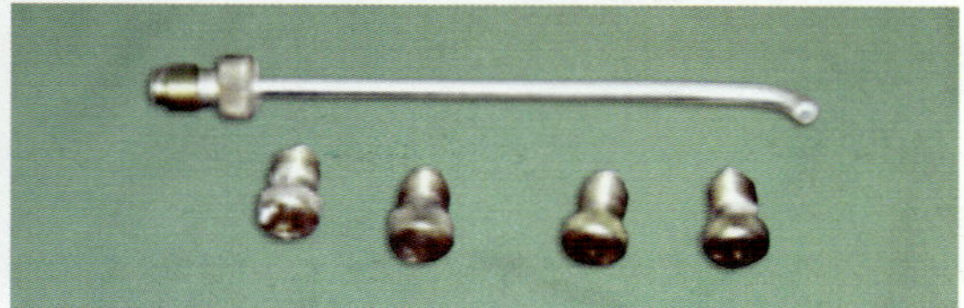

Fig. 1: Cryosurgery equipments—Cryogen storage cylinder, handheld cryogen-spray canister, cryoprobes, cryospray nozzles.

3. *Cryoprobe*: They are available in various shapes and sizes that get attached to the cryogen. They are cooled by the spray of the cryogen.
4. *Cryogen storage device*: They are metal cylinders/containers that store gaseous cryogens as compressed gas and have inbuilt internal pressure equalization mechanism, e.g. Dewar's gas container. The cryogen is transferred to the cryogun before the procedure by using a siphon or tilting the container to pour the cryogen into the gun via a funnel. Insulated gloves must be worn while transferring the cryogen, e.g. Brymill cryogenic system.

METHODOLOGY OF CRYOSURGERY

Counseling and Consent

A written informed consent is obtained from the patient after explaining the procedure, the achievable results, recurrence rate and various complications of the procedure. The consent form should mention the possibility of temporary postinflammatory blister formation and pigmentation alterations.

History Taking and Examination

A detailed history of general medical condition, previous treatment received for the condition with results and whether it is a primary or recurrent lesion, is taken. History of sensitivity to cold, cold urticaria, Raynaud's phenomenon or vascular insufficiency may be recorded. Physical examination to assess the skin type of the patient, lesional characteristics such as size, margin, location, depth, biological behavior and approximation to superficial nerves and previous treatment sites should be undertaken.

PREOPERATIVE PREPARATION

The area to be treated is exposed adequately and cleaned thoroughly with spirit or povidone-iodine. Usually, intralesional or topical anesthesia is not required. It may be used for malignant lesions since longer freeze time required to ablate deeper malignant tissue may produce severe pain. An anxious patient is counseled and an analgesic or antianxiety drug may be administered. The surrounding normal skin may be insulated to prevent spray of surrounding areas. Sites such as the eyes, nares and ears must be protected with goggles, gauze or padding.

TREATMENT

Different methods of applying the cryogen to the skin lesion include:

1. *Timed spot freeze technique*: The cryogen is sprayed directly on the lesion through an appropriate sized nozzle, which is chosen according to the size of the lesion. The nozzle is held 1 cm away from the skin surface and the cryogen sprayed in the center of the lesion until an ice ball forms that completely encompasses the lesion (confirmed by palpating between the fingers) and the desired margin is reached (Fig. 2). For adequate treatment, the lateral spread of freeze should extend at least 2 mm beyond the margin in benign lesion and 5 mm or more for malignant lesion. The spraying is continued for adequate duration (holding time) after which the lesion is allowed to thaw to complete one freeze-thaw (FT) cycle. Complete thawing is suggested by the disappearance of frozen white surface. For larger lesions (> 2 cm in diameter), different parts of the lesion are treated separately with overlapping margins.

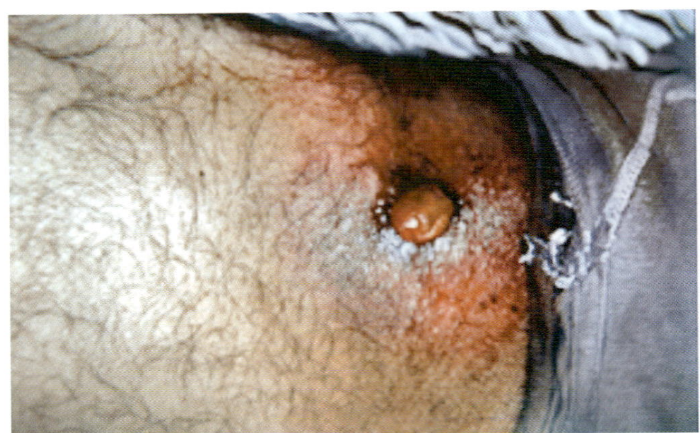

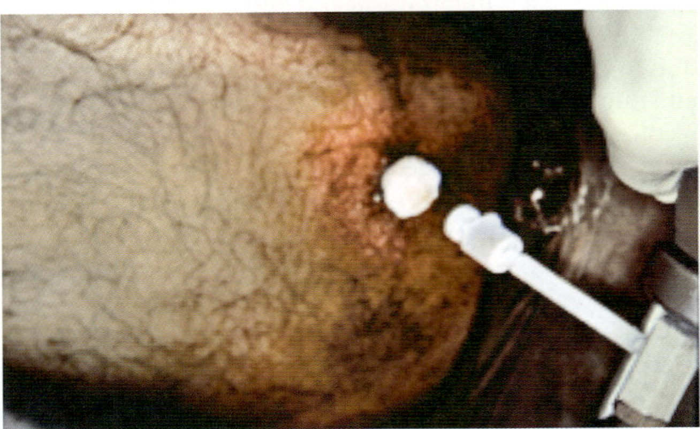

Fig. 2: Pyogenic granuloma precryotherapy. Pyogenic granuloma being frozen with ice ball formation.

Spot freeze can be carried out in two ways:

a. Open spray technique: It is useful for large, superficial, irregular lesions, those on curved surfaces or when light superficial freeze is desired. There are two methods for open spray:
   i. *Paint brush method*: The lesion is treated by spraying from one side of the lesion and moving up and down across the lesion.
   ii. *Spiral method*: The cryogen is sprayed initially in the center of the lesion and then moved outwards in concentric circles (Figs. 3A to C).
b. Confined-spray technique: It is preferred for round, small, discrete lesions or those close to vital structures.

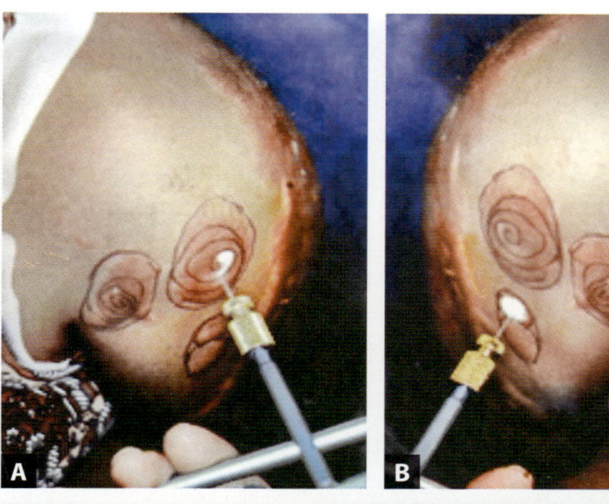

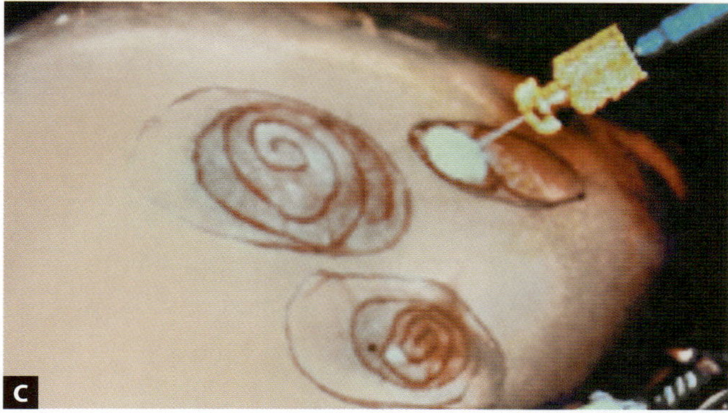

Figs. 3A to C: Spiral method of open spray freeze of cryotherapy.

In this, the range of spray is limited to a discrete area by use of neoprene or polystyrene cones.

2. *Use of cryoprobe*: An appropriate sized cryoprobe attached to the cryogun is directly applied to the lesion before spraying the cryogen. A thin layer of vaseline or petrolatum is applied to the probe tip to allow smooth contact with the lesion. While the cooling is occurring, the lesion gets attached to the probe which should be raised above the surrounding normal skin by few millimeters to prevent damage to the surrounding skin. Once the lesion is frozen, it is allowed to thaw. The probe should be allowed to release spontaneously from the lesion during the thawing process and must not be pulled earlier. In this technique, longer freezing time is required as compared to open spray technique.

This technique is preferred in vascular lesions, since direct application of the cryoprobe blanches the lesion and reduces the lesional temperature, thus increasing the depth of the freeze. With this method, there is uniformity of cooling over area of contact and a narrow rim around including the deeper tissue.

3. *Dipstick method*: A cotton bud is dipped into the cryogen (liquid nitrogen slush or dry ice) placed in a disposable container and then applied firmly on the lesion until a halo of ice forms around the bud. The size of the bud should be smaller than the lesion. The depth of freeze can be increased by applying pressure on the lesion. It is used to treat benign lesions and not recommended for malignant lesions. The method has the advantage of not needing a spray or probe equipment and is therefore cheap. However, repeated applications may be necessary to achieve proper freeze thaw.

4. *Histofreezer*: It has been primarily advocated for treatment of warts. It is a gentler treatment than liquid nitrogen because higher temperature is achieved, is less expensive and easy to store. It is a small unit containing a liquid-gas mixture of dimethyl ether and propane in an aerosol spray can. The mixture is sprayed through a narrow tube to a cotton applicator, which is applied to the wart. The mixture evaporates and freezes the wart. A temperature of –50°C is reached at the cotton tip, that freezes the wart. In a randomized trial comparing liquid nitrogen cryotherapy and histofreezer for the treatment of hand warts, patients cured of warts were 67% and 35% ($p = 0.01$) and the number of warts that resolved were 66% and 49% ($p = 0.08$) with the two modalities respectively.[1] The treatments were about equally effective in dorsal non-protuberant and small (less than 5 mm) warts but the overall results of liquid nitrogen were better. It is not available in India.

5. *Intralesional cryotherapy*: This is a method of applying cryotherapy to large and deep lesions to achieve more effectiveness and avoid many disadvantages of conventional techniques including surface complications. In this, a needle is introduced into the skin from one point that runs through the deeper tissues of the lesion and appears at the surface on the opposite border. A cryogen is then passed through one end of the needle which gets released into the atmosphere from the opposite end. An ice cylinder is formed around the embedded part of the needle within the deeper tissues. Many types of needles have been developed to facilitate greater efficacy by achieving better depth of freeze. These needles are angled, curved and hook-shaped. Lumbar puncture needles have also been used. This procedure has been used to treat both epidermal and deep dermal lesions, but is useful to treat large and deep dermal lesions such as keloids.

It is important to determine the depth of tissue to be frozen. The depth of freezing can be estimated by insertion of thermocouples mounted on needles, with their tips lying beneath or lateral to the lesion. Ultrasound machines like DermaScan® C ver. 3 fitted with a sharp focus probe, frequency of 20 mHz and a scan length of 12.1 mm have been used to locate thermocouples.

POST-TREATMENT CARE

The patient is explained about the immediate skin reactions that occur post-cryotherapy. There is peripheral erythema occurring immediately to 30 minutes after therapy, with edema setting within a few minutes to few hours. There may be blister formation 1–3 days later, followed by crusting that lasts for up to 2 weeks. The crust falls off leaving behind mild pinkish discoloration or erythematous atrophic scar. The patient is asked to apply a mild to moderately potent topical steroid and antibiotic combination. If the blister is large, it may be punctured with a sterile needle, or aspirated with its roof left in position as a natural protective film. A nonsteroidal anti-inflammatory drug (NSAID) is concomitantly administered. The treated area is best left open, washed gently with soap and water and patted dry.

INDICATIONS OF CRYOTHERAPY

This procedure has been used to treat a wide variety of skin conditions (Table 1):

1. Vascular lesions
2. Benign tumors
3. Acne
4. Pigmented lesions
5. Viral infections
6. Inflammatory dermatoses
7. Infectious dermatoses
8. Premalignant and malignant tumors.

Most of the evidence on the effectiveness of cryosurgery comes from uncontrolled trials. With the advent of several sophisticated ablative procedures like radiofrequency ablation or lasers, cryosurgery may be reserved for the following conditions:

- Genital warts in HIV positive patients or during pregnancy.[2]
- Hemangiomas/vascular malformations: Macular, flat-topped, superficial lesions, exophytic lesions or those with subcutaneous component (deep or mixed hemangiomas and malformations).[3]
- Well-defined, superficial non-melanoma skin cancers (basal and squamous cell carcinoma) especially located on trunk.[4]
- As combination therapy for lesions located on covered sites, e.g. plantar warts in combination with keratolytics, keloids (Figs. 4A to E) in combination with intralesional steroids.[5,6]

In other dermatoses, it may be used as alternate therapy especially under the following circumstances:

- In old patients with pacemakers in whom electrocautery is contraindicated.
- In patients on anticoagulants.
- In subjects allergic to anesthetic agents.
- Patients with transmissible conditions such as HIV and hepatitis.
- For genital lesions during pregnancy.
- If other ablative modalities are not available.

COMPLICATIONS

Complications are associated with inappropriate patient selection, the duration of freezing and the number of FT cycles undertaken.[7,8]

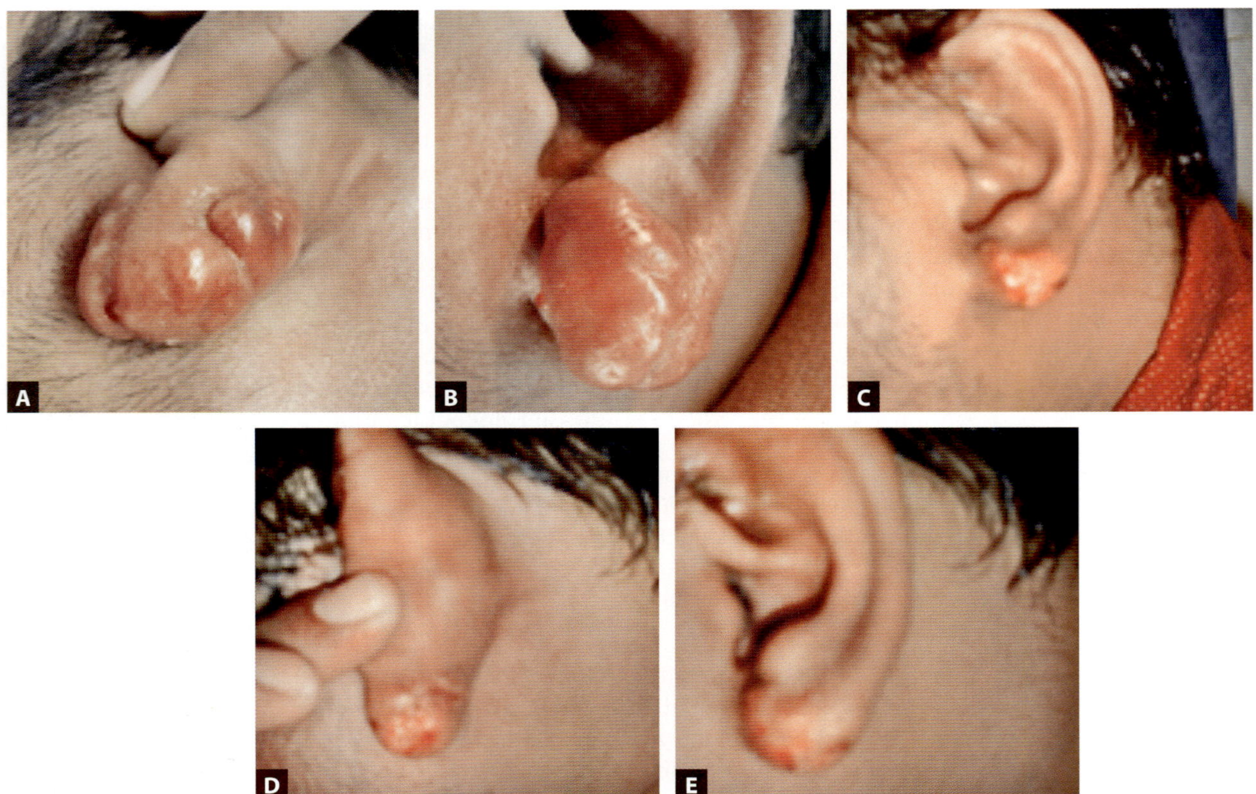

Figs. 4A to E: Pre- and post-treatment photographs of treatment of ear lobe keloids with cryotherapy.

Table 1: List of dermatoses where cryotherapy has been used.

Lesion	Technique	Freeze time (seconds)	Number of freeze-thaw cycles	Margin (mm)	Number of treatment sessions	Comments
Vascular lesions						Cryotherapy is considered to be superior to pulsed dye laser in hemangiomas with elevated and/or subcutaneous component[3]
Capillary hemangioma[9]	Cp	5–30	1–2	1	1–4 at 8 weeks interval	Cryosurgery done in areas where immediate treatment is indicated like periocular area, nose, lips, anogenital area
Cavernous hemangioma[10]	Cp	5–30	2	1	2–4 at 8 weeks interval	
Spider nevus[9]	Cp	5	1		1	
Angiokeratoma of Mibelli[11]	Cp or os	10	1	1	3 at 8 weeks interval	
Angiokeratoma of Fordyce[11]	Cp or os	10	1	1	3 at 8 weeks interval	
Venous lake[12]	Cp	10	1	1	1	Ice ball should not extend beyond vermilion border to prevent unsightly hypopigmentation
Cherry angioma[11]	Cp	10	1	< 1	1	
Pyogenic granuloma[13]	os	15	1	< 1	1	
AIDS-related Kaposi's sarcoma[14]	os	15–30	1–2	3	3 at 3 weeks interval	
Benign tumors Cryotherapy is a valuable alternative or adjuvant to other ablative procedures in certain situations (see Introduction)	os or Cp	3–60	1	2–3		
Milia[15]	Cp	Ice formation	1	1	1	
Myxoid cyst[11]	Cp or os	30	2	1	1–3 at 8 weeks interval	
Syringoma[16]	Cp	Ice formation	1	1	2–3 at 4–8 weeks interval	
Trichoepithelioma[17]	Cp	Ice formation	1	1	2–3 at 4–8 weeks interval	
Trichilemmal cyst[17]	os	Ice formation	1	1	2–3 at 4–8 weeks interval	
Steatocystoma multiplex[18]	os	Ice formation	1	1	2–3 at 4–8 weeks interval	
Skin tag[19]	os	5–10	1	1	1	
Dermatofibroma[20]	Cp or os	30	1	2	1–3 at 4–8 weeks interval	
Seborrheic keratosis[21]	os/Cp/d	Flat lesions: 5s Hyperkeratotic lesions: 30 s	12	1	1	
Sebaceous hyperplasia[20]	os/Cp	5–15	1	1	1	
Verrucous epidermal nevus[22]	os	5	1	1	Up to 5 at 4–8 weeks interval	
Acrokeratosis verruciformis[11]	os	5	1	1	Several at 6–8 weeks interval	
Dermatosis papulosa nigra[21]	os/Cp	Ice formation	1	Nil	Several at 6–8 weeks interval	
Adenoma sebaceum[23]	os	5–20	1	1	3–6 at 3 weeks interval	
Rhinophyma[9]	os	30	2	Entire nose	4–6 at 8 weeks interval	
Xanthelasma[24]	os	5	1	1	2–3 at 4–8 weeks interval	

Contd...

Contd...

Lesion	Technique	Freeze time (seconds)	Number of freeze-thaw cycles	Margin (mm)	Number of treatment sessions	Comments
Porokeratosis[25]	os	Ice formation	1	2	2 at 2 weeks interval	
Elastosis perforans serpiginosa[26]	os	10	1	1–2	2 at weekly interval	
Cutaneous horn[21]	os	10–15	1	2	1	
Keloids[5] (*see* Figure 26.4)	os/Cp	15–30	1	1	5–10 at 4–8 weeks interval	Significant to complete remission reported in 51–85% cases.[5] Better results in combination with I/L steroids. Lesions < 2 years duration show better results
Granuloma annulare[27]	Cp	10–20	1	1		Some physicians prefer nitrous oxide since liquid nitrogen causes permanent atrophic scars
Necrobiosis lipoidica[9]	Cp	20–30	1	1		
Acne[28] Alternate therapy to other physical modalities for lesions unresponsive to medical treatment						
Papulopustules	os	2–5	1			
Acne cyst	os/d	5–15	1		2–3 at 4 weeks interval	
Acne scars	os. Paint brush technique for diffuse acne scars (cryoabrasion)	Face: 5 Back: 5–15	1	-	Monthly	Useful for small, shallow pits than deep pitted scars. For acne keloidalis: Cryo+ I/L steroid. Moderate to good response (flattening) in 85% cases with early and in particular, vascular acne keloids as compared to I/L steroid[29]
Viral infections Common warts[6] cryotherapy is standard therapy for warts and an alternative to other ablative modalities	os/d	10. A 10s sustained freeze was found more effective than traditional freeze (treating until here is a halo of ice around the wart) but carried significantly greater morbidity in terms of pain and blistering[30]—plantar warts: 30–60	1 2: plantar warts	2	13 at weekly interval	Combination therapy with keratolytics better Pretreatment pairing of excess verrucosity before cryotherapy is effective for plantar but not hand warts
Genital warts/Condyloma acuminata[31]	os	10	1	1	1–3	Standard therapy for this condition Useful in podophyllin-resistant or podophyllin- undesirable lesions Better cure rates than TCA or podophyllin but less effective than electrodessication[31]

Contd...

Contd...

Lesion	Technique	Freeze time (seconds)	Number of freeze-thaw cycles	Margin (mm)	Number of treatment sessions	Comments
						Combination with podophyllin or TCA provides significantly faster clearance than single modality[32] Safest treatment in pregnancy[2]
Molluscum contagiosum[9]	os	Ice ball formation	1	-		
Pigmented lesions						
Melasma[11]	os	Ice formation	1	Feathering: Spraying lightly the border of ice field to prevent sharp demarcation between post-treatment hypopigmentation and surrounding skin and reduce contrast	At 4–6 weeks interval	Cryotherapy may be an option especially in fair-skinned individuals
Freckles[11]	Cp	Ice formation	1	Feathering	1	Cryotherapy may be an option especially in fair skinned individuals.
Idiopathic guttate hypomelanosis[11]	os	5	1	1	At 4–6 weeks interval	Lesions gently frozen with liquid nitrogen have been shown to repigment in 6–8 weeks[33,34]
Tattoo[35]	os	30	2	1	At 4–6 weeks interval	Few reports have shown good efficacy in this condition[35]
Solar lentigo[36]	os/Cp	5–10	1	Feathering	1	A study showed comparable efficacy with dermabrasion but with higher rates of hypopigmentation[37]
Lentigo simplex[11]	os/Cp	Light	1	Feathering	1	In one RCT, cryotherapy found twice as effective than CO_2 or argon laser[38]
Inflammatory conditions Psoriasis, lichen simplex chronicus, hypertrophic lichen planus, prurigo nodularis, chronic DLE[15]	os	10–15 to 20–30	1			Mild resolution of psoriasis or lichen planus by inducing normal reepithelization following physical destruction of lesions via reverse Koebner phenomenon. Efficacy is limited
Oral lesions[39] Benign lesions—hemangioma, lymphangioma, pyogenic granuloma, mucocele, papilloma Precancerous and cancerous lesions—leucoplakia, lichen planus, frictional leucokeratosis, erythroplasia, SCC	os: In most lesions Cp-deep and fluid-filled lesions					Caution to be maintained while performing cryosurgery over base of tongue, posterior wall of pharynx or tonsils as ventilatory impairment may occur - 20% recurrence after cryosurgery for leukoplakia

Contd...

Contd...

Lesion	Technique	Freeze time (seconds)	Number of freeze-thaw cycles	Margin (mm)	Number of treatment sessions	Comments
Infections Cutaneous leishmaniasis, chromoblastomycosis, larva migrans[40,41]	os/d	15–20	2		3 at 3 weeks interval	In a large series, cutaneous leishmaniasis was successfully treated with a simple protocol of cryosurgery with minor side-effects[40] Cryosurgery was found useful for small lesions (< 15 cm^2) of chromoblas tomycosis[41]
Premalignant skin lesions Actinic keratosis, actinic cheilitis, LSA[36,42] Bowen's disease[43]	os/Cp os/Cp	20–30 20–30	1 2	3		
Malignant skin lesions BCC, superficial SCC, lentigo maligna[44–46]	os Fractional cryotherapy for tumors > 10 mm: Initially center of lesion is frozen and the procedure repeated until tumor size <10 mm; followed by standard cryotherapy	30	2 In RCT, for BCC: 1 FT cycle-79.4% cure rate 2 FT cycle-95.3% cure rate[44]	BCC: 5 mm SCC: 1 cm Lentigo maligna: 1 cm		Good prognosis after cryotherapy: Superficial tumors, lesions on trunk Bad prognosis: Recurrent tumors, lesions without defined margin, large lesions, tumors localized to folds of central face, morpheform BCC Precryo shave excision or curettage improves results of cryosurgery In a case series, overall cure rate for NMSC with cryotherapy was 97% with very few recurrences[47] During 30-year treatment period, cure rate for NMSC was 98.6%[48]
Malignant melanoma[49]	os	30	2			Palliative therapy for multiple cutaneous metastases in disseminated stage
Recalcitrant alopecia areata[50]	Liquid nitrogen spray	15 seconds	Dual freeze-thaw cycles of 15 seconds each		Maximum 5 sessions 2 weeks apart	10 patients included. 50% showed excellent response, 30% satisfactory, 10% fair, and 10% had poor response. No serious adverse effects seen. Sustained hair regrowth in 80% cases at16(th) week.
Tache noire on scapular region[51]	Liquid nitrogen spray	15 s of freezing and 3 min of thawing	Two		Single	One patient treated, complete tick removed
Oral lichen planus[52]	nitrous oxide with cryoprobe	one session of 20-25 s freeze-thaw cycles with N_2O gas under local anesthesia	One	Entire lesion or center of large lesion	Single	Cryotherapy reduced severity of lesions significantly but response similar to topical steroid. 57% cases had minor swelling at cryotherapy site and 40% had pain in first 7-10 days after cryotherapy

Key: Cp, cryoprobe; os, open spray technique; d, dipstick; I/L steroids, intralesional steroids; TCA, trichloroacetic acid; RCT, randomized controlled trial; SCC, squamous cell carcinoma; LSA, lichen sclerosus et atrophicus; BCC, basal cell carcinoma; FT cycle, freeze-thaw cycle; NMSC, non-melanoma skin cancer

Acute

- Local pain: More in periungual area, temple, plantar areas, eyelids, lips, mucous membranes. Tingling and numbness is common, especially on the fingers.
- Edema, especially on eyelids, lips, labia, prepuce; more in infants and elderly.
- Cryoblister formation.
- Syncope (vasovagal reaction) in anxious patients.
- Headache (migraine type) after treatment of head and neck area.

Subacute

- Hemorrhagic necrosis.
- Wound infection: Due to use of infected cryoprobes or redipping cotton swabs into the cryogen.
- Delayed wound healing after treatment over extremities.
- Temporary scar hypertrophy.
- Subcutaneous emphysema due to insufflation of underlying tissue on spraying over broken skin.

Protracted

Common

- Hypopigmentation especially in dark-skinned individuals. Can be minimized by freezing for < 30 sec.
- Atrophic scar: Occurs when freezing time > 30 sec.
- Local hypoesthesia due to nerve damage especially in areas where nerves lie superficially such as sides of fingers, angle of jaw, postauricular area, sides of tongue, ulnar fossa of elbow.
- Milia formation.
- Cicatricial alopecia: Can be minimized by freezing for < 30 sec.

Uncommon

- Cartilage damage.
- Traumatic neuroma.
- Pyogenic granuloma.
- Fibroxanthoma.

CONTRAINDICATIONS TO CRYOTHERAPY

Absolute

- Blood dyscrasias of unknown origin.
- Cold intolerance.
- Raynaud's disease.
- Cold urticaria.
- Cryoglobulinemia.
- Lesions in which tissue pathology is required.
- Lesions in areas of compromised circulation.
- Sclerosing basal cell carcinoma (BCC) or recurrent BCC or squamous cell carcinoma (SCC) located in high risk areas like temple or nasolabial folds.

Relative

- Keloidal tendency.
- Collagen vascular diseases.
- Dark-skinned individuals due to high risk of developing cosmetically inacceptable protracted hypopigmentation.
- Lesions over nasolabial fold, eyelid margins, ala nasi and hair-bearing areas (high risk of developing alopecia especially cicatricial alopecia).
- Patients with sensory loss at lesional sites.
- Pyoderma gangrenosum.

Tips and Pitfalls

- Cryosurgery is particularly useful for patients with lesions on mucosae, inaccessible areas, multiple lesions, with pacemakers, pregnant and lactating women, small children as well as in the elderly.
- In Indian skin, pigmentary changes are common after cryosurgery.
- Likewise, the cryoblister may be very painful. Patient should be properly counseled about this.
- Cryosurgery for palmar and plantar warts, can lead to necrosis and delayed healing, particularly over weight bearing areas.
- Cryosurgery on tips of fingers should be avoided in patients with vascular compromise.
- Recurrences may need repeated treatments.

CONCLUSION

Cryotherapy is a simple, safe and inexpensive office procedure for the treatment of various benign, premalignant and well-circumscribed malignant tumors. The list of indications where cryotherapy has been used, along with levels of evidence are listed in Table 1. It provides satisfactory cosmetic results with minimal complications if patient selection is proper and if it is undertaken by a trained and experienced dermatologist.

ACKNOWLEDGMENT

We thank Dr Vinay Saraf, Senior Consultant Dermatologist, Nanavati Hospital, Mumbai for providing the photographs for this chapter.

REFERENCES

1. Erkens AM, Kuijpers RJ, Knottnerus JA. [An end to office hours for warts? A randomized study of the effectiveness of liquid nitrogen and of the Histofreezer. Ned Tijdschr Geneeskd. 1991;135:171-4.

2. Mayeaux EJ, Harper MB, Barksdale W, et al. Noncervical human papillomavirus genital infections. Am Fam Physician. 1995;52:1137-46.
3. Michel S, Wlotzke U, Hohenleutner U, et al. Laser and cryotherapy of hemangioma in infants in a direct comparison. Hautarzt. 1998;49:192-6.
4. Mallon E, Dawber R. Cryosurgery in the treatment of basal cell carcinoma. Assessment of one and two freeze-thaw cycle schedules. Dermatol Surg. 1996;22:854-8.
5. Zouboulis CC, Blume U, Buttner P, et al. Outcome of cryosurgical treatment in patients with keloids and hypertrophic scars. Arch Dermatol. 1993;129:1146-51.
6. Scheinfeld NS. Treatment of verruca vulgaris. Skinmed. 2006;5:37-8.
7. Elton RF. Complications of cutaneous cryosurgery. J Am Acad Dermatol. 1983;8:513-9.
8. Dawber RP. Cryosurgery: complications and contraindications. Clin Dermatol. 1990;8:108-14.
9. Thai KE, Sinclair RD. Cryosurgery of benign skin lesions. Australas J Dermatol. 1999;40:175-84.
10. Reischle S, Schuller-Petrovic S. Treatment of capillary hemangiomas of early childhood with a new method of cryosurgery. J Am Acad Dermatol. 2000;42:809-13.
11. Sinclair RD, Tzermias C, Dawber RP. Cosmetic cryosurgery. In: Baran R, Maibach HI (Eds). Textbook of Cosmetic Dermatology. London: Martin Dunitz; 1998;691-700.
12. Suhonen R, Kuflik EG. Venous lakes treated by liquid nitrogen cryosurgery. Br J Dermatol. 1997;137:1018-9.
13. Mirshams M, Daneshpazhooh M, Mirshekari A, et al. Cryotherapy in the treatment of pyogenic granuloma. J Eur Acad Dermatol Venereol. 2006;20:788-90.
14. Serfling U, Hood AF. Local therapies for Kaposi's sarcoma in patients with acquired immunodeficiency syndrome. Arch Dermatol. 1991;127:1479-81.
15. Drake LA, Ceilley RI, Cornelison RL. Guidelines for care for cryosurgery. American Academy of Dermatology Committee on Guidelines of Care. J Am Acad Dermatol. 1994;31:648-53.
16. Kuflik EG. Cryosurgery updated. J Am Acad Dermatol. 1994;31:925-44.
17. Graham GF. Cryosurgery. Clin Plast Surg. 1993;20:131-47.
18. Apaydin R, Bilen N, Bayramgürler D, et al. Steatocystoma multiplex suppurativum: oral isotretinoin treatment combined with cryotherapy. Australas J Dermatol. 2000;41:98-100.
19. Luba MC, Bangs SA, Mohler AM, et al. Common benign skin tumors. Am Fam Physician. 2003;67:729-38.
20. Lanigan SW, Robinson TW. Cryosurgery for dermatofibromas. Clin Exp Dermatol. 1987;12:121-3.
21. Andrews MD. Cryosurgery for common skin conditions. Am Fam Physician. 2004;69:2365-72.
22. Kosann MK. Inflammatory linear verrucous epidermal nevus. Dermatol Online J. 2003;9:15.
23. Shroff HJ. Current approach to the management of nevi. Indian J Pediatr. 1983;50:545-6.
24. Hawk JL. Cryotherapy may be effective for eyelid xanthelasma. Clin Exp Dermatol. 2000;25:351.
25. Bhushan M, Craven NM, Beck MH, et al. Linear porokeratosis of mibelli: successful treatment with cryotherapy. Br J Dermatol. 1999;141:389.
26. Rosenblum GA. Liquid nitrogen cryotherapy in a case of elastosis perforans serpiginosa. J Am Acad Dermatol. 1983;8:718-21.
27. Blume-Peytavi U, Zouboulis CC, Jacobi H, et al. Successful outcome of cryosurgery in patients with granuloma annulare. Br J Dermatol. 1994;130:494-7.
28. Graham GF. Cryosurgery for acne. In: Zacarian SA (Ed). Cryosurgery for Skin Cancer and Cutaneous Disorders. St Louis: Mosby Press; 1985;59-76.
29. Layton AM. A comparison of intralesional triamcinolone and cryosurgery in the treatment of acne keloids. Br J Dermatol. 1994;130:498-501.
30. Connolly M, Bazmi K, O'Connell M, et al. Cryotherapy of viral warts: a sustained 10-s freeze is more effective than the traditional method. Br J Dermatol. 2001;145:554-7.
31. Stone KM, Becker TM, Hadgu A, et al. Treatment of external genital warts: a randomised clinical trial comparing podophyllin, cryotherapy, and electrodessication. Genitourin Med. 1990;66:16-9.
32. Sherrard J, Riddell L. Comparison of the effectiveness of commonly used clinic-based treatments for external genital warts. Int J STD AIDS. 2007;18:365-8.
33. Kumarasinghe SP. 3-5 second cryotherapy is effective in idiopathic guttate hypomelanosis. J Dermatol. 2004;31:437-9.
34. Ploysangam T, Dee-Ananlap S, Suvanprakorn P. Treatment of idiopathic guttate hypomelanosis with liquid nitrogen: light and electron microscopic studies. J Am Acad Dermatol. 1990;23:681-4.
35. Colver GB, Dawber RP. Tattoo removal using a liquid nitrogen cryospray. Clin Exp Dermatol. 1984;9:364-6.
36. Dawber R, Graham C, Jackson A. Benign lesions. Cutaneous Cryosurgery: Principles and Clinical Practice. London: Martin Dunitz Ltd; 1992;29-76.
37. Hexsel DM, Mazzuco R, Bohn J, et al. Clinical comparative study between cryotherapy and local dermabrasion for the treatment of solar lentigo on the back of the hands. Dermatol Surg. 2000;26:457-62.
38. Stern RS, Dover JS, Levin JA, et al. Laser therapy versus cryotherapy of lentigines: a comparative trial. J Am Acad Dermatol. 1994;30:985-7.
39. Ishida CE, Ramos-e-Silva M. Cryosurgery in oral lesions. Int J Dermatol. 1998;37:283-5.
40. Al-Majali O, Routh HB, Abuloham O, et al. A 2-year study of liquid nitrogen therapy in cutaneous leishmaniasis. Int J Dermatol. 1997;36:460-2.
41. Bonifaz A, Martinez-Soto E, Carrasco-Gerard E, et al. Treatment of chromoblastomycosis with itraconazole, cryosurgery, and a combination of both. Int J Dermatol. 1997;36:542-7.
42. Lubritz RR, Smolewski SA. Cryosurgery cure rate of actinic keratoses. J Am Acad Dermatol. 1982;7:631-2.
43. Sinclair RD, Dawber RP. Cryosurgery of malignant and premalignant diseases of the skin: a simple approach. Australas J Dermatol. 1995;36:133-42.

44. Zacarian SA. Cryosurgery of cutaneous carcinomas. An 18-year study of 3,022 patients with 4,288 carcinomas. J Am Acad Dermatol. 1983;9:947-56.
45. Kuflik EG, Gage AA. The five-year cure rate achieved by cryosurgery for skin cancer. J Am Acad Dermatol. 1991;24: 1002-4.
46. Graham GF, Clark LC. Statistical analysis in cryosurgery of skin cancer. Clin Dermatol. 1990;8:101-7.
47. Holt PJ. Cryotherapy for skin cancer: results over a 5-year period using liquid nitrogen spray cryosurgery. Br J Dermatol. 1988;119:231-40.
48. Kuflik EG. Cryosurgery for skin cancer: 30-year experience and cure rates. Dermatol Surg. 2004;30:297-300.
49. Weyer U, Petersen I, Ehrke C, et al. Immunomodulation by cryosurgery in malignant melanoma. Onkologie. 1989; 12: 291-6.
50. Zawar VP, Karad GM. Liquid Nitrogen Cryotherapy in Recalcitrant Alopecia Areata: A Study of 11 Patients. Int J Trichology. 2016;8(1):15-20
51. Zawar V, Karad G, Chuh A. Tâche Noire: A Classic Case Treated with Dual Freeze Cycles of Liquid Nitrogen Cryotherapy and Clasped Manoeuvre. J Cutan Aesthet Surg 2015;8:184-6.
52. Amanat D, Ebrahimi H, Zahedani MZ, Zeini N, Pourshahidi S, Ranjbar Z. Comparing the effects of cryotherapy with nitrous oxide gas versus topical corticosteroids in the treatment of oral lichen planus. Indian J Dent Res. 2014;25:711-6.

Chapter

27

Surgical Management of Cutaneous Cysts and Lipomas

Vinay Saraf, Ragunatha S

Key Messages

- Cutaneous cysts and lipomas are most common benign tumors of skin and subcutaneous tissue.
- Depending on type, size and location of the lesions appropriate surgical procedures are used.
- Minimal invasive techniques assisted with suction or laser punch result in complete removal of cysts with better cosmetic outcome compared to conventional surgical excision.
- Tumescent liposuction and lipolysis either by laser or injection of phosphatidylcholine/sodium deoxycholate followed by conventional excisions are the newer methods in surgical removal of lipomas.
- These procedures should be done by experienced dermatologists because of potential complications associated with lasers and injections.

SURGICAL MANAGEMENT OF CUTANEOUS CYSTS

INTRODUCTION

Cutaneous cysts are very common, and epidermoid cysts constitute 80% of the cutaneous cysts. Epidermoid cysts should always be subjected to histopathological examination, since it has been suggested that 1% of the epithelial cysts may have a basal or squamous cell carcinoma in their wall.[1]

Different surgical techniques for cutaneous cysts include punch removal, incisional excision, elliptical excision, excision with secondary healing.

PUNCH REMOVAL TECHNIQUE

This is a rapid and easy technique (Figs. 1A to D) to remove cysts up to one centimeter in diameter using only 2–4 mm skin punch. The punch is held over the visible central punctum and the skin is held taut perpendicularly to the relaxed skin tension lines (RSTLs). The punch is advanced through the overlying skin into the cyst cavity. The contents are then evacuated with firm lateral pressure, carefully removing all the keratinous debris and the entire cyst wall. The edge of the wall usually presents itself at the wound margin, as the contents are evacuated. After evacuation of the cyst, a small 3–5 mm curette is used to curette and extract the cyst wall with gentle traction. Alternatively, small curved scissors can be used to dissect around the cyst wall and then gently pulling the cyst wall with Adson forceps till the base of the cyst is reached which is identified by observing its blood supply at the base. The base is clamped with artery forceps and cut with scissors. The wound is cleaned with hydrogen peroxide and closed with simple suture technique after achieving good hemostasis with pressure.[2]

INCISIONAL SURGICAL TECHNIQUE

In this technique (Figs. 2A to J), a single linear incision aligned with the RSTLs or existing wrinkles over the cyst is made. The incision is stopped at the level of glistening white cyst wall. The cyst is then dissected out bluntly using mosquito forceps. The base is clamped and cut. After cleaning the wound with hydrogen peroxide, simple suturing technique is used to close the wound.[2-4]

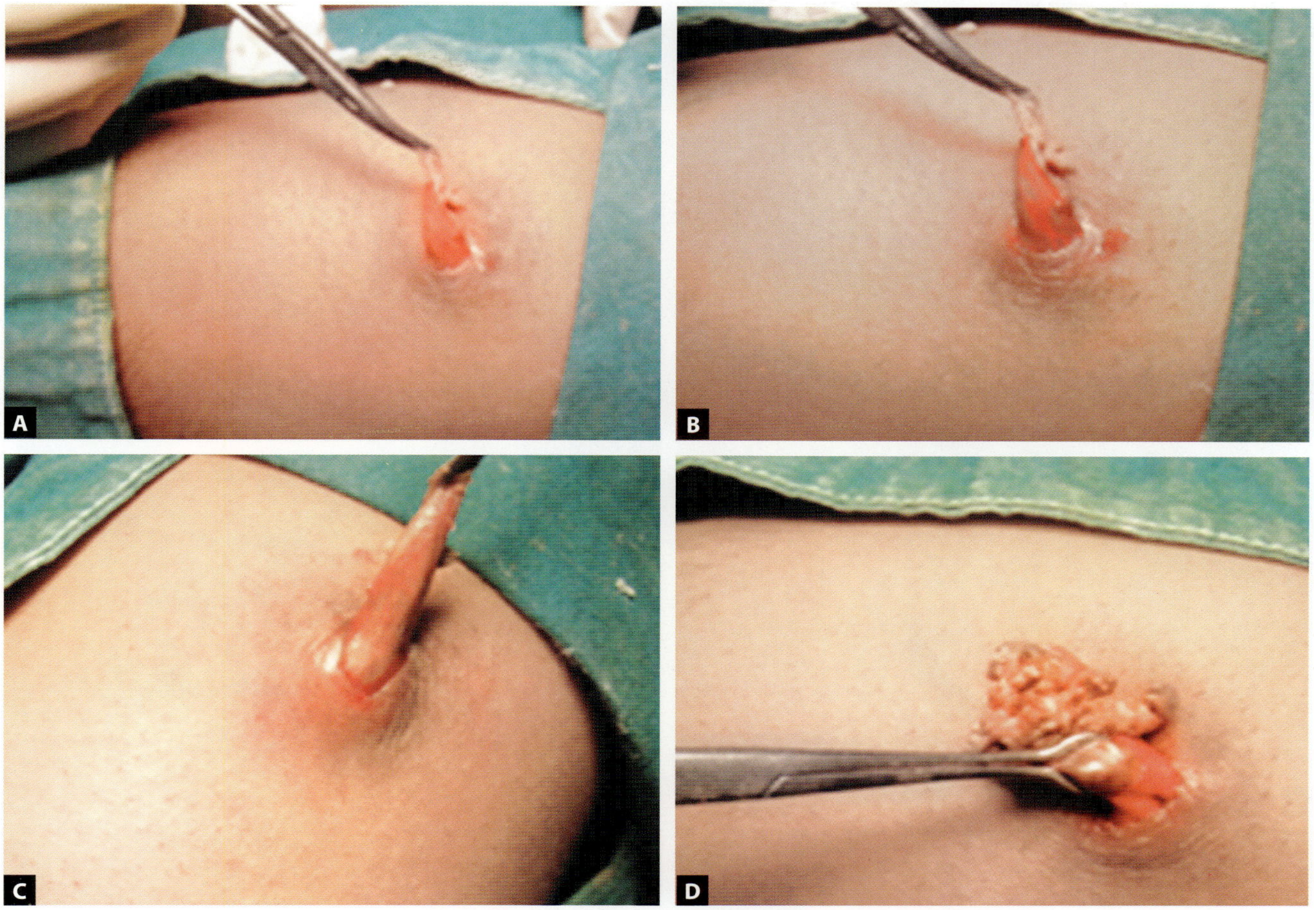

Figs. 1A to D: Cyst with avulsion of cyst wall through a small incision.

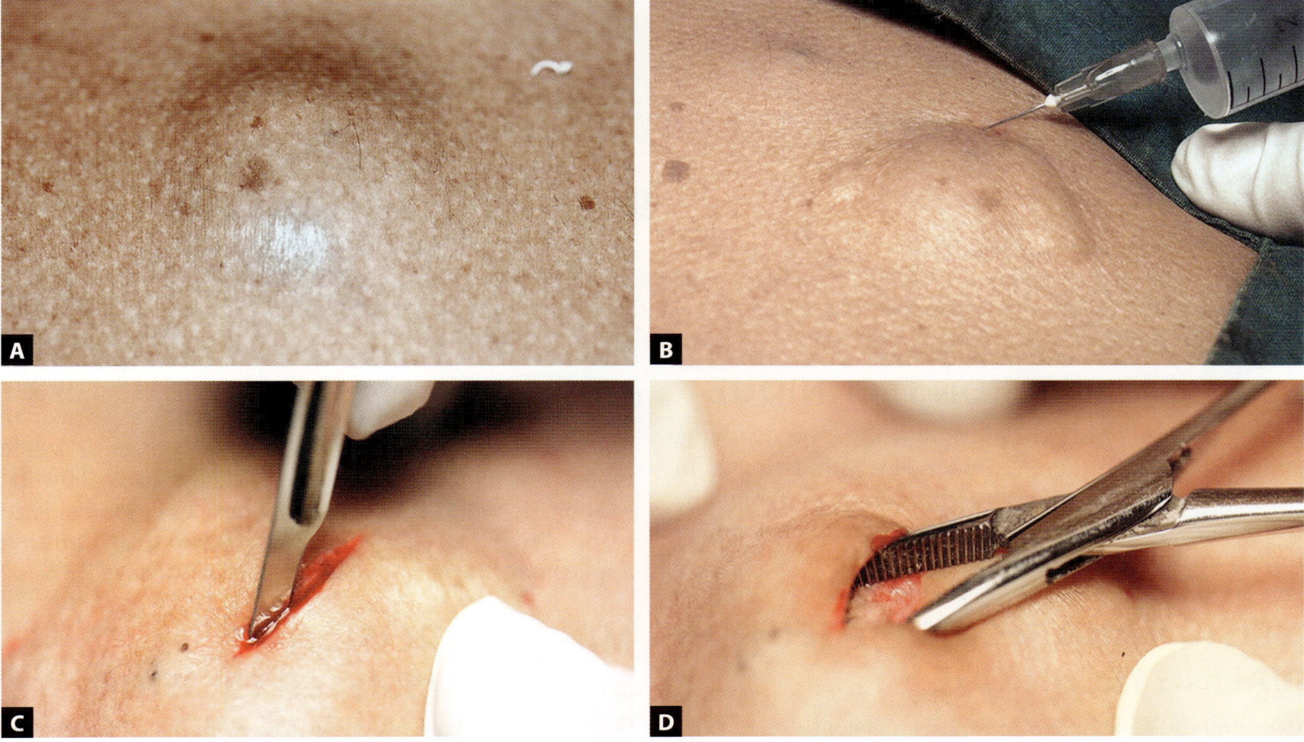

Figs. 2A to D

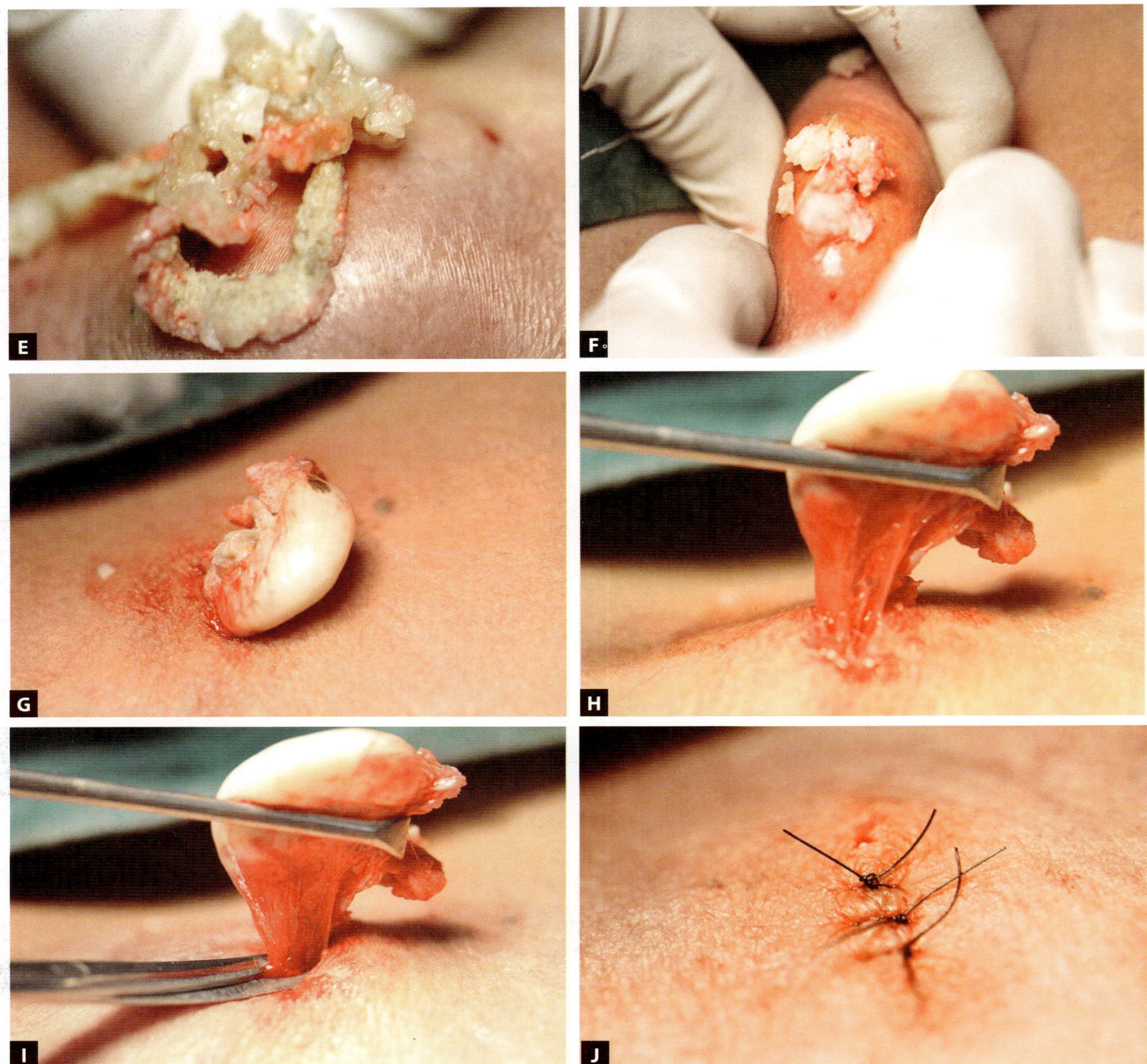

Figs. 2A to J: (A) Sebaceous cyst; (B) Giving field block; (C) Incision with 15 no. Blade; (D) Blunt dissection with artery forceps; (E and F) Manual extraction of sebaceous material; (G) Cyst partially extracted; (H) Further extraction and clamping of the base of the cyst; (I) Cutting the fibrous strands and blood supply of the cyst; (J) Wound sutured with 3-0 ethilon suture.

ELLIPTICAL EXCISION TECHNIQUE

In this technique, fusiform incision is done on overlying skin to include the punctum. Undermining and dissection is done all around the cyst. The cyst is removed intact by cutting at its base. The wound is cleaned and closed with simple suturing technique (Figs. 3 to 6).[1]

EXCISION AND SECOND-INTENTION HEALING TECHNIQUE

This technique is used for numerous small epidermoid cysts commonly seen in male patients with acne on the lower posterior auricular skin, the earlobe, the posterior auricular sulcus and the posterior auricular scalp skin over the mastoid. Simple selective incision and drainage, or isolated excisions is the method of choice. The wound is allowed to heal by second intention over the next 1–2 months period using daily hydrogen peroxide and topical antibiotic application. The cosmetic results are satisfactory.[2,3]

MINIMAL INCISION SUCTION-ASSISTED EXCISION

In minimal incision excisions, the contents of the cysts are squeezed out through incision site manually by applying

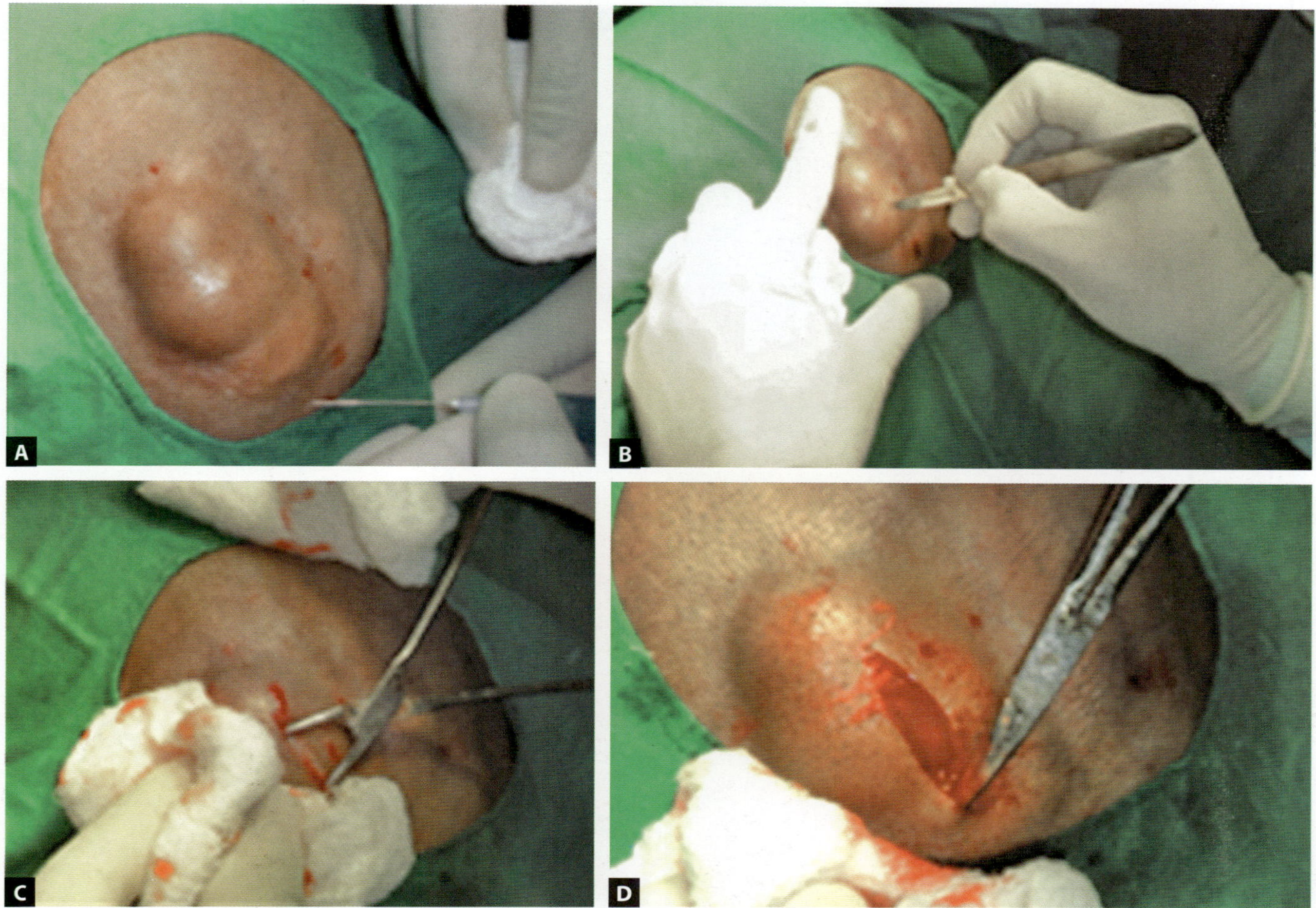

Figs. 3A to D: Excision of pilar cysts on scalp after undermining with blunt dissection incision over the cyst.

lateral pressure. However, lateral pressure, sometimes, causes intracavitary rupture, fragmentation, infections and recurrences. Hence, negative-pressure suction can be used instead of lateral pressure to completely remove the cysts measuring >2 cm.[5]

LASER PUNCH WITH POSTPONED MINIMAL EXCISION

It is a two-step procedure where carbon dioxide laser is used initially to make multiple punctures in the cyst to form a hole of 2–4 mm. The contents of the cysts are partially evacuated through hole with gentle pressure. Any remnants in the cyst are removed by washing with normal saline. The hole is sealed with a suture or glue and standard postoperative care is advised. After one month, once the cyst has become small, minimal excision technique is performed to remove the cyst wall completely. This method is suitable for large cyst or cyst over thick skin where the cyst wall is more friable or expression of the contents is difficult.[6]

Carbon dioxide laser has also been used to make a small hole as a part of minimal invasive excision of epidermal cysts. Small, freely mobile and non-inflammed epidermal cysts measuring 0.5 to 1.5 cm have been treated successfully with this method.[7]

SPECIFIC TECHNIQUES FOR DIFFERENT TYPES OF CYSTS

a. Epidermoid Cysts

Epidermoid cysts can be managed by any of the above techniques.

b. Infected or Inflamed Cysts

These cysts are preferably treated with systemic antibiotics with small amount (5 mg/mL) of intralesional triamcinolone acetonide into the cyst cavity along with warm compresses. For fluctuant cysts, incision and drainage is best option. Finally, excision is done.[3,4]

c. Milia

Surgical evacuation is the best option using a number 11 blade with comedone extractor. A fine tip cautery with very low current electrodesiccation is another option. In both techniques, cosmetic results are good.[1]

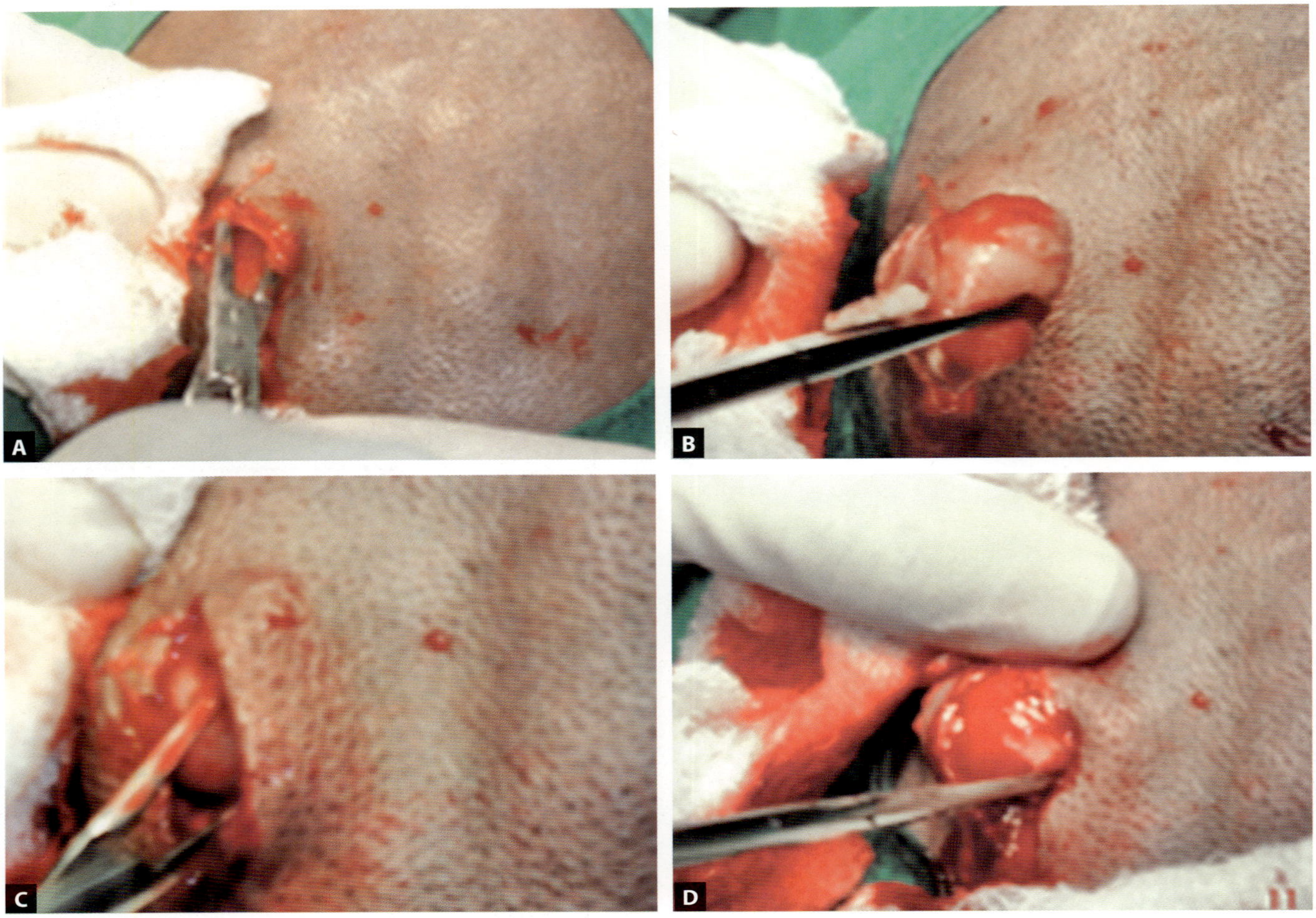

Figs. 4A to D: Undermining and extrusion of the cyst with intact cyst wall. (A) Multiple pilar cysts on scalp; (B) Removal with simple excision; (C) Blunt dissection with artery forceps; (D) Cysts removal with intact wall.

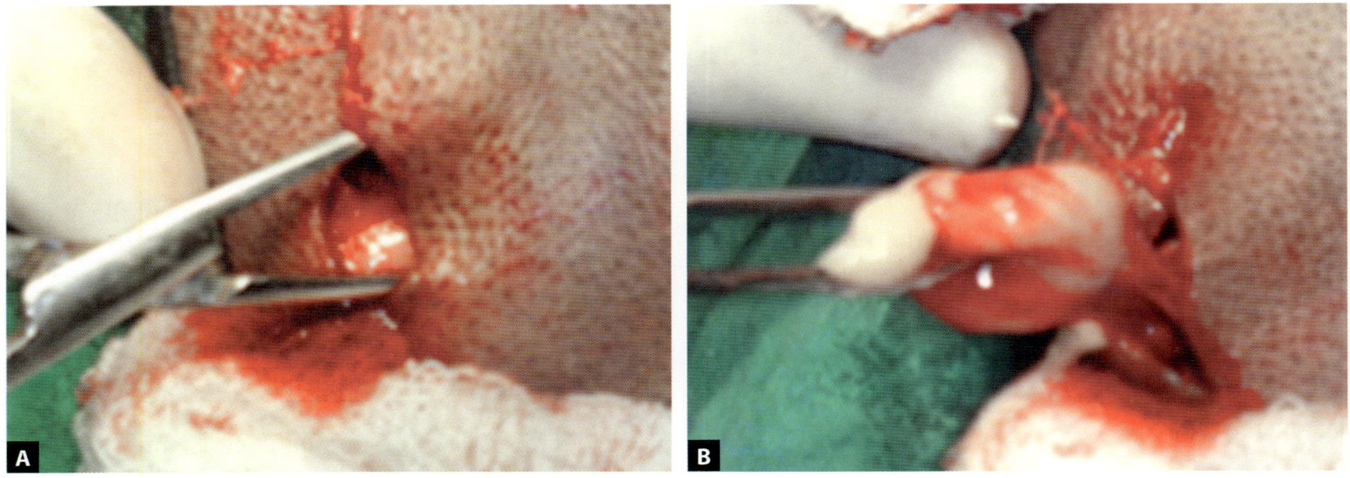

Figs. 5A and B: Excision of cyst—final step.

d. Steatocystoma Multiplex

The therapeutic option is same as that for the treatment of epidermoid cysts.[2]

e. Mucous Cysts

Excision is the standard treatment approach. Care must be taken to orient the excision so as not to alter the appearance

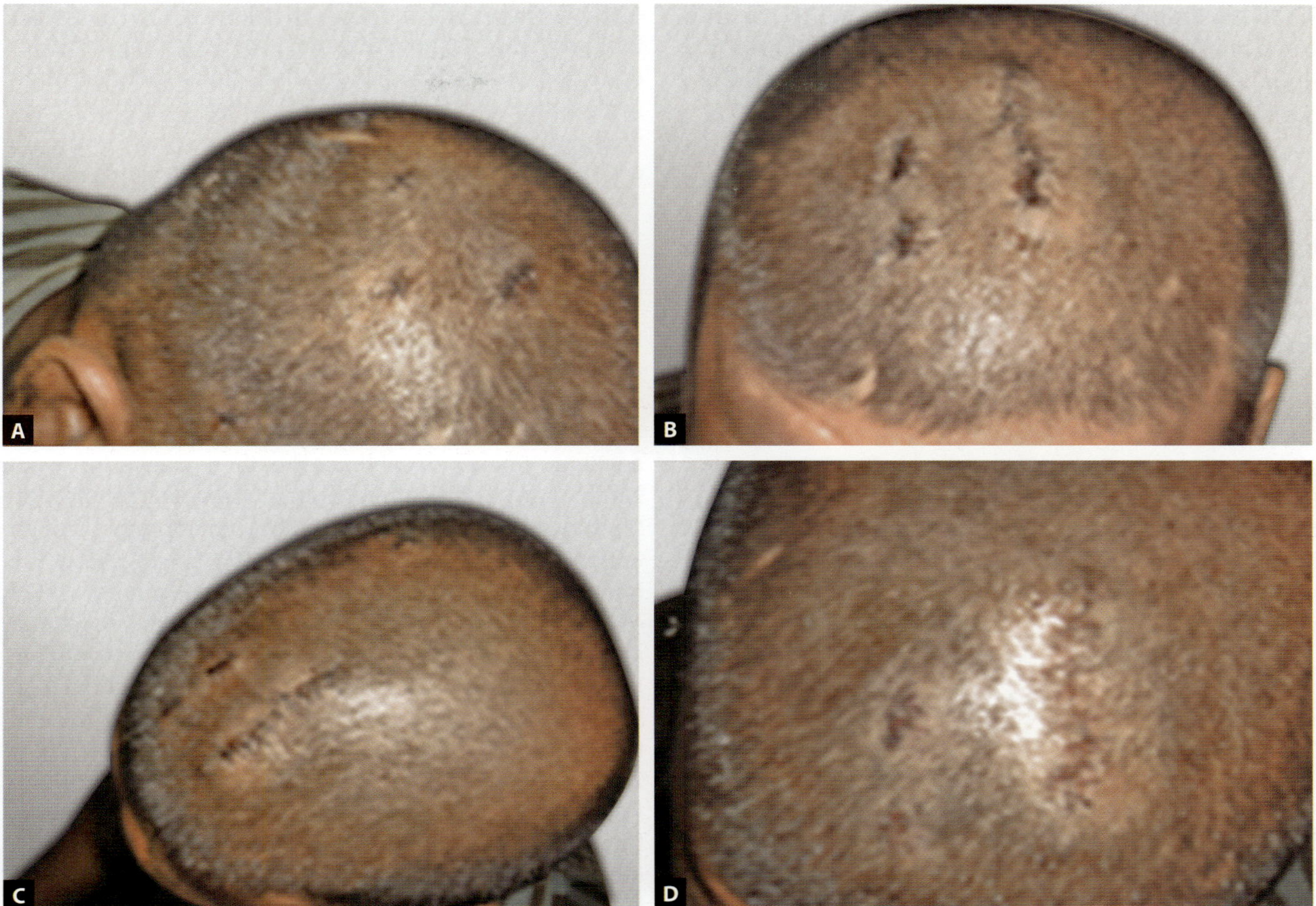

Figs. 6A to D: Simple interruted suturing after suture removal good healing with minimal scarring.

of the vermillion. Simple incising and draining the cyst is not enough to prevent recurrences. The underlying mucous or minor salivary glands must be removed down to the orbicularis oris muscle. The wound is closed with chromic catgut so no suture removal is required. Chalazion clamp can be used to fix the mucous cyst.[1,3]

f. Dermoid Cyst

Therapy consists of complete surgical excision. Skull films, CT scans and MRI must be used to evaluate the dermoid and its potential intracranial extensions before surgery.[1,4]

CONCLUSION

A vast variety of cysts are encountered in the skin, and the dermatosurgeon must be well versed with both the common and uncommon types. With proper excision, evacuation and closure techniques, good cosmetic results can be achieved.

SURGICAL MANAGEMENT OF LIPOMAS

Lipomas are the benign tumors of mature adipocytes. Several types of lipoma are described. These include, simple, fibrolipoma, angiolipoma, pleomorphic, spindle cell and myolipoma. Lipoma can be a part of associated syndrome, e.g. Madelung syndrome, Gardner's syndrome, Cowden's syndrome, Bannayan-Riley-Ruvalcaba syndrome and familial multiple lipomatosis.[8] Clinically, lipoma is a slow-growing, asymptomatic mobile swelling with characteristic doughy consistency. The lesion is usually located in the subcutaneous tissue but can be found in intermuscular septa, abdominal viscera, oral cavity, internal auditory canal, cerebellopontine angle and thorax.[9] However, subcutaneous lipoma is of concern for dermatologists. The size of lipoma may vary from a small swelling to a large tumor measuring >15 cm and can occur anywhere on the body.[10] Hence, appropriate lipoma removal techniques need to be used for better cosmetic result.

Depending on the size, type and location of lipoma several lipoma removal techniques have been used successfully. These include conventional surgical excision, minimal invasive techniques like stab incision squeeze technique (SIST) and distant incision technique, injection lipolysis, tumescent liposuction and laser lipolysis.

Small lipomas can be easily excised surgically with good cosmetic outcome. However, excision of larger lesions measuring >10 cm can result in significant scarring. In such situation, tumescent local anaesthesia (TLA) with liposuction has been used successfully. This technique may not be feasible for extensive fibrous lesions. Laser lipolysis, a minimally invasive and effective method of removal of such lesions has been proposed. It can be used alone or before liposuction.[11]

STAB INCISION SQUEEZE TECHNIQUE

The stab incision squeeze technique (SIST) is suitable for small, superficial, encapsulated lipomas. Normal saline is injected preoperatively into the subcutaneous tissue immediately surrounding the lipoma to facilitate enucleation. A single linear stab incision, as short as 1/4th to 1/3rd of the palpable diameter of the lipoma, is made. Blunt undermining and dissection with mosquito forceps is done to disrupt the fibrous tethers between the capsule and surrounding subcutaneous tissue. Pressure on the lateral aspects of the incision is exerted adequately to express the entire tumor (squeeze technique). The wound is closed with subcutaneous and surface sutures and pressure dressing (Figs. 7A to F).[12]

DISTANT INCISION TECHNIQUE

This technique is used for lipomas of the forehead, lower eyelids, cheeks, lips and sternal areas. Good cosmetic results are obtained by making the incision at a somewhat distant site. Incision may be hidden in the scalp, eyelids or nasolabial folds, preauricular skin, oral mucosa or inframammary folds.[12-18]

TUMESCENT LIPOSUCTION

Tumescent anesthesia is infused directly into the lesion and after 20 minutes, two to three small incisions are made for liposuction cannulas. One of the incision is made at the dependent part of lipoma for drainage. A 3 mm diameter cannula with 10 mL Luer-lock syringe is enough for liposuction. Complete removal of remaining stroma is done by a hemostat with blunt dissection. A penrose drain is placed for one day and after 5–7 days wound is closed with suture. Tumescent liposuction is associated with ecchymosis, hematoma and acute dimpling which resolve over a period of time.[10]

LASER LIPOLYSIS

In this technique, following TLA of lipoma and surrounding area, a small incision of 2 mm is made at the lateral edge of treatment area. Laser lipolysis is performed with continuous wave 980-nm diode laser delivered through a 600 μm fiberoptic cable, ensheathed, except for distal 2 mm, in a 1.2 mm diameter stainless steel cannula. The fiberoptic canula is introduced into the lipoma through 2 mm incision and laser is delivered once the tip of the fiberoptic is localized inside the lesion. A total of 7000 J of laser at 20 W power can be delivered in the deep, mid and superficial planes of the lesion to ensure complete lipolysis and lysis of fibrous attachments and capsule. Adequate lipolysis is indicated by minimal resistance to the motion of cannula which is advanced approximately 2 mm/sec. The laser is moved in a fan-like movement. The fragmented and partially liquefied contents of lipoma, fibrous tissue and capsule are expressed through the incision site by applying lateral pressure. The incision site is left open for drainage, and for prevention of formation of seroma or hematoma. Approximately 90% of lipomas can be removed completely with this technique. The retreatment of incompletely removed lipomas is generally well tolerated considering minimal invasive nature of the procedure.[11]

INJECTION LIPOLYSIS

Injection of detergents like phosphatidylcholine (PDC)/sodium deoxycholate (DC) into the subcutaneous fat is usually done for non-surgical contouring of body and removal of localized collection of excess fat. PDC/DC when injected into lipoma causes fat necrosis. Same technique and agents have been used successfully in the significant reduction of size of lipoma. However, there is lack of long-term efficacy, safety and recurrences.[19-21]

Similarly intralesional triamcinolone acetonide with equal amount of 1% lignocaine can be injected at the center of the lesion. Injection can be repeated several times every month for significant reduction in size of the lesion. It is used for the treatment of lipoma measuring <1 inch.[2]

Injection lipolysis is not an appropriate technique for complete removal of lipoma. But can be used preoperatively to reduce the size of the lesion.

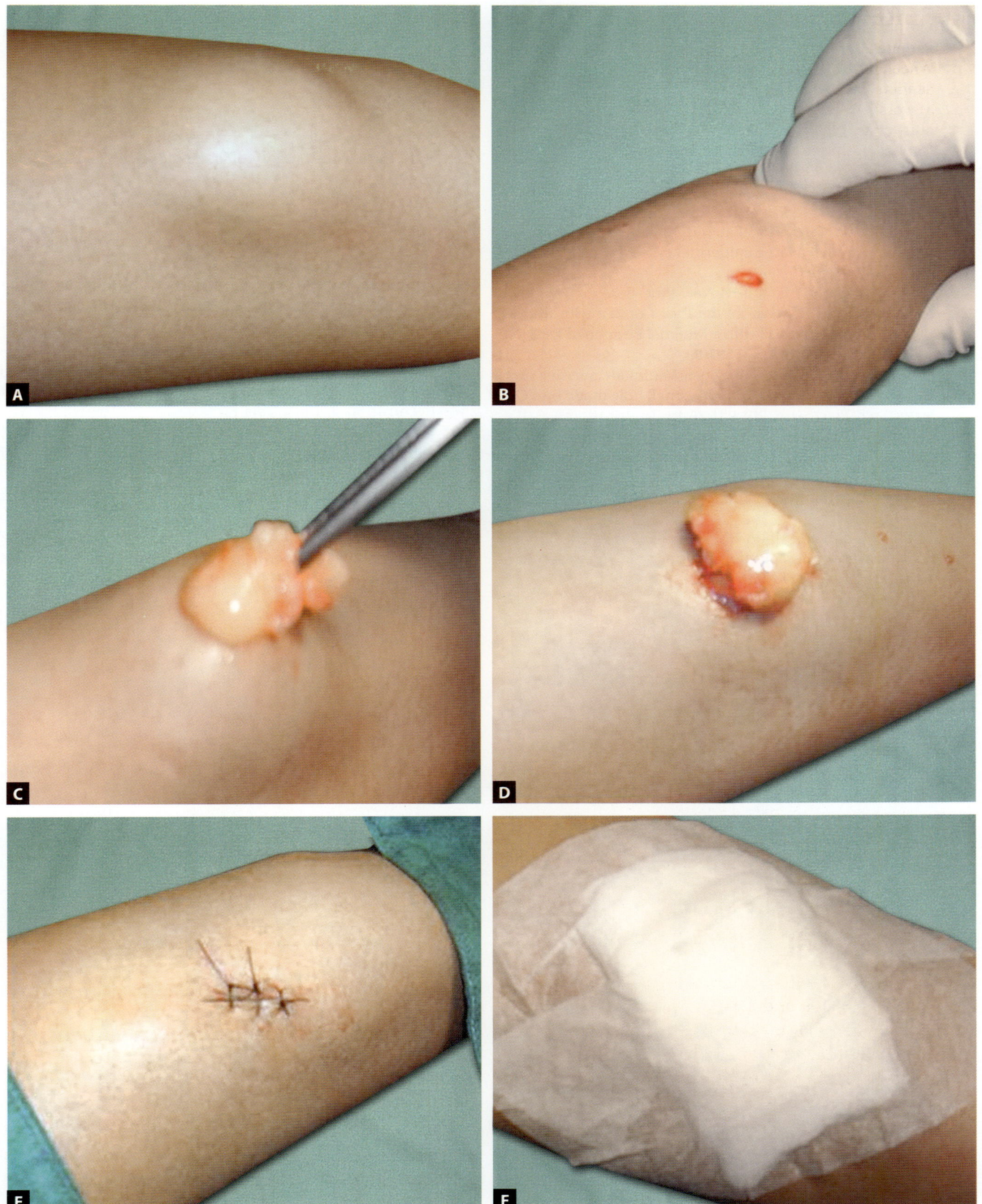

Figs. 7A to F: Lipoma removed through a small incision. (A) Large lipoma; (B) Small incision; (C and D) Fat removal with squeeze technique; (E) Wound closure with simple interrupted sutures; (F) Three layer dressing.

REFERENCES

1. Parlette III HL. Management of cutaneous cysts. In: Wheeland RG (Ed). Cutaneous Surgery. Philadelphia: WB Sanders. 1994; p. 647-63.
2. Mevorah B, Bovet R. Treatment of retro-auricular keratinous cysts. J Dermatol Surg Oncol. 1984;10:40-4.
3. Danna J. A simple treatment for sebaceous cysts. N Orleans Med Sci J. 194;98:528.
4. Robertson TM. Treatment of sebaceous cysts. Practitioner. 1989;233:700-1.
5. Park SW, Choi J, Lee HS, et al. Minimal incision suction-assisted excision of a large epidermal cyst. Aesthet Plast Surg. 2015;39:570-3.
6. Wu H, Wang S, Wu L, et al. A New Procedure for Treating a Sebaceous Cyst: Removal of the Cyst Content with a Laser Punch and the Cyst Wall with a Minimal Postponed Excision. Aesthet Plast Surg. 2009;33: 597-9.
7. Song SW, Burm JS, Yang WY, et al. Minimally invasive excision of epidermal cysts through a small hole made by a CO_2 laser. Arch Plast Surg. 2014;41:85-8.
8. Pandya KA, Radke F. Benign skin lesions: lipomas, epidermal inclusion cysts, muscle and nerve biopsies. Surg Clin North Am. 2009:89:677-87.
9. Salam GA. Lipoma excision. Am Fam Physician. 2002;65: 901-4
10. Choi CW, Kim BJ, Moon SE, et al. Treatment of lipomas assisted with tumescent liposuction. J Eur Acad Dermatol Venereol. 2007;21:243-6.
11. Stebbins WG, Hanke W, Petersen J. Novel method of minimally invasive removal of a large lipoma after laser lipolysis with 980 nm diode laser. Dermatol Ther. 2011;24: 125-30.
12. Shelley ED, Shelley WB. Piezosurgery: a conservative approach to encapsulated skin lesions. Cutis. 1986;38:123-6.
13. Vidimos AT. Management of Lipomas. In: Wheeland RG (Ed). Cutaneous Surgery. Philadelphia: WB Sanders. 1994; p. 675-83.
14. Fabri PJ, Adams JR. Simplified excision of lipomas. Surg Cynecol Obstet. 1987;165:173-4.
15. Hardin FF. A simple technique for removing lipomas. J Dermatol Surg Oncol. 1982;8:316-7.
16. Powell B, McLean NR. The treatment of lipomas by the "squeeze" technique. JR Coll Surg Edinb. 1985;30:391-2.
17. Harris WG. Treatment of lipomas by the squeeze technique. Letter JR Coll Surg Edinb. 1986;31:258.
18. Peinert RA, Courtiss EH. Excision from a distance: a technique for removal of benign subcutaneous lesions. Plast Reconstr Surg. 1983;72:94-6.
19. Rotunda AM, Albon G, Kolodney MS. Lipomas treated with subcutaneous deoxycholate injections. J Am Acad Dermatol. 2005;53:973-8.
20. Nanda S. Treatment of lipomas by injection lipolysis. J Cut Aesthet Surg. 2011;4:135-7.
21. Amber KT, Ovadia S, Camacho I. Injection therapy for the management of superficial subcutaneous lipomas. J Clin Aesthet Dermatol. 2014;7(6):46-8.

Chapter

28

Flaps for Facial Reconstruction

Vishwanath Jigjinni

Key Messages

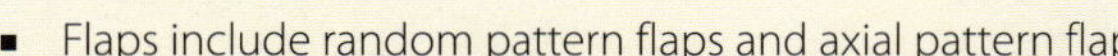

- Flaps include random pattern flaps and axial pattern flaps.
- Flaps are useful for closure of surgical wounds which cannot be closed by direct closure.
- Design of flap is vital to ensure proper reconstruction.
- Axial pattern flaps are more advanced flaps containing a specific vessel.
- Axial pattern flaps are preferred for better aesthetic results on face.
- Proper knowledge of anatomy, esthetic sense and training are needed for proper results.

INTRODUCTION

The fundamental techniques of dermatosurgery are most commonly applied in the treatment of the lesions of skin and soft tissues. These lesions are more commonly seen in the face due to its exposure to ultraviolet (UV) light and a dermatosurgeon is frequently consulted for these facial lesions.

Patients are often concerned about facial lesions as face is always the most exposed region of the body barring few cultures. Facial expressions are the essential ingredients of social interaction. The patients with facial lesions are very anxious about scars and disfigurement following the treatment. Fortunately in the facial region, due to an excellent blood supply, a dermatosurgeon has more reconstructive options than any other part of the body. The facial scars heal well with good esthetic outcome. These facts should always be stressed by the surgeon to patients seeking consultation for facial lesions to alleviate their anxiety.

Understanding the anatomy of the facial skin, its esthetic subunits, blood supply as well as physiological and anatomical changes associated with aging are important for a dermatosurgeon treating facial lesions.

Comprehensive knowledge of skin flaps, in terms of anatomy, design and blood supply has evolved mainly due to their application in the reconstruction of facial defects. Hence, it is important to understand the basic concepts of skin flap surgery in order to treat facial lesions more comprehensively.

HISTORICAL BACKGROUND[1]

The application of flaps in reconstructive surgery is recorded in Sushrut Samhita which dates back to 600 BC, where in pedicled flaps for nasal reconstruction were described. In 16th century Tagliocozzi used an arm flap for nasal reconstruction. In 1794 a letter was published in a British magazine which described a potters' tribe in India which was using forehead flap for nasal reconstruction.

Advancement flaps were first used by Celsius in Roman era. Later they were popularized by French surgeons.

Limberg in 1946[2] described a rhomboid transposition flap while the bilobed flap was described by Esser in 1918. He also popularized rotation flaps with back cut to increase the mobility of the flap.

All the flaps described above were random pattern flaps. But with the increased knowledge of cutaneous vascular anatomy, various axial pattern flaps (vide infra) were designed such as forehead flap by McGregor (1963), deltopectoral flap by Bakamjian (1965), groin flap by McGregor and Jackson (1972) and fasciocutaneous flaps in lower limbs by Ponten (1981).

The advances in anatomy, physiology lead to the application of composite flaps like muscle, musculocutaneous, osteocutaneous and microvasular flaps which

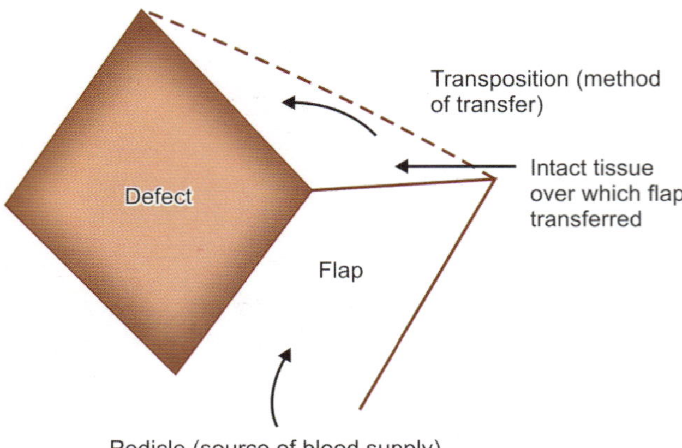

Fig. 1: Basics of flap.

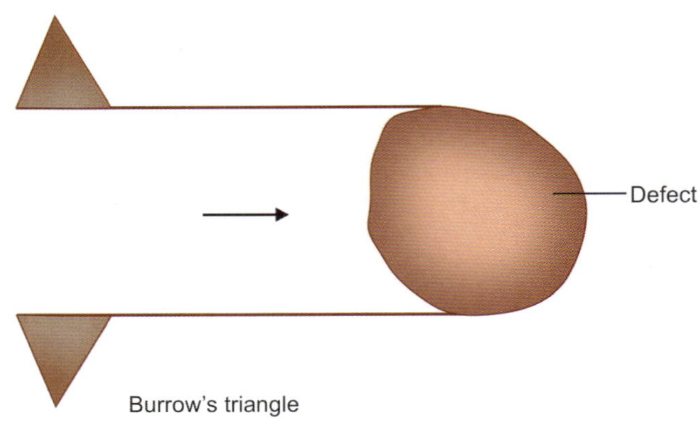

Fig. 2: Advancement flap.

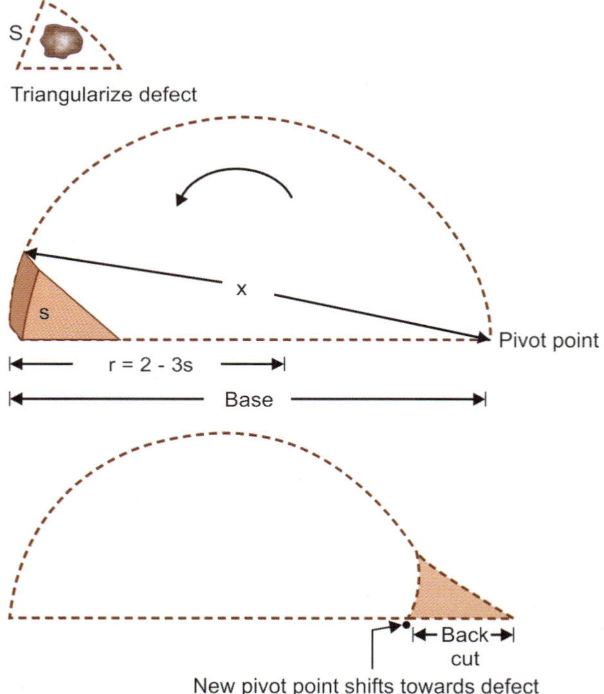

Fig. 3: Rotation flap.

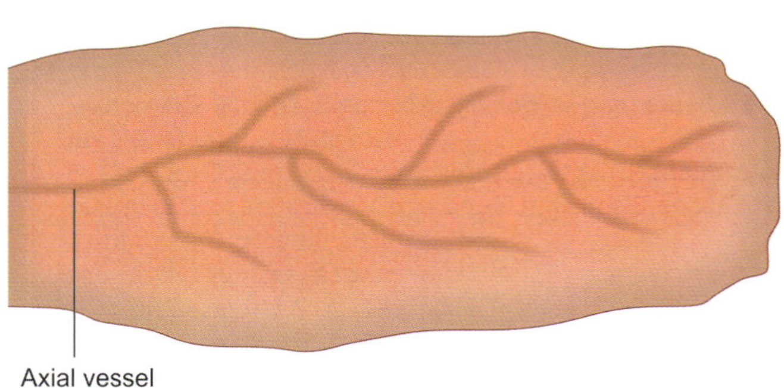

Fig. 4: Axial pattern flap.

is beyond the scope of this chapter. Furthermore the introduction of tissue expander has made available larger segment local tissue for reconstruction.

BASIC CONCEPTS OF FLAPS

Definition

The origin of term **flap** is derived from Dutch word *flappe* which means a broad and loose structure hung and fastened only by one side. The flap in medical term is defined as a unit of tissue of variable composition that is transferred from one site (donor) to another (recipient) while maintaining its blood supply (Fig. 1).

Classification

1. **On the basis of blood supply** flaps can be classified as Random pattern or axial pattern.

   Random pattern flaps

   The blood supply of random pattern flaps is derived from unnamed microscopic vessels present in the contiguous tissues. Three types of random pattern flaps are:

   a. **Advancement flaps:** In this type of flap a segment of tissue is moved in a linear axis to reconstruct the defect (Fig. 2).
   b. **Transposition flap:** In this type of flap a segment of tissue is transferred over an intervening area of normal skin to the defect (Fig. 1).
   c. **Rotation flap:** In this flap the tissue is rotated around a pivot point to reconstruct the defect (Fig. 3).

   Non-random flaps

   a. *Axial pattern flaps*: In axial pattern flaps there is a known blood vessel supplying a segment of tissue making these flaps more reliable in terms of the blood supply. Generally in random pattern flap the length to breadth ratio is 1:1 which can be extended to 3:1 in face due to its rich blood supply. But this ratio is much higher in axial pattern flaps depending on the region of the body (Fig. 4).

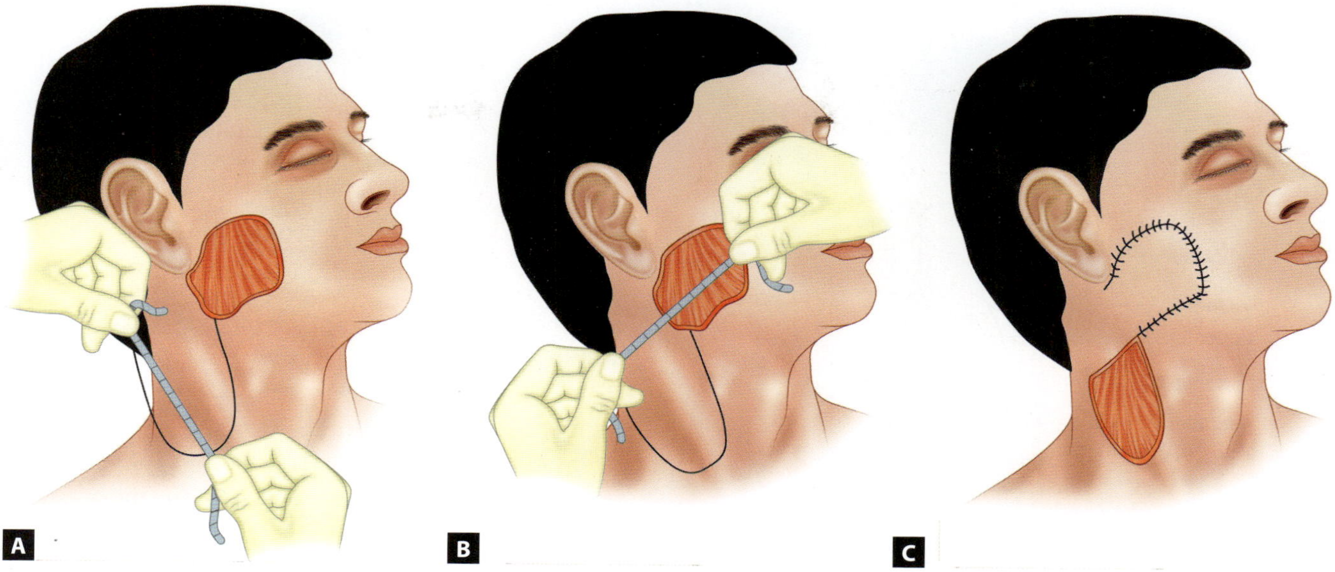

Figs. 5A to C: Planning in reverse.

b. *Other non-random flaps*: Other non-random flaps like fasciocutaneous, septocutaneous, perforator flaps are used in reconstruction of extremities and are beyond the scope of this textbook.

2. **On the basis of tissue transferred** the flaps may be:
   a. *Simple*: Where a single type of tissue is transferred e.g. skin, muscle.
   b. *Composite*: Where a combination of tissue is transferred, e.g. skin and muscle (e.g. myocutaneous).
3. **On the basis of location of the defect** the flap may be:
   a. *Local*: Where the defect is adjacent to the donor site.
   b. *Distant*: Where the defect is in a different region than the donor site.

The distant flap may be **pedicled** where the blood supply is preserved through an intact tissue bridge; or it may be **free flap** where the donor tissue is separated from the donor site along with the vascular pedicle and the blood supply is re-established in the recipient area by anastomosis of vascular pedicle to the vessels in the recipient region.

FLAP ANATOMY AND FLAP DESIGN

As described earlier and shown in Figure 1 a flap is a segment of tissue harvested from a donor area and transferred into the defect keeping its blood supply intact. This is the basis of flap design, which in turn, forms the basis of good reconstruction. The important considerations in flap design are:

a. **Defect**: Always assess the defect carefully in terms of size, shape, tissues in the floor and special tissue requirement such as hair-bearing tissue, etc.
b. **Reconstructive options:** There are many reconstructive methods available to repair a defect. It is a good dictum to think of the simplest options first and go up the reconstructive ladder to more complex method if the simpler options will not fulfill the reconstructive requirements.
c. **Planning in reverse:** The surgeon should measure the defect carefully and make a template of the defect and transfer these measurements or the template to the donor site to mark the flap outline (Figs. 5A to C).
d. **Donor site:** It is very important to choose the donor site carefully to get a good result in the flap reconstruction.

The basic principle applied is "Stealing from Peter to pay Paul". Hence the donor site should have relatively *excess tissue* which can be transferred to the defect. This is best tested by pinching the skin and subcutaneous tissue in various areas and direction in the potential donor site.

In facial reconstruction the *esthetic appearance* is of prime importance. The tissue transferred should be optimum in terms of:

- Colour match
- Texture

Special considerations are necessary in terms of sensation in some areas, hair-bearing skin in eyebrow and moustache area and function in certain areas like eyelid and lips.

While designing a facial flap a special consideration should be given to *esthetic subunits* of the face (Fig. 6). Such refinement improves the esthetic results of flap reconstruction. It is also important to design flaps in such a way that the resulting donor scar falls in the line of junction of esthetic unit such as nasolabial groove or in the line of relaxed skin tension lines (RSTLs) (Fig. 7). Older patients are good candidates for flap surgery due to laxity, inherently seen in aging skin, which is useful for flap harvesting. This age group also has very evident RSTL which makes flap designing easier. Coincidently this age group also has more prevalence of facial skin lesions.

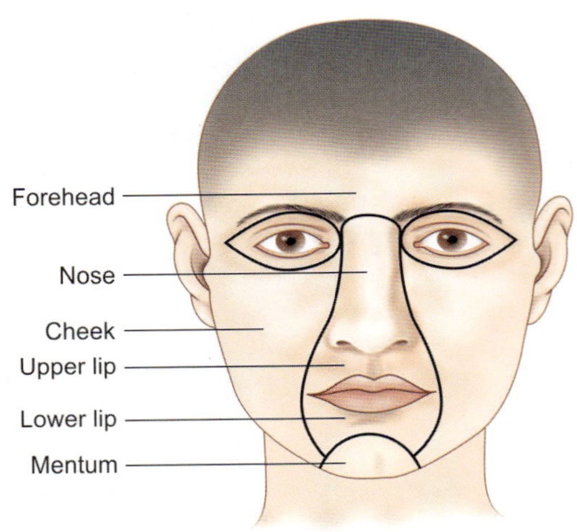

Fig. 6: Esthetic subunits of face.

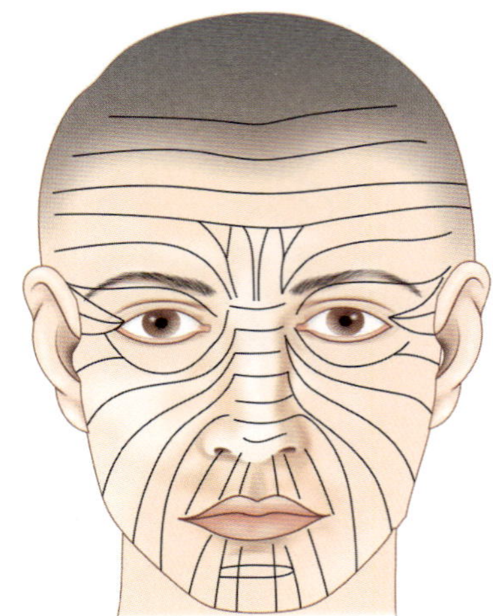

Fig. 7: Resting skin tension lines (RSTLs) of the face.

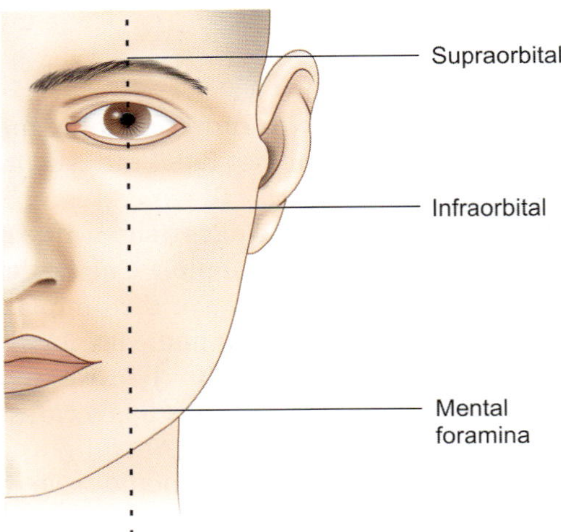

Fig. 8: Anatomy of foramina for nerve blocks.

Blood Supply of Face

Blood supply of face is important in axial pattern flaps such as lateral forehead flap (anterior branch of superficial temporal artery), nasolabial flap (facial artery which terminates as angular artery). The length-to-breadth ratio of such flap is high and the flap can be designed to reach a defect farther away from the donor site. The facial skin gets its vascular supply through terminal branches of external carotid artery, namely facial and superficial temporal arteries. The forehead gets its blood supply from branches of ophthalmic artery namely supratrochlear and supraorbital arteries.

Nerve Supply of Face

Nerve supply of face is important as regards preserving sensation in areas such as lips and eyelids. It is also useful in giving nerve blocks (Fig. 8). It is important to note that all three nerves namely supraorbital, infraorbital and mental nerve emerge from bony canals which lie in a vertical line that passes through pupil on that side. All nerves mentioned are branches of three divisions of trigeminal nerve respectively. The ear is supplied in its lower half by greater auricular nerve, which arises from cervical plexus.

FLAP PHYSIOLOGY

The viability of a flap is based on the tissue perfusion which is derived through an intact blood supply. This is possible through careful planning of the flap. Any segment of skin derives its blood supply from periphery and through deeper tissues. In a flap design it is imperative to keep an intact tissue bridge while other incisions are made to mobilize the flap and transfer it into the defect. The perfusion pressure in the capillaries has to be maintained above the critical capillary closure pressure to ensure the tissue is adequately perfused and kept viable. This is related to the anatomy of local vasculature, i.e. axial or random pattern and also to the density of capillary network which varies in different areas of the body. In any flap this perfusion is insured by:

a. **Length-to-breadth ratio:** As described earlier in a random pattern flap this ratio is 1:1 but can be extended in face to 4:1 or 5:1 due to its rich blood supply. But 3:1 ration is a good safe limit in the face. In axial pattern flap this ratio can be 6:1.
b. **Delay phenomenon:** In some regions of body where there is an inadequate blood supply the length-to-breadth ratio can be increased by making partial incisions, e.g. only lateral incisions. After a delay of 2 weeks all incisions are made and the flap is transferred. The initial partial incisions help induct blood supply from non-incised tissues thereby increasing the L:B ratio. This is applied mainly for the flaps in lower extremities and is rarely used in facial reconstruction.
c. **Tissue tension:** The tissue tension reduces tissue perfusion by stretching and collapse of capillaries. Hence the flaps should be designed such that there

is no tissue tension when the flap is sutured into the defect. The common mistake is underestimating the size of the flap which should ideally be larger (in length and breadth) than the defect to avoid the tension.

Finally **tissue handling** is also important for good result. The surgeon should familiarize with the use of skin hooks instead of handling the flap with tissue forceps which, if not used carefully, can damage the tissue. The **undermining** of edges should be limited. This procedure mobilizes a tissue at the expense of interrupting its blood supply. The importance of **hemostasis** cannot be overemphasized. A hematoma increases the tissue tension and interferes with blood supply of the flap leading to flap necrosis and infection. The vitality of tissue is preserved by avoiding **desiccation** of tissues during surgery.

PREOPERATIVE CARE

When a patient is seen in a consulting room, a detailed history is taken and a comprehensive physical examination is done. It is important to note history of hypertension, diabetes and cardiac diseases. The history should include an enquiry about previous surgeries, dental procedures (especially under local anesthesia), regular medications including nonsteroidal anti-inflammatory drugs (NSAIDs) like aspirin and known allergies.

Physical examination should include checking for anemia, high blood pressure and systematic examination of heart, lungs, abdomen, extremities and neck. The local lesion is examined for its size, site, mobility and consistency. The regional lymph nodes are checked for enlargement.

Preoperative investigations are planned according to the general health and the age of the patient, but should include hemogram and routine urine test. The older patients may need more comprehensive investigations such as blood sugar, urea, creatinine, electrolyte, liver function tests, chest X-ray and electrocardiogram. The patients with poor health may require a consultation with physician before the surgery is planned. Coagulation profile is checked in patient suspected of bleeding diathesis.

The patients on antiplatelet drugs such as aspirin are instructed to stop their use 2–3 weeks before the scheduled date of surgery. Smokers are advised to stop smoking 1–2 weeks prior to surgery. On the day of the surgery appropriate instructions are given about starvation and taking essential medications like antihypertensive drugs. The diabetic patients are managed as per the planned anesthesia, e.g. local or general. The patient is instructed about the shaving and shower and instructed to visit the hospital along with the results of investigations and a responsible accompanying person.

ANESTHESIA AND SURGICAL TECHNIQUES

Most of the small flaps can be done on outpatient basis. As described earlier the lesion should be marked with indelible ink. Then proposed margin of resection is drawn around the lesion. The flap to be utilized for reconstruction is decided and its outline is marked using the planning in reverse method (*See* Figs. 5A to C).

Local anaesthesia is sufficient in majority of cases. Lignocaine 2% with adrenaline in 1:200,000 is commonly used local anesthetic agent. It can be diluted with equal amount of water for injection to increase the volume where a larger field of surgery is planned. Addition of bupivacaine (0.25% or 0.5%) helps prolong the anesthesia and also gives good postoperative analgesia. Sodium bicarbonate solution (7.5%) added to lignocaine in 1:5 dilution increases the pH of the latter and helps reduce the pain during the infiltration. It is good practice to inject local anesthetic drug 10–15 minutes before the incision to allow the anesthetic and vasoconstrictive effect of the injected solution to take place. This time can be utilized for hand scrub and the preparation of the operative part. The patient is made to lie comfortably on the operation table. It is a good practice to cover the eyes of the patient with a moist gauze to shield them from bright operating lights unless the surgical field includes eyelids or eyebrows. For elderly patients and those with coexisting medical condition, it is safe to have an anesthesiologist be present during the surgery either to monitor the patient or to give sedation as an adjunct to local anesthesia.

Incisions are made as per the markings. The lesion is excised taking care not to crush the specimen with toothed forceps. The open wound is covered with moist gauze and firm pressure is applied to get hemostasis. After waiting for 2–3 minutes the gauze is removed and the bleeding is controlled with bipolar diathermy.

Next the flap margins are incised and the flap to be transposed is undermined minimally to allow it some mobility. The undermining is done in the subdermal fat layer protecting the rich dermal vascular plexus. Hemostasis is achieved again and the flap is ready to be transferred into the defect.

Always begin by closing the donor defect which releases any tension on the flap. 4-0 or 5-0 absorbable sutures like Polyglactin (Vicryl) for deeper layers and 4-0 or 5-0 Nylon (Ethilon) or Polypopylene (Prolene) for skin are good suture materials. The subcutaneous tissue is approximated with interrupted and inverted sutures, taking a small bite of dermis to achieve good approximation of the wound edges and wound strength. The skin is approximated with interrupted sutures either simple or vertical mattress, depending how easily the skin gets approximated. The most important point in skin closure is to ensure that the skin edges approximate well with eversion. The finer suture like 6-0 Polypropylene may be used for eyelid skin.

With good hemostasis there is rarely any need for wound drainage. Light dressing is applied after the wound closure without using excessive compression.

POSTOPERATIVE CARE

Most of the patients are treated on outpatient basis. They should be given adequate pain relief. The use of NSAID should be minimal to prevent hematoma formation. Routine prophylactic antibiotics are not indicated. The patients are instructed to remove dressing on the first or second postoperative day and to wash area with lukewarm water and soap. It helps to apply nonstaining ointment like neosporin or chloromycetin on the wound which acts like water impermeable barrier and helps reassure patients. The patients are also warned that there is a possibility of some tissue swelling and ecchymosis which will subside in 2–3 weeks. In the event of small bleeding, the patient is instructed to sit upright and told to apply firm pressure on the wound with a clean gauze piece for 15 minutes. The patient may be handed over a few of these at the time of discharge. The sutures are removed on 5th to 7th postoperative day. The patient is instructed to massage the scar with vitamin E based moisturizing cream or in some patients silicone gel may be applied to facilitate the scar maturation. Patients are advised to use UV protection for a year after the surgery.

COMPLICATIONS OF FLAPS

a. **Hematoma:** The face has excellent blood supply which helps in better survival of flaps. But the disadvantage of the good blood supply is that there are more possibilities of hematoma formation. The hematoma increases tissue tension jeopardizing the blood supply to the flap. Prevention is always better as in any other field of medicine. Meticulous hemastasis, withdrawal of drugs like aspirin, vitamin E, clopidogrel is important in prevention of the hematoma. The hematoma cannot be prevented by tight dressing; on the contrary this excessive pressure may lead to flap necrosis. It is best to drain the wound in cases where there is a possibility of postoperative bleeding.
b. **Flap necrosis:** A good flap design in terms of suitability of the donor site (adequate tissue), L:B ratio, tissue tension is important in prevention of this complication. Smokers are advised to stop smoking 1 to 2 weeks prior to surgery.
c. **Infection:** Infection is a relatively rare complication due to excellent blood supply in the face. Prophylactic antibiotics are not routinely used for such surgery. Meticulous design and planning and good tissue handling help prevent complications such as tissue necrosis, flap necrosis and hematoma which are precursors of infection. The infection manifests as pain, discharge and the local signs of inflammation are evident. The treatment consist of wound drainage where possible and antibiotics.
d. **Scars:** Scars are inevitable sequel of any surgery. It is important to design the flaps carefully with due consideration of the esthetic units, the borders between these units and RSTLs as described earlier. Unacceptable scars may be revised 6–12 months after surgery once the scar maturation is complete.
e. **Nerve damage:** Nerve damage is a rare complication of cutaneous surgery and any anesthesia or paresthesia due to division of terminal sensory branches usually resolves in 6–12 months. But care should be taken in the area lateral to the lateral end of eyebrow where the temporal branch of facial nerve is superficial and the damage to the nerve in this region will cause the paralysis of the frontalis muscle leading to brow ptosis.

THE DETAILS OF BASIC FLAPS AND THEIR APPLICATION (TABLE 1)

Advancement Flaps

Advancement flap is one where a tissue is moved in a linear direction to fill a defect. In fact undermining that is commonly done during wound closure is a type of advancement flap. Advancement flaps are useful in defects where closure with undermining will distort contours or hair line, e.g. forehead, eyebrows, cheek close to eyelid, nasal dorsum, vermillion of lip or ala of nose. A defect in these areas can be reconstructed with advancement flap from adjacent area rather than by undermining the edges and direct closure of the wound which will cause distortion of hair line, eyebrow position, lid margin, vermillion or alar rim. The advancement flap can be single pedicled where tissue is moved from one side of the defect (U-plasty) or it can be bi-pedicled where tissue is obtained from both

Table 1: Choice of flaps for regional defects

Scalp	
Small defects ≤6 cm	Single or multiple rotation flaps
Larger defects	Pericranium intact: Skin graft No pericranium: Transposition flap + skin graft
Forehead	Bilateral advancement flaps
Cheek	
Medial	▪ Cheek advancement ▪ Transposition flap ▪ V-Y advancement flap especially near ala
Lateral	▪ Transposition flap ▪ Rotation flap for larger defect
Lip	
Central	Bilateral advancement flap
Lateral	Rotation
Nose	Advancement of dorsal nasal skin, bilobed flap or nasolabial flap, forehead flap for large defects

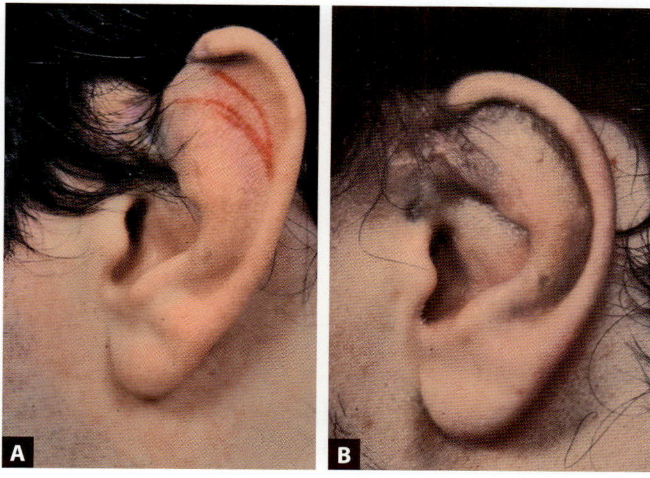

Figs. 9A and B: Helical advancement flap.

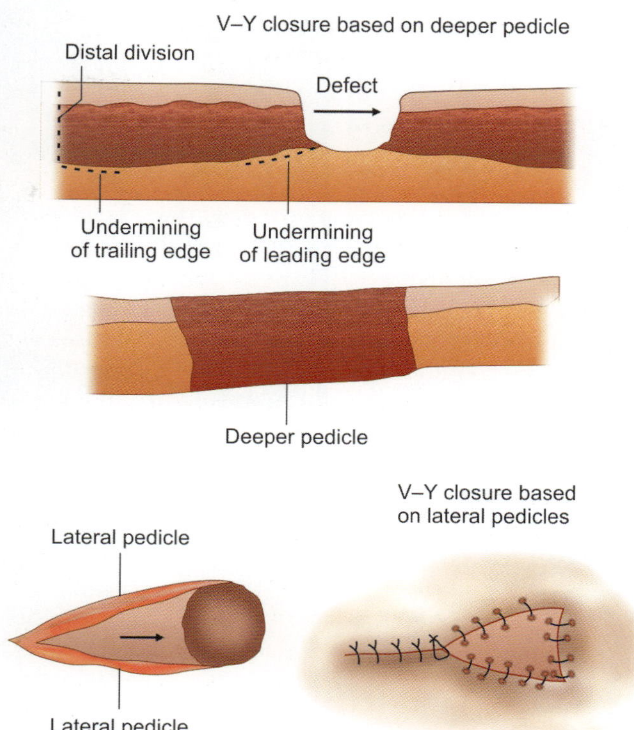

Fig. 10: V-Y advancement flap.

sides of the defect (H-plasty). When advancement flaps are used, one creates discrepancy in the length of the two sides of the skin edges which is corrected either by cutting out a tissue at the base as Burrow's triangle or by a Z-plasty in the trailing end of the wound (see Fig. 2).

The classical examples of unipedicled advancement flaps are seen in the closure of defects near ala of the nose where the defect is cut as a crescent and the cheek skin is advanced to close the defect giving an excellent result. The skin is undermined through a plane in the subcutaneous fat just below dermis thus avoiding injury to deeper vessels and nerves while preserving the dermal vascular plexus which is vital to its perfusion.

The mucosal advancement flap is used to resurface the vermillion of the lip especially after excision of a lesion or after excision of segments affected by vitiligo. The undermining is done through submucosal plane and the approximation of the edges is done using an absorbable suture like undyed Polyglactin (Vicryl) or catgut (4-0 or 5-0). I prefer not to use Polyglecaprone (Monocryl) as it gives a troublesome pricking sensation although the sutures are less visible because Monocryl is a transparent material.

Full thickness of tissue can also be advanced to reconstruct defect especially in lip or helical rim. The advanced tissue unit is based on intact bridge of tissue, e.g. posterior skin in case of helical advancement (Figs. 9A and B).

V-Y Advancement Flap

Another useful advancement flap is V-Y advancement flap which is versatile and uses matching tissue from the contiguous area. Although more commonly used in hand surgery this flap is useful for reconstruction in forehead, lower part of nose and upper lip areas. This flap derives its perfusion through the intact bridge of subcutaneous tissue which can be either deep to the flap or lateral to it. The advancement is obtained due to laxity in the subcutaneous plane and closure is helped by the tissue laxity on either side of the flap (Fig. 10).

When V-Y advancement is done based on a deep pedicle the flap is cut as per the markings. The flap is advanced into the defect. If there is lack of adequate mobility then the leading edge and also the trailing edges can be undermined minimally to achieve a greater mobility.

In a lateral pedicle V-Y flap the entire undersurface of the flap is undermined. Gentle dissection of the connective tissue septae in the lateral tissue achieves the desired advancement. The closure starts in the donor area which helps to propel flap into the defect. It is useful in many regions of the face (Figs. 11 to 14).

The versatility of V-Y advancement is used even as an adjunct to other flaps especially for closing the donor defect.

Transposition Flaps

The transposition flaps are more commonly used in the facial reconstruction due to availability of donor sites with adequate tissue laxity. They are used in forehead, cheek, temporal area, ear and nasal tip. Many modifications have been done to suit a particular reconstructive requirement (Fig. 15).[3]

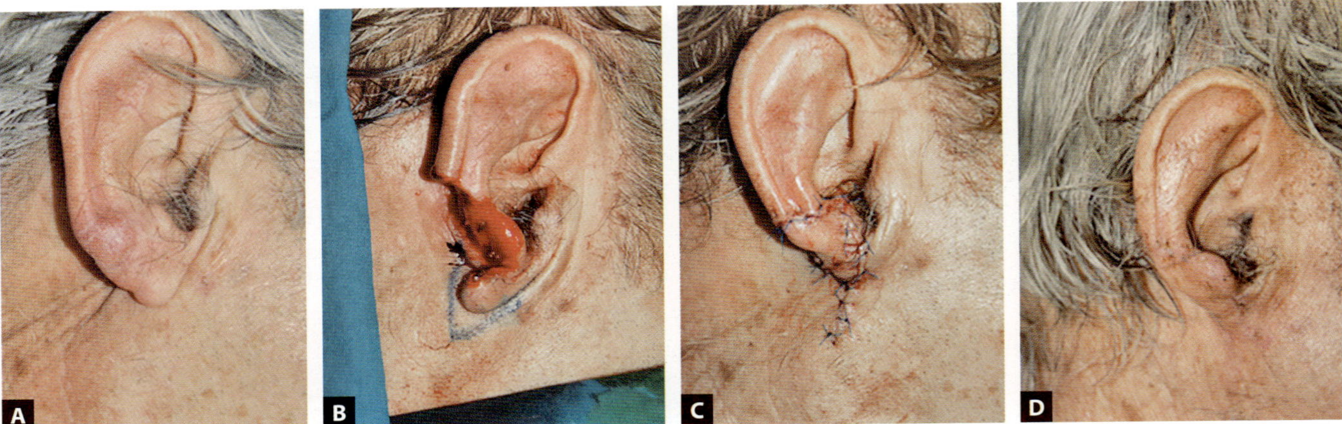

Figs. 11A to D: V-Y advancement flap for ear.

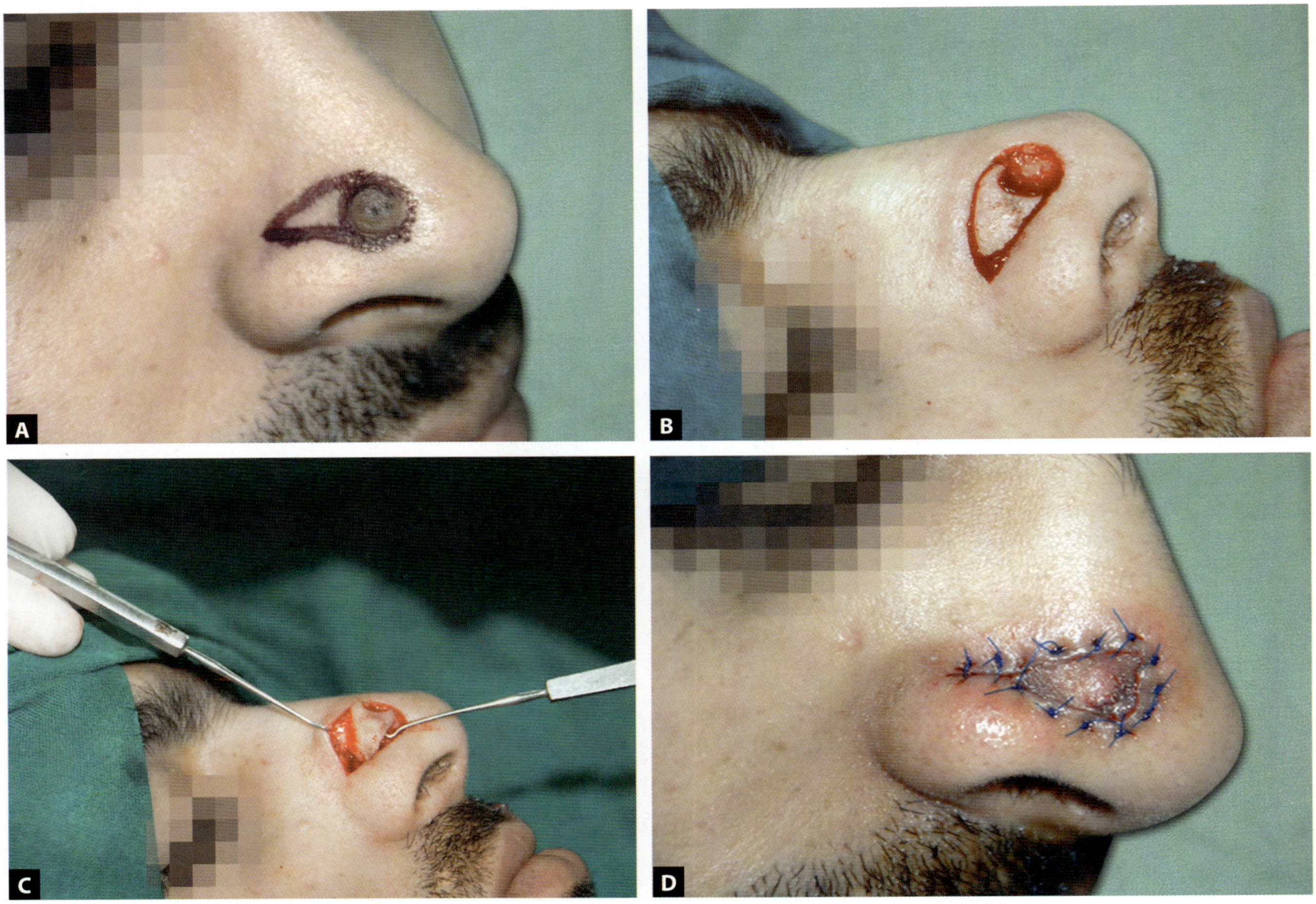

Figs. 12A to D: V-Y flap for nose.

THE DETAILS OF FLAP DESIGN AND RECONSTRUCTION

The lesion to be excised is demarcated with marking ink and the margin of excision is also marked. Then the direction of RSTLs or skin creases or maximum skin laxity is noted. The defect is now marked as a rhomboid with all sides equal and the angles as 60°, 120°. A V-shaped flap is marked starting from a point which is adjacent to the angle of 120°. Both the lines of V are of the same length as the rhomboid and they form an angle of 60°. The lesion is excised and the flap is undermined in the subcutaneous plane. The hemostasis, flap transfer and the closure is done as described earlier.

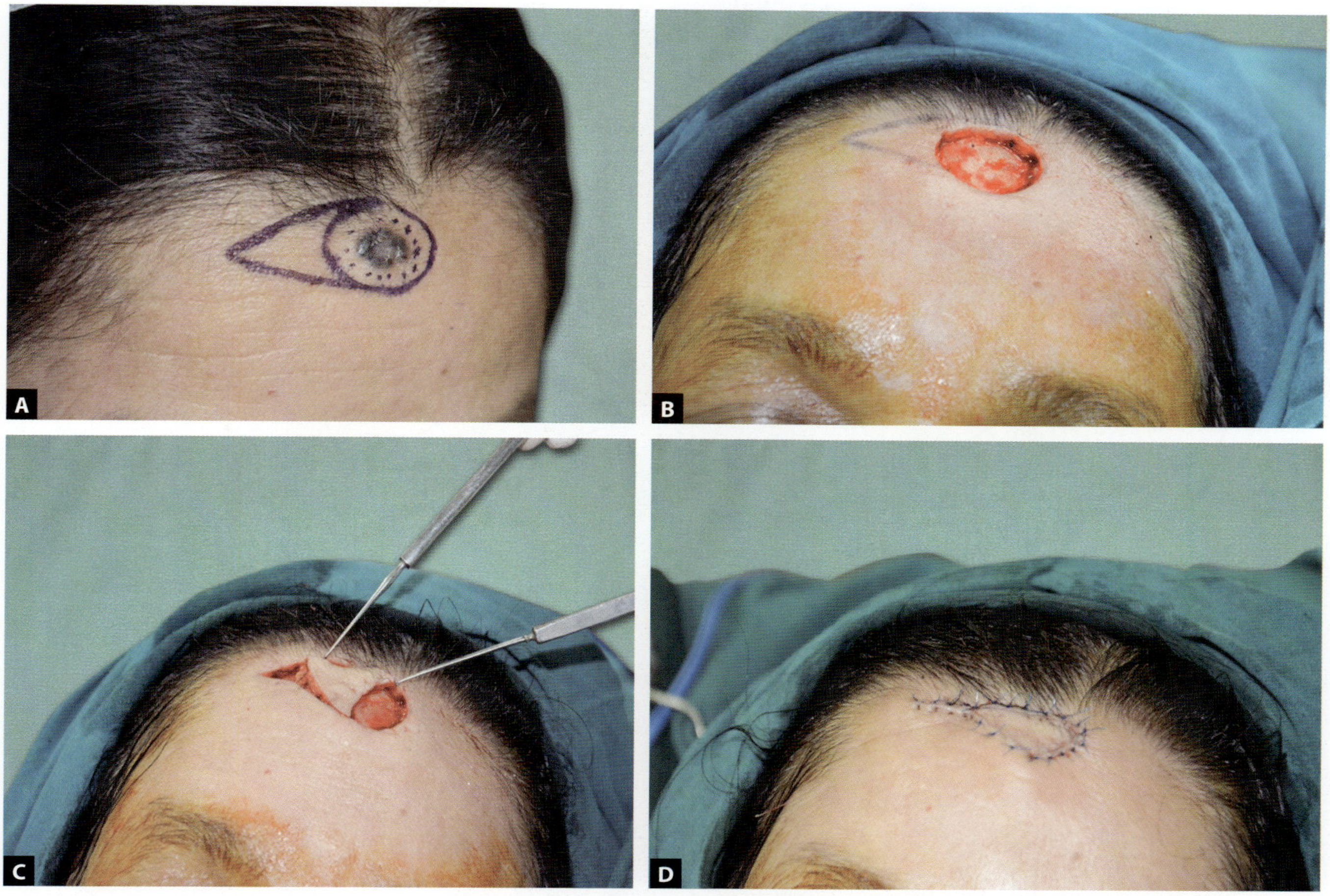

Figs. 13A to D: V-Y flap for forehead.

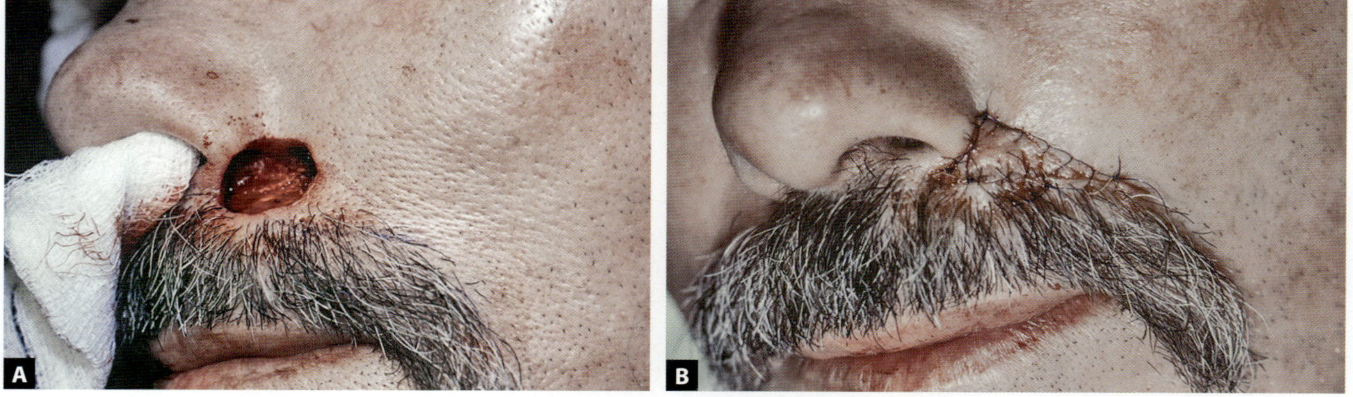

Figs. 14A and B: V-Y flap for upper lip.

Surgeons rarely excise the lesion to make a rhomboid shaped defect. Hence the rhomboid flap may be cut as rhomboid or as an arc of circle or as a triangle to fit the defect with some adjustments.

A useful modification of the rhomboid flap is called **'square peg in a round hole'**.[4] Most of the lesions are excised as a circle. The flap is then drawn from the periphery of the defect noting the area of maximum skin laxity. AV-shaped flap is marked and cut to fit the defect, excising the angles of the flap when necessary. The main disadvantage of this flap is that it leaves a small dog-ear at the pivot point. This usually becomes less obvious with passage of time or may need a small revision surgery. But this flap certainly adds versatility to reconstruction of facial defects (Figs. 16 to 18).

Bilobed flap is another useful modification where two transposition flaps with a common pedicle are used to fill the successive defects and the most distal donor site is

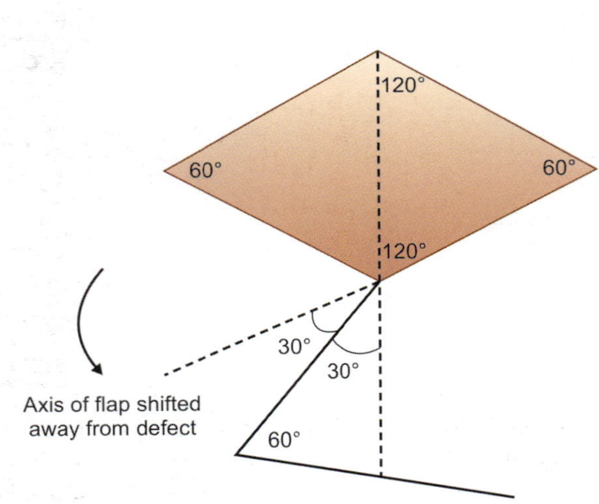

Fig. 15: Dufourmentel flap.

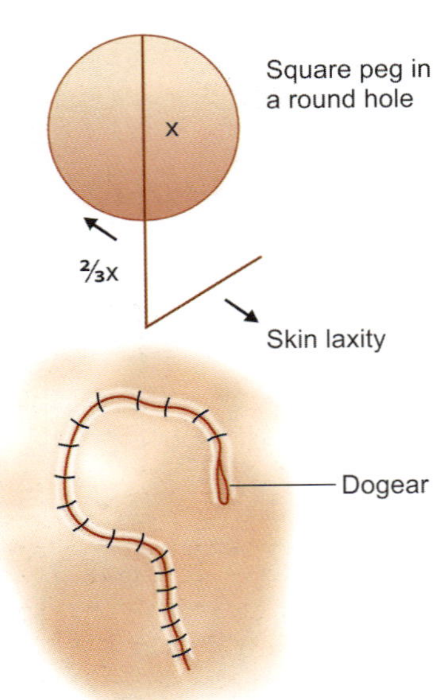

Fig. 16: Square peg in a round hole flap.

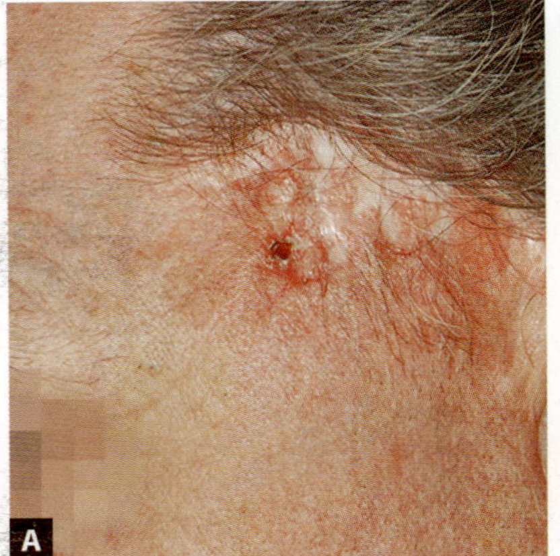
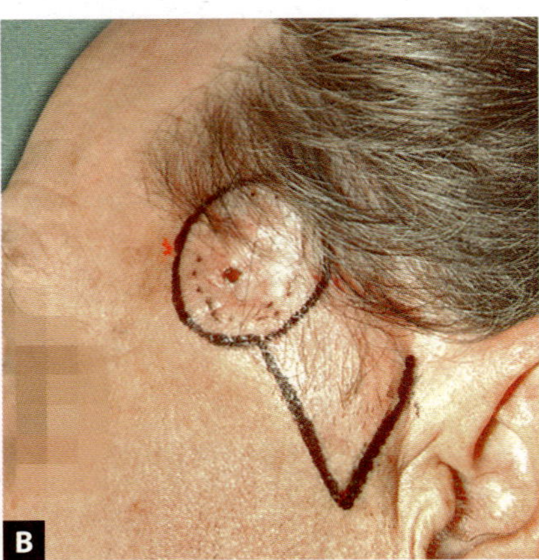
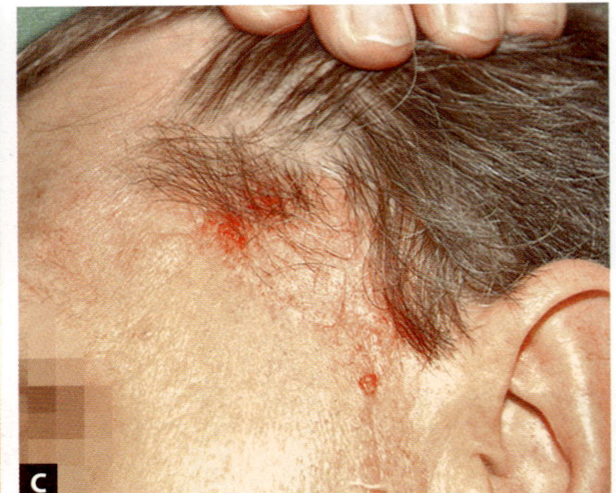

Figs. 17A to C: Square peg in a round hole flap.

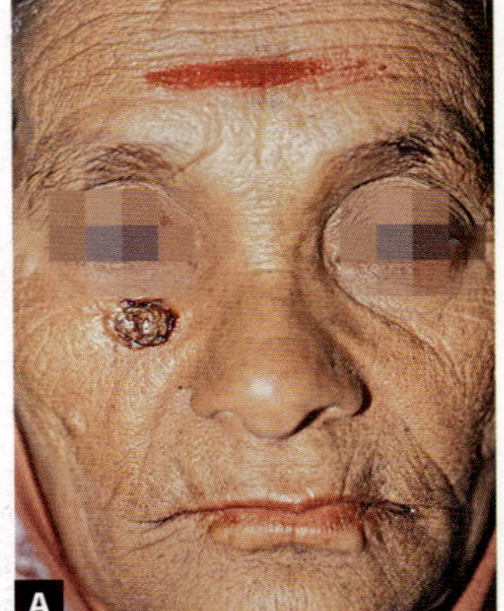
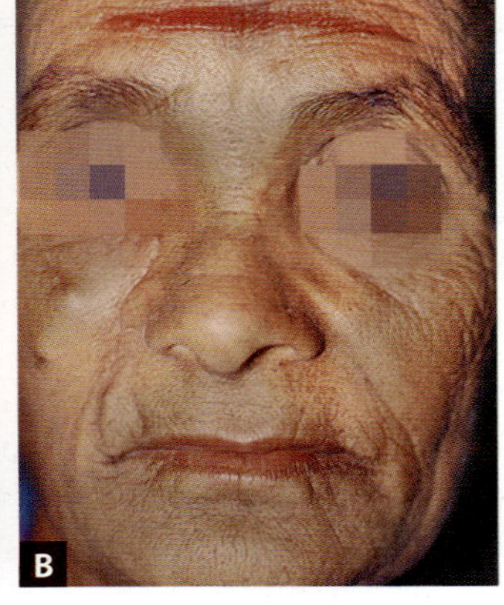

Fig. 18: Transposition flap from nasolabial area.

closed primarily.[4] It is useful for reconstruction of defects where tissue laxity in the contiguous area is deficient as to be closed primarily, e.g. nasal tip and ala.[5]

The defect is assessed for its size and location. The area where there is maximum skin laxity from where the second flap will be designed is assessed. A vertical line through the defect is drawn. The pivotal point is about one radius distance from the defect. The primary flap adjacent to the defect and slightly smaller than the defect with long axis 30–45° to the line drawn through the defect is marked. Then the second flap adjacent to primary flap and again smaller (about half the size of the first) than the primary at an angle 60–180° to the line through the defect is marked. The flaps are dissected through a subdermal plane, rotated into the successive defects. The defect of the second flap is closed primarily. It is important to base flaps on lateral side while reconstructing defects of the nasal tip and base them on medial side for the defects of the ala of nose. It is important not to cross the midline while designing the flaps (Figs. 19 to 21).[6]

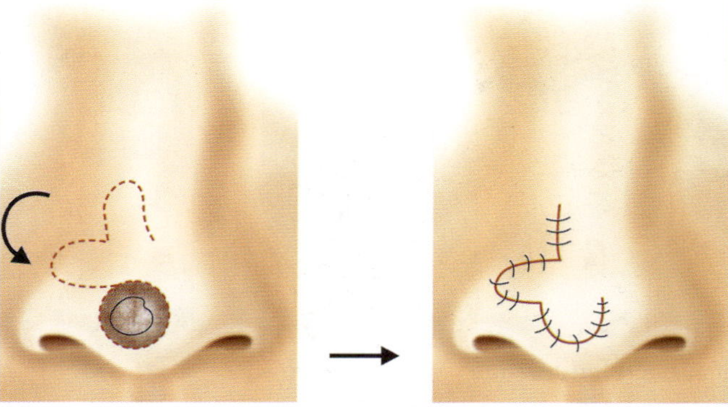

Fig. 19: Bilobed flap.

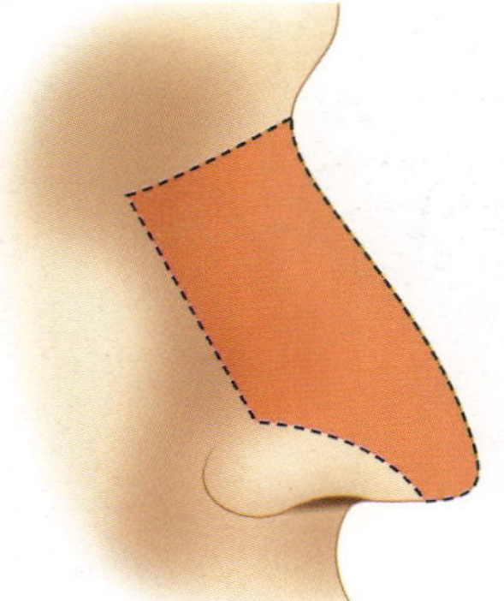

Fig. 20: Area for bilobed flap reconstruction.

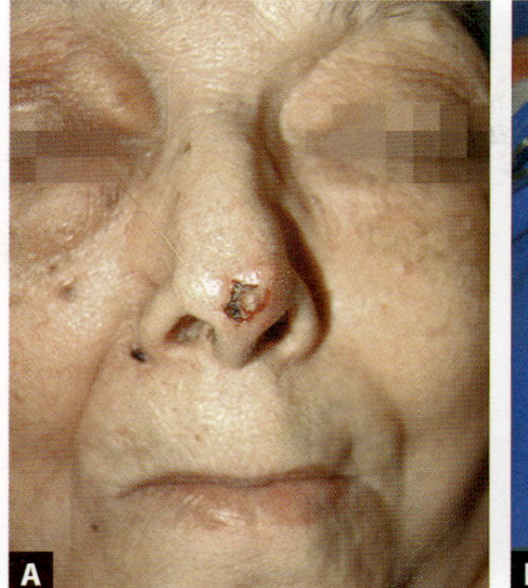
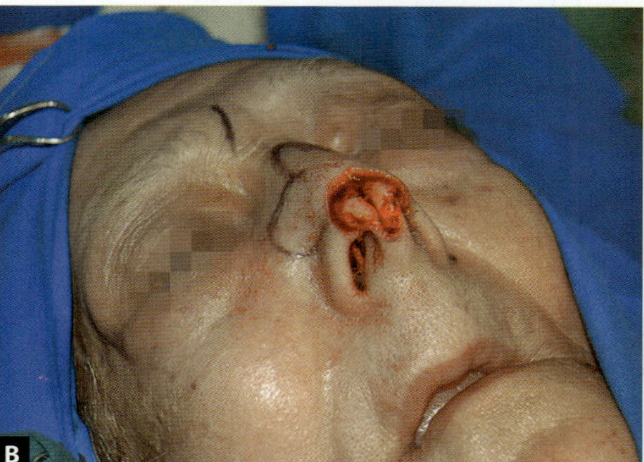
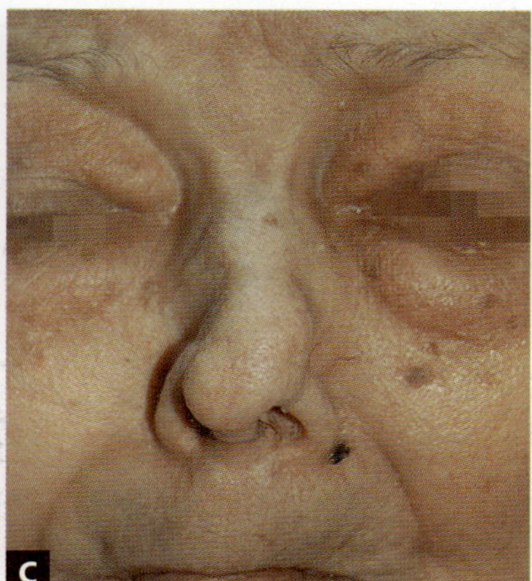

Figs. 21A to C: Bilobed flap.

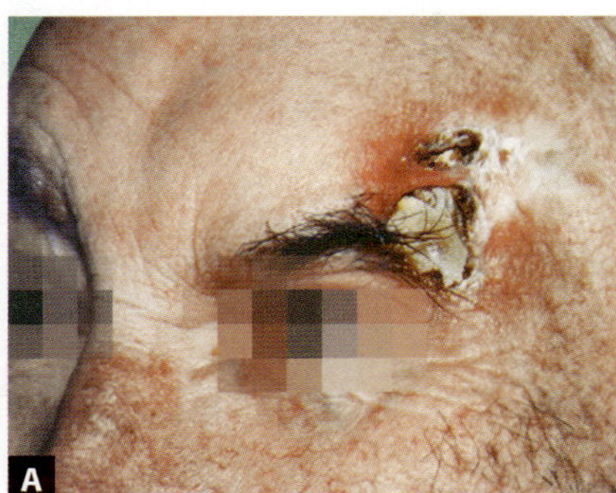
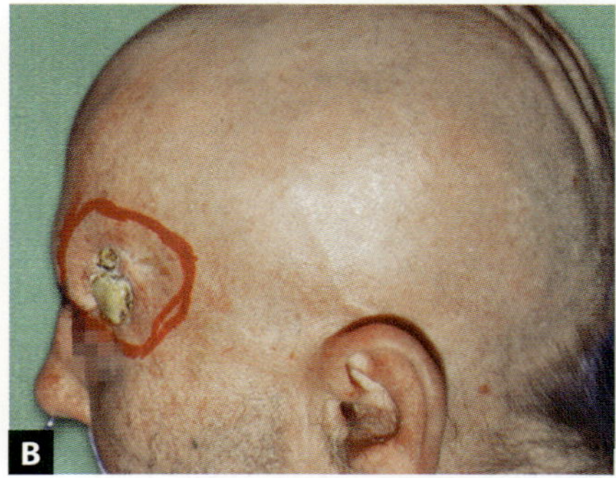
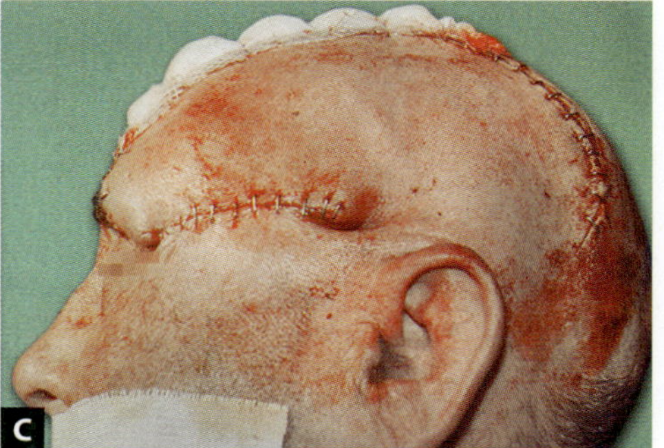

Figs. 22A to C: Rotation flap in scalp.

Rotation Flaps

The rotation flaps are more useful in areas with uniform laxity that does not allow harvest of a flap and closure of the defect, e.g. scalp (Figs. 22A to C). The flaps are most useful in areas where there are no significant anatomical landmarks to obstruct the rotational movement of the flap. The large segment of tissue is rotated around a pivot point into the defect. The donor defect is usually repaired by direct closure (Tenzel flap) (Figs. 23A to C) or by local Z-plasty (Mustarde flap) (Figs. 24A to C) or by using a small skin graft. The mobility of this flap can increased by a back cut or by cutting a Burrows triangle near the pivot point, the latter also helps reducing tension in the flap.[7] The long incisions are required to mobilize tissue sufficiently. The rotation flaps are generally inferiorly based to allow lymphatic drainage. These flaps are mainly used in scalp and cheeks where the long scars can be more easily concealed (Figs. 25A to C).

It is important to triangularize the defect. The diameter of the semicircle should be 3 times the length of the defect and the circumference of the flap should be 5–8 times the width of the defect. Always ensure that the length from the pivot point to the apex of the flap is greater than the

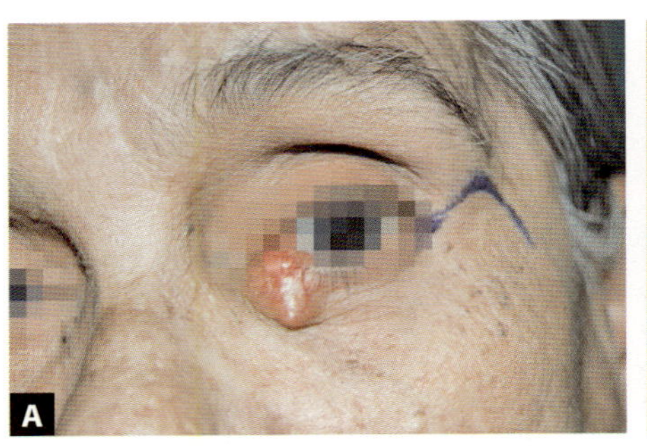
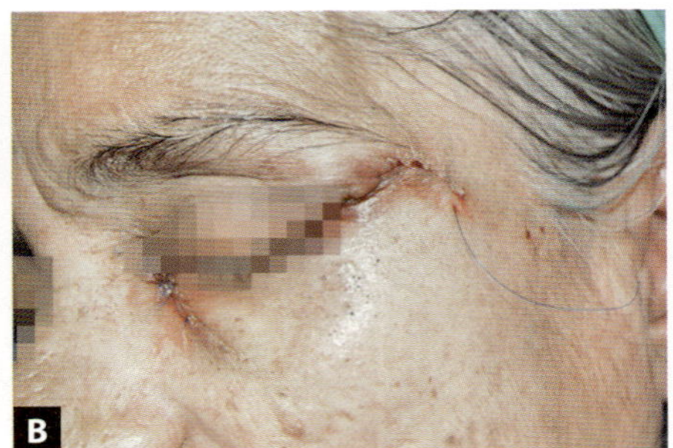
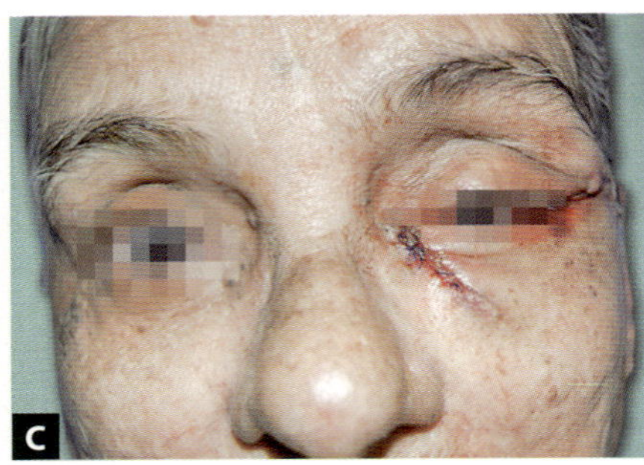

Figs. 23A to C: Tenzel flap for eyelid reconstruction.

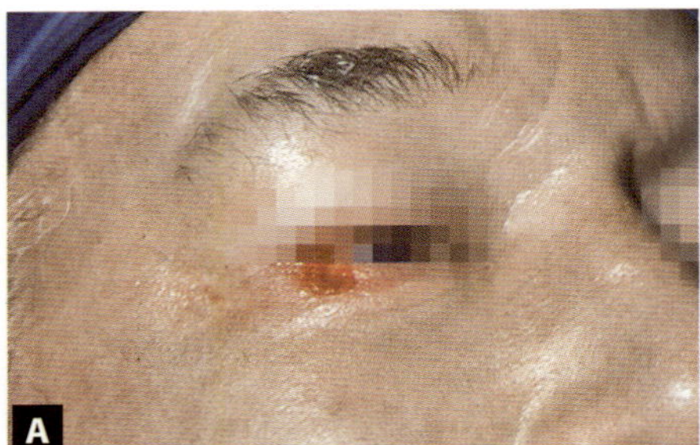
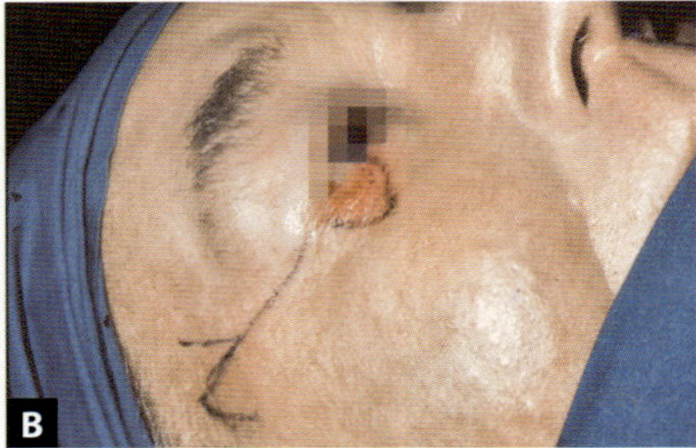
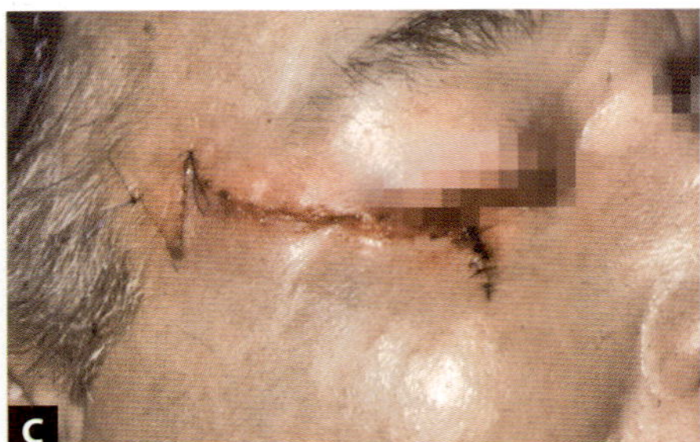

Figs. 24A to C: Mustarde flap for eyelid reconstruction.

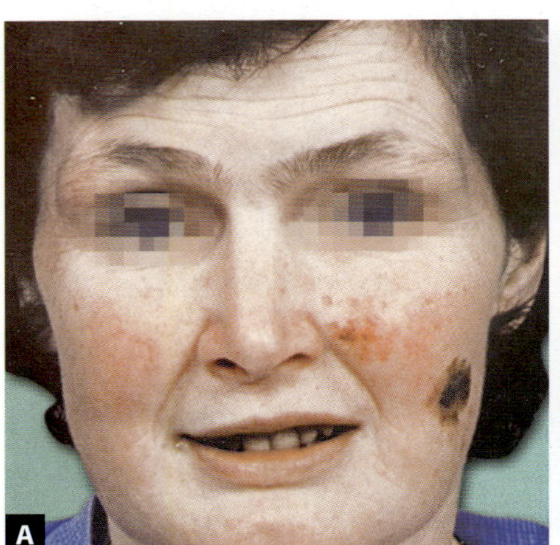
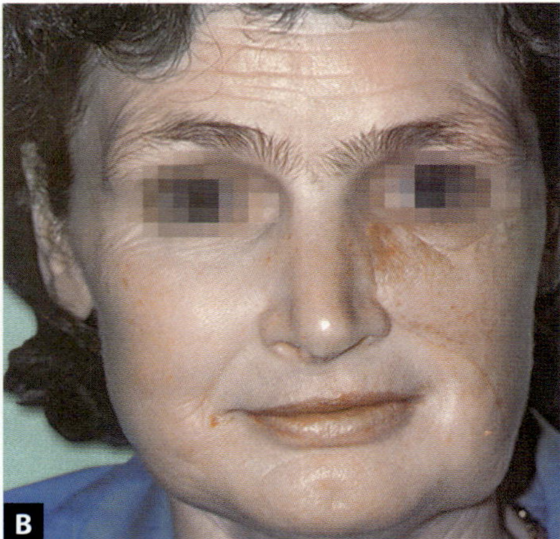
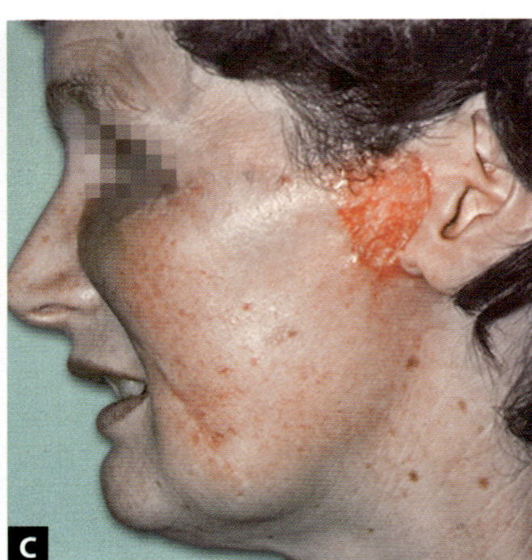

Figs. 25A to C: Cheek rotation flap.

distance to the apex of the defect so the flap can inset easily into it without excessive tension. Also note that the length of the leading edge of the flap is greater than the farthest point of the defect.

The flap is marked and incised. In the scalp it is raised in the subgaleal plane and in cheek it is raised in the subdermal plane. The flap is rotated and sutured into the defect. The donor defect is either closed primarily or grafted or repaired with another local flap.

AXIAL PATTERN FLAPS

Nasolabial Flap

The nasolabial flap is based on the angular artery which courses along the nasolabial groove. The flap can be harvested with the pedicle being proximal or distal. It is useful for the defects of lower part of nose, lower eyelid, upper cheek (distally based) and upper lip (proximally based). The distally based flap is perfused through anastomotic vessels between angular artery and the branches of ophthalmic artery near the medial orbital margin. The flap is marked with margins along the junction between esthetic subunits or parallel to it which ensures that the resulting scar lies in the junctional area giving excellent esthetic result (Figs. 26A to F). The flap is dissected in a plane between subcutaneous fat and facial muscle which ensures incorporation of the axial vessels in the flap. The flap is then transferred into the defect and sutured in two layers as described earlier. The donor

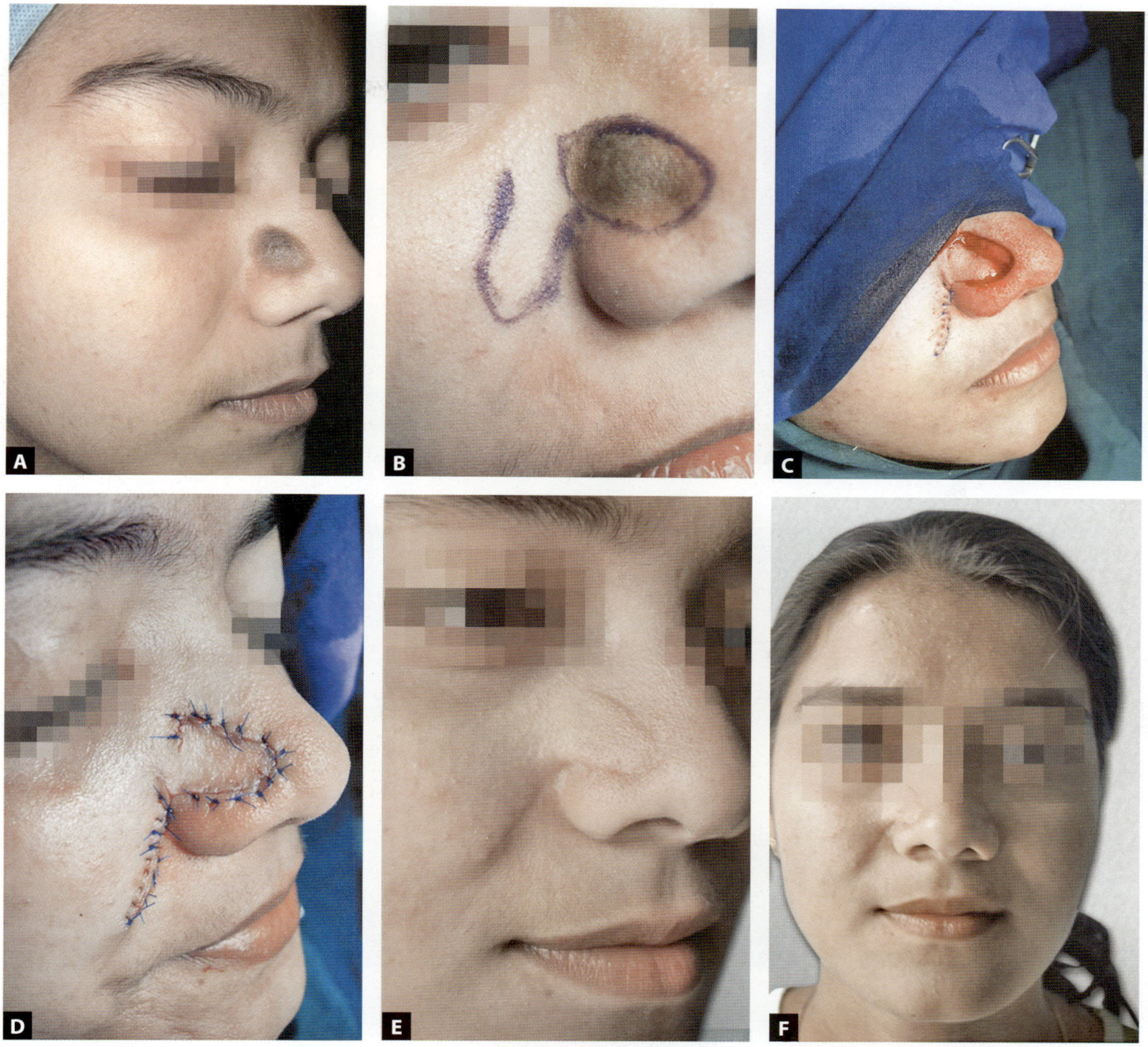

Figs. 26A to F: Nasolabial flap.

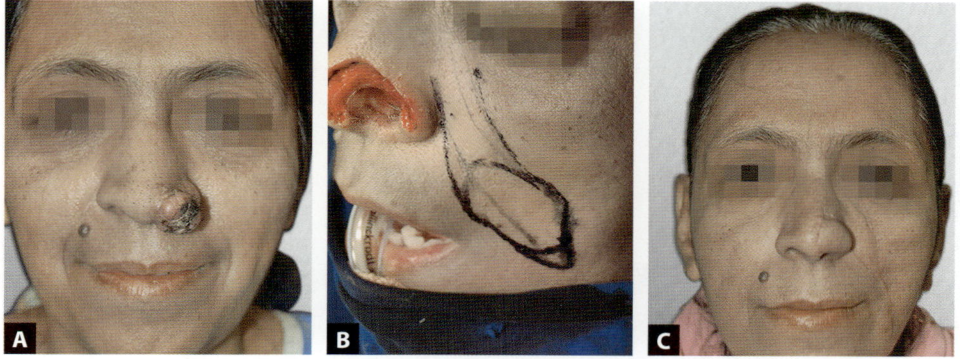

Figs. 27A to C:: Alar reconstruction with nasolabial flap.

site is too closed in two layers. A long flap can be used to reconstruct the full thickness defects in the lower region of nose by folding the flap on itself. The disadvantage of this flap is that it may require further surgeries to divide the pedicle or to reduce the bulk of the flap (Figs. 27A to C).

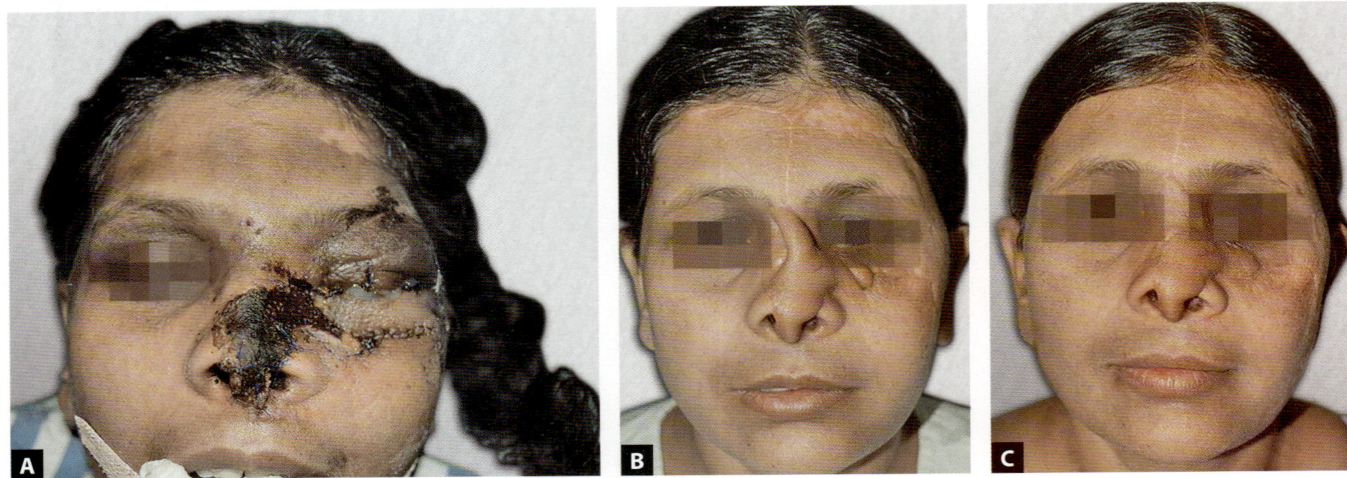

Figs. 28A to C: Median forehead flap for nasal reconstruction.

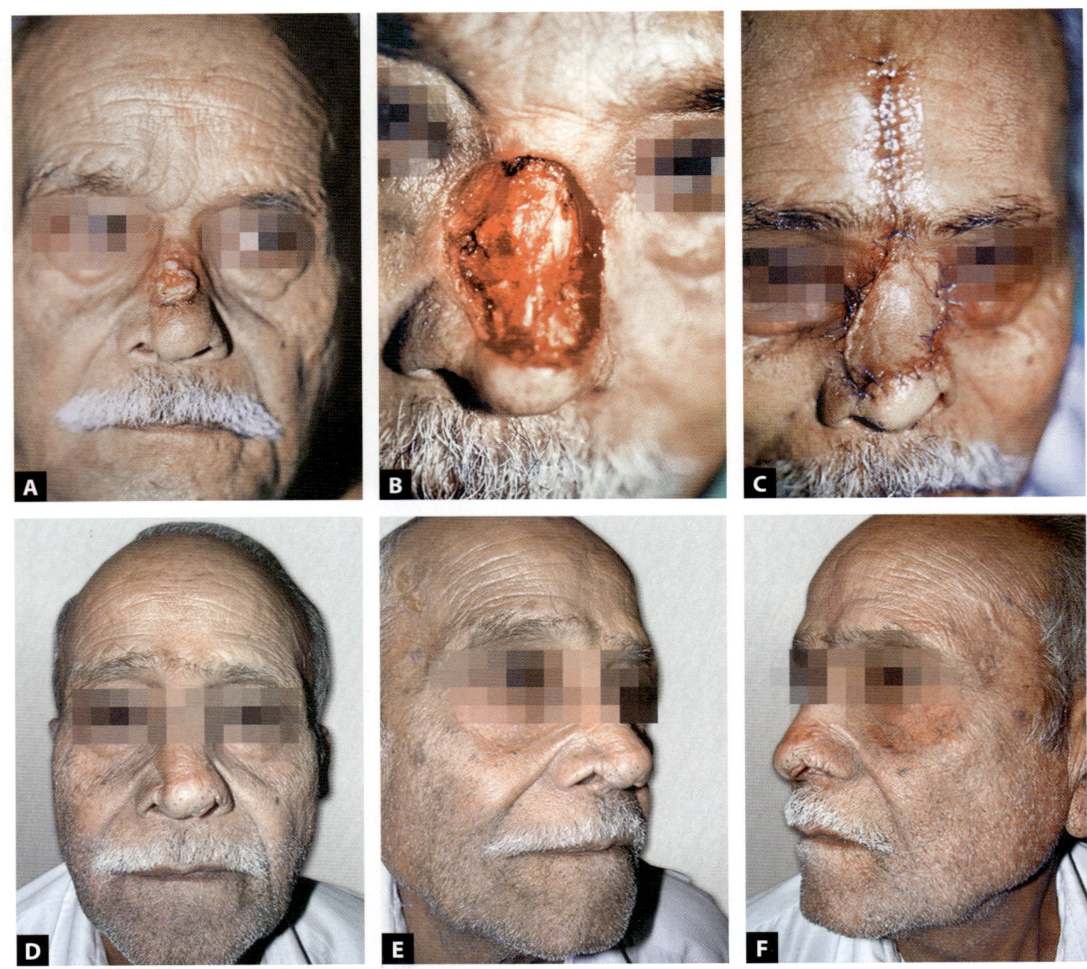

Figs. 29A to F: Forehead flap.

Midline Forehead Flap

The midline forehead flap is based on the terminal branches of angular artery and supratrochlear vessels. Being one of the earliest flaps that have been described, this is the most commonly utilized flap for the reconstruction of nose, upper eyelid and inner canthus. In the midline the frontalis muscle is absent and the flap is raised in the subcutaneous plane superficial to the periosteum. The donor site is closed in layers and the flap is inset into the defect.

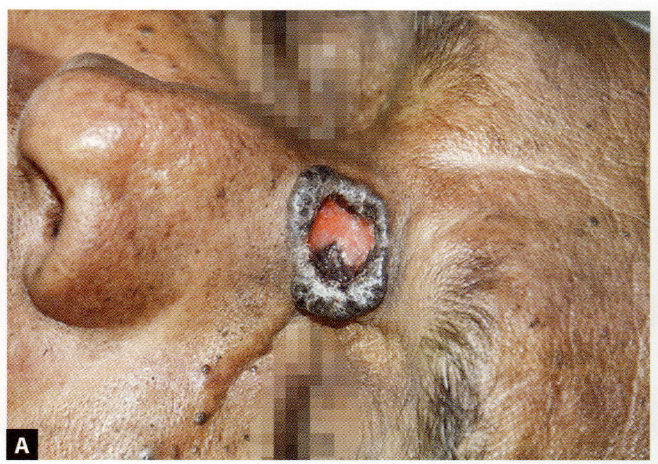

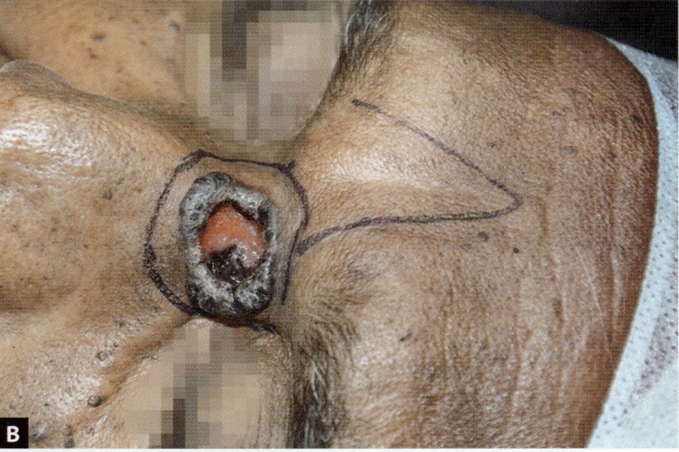

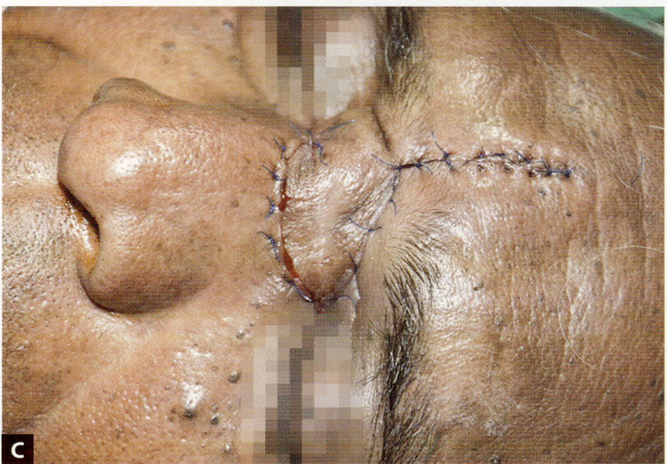

Figs. 30A to C: Glabellar flap for inner canthal defect.

In the design of the flap and the reconstruction of the primary defect it is important to consider the esthetic units of nose taking care not to transgress the boundaries (Figs. 28 and 29). The disadvantage of this flap is that second surgery is needed to divide the pedicle which can be safely done after a delay of three weeks. The glabellar flap is smaller flap and is useful for the smaller defects in the contiguous area (Figs. 30A to C).

PEARLS AND PITFALLS

Pearls

- Always assess the defect before flap design
- Consider the esthetic units while designing the flap
- Design flap slightly larger than the assessment
- Plan in reverse
- Meticulous hemostasis and gentle tissue handling

Pitfalls

- Poor design in terms of SIZE
- Tissue tension, poor hemostasis and improper tissue handling leading to flap necrosis
- Damage to Facial nerve near lateral end of eyebrow and lower margin of mandible

REFERENCES

1. Converse JM, McCarthy JG, Brauer RO, Ballantyne DL. Transplantation of skin: Grafts and flaps. In: Converse JM (Ed): Reconstructive Plastic Surgery, 2nd edition Philadelphia: WB Saunders; 1977. pp. 152-239.
2. Limberg AA. Mathematical principles of local plastic procedures on the surface of the human body. Leningrad: Medgriz; 1946.
3. Dufourmentel C. An L-shaped flap for lozenge-shaped defect. Transactions of the third international congress of plastic surgeons. Amsterdam: Excerpta Medical Foundation; 1963. p. 772.
4. Quaba AA, Sommerlad BC. A square peg into a round hole: a modified rhomboid flap and its clinical application. Br J Plast Surg. 1987;40(2):163-70.
5. Zimany A. The bilobed flap. Plast Reconstr Surg. 1953; 11(6):424-34.
6. Khouri R. Skin flaps. In: Nouri K, Leal-Khouri S (Eds). Techniques in dermatologic surgery. St Lois: Mosby; 2003. pp. 141-51.
7. Baker SR. Local flaps in facial reconstruction. 2nd edition Philadelphia: Mosby; 2007.

Chapter 29

Flap Surgeries: A Dermatologist's Perspective

Biju Vasudevan, Divya Gorur, Shilpa K

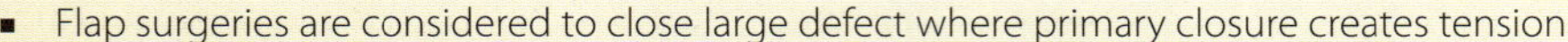

Key Messages

- Flap surgeries are considered to close large defect where primary closure creates tension.
- Plan in reverse.
- Size of the defect, site, and mobility of surrounding tissue are important factors to be considered while planning for the type of local flap surgery.
- The final lines of closure along the RSTL ensure reduced wound tension and better cosmetic outcome.
- A thorough knowledge of the anatomy is essential for optimal outcome and to avoid complications.
- Aseptic precaution, intraoperative hemostasis, and minimal tissue-handling reduce complications.

INTRODUCTION

Closure of a large surgical defect is one of the most challenging hurdles which have to be overcome by any surgeon. The concept of flap surgery evolved to overcome this challenge. The history of flap surgery dates back to 600 BC, when Sushruta performed cheek flaps for nose and earlobe reconstruction. The forehead pedicle flap performed by him is even today referred to as "the Indian flap". During Roman times, Celsus (25 AD) and Oribasius (325–403 AD) described random circulation pedicled flaps and local tissue rearrangements for the lips, nose, ears and forehead.[1,2]

DEFINITION

A flap is a unit of tissue that is transferred from one site (donor site) to another (recipient site) while maintaining its own blood supply.

The skin color and thickness, tissue composition, location, and subunits involved are the important factors that have to be considered while planning for the flap surgery. All layers absent must be reconstructed to receive optimal functional and aesthetic outcomes. Areas that provide a good source of tissue for recruitment include: the forehead, cheek, chin, submenton and neck.[3,4]

Flaps may range from simple advancements of skin to composite ones made up of different types of tissue. A local cutaneous flap is described as skin and subcutaneous tissue transferred from an area adjacent to the defect and having direct blood supply to cover the primary defect. A composite flap may include: skin, muscle, bone, fat, or fascia and is more complex to deliver.

CLASSIFICATION OF FLAPS (FIG. 1)

Flaps are classically categorized based on the following:

- Vascular supply
- Composition
- Method of transfer, and design.

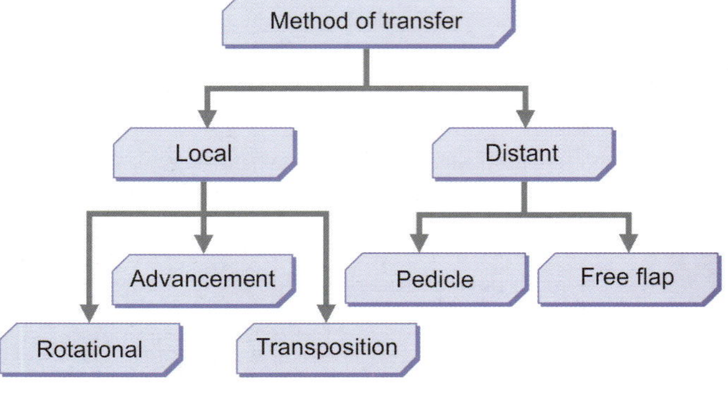

Fig. 1: Classification of flaps.

Based on blood supply, they are classified as random (no named blood vessel) and axial (named blood vessel) flaps.

Composite flaps include cutaneous, fasciocutaneous, musculocutaneous, and osteomusculocutaneous flaps.

Flaps based on method of transfer and design are:

- Local
  - Rotational
  - Advancement and
  - Transposition flaps
- Distant
  - Pedicle
  - Free flap

GENERAL PRINCIPLES WHILE PLANNING FOR FLAP SURGERY

- Ideal areas for tissue recruitment should be chosen, based on the size of defect and surrounding tissue mobility.
- Location of the defect is an important factor while designing the type of flap. Important facial landmarks to be considered to avoid distortion are angle of the mouth, philtrum, defects around the eyes, canthi, hairline, nasal ala, and tip of the nose.
- Incision is marked such that the scars rest within the relaxed skin tension lines and should be closed parallel to the lines of maximal extensibility.[5] Incisions designed along subunit borders will fall within the relaxed skin tension lines.
- If more than 50% of the cosmetic subunit is involved then consider resection of entire subunit.
- Ideal borders to camouflage scars include the nasolabial creases, supratarsal creases, mental crease, vermilion borders, and anterior hairline.
- Use of tumescent anesthesia reduces intraoperative bleeding and prolongs the duration of anesthesia, also at the same time increasing the safe upper limit of anesthetic agent especially when large flaps are planned. A regional nerve block can be considered while operating on a large area.
- Once the defect is created, it is kept hydrated by placing wet saline gauze over the defect.
- Undermining reduces the tension during wound closure. This has to be done in avascular plane.
- A corner stitch is applied in most of the flap surgeries near the tip of flap which is usually angulated to close the defect with the flap tissue, a half-buried horizontal suture (corner suture) is placed, to secure the angled tip to the tissue. The needle enters vertically 5–6 mm away from wound margin; it is then passed horizontally from one side of flap tip to the other, at the level of deep dermis into the tip of flap. The needle exits the skin adjacent to the point of entry.

PREOPERATIVE EVALUATION

History of radiation, smoking, keloidal tendency, immunocompromised state and diabetes are to be taken; since these factors may increase the risk of complications. Since one of the common indications for flap surgery is carcinoma, usually in elderly population, thorough investigation including complete hemogram, liver and renal function test, chest X-ray and electrocardiogram (ECG) is essential for such patients, along with fitness certified by a physician.

TYPE OF ANESTHESIA

Most of the local flap surgery can be done under local anesthesia using 1% lignocaine with adrenaline. Sodium bicarbonate in the ratio of 1:4 can be used to reduce the burning sensation.

Tumescent anesthesia gives the added advantage of reduced bleeding and better undermining during the procedure. Nerve blocks also can be utilized while operating on large areas.

The composite flap and axial-pattern flap are complex procedures performed by plastic surgeons. Local flap surgeries are simpler as the tissue is recruited from the area surrounding the defect. These surgeries can be performed by a well-trained dermatosurgeon. Here we have described few simple local flap surgeries which can be done by dermatosurgeons with proper preoperative planning and thorough knowledge of anatomy.

ROTATIONAL FLAP

Indication

Rotation flaps are ideal to close spherical defects on the scalp. Other preferred sites are cheek defects 3–4 cm in diameter and defects less than 2 cm over lateral forehead and temple.

Technique

Rotational flaps are pivoted around a fixed point at the base of the flap and rotated along an arc towards the defect. Classically, rotation flaps are designed to move along an arc of 30° or less with the radius approximately 2–3 times the diameter of the defect and the length approximately four to five times the width of the defect (Figs. 2A to C). Most rotational flaps may invariably possess a component of advancement in them and are termed rotation-advancement flaps.[6] Flaps that rotate or transpose around a cutaneous pedicle are restrained by the tethering effect of the base of that tissue. Flap design that fails to adjust for this force may end up with unwanted degrees of tension and/or surrounding tissue displacement.[6]

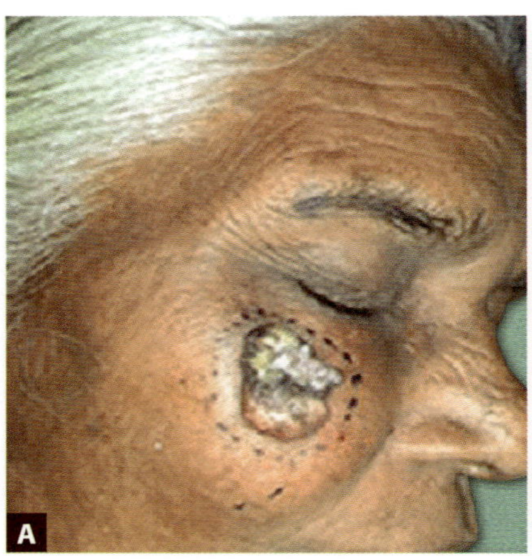

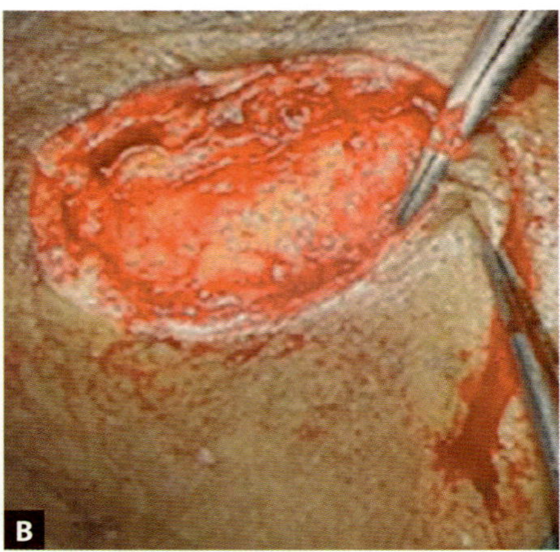

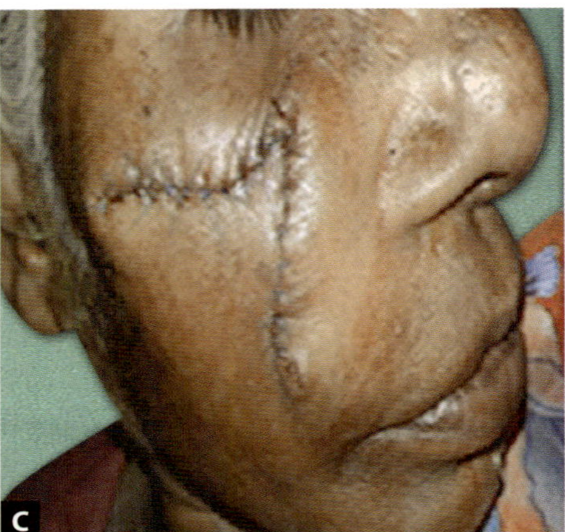

Figs. 2A to C: Classic rotation flap.

Variations of Rotation Flap

O-Z reconstruction is a double rotation flap, where two rotation flaps are designed in opposite orientation on both sides of the defect. The two flaps are opposed with a Z-shaped repair. The optimum design for wound closure is an acute angled-flap closure with length four times the radius of the defect. This type of double rotation is especially useful in scalp for recruitment of tissue from different locations. When two or more rotation flaps are designed together, the defect should preferably be located in the center of the scalp.[7]

Variations of O-Z plasty to close large scalp defect are triple rotation, pinwheel flap and double hatchet flap, which have both rotational and advancement component.[8]

Tips

- The angle of rotation should be 30° to prevent tip necrosis.
- Width of the pedicle should be double the size of defect, length of the pedicle 3–4 times the size of defect.
- Scalp incisions should be parallel to the hair shafts to avoid a linear hairless scar. The level of undermining in scalp is the galea aponeurotica.

ADVANCEMENT FLAPS

Indications

Defects on forehead, medial cheek, eyebrows, lip margins, lower eyelid and chin can be closed with this flap technique.

Types

The advancement flap can be following:

- Single pedicle
- Bipedicle which includes the H-plasty, A-T plasty or V-Y plasty
- Subcutaneous tissue pedicle flap.

Defects on forehead, medial cheek and eyebrows can be closed by unipedicle flap and H-plasty. O-T and A-T plasty are preferred on forehead, lip margins, lower eyelid and chin.

Technique

Advancement flaps depend on the advancement of the surrounding tissue along a linear axis to close a defect. It is moved primarily in a straight line from the donor site to the recipient site. No rotational or lateral movement is applied. The advancement of two skin edges from a fusiform skin excision represents the simplest of advancement flap design (Figs. 3A to D). Classically, advancement flaps have a length-to-width ratio of 1:1 or 2:1.[9] The defect can also be closed by a T- or H-plasty, where depending on the size of defect and incision taken, the line of closure will be T or H-shaped.

Unipedicle Advancement Flap

Unipedicle advancement flaps have single cutaneous pedicle, incision is placed parallel to the defect, with movement of flap being unidirectional towards the defect. Thorough undermining of the flap and surrounding tissue is necessary to allow easy movement of the tissue. The thickness of the flap should be equivalent or proportional to that of the defect, ideally including a thin layer of fat to ensure adequate vascularity. Unipedicle advancement is designed with defect width to flap-width ratio of 1:3, which will ensure adequate flap perfusion.[10,11] Pinch in various directions around the defect to access the tissue reservoir for the flap. If the axis of greatest laxity lies along the short axis of the defect, then an advancement flap is appropriate. The standing cone deformities can be prevented by excising Burrow's triangle.

H-Plasty Bipedicle Advancement Flap

H-plasty is a bipedicle advancement flap; here the incision is extended on both sides of the defect and advanced towards each other. Each portion of flap on both sides is responsible for covering a portion of the defect (Figs. 4A to D). The flap length need not be equal on both sides; it can be altered based on elasticity and redundancy of adjacent tissue.[12,13]

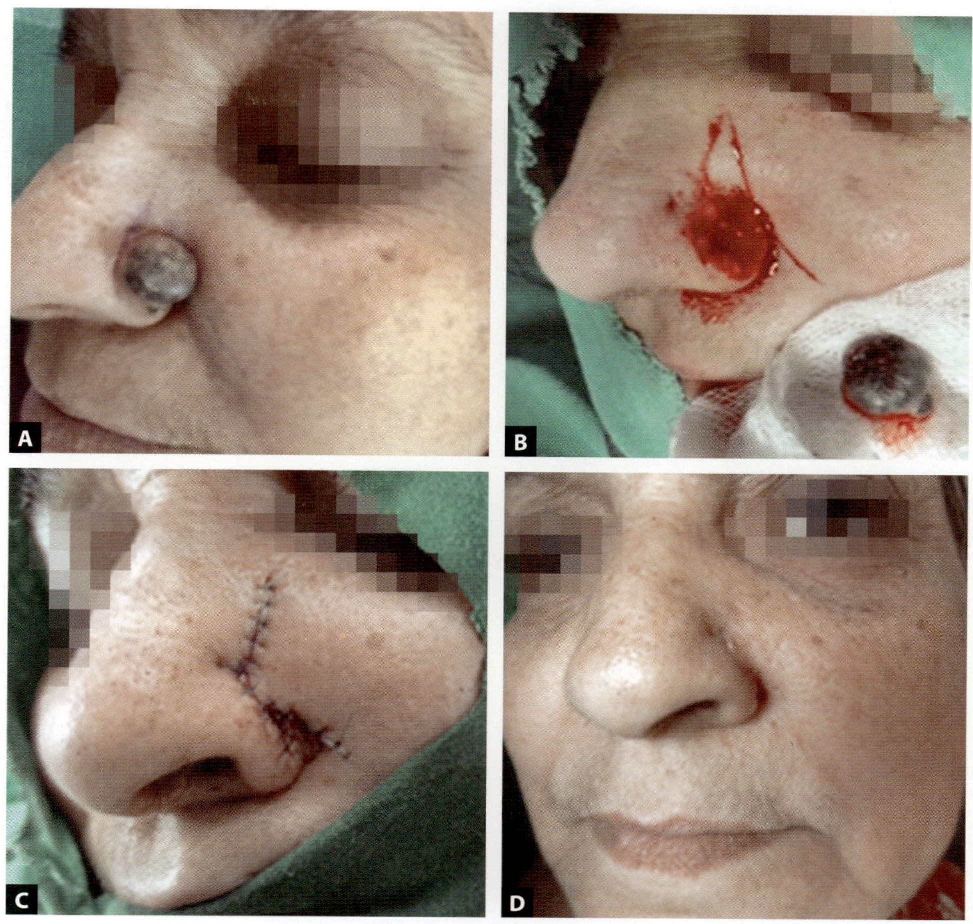

Figs. 3A to D: Advancement flap on the nose.

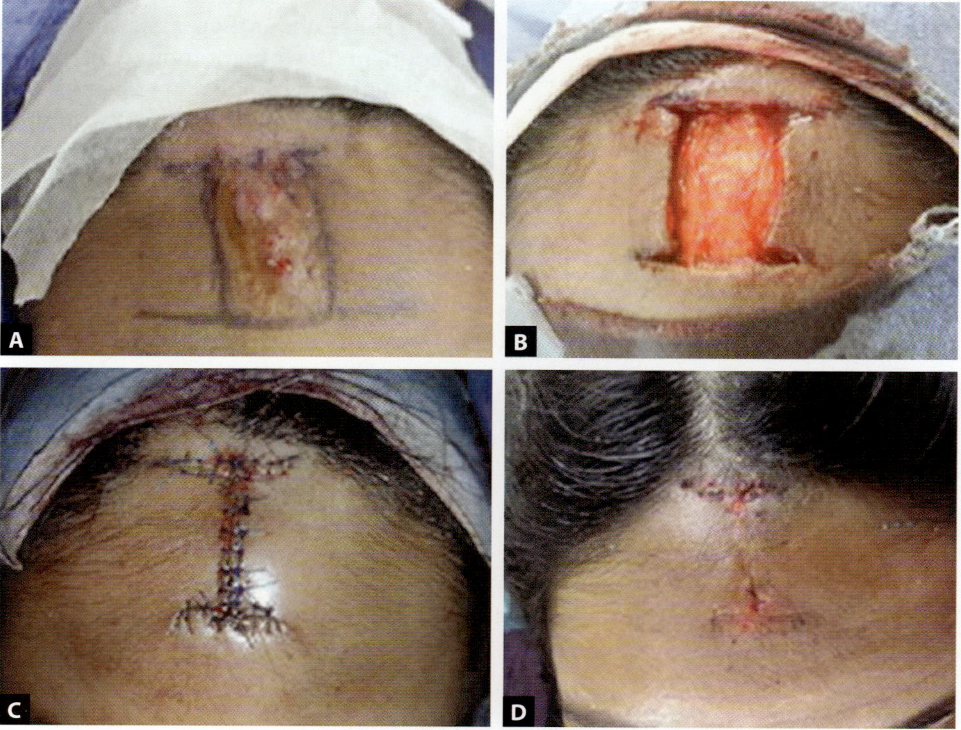

Figs. 4A to D: H-flap on forehead.

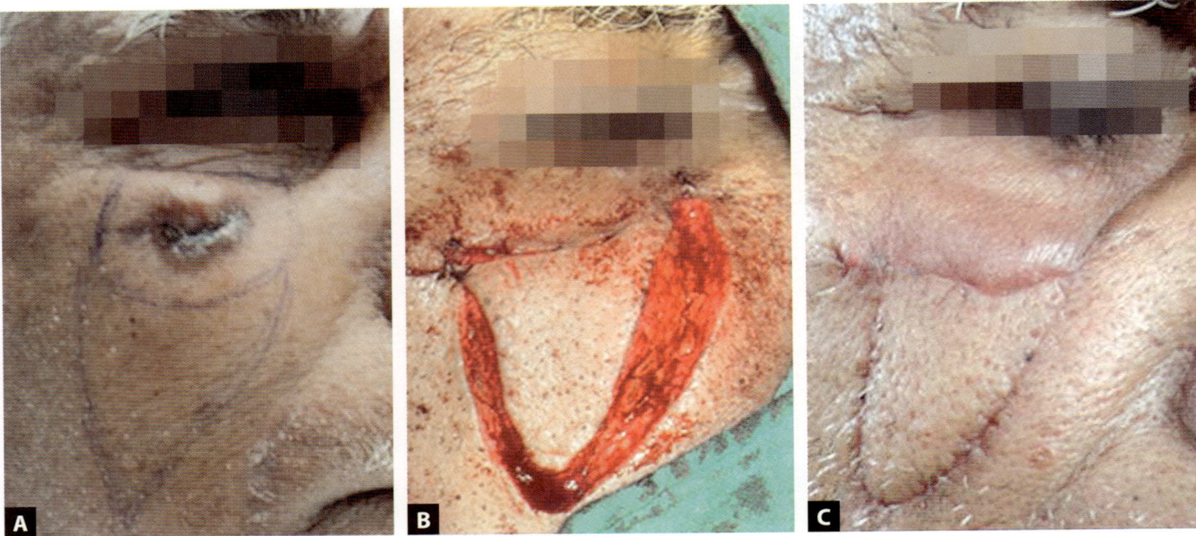

Figs. 5A to C: V-Y flap on the cheek.

A-T Plasty

In A-T plasty, a triangular defect is transformed into a T-shaped scar. Here instead of placing two incisions parallel to the defect, a single incision on the opposing side of defect is made. A standing cutaneous deformity develops at the defect site opposite the two incisions made, which can be excised and closed; the final suture line is in a T configuration. The advantage of this design is that it creates two small defects instead of a single large defect, which may be difficult to harvest in area of limited mobility. These flaps can also be performed above the eyebrow, vermilion border of the lip and eyes.[14-16]

V-Y Plasty

The island pedicle flap is also called as V-Y plasty, owing to its final configuration of closure.[17,18] After the dermal margins are severed, the flap can be advanced as far as the deep pedicle allows (Figs. 5A to C). The flap has a rich vascular supply from underlying vessels, hence chances of necrosis is minimal with this reconstruction. The island pedicle flap can be utilized to close defects on the upper lip and nose-lip-cheek junction.[19-22]

TRANSPOSITION FLAPS

Transposition flaps are versatile flaps whose design creates a second defect. The flap is raised from a donor site and rotated over an incomplete bridge of skin to be placed into the defect site. The donor site must also be closed as part of the design. The three classic transposition flaps include the (1) rhombic flap, (2) bilobed flap and, (3) Z-plasty. The other common configurations of transposition flap are triangle, rectangle, parabola, note and island flap.

Rhombic Flap

The rhombus flap is a cutaneous random-pattern flap which is dependent on the dermal and subdermal plexus for its survival.

Indications

It is used for reconstruction of the defect on cheek, chin, nose, neck and small defects on the trunk.

Technique

The classic Limberg flap is used to repair a defect which has a configuration of a rhombus with two opposing 60° angles and another two opposing 120° interior angles. The 60° and 120° rhombus can be taken as two equilateral triangle base to base. The short diagonal of the rhombus is equal to the sides of the rhombus. The flap is designed by extending the line of short diagonal to the length equal to that of diagonal, which is also the length of side of the defect. The majority of wound closure tension is at the donor site and has been calculated to be 20° to the short diagonal of the rhombus defect.[23] Skin mobility and extensibility are the important factors to be considered to minimize wound closure tension to avoid distortion of surrounding facial structures (Figs. 6A to C). The rhomboid flap is a safe and versatile flap which can be used in every area of the human body and in various surgical specialties.[8,24,25]

The dufourmentel modification of this flap design can be used for rhomboid shaped defects that have any combination of interior angles, not just those of 60° and 120°.

COMPLICATIONS

Bleeding, secondary infection, failure of flap, pin-cushioning and flap necrosis are the common side

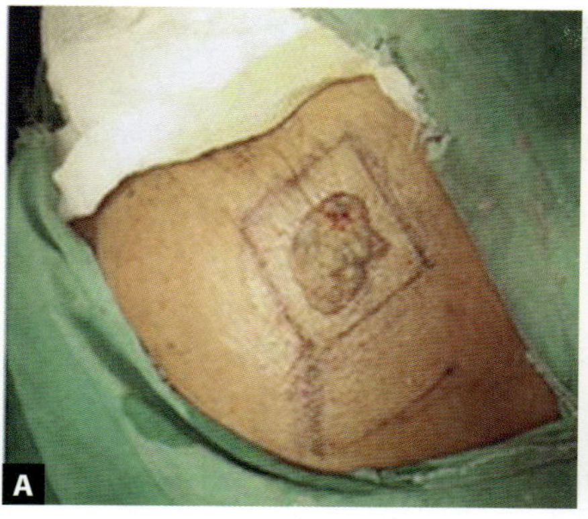

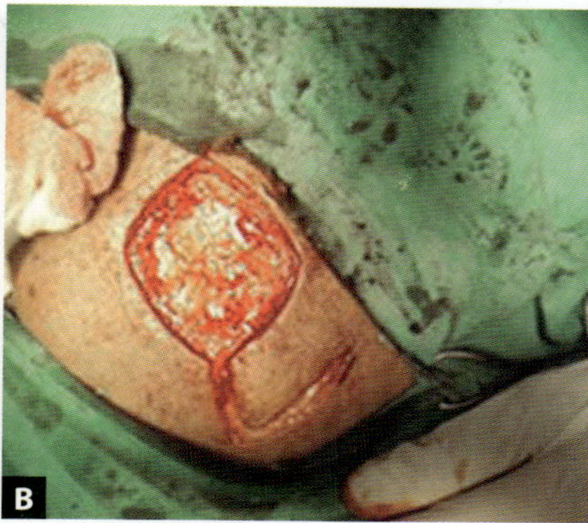

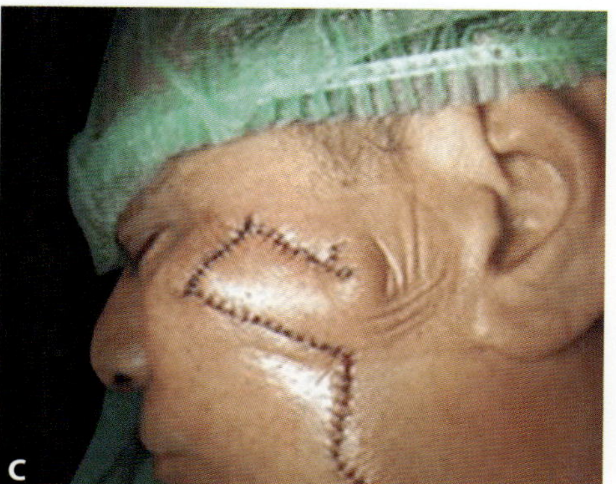

Figs. 6A to C: Classical rhomboid flap.

Table 1: Flap surgeries and their applications at various sites.

Rotation flap	
Double rotation flap	Cheek defects in lower preauricular area and scalp Scalp
Advancement flap	
▪ Unipedicle	Forehead, medial cheek, eyebrows
▪ H-plasty	Forehead, lip margins, lower eyelid and chin
▪ O-T and A-T plasty	Cheek, lateral canthus of eye
▪ V-Y plasty	Sides of face
Transposition flap	
▪ Rhombic	Cheeks, back, buttocks
▪ Island	Forehead, cheeks, upper nasal dorsum
▪ Z-plasty	Scars ≤2 cm against relaxed skin tension lines (RSTL)

effects encountered. A well-designed flap with through undermining of the tissue before closing reduces wound tension and hence decreases chances of flap necrosis and failure. Intraoperative bleeding can be controlled by electrocautery or ligation. Placing of drains are usually not required in a local flap, a penrose drain can be kept if there is significantly large dead space. Postoperative pressure dressing for 24–48 hours prevents formation of hematoma, which can compromise the local flap by inducing vasospasm and by creating a space between the flap and recipient bed. Strict aseptic precautions during surgery and giving postoperative systemic antibiotics reduces secondary infection.[26]

Late Complications

Pincushioning or trap door deformity is commonly seen after transposition flaps, which develops 2–3 months postoperatively. The flap appears bulky, protruding above the surface of surrounding normal skin. This can be due to curvilinear incision or failure to undermine the surrounding area during surgery. Hence, this complication can be avoided by overcoming these factors and also matching the depth of defect and the depth of donor flap. Once the trap door deformity does occur, it can be corrected by injecting 10 mg/mL of triamcinolone into the base of the flap 2–3 times in 4–6 weeks apart.

SUMMARY

Table 1 depicts the application of flap surgeries at various sites.

REFERENCES

1. Champoneria MC, Workman AD, Gupta SC. Sushruta: father of plastic surgery. Ann Plast Surg. 2014;73(1):2-7.
2. Fang F, Chung KC. An evolutionary perspective on the history of flap reconstruction in the upper extremity. Hand Clin. 2014;30(2):109.
3. Burget GC, Menick FJ. The subunit principle in nasal reconstruction. Plast Reconstr Surg. 1985;76:239-47.
4. Larrabee WF Jr. Design of local skin flaps. Otolaryngol Clin North Am. 1990;23:899-923.
5. Murakami CS, Nishioka GJ. Essential concepts in the design of local skin flaps. Facial Plast Surg Clin North Am. 1996;4:455-68.
6. Baker SA. Rotation flap. In: Baker SA (Ed). Local Flaps and Reconstruction, 2nd edition. Philadelphia: Elsevier; 2007. pp. 107-11.
7. Baker SA. Advancement flap. In: Baker SA (Ed). Local Flaps and Reconstruction, 2nd edition. Philadelphia: Elsevier; 2007. pp. 157-62.
8. Baker SA. Transposition flap. In: Baker SA (Ed). Local Flaps and Reconstruction, 2nd edition. Philadelphia: Elsevier; 2007. pp. 134-9.
9. Fernández-Calderón M, Casado-Sánchez C, Cabrera-Sánchez E, et al. Versatility of hatchet flaps for the repair of scalp defects. Actas Dermosifiliogr. 2012;103(7):629-31.
10. Redondo P. Repair of large defects in the forehead using a median forehead rotation flap and advancement lateral U-shaped flap. Dermatol Surg. 2006;32(6):843-6.
11. Krishnan R, Garman M, Nunez-Gussman J, et al. Advancement flaps: a basic theme with many variations. Dermatol Surg. 2005;31(8 Pt 2):986-94.
12. Cook JL, Goldman GD. Random pattern cutaneous flap. Robinson JK (Ed.) Surgery of the skin: procedural dermatology, 2nd edition. Philadelphia: Elsevier; 2010. pp. 257-8.
13. Hirshowitz B, Mahler D. T-plasty technique for excisions in the face. Plast Reconstr Surg. 1966;37:453-8.
14. Moody BR, Sengelmann RD. Standing cone avoidance via advancement flap modification. Dermatol Surg. 2002; 28: 632-5.

15. Stevens C, Tan L, Kassir R, Calhoun K. Biomechanics of A-TO-T flap design. Laryngoscope. 1999;109:113-7.
16. Jackson IT. Local flap reconstruction of defects after excision of nonmelanoma skin cancer. Clin Plast Surg. 1997;24:747-67.
17. Gormley DE. Use of Burow's wedge principle for repair of wounds in or near the eyebrow. J Am Acad Dermatol. 1985;12:344-9.
18. O'Donnell M, Briggs C, Condon KC. The horn flap: a curved V-Y advancement flap with lateral pedicle. Br J Plast Surg. 1992;45:42-3.
19. Dini M, Innocenti A, Lo Russo G, et al. The use of the V-Y fasciocutaneous island advancement flap in reconstructing postsurgical defects of the leg. Dermatol Surg. 2001;27:44-6.
20. Robbins TH. The "deep pedicle" V-Y advancement flap. Plast Reconstr Surg. 2004;113:463-4.
21. Zook EG, Van Beek AL, Russell RC, et al. V–Y advancement flap for facial defects. Plast Reconstr Surg. 1980;65:786-97.
22. Cook J. Commentary on V–Y nasolabial advancement flaps in the repair of central facial defects. Dermatol Surg. 2001;27:659-60.
23. Lister GD, Gibson T. Closure of rhomboid skin defects: the flap of limberg and dufourmentel. Br J Plast Surg. 1972;25:300-14.
24. Limberg A. Mathematical principles of local plastic procedures on the surface of the human body. Leningrad: Medgis; 1946.
25. Turan T, Kuran I, Ozcan H, et al. Geometric limit of multiple local Limberg flaps: a flap design. Plast Reconstr Surg. 1999;104(6):1675-8.
26. Jewett BS. Complications of flap surgery. In: Baker SA (Ed). Local Flaps and Reconstruction, 2nd edition. Philadelphia: Elsevier; 2007. pp. 691-9.

Chapter 30

Scar Revision

Raghunatha Reddy R, Shashikumar BM, Savitha AS

Key Messages

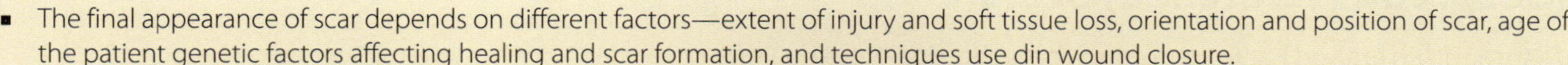

- The final appearance of scar depends on different factors—extent of injury and soft tissue loss, orientation and position of scar, age of the patient genetic factors affecting healing and scar formation, and techniques use din wound closure.
- Patient expectations have to be realistic, there is no perfect scar that can be designed.
- Proper knowledge of anatomic and cosmetic units is important in scar analysis.

INTRODUCTION

Scar formation is an inevitable result of surgery or trauma that results in full thickness epidermal loss and breach in dermis. Scars, especially those over face and other exposed sites can be cosmetically, functionally, psychologically and socially disturbing.[1] An ideal scar is one that has matured rapidly without contracture or increase in width or formation of more collagen than is necessary for its strength.[2] It is nearly impossible to have such an ideal scar despite adopting the best surgical technique and utmost wound care. The final appearance of the scar can vary greatly based on the extent of injury and soft tissue loss, orientation and position of the scar, age of the patient, genetic factors affecting healing and scar formation, and techniques used in wound closure.[3] Scars which are wide, raised, depressed, hyperpigmented and those that are against the relaxed skin tension lines (RSTLs) give poor cosmetic results.[1] Successful outcomes of scar revision surgery are reflected in matching the patient's expectations with technical achievability.

Scar revision is one of the most commonly requested procedures particularly for the scars over the exposed and cosmetically important areas such as the face. A holistic approach to the patient undergoing scar revision is desirable and requires extensive preoperative assessment including that of patients psychological state, technical skills and expertise, realistic expectations for achieving satisfactory outcome. As scars will have unique characteristics, therapeutic options should be tailored to the patient's requirements and the area affected.[2]

DEFINITION

The Oxford English dictionary defines scar as "the trace of a healed wound, sore or burn, a fault or a blemish remaining as a trace of some former condition or resulting from some particular scar." Dorland's medical dictionary defines scar as "mark remaining after the healing of the wound or other morbid process". The lay population refers to scar as an unsightly healed wound. Conversely surgeons tend to think of surgical scar as an expected outcome of violation of the dermis. In etiopathological medical terminology a scar is defined as 'a non regenerative wound healing as a result of surgery, laceration, burns, chronic wounds, acne, etc.'[2]

PATIENT EXPECTATION

Individuals bearing scars deemed functionally or cosmetically undesirable often seek the services of a surgeon to eliminate the scars and to restore the tissue to its pre-injury state. In counselling patients about scar revision, it is important to emphasize that the procedure is designed to trade a poor scar for a better scar. Misconceptions about creating an invisible scar must be corrected.[4] The physician must educate the patient about the nature of scars and scar revision. It is equally important that the physician tries to understand what impact the scar has on the patient within his or her social context or from a functional stand point. Only then can the physician adequately explore the different options and properly prepare the patient for a realistic outcome.[5]

It has to be made understood to the patient that "***Once a scar—its a scar forever, it cannot be removed or restored to total normalcy—It can be improved to look better both functionally and aesthetically to the best possible with combination of all therapeutic modalities***".

IDEAL SCAR

An ideal scar is one that is nearly imperceptible and is level with the skin and blends in the RSTLs. Scar appearance can vary greatly due to surgical technique, final orientation of the scar, shape of the scar and its location on the body.[1] A scar may be deemed cosmetically acceptable depending on its color, width, depth or height, location and orientation.[5]

SCAR CLASSIFICATION (TABLE 1)[6]

Widespread (Stretched) Scars

Widespread (stretched) scars appear when the fine lines of surgical scars gradually become stretched and widened, which usually happens within 3 weeks after surgery. They are typically flat, pale, soft, symptomless scars. Stretch marks (abdominal striae) after pregnancy are variants of widespread scars in which there has been injury to the dermis and subcutaneous tissues but the epidermis is unbreached. There is no elevation, thickening, or nodularity in mature widespread scars, which distinguishes them from hypertrophic scars.

Scar Contractures

Scars that cross joints or skin creases at right angles are prone to develop shortening or contracture. Scar contractures occur when the scar is not fully matured, often tend to be hypertrophic, and are typically disabling and dysfunctional. They are common after burn injury across joints or skin concavities.

Table 1: Classification of scar.

Mature scar	A light colored flat scar
Immature scar	A red, sometimes itchy or painful, and slightly elevated scar in the process of remodelling. Many of these will mature normally over time
Linear hypertrophic scar	A red, raised, sometimes itchy scar confined to the border of the original incision. These scars may increase in size rapidly for 3–6 months and then, after a static phase, begin to regress. After maturation, they may have an elevated, slightly rope like appearance with the increased width
Widespread hypertrophic scar	A widespread red, raised, sometimes itchy scar that remains within the borders of the original injury
Minor keloid	A focally raised, itchy scar extending over normal tissue. This may develop up to 1 year after injury and does not regress on its own
Major keloid	A large raised (>0.5 cm) scar, possibly painful or pruritic and extending over normal tissue. This may result from minor trauma and can continue to spread over years

FACTORS AFFECTING WOUND HEALING (TABLE 2)[2,7]

Table 2: Factors affecting wound healing.

Systemic factors	*Local factors*
▪ Malnutrition–protein, vitamin A, vitamin C deficiency ▪ Drugs-steroids, penicillamine, nicotine, NSAIDs, and anticancer drugs ▪ Chronic debilitating illness and infections ▪ Endocrinological disorders ▪ Systemic vascular disorders ▪ Connective tissue disorders ▪ Old age	▪ Poor surgical technique ▪ Vascular disorders—arteriosclerosis, venous insufficiency ▪ Tissue ischemia ▪ Infections ▪ Drugs ▪ Foreign bodies

Abbreviations: NSAIDS, nonsteroidal anti-inflammatory drugs

ASSESSMENT OF SCARS

Quantitative and qualitative measurement modalities are needed to effectively evaluate and monitor treatments of scars. Scar assessment is very important for the management and counselling purposes.

Objective Assessment of Scars

Scar-measuring devices should be non invasive, accurate, reproducible, and easy-to-use to facilitate objective data collection and have clinical utility. Existing devices assess parameters such as pliability, firmness, color, perfusion, thickness, and Three-dimensional (3D) topography.[8]

a. **Pliability**: The pneumatonometer uses pressure to objectively measure skin pliability. It is composed of a sensor, a membrane, and an air-flow system that measures the amount of pressure needed to lock the system.[9] The cutometer is a non invasive suction device that has been applied to the objective and quantitative measurement of skin elasticity. It measures the viscoelasticity of the skin by analyzing its vertical deformation in response to negative pressure.[10]
b. **Firmness:** The durometer applies a vertically directed indentation load on the scar to measure tissue firmness.[11]
c. **Color:** Spectrophotometric color analysis to calculate erythema and melanin index.
d. **Thickness:** Tissue ultrasound palpation system (TUPS) have been used to quantify scar thickness. [12]
e. **Perfusion:** Laser Doppler perfusion imaging is an established technique for the measurement of burn scar perfusion. It aids in early determination of burn depth and subsequent treatment course.[13]

f. **Three-dimensional topography**: These can capture scar surface characteristics with high definition and reproducibility.

Subjective Scar Assessment

Scar scales have been devised to quantify scar appearance in response to treatment.

a. **The Vancouver scar scale (VSS):**[14] It is used mainly for burn scars.
b. **Patient and observer scar assessment scale (POSAS)**: The POSAS includes subjective symptoms of pain and pruritus and expands on the objective data captured in the VSS.[15]
c. **Visual analog scale (VAS)**: The multidimensional VAS is a photograph-based scale derived from evaluating standardized digital photographs in 4 dimensions (pigmentation, vascularity, acceptability, and observer comfort) plus contour.[16]
d. **Manchester scar scale (MSS):** The manchester scar scale, proposed by Beausang et al. in 1998, differs from the POSAS in that it includes an overall VAS that is added to the individual attribute scores.[17]
e. **Stony brook scar evaluation scale (SBSES):** This is a 6-item ordinal wound evaluation scale developed to measure short-term cosmetic outcome of wounds 5–10 days after injury up to the time of suture removal.[18]

These observer-dependent scales consider factors such as scar height or thickness, pliability, surface area, texture, pigmentation, and vascularity.[8]

TIMING OF THE SCAR REVISION SURGERY[1,2,4,5]

Scars tend to improve spontaneously as they mature. The timing of scar revision has traditionally been in the range of 6–12 months. However, some scars cause enough deformity that they should be considered for scar revision earlier. One rule of thumb is the "plateau phenomenon". That is, if the patient and the physician observe the scar over a 6- to 8-week period and there is no significant improvement, then a decision can be made as to whether scar revision is indicated. Typically, scar revision is not performed before 3 months following the injury. It is important to note resolution of the acute inflammatory changes in the tissues surrounding the scar. The skin should be soft, supple, and non-tender, demonstrating no significant residual erythema, edema, or induration. The necessity and timing of scar revision are a joint decision made by the patient and the physician. One of the roles of the physician is to inform and educate the patient about the available options and level of improvement that can be expected.

SCAR ANALYSIS AND PLANNING

A complete and proper examination of the scar and its surrounding tissue is essential to plan for an appropriate therapeutic modality. A thorough knowledge of vital anatomical structures like vessels and nerves of significance and the implication of the procedure to the surrounding structures is also important. ***"Surgery without the above knowledge and planning is like diving into water without the knowledge of depth and what lies underneath".***

Factors which are to be considered are as follows:[7,19]

- **Physical examination:** Anatomical location and its proximity to vital structures, its directions with respect to local RSTL, length, width and shape, its contour (elevated, depressed, atrophic, hypertrophic or keloidal), color (hyper- or hypo- and depigmented), blanching effect as well as presence of small vessels would reveal the vascularity, thus determining the maturity of scar and total number of scars.
- Physical examination of the surrounding tissue is vital since local landmarks may be distorted, e.g. angle of eyes, around the lips, scalp margins. Care should be taken to avoid this complication.
- **Cosmetic units and cosmetic unit junctions** are two most important landmarks to be considered during the scar revision surgeries involving the face. An incision should be restricted to a cosmetic unit without crossing the cosmetic unit junction. The incision and ensuing suture lines and resultant scar should ideally be placed in a cosmetic unit junction wherever possible.
- For scars that are not oriented along the RSTL and are oriented at an angle of 30° or more, the scar revision techniques like Z-plasty may be essential to orient the ensuing scar along the direction of RSTL or with a less acute angle.
- Psychological and cosmetic evaluation of the patient is of utmost importance. One must evaluate patient's expectation which must be realistic and assess the psychological impact of the scar on the patient. If a scar is inducing a disproportionate psychological impact and if the expectation of the patient from the scar revision surgery is higher, it would be wiser to seek psychological assessment and proper counselling before proceeding with scar revision surgery. It should be stressed that ***"no scar can ever be made to disappear but it can only be altered or modified by scar revision procedures."***
- Invariably patients with scars over the face will have greater expectation and seek the corrective measures with urgency. However, the results of scar revision surgery are at its best after 3–6 months with massage and other corrective invasive methods. Scar revision surgery should always be discouraged if the patient seeks the same with expectation of immediate results.

PREOPERATIVE PLANNING

As with any procedure, preoperative planning is of critical importance. Photographs should be taken and the deformity carefully analyzed. There may be several reconstructive options, but after thoughtful planning one should choose the ideal procedure for an individual patient's scar. Appropriate knowledge of the local anatomy is essential to achieve the desired outcome and to avoid undesirable side-effects. Facial landmarks, such as cosmetic units and their junctions, free margins like eye lids, lips and nostrils, relation of the scar to the scalp and hairline and orientation of the scar to the RSTL is very essential. Limiting the incision within the cosmetic unit and placing the incision in the cosmetic unit junction is important for achieving satisfactory outcome. One should draw the planned incision lines prior to injecting local anesthesia.

Infiltrate local anesthetic agent such as 1–2% xylocaine with epinephrine 1:100000 to 1:200000 solutions into the mid dermis at least 10 minutes prior to the procedure to create vasoconstriction and to enhance tissue turgor. This will aid in achieving a bloodless field and maximal anesthesia. If the requirement for the quantity of local anesthetic is more than the safe permissible limit, in such situation it is ideal to use the tumescent anesthesia. Always identify the RSTLs and mark as well, since their directions over the face can be confusing to the best of the esthetic surgeons. It is ideal to have a picture depicting RSTLs over the face pasted in the vicinity since the RSTLs run in multiple directions over the face. In a situation where it is difficult to identify RSTL's, one may perform pinch technique or make a punch biopsy and wait for few minutes as the long axis of the punched wound gets oriented along the RSTLs.

PREOPERATIVE PREPARATION

- Proper assessment and analysis of the scar.
- Planning for ideal procedure/surgery, shortlist two or three plans and list on priority
- Counsel the patient by explaining in detail about the scar, planning and the possible outcome by explaining the realistic outcome.
- Preoperative photographs of the scar from different angles.
- Obtain a proper history of any relevant illness and the medications the patient is taking which may have influence on the outcome of the surgery.
- Elicit history of allergic reactions to drugs and history of vasovagal syncope.
- Perform appropriate routine investigations, and specific investigations if any required.
- Obtain informed consent for the surgery, anesthesia and also for change of plan of surgery on the operating table if the need arises.
- Advice to stop smoking a week before surgery.
- Advice to stop medications, which may interfere with healing and antiplatelets and anticoagulants at least a week prior to the surgery.
- Test dose of medications like local anesthetic and antibiotics.
- Start appropriate antibiotic prophylaxis.
- Anxiolytics and if required mild sedation may be considered as per the patient assessment.

TECHNIQUES[2,7]

Nonsurgical

Several noninvasive procedures and medications have been described for the enhancement of healing process and to improve the outcome of resultant scar.

- Massage
- Silicone gel or sheeting
- Pressure dressings suitable to the scar and its anatomical location.
- Vitamin E and A
- Herbal extract (Allium cepa, madecassol)
- Steroid injections
- Antimitotics
- Laser
- Soft tissue augmentation
- Radiotherapy
- Cryotherapy
- Interferon
- Makeup camouflage
- Electrical stimulation of skin (ESS) for depressed scars.

Individually, the above-mentioned procedures and medications do not provide complete and satisfactory results and the available evidence to support their use is sparse. A combination of the above procedures and their appropriate utilization postoperatively can help achieve desirable results.

Topical silicone gel or sheeting has been reported to improve the scar contour, color and texture.[20] The mechanism of action of silicone on scar improvement is not well understood. One theory is that hydration of subcutaneous tissue may have an effect on fibroblast activity.[21] Another theory postulates that there will be decreased fibroblastic activity due to the negatively charged static-electrical field created under the silicone.[21] However, silicone gel or sheets have not been shown to be superior to massaging with lubricating gels or oils. Silicone sheets or gels have not been shown microscopically to penetrate the scar tissue to substantiate the therapeutic effect of scar remodeling or prevention of hypertrophic scars or keloids. Gels or self-adhesive sheets should be applied to the wound after suture removal and, ideally, continued for 3 months. The recommendation for silicone gel sheeting is a minimum 12-hour daily wear. The sheet should be snugly fit on the scar, a pressure garment be worn as per the suitability of the site. The heat generated while massaging has been postulated to be responsible for the scar remodeling by enhancing collagen synthesis. In the author's own observations there was no significant difference with reference to remodeling between massaging with a drop of vegetable oil and that of silicone gel. However, massaging along the direction of the scar either with a lubricating gel or oil or silicone gel, starting 2–3 weeks after the suture removal or wound healing twice daily for 30–60 seconds each time have shown to flatten the edges, smoothen the irregularities, remodel the scars faster and prevents possibilities of hypertrophic scar formation.

Pressure dressing yielding constant pressure has been found useful in scar remodeling and preventing hypertrophic scaring and keloid. Ready to use pressure garments are available in various sizes and are ideal for use over the chest, trunk and limbs and are particularly useful for post-burns scars.

Hyperpigmented scars can be treated with pigment lightening agents such as hydroquinone, kojic acid, retinoic acid, topical steroids and alpha hydroxy acids.[5] Improvement in the pigmentation is an important aspect of management of any scar.

There have been reports of herbal preparations and miscellaneous agents being useful for the above purposes but substantial evidence is lacking.[2]

Hair cover, make up and accessories can sometime offer excellent coverage for the scar. Newer make up lines and techniques have improved and allow for more natural looking and for better coverage. Tattooing also has been used as a permanent camouflage technique that can be useful for hyperpigmented or abnormally pigmented scars especially those which cover a large area or are in an area less amenable to surgical revision.

A number of measures like intralesional agents, soft tissue fillers and pulsed dye lasers have been practiced for treating, camouflaging and remodeling scars. Of these, intralesional injections of triamcinolone acetonide in strength of 10 mg/mL or 40mg/ml diluted to 20 mg/mL alone or in combination with cryotherapy (Figs. 1A and B) has been most widely practiced with satisfactory results for both prevention and treatment of hypertrophic and keloid scars.

Soft tissue augmentation using injectable fillers is very effective for depressed or pitted scars. These agents include bovine collagen (collagen), homologous human collagen (Dermologen), autologous fat transplantation and freshly prepared autologous dermal grafts. Hyaluronic acid fillers are temporary and have been used successfully with good cosmetic acceptability but the disadvantage being their short lived results and prohibitive cost. However, they can be used with great satisfaction in situations warranting immediate cosmetic improvement of the depressed scars over cosmetically important areas.

Microneedling Therapy

Microneedling therapy is also known as collagen induction therapy. The treatment is performed as an office procedure after application of a local anesthetic cream, by means of an instrument known as a dermaroller. A dermaroller is a simple, hand-held instrument consisting of a handle with a cylinder studded all around with fine, stainless steel needles 0.5–2 mm in length. This needle-studded cylinder is rolled on the skin in multiple directions to achieve a therapeutic benefit and hence the name 'Dermaroller'. These needles cause small pinpoint injuries on the treated skin, which apparently heal within 2–3 days with no post-treatment sequelae. Treatment with dermaroller is performed at 4–8 week intervals and multiple sittings are needed to achieve the desired effect on the skin.

There are certain advantages with dermaroller or microneedling therapy over laser resurfacing; former does not lead to any epidermal injury as is seen with lasers, there is minimal downtime associated with the procedure unlike ablative laser resurfacing and the treatment is far cheaper as compared to lasers. The treatment can be performed in an office setting and does not need any extensive special training or expensive instruments.[22]

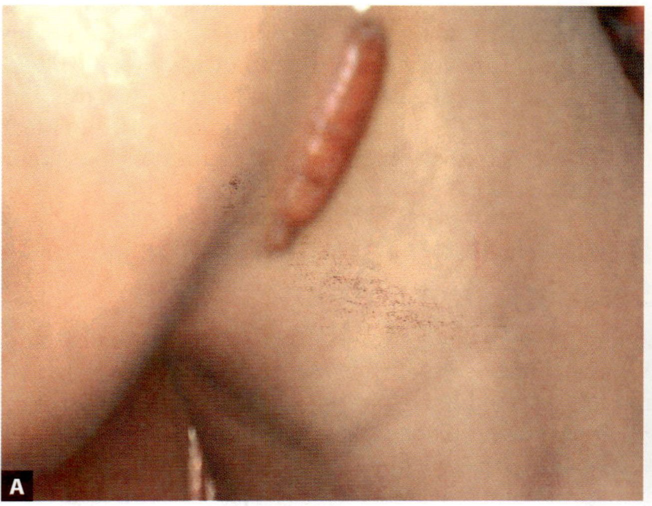

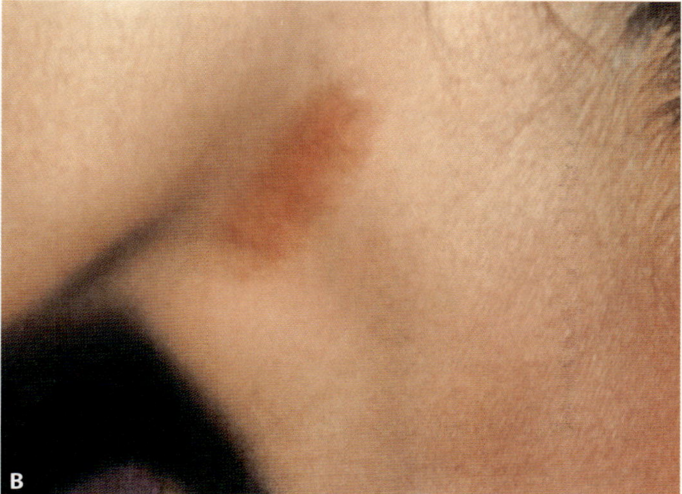

Figs. 1A and B: Hypertrophic scar over the neck, treated with cryotherapy and intralesional steroid. (A) Pretreatment; (B) After single treatment session.

Lasers

Different lasers have been used for the treatment of hypertrophic scar and keloids, but only pulsed dye lasers are proven to be of significant benefit in both reducing the size and prevention of formation of hypertrophic scar and keloid scar. Early and more vascular the lesion, better the results with pulsed dye laser. Various other lasers like carbon dioxide lasers and Erbium:YAG lasers have been used with varying success, but their benefits are limited due to the ablative nature and recurrences are common.

SURGICAL METHODS

Meticulous planning, atraumatic surgical technique, careful handling of the tissue, use of appropriate suture materials and suturing techniques are essential components of surgical scar revision technique. Appropriate surgical instruments like fine needle holder with dissecting scissors, thumb forceps and surgical hooks do play an important role in the surgical outcome. The incisions have to be perpendicular without any beveling. Accurate skin opposition and eversion should be achieved by giving importance to wound closure in multiple layers like buried intradermal suturing for achieving finely approximated wound edges. Skin opposition can be achieved with either interrupted percutaneous or subcuticular sutures with minimal skin tension to avoid suture indentation marks. Interrupted sutures are recommended as they can be used to correct the irregular wound margins and if a hematoma develops it is possible to drain the hematoma by removing individual sutures as required, whereas this advantage is lacking with continuous intradermal suturing. If intradermal suturing has been done with care with approximation of edges, skin opposition can also be achieved with tissue glues supported by steristrip adhesive plaster over the intact sutures and to be continued for 3–4 weeks after suture removal. Buried vertical mattress sutures are ideal for wound edge eversion, especially for deep defects.[23] The placement of tension suture in the middle of the wound and then the others at each end allows redundancy to be worked out into the middle.[2] The sutures must be removed at an appropriate time to reduce the risk of permanent suture marks, it varies from 5–10 days depending on the site and inversely proportional to the tension on the wound edges.

The routinely formed scar revision techniques comprises of fusiform (elliptical) scar revision, Z-plasty, W-plasty, VY-plasty and serial partial excision with fusiform scar revision, of which the most commonly performed are fusiform scar revision and Z-plasty techniques.

Restoration of Anatomical Landmarks

If an eyebrow, vermillion border, or other anatomical landmarks have been displaced by initial injury, relocation of these structures to their normal position is more important than simple scar revision, even if this results in new scars or the use of flaps or grafts which might result in poor color match.[2]

Direct Excision (Simple Excision) (Figs. 2 to 4)

When possible, completely excise the scar tissue with an elliptical incision and close the wound primarily by advancement of the adjacent normal tissue. Undermining is very important and should be done symmetrically on either side to avoid wound tension. The fine scars should be aligned along or as much as possible in line with RSTLs.[2] Fusiform scar revision is indicated for the scars that follow RSTLs. If required fusiform scar revision may be modified as per the needs with a ***slightly curvilinear incision***[1] or by two curvilinear incisions in continuation making it as ***lazy S-shaped incision***. Scarring can be minimized by beveling one edge and counter beveling the other, creating a tongue and groove effect when sutured, this is ideal for scars over seborrhoeic areas. A re-excised scar will always be longer than the original scars, and this factor should be made clear to the patient.[1]

Serial Excision (Figs. 5A and B)

It is recommended when the scar is too large for a single fusiform excision without excessive tension on the skin closure.[2] It can be carried out in two or more stages as per the requirement related to the size and site of the scar, carries less risk and requires longer interval with minimal care between the stages. Serial partial excision when judicially executed serves as an alternative to tissue expansion techniques with good results. Both tissue expansion and serial excision make use of similar biochemical properties of the skin to make greater quantities of normal tissue. Tissue expansion techniques carry higher risks and complication rates. It needs weeks and months between operations, requires multiple visits to the surgeons, induces more discomfort during expansion, prone for infections, and in addition may lead to mechanical failure of the implants. As a result of this and prohibitive cost, tissue expansion techniques are not ideal for routine scar revision except for certain sites like larger scars over scalp.

Reorientation Techniques for Scar Revision Surgeries

Z and W-plasties, geometric broken line closure and VY-plasty are some of the scar revision surgeries which require reorientation of scars.

Optimal scar placement follows skin tension lines. On the face the margins of the cosmetic units (cosmetic unit junctions) generally follow RSTL. Where the orientation of the scar is unfavorable, the principle should be to reorient rather than to simply excise and resuture. The changes

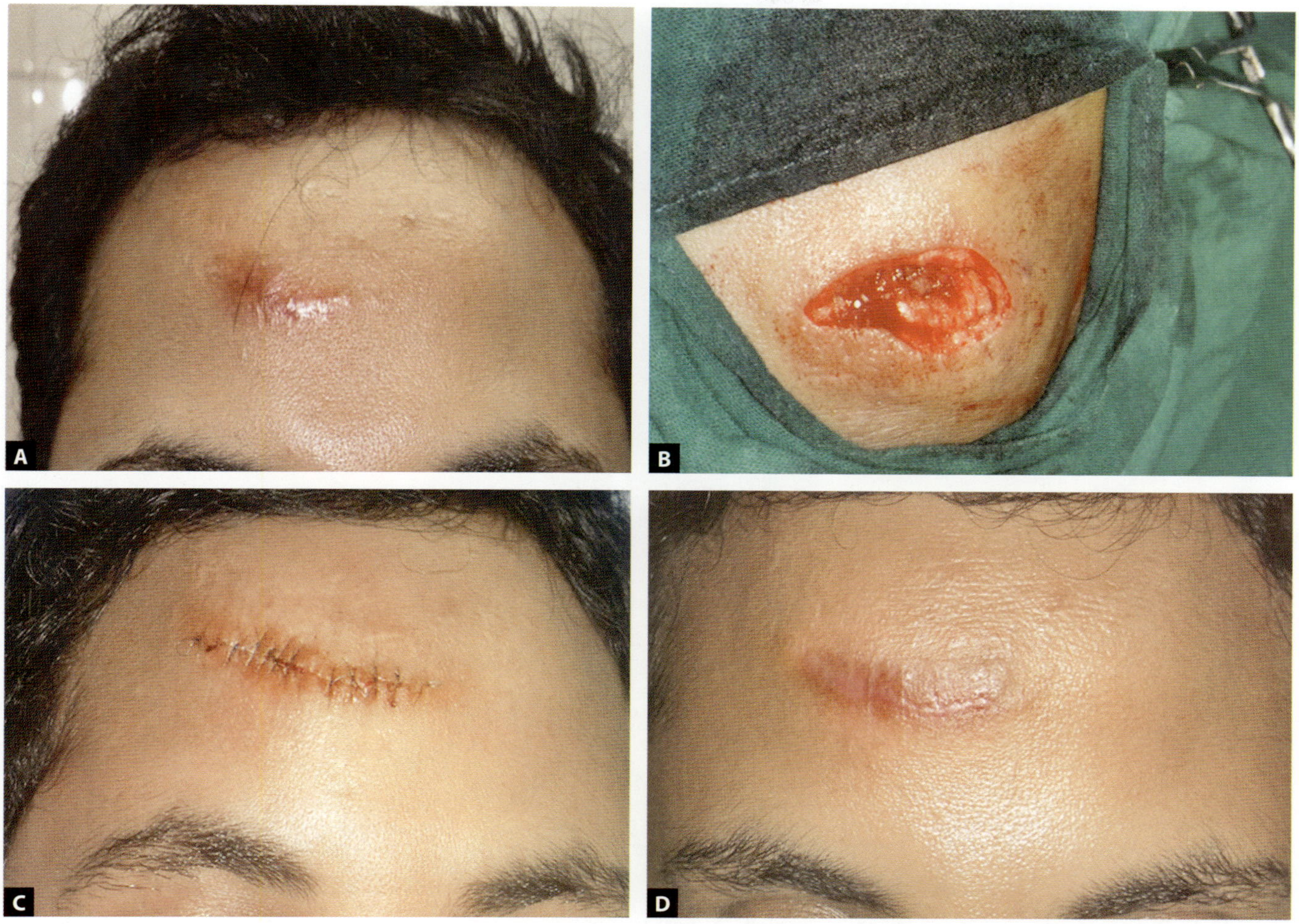

Figs. 2A to D: Scar revision by elliptical excision. (A) Post-traumatic scar over forehead; (B) Intraoperative elliptical excision; (C) Postsurgery immediately after suture removal; (D) Five months postsurgery.

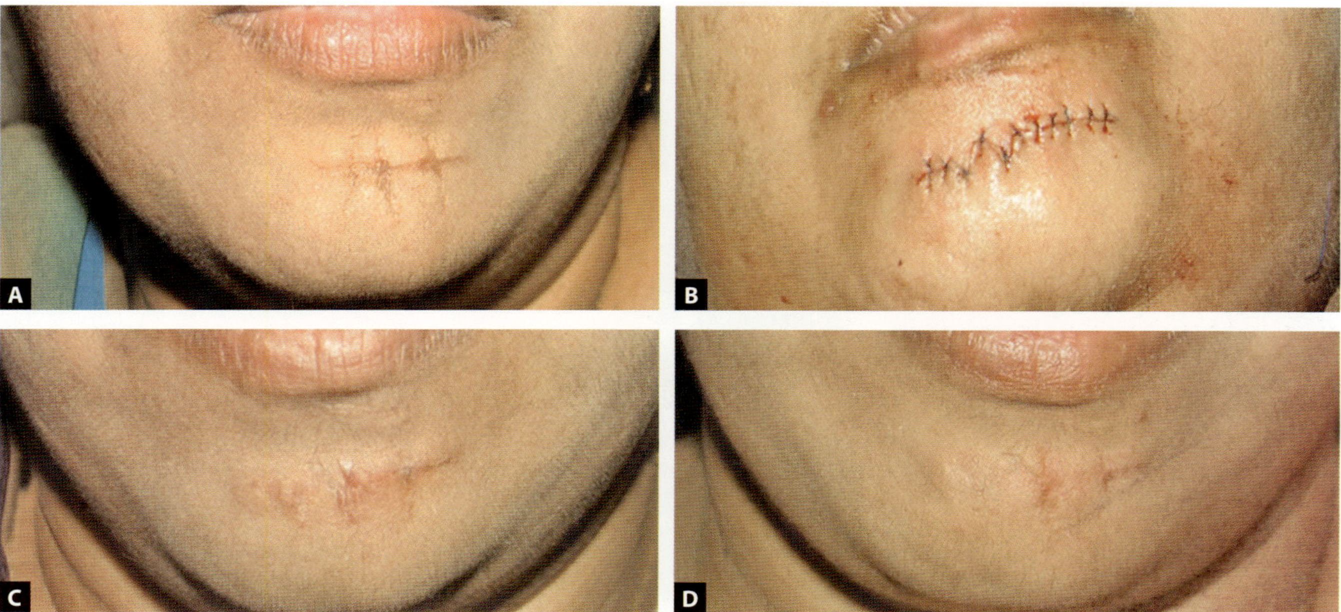

Figs. 3A to D: Scar revision by elliptical excision. (A) Postsurgical scar with suture indentation scars; (B) Elliptical excision with excision of vertical suture indentation scars, immediately after surgery; (C) Three month postsurgery; (D) Six months postsurgery.

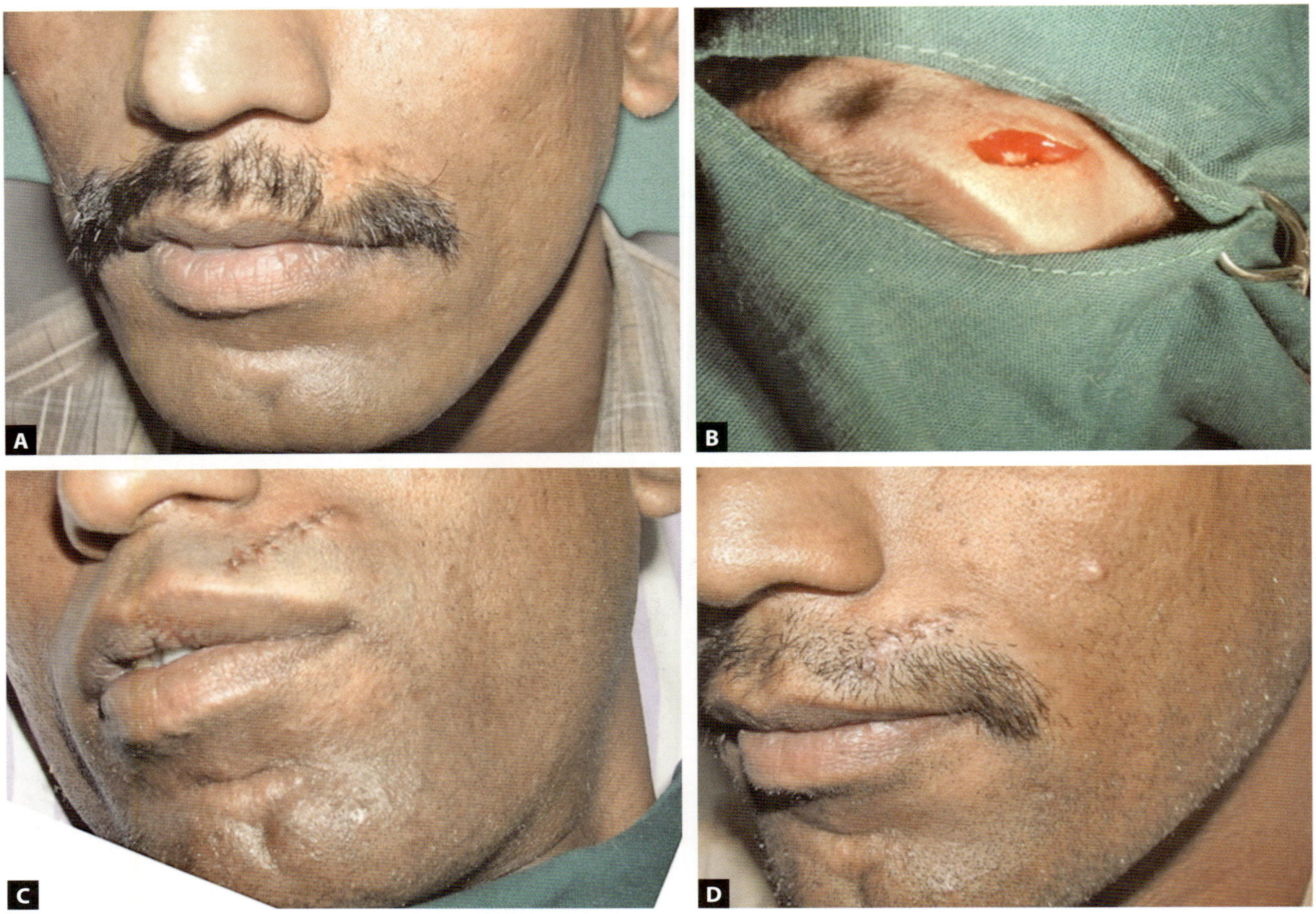

Figs. 4A to D: Scar revision by simple, elliptical excision. (A) Post-traumatic scar with cicatricial alopecia over mustache; (B) Elliptical excision, intraoperative; (C) Immediate postexcision and suturing; (D) Two months postsurgical, reduction in scar size, with few hairs over the scar.

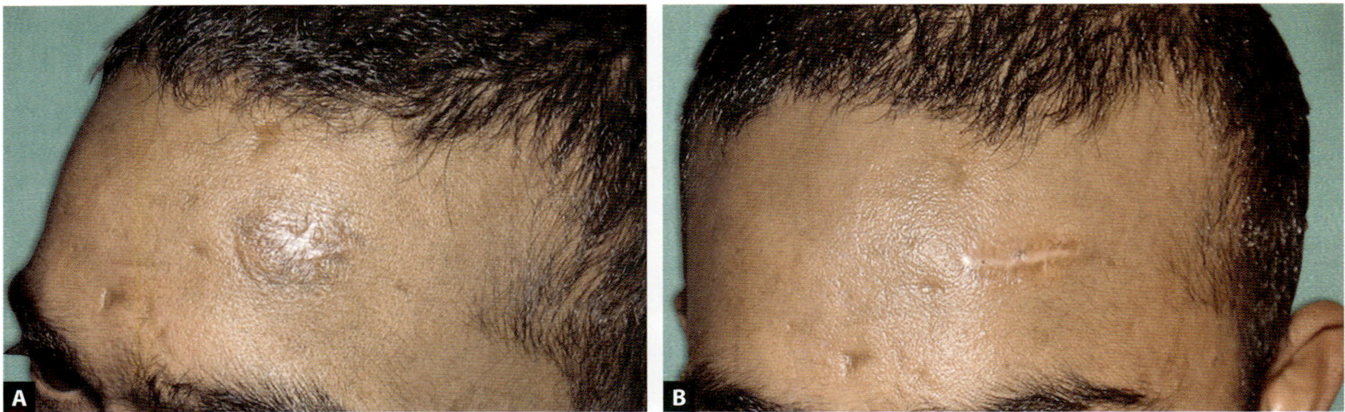

Figs. 5A and B: Scar revision by serial excision. (A) Post-traumatic scar for elliptical excision; (B) Post-traumatic scar 3 months after second session of elliptical excision by serial partial excision.

in local stress with facial muscle movements results in creases making it difficult to assess optimal angle for scar placement over the face, for example, labiomental fold, necessitating to change the plan of action as against the original and an informed consent for the same should be obtained. Despite the expertise it may be difficult to assess the exact direction of RSTLs over the face and it is advisable to always have a pictorial diagram of facial RSTLs, cosmetic units and cosmetic unit junctions in the operation theater. In a difficult situation alternative method is to excise the lesion circumferentially and to wait for few minutes for the defects to get oriented along the RSTLs.[19]

Z-plasty

Z-plasty is one of the oldest yet most useful techniques for scar revision. Z-plasty creates irregular lines making the scar less visible. In addition to other benefits it alters direction of prominent scar placed perpendicular to RSTLs by reorienting parallel to RSTLs. Furthermore, it has the advantage of lengthening a contracted scar which is ideal in situation of visible deformation of free margin, including the eyes, nasal ala, or lip.[1]

In principle, Z-plasty is two zigzag triangular flaps (Fig. 6) that are transposed into the shape of a 'Z'. Two points in the construction of Z-plasty are critical to its understanding and performance: angle magnitude and length of common diagonal (also referred to as common limb or the common member). The central diagonal refers to the scar, two arms that are of the same length as common diagonal are extended from the ends in opposite directions. The angle of designed triangle determines the degree of tissue lengthening, whereby greater angle results in greater gains. The classic 60° Z-plasty angle result in 90° change in scar direction and 75% gain in tissue length. An incision is made along or around the scar and the outlined arms in opposite directions at each ends but at the same length as that of the central limb. The skin is widely undermined and the flap is loosened. The tips of the triangular flaps are then transposed to change the direction of the common diagonal into the transverse diagonal (Figs. 7 and 8). Thus a single Z-plasty effectively changes the direction of the scars and lengthens the scars simultaneously and the tension placed across the transverse diagonal critically increases. The resultant scars can be quite noticeable because of large 'Z' configuration. In these cases, multiple Z-plasty has the advantage of better hiding the 'Z' shape by using multiple smaller 'Z' shapes along the scar lines, as well distributing the tension across the multiple smaller transverse diagonal.[1]

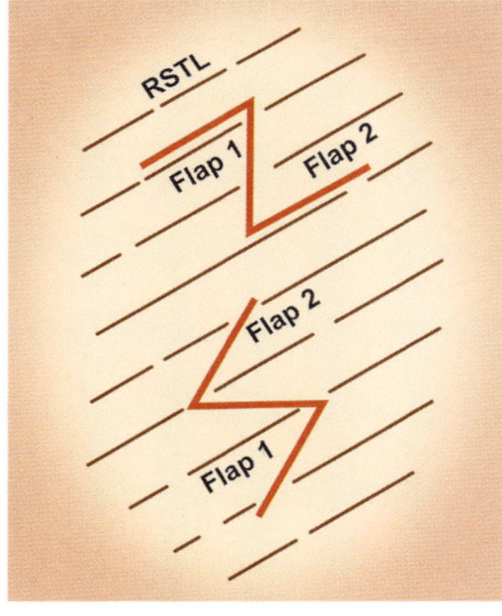

Fig. 6: Schematic diagram of Z-plasty.

Multiple Z-plasties

Z-plasties can be combined in series to reduce tissue contraction (Fig. 9)

Z-plasties are frequently used to correct contracted or asymmetrical anatomical landmark such as elevated or depressed oral commisure,[1] to reorient scars which are placed perpendicular to the RSTLs, to make the resultant scar more stronger at places where there are pulling forces on either sides, e.g. over the angle of the mandible. Z-plasties either single or multiple are practised in contracted scars for releasing the contracture at places such as neck, axillae and other such places where movements are essential. Apart from the advantages of reorienting the scar parallel to RSTLs it has psychological advantage of breaking the monotony of appearance of pre-existing scar, which in other terms can be described as ***cheating the scar.***

Variations in Z-plasty[24]

Double opposing Z-plasties (Fig. 10): In this mirror images of Z-plasty incision are made back to back and flaps

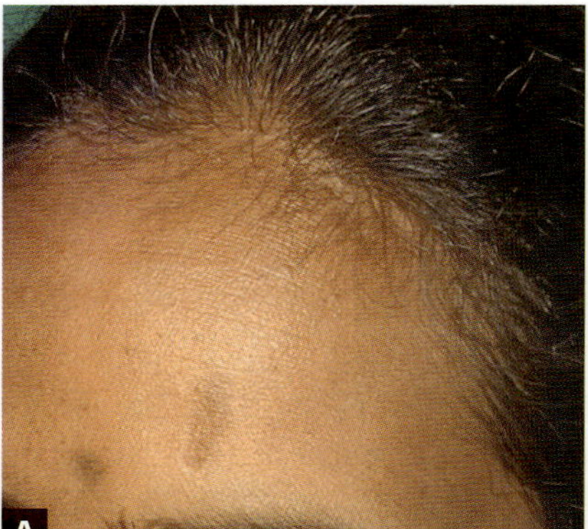

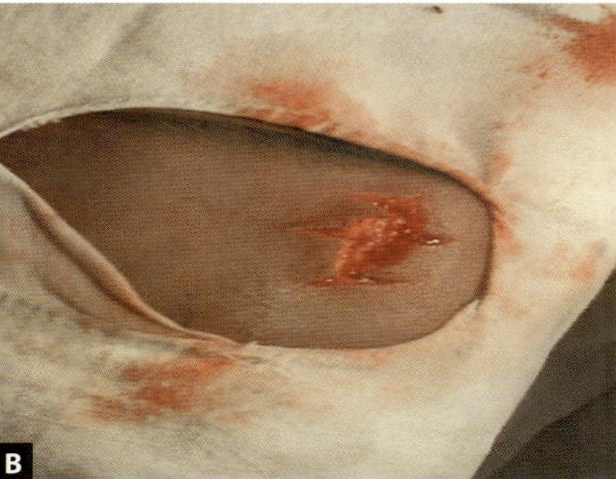

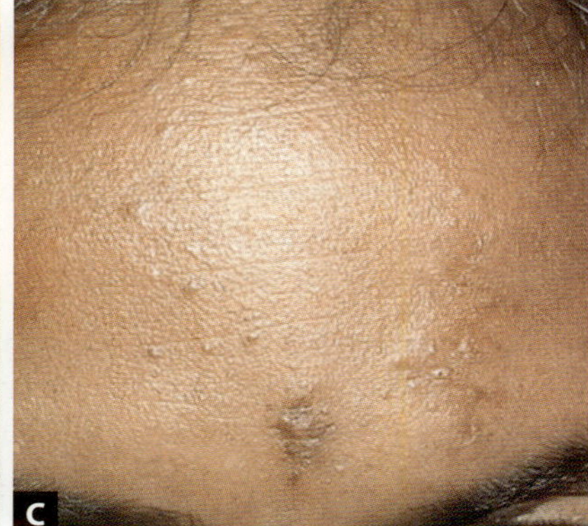

Figs. 7A to C: Z-plasty for vertical forehead scar. (A) Post-traumatic scar over the forehead; (B) Intraoperative, showing limbs of Z-plasty; (C) Postoperative after 3 months of surgery.

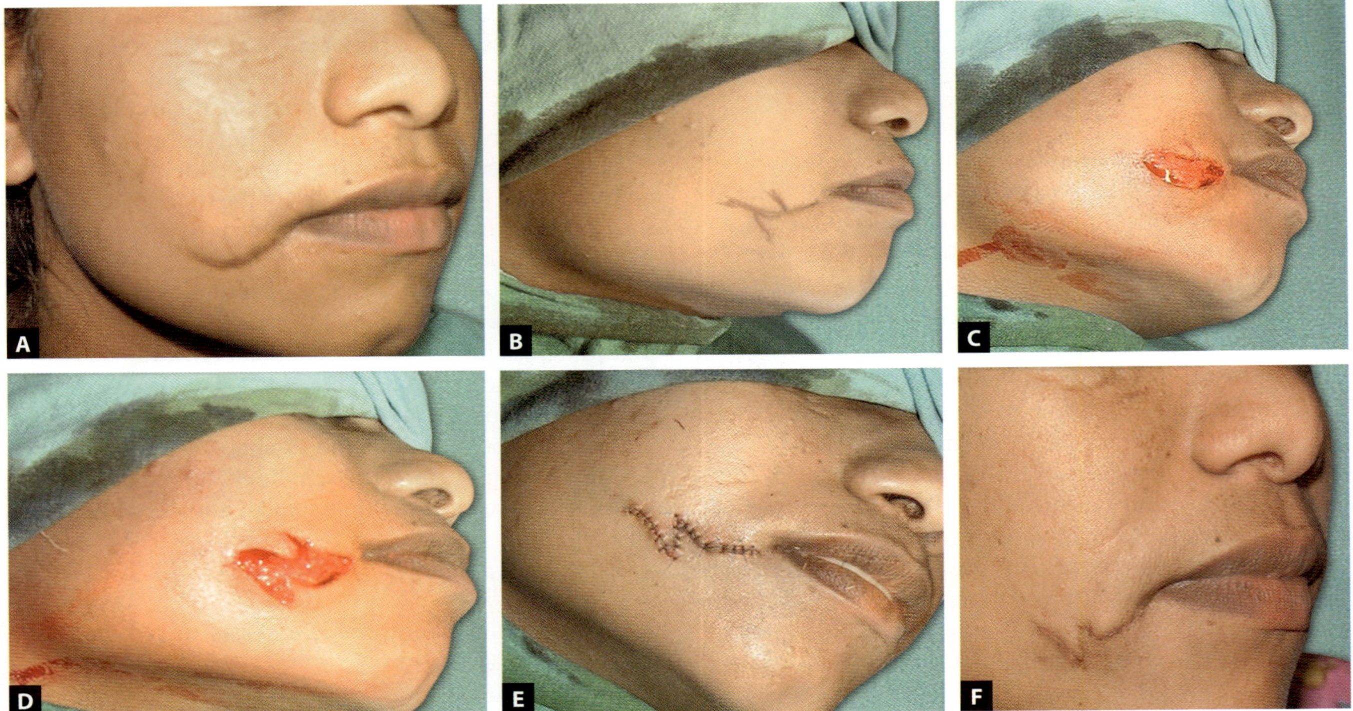

Figs. 8A to F: Z-plasty. (A) Curvilinear trap door scar over the angle of mouth; (B) Marking before surgery showing the limbs of Z-plasty; (C) Excision of ellipse; (D) Intraoperative showing the incision for limbs of "Z"; (E) After suturing; (F) Three months after surgery.

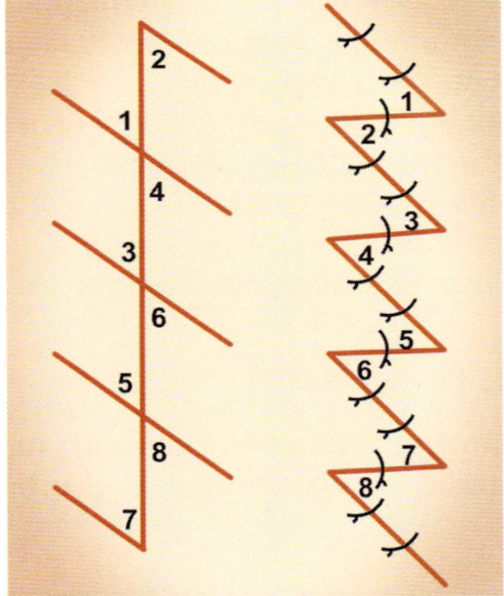

Fig. 9: Schematic diagram of multiple Z-plasties.

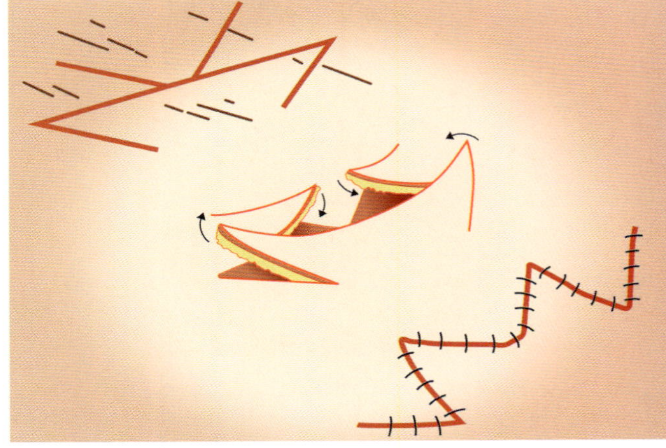

Fig. 10: Double opposing Z-plasty. Mirror images of Z-plasty incisions are drawn back to back. The flaps of each Z-plasty are interposed.

of each are interposed. It offers the advantage of significant lengthening in areas with limited skin availability such as release of a medial canthal web or scar contracture.

Unequal triangles (skew Z-plasty) (Fig. 11): Areas of varying skin elasticity such as the scar edges can be revised using unequal triangular flaps by changing the angle. The limb of 'Z' on the less elastic side is kept longer than the other one.

Half Z-plasty: It is used when the surrounding skin on one side of the scar is elastic and the other side is inelastic. Here the inelastic side is incised to release the scar and a triangular flap from the normal side is transposed to fill the defect created. This is especially useful to release scar contractures at the burn-normal skin interface.

Four flap Z-plasty (Limberg flap) (Fig. 12): The angles of the 'Z' at both ends of the scar are kept at 90° and then each flap is subdivided into 45° angled flaps. This 4 flap Z-plasty gives an advantage of good gain in length and is particularly helpful for releasing severe scar contractures that tether or restrict normal flexion like first web space

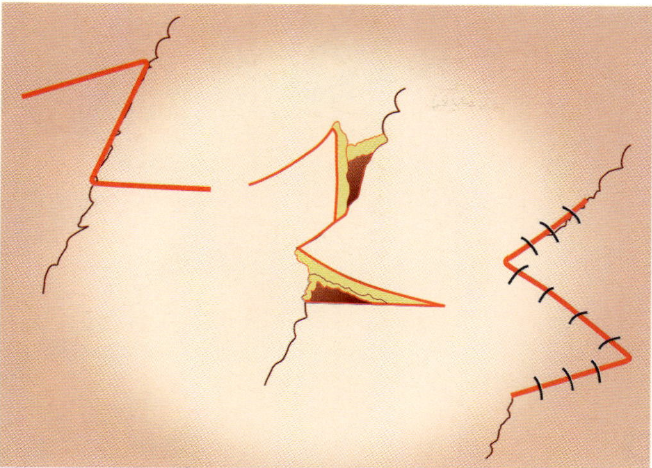

Fig. 11: Unequal triangle Z-plasty.

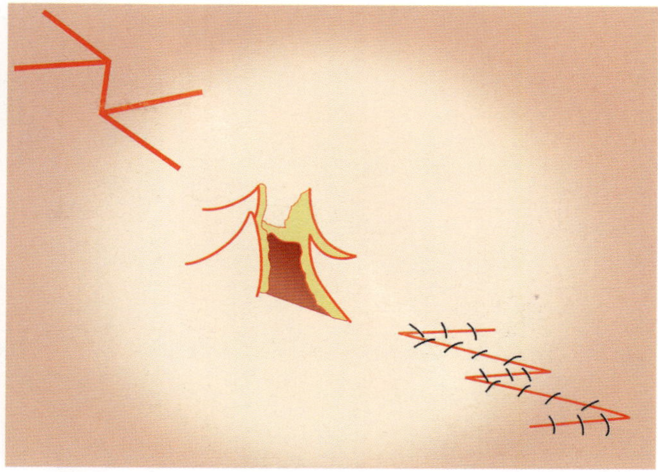

Fig. 12: Four flap Z-plasty.

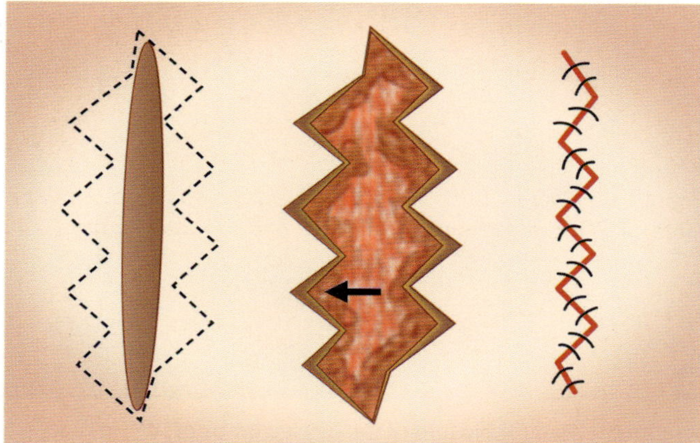

Fig. 13: Schematic diagram of W-plasty.

contracture and post-burn axillary contractures.

Planimetric Z-plasty: In this the central incision of the Z-plasty is extended. It is used for scar interruption and elongation of skin on a planer surface.

S-plasty

It is used for managing oval contracted scar (e.g. tracheostomy scar) when large triangular flaps are required to be transposed. Rounding of the flap ends ensure better survival.

W-plasty and Geometric Broken Line Closure

Both W-plasty and geometric broken line closure techniques relay on similar principle that an irregular line is less visible then a straight line. This is especially advantageous when the scar is not along the RSTL, and therefore may be more visible. W-plasty is ideally indicated for scars which are perpendicular to RSTLs and those which are longer than 2 cm and located on the face. W-plasty (Fig. 13) consists of series of small triangular advancement flaps on either side of the scar.[25] W-plasty is performed by outlining a zigzag line on one side of the scar and a mirror image of the same on the other side. The tips of the 'W' should run parallel to RSTLs as the scar is running perpendicular to it. The scar is excised along the lines then approximated so that the mirror image is coinciding and forms a single zigzag line. The incision is carefully re-approximated by using a combination of dermal three-point tip suture (half buried intradermal suture) and interrupted percutaneous suture (Figs. 14A to D). The advantage of W-plasty is reduced with longer scars because the resultant scar appears monotonous and noticeable. In such a situation geometric broken line closure is more apt[1].

V-to-Y Repair and Y-to-V Repair

In a situation of scars near the free margins such as around the eyes and mouth causing contracture and leading to ectropion or eclabion, V-to-Y repair is an ideal procedure to lengthen the scar and to relieve the contracture. This technique is ideal for small scars.

The technique involves making a V-shaped incision along the length of the contracted scar. The scar is released by undermining the wound sufficiently and pushing it up away from the incision. The newly created defect is then closed such that the two sides of the defect are brought together to form a straight line along the initial scar line and the resultant suture line resembles the letter Y. Just as the V-to-Y repair can raise an anatomic point, a Y-to-V repair can be used to lower it. The incision is made in a Y shape and similarly sutured to form a V.[1]

Jumping Man Procedure[24]

It is a combination of Z-plasty with V-Y advancement described to manage epicanthal fold.

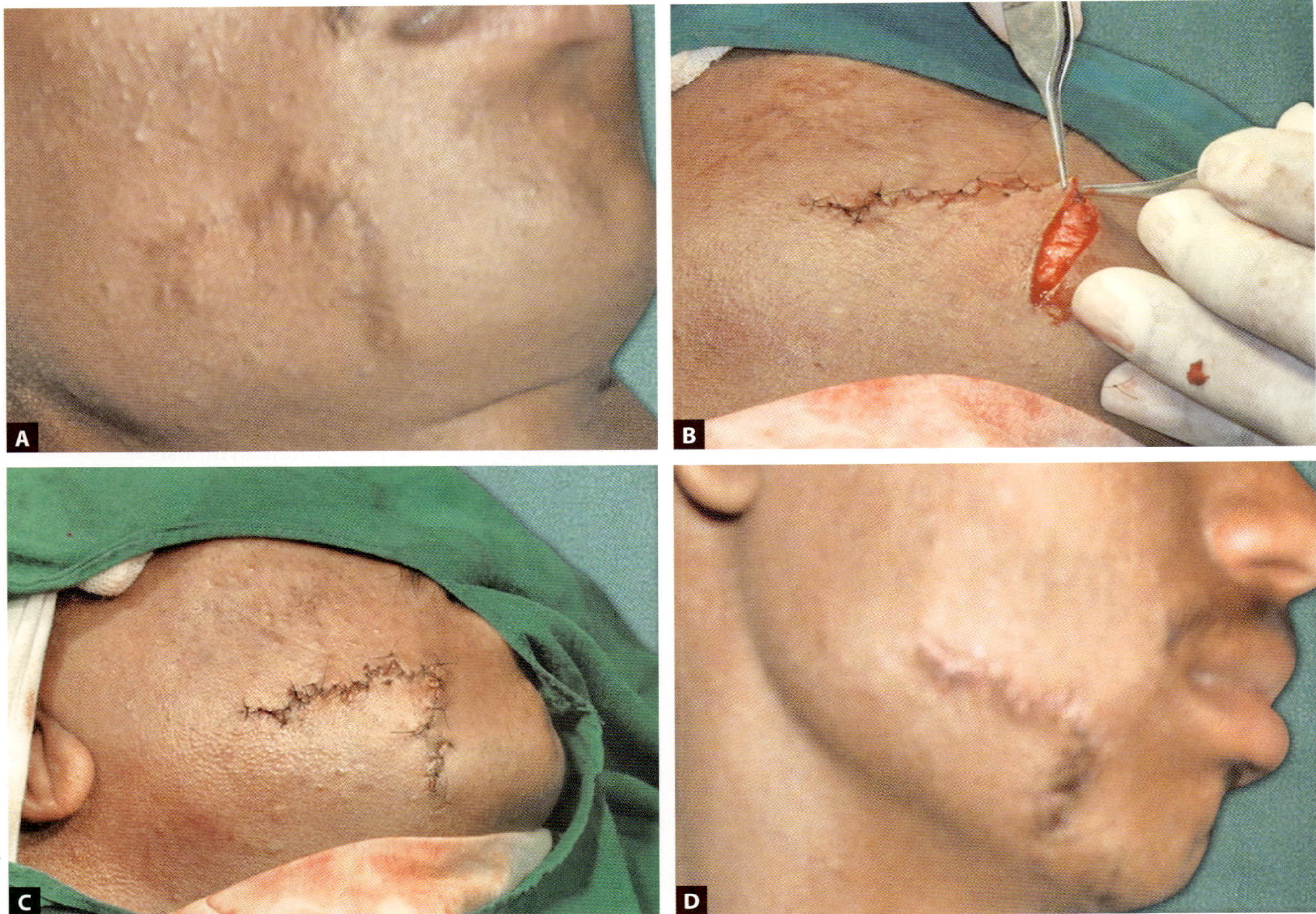

Figs. 14A to D: W-plasty. (A) Irregular, vertical and transverse, post-traumatic scar; (B) Closure of the incised limbs of "W" incision; (C) One week after surgery; (D) Two months after the surgery.

Trapdoor Deformity Repair

A mild trapdoor deformity can usually be managed with intralesional steroids administered 4 weeks postoperatively. If the deformity is not corrected by the intralesional steroids, surgical revision may be required. An incision is made along the curvature of the flap to excise the most uneven or spread scar. The incised flap is then reflected back. The under surface is thinned and the base of the defect deepened. The flap can be thinned to a greater extent than it was. The excess flap tissue is trimmed. The wound edges are undermined sufficiently. The flap is then gently draped back and placed slightly inset to the surrounding skin and sutured appropriately.

Dermal Grafts

Autologous dermal grafts are used as fillers in the management of depressed scars. They have a long-term survival and are cost effective. The advantages of dermal graft over other techniques are no allergic reactions as it is autologous, readily available, easily contoured to fit the defect and is firm.

Procedure

The graft is harvested using skin biopsy punches from postauricular area as it relatively lacks appendages. The epidermis and excess of fat is trimmed off. The epidermis can also be abraded either manually or using a motor before excision of graft. Subcision is carried out in the recipient area to create a pocket where the graft is to be placed. The donor graft should be 3–5 mm more than the recipient area dimensions. Trypsinization of the grafts helps in better handling. A method of insertion of dermal grafts for linear scars is railroading technique. Here the excised graft is trimmed to the required dimensions and one end is tied with 3-0 polyglactin 910. A 16-G needle with syringe attached for grip is inserted through one edge of the scar (recipient area). The sharp bevel of the needle exits from the other end of the scar. The needle is kept in the same position and moved side to side within the confines of the scar creating only one tunnel. The free end of the suture material tied to one end of the dermal graft is threaded into the bevel of the needle till the suture's free end exits through the hub of the needle. Sutured end of the dermal graft is at the level of bevel of the needle.

The dermal graft is now railroaded through the tunnel till the other edge of the linear scar. Suture at one edge of the scar is cut and the graft is left in place. As only one tunnel is created, the possibility of graft losing track is less and pre-trypsinization facilitates easy sliding of the graft in the tunnel. The edges of the scar can be secured with tapes or sutured with 5-0 polypropylene. The lift of the atrophic scar along with decrease in shadow effect can be visualized immediately . The sutures are removed after 5 days.[26]

Role of Botulinum Toxin[27]

Botulinum toxin has been utilized successfully in many facial and extra facial regions to limit superfluous movement. In addition to botulinum toxin's well-known effect on reducing muscular activity there also appears to be an inhibitory effect of botulinum toxin itself on fibroblasts, thereby, offering another potential mechanism for producing a more satisfactory outcome for problematic scar revision and lesion removal.

Prevention of Scars

A scar may not naturally conform to the best direction of the relaxed skin tension lines of the face or body. Although excision techniques such as Z or W plasty are useful in reorientation of scar direction, they are not always completely effective alternatives and may create extra scarring on the patient. In such situations, botulinum toxin may be used to eliminate the tension produced by muscular forces surrounding the scar. It would probably be the best practice in these circumstances to inject superficially at the time of the procedure or at suture removal and in a low dose.

In an Established Scar

Occasionally, scarring will appear in areas that are amplified by movement. This may be less obvious when one is young. However, as one ages, tissues become less supple and the skin diminishes in thickness allowing the underlying muscular activity to become more apparent as wrinkles and lines. In such areas, botulinum toxin may be employed to the cosmetic advantage of the patient.

Autologous Fat Graft

Adipose tissue has recently been identified as a source of processed lipoaspirate cells or adipose-derived stem cells (ADSCs).[28] Hence, fat grafts may not only serve as fillers, but also improve the quality of aged and scarred skin. The fat is harvested from the donor area preferably the thigh, processed and the injected into recipient area. The fat grafts can be combined with platelet rich plasma for better results.[29]

PLATELET-RICH PLASMA

It has been postulated that autologous platelet-rich plasma (PRP) could be used for the treatment of depressed facial scars, because it can enhance wound healing, which has been shown to accelerate tissue repair.[30] PRP in combination with laser has been reported to work well in depressed scars. The possible mechanism of PRP in the reconstruction of a depressed scar is by promoting the recovery of laser-damaged skin through the numerous growth factors present in PRP, especially platelet-derived growth factor. This growth factor may help stimulate the production of other growth factors important in tissue remodeling, which promote connective tissue healing by up regulating collagen and protein synthesis.[31]

Platelet-rich plasma (PRP) has been used in combination with microneedling for management of acne scars for better results.[32]

DERMABRASION AND ABLATIVE LASERS

If there are texture abnormalities and irregular elevated wound edges which could not be corrected by massaging for 2–3 months following the surgery, spot dermabrasion is an ideal technique either used alone or in combination with re-excision. Importance should be given to prevent post-inflammatory hyperpigmentation by sun avoidance and with topical depigmenting agents. Dermabrasion can be carried out by a motorized dermabrader with diamond fraises or with a dental micro-motor apparatus attached with different shape and sizes of dental burs.

NONABLATIVE LASERS

Nonablative lasers like long-pulsed frequency doubled Nd:YAG laser and pulsed dye lasers are useful mainly in hyperpigmented and hypervascular mature scars. They are effective in eliminating the unsightly vascular and pigmented components of the scar without compromising the integrity of the skin.[33]

Table 3 gives the practical guidelines for scar revision.

POSTOPERATIVE CARE

- Postoperatively look for appropriate hemostasis immediately and possibility of hematoma if any.
- Appropriate and esthetic dressings play an important role particularly over-exposed areas.
- Keep the patient under observation for at least one hour or inpatient care may be considered as per the requirement of the individual patient.
- Restricting the mobility of the limb or part may be required, especially if the surgical site is in the vicinity of a joint.

Table 3: Practical guidelines for the management of various types of scars.

Type of scar	Up to 6 weeks	6 weeks to 3 months	After 6 months	After year
Linear scar Normal scar maturation	Avoid sun exposure **Preventive measures** Moisturizing Taping Silicone Reevaluate after 6 weeks	Preventive measures up to 3 months	▪ Further scar maturation - continue silicon as long as necessary	
Hypertrophic scar		▪ Continue preventive therapy ▪ Pressure/massage therapy	▪ Continue preventive and pressure therapy ▪ Intralesional corticosteroid ▪ Surgery to release contracture	▪ Surgical scar revision ▪ Resurfacing with supportive or preventive therapy
Widespread hypertrophic scar	Avoid sun exposure **Preventive measures** Silicone + Compression Moisturizing Taping Silicone Reevaluate after 6 weeks	▪ Custom made pressure garments with silicone inlays or garments ▪ Intralesional corticosteroid ▪ Surgery to release contracture	▪ Continue or intensify previous treatments ▪ Custom made pressure garments with silicone inlays or garments ▪ Intralesional corticosteroid, Bleomycin, 5-fluorouracil and/or verapamil ▪ Surgery to release contracture	▪ Surgical scar revision ▪ Resurfacing with supportive or preventive therapy
Keloid	Avoid sun exposure Silicone + Compression Moisturizing	▪ Silicone ▪ Compression ▪ Intralesional corticosteroid, Bleomycin, 5-fluorouracil and/or verapamil		▪ Surgical excision - with electron beam irradiation/ brachytherapy (iridium 192) ▪ Intralesional Cryotherapy

- Appropriate antibiotics and anti-inflammatory drugs to be given for a required duration.
- Inspect the wound to look for any hematoma or early signs of infection and change the dressing ideally on the 3rd postoperative day.
- Percutaneous sutures may be removed as early as the 5th day over the face to avoid suture indentation marks or may be as late as 10 days depending on the site and tension on the wound edges. Consider removal of alternate sutures on 5th day if there is a possibility of dehiscence.
- Steri-strips may be applied immediately following suture removal and to be continued for at least for 3–4 weeks, especially over cosmetically important areas.
- Avoidance of sun exposure and use of sun screens and other physical modes of sun protection should be advised to prevent postinflammatory hyperpigmentation.
- Mild pressure massage along the long axis of the scar with any lubricating agent like olive or mineral oil, twice or thrice daily for a period of 1–2 minutes each time for up to 1–3 months facilitates flattening of rough edges of the scar. This may also help in preventing hypertrophic scar formation.
- Therapeutic spot dermabrasion may be considered to flatten the edges.
- Procedures like intralesional steroid injections and topical 5-fluorouarcil may be considered in a patient prone to develop keloids and if there is any early indication for the same.
- Follow-up photographs should be taken ideally for at least 6 months postoperative period.

Tips

For getting best results and pitfalls to be avoided

- Attempt scar revision on a mature scar – since the scars continue to remodel, at least wait for 6 months before attempting any kind of surgical intervention.
- Do not attempt scar revision surgery in a patient who expects faster results, the best results of the scar revision surgery are obtained at least after 6 months.
- Counsel the patient thoroughly to make them understand possible results with best efforts, and it should be clear that no scar can be made to disappear, but can be made better, with reference to size, shape orientation, color and anatomical function.
- Plan properly, and apply the best possible procedure to the individual patients requirements.
- Meticulously follow the principle of esthetic surgery to give best possible results, with reference to marking, the incision, suturing techniques, suture removal and application of steri-strips after suture removal.
- Informed consent and pre- intra- and postoperative photography should be obtained.
- Postoperative care with regular massaging and if required other interventions like, physiotherapy, dermabrasion, intralesional steroids are very essential for the best outcome.
- Do not over promise the patient, always under promise and deliver better results.
- Avoid wound infection and other possible causes for delayed wound healing.
- Do not compromise with the standard surgical prerequisites like, sterilization, proper operation theater set up, good instruments, good lighting, assistance, and resuscitation measures.
- Always seek the help of the plastic or esthetic surgeons when required.

SUMMARY

- Scars over the exposed and cosmetically important areas commonly present to dermatologists.
- Scars that cause contractures and limitation of joint movement or cause distortion of vital anatomical structures like eyes, mouth, etc. usually present to plastic and reconstructive surgeons.
- Treatments such as chemical or surgical scar revisions may vary greatly as do the scars and patient characteristics. The treating physician should therefore be well versed in all procedures and should choose the procedure or combination of procedures best suited to the individual scar/patient.
- Examination and physical analysis of the scar, psychological assessment and thorough counseling of the patient with assessment of patient expectation are vital before scar revision surgery.
- Patient should be informed of the proposed plan and possible deviations from the proposed plan and informed consent should be sought. The patient should understand that ***" no scar can ever made to disappear but can be significantly modified to look better cosmetically and or functionally".***
- Treatment options for scars vary from medical lines of management like, TCA CROSS, phenolization, topical and intralesional steroids to physical modalities like massage, pressure garments, augmentation by dermal fillers like, collagen, silicone, fat, etc. to surgical interventions such as elliptical excision, "Z" plasty, "W" plasty, Geometric broken line closure, V-to-Y or Y-to-V repair, or excision with either split or full thickness grafts and complex closures involving flaps.
- Fractional and pixel lasers may play an important role in the treatment of post-acne scars. Scar resurfacing can be achieved with Er:YAG and CO_2 lasers and pulsed dye lasers can improve fresh and vascular scars and keloids.
- All patients seeking scar revision surgery should be explained that the results are not instantaneous and that it may take 6 months to 1 year to achieve best results.

REFERENCES

1. Lee KK, Gorman AK, Swanson NA. Scar revision. In: Robinson JK, Hanke CW, Sengelmann RD, Siegel DM (Eds). Surgery of the skin—procedural dermatology, 1st edition. Philadelphia, Mosby; 2005. pp.401-10.
2. Parkhouse N, Cubison TCS, Hmzah MD. Scar revision. In: Mathes SJ (Ed). Plastic surgery, 2nd edition. Philadelphia, Saunders; 2006. pp.235-67.
3. Kokoska MS, Thomas JR. Scar revision. In: Papel ID (Ed). Facial Plastic and Reconstructive Surgery, 3rd edition. New York, Thieme; 2009. pp.59-65.
4. Shockley WW. Scar revision techniques. Operative Techniques in Otolaryngology. 2011;22:84-93.
5. Moran ML. Scar revision; management of facial cutaneous defects. Otolarynlogical Clinics of North America. 2001;34:767-80.
6. Mustoe TA, Cooter RD, Gold MH, et al. International clinical recommendations on scar management. International Advisory Panel on Scar Management. Plast Reconstr Surg. 2002;110(2):560-71.
7. Savant SS. Scar revision. In: Savant SS (Ed). Textbook of dermatosurgery and cosmetology. 2nd edition. Mumbai, ASCAD; 2005. pp.202-7.
8. Fearmonti R, Bond J, Erdmann D, et al. A Review of Scar Scales and Scar Measuring Devices. Eplasty. 2010;10:e43.
9. Spann K, Mileski WJ, Atiles L, et al. Use of a pneumatonometer in burn scar assessment. J Burn Care Rehabil. 1996;17:515-7.
10. Fong S, Hung L, Cheng J. The cutometer and ultrasonography in the assessment of postburn hypertrophic scar: a preliminary study. Burns. 1997;23(1):S12-8.
11. Falanga V, Bucalo B. Use of the durometer to assess skin hardness. J Am Acad Dermatol. 1993;29(1):47-51.
12. Fong S, Hung L, Cheng J. The cutometer and ultrasonography in the assessment of postburn hypertrophic scar: a preliminary study. Burns. 1997;23(1):S12-8.
13. Bray R, Forrester K, Leonard C, et al. Laser Doppler imaging of burn scars: a comparison of wavelength and scanning methods. Burns. 2003;29:199-206.
14. Nedelec B, Shankowsky HA, Tredget EE. Rating the resolving hypertrophic scar: comparison of the Vancouver Scar Scale and scar volume. J Burn Care Rehabil. 2000;21(3): 205-12.
15. Draaijers LJ, Tempelman FR, Botman YA, et al. The patient and observer scar assessment scale: a reliable and feasible tool for scar evaluation. Plast Reconstr Surg. 2004;113(7):1960-5; discussion 1966-7.
16. Duncan JA, Bond JS, Mason T, et al. Visual analogue scale scoring and ranking: a suitable and sensitive method for assessing scar quality? Plast Reconstr Surg. 2006;118(4): 909-18.
17. Beausang E, Floyd H, Dunn KW, et al. A new quantitative scale for clinical scar assessment. Plast Reconstr Surg. 1998;102(6):1954-61.
18. Singer AJ, Arora B, Dagum A, et al. Development and validation of a novel scar evaluation scale. Plast Reconstr Surg. 2007;120(7):1892-7.
19. Borges AF. Relaxed skin tension lines. Dermatol Clin. 1989;7:169-77.
20. Fulton VE. Silicone gel sheeting for the prevention and management of evolving hypertrophic and keloid scar. Dermatol Surg. 1995;21:947-51.
21. Hirshowitz B, Lindenbaum E, Har-Shai Y, et al. Static-electric field induction by a silicone cushion for the treatment of hypertrophic and keloid scars. Plast Reconstr Surg. 1998;101:1178-83.
22. Majid I. Microneedling therapy in atrophic facial scars: An objective assessment. J Cutan Aesthet Surg. 2009;2:26-30.
23. Kaplan B, Potter T, Moy RL. Scar revision. Dermatol Surg. 1997;23:435-42.

24. Garg S, Dahiya N, Gupta S. Surgical scar revision: An overview. J Cutan Aesthet Surg. 2014:7:3-13.
25. Park SS. Scar revision through W-plasty. Facial Plast Surg Clin North Am. 1998;6:157-61.
26. Nirmal B, Somiah S, Sacchidanand SA. Railroading technique of dermal grafting for linear atrophic scarring. J Cutan Aesthet Surg. 2014;7:224-6.
27. Goodman GJ. The use of botulinum toxin as primary or adjunctive treatment for post-acne and traumatic scarring. J Cutan Aesthet Surg. 2010;3:90-2.
28. Zuk PA, Zhu M, Mizuno H, et al. Multilineage cells from human adipose tissue: Implications for cell-based therapies. Tissue Eng. 2001;7:211-28.
29. Cervelli VI, Nicoli F, Spallone D, et al. Treatment of traumatic scars using fat grafts mixed with platelet-rich plasma, and resurfacing of skin with the 1540 nm nonablative laser. Clin Exp Dermatol. 2012;37(1):55-61.
30. Ganio C, Tenewitz FE, Wilson RC, et al. The treatment of chronic nonhealing wounds using autologous platelet-derived growth factors. J Foot Ankle Surg. 1993;32(3):263-8.
31. Young Oh, Kim BJ, Kim MN (Eds). Depressed Facial Scars Successfully Treated with Autologous Platelet-rich Plasma and Light-emitting Diode Phototherapy at 830 nm. Ann Dermatol. 2014;26(3):417-8.
32. Chawla S. Split face comparative study of microneedling with PRP versus microneedling with vitamin C in treating atrophic post acne scars. J Cutan Aesthet Surg. 2014;7: 209-12.
33. Cassuto DA, Emanuelli G. Non-ablative scar revision using along pulsed frequency doubled Nd:YAG laser. J Cosmetic and Laser Ther. 2003;5:1-5.

Chapter

31

Dermabrasion

Satish S Savant, Sandeep Savant, Behroze M Deputy

Key Messages

- Dermabrasion is an effective way of resurfacing.
- It needs surgical skill and training.
- It can be used in both cosmetic and non-cosmetic indications.
- Prolonged healing time and complications attributed to full face dermabrasion, has increased the popularity of fractional lasers; however multiple sessions of fractional lasers can never achieve the aesthetically superior results of full face dermabrasion.
- Spot dermabrasion is use full treatment modality in vitiligo surgeries, tumors of face including syringoma, trichoepithelioma, adenoma sebaceum, seborrheic keratosis, Darier's disease, etc.

INTRODUCTION

Dermabrasion is defined as sequential planing of the raised, altered or otherwise normal skin from the epidermis through the papillary dermis to the desired level (up to the junction of upper and mid-reticular dermis) with either manual and/or electrical motorized abraders and further allowing this wound to heal by secondary intention so as to achieve leveling (resurfacing) effect to make the cutaneous lesions and/or scars less conspicuous.

Dermabrasion involves mechanical removal of layers of skin. Dermabrasion restricted up to upper reticular to mid-reticular dermis creates a superficial wound and initiates a secondary intention wound healing process. The epidermis then regenerates from the epidermal appendages (hair follicles, pilosebaceous and sweat glands) and from the margins. This process begins within 24 hours of dermabrasion and takes about 7–12 days to complete. The new epidermis shows greater organization and vertical polarity. Dermal regeneration is a slow process taking several months. The regenerated dermis demonstrates less elastosis and improved organization, with compact horizontally arranged bundles of collagen interspersed with elastic fibers (collagen remodeling). Ground substance is decreased and telangiectasias are absent. The overall result is soft supple skin that appears more youthful and has fewer rhytids and dyschromias.

The objective of every dermabrasion should be to reorganize and restructure the collagen of the papillary dermis without causing injury beyond the upper reticular dermis as any abrasion below this plane is likely to result in scarring.

Cryoanesthesia has been advocated to make the skin firmer as an aid to even dermabrasion. However, in India, cryoanesthesia is not available and hence facial dermabrasions are performed under general anesthesia (GA). Further, we have to dermabrade the skin in "as is where is condition" as per the pattern of various dermal layers. Hence, it is important to be aware of the markers for identification of the different layers which are described in Box 1.

HISTORY

Dermabrasion is a technique for skin resurfacing that has been in use for nearly 100 years.[1,2] In 1905, Kromeyer, a German dermatologist, reported the use of power driven abrading instruments on skin chilled with ether spray and CO_2 snow for the treatment of post-acne scarring.[2] He studied the effect of dermabrasion to various depths and established that the wounds healed without scars if the surgical injury did not penetrate through the reticular dermis, thus laying down the basic guideline for the depth of abrasion.[1,3]

Box 1: Guidelines for assessing depth of dermabrasion as one progresses through the skin (Author's original work).[3]

- Removal of skin pigment (epidermis)
- Appearance of multiple, tiny punctate bleeding points with high-field density (superficial papillary dermis)
- Change in the pattern of bleeding: Appearance of larger, rapidly bleeding points with low-field density and increased splattering (junction of mid to deep papillary dermis)
- Appearance of faintly visible pinkish or whitish to grayish parallel lines and ridges (junction of deep papillary to upper reticular dermis)
- Excessive bleeding with fraying or appearance of breaks in the parallel lines and ridges with a feeling of resistance: Optimal level and adequate depth of dermabrasion (junction of upper and mid-reticular dermis)
- Herniation of tiny yellow bits of fat (lower reticular dermis ruptured at places): Not a good sign, stop dermabrading at this level.

Kurtin, a dermatologist at Mount Sinai Hospital in New York, was the first to present a series of patients who underwent dermabrasion with modified dental equipment in 1953.[4-6] Various abrasive end pieces were described such as rasps, burrs and wire-brushes. Black coined the term 'Dermabrasion' in 1954. Alt and Yarborough further contributed to this field by advocating use of the diamond fraise and wire-brush end pieces respectively. Lowenthal reported that better results were obtained when ice pick scars were punch grafted prior to dermabrasion.[7,8]

In India, Maneksha in 1955 used sand paper for treating smallpox scars, acne scars, tattoos and allied defects.[2,9] The manual metallic dermabraders were introduced by him mainly to treat smallpox scars and till today, these form one of the essential instruments for performing controlled dermabrasion.

The authors introduced techniques to achieve safe dermabrasion at various levels of depth with therapeutic spot as well as dermabrasion procedures for treating a variety of skin conditions like papular lichen amyloidosis (PLA),[1-5] stable vitiligo,[6] acne scars and genodermatoses[2] such as adenoma sebaceum, multiple trichoepitheliomas, Darier's disease, etc. Dermabrasion has been used for treating many cutaneous conditions varying from acne scars to the removal of tattoos or tumors or scar revisions.[9-21] It is possible to dermabrade skin in any area of the body by altering the methodology according to the anatomical features of the region.

The popularity of this procedure has diminished with the advent of newer procedures including chemical exfoliation, laser resurfacing, nonablative laser resurfacing and microdermabrasion because of the invasiveness and longer downtime for dermabrasion. However, dermabrasion in hands of a skilled and experienced surgeon is a cheaper and effective remedy, especially for deep scars and rhytids.

INDICATIONS[9-32]

Conditions for which dermabrasion has been used are shown in Table 1.

Table 1: Conditions for the use of dermabrasion.[9-21]

1. Facial scars	Post-acne scars, chickenpox, herpes zoster, smallpox, traumatic scars
2. Acne	Chronic resistant acne (reduces size of sebaceous duct with better sebum drainage, prophylactic use), acne rosacea and enlarged pores
3. Stable vitiligo	Therapeutic spot wounding, preparation of recipient area prior to grafting in all types of grafting methods: suction blister technique (SBT), ultra thin skin grafting, melanocyte and keratinocyte suspension method
4. Hyperkeratotic lesions	Lichen simplex chronicus (LSC), hypertrophic lichen planus (HLP), papular lichen amyloidosis (PLA), porokeratosis, linear verrucous nevus (LVN), prurigo nodularis
5. Pigmentation	Melasma, freckles, post inflammatory hyperpigmentation (PIH), tattoos, periorbital hypermelanosis
6. Tumors	Syringoma, trichoepithelioma, adenoma sebaceum, seborrheic keratosis, Darier's disease, nevus depigmentosus, congenital nevi, neurofibromatosis, Bowen's disease, basal cell carcinoma
7. Actinic	Actinic keratosis, actinic cheilitis, photoaging
8. Miscellaneous	Pyogenic granuloma, fine wrinkling, rejuvenation, rhinophyma, xeroderma pigmentosa (prophylactic)

CONTRAINDICATIONS[1-7,9,13-16,33-37]

Contraindications include keloidal tendency, atrophic hairless scars of burns and trauma, bleeding disorders, active infection, history of taking isotretinoin (wait for 12–18 months). Patients with types 4–6 skin need special counseling.

PREOPERATIVE PROCEDURES[1-3,8,13,38-43]

The following techniques can be adopted 6–8 weeks before the planned date of dermabrasion, depending on the indication, for better end results.

- *Scar-revision techniques*: Undermining (subcision), punch excision and closure, punch elevation, punch excision and graft replacement.
- *Electrocauterization, radiosurgery*: For raised lesions and borders.

PATIENT INFORMATION

Patient counseling should include special emphasis on the following aspects:

- Realistic expectation of surgical outcome (50–70% improvement and not complete elimination).
- Multiple sittings may be required.

- Postoperative sequelae, side effects and complications. Postoperative sun avoidance and sun protection for 3 months.
- If possible, the procedure should be deferred till beginning of monsoons (lesser chances of PIH) as per author's experience.

EQUIPMENT

- Mechanical (manual) (Fig. 1).
  - Sand papers (water paper No. 80, 110).
  - Hand held metallic dermabraders (*Source:* Dr. Maneksha).
- Electrical
  - Wire-brushes, burrs and diamond fraises (various sizes and shapes) (Fig. 2).
  - Cable: Unit or hand machine (average 15,000 rpm) (Fig. 3).

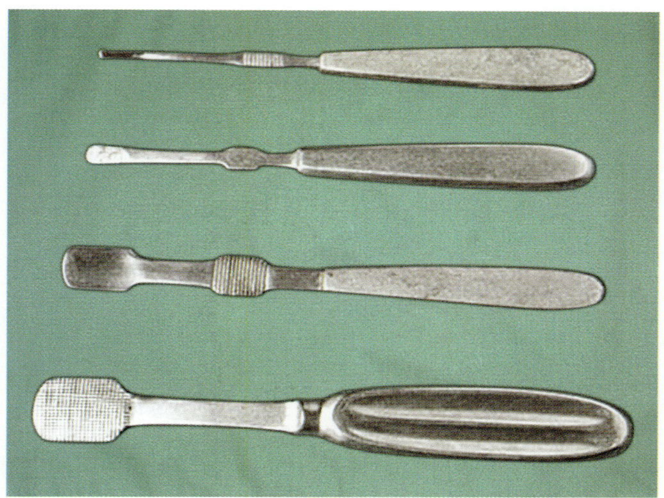

Fig. 1: Manual dermabraders.

PREOPERATIVE WORKUP

This is performed as per any surgical procedure. Since facial dermabrasion is done under general anesthesia, preanesthetic checkup and clearance are needed. Informed consent and photographs are mandatory. In selected cases, particularly, full face dermabrasion, test spot dermabrasion at postauricular site may be done 4–6 weeks prior to planned date of surgery, to study healing pattern and possibility of complications in a given case. Thus, it also carries medicolegal significance. Close shave, removal of excess hair is done just before operation. Injection of vitamin K (1 mL containing 10 mg) is given 1 day before surgery in cases of extensive dermabrasion.

FACIAL DERMABRASION

Operative Procedure[44-48]

The important steps in this major procedure are as follows:

1. *Use of protective gear by operating staff*: Cap, mask, gown, gloves and face shield (Universal precautions as splattering of blood often occurs during the procedure).
2. *Mark the submandibular margin*: Just beneath and parallel to the inferior border of the mandibular ramus from infra-auricular area to the center of the chin on both the sides.
3. Induction of GA with endotracheal intubation (if using halothane), supine position with posterior tilting of head with head ring, hair taped with micropore tape and tucked under the cap, ears plugged with cotton, antibiotic ointment in eyes, roller gauze in mouth for cheek protrusion, IV fluids as required.
4. Surgical preparation and marking the pitted scars/lesions individually with marker pen.
5. *Anesthesia*: The procedure can be done under different types of anesthesia—local, regional or general. Spot dermabrasion can be done under local anesthesia

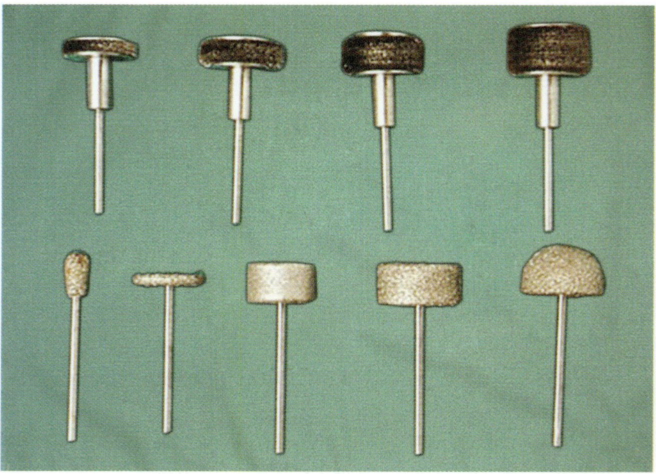

Fig. 2: Diamond fraises and wire brushes.

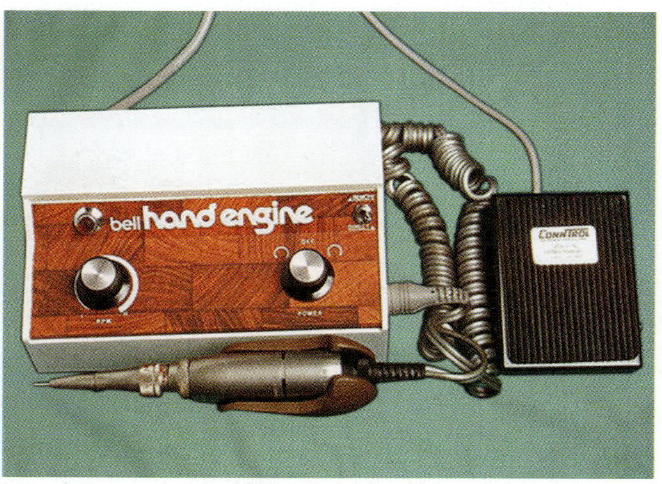

Fig. 3: Dermabrasion machine.

(LA). Full face dermabrasion needs to be performed under GA. Tumescent anesthesia too has been used to perform dermabrasion.[45]

6. *Technique*
   a. Face is turned to one side and skin stretched by an assistant, so as to provide a flat and taut surface for planing.
   b. Using either wire brush or diamond fraise end piece, hold the hand piece in safety razor grip. Direction of pull should be towards the handle of hand piece, i.e. perpendicular to the axis of the direction of rotating end piece. First establish the submandibular border, by smooth strokes along the marked line from either ear to the chin. Ipsilateral sides are abraded from the temporal hairline to coalesce with the submandibular border. Feather the established inferior edge of the submandibular border, by light perpendicular short strokes going 1 cm beneath it, either with electrical or manual abraders. Establish the submandibular margin on the other side in a similar manner.
   c. Individual pitted marked out scar surface is moderately stretched. Using a pear-shaped diamond fraise end piece and with pencil-like vertical grip of hand machine, gently rotate the hand piece clockwise in small circles to lightly abrade the base of the scar and firmly abrade its edges (shouldering). Smoothen out all the marked scars individually in a similar fashion.
   Raised lesions of trichoepitheliomas, adenoma sebaceum, Darier's, etc. are flattened out by abrading them individually with pear-shaped dermabraders or by sculpting with No. 15 blades or by radiosurgery to the level of the surrounding skin.
   e. Segmental electrical cosmetic facial unit wise dermabrasion (Fig. 4): With wire-brush or disc diamond fraise attached to hand piece held in a razor grip, head is turned to one side and skin stretched. Establish the infraorbital margin by dermabrading downward on the cheeks and sideways on the temporal region along the bony margin in a curvilinear manner leaving 2–3 cm of normal skin around the eyes unabraded. Further, dermabrade segmentally in the following order of preference: right cheek, chin, left cheek, forehead, glabella, nose and upper lip. Segmental abrasion should always either overlap or feather into the adjoining segments at the natural folds like vermillion borders, nasolabial folds, etc. or peripheral regional boundaries like the hairline and ear to ear submandibular line inferiorly. Abrade evenly up to adequate depth, i.e. up to the junction of mid and deep papillary dermis. This is followed by mechanical dermabrasion which gives better control thus providing safety.
   f. Manual dermabrasion: Manual metallic dermabraders yield better depth control. Large abraders are used for flatter surfaces and smaller ones for narrow surfaces and curvatures. Dermabrade till optimum depth is reached, i.e. up to the junction of upper and mid-reticular dermis or as per the requirement. It is better to under-abrade to avoid complications. In between the procedure, hemostasis is achieved with ice-cold sponges.
   g. Termination: Finally, two quick face rubs with No. 80, followed by No. 110 sand papers (water papers) are done in the same segmental, sequential order to smoothen out the surface. Hemostasis is achieved with ice-cold sponges.
   h. For patients under GA with endotracheal intubation, abrade one side of the face fully in similar fashion going stepwise from steps (a) to (g). Other side is then abraded similarly after changing the direction of the endotracheal tube to the opposite side. Lastly, remove the tube and abrade the remaining area of chin and upper lip first electrically and then mechanically. Two quick rubs with sand paper are given and hemostasis achieved with ice-cold sponges.

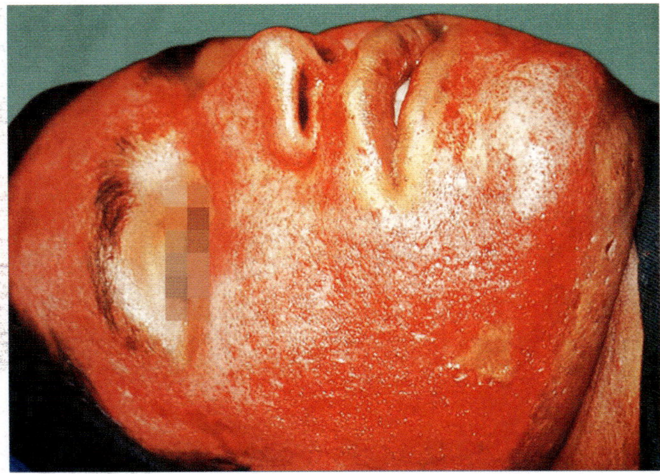

Fig. 4: Immediately following dermabrasion.

Postoperative Management[47]

The guidelines for postoperative management are as follows:

a. Intravenous (IV) fluids.
b. Admit the patient and discharge only when oozing stops (about 7 days).
c. Dressing: Two methods
   i. Face is dressed only with double layer of framycetin tulle (Fig. 5).
   ii. Face is not dressed at all allowing the serum to ooze continuously.
d. Towel is lightly wrapped around the neck to absorb the oozing serum. Two fans are placed across either cheek for faster drying of the secretions.

e. *Medications*: Antibiotics, analgesics, short course of tapering steroids (IV first day, changed to oral from day 2) usually 8 mg IV dexamethasone on day 1 and tapered fast. Injection of vitamin K (1 mL) should be continued from a day before surgery, followed by on the day and the next day after dermabrasion (total of 3 consecutive days).
f. Serous discharge oozes for 2–3 days and then dries to form crusts, either directly on the face or on the stuck framycetin gauzes. Both fall off by 10–15 days.
g. Emollients and sunscreens for next 3 months.
h. Patient remains indoor for 4 weeks and avoids direct sunlight for further 2–3 months.

Figures 6 and 7 show pre- and postoperative results after dermabrasion in a patient with post-acne scarring.

Side Effects

Side effects are many and include pain, edema, exudation, discomfort, crusting, erythema, milia, hyperpigmentation (reversible), persistent erythema, permanent hypopigmentation, and exacerbation of acne (reversible).

Complications

Bleeding, telangiectasia, gouging, infection, scarring, keloid, allergic contact dermatitis, complications of LA or GA.[48,49]

Advantages and Disadvantages

Relative advantages and disadvantages of the procedure are shown in Table 2.

REGIONAL/SPOT DERMABRASION

Apart from face, dermabrasion can be done on any portion of the body (regional) or only the lesion (spot), according to the location and the clinical features of the lesion, after taking into consideration the side effects and complications.

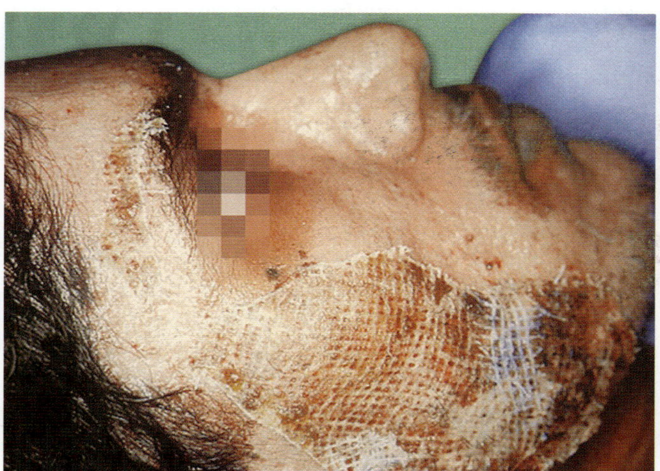

Fig. 5: Healing phase.

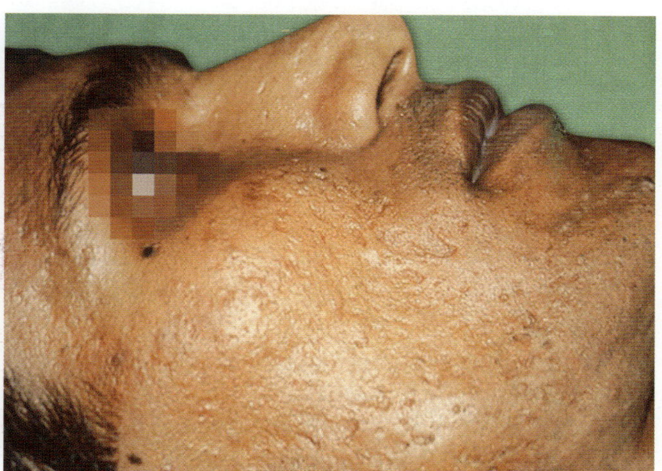

Fig. 6: Acne scars before dermabrasion.

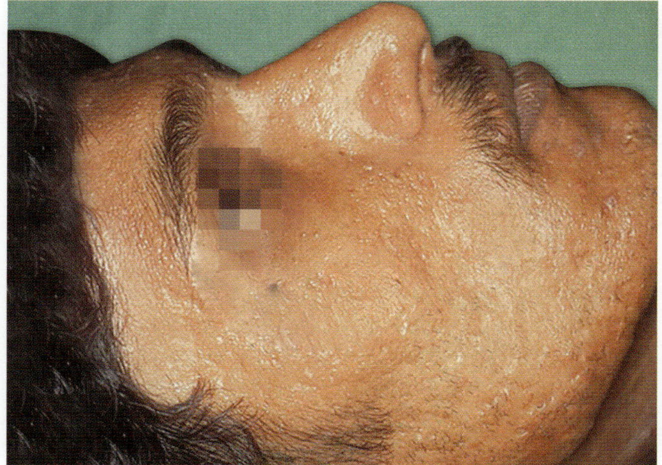

Fig. 7: Acne scars after dermabrasion.

Table 2: Full face dermabrasion: advantages and disadvantages.

Advantages	*Disadvantages*
▪ Excellent cosmetic improvement—50–80% even in cases of deep scars ▪ Multiple roles: Cosmetic/therapeutic/prophylactic (for actinic keratoses/xeroderma pigmentosa to prevent malignancy) ▪ All the scars and lesions treated at one time ▪ Can be combined with scar revision/electrocauterization, radiosurgery, chemical peeling, etc. ▪ Better control over depth than other ablative procedures as one can visually assess the various skin layers	▪ Hospital admission ▪ Prolonged postoperative rest ▪ Need for GA ▪ Avoidance of sunlight for 3 months ▪ Multiple sittings may be required for better cosmetic results ▪ Deep ice-pick scars cannot be corrected by dermabrasion alone ▪ Permanent hypopigmentation may occur

The methodology for regional or spot dermabrasion is essentially the same; however, one may have to make a few modifications as described below:

a. *Vitiligo*: Superficial spot dermabrasion till pinpoint bleeding (epidermabrasion) can be done for stable vitiligo in hairy area for faster repigmentation and as an adjuvant to medical line of treatment, prior to grafting by SBT or ultrathin split-thickness skin graft (STSG) or application of melanocyte keratinocyte suspension. Prior to grafting by thin Thiersch's STSG, slightly deeper dermabrasion is done till change in bleeding pattern (junction of mid to deep papillary dermis).
b. *Hypertrophic lichen planus (HLP):* Two sittings of deep spot dermabrasion are usually required.
c. *Papular lichen amyloidosis (PLA)*: Leave island strips of normal skin in between the abraded area, lest large wounds created may delay healing.
d. *Tattoo*: Deeper abrasion, multiple sittings may be required.
e. *Striae, scars*: Abrade superficially and linearly along the lesion.
f. *Lichen simplex chronicus (LSC), linear verrucous epidermal nevus, prurigo nodularis*: Abrade deep, multiple sittings may be required depending on the depth and number of lesions.

Manual spot dermabrasion can also be performed with disposable presterilized scratch pads having roughened surfaces and commonly used to clean cautery tips.[50]

Advantages

- Quick, symptomatic relief in HLP, LSC, PLA, prurigo nodularis.
- Faster results compared to other modalities in LSC, PLA, HLP, prurigo nodularis.
- An adjuvant to medical treatment in vitiligo.
- Inexpensive, simple office procedure.
- Can be done under LA.

Disadvantages

- It can be used only where cosmetic importance is secondary to functional importance: Patient acceptance is vital.
- Abrasion may have to be carried to a deeper level for results and prevention of recurrence, and may lead to scarring.
- Multiple sittings may be required.

COMBINATION TECHNIQUE (AUTHOR'S MODIFICATION)[51]

Dermabrasion can be combined with CO_2 laser for deep facial acne scars described as follows:

a. First pass of CO_2 laser to abrade the epidermis after treating individual scars.
b. Regular dermabrasion with diamond fraise/wire-brush electrical and manual metallic dermabraders.
c. Finally, one or two CO_2 laser passes for tightening effect.

However, the disadvantage is the persistent erythema and transient PIH which can last up to 6 months post-laser procedure.

SUMMARY

As stated earlier, dermabrasion is largely being replaced by lasers, particularly after the advent of fractional lasers. Facial dermabrasion is technically a difficult procedure and requires plenty of experience and training. Proper patient selection, recognition of planing depth, greater surgical skill and technique, good postoperative care are all essential for its successful outcome. Despite recent publications that dermabrasion can be performed safely on patients taking systemic isotretinoin,[52,53] the author believes it is prudent to stop isotretinoin atleast 6–12 months prior to dermabrasion.The author is of the opinion that elective full face dermabrasion is a major invasive procedure where any preventable side effect should be avoided in the vital cosmetic facial area. It is useful to treat variety of conditions from acne scars to genodermatoses to facial rejuvenation. It can also be combined with other dermatosurgical modalities like chemical peeling, soft tissue augmentation, face lifts and lasers. The author feels that it is still useful in the current scenario in the following situations:

- Therapeutic spot dermabrasion is a simple and useful modality to treat various skin conditions as an office procedure. It can be curative by itself or used as an adjuvant to medical line of treatment.
- It also gives faster results and since the technique is simple, many of the dermatologists can easily undertake it.
- As compared to fully ablative resurfacing with the carbon dioxide and Er:YAG lasers, dermabrasion demonstrates similar or greater efficacy for the treatment of scars, rhytids, genodermatoses, etc. with less postoperative erythema and more rapid re-epithelialization. The most significant difference as compared to other modalities is that in dermabrasion you know the exact depth which you have reached whereas in other resurfacing modalities, it is a blind alley as you do not know how deep your chemical peel is going to sink or to what level your last laser pass is going to reach.

Although experience and skill are necessary in order to avoid complications with full-face dermabrasion, its efficacy remains unmatched for the patient who is willing to endure the resultant recovery period. While new technologies continue to emerge, dermabrasion will likely remain an essential and unmatched modality for scar improvement.

Tips

- In acne scars, it is mainly the surrounding skin which has to be abraded to the depth of the scar to obtain the leveling effect.
- However, in case of elevated lesions such as benign tumors, lesions are abraded so as to bring them to the level of surrounding skin thus achieving the contouring effect. This is far easier than that for acne scars and chances of scarring are less.
- For facial dermabrasion a test patch can be done 6 weeks prior to study healing patterns and complications.
- Beginners can start with abrading lesions over trunk and extremities, which have lesser cosmetic significance, to get a hang of the procedure before attempting facial abrasion.
- Sterilized disposable scratch pads can be used for mild to moderate manual dermabrasion, however authors have no personal experience using disposable scratch pads.

REFERENCES

1. Coleman WP, Lawrence N. The history of skin resurfacing. In: Coleman WP, Lawrence N (Eds). Skin Resurfacing, 1st edition. Baltimore: Williams and Wilkins; 1998.pp.3-6.
2. Padilla RS. Dermabrasion. In: Wheeland RG (Ed). Cutaneous Surgery, 1st edition. Philadelphia: WB Saunders Co.; 1994.pp.470-90.
3. Savant SS. Dermabrasion. In: Savant SS, Shah RA, Gore D (Eds). Textbook and Atlas of Dermatosurgery and Cosmetology, 2nd edition. Mumbai: ASCAD; 2005.pp.217-34.
4. Iverson PC. Surgical removal of traumatic tattoos of face. Plast Reconstr Surg. 1947;2:427-30.
5. Kurtin A. Corrective surgical planing of skin; new technique for treatment of acne scars and other skin defects. AMA Arch Derm Syphil. 1953;68:389-94.
6. Mandy SH. Dermabrasion. In: Lask GP, Moy RL (Eds). Principles and Techniques of Cutaneous Surgery, 1st edition. New York: McGraw-Hill; 1996.pp.495-503.
7. Burks JW. Technique of surgical abrasion. In: Burks JW (Ed). Dermabrasion and Chemical Peeling, 1st edition. Springfield: Charles C Thomas; 1956;94-103.
8. Lowenthal LJA. Punch biopsy with autografts. AMA Arch Derm Syphil. 1953;67:629.
9. Maneksha RJ. Scars. In: Maneksha RJ (Ed). Plastic Surgery in the Tropics, 1st edition. Mumbai: Bombay Popular Prakashan; 1965;20-31.
10. Savant SS. Therapeutic regional dermabrasion in papular lichen amyloidosis of shin. Indian J Dermatol Venereol Leprol. 1995;61:196-201.
11. Savant SS. Therapeutic spot dermabrasion. Study of 197 sites in 11 skin conditions. Indian J Dermatol Surg. 1999; 1:5-15.
12. Savant SS. Therapeutic spot and regional dermabrasion in stable vitiligo. Indian J Dermatol Venereol Leprol. 1996;62: 139-45.
13. Savant SS. Facial dermabrasion in acne scar and genodermatoses—A study of 65 patients. Indian J Dermatol Venereol Leprol. 2000;66:79-84.
14. Roenigk HH. Dermabrasion for miscellaneous cutaneous lesions (exclusive of scarring for acne). J Dermatol Surg Oncol. 1977;3:322-8.
15. Epstein E. Dermabrasion for therapeutic purposes. In: Epstein E, Epstein E Jr (Eds). Skin Surgery, 6th edition. Philadelphia: WB Saunders Co; 1987.pp.344-7.
16. Roenigk HH Jr. Dermabrasion. In: Roenigk RK, Roenigk HH Jr (Eds). Dermatologic Surgery-Principles and Practice, 1st edition. New York: Marcel Dekker Inc.; 1989.pp.959-78.
17. Katz BE. Dermabrasion for scar revision. In: Roenigk RK, Roenigk HH Jr (Eds). Surgical Dermatology, 1st edition. UK: Martin Dunitz; 1993.pp.385-94.
18. Clabough W. Removal of tattoos by superficial dermabrasion. Arch Dermatol. 1968.pp.98:515-21.
19. Matarasso SL. Indications for skin resurfacing. In: Coleman WP, Lawrence N (Eds). Skin Resurfacing, 1st edition. Baltimore: Williams and Wilkins; 1998.pp.7-16.
20. Verheyden CN. Treatment of facial angiofibromas of tuberous sclerosis. Plast Reconstr. Surg. 1996;98:777-83.
21. Yarborangh JM. Ablation of facial scars by programmed dermabrasion. J Dermatol Surg Oncol. 1988;12:292-4.
22. Hruza GJ. Dermabrasion. Facial Plast Surg Clin North Am. 2001;9:267-81.
23. Bohn J, Stevenson H, Aberg M. Dermabrasion of large congenital melanocylic naevi in neonates. Scand J Plast Reconstr Surg Hand Surg. 2000;34:321-6.
24. Aronsson A, Eriksson T, Jacobsson S, et al. Effects of dermabrasion on acne scarring. A review and study of 25 cases. Acta Dermat Venereol. 1977;77:39-42.
25. Kim EK, Hovsepian RV, Mathew P, Paul MD. Dermabrasion. Clin Plast Surg. 2011;38:391-5.
26. Surowitz JB, Shockley WW. Enhancement of facial scars with dermabrasion. Facial Plast Surg Clin North Am. 2011; 19:517-25.
27. Harmon CB, Zelickson BD, Roenigk RK, et al. Dermabrasive scar revision. Immunohistochemical and ultrastructural evaluation. J Dermatol Surg. 1995;21:503-8.
28. Gold MH. Dermabrasion in dermatology. Am J Clin Dermatol. 2003;4:467-71.
29. Poulos E, Taylor C, Solish N. Effectiveness of dermasanding (manual dermabrasion) on the appearance of surgical scars: a prospective, randomized, blinded study. J Am Acad Dermatol. 2003;48:897-900.
30. Roxo RF, Sarmento OF, Kausalek AZ, et al. Successful treatment of a hypochromic scar with manual dermabrasion. J Dermatol Surg. 2003;29:189-91.
31. Gillard M, et al. Conventional diamond fraise vs manual spot dermabrasion with dry well sanding screen for scars from skin cancer surgery. Arch Dermatol. 2002;138:1035-9.
32. Harmon CB. Dermabrasion. Derm Clinics. 2001;19:439-42.
33. McGregor IA. Free skin grafts. In: McGregor IA (Ed). Fundamental Techniques of Plastic Surgery and their Surgical Applications, 8th edition. Edinburgh: Churchill Livingstone; 1989.pp.39-63.
34. Hung VC, Lee JY, Zitelli JA, et al. Topical tretinoin and epithelial wound healing. Arch Dermatol. 1989;125:65-9.
35. Hevia O, Nemeth AJ, Taylor JR. Tretinoin accelerates healing after trichloroacetic acid chemical peel. Arch Dermatol. 1991;127:678-82.
36. Mandy SH. Tretinoin in the preoperative and postoperative management of dermabrasion. J Am Acad Dermatol 1986;15:878-9, 888-9.
37. Clark RA. Cutaneous tissue repair: basic biologic considerations. I. J Am Acad Dermatol. 1985;13:701-25.
38. Koranda FC. Treatment and modalities in facial acne scars. In: Thomas JR, Holt GR (Eds). Facial Scars Incision, Revision and Camouflage, 1st edition. St. Louis: The CV Mosby Co.; 1989.pp.278-89.

39. Savant SS, Gore D. Acne scar revision surgery. A study of 350 cases with pitted scars. Indian J Dermatol Surg. 1999;1:11-2.
40. Johnson WC. Treatment of pitted scars: punch transport technique. J Dermatol Surg Oncol. 1976;2:337-9.
41. Orentreich DS, Orentriech N. Subcutaneous incision less (subcision) surgery for the correction of depressed scars and wrinkles. J Dermatol Surg Oncol. 1995;21:543-9.
42. Solotoff SA. Treatment for pitted acne scarring—postauricular punch grafts followed by dermabrasion. J Dermatol Surg Oncol. 1986;12;1079-84.
43. Mancuso A, Farber GA. The abraded punch graft for pitted facial scars. J Dermatol Surg Oncol. 1991;17:32-4.
44. Coleman WP, Klein JA. Use of tumescent technique for scalp surgery, dermabrasion and tissue augmentation. J Dermatol Surg Oncol. 1992;18:130-5.
45. Goodman G. Dermabrasion using tumescent anaesthesia. J Dermatol Surg Oncol. 1994;20:802-7.
46. Baker TM. Dermabrasion as a complement to aesthetic surgery. Clin Plast Surg. 1998;25:81-8.
47. Campbell RM, Harmon CB. Dermabrasion in our practice. J Drugs Dermatol. 2008;7:124-8.
48. Goldman MP, Fitzpatrick RE, Smith SR. Resurfacing complications and their management. In: Coleman WP, Lawrence N (Eds). Skin Resurfacing, 1st edition. Baltimore: Williams and Wilkins Co.; 1998.pp.295-301s.
49. Branham GH, Thomas JR. Rejuvenation of the skin surface: chemical peel and dermabrasion. Facial Plast Surg. 1996;12:125-33.
50. Ina Z, Romanzi A, Gherardini G. Tricks and Tips for Manual Dermabrasion. Dermatologic Surgery. 2016;42(12):1393-4.
51. Savant SS. The carbon dioxide and erbium: YAG lasers. In: Savant SS, Shah RA, Gore D (Eds). Textbook and Atlas of Dermatosurgery and Cosmetology, 2nd edition. Mumbai: ASCAD; 2005.pp.461-76.
52. Bagatin E, dos Santos Guadanhim LR, Yarak S, et al. Dermabrasion for acne scars during treatment with oral isotretinoin. Dermatol Surg. 2010;36(4):483-9.
53. Chandrashekar BS, Varsha DV, Vasanth V, et al. Safety of performing invasive acne scar treatment and laser hair removal in patients on oral isotretinoin: a retrospective study of 110 patients. Int J Dermatol. 2014;53(10):1281-5.

Chapter

32

Keloids and Hypertrophic Scars

Sanjay Singh, Savita Yadav,
Sangeeta Varma, Somesh Gupta

Key Messages

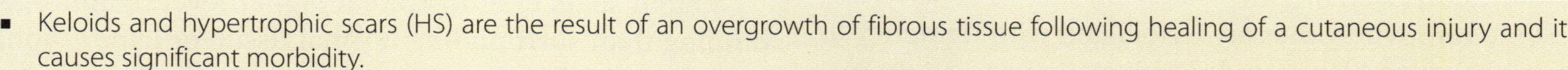

- Keloids and hypertrophic scars (HS) are the result of an overgrowth of fibrous tissue following healing of a cutaneous injury and it causes significant morbidity.
- There are important differences between keloid and HS.
- There are several treatment modalities which are useful for the management of keloids, though no single modality is completely effective.
- The most commonly used modalities are pressure, silicone gel sheets, intralesional steroids, 5-fluoro-uracil (5-FU), cryotherapy, surgical excision, radiation therapy and lasers.
- These may be used singly or more commonly in combination.
- Once established, however, keloids are difficult to treat, with a high recurrence rate regardless of therapy.
- One should realize that keloids will only improve and not disappear completely.
- Patients with a tendency for keloids should be advised about preventive measures.

INTRODUCTION

Keloids and hypertrophic scars (HS) are the result of an overgrowth of fibrous tissue following healing of a cutaneous injury. Keloids extend beyond the margins of the original wound, do not usually regress spontaneously and tend to recur after excision, while hypertrophic scars do not expand beyond the boundaries of the initial injury and may undergo partial spontaneous resolution.[1] Keloids and hypertrophic scars may cause functional impairment and cosmetic disfigurement and are often associated with morbidity.

HISTORY

The first description of keloids was given by Smith Papyrus in 3000 BC.[2] Subsequently, in 1806, Jean Louis Alibert used the term cheloide, derived from the Greek word chele, meaning crab's claw, to describe the lateral growth of tissue into unaffected skin and added oid, meaning 'Like'.[3] In 1825, he wrote a chapter entitled "Les cancroidesou Keloides" which established the current term Keloid. Unfortunately, in over 3000 years history of keloids, there is no satisfactory treatment available for this troublesome disease. The research on keloids faces several hurdles including absence of animal models and lack of interest of funding agencies and industry.

EPIDEMIOLOGY

Keloids mostly arise at puberty with peak age of onset between 10 and 30 years of age.[2] Keloids have been observed in infants and adults over the age of 70. Keloid was identified in 0.6% of the children aged between 6 and 11 in Taiwan in a cross-sectional study. It was mostly seen following BCG vaccination.[4]

There exists an equal risk between men and women. But female predominance may be due to the number of ear lobe keloids secondary to piercing among women.[5,6] It is mostly sporadic, though familial cases have been described. It is mostly autosomal dominant with incomplete penetrance and variable expression, though autosomal recessive cases have also been described.[7] The increased risk of developing keloids in identical twins strongly supports a role for genetics.[8]

The exact prevalence of keloids is not known and the data may be underestimation of its actual occurrence. According to various population based data, it ranges from 4% to 16% in Black and Hispanic.[9] The prevalence in England is as low as 0.9%.[7] It is most common in darker racial ethnic group with reported incidence ratios ranging from 2 to 1 and from 19 to 1 between Blacks and Whites.[10] It is most prevalent in African American, Hispanic and Asian population and least common in Caucasians and albinos.[11] Its absence in albinos have led to speculation of role of melanocytes. Among the Asians, it is more common in Chinese population.[11] Why certain races are more susceptible is not known. Its predisposition has been associated with certain HLA haplotypes; B4, B21, BW16, BW35, DR5 and DQW3 as well as blood group type A.[7] Recently, positive association of HLA DQA1 and DQB1 alleles with keloids in Chinese Han people have been demonstrated using PCR-SSP method.[12] HLA-DRB1*15 is associated with risk of developing keloid in Caucasians of Northern European origin.[13]

Some rare syndromes are associated with tendency to develop keloids which include Rubinstein-Taybi syndrome, Geominne syndrome, Ehlers-Danlos syndrome, Leigh necrotizing encephalomyelopathy, Ullrich congenital muscular dystrophy and pachydermoperiostosis.[14,15]

PATHOPHYSIOLOGY

The exact pathophysiology of keloid is not fully understood. There is enormous number of studies and postulates trying to explain the etiology. There are number of hypotheses which have been postulated as shown in the Box 1.

Box 1: Various hypotheses of keloid formation.

- Sebum autoimmune hypothesis
- Hypoxia hypothesis
- Tension hypothesis
- Hormonal hypothesis
- Essential fatty acid hypothesis

According to the sebum autoimmune hypothesis, keloids are a result of immune reaction to sebum which acts as antigen after being secreted intradermally following trauma. This is supported by the clinical characteristics highlighted by some researchers.[16,17] Only humans develop true keloids and are the only animals with sebaceous glands. Keloids are common on seborrheic areas mostly. Interestingly, keloids are rarely described on volar skin which lacks sebaceous glands. Keloids are seen more frequently after puberty when the sebaceous glands are most active and its incidence decrease in the later decades of life when sebum production fall down. Also, after puberty, keloids can be activated from older wounds incurred during childhood, for example, earlobe keloids and keloids at vaccination sites.[18]

Hypoxia hypothesis asserts that hypoxia present in keloid and hypertrophic scar stimulate excessive collagen production. Transmission electron microscopy have demonstrated that the microvessels are occluded because of excessive endothelial tissue which leads to hypoxia.[19,20] Hypoxia/Hypoxia inducible factor-1α has been found to provide a favorable microenvironment for keloidal keratinocytes to adopt a fibroblast-like appearance through epithelial-to-mesenchymal transition. This might lead to enhanced capacity of keloidal keratinocytes to invade in adjacent normal area beyond the wound margin.[21] According to tension hypothesis, keloids are caused and exacerbated by tension in wounds. This is supported by the occurrence of keloids and its recurrence in areas of highest tension on the body (chest wall, scapular region and suprapubic regions) and lowest recurrence in areas of low tension (neck, earlobes and lower limbs).[22,23]

Influence of hormones has been speculated due to its occurrence at puberty and pregnancy, worsening during pregnancy and rarity in postmenopausal women.[11,24,25]

Acromegalics are highly susceptible to keloid formation.[11]

Keloid scars demonstrate a higher level of androgen binding than surrounding normal tissue or hypertrophic scars.[7] It is also interesting to note that circulating androgen concentrations rise during pregnancy. The chest, upper back and neck are areas predisposed to keloids and these areas have a higher rate of dihydrotestosterone metabolism.[26]

According to essential fatty acid hypothesis, an essential fatty acid deficiency of precursors and inflammatory competitors for arachidonic acid may be a factor in the multifactorial etiology of keloid formations. Nutrition may also be a contributing factor in rural black South Africans.[27-29]

Irrespective of the above different hypotheses, the primary biochemical abnormality is the imbalance between matrix degradation and collagen synthesis, resulting in excess accumulation of collagen in the wound. One of the limiting factors in keloid research is the lack of a good laboratory model for study, though various animal models have been studied. Human skin graft on athymic mice and porcine model appear promising. These can probably help in better understanding of pathogenesis and thus helping in better treatment.[30]

In most patients, trauma is the main provoking factor which may occur in any form: abrasions, incisions, insect bites, chemical and thermal burns, acne, chickenpox, bacterial or viral infections and vaccination. Many a times, patients do not recall an inciting event and these are known as "spontaneous keloids". The most important risk factor for the development of keloids is a wound healing by secondary intention, especially if healing time is increased. It is widely accepted that keloids develop subsequent injury or inflammation of skin but the exact pathogenesis is unknown. Normal scars seem to have a negative feedback mechanism whereby fibroblasts are mobilized to repair a cutaneous defect and their activity is appropriately dampened to prevent excessive repair. Negative feedback mechanism is somehow defective in keloidal fibroblasts ultimately resulting in exuberant scar formation with the propensity to recur.[31]

The metabolic aberration which leads to keloid formation occurs in the final phase of wound healing when keloids fail to mature and become compact.[32] Aberrant expression of various growth factors and their receptors has been described for keloid-derived fibroblasts. For example, keloidal fibroblasts have been shown to over express the growth factors: VEGF, TGF-β1, TGF-β2, CTGF, as well as the PDGF-α receptor.[33-37] The key role of TGF-β has been extensively studied. It has been found that TGF-β1 and β2 are profibrotic and promote scar formation.[36] In one study, keloidal fibroblasts were found to have lower rates of apoptosis, thought to be related to a down-regulation of apoptosis-related genes.[38]

Various polymorphisms of genes encoding TGF-β1, β2, β3 as well as the TGF-β receptor have been evaluated, but no statistically significant associations with keloids have been identified.[39-42] Thus, there is possibility of role of multiple genes that impart susceptibility to keloid development, with different genes contributing to keloid formation in different families. Seifert et al. studied the gene expression profiles of fibroblasts from different sites of the keloids; 105 genes were identified that were differentially regulated (79 genes were upregulated and 26 downregulated). The apoptosis inhibitor AVEN was found to be upregulated at the active margin of keloids, while apoptosis-inducing genes such as ADAM12 and genes inducing extracellular matrix (ECM) degradation such as matrix metalloproteinase-19 were upregulated in the regressing keloid center[9]. p53 gene codon 72 polymorphism may play a role in susceptibility to keloid in Chinese population.[43]

Risk factors that increase the chances of keloids include:[44,45]

- African, American, Asian or Hispanic ethnicity
- Between 10–30 years age
- Deep skin wounds such as those from burns or surgical scars
- Scars from acne, vaccination or chicken pox
- Family history
- In darkly pigmented skin, the risk increases 15–20 folds
- People with blood group A
- Surgical intervention of pre-existing keloid.

CLINICAL FEATURES

Keloids occur most commonly on the chest, shoulders, upper back, back of the neck, cheeks and earlobes.[46,47] Unusual formation of keloid after recurrent episodes of herpes zoster can be seen.[48] Genital keloids have been reported to occur subsequent to circumcision or following trauma.[49,50] In addition, multiple cases of corneal keloids including giant ones following corneal trauma have been described.[51,52] Eyelids, mucous membranes, palms and soles can also be affected.[47] Clinically, keloids range in consistency from soft and doughy to rubbery and firm nodules, which can be skin colored, hypopigmented or erythematous secondary to telangiectasias. Lesions are usually devoid of hair follicles and other functioning adnexal glands. Earlobe keloid can assume several clinical forms: button-shaped keloid, dumb-bell shaped keloid, fibrotic intralobular type and a more destructive lesion that involves the whole lobe.[11] Park et al. have classified ear lobe keloid in 5 types: (1) Pedunculated, (2) sessile (single nodular), (3) sessile (multinodular), (4) buried and mixed.[53]

By examining the keloid scars of 211 Afro-Caribbean patients in Jamaica, Bayat and colleagues described site-specific morphologies of keloid: trunk scars were geometrically-shaped with clear margins or irregular in outline, surface and margin; back single scars were well-demarcated botryoid but multiple scars were butterfly-shaped, spheroidal and irregular; chest scars were butterfly or non-butterfly shaped, found most commonly in the midsternal line; upper limb scars mostly in the deltoid region (propeller-shaped) or elsewhere nodular, linear to irregular; on ear the most common site being the lobe, having reniform to bulbous shape; face and neck keloids were firm nodular to hard; posterior auricular keloids were either horizontal and oblong-shaped or vertical and reniform in outline; scalp keloids were most common in the occipital area varying from small papules to large plaques; lower limb keloids varied from propeller, butterfly, petalloid to dumbbell-shaped. Three plantar and eight pubic keloids were rare findings.[54]

Keloids are frequently symptomatic, with most patients reporting tenderness or pruritus. Lee et al.[48] evaluated 28 patients with keloids and found that more than 80% of patients experienced keloid associated pruritus and about half experienced pain.[55] Most patients present with 1 or 2 keloids; but a few patients have multiple lesions such as in case of spontaneous keloids or keloids as a consequence of acne or chickenpox. Female sex, younger age at presentation and the presence of a positive family history were associated with the development of keloid scars in multiple anatomical sites in Afro-Caribbean individuals in one study.[6] There are no well-documented cases of malignant degeneration of an unirradiated keloid except one recently reported case of basal cell carcinoma developing in the ear lobe keloid.[56] Keloids and hypertrophic scars are among the common cause of functional and aesthetic deformities leading to psychosocial stress to the patient and thus impairing the quality of life. Interestingly, keloids and HS can have severe negative psychosocial impact on the patients where keloids are not common as shown by Bock and associates in Germany, while a study by Oliatan did not show any negative impact in keloid endemic population of Nigeria.[57,58]

HISTOPATHOLOGY

Keloid is a clinical diagnosis and routine histological analysis is unnecessary.[59] However, several malignant tumors i.e. dermatofibrosarcoma protuberans, trichilemmal carcinoma and keloidal basal cell carcinoma and, deep fungal infections such as lobomycosis resemble keloids. Hence, several authors recommend biopsy to rule out such cases.[60]

Keloids have a normal epidermal layer and thickened dermis. Collagen bundles are thicker, more eosinophilic, glassy, closely arranged and more abundant in keloids, yielding acellular, node-like structures in the deep dermal region. In addition to collagen, proteoglycans are another major ECM component deposited in excess amounts in keloid scars. There is decreased concentration of adnexal structures.[61] The four histologic features that are considered pathognomonic for their diagnosis include (1) the presence of keloidal:hyalinized collagen, (2) a tongue-like advancing edge underneath normal-appearing epidermis and papillary dermis, (3) horizontal cellular fibrous bands in the upper reticular dermis and (4) prominent fascia-like fibrous bands.[61,62]

Hypertrophic scar contains nodules of highly compact collagen, often with a capsule-like band at their periphery. Blood vessels are frequently observed at the periphery. In the early stage, bundles or tracts may be in curvilinear form demonstrating a whorl-like arrangement. By electron microscopy, the nodule is seen to contain highly stellate fibroblasts with dilated rough endoplasmic reticulum and few other organelles.[63]

Table 1 outlines the differentiating features of keloids and hypertrophic scars.

TREATMENT

It is difficult to eradicate keloids and hypertrophic scars, and most of the modalities used for treatment are associated with side effects. Counseling should be done regarding treatment options, side effects and cost and the final decision to undertake treatment should lie with patients. As will be evident from subsequent reading, there is a vast armamentarium of treatment options. This suggests that none of the treatments is satisfactory in all patients and there is no universally accepted protocol. In general, keloids are more unresponsive, resistant and have higher rate of recurrence as compared to hypertrophic scar. The treatment of hypertrophic scar and keloid is not very distinct and often overlap. Reported clinical trials suffer from lack of uniformity in case selection (no distinction of keloids and hypertrophic scars), subjective evaluation of treatment outcome and limited follow-up. Blinding is often difficult with many surgical procedures. It is important to realize that even keloids at different sites behave differently in response to treatment. For example, recurrence is less common after excision of an earlobe keloid (Figs. 1 and 2) while keloids in presternal region are resistant to most of the treatment modalities (Figs. 3A and B).[64]

All the different treatments available for management of keloids and HS are listed in Box 2.

Several factors need to be assessed while choosing therapy in a given patient. These include size of keloid, its location, duration, previous treatments and morphology. An international advisory panel on scar management recommended a combination of silicone gel sheet and intralesional corticosteroids as first line therapy (Figs. 4A and B). Second line therapy for resistant cases included laser therapy followed by surgery with adjunctive silicone gel sheet, if required.[65] The treatment modalities have been used with variable success rates and recurrence rates. In general, there is approximately 70% chance of

Table 1: Differentiating features between hypertrophic scars and keloids.

	Hypertrophic scars	*Keloids*
Clinical features	Raised red or pink in color but do not extend beyond margins of original wound be it either traumatic or surgical	Continue to evolve over time without a quiescent or regressive phase
	Generally appear within 4 weeks after trauma	Take up to 1 year to appear
	Often observed in extensor surfaces such as knees and elbows	Do not affect the joint areas of the body generally and affect sebaceous areas (upper part of body)
	Rarely elevate more than 4 mm above skin surface	Grow larger into nodular appearances
Biochemical and molecular differences[46]		
Collagen bundles	Fine, well-organized, wavy parallel to epidermis	Large, thick, closely packed random to epidermis
Myofibroblast	Present	Absent
(α-sm actin expressing)	Nodular formation	Around blood vessel walls
PCNA expressing	Low expression	High expression
Mucin deposition	Negative	Focal expression in dermis
ATP level	Low expression	High expression
Hyaluronic acid localization	Major component papillary dermis	Thickened, granular/spinous layer
Amorphous substance on electron microscopy	Absent	Diffuse pattern
Apoptosis	Decreased	Increased/Decreased
p53 level	Low	High

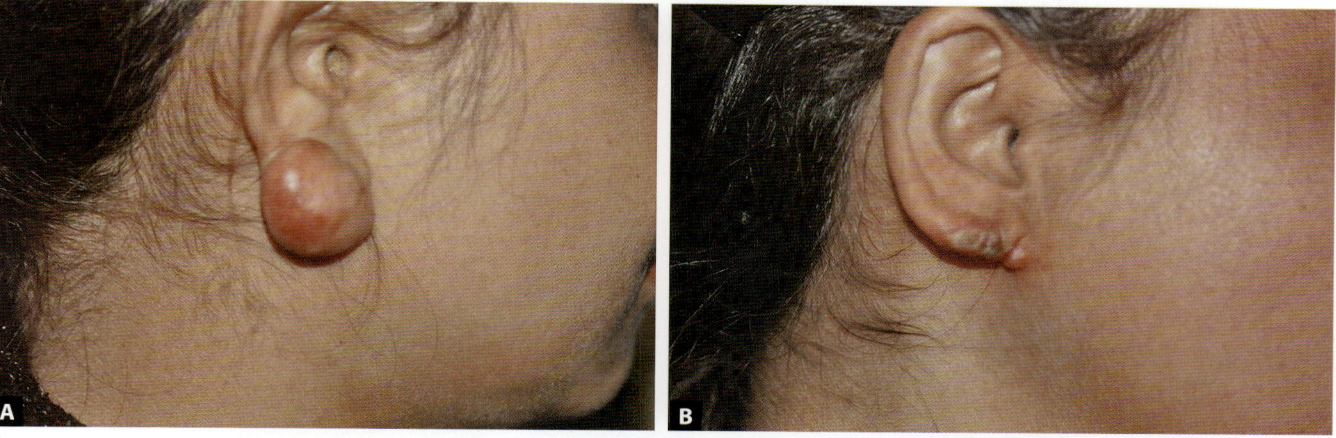

Figs. 1A and B: (A) Earlobe keloid before excision; (B) No recurrence one month later.

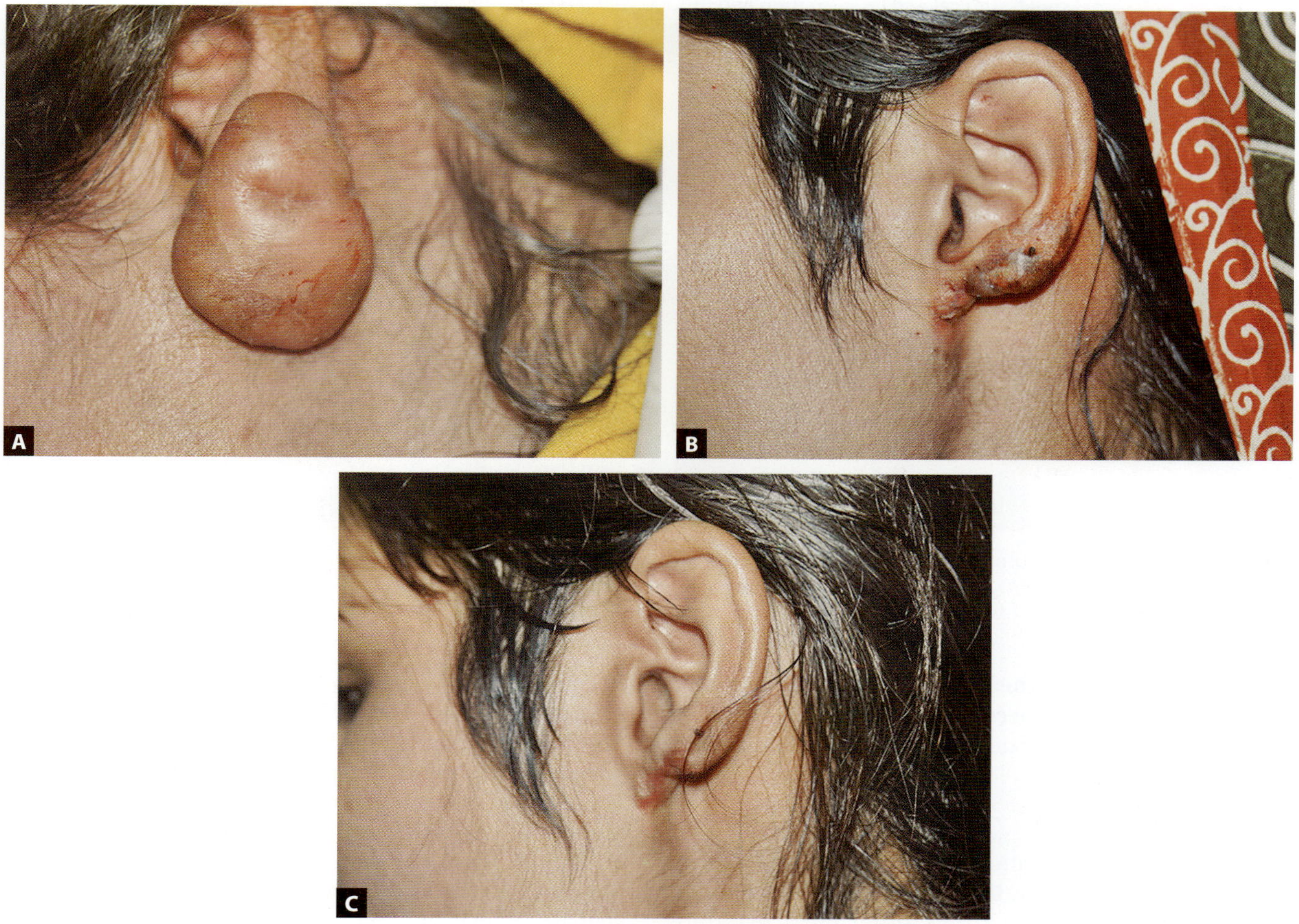

Figs. 2A to C: (A) A large earlobe keloid treated with excision and closure, (B) One week later and (C) One month later.

Box 2: Different treatments available for management of keloids and HS.

- Local treatments: Corticosteroids, retinoic acid, imiquimod, silicone gel
- Intralesional therapies: Corticosteroids, bleomycin, 5-flurouracil, interferon, verapamil
- Surgical therapies: Surgical excisions, radiofrequency debulking, laser debulking
- Physical therapies: Cryotherapy, radiofrequency, lasers (CO_2, pulsed dye lasers), radiation
- Others: Compression therapy, miscellaneous

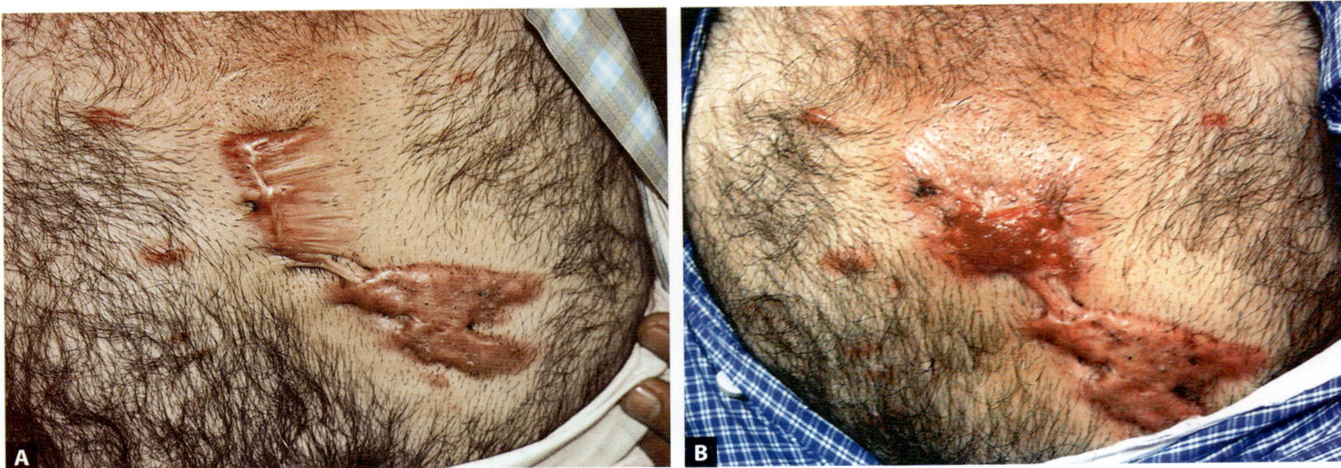

Figs. 3A and B: (A) Presternal keloid treated with different modalities including intralesional steroids, 5-FU, pressure therapy, silicone gel sheet, surgical and laser excision and (B) One year later—the lesion is worse than the baseli.

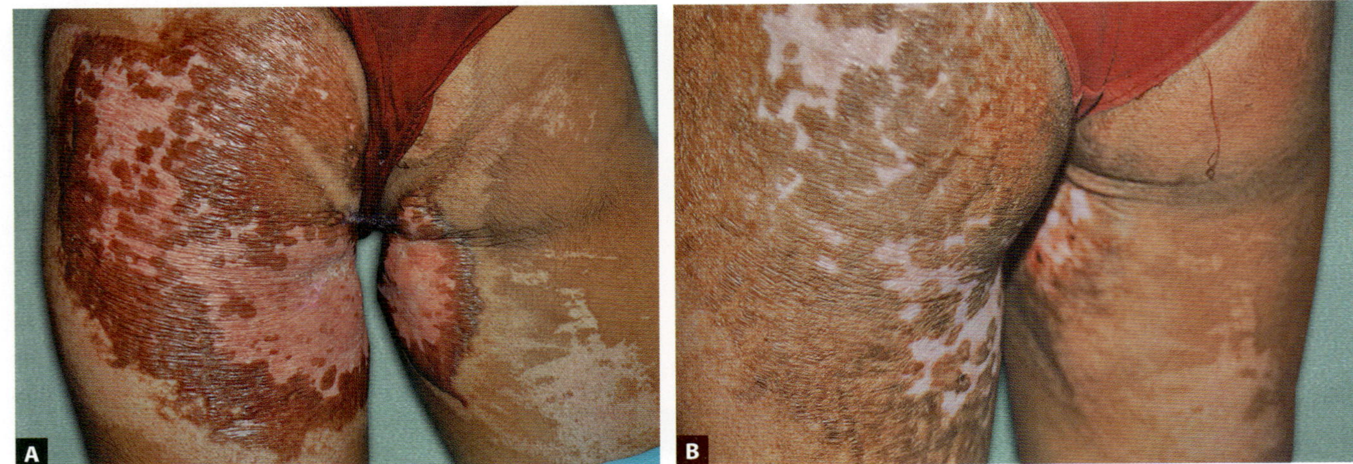

Figs. 4A and B: (A) Post burn keloid and (B) Good improvement in color, texture and thickening with a combination of intralesional steroids, silicone gel sheet and pressure garment.

improvement with treatment; however, the mean amount of improvement to be expected was around 60%. There was no statistically significant difference between treatments.[66]

Corticosteroids

Corticosteroids are the most frequently used treatment modality, most commonly being triamcinolone acetonide. Besides triamcinolone, various other corticosteroids has been used for raised dermal scarring, such as dexamethasone, hydrocortisone acetate, and methyl prednisolone. It is the first line therapy for the treatment of keloids and second line for hypertrophic scars.[8] The concentration of triamcinolone depends upon the amount of scar formation, the body area involved and individual lesion. There is considerable variation among practitioners regarding the protocol for therapy. Mostly, it is given at a dose of 5–10 mg/mL, injected into the upper dermis in hypertrophic scar every 3–6 weeks. In keloids, it can be given at a dose up to 40 mg/mL.[67] It also stimulates fibroblast degeneration.[68] It may also reduce plasma protease inhibitors so that collagenase degrades collagen. There is an increase in production of basic fibroblast growth factor (bFGF) and a decrease in the production of TGF-b1 by human dermal fibroblasts, endogenous vascular endothelial growth factor and insulin-like growth factor-1. There is 50–100% reduction and 9–50% recurrence in keloid.[65] Adverse effects of treatment include: Pain, skin and subcutaneous fat atrophy, telangiectasia, necrosis, ulcerations and hypopigmentation.Cushing's syndrome resulting from intralesional triamcinolone has been reported in the literature. Most recent recommendations does not find adult patients at increased risk for developing Cushing's syndrome although children appear to be at risk for developing Cushing's syndrome.[69] Various measures has been used to reduce the pain due to intralesional injection. A mixture of 2% plain lignocaine and 0.5% bupivacaine in equal volumes injected subcutaneously, either beneath the keloid or around it as a field block leads to painless intralesional injection and prolongs postinjection analgesia.[70] Besides this, lidocaine tape has been found to significantly reduce the pain.[71] Results can be improved when intralesional steroid is combined with other therapies such as surgery, pulsed dye laser (PDL) irradiation, intralesional 5-FU, IFN-α2b,cryotherapy or intralesional bleomycin.[68,72,73] Intralesional steroids can be given by any syringe depending upon the thickness of the lesion. Use of a dental syringe is preferred by many physicians. Many treatments, once/twice a month may be followed to achieve the goals.

Topical steroid creams have been used but dermal absorption is limited. Hyaluronidase may be mixed with the steroids in some cases and given intralesionally in 1:1 ratio. Recently, a study has used triple combination of 5-fluoruracil, triamcinolone acetonide, and hyaluronidase with good tolerability and result.[74] Steroids can be continued for prevention after remission unless side effects appear.

Surgical Excision

Surgical excision is one of the earliest forms of treatment, with the major limitation being very high recurrence rate. Cure rates for surgery alone ranged from 7% to 55%.[75] So, various other complementary modalities, such as intralesional corticosteroids,bleomycin, interferon, radiotherapy or cryotherapy is used to avoid recurrence. Intramarginal excision is advised to prevent additional collagen synthesis.[75] A novel technique of keloid core extirpation was advised without any adjuvant by Lee et al.[76] In this technique, they excised the inner fibrous core from the keloid and covered the defect with a keloid rind flap, which was arterialized by the subcapsular vascular plexus. About 24 keloids of the ear, trunk, face and genitalia were treated. Of these, 20 patients who healed primarily after surgery showed no evidence of keloid recurrence during the follow-up. Scars can also be excised and resurfaced with a skin graft, a flap or normal skin that has been stretched by tissue expander. In hypertrophic scars, besides simple excision, Z-plasty for scars crossing joints or wrinkle creases at right angles, or W-plasty for facial scars can be done, so that the new scar is formed within the relaxed skin tension lines.[77] In general, earlobe keloids are less likely to recur (Figs. 1 and 2).[78] Multimodal therapy in form of intramarginal keloid excision followed by intralesional corticosteroid injections and individually customized pressure splints for management of earlobe keloids have shown good results with less recurrences.[79]

Cryotherapy

Cryotherapy is an easy, cheap and safe mode of treatment. It induces vascular damage that may lead to hypoxia and ultimately tissue necrosis. Repeat sessions of cryotherapy is usually required for beneficial outcome and to prevent recurrences. Thaw cycles of 20 to 30 seconds is used and this should be repeated 1 to 12 times in total, depending on the size of the scar.[8] While many studies have documented the efficacy of contact or spray cryotherapy, the authors' found that the safety and efficacy of intralesional needle cryoprobe seems to be more than the contact or spray cryosurgery.[80,81] A wide bore spinal needle or 18-gauge hypodermic needle is introduced into the lesion parallel to skin surface and the nozzle of cryogen is connected to this needle. Liquid nitrogen runs through the needle to freeze the deeper pathological tissue. When the scar becomes white, irrespective of the duration of the freezing process, the valve of the cryogun is closed and the needle is left to thaw for 2–3 minutes and is then withdrawn. With this, fewer treatment sessions are needed as compared to the contact/spray in which up to 20 sessions are required. The side effects are milder and include pain, local edema, epidermolysis and transient hypopigmentation. Hypopigmentation is common and in dark skinned patients, may be striking and hence patients need to be properly counselled. The re-epithelialization period is short, so the treatment intervals can be shortened to 2–3 weeks. The main advantage of intralesional therapy is that it causes minimal surface destruction and the volume of keloid can be frozen, increasing the success rate with less depigmentation, which makes it a useful technique in dark skinned individuals.[82] In surface cryosurgery, the lethal zone also involves the surface epithelium which is not involved in keloids and deeper pathological tissue in the dermis may be spared. On histomorphometric analysis, the treated scars have more organized and parallel collagen fibers as compared to the pretreated scars. Better results are reported when cryosurgery is combined with intralesional triamcinolone than either of them alone.[68] Cryotherapy induces edema and cellular breakdown causing a decrease in density of fibrous tissue so that injection can be given easily. It may also provide anesthesia before infiltrating steroid. Response to treatment varies in different studies ranging from 32% to 80%.[83,84]

Laser Therapy

Lasers were introduced for hypertrophic scars and keloids in mid-eighties. Argon laser was first to be used, but discontinued due to its poor response rate.[65] Carbon dioxide laser (CO_2) monotherapy also had recurrence rate as high as 90% or more.[85-87] Few authors have found CO_2 laser as effective and well-tolerable modality for managing keloid.[88,89] Recent literature support good efficacy of neodymium: yttrium-aluminium-garnet (Nd: YAG) laser in management of keloids.[90,91] Of all, PDL proved to be most effective in the improvement of scar texture, redness, size, reduction in itching and pain and pliability.[92,93] The PDL wavelengths 585 and 595 nm are most frequently used with pulse duration of 0.45 ms and a fluence of 6.5–7.25 J/cm^2. They are effective not only in the treatment but also in the prevention of hypertrophic scars and early the intervention, better the results.[93,94] Other modalities such as steroids and silicone gel sheeting can be used along with the laser. Two laser combinations are also being tried by some people as combination of the CO_2 laser with erbium: yttrium-aluminium garnet (Er: YAG) laser or PDL.[95-97]

It is based on the principle of selective photothermolysis causing heat and coagulation necrosis. This leads to hypoxia, dissociation of disulfide bonds due to heating and subsequent collagen fiber realignment.[98] There is also a hypothesis that laser causes regression of keloid due to induction of apoptosis and upregulation of extracellular signal regulated kinase and p38 mitogen-activated protein kinase activity. PDL causes decrease in fibroblast proliferation, collagen III deposition, downregulation of TGF-β1 expression and decrease in the number of mast cells.[99,100] Side effects of laser treatment are postoperative purpura, hyperpigmentation or hypopigmentation and blister formation.

Pressure Therapy

Though, it has been popular for treatment and prevention of raised scars for past four decades, exact mechanism by which it works remains unknown, though several theories have been proposed. Various hypotheses include fibroblast degeneration due to localized hypoxia, reduced chondroitin-4-sulfate and decreased activity of MMP-28.[101] Change in glycosaminoglycan levels due to mechanical pressure and capillary permeability during the early phase of wound healing decrease the scar formation time.[101,102] Role for prostaglandin E2 is also postulated.[103,104] Theoretically, pressure will be effective when it is above the arterial capillary closing pressure of 25 mm Hg. Thus, the recommendation is that pressure should be around 20–40 mm Hg, but not above 40 mm Hg, otherwise it will reduce the peripheral blood circulation.[93] The pressure should be applied 24 hours a day for a period of 20–25 weeks.[65] Custom-made garments is preferable as they apply uniform and controlled pressure to the scar only.[105-107] They are the preferred first line treatment for hypertrophic burnt scars in many places as they mature rapidly with less erythema and thickness. Thus, pressure may alleviate itching and pain and may cause early scar maturation, decreasing contractures and avoiding the need for surgical intervention.[102,108] A meta-analysis has found no difference in the results after pressure therapy[109] The pressure loss of the custom-made garments; discomfort from heat and sweating, swelling of limbs, rashes, eczema, excessive friction, blistering, breakdown of scar and the compliance of the patient using the garment are other factors which can discourage the use of pressure therapy.[8,102]

Silicone Material

Silicone is a popular method for prevention and treatment of raised scars. Silicone is available in the forms of gel sheets, gel cushion, liquid, creams, spray, vitamin-supplemented silicone silastic sheets and orthosis garments[8] It is suggested that silicone affects hydration of the skin by decreasing the water vapour transmission rate, which is responsible for decrease in capillary permeability, reduced hyperemia and reduced collagen deposition.[110] Hydration also affects keratinocytes of the lesion to alter growth factor secretion which affects the fibroblasts.[111] A patient who is prone to form hypertrophic scars after surgical excisions should apply the sheets as soon as re-epithelialization is over. It is to be applied daily for at least 12 hours till the results achieved or for a minimum of 2 months. The time is hypothetical as the exact duration of application for the improvement of lesions is not known.[67] The sheet results in flattening of the lesion, increased malleability and softening of the scar.[112-114] The side effects include itching, rash, bad smell from the sheet/gel, fragility of the sheet, skin maceration due to accumulation of water below the sheet, poor compliance of the patient as it has to be used for long duration and for long hours.[115-117] Various combinations of therapies such as pressure therapy with silicone sheets have been applied especially in anatomic areas that do not respond to sheet due to difficulty in maintaining the sheet in position as chin, breast, clavicle, neck, face though complications increase with such combinations.

Radiotherapy

Radiation therapy can be used as monotherapy or as an adjunctive to surgical excision. It is an increasingly popular post-surgical excision therapy of keloids and hypertrophic scars, due to low recurrence rates. The exact mechanism of its effect is still not known. Proposed mechanisms include effect on fibroblasts, including prevention of fibroblast repopulation after excision or modulation of humoral or cellular immunity leading to inhibition of fibroblasts, or by inhibiting angiogenesis.[118] Two type of modality has been used, i.e. external beam therapy, or brachytherapy. Shen et al. in their retrospective study on 834 keloids that were treated with electron beam therapy over a 14-year period found a recurrence rate of 9.59%. Time to recurrence ranged from 6 to 28 months, and adverse effects were seen in 9.83% of subjects, most commonly with dyspigmentation.[118] Van Leeuwen and colleagues conducted a systematic review including 33 studies using radiation therapy, as adjuvant treatment for post-excision keloids. They found lowest recurrence rates with high dose radiation brachytherapy (10.5%) as compared with low dose radiation brachytherapy (21.3%) and external beam radiation (22.2%). Also, lower recurrence rates were found with shorter time interval (<7 hours) between excision and radiation, as compared with longer time intervals (>24 hours). It has been found that presternal keloids show higher recurrence rates with low irradiation dose in comparison to higher radiation dose.[118] External beam radiation reaches the border of the papillary layer and the reticular dermis, where the keloid is generated whereas the soft X-rays cannot reach to that level.[119] Postoperative radiation therapy has been found to be more effective than intralesional corticosteroid in a randomized study of ear lobe keloid.[120] The dosage according to Ogawa et al. is 20 Gy in 4 fractions over 4 days on anterior chest wall, scapular region, and suprapubic region and 10 Gy in 2 fractions over 2 days on earlobes, 15 Gy in 3 fractions over 3 days on other sites.[121] Hyperpigmentation, hypopigmentation, transient erythema are some of the side effects after irradiation. Risk of causation of malignant tumor by irradiation is an exaggeration; only few patients have reported to have developed the malignancy in several large series.[122] It is contraindicated in children and areas of breast and thyroid which are prone to malignancies.[47,118]

5-Fluorouracil

5-fluorouracil (5-FU) is a fluorinated pyrimidine, an antimetabolite, which inhibits thymidylate synthase and interferes with RNA synthesis and function. It is used in malignancies as it affects rapidly proliferating cells. In keloids, it blocks collagen synthesis and has shown in tissue culture to inhibit fibroblast proliferation. It also has an inhibitory effect on TGF-β induced type I collagen gene expression in human fibroblasts.[123] Fibroblast regression depends on the duration of exposure to the drug and the dose given. It is usually given in the dose of 50 mg/mL. 5-FU given intralesionally once in a week or once in every 2 weeks is effective.[73] Symptomatic and inflamed lesions tend to respond most while the older, non-inflamed, asymptomatic scars respond less.[73]

On an average, 5–10 injection sessions are required to achieve complete flattening of the lesions. A retrospective study found that 5-FU/steroid combination with excision had a 92% average reduction in lesion size compared with 73% in the group of patients who did not receive 5-FU and patients who received 5-FU/steroid without excision had an average lesion size reduction of 81%. Thus, it was concluded that combination of 5-FU/triamcinolone is superior to intralesional steroid therapy alone.[124] Similar result was seen by another group from Iran.[125] The risk associated with the 5-FU were pain, urticaria, skin breakdown, purpura, localized hair loss, pigment changes, systemic absorption.[126]

Bleomycin

It was originally isolated from fungus, *Streptomyces verticillus* and has antitumor, antibacterial and antiviral activity. It causes necrosis of keratinocytes. Mainly, it inhibits DNA synthesis but can inhibit RNA and protein synthesis. It is known to induce apoptosis also.[73] The activity/concentration of enzyme TGF-β lysyl oxidase is increased in keloid and hypertrophic scars which is noticed to decrease after bleomycin injections.[73] It is administered either by intradermal injections or multiple punctures are made in the form of 40 punctures per 1 cm^2 with the help of 22 G needle or 0.1 mL (1.5 IU/mL) at a maximum dose of 6 mL is used.[127-130] In one study, there were four therapeutic sessions at 1-month intervals.[131] In another study, three applications were given at 15 days interval.[128] In short, the therapy can have 2–6 sessions for complete flattening of scars.[130] It is seen that the response of bleomycin is better if the lesion is more than 100 mm^2.[132] Bleomycin is easy to administer, high regression rate with less complications and low recurrence rate.[128] Caution is required in pregnant women and children. Complications can be hyperpigmentation, pain, ulceration, Raynaud's phenomenon, gangrene, fibrosis, neutrophilic eccrine hidradenitis, alopecia, edema and nail changes but cutaneous toxicity occurs only when the dose is 200–300 units or above. It should not be combined with radiotherapy as both emit free radicals.[127]

Imiquimod

It is therapeutically safe and effective in the treatment of keloid.[133] It inhibits the collagen production by interferon (IFN) release (IFN-α and IFN-γ) and alters expression of an apoptotic gene which is important for the progression of the disease.[73] It can be applied every night for 5 days a week, with 2 days off and can be continued for a total of 8 weeks. Common side effects are itching, burning, pain, blister/ulceration, localized hyperpigmentation and flu-like symptoms—fever, headache, nausea, fatigue, muscle pain, bone pain. The authors'found that after excision, suppression of keloids with imiquimod is only temporary and the disease recur after discontinuation of imiquimod.[134] Similarly, a prospective, double blind, placebo-controlled did not find any significant reduction in recurrence rates when using imiquimod versus placebo after keloid excision.[135]

Chandawarkar et al. carried out treatment of recurrent keloid in three steps:

- First step was excision of keloid, application of dermal replacement materials and immobilization and dressing with a vacuum-assisted wound dressing.
- Second step was application of autologous split thickness skin graft and
- Third step was the local application of 5% imiquimod cream for 8 weeks. The patient was asymptomatic after 15 months of surgery.[136]

Although this is an interesting therapeutic approach, it is of a low-level evidence since it is based on one case report.

Radiofrequency Device

By the use of ThermaCool® radiofrequency device, the changes in collagen fibril morphology and production changes were seen, but did not show any clinical improvement in hypertrophic scars and keloid.[137] It has been found to be very effective modality with good cosmetic outcome in ear keloids with less recurrence.[138,139]

Verapamil

It is a calcium channel antagonist used as an antiarrhythmic drug. In a study, it has shown to stimulate the synthesis of procollagenase increasing collagenase activity leading to reduction in fibrous tissue production.[118] Verapamil blocks the synthesis and secretion of ECM molecules and increase fibrinase.[140] It also reduces the basal IL-6 and vascular endothelial growth factor production in the keloidal fibroblasts culture leading to inhibition of cell growth and proliferation by 29%.[141] It has been tried in combination with other modalities such as surgical excision alone or with W-plasty or skin grafting, pressure therapy and topical silicone.[142-144] Wang et al. conducted a meta-analysis and found efficacy of intralesional verapamil similar to conventional corticosteroid injections with fewer side effects.[145]

Onion Extract and Heparin

The topical preparation (Contractubex®) containing onion extract, heparin and allantoin are being used for many years to treat wounds and keloid. The exact mechanism of onion extract is unclear. In vitro studies has shown a dose-dependent inhibitory effect on fibroblasts proliferation. Besides this, it has been found to inhibit histamine and upregulate the expression of matrix metalloproteinase-1.[146] Overall, it works by reducing inflammation and fibroblast proliferation. In an open randomized study comparing intralesional TAC and onion extract gel with intralesional triamcinolone alone, TAC with onion extract was more effective in terms of pain sensitiveness, itching and elevation but not in erythema and in duration. The gel was given 3 times daily for 3 months and intralesional triamcinolone every 4 weeks for a total of 4 treatments. All patients were treated for 3 months, and followed up to 2 months.[147] There are contradictory reports in other studies. Combination of onion extract and petrolatum-based ointments found no improvement in scar, but onion extract and silicone sheet gel was found to be more effective.[148] Presently, there is no conclusive evidence of its efficacy in keloids.[146]

Botulinum Toxin

Various studies have assessed effect of botulinum toxin type A (BTA) on scar. Reduction in tensile force leading to decreased cell proliferation and collagen deposition when BTA injected adjacent to the primary wound margins has been hypothesized as mechanism of action.[149] Elhefnawy in his prospective study have assessed effect of intralesional botulinum toxin type A in 20 patients with hypertrophic scars. It was given once a month for 3 months with a follow-up period of 6 month. Author has noticed significant improvement in all three parameters assessed, i.e. erythema, itching and pliability.[150] Similarly, a randomized controlled trial has documented efficacy of BTA almost similar to intralesional steroid.[151] However, further randomized trials are still required to fully establish the efficacy.

EMERGING DRUGS FOR SCAR REDUCTION

GROWTH FACTORS AND CYTOKINES

Basic Fibroblast Growth Factor

Delayed wound healing is a known risk factor for keloid formation and acceleration of wound healing should improve scarring. Basic fibroblast growth factor (bFGF) has been proven clinically to accelerate acute and chronic wound healing in pediatric burn scars. It activates the local macrophages up to the remodelling phase which occurs after several weeks of injury. There was a higher rate of developing hypertrophic scars in those who received conventional treatment than those who received bFGF which was evaluated by pigmentation, pliability, height and vascularity of the lesion.[152]

Transforming Growth Factor-beta-3

Transforming Growth Factor-beta-3 (TGF-β3) is antifibrotic and its administration may lead to the reduction in scars.[153-155] Mannose-6-phosphate inhibits the associated peptide, preventing the activation of TGF-β1 and 2, thus reducing scarring in both animal and human wounds. The efficacy can be increased by adding TGF-β3 isoform. Role of avotermin (recombinant, active human TGF-β3) as potential therapy for accelerating wound healing and improving scar appearance is well-documented in many studies.[156,157]

Interferon

Interferon alpha, beta and gamma have shown to increase the collagen breakdown and interfere with collagen synthesis and cross-linking. The TGF-β is also antagonized by systemic interferon therapy.[158] Intralesional interferon alpha-2b (IFN) α-2b in dose of 1.5 million IU, given twice over 4 days, reduced keloid to half its size by day 9.[159] The disadvantages include decreased wound strength, delayed re-epithelialization and the pain associated. Studies have shown significant benefits over TAC and low recurrence rate of 19% as compared to 51% with steroid in postoperative cases.[160] Lee et al. have assessed efficacy of intralesional IFNα-2b given along with intralesional triamcinolone acetonide in the treatment of keloid. They found significant decrease in depth and volume of keloids with combination therapy of intralesional IFNα-2b and triamcinolone acetonide when compared with intralesional triamcinolone acetonide alone.[161]

Interleukin-10

It has anti-inflammatory properties and decreases the levels of IL-6 and IL-8 which are thought to rise rapidly in wounds and have role in adult scar formation.[162]

Extracellular Matrix Modulators

- **Prolyl 4-hydroxylase inhibitors**: Prolyl 4-hydroxylase is an enzyme required for the formation of procollagen bundles. Its inhibition by agents like FG-1648 (a topically active phenanthroline derivative), doxorubicin (commonly used chemotherapeutic agent) and mimosine (an analogue of catechol) can reduce collagen synthesis.[163-165]
- **Cis-hydroxyproline**: It can be given in a microsphere form with a magnetic field directed to the target tissue. It resulted in a 16% decrease in a collagen content in an animal model.
- **Tissue transglutaminase inhibitors**: Tissue transglutaminase (TTG) has role in cross-linking of Type III procollagen in hypertrophic scars and keloids.
- **Putrescine inhibits TTG**: In phase II clinical trials, it showed significant improvement in hypertrophic scars with minimal side effects.[166]

OTHER PRODUCTS AND THERAPIES

Topical Tamoxifen

It is a nonsteroidal antiestrogenic drug used in breast cancer. It decreases the expression of TGF-β which causes the proliferation of fibroblast and collagen production.[73]

Tranilast

The mechanism by which it inhibits the collagen is not known but in the dosage of 3–300 μM, it inhibits the collagen synthesis of fibroblasts and TGF-β1 in keloid. It is an antiallergic medicine which inhibits the release of histamine and prostaglandins from mast cells.[167]

Prostaglandin

Prostaglandin decreases keloid fibroblast migration and contraction through EP2/EP4—cAMP mechanism.[168]

Tacrolimus and Rapamycin

Tacrolimus is a potent immunosuppressive medication that act on FKBP12 receptor. It suppresses production of IL-2 by inhibiting calcineurin. An open-label pilot study noticed decrease in erythema, induration, tenderness, and pruritus in most of the patients with keloid using tacrolimus 0.1% ointment twice daily for 12 weeks.[169] At molecular level, rapamycin has been found to be dose- and time-dependent downregulating the expression of cytoplasmic PCNA, cyclin D1, fibronectin, collagen and alpha-SMA, leading to anti-proliferative effect on fibroblast.[170]

Pentoxifylline

In a study by Berman and Duncan, pentoxyiflline was found to inhibit the fibroblasts and collagen, glycosaminoglycans and fibronectin activity but had no effect on collagenase activity in the skin of patients with keloid, scleroderma and morphea.[171]

Retinoic Acid

Tretinoin may improve chronic inflammation and prevent expansion of keloid tissues into the normal skin. They are potent inhibitors of Matrix metalloproteinases (MMP's) and the study showed that significant upregulation if MMP-13 and significant downregulation of MMP-1 and MMP-8 in keloid derived fibroblasts at both mRNA and protein levels.[172] Retinoid (0.05% tretinoin) was applied locally on 11patients of keloid for 12 weeks. About 2 patients developed contact dermatitis. At the end of the study, significant decrease in weight and size was found.[173] Kwon et al. in their study noticed similar efficacy of tretinoin to that of silicone gel in preventing development of hypertrophic scars and keloids and also improving appearance of scar after surgery.[174]

Collagenase

Intralesional injection of collagenase based on the principle of enzymic digestion resulted in temporary reduction in scar volume, returning to the same (or greater) levels after 6 months of follow-up. Side effects were numerous and severe including pain, swelling, blistering, ulceration and ecchymosis at the site of injection.[175] Bae-Harboe et al. have found intralesional collagenase followed by compression as a safe and effective treatment for earlobe keloids.[176]

Collagenase D (derived from the larvae Dermestes frischii) was found to be more effective as compared to other types of collagenase such as *Clostridium histolyticum* collagenase and Collagensase PC from paralithodes camtschatica(red king crab).[177]

Hyaluronic Acid

Hyaluronic acid can normalize hyperproliferation, growth factor production and extracellular matrix deposition in keloid.[178] When used in high concentration, it has shown good results in reduction of scar thickness.[179]

The list of treatment modalities tried is extensive and includes adhesive tape support, massage therapy,

Flowchart 1: Management algorithm for small keloids.

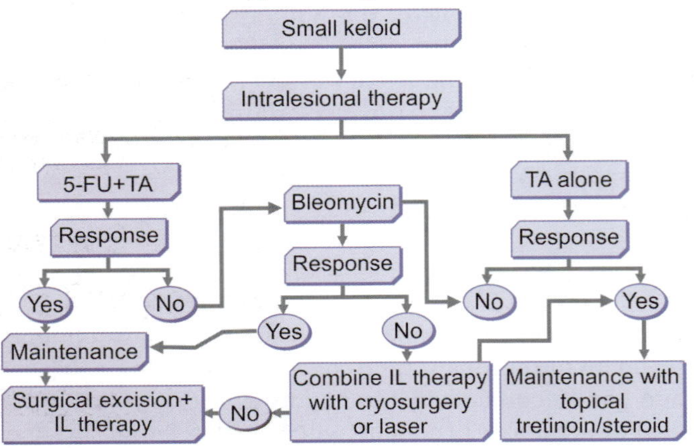

Flowchart 2: Management algorithm for large, bulky keloids.

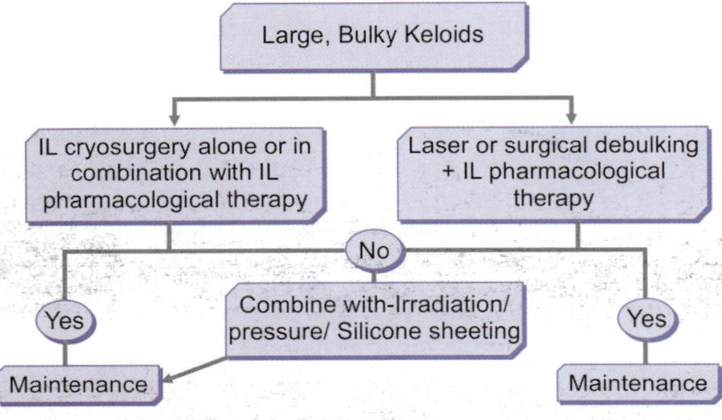

Flowchart 3: Management algorithm for extensive keloids.

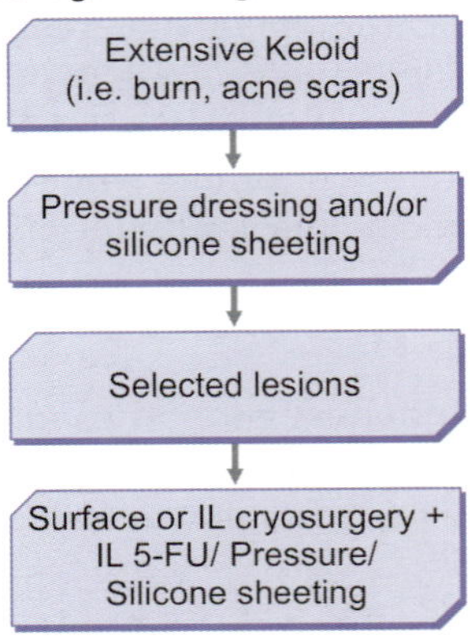

Flowchart 4: Management algorithm for earlobe keloids.

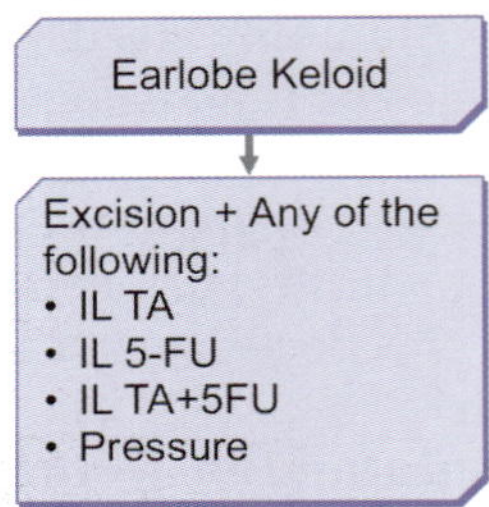

topical vitamin E, topical cyanoacrylates, allantoin-sulfomucopolysaccharide gel, glycosaminoglycan gel, moist exposed burn ointment, extracts from plants (made cassol from *Centella asiatica*, alpha centella cream from *Bulbine frutescens*, leucyanidin and ellagic from *Anogeissus latifolia*, extract of *Butea monosperma* bark), which may improve the wound epithelialization and increase wound tensile strength. Topical tocoretinate was reported to improve skin stiffness and glossy appearance of hypertropic scars.[68]

Catechins (Epicatechin gallate) resulted in improvement in quality of scar formation in a rat incisional wound model. Dermatography can be done in flat or slightly elevated scars, which includes microsurgical needle tattooing. This procedure can provide camouflage pigmentation along with the benefit of inducing atrophy of scars due to the cutting action of the needles.[68]

Flowcharts 1 to 4 depict suggested guidelines for management of keloids; however, it is important to note that management of keloids has to be individualized.

PREVENTION

As is evident from the long list of treatment modalities, it is difficult to treat keloids. Also the long duration of therapy, recurrence and psychosocial aspect add to the cost of treatment. Thus, prevention is the optimal approach. Patients with a family history of keloids should consider not having ear piercings. If piercing is mandatory, it should be done in early childhood. Principles of prevention in keloid on the head and neck include: Withholding nonessential cosmetic surgery, closing all wounds with minimal tension (i.e. making incisions along Langer's lines) and the use of pressure garments for 4–6 months after injury. We should always aim for primary closure of wounds. Adequate debridement of contaminated wounds, good hemostasis, gentle handling of tissues and limiting foreign bodies are other precautions to be taken. Adequate nutrition should be provided, so normal tissue substrates can be synthesized efficiently.[176] Foremost is the avoidance of all unnecessary procedures. The best way to deal with a keloid is not to get one. A person who has had keloid should not undergo elective skin surgeries or procedures such as piercing. When it comes to keloids, prevention is crucial because current treatments are often not completely successful and may not work at all.

REFERENCES

1. Bayat A, McGrouther DA, Ferguson MWJ. Skin scarring. BMJ. 2003;326(7380):88-92.
2. Davidson S, Aziz N, Rashid RM, Khachemoune A. A primary care perspective on keloids. Medscape J Med. 2009;11(1):18.

3. Wittenberg GP, Fabian BG, Bogomilsky JL, et al. Prospective, single-blind, randomized, controlled study to assess the efficacy of the 585-nm flashlamp-pumped pulsed-dye laser and silicone gel sheeting in hypertrophic scar treatment. Arch Dermatol. 1999;135(9):1049-55.
4. Yang Y-C, Cheng Y-W, Lai C-S, Chen W. Prevalence of childhood acne, ephelides, warts, atopic dermatitis, psoriasis, alopecia areata and keloid in Kaohsiung County, Taiwan: a community-based clinical survey. JEADV. 2007;21(5):643-9.
5. Kelly AP. Medical and surgical therapies for keloids. Dermatol Ther. 2004;17(2):212-8.
6. Bayat A, Arscott G, Ollier WER, et al. Keloid disease: clinical relevance of single versus multiple site scars. Br J Plast Surg. 2005;58(1):28-37.
7. Marneros AG, Norris JE, Olsen BR, Reichenberger E. Clinical genetics of familial keloids. Arch Dermatol. 2001; 137(11):1429-34.
8. Ud-Din S, Bayat A. New insights on keloids, hypertrophic scars, and striae. Dermatol Clin. 2014;32(2):193-209.
9. Seifert O, Bayat A, Geffers R, et al. Identification of unique gene expression patterns within different lesional sites of keloids. Wound Repair Regen. 2008;16(2):254-65.
10. Kelly AP. Keloids. Dermatol Clin. 1988;6(3):413-24.
11. Textbook of Cosmetic Dermatology, 3rd edition, by Maibach [Internet]. [cited 2016 Dec 12]. Available from: http://chipsbooks.com/txtcosm3.htm
12. Lu W-S, Wang J-F, Yang S, et al. Association of HLA-DQA1 and DQB1 alleles with keloids in Chinese Hans. J Dermatol Sci. 2008;52(2):108-17.
13. Brown JJ, Ollier WER, Thomson W, Bayat A. Positive association of HLA-DRB1*15 with keloid disease in Caucasians. Int J Immunogenet. 2008;35(4-5):303-7.
14. Halim AS, Emami A, Salahshourifar I, Kannan TP. Keloid scarring: Understanding the genetic basis, advances, and prospects. Arch Plast Surg. 2012;39(3):184-9.
15. Ghatnatti V, Sarma D, Saikia U. Enlarged hands and feet - Not always acromegaly. Indian J Endocrinol Metab. 2012;16(Suppl 2):S318-20.
16. Fong EP, Chye LT, Tan WT. Keloids: time to dispel the myths? Plast Reconstr Surg. 1999;104(4):1199-202.
17. Fong EP, Bay BH. Keloids - the sebum hypothesis revisited. Med Hypotheses. 2002;58(4):264-9.
18. Coop CA, Schaefer SM, England RW. Extensive keloid formation and progression after each vaccination. Hum Vaccin. 2007;3(4):127-9.
19. Kischer CW, Shetlar MR, Chvapil M. Hypertrophic scars and keloids: a review and new concept concerning their origin. Scan Electron Microsc. 1981;(Pt 4):1699-713.
20. Cw K. The microvessels in hypertrophic scars, keloids and related lesions: a review. J Submicrosc Cytol Pathol. 1992;24(2):281-96.
21. Ma X, Chen J, Xu B, et al. Keloid-derived keratinocytes acquire a fibroblast-like appearance and an enhanced invasive capacity in a hypoxic microenvironment in vitro. Int J Mol Med. 2015;35(5):1246-56.
22. Akaishi S, Akimoto M, Ogawa R, Hyakusoku H. The relationship between keloid growth pattern and stretching tension: visual analysis using the finite element method. Ann Plast Surg. 2008;60(4):445-51.
23. Viera MH, Amini S, Konda S, Berman B. Do postsurgical interventions optimize ultimate scar cosmesis. G Ital Dermatol E Venereol Organo Uff Soc Ital Dermatol E Sifilogr. 2009;144(3):243-57.
24. Park TH, Chang CH. Keloid recurrence in pregnancy. Aesthetic Plast Surg. 2012;36(5):1271-2.
25. Kim H-D, Hwang S-M, Lim K-R, et al. Recurrent auricular keloids during pregnancy. Arch Plast Surg. 2013;40(1):70-2.
26. Schierle HP, Scholz D, Lemperle G. Elevated levels of testosterone receptors in keloid tissue: an experimental investigation. Plast Reconstr Surg. 1997;100(2):390-5; discussion 396.
27. Louw L. Keloids in rural black South Africans. Part 1: general overview and essential fatty acid hypotheses for keloid formation and prevention. Prostaglandins Leukot Essent Fatty Acids. 2000;63(5):237-45.
28. Louw L, Dannhauser A. Keloids in rural black South Africans. Part 2: dietary fatty acid intake and total phospholipid fatty acid profile in the blood of keloid patients. Prostaglandins Leukot Essent Fatty Acids. 2000;63(5):247-53.
29. Louw L. Keloids in rural black South Africans. Part 3: a lipid model for the prevention and treatment of keloid formations. Prostaglandins Leukot Essent Fatty Acids. 2000;63(5):255-62.
30. Ramos MLC, Gragnani A, Ferreira LM. Is there an ideal animal model to study hypertrophic scarring? J Burn Care Res Off Publ Am Burn Assoc. 2008;29(2):363-8.
31. Robles DT, Moore E, Draznin M, Berg D. Keloids: pathophysiology and management. Dermatol Online J. 2007;13(3):9.
32. Wolfram D, Tzankov A, Pülzl P, Piza-Katzer H. Hypertrophic scars and keloids: a review of their pathophysiology, risk factors, and therapeutic management. Dermatol Surg. 2009;35(2):171-81.
33. Marneros AG, Krieg T. Keloids-clinical diagnosis, pathogenesis, and treatment options. J Dtsch Dermatol Ges J. 2004;2(11):905-13.
34. Khoo YT, Ong CT, Mukhopadhyay A, et al. Upregulation of secretory connective tissue growth factor (CTGF) in keratinocyte-fibroblast coculture contributes to keloid pathogenesis. J Cell Physiol. 2006;208(2):336-43.
35. Whitby DJ, Ferguson MW. Immunohistochemical localization of growth factors in fetal wound healing. Dev Biol. 1991;147(1):207-15.
36. Haisa M, Okochi H, Grotendorst GR. Elevated levels of PDGF alpha receptors in keloid fibroblasts contribute to an enhanced response to PDGF. J Invest Dermatol. 1994;103(4):560-3.
37. Chin GS, Liu W, Peled Z, et al. Differential expression of transforming growth factor-beta receptors I and II and activation of Smad 3 in keloid fibroblasts. Plast Reconstr Surg. 2001;108(2):423-9.
38. Sayah DN, Soo C, Shaw WW, et al. Downregulation of apoptosis-related genes in keloid tissues. J Surg Res. 1999;87(2):209-16.
39. Bayat A, Bock O, Mrowietz U, et al. Genetic susceptibility to keloid disease and hypertrophic scarring: transforming growth factor beta1 common polymorphisms and plasma levels. Plast Reconstr Surg. 2003;111(2):535-543; discussin 544-6.
40. Bayat A, Bock O, Mrowietz U, et al. Genetic susceptibility to keloid disease: transforming growth factor beta receptor gene polymorphisms are not associated with keloid disease. Exp Dermatol. 2004;13(2):120-4.
41. Bayat A, Bock O, Mrowietz U, et al. Genetic susceptibility to keloid disease and transforming growth factor beta 2 polymorphisms. Br J Plast Surg. 2002;55(4):283-6.

42. Bayat A, Walter JM, Bock O, et al. Genetic susceptibility to keloid disease: mutation screening of the TGF beta3 gene. Br J Plast Surg. 2005;58(7):914-21.
43. Zhuo Y, Gao J, Luo S, et al. p53 gene codon 72 polymorphism and susceptibility to keloid in Chinese population. Zhongguo Xiu Fu Chong Jian Wai Ke Za Zhi. 2005;19(1):28-30.
44. Shaheen A, Khaddam J, Kesh F. Risk factors of keloids in Syrians. BMC Dermatol. 2016;16(1):13.
45. Tirgan MH, Tirgan MH. Neck keloids: evaluation of risk factors and recommendation for keloid staging system. F1000Research [Internet]. 2016 Aug 19 [cited 2016 Dec 20];5. Available from: /articles/5-1528/v2.
46. Köse O, Waseem A. Keloids and hypertrophic scars: are they two different sides of the same coin? Dermatol Surg. 2008;34(3):336-46.
47. Gauglitz GG, Korting HC, Pavicic T, et al. Hypertrophic scarring and keloids: pathomechanisms and current and emerging treatment strategies. Mol Med Camb Mass. 2011;17(1-2):113-25.
48. Koley S, Saoji V, Salodkar A. Unusual formation of keloids after each episode of recurrent herpes zoster in an HIV positive patient. Indian J Sex Transm Dis. 2009;30(2):109-11.
49. Xie L-H, Li S-K, Li Q. Combined treatment of penile keloid: a troublesome complication after circumcision. Asian J Androl. 2013;15(4):575-6.
50. Shrotriya R, Thorat T, Puri V, Kulkarni S. Labial keloid: rare presentation of a common malady. Indian J Burns. 2015;23(1):92.
51. Chawla B, Agarwal A, Kashyap S, Tandon R. Diagnosis and management of corneal keloid. Clin Experiment Ophthalmol. 2007;35(9):855-7.
52. Jung JJ, Wojno TH, Grossniklaus HE. Giant corneal keloid: case report and review of the literature. Cornea. 2010;29(12):1455-8.
53. Park TH, Seo SW, Kim JK, Chang CH. Earlobe keloids: classification according to gross morphology determines proper surgical approach. Dermatol Surg. 2012;38(3): 406-12.
54. Bayat A, Arscott G, Ollier WER, et al. Description of site-specific morphology of keloid phenotypes in an Afrocaribbean population. Br J Plast Surg. 2004;57(2):122-33.
55. Lee S-S, Yosipovitch G, Chan Y-H, Goh C-L. Pruritus, pain, and small nerve fiber function in keloids: a controlled study. J Am Acad Dermatol. 2004;51(6):1002-6.
56. Goder M, Kornhaber R, Bordoni D, et al. Cutaneous basal cell carcinoma arising within a keloid scar: a case report. Onco Targets Ther. 2016;9:4793-6.
57. Bock O, Schmid-Ott G, Malewski P, Mrowietz U. Quality of life of patients with keloid and hypertrophic scarring. Arch Dermatol Res. 2006;297(10):433-8.
58. Olaitan PB. Keloids: assessment of effects and psychosocial-impacts on subjects in a black African population. Indian J Dermatol Venereol Leprol. 2009;75(4):368-72.
59. Gulamhuseinwala N, Mackey S, Meagher P, Powell B. Should excised keloid scars be sent for routine histologic analysis? Ann Plast Surg. 2008;60(2):186-7.
60. Ogawa R, Akaishi S, Hyakusoku H. Differential and exclusive diagnosis of diseases that resemble keloids and hypertrophic scars. Ann Plast Surg. 2009;62(6):660-4.
61. Jumper N, Paus R, Bayat A. Functional histopathology of keloid disease. Histol Histopathol. 2015;30(9):1033-57.
62. Lee JY-Y, Yang C-C, Chao S-C, Wong T-W. Histopathological differential diagnosis of keloid and hypertrophic scar. Am J Dermatopathol. 2004;26(5):379-84.
63. Linares HA, Kischer CW, Dobrkovsky M, Larson DL. The histiotypic organization of the hypertrophic scar in humans. J Invest Dermatol. 1972;59(4):323-31.
64. Chuangsuwanich A, Gunjittisomram S. The efficacy of 5% imiquimod cream in the prevention of recurrence of excised keloids. J Med Assoc Thail. 2007;90(7):1363-7.
65. Mustoe TA, Cooter RD, Gold MH, et al. International clinical recommendations on scar management. Plast Reconstr Surg. 2002;110(2):560-71.
66. Leventhal D, Furr M, Reiter D. Treatment of keloids and hypertrophic scars: a meta-analysis and review of the literature. Arch Facial Plast Surg. 2006;8(6):362-8.
67. Brissett AE, Sherris DA. Scar contractures, hypertrophic scars, and keloids. Facial Plast Surg FPS. 2001;17(4):263-72.
68. Atiyeh BS. Nonsurgical management of hypertrophic scars: evidence-based therapies, standard practices, and emerging methods. Aesthetic Plast Surg. 2007;31(5):468-92; discussion 493-4.
69. Fredman R, Tenenhaus M. Cushing's syndrome after intralesional triamcinolone acetonide: a systematic review of the literature and multinational survey. Burns J Int Soc Burn Inj. 2013;39(4):549-57.
70. Mishra S. Safe and less painful injection of triamcenolone acetonide into a keloid--a technique. J Plast Reconstr Aesthetic Surg. 2010;63(2):e205.
71. Tosa M, Murakami M, Hyakusoku H. Effect of lidocaine tape on pain during intralesional injection of triamcinolone acetonide for the treatment of keloid. J Nippon Med Sch. 2009;76(1):9-12.
72. Camacho-Martínez FM, Rey ER, Serrano FC, Wagner A. Results of a combination of bleomycin and triamcinolone acetonide in the treatment of keloids and hypertrophic scars. An Bras Dermatol. 2013;88(3):387-94.
73. Jones CD, Guiot L, Samy M, et al. The Use of chemotherapeutics for the treatment of keloid scars. Dermatol Rep [Internet]. 2015 May 21 [cited 2017 Jan 13];7(2). Available from: http://www.ncbi.nlm.nih.gov/pmc/articles/PMC4500869/
74. Goyal NN, Gold MH. A novel triple medicine combination injection for the resolution of keloids and hypertrophic scars. J Clin Aesthetic Dermatol. 2014;7(11):31-4.
75. Engrav LH, Gottlieb JR, Millard SP, et al. A comparison of intramarginal and extramarginal excision of hypertrophic burn scars. Plast Reconstr Surg. 1988;81(1):40-5.
76. Lee Y, Minn KW, Baek RM, Hong JJ. A new surgical treatment of keloid: keloid core excision. Ann Plast Surg. 2001;46(2):135-40.
77. Arno AI, Gauglitz GG, Barret JP, Jeschke MG. Up-to-date approach to manage keloids and hypertrophic scars: a useful guide. Burns J Int Soc Burn Inj. 2014;40(7):1255-66.
78. Mutalik S. Treatment of keloids and hypertrophic scars. Indian J Dermatol Venereol Leprol. 2005;71(1):3-8.
79. Walliczek U, Engel S, Weiss C, et al. Clinical outcome and quality of life after a multimodal therapy approach to ear keloids. JAMA Facial Plast Surg. 2015;17(5):333-9.
80. Gupta S, Kumar B. Intralesional cryosurgery using lumbar puncture and/or hypodermic needles for large, bulky, recalcitrant keloids. Int J Dermatol. 2001;40(5): 349-53.

81. Har-Shai Y, Dujovny E, Rohde E, Zouboulis CC. Effect of skin surface temperature on skin pigmentation during contact and intralesional cryosurgery of keloids. J Eur Acad Dermatol Venereol. 2007;21(2):191-8.
82. Har-Shai Y, Amar M, Sabo E. Intralesional cryotherapy for enhancing the involution of hypertrophic scars and keloids. Plast Reconstr Surg. 2003;111(6):1841-52.
83. Zouboulis CC, Blume U, Büttner P, Orfanos CE. Outcomes of cryosurgery in keloids and hypertrophic scars. A prospective consecutive trial of case series. Arch Dermatol. 1993;129(9):1146-51.
84. Rusciani L, Paradisi A, Alfano C, et al. Cryotherapy in the treatment of keloids. J Drugs Dermatol. 2006;5(7):591-5.
85. Apfelberg DB, Maser MR, White DN, Lash H. Failure of carbon dioxide laser excision of keloids. Lasers Surg Med. 1989;9(4):382-8.
86. Norris JE. The effect of carbon dioxide laser surgery on the recurrence of keloids. Plast Reconstr Surg. 1991;87(1): 44-49; discussion 50-3.
87. Ang CC, Tay YK, Kwok C. Retrospective analysis of earlobe keloids treated with the carbon dioxide laser ablation or cold steel debulking surgery. J Cosmet Laser. 2013;15(5):271-3.
88. Nicoletti G, De Francesco F, Mele CM, et al. Clinical and histologic effects from CO2 laser treatment of keloids. Lasers Med Sci. 2013;28(3):957-64.
89. Scrimali L, Lomeo G, Nolfo C, et al. Treatment of hypertrophic scars and keloids with a fractional CO_2 laser: a personal experience. J Cosmet Laser Ther. 2010;12(5):218-21.
90. Al-Mohamady AE-SAE-H, Ibrahim SMA, Muhammad MM. Pulsed dye laser versus long-pulsed Nd:YAG laser in the treatment of hypertrophic scars and keloid: A comparative randomized split-scar trial. J Cosmet Laser Ther. 2016;18(4):208-12.
91. Rossi A, Lu R, Frey MK, et al. The use of the 300 microsecond 1064 nm Nd:YAG laser in the treatment of keloids. J Drugs Dermatol. 2013;12(11):1256–62.
92. Alster TS. Improvement of erythematous and hypertrophic scars by the 585-nm flashlamp-pumped pulsed dye laser. Ann Plast Surg. 1994;32(2):186-90.
93. de las Alas JMG, Siripunvarapon AH, Dofitas BL. Pulsed dye laser for the treatment of keloid and hypertrophic scars: a systematic review. Expert Rev Med Devices. 2012;9(6):641-50.
94. Gaston P, Humzah MD, Quaba AA. The pulsed tuneable dye laser as an aid in the management of postburn scarring. Burns J Int Soc Burn Inj. 1996;22(3):203-5.
95. Alster TS, Lewis AB, Rosenbach A. Laser scar revision: comparison of CO_2 laser vaporization with and without simultaneous pulsed dye laser treatment. Dermatol Surg. 1998;24(12):1299-302.
96. Cheng ET, Nowak KC, Koch RJ. Effect of blended carbon dioxide and erbium:YAG laser energy on preauricular and ear lobule keloid fibroblast secretion of growth factors: a serum-free study. Arch Facial Plast Surg. 2001;3(4):252-7.
97. Cheng ET, Pollard JD, Koch RJ. Effect of blended CO_2 and erbium:YAG laser irradiation on normal and keloid fibroblasts: a serum-free study. J Clin Laser Med Surg. 2003;21(6):337-43.
98. Alster TS, Williams CM. Treatment of keloid sternotomy scars with 585 nm flashlamp-pumped pulsed-dye laser. Lancet Lond Engl. 1995;345(8959):1198-200.
99. Kuo YR, Wu WS, Jeng SF, et al. Activation of ERK and p38 kinase mediated keloid fibroblast apoptosis after flashlamp pulsed-dye laser treatment. Lasers Surg Med. 2005;36(1):31-7.
100. Bettinger DA, Yager DR, Diegelmann RF, Cohen IK. The effect of TGF-beta on keloid fibroblast proliferation and collagen synthesis. Plast Reconstr Surg. 1996;98(5):827-33.
101. Hambleton J, Shakespeare PG, Pratt BJ. The progress of hypertrophic scars monitored by ultrasound measurements of thickness. Burns. 1992;18(4):301-7.
102. Macintyre L, Baird M. Pressure garments for use in the treatment of hypertrophic scars--a review of the problems associated with their use. Burns. 2006;32(1):10-5.
103. Renò F, Sabbatini M, Stella M, et al. Effect of in vitro mechanical compression on Epilysin (matrix metalloproteinase-28) expression in hypertrophic scars. Wound Repair Regen. 2005;13(3):255-61.
104. Renò F, Grazianetti P, Cannas M. Effects of mechanical compression on hypertrophic scars: prostaglandin E2 release. Burns J Int Soc Burn Inj. 2001;(3):215-8.
105. Rayner K. The use of pressure therapy to treat hypertrophic scarring. J Wound Care. 2000;9(3):151-3.
106. Puzey G. The use of pressure garments on hypertrophic scars. J Tissue Viability. 2002;12(1):11-5.
107. Macintyre L. Designing pressure garments capable of exerting specific pressures on limbs. Burns. 2007;33(5): 579-86.
108. Leung PC, Ng M. Pressure treatment for hypertrophic scars resulting from burns. Burns. 1980;6(4):244-50.
109. Anzarut A, Olson J, Singh P, et al. The effectiveness of pressure garment therapy for the prevention of abnormal scarring after burn injury: a meta-analysis. J Plast Reconstr Aesthetic Surg. 2009;62(1):77-84.
110. Niessen FB, Spauwen PH, Robinson PH, et al. The use of silicone occlusive sheeting (Sil-K) and silicone occlusive gel (Epiderm) in the prevention of hypertrophic scar formation. Plast Reconstr Surg. 1998;102(6):1962-72.
111. McCarty M. An evaluation of evidence regarding application of silicone gel sheeting for the management of hypertrophic scars and keloids. J Clin Aesthetic Dermatol. 2010;3(11):39-43.
112. Carney SA, Cason CG, Gowar JP, et al. Cica-Care gel sheeting in the management of hypertrophic scarring. Burns. 1994;20(2):163-7.
113. Chan KY, Lau CL, Adeeb SM, et al. A randomized, placebo-controlled, double-blind, prospective clinical trial of silicone gel in prevention of hypertrophic scar development in median sternotomy wound. Plast Reconstr Surg. 2005;116(4):1013-20; discussion 1021-2.
114. Gold MH. A controlled clinical trial of topical silicone gel sheeting in the treatment of hypertrophic scars and keloids. J Am Acad Dermatol. 1994;30(3):506-7.
115. Musgrave MA, Umraw N, Fish JS, Gomez M, Cartotto RC. The effect of silicone gel sheets on perfusion of hypertrophic burn scars. J Burn Care Rehabil. 2002;23(3):208-14.
116. Nikkonen MM, Pitkanen JM, Al-Qattan MM. Problems associated with the use of silicone gel sheeting for hypertrophic scars in the hot climate of Saudi Arabia. Burns 2001;27(5):498-501.
117. Van den Kerckhove E, Stappaerts K, Boeckx W, et al. Silicones in the rehabilitation of burns: a review and overview. Burns. 2001;27(3):205-14.

118. Berman B, Maderal A, Raphael B. Keloids and hypertrophic scars: pathophysiology, classification, and treatment. Dermatol Surg. 2017;43(Suppl 1):S3-18.
119. Ogawa R, Mitsuhashi K, Hyakusoku H, Miyashita T. Postoperative electron-beam irradiation therapy for keloids and hypertrophic scars: retrospective study of 147 cases followed for more than 18 months. Plast Reconstr Surg. 2003;(2):547-53; discussion 554-5.
120. Sclafani AP, Gordon L, Chadha M, Romo T. Prevention of earlobe keloid recurrence with postoperative corticosteroid injections versus radiation therapy: a randomized, prospective study and review of the literature. Dermatol Surg. 1996;22(6):569-74.
121. Ogawa R, Miyashita T, Hyakusoku H, et al. Postoperative radiation protocol for keloids and hypertrophic scars: statistical analysis of 370 sites followed for over 18 months. Ann Plast Surg. 2007;59(6):688-91.
122. Ogawa R, Yoshitatsu S, Yoshida K, Miyashita T. Is radiation therapy for keloids acceptable? The risk of radiation-induced carcinogenesis. Plast Reconstr Surg. 2009;124(4):1196-201.
123. Asilian A, Darougheh A, Shariati F. New combination of triamcinolone, 5-Fluorouracil, and pulsed-dye laser for treatment of keloid and hypertrophic scars. Dermatol Surg. 2006;32(7):907-15.
124. Davison SP, Dayan JH, Clemens MW, et al. Efficacy of intralesional 5-fluorouracil and triamcinolone in the treatment of keloids. Aesthet Surg J. 2009;29(1):40-6.
125. Darougheh A, Asilian A, Shariati F. Intralesional triamcinolone alone or in combination with 5-fluorouracil for the treatment of keloid and hypertrophic scars. Clin Exp Dermatol. 2009;34(2):219-23.
126. Atiyeh BS, Costagliola M, Hayek SN. Keloid or hypertrophic scar: the controversy: review of the literature. Ann Plast Surg. 2005;54(6):676-80.
127. Yamamoto T. Bleomycin and the skin. Br J Dermatol. 2006;155(5):869-75.
128. Aggarwal H, Saxena A, Lubana PS, et al. Treatment of keloids and hypertrophic scars using bleom. J Cosmet Dermatol. 2008;7(1):43-9.
129. España A, Solano T, Quintanilla E. Bleomycin in the treatment of keloids and hypertrophic scars by multiple needle punctures. Dermatol Surg. 2001;27(1):23-7.
130. Saray Y, Güleç AT. Treatment of keloids and hypertrophic scars with dermojet injections of bleomycin: a preliminary study. Int J Dermatol. 2005;44(9):777-84.
131. Yeowell HN, Marshall MK, Walker LC, et al. Regulation of lysyl oxidase mRNA in dermal fibroblasts from normal donors and patients with inherited connective tissue disorders. Arch Biochem Biophys. 1994;308(1):299-305.
132. Naeini FF, Najafian J, Ahmadpour K. Bleomycin tattooing as a promising therapeutic modality in large keloids and hypertrophic scars. Dermatol Surg. 2006;32(8):1023-30.
133. Berman B, Harrison-Balestra C, Perez OA, et al. Treatment of keloid scars post-shave excision with imiquimod 5% cream: a prospective, double-blind, placebo-controlled pilot study. J Drugs Dermatol. 2009;8(5):455-8.
134. Malhotra AK, Gupta S, Khaitan BK, Sharma VK. Imiquimod 5% cream for the prevention of recurrence after excision of presternal keloids. Dermatol Basel Switz. 2007;215(1):63-5.
135. Block L, Gosain A, King TW. Emerging therapies for scar prevention. Adv Wound Care. 2015;4(10):607-14.
136. Chandawarkar RY, Piorkowski J, Amjad I, Deckers PJ. Combination therapy of a large, recurrent keloid. Dermatol Surg. 2007;33(2):229-35.
137. Meshkinpour A, Ghasri P, Pope K, et al. Treatment of hypertrophic scars and keloids with a radiofrequency device: a study of collagen effects. Lasers Surg Med. 2005;37(5):343-9.
138. Fruth K, Gouveris H, Kuelkens C, Mann WJ. Radiofrequency tissue volume reduction for treatment of auricle keloids. The Laryngoscope. 2011;121(6):1233-6.
139. Klockars T, Bäck LJ, Sinkkonen ST. Radiofrequency ablation for treatment of auricular keloids: our experience in eleven patients. Clin Otolaryngol 2013;38(5):381-5.
140. Xu S, Teng J, Xie J, Shen M, Chen D. Comparison of the mechanisms of intralesional steroid, interferon or verapamil injection in the treatment of proliferative scars. Zhonghua Zheng Xing Wai KeZaZhi. 2009;25(1):37-40.
141. Giugliano G, Pasquali D, Notaro A, et al. Verapamil inhibits interleukin-6 and vascular endothelial growth factor production in primary cultures of keloid fibroblasts. Br J Plast Surg. 2003;56(8):804-9.
142. Copcu E, Sivrioglu N, Oztan Y. Combination of surgery and intralesional verapamil injection in the treatment of the keloid. J Burn Care Rehabil. 2004;25(1):1-7.
143. Lawrence WT. Treatment of earlobe keloids with surgery plus adjuvant intralesional verapamil and pressure earrings. Ann Plast Surg. 1996;37(2):167-9.
144. D'Andrea F, Brongo S, Ferraro G, Baroni A. Prevention and treatment of keloids with intralesional verapamil. Dermatol Basel Switz. 2002;204(1):60-2.
145. Wang R, Mao Y, Zhang Z, et al. Role of verapamil in preventing and treating hypertrophic scars and keloids. Int Wound J. 2016;13(4):461-8.
146. Khansa I, Harrison B, Janis JE. Evidence-based scar management: how to improve results with technique and technology. Plast Reconstr Surg. 2016;138(3 Suppl):165S-78S.
147. Koc E, Arca E, Surucu B, Kurumlu Z. An open, randomized, controlled, comparative study of the combined effect of intralesional triamcinolone acetonide and onion extract gel and intralesional triamcinolone acetonide alone in the treatment of hypertrophic scars and keloids. Dermatol Surg. 2008;34(11):1507-14.
148. Hosnuter M, Payasli C, Isikdemir A, Tekerekoglu B. The effects of onion extract on hypertrophic and keloid scars. J Wound Care. 2007;16(6):251-4.
149. Heppt MV, Breuninger H, Reinholz M, et al. Current strategies in the treatment of scars and keloids. Facial Plast Surg. 2015;31(4):386-95.
150. Elhefnawy AM. Assessment of intralesional injection of botulinum toxin type A injection for hypertrophic scars. Indian J Dermatol Venereol Leprol. 2016;82(3):279-83.
151. Shaarawy E, Hegazy RA, Hay RMA. Intralesional botulinum toxin type A equally effective and better tolerated than intralesional steroid in the treatment of keloids: a randomized controlled trial. J Cosmet Dermatol. 2015;14(2):161-6.
152. Akita S, Akino K, Imaizumi T, et al. The quality of pediatric burn scars is improved by early administration of basic fibroblast growth factor. J Burn Care Res. 2006;27(3): 333-8.
153. Rumalla VK, Borah GL. Cytokines, growth factors, and plastic surgery. Plast Reconstr Surg. 2001;108(3):719-33.

154. Border WA, Noble NA. Transforming growth factor beta in tissue fibrosis. N Engl J Med. 1994;331(19):1286-92.
155. Robson MC. Proliferative scarring. Surg Clin North Am. 2003;83(3):557-69.
156. Ferguson MWJ, Duncan J, Bond J, et al. Prophylactic administration of avotermin for improvement of skin scarring: three double-blind, placebo-controlled, phase I/II studies. Lancet Lond Engl. 2009;373(9671):1264-74.
157. McCollum PT, Bush JA, James G, et al. Randomized phase II clinical trial of avotermin versus placebo for scar improvement. Br J Surg. 2011;98(7):925-34.
158. Tredget EE, Shankowsky HA, Pannu R, et al. Transforming growth factor-beta in thermally injured patients with hypertrophic scars: effects of interferon alpha-2b. Plast Reconstr Surg. 1998;102(5):1317-28; discussion:329-30.
159. Berman B, Duncan MR. Short-term keloid treatment in vivo with human interferon alfa-2b results in a selective and persistent normalization of keloidal fibroblast collagen, glycosaminoglycan, and collagenase production in vitro. J Am Acad Dermatol. 1989;21(4 Pt 1):694-702.
160. Berman B, Flores F. Recurrence rates of excised keloids treated with postoperative triamcinolone acetonide injections or interferon alfa-2b injections. J Am Acad Dermatol. 1997;37(5 Pt 1):755-7.
161. Lee JH, Kim SE, Lee A-Y. Effects of interferon-alpha2b on keloid treatment with triamcinolone acetonide intralesional injection. Int J Dermatol. 2008;47(2):183-6.
162. Yang GP, Lim IJ, Phan TT, et al. From scarlessfetal wounds to keloids: molecular studies in wound healing. Wound Repair Regen. 2003;11(6):411-8.
163. Kim I, Mogford JE, Witschi C, et al. Inhibition of prolyl 4-hydroxylase reduces scar hypertrophy in a rabbit model of cutaneous scarring. Wound Repair Regen. 2003; 11(5):368-72.
164. Sasaki T, Majamaa K, Uitto J. Reduction of collagen production in keloid fibroblast cultures by ethyl-3,4-dihydroxybenzoate. Inhibition of prolyl hydroxylase activity as a mechanism of action. J Biol Chem. 1987;262(19): 9397-403.
165. Ju H, Hao J, Zhao S, Dixon IMC. Antiproliferative and antifibrotic effects of mimosine on adult cardiac fibroblasts1. Biochim Biophys Acta. 1998;1448(1):51-60.
166. Dolynchuk KN, Ziesmann M, Serletti JM. Topical p utrescine (Fibrostat) in treatment of hypertrophic scars: phase II study. Plast Reconstr Surg. 1996;97(1):117-23; discussion 124-5.
167. Suzawa H, Kikuchi S, Arai N, Koda A. The mechanism involved in the inhibitory action of tranilast on collagen biosynthesis of keloid fibroblasts. Jpn J Pharmacol. 1992;60(2):91-6.
168. Sandulache VC, Parekh A, Li-Korotky H, et al. Prostaglandin E2 inhibition of keloid fibroblast migration, contraction, and transforming growth factor (TGF)-beta1-induced collagen synthesis. Wound Repair Regen. 2007;15(1):122-33.
169. Viera MH, Amini S, Valins W, Berman B. Innovative therapies in the treatment of keloids and hypertrophic scars. J Clin Aesthetic Dermatol. 2010;3(5):20-6.
170. Ong CT, Khoo YT, Mukhopadhyay A, et al. mTOR as a potential therapeutic target for treatment of keloids and excessive scars. Exp Dermatol. 2007;16(5):394-404.
171. Berman B, Duncan MR. Pentoxifylline inhibits the proliferation of human fibroblasts derived from keloid, scleroderma and morphoea skin and their production of collagen, glycosaminoglycans and fibronectin. Br J Dermatol. 1990;123(3):339-46.
172. Uchida G, Yoshimura K, Kitano Y, et al. Tretinoin reverses upregulation of matrix metalloproteinase-13 in human keloid-derived fibroblasts. Exp Dermatol. 2003;12(Suppl 2): 35-42.
173. Panabiere-Castaings MH. Retinoic acid in the treatment of keloids. J Dermatol Surg Oncol. 1988;14(11):1275-6.
174. Kwon SY, Park SD, Park K. Comparative effect of topical silicone gel and topical tretinoin cream for the prevention of hypertrophic scar and keloid formation and the improvement of scars. J Eur Acad Dermatol Venereol. 2014;28(8):1025-33.
175. Kang N, Sivakumar B, Sanders R, et al. Intra-lesional injections of collagenase are ineffective in the treatment of keloid and hypertrophic scars. J Plast Reconstr Aesthetic Surg. 2006;59(7):693-9.
176. Bae-Harboe Y-SC, Harboe-Schmidt JE, Graber E, Gilchrest BA. Collagenase followed by compression for the treatment of earlobe keloids. Dermatol Surg. 2014;40(5):519-24.
177. Shmoilov AM, Rudenskaya GN, Isaev VA, et al. A comparative study of collagenase complex and new homogeneous collagenase preparations for scar treatment. J Drug Deliv Sci Technol. 2006;16(4):285-92.
178. Hoffmann A, Hoing JL, Newman M, Simman R. Role of hyaluronic acid treatment in the prevention of keloid scarring. J Am Coll Clin Wound Spec. 2013;4(2):23-31.
179. Borgognoni L, Reali UM. Intralesional hyaluronic acid treatment of pathological scars. Ann Plast Surg. 1997;38(3): 308, 7A.

Section 3

Special Cutaneous Surgical Procedures

Section Outline

Chapter

33

Overview of Vitiligo Surgery

Mysore Venkataram, Koushik Lahiri

Key Messages

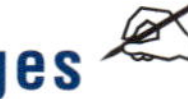

- Surgery for vitiligo is useful in resistant areas and residual lesions.
- The choice of surgical treatment depends on the type of vitiligo, extent and site of lesions, the availability of equipment and expertise of the treating surgeon. Sometimes, more than one procedure may be required.
- Currently available methods are classified as grafting and nongrafting techniques. The grafting techniques, which are the more commonly used, include both tissue grafts and the more recent cellular methods.
- Methods of assessing stability include duration of stability by history, presence of Keobner's phenomenon, test grafting; however, none of these methods are fully accurate.
- IADVL Task Force recommends 1 year of absence of spread or absence of new lesions as the required duration of stability before surgery can be considered.

INTRODUCTION

Vitiligo is a common acquired depigmenting disorder, characterized clinically by white patches and histologically by an absence or near absence of functional melanocytes in the affected areas. Different clinical types of vitiligo include localized, generalized and segmental patterns. The disease is of great cosmetic importance in brown or black skin and causes much social stigma. It runs a variable course, with many lesions achieving stability either with or without treatment. The pathogenesis of vitiligo is only partially understood; the destruction of melanocytes occurs due to a complex interaction of environmental, genetic and immunologic factors. Conventional medical treatments (topical and systemic corticosteroids, immunomodulators) and physical therapies (phototherapy, lasers) are effective only in 50–60% of cases. Certain areas such as acral, bony and nonhairy areas are resistant to these treatments. Surgical treatment is useful in such resistant areas and residual lesions. Figure 1 shows an overview of current treatment modalities in vitiligo.

HISTORY

Different corrective surgical methods have evolved during the last 4 decades. Important milestones in the historical evolution of vitiligo surgery are: Thin Thiersch's graft[1] epidermal grafting by suction blister[2] punch grafting[3] minipunch grafting[4,5] cultured melanocytes grafting[6,7] grafting of cultured epidermis[8] autografting and PUVA[9,10] transplantation of autologous cultured melanocytes[11] single hair transplant[12] ultrathin epidermal sheets and basal cell layer suspension[13] minigrafting and NB-UVB.[14]

PRINCIPLE OF SURGICAL TREATMENT

The basic objective of surgical treatment in vitiligo is to produce cosmetically acceptable repigmentation of the vitiliginous lesions. The basic principle is to introduce melanocytes into the lesional skin, which will then establish and function as epidermal melanin units. The cells survive and function if the stability has been achieved, and the disease is in a state of donor dominance. The melanocytes may be introduced through either tissue grafts or through cellular grafts.

METHODS OF SURGERY

The ideal surgical treatment modality for vitiligo should provide complete or near complete repigmentation, in

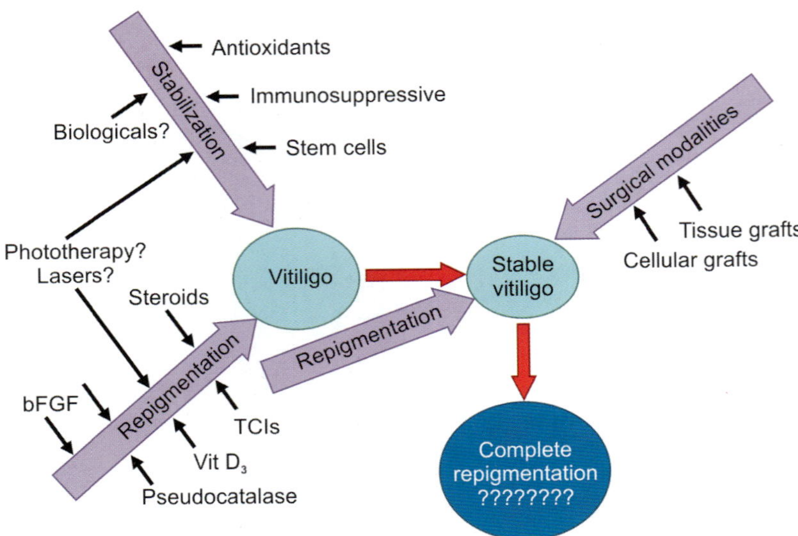

Fig. 1: Overview of management of vitiligo.
Courtesy: Dr Davinder Prasad.

Table 1: Techniques in vitiligo surgery.

Grafting techniques		***Nongrafting techniques***
Tissue grafts Minipunch grafting	*Cellular grafts* Noncultured cell suspensions—epidermal cell and follicular cell	Micropigmentation
Suction blister grafting	Cultured melanocytes/keratinocytes grafts	Excision/closure
Thin split thickness grafting		Dermabrasion, chemabrasion
Hair follicle grafts, smash grafts, mesh grafts		Lasers and light therapy systems—excimer laser, excimer light, targeted phototherapy

the shortest possible time, with minimal discomfort to the patient, have no or minimal side effects and is cheap. However, such an ideal treatment is not available. The choice of surgical treatment depends on the type of vitiligo, extent and site of lesions, the availability of equipment and expertise of the treating cutaneous surgeon. Sometimes, more than one procedure may be required. Currently available methods are classified as grafting and nongrafting techniques. The grafting techniques, which are the more commonly used, include both tissue grafts and the more recent cellular methods (Table 1).

Factors to be Considered for Patient Selection

For any surgical method to yield good results, proper selection of cases is of paramount importance. Stability of vitiligo is considered as the most important parameter while opting for any transplantation technique to treat vitiligo.

Concept of Stability in Vitiligo

Stability indicates absence of new lesions and absence of spread of existing lesions. An additional feature can be evidence of repigmentation and absence of Koebner's phenomenon.[15] However, there are several aspects which need consideration while considering surgery:

- What should be the minimum duration of stability?
- Is stability patient specific or area specific or lesion specific?
- Validity of test grafting (TG).
- Importance of Koebner's phenomenon.
- How long does stability last?
- Induced versus spontaneous stability.
- Concept of cellular stability.

Each of these aspects is discussed below in detail.

Duration of Stability

Despite the fact that surgery in vitiligo has been practiced for decades, it is important to note that consensus does not exist regarding the optimal required period of stability. The total lack of agreement amongst different workers can be striking, as seen in Table 2. Recently in their consensus recommendations, the IADVL Task Force for standard guidelines of care for dermatosurgical procedures attempted to provide a clear definition of stability—a patient reporting no new lesions, no progression of existing lesions and absence of Koebner phenomenon during

Table 2: Minimum period of stability in different studies.

Author	Year	Period of stability
Das SS, Pasricha JS	1992	4 months
Boersma BR, Westerhof W	1995	6 months
Jha AK, Pandey SS, Shukla VK	1992	1 year
Savant SS	1992	2 years
Falabella R	2003	2 years
Falabella R	1995	2 years
Falabella R	1992	3 years

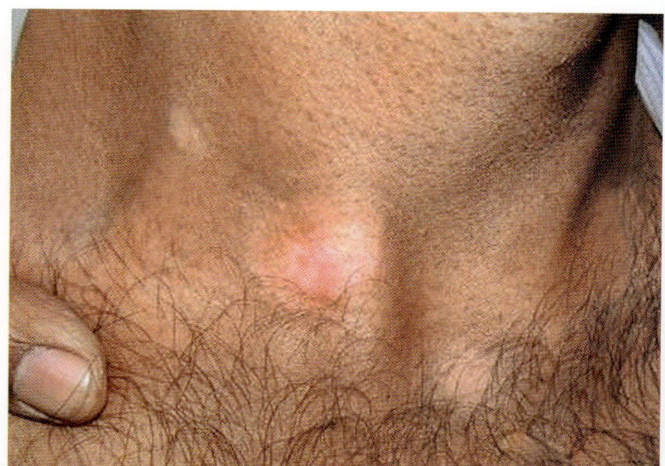

Fig. 3: Unstable vitiligo.

the past 1 year.[16] Spontaneous repigmentation is also considered as favorable signs for vitiligo surgery.

Stability

Stability may be lesion-specific in many patients. Due to poorly understood reasons, simultaneous depigmentation and repigmentation have been noticed in different areas of the same patient.[17] Variable results have been obtained over the donor site and recipient site of the same patient.[17-20] A stable lesion has a well-defined, sometimes pigmented border, shows spotty pigmentation (Fig. 2). An unstable vitiligo lesion has ill-defined border (Fig. 3).

Test Grafting

In view of the above lack of consensus about the minimal period of stability, objective criteria are needed for defining stability. One such test was the introduction of TG or minigrafts test by Falabella in 1995.[19] Test grafting (TG) consists of placing six to eight punch grafts within a vitiligo lesion and observing over the next 12 weeks (read the Chapter on punch grafting for details). Unequivocal repigmentation occurring beyond 1 mm from the border of the test graft indicates a positive test and therefore is an indicator of stability (Fig. 4). This TG has been found to be a more reliable exercise than the arbitrarily defined period

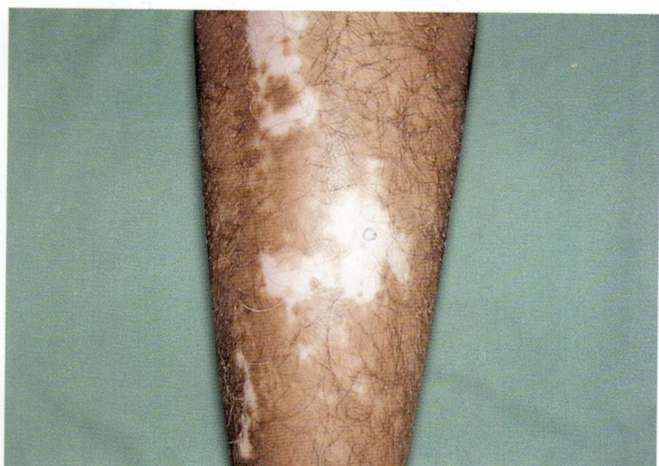

Fig. 2: Stable vitiligo.

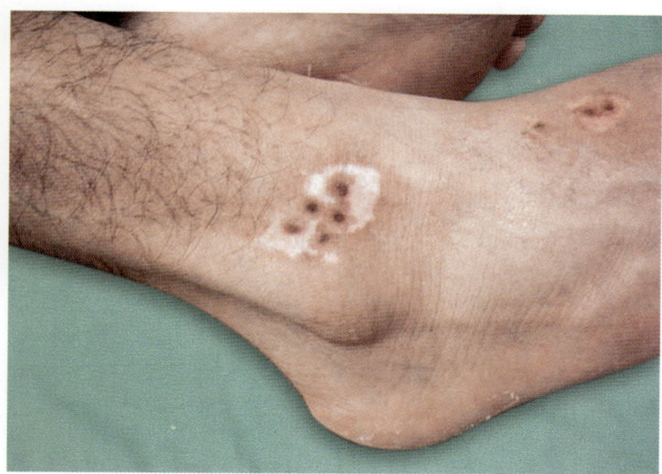

Fig. 4: Test grafting.

of stability alone.[21-23] However, the concept of TG too has been subjected to scrutiny.[17,21]

- It has been suggested that behavior of donor area, from where punches are taken, too should be taken into consideration, concurrently, in addition to the behavior of the minigrafts in the recipient site, while testing for stability. This is because donor area stability may be different from recipient area stability.
- TG positivity does not necessarily guarantee a favorable outcome in all cases even after perfect graft take up.
- Encouraging results have been obtained even after grafting in some TG negative cases.
- Simultaneous donor site repigmentation and depigmentation of grafts at the recipient site or donor site depigmentation with complete repigmentation of the recipient area have been observed.

Juhlin emphasized and observed, "neither the history nor test graft is a complete help to obtain good effect. It seems we have to wait until the method of identification and isolation of skin-homing melanocyte-specific cytotoxic T lymphocytes is available".[24] Falabella himself expressed

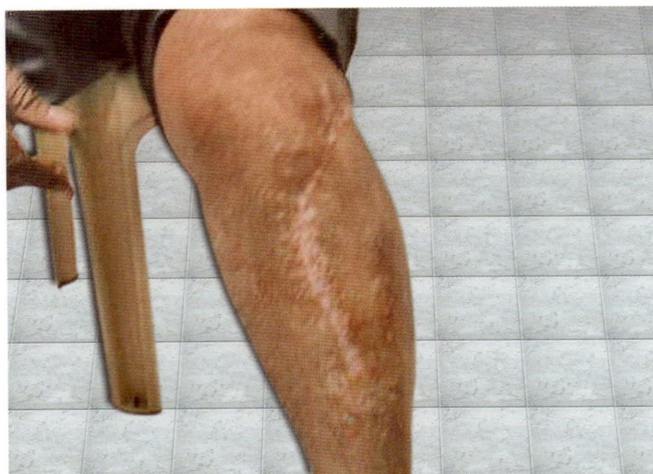

Fig. 5: Koebner's phenomenon.

his doubts about the comprehensiveness of minigraft test. He observed, "even when the minigrafting test is positive, 'depigmenting activity' may still be present and prevent satisfactory repigmentation".[25]

Koebner's Phenomenon (KP)

Koebner's phenomenon (KP) indicates active disease (Fig. 5). More recently Njoo et al. explored the association between the experimentally induced Koebner phenomenon (KP-e) and the Kobner phenomenon by history (KP-h), disease activity and therapeutic responsiveness in vitiligo vulgaris.[15] They proposed a scoring system to measure disease activity on a 6-point scale from –1 to +4 [vitiligo disease activity (VIDA) score (Table 3)]. It is suggested that surgery for vitiligo may be performed only in patients with VIDA scores of –1 or 0. The KP-e may function well as a clinical factor to assess present disease activity and may also predict the responsiveness to phototherapy. But despite the more comprehensive nature of the scoring system, VIDA scoring system was found lacking as VIDA score did not always predict a positive KP-e.

Hence, it can be concluded that, overdependence on KP or TG may be sometimes misleading in this enigmatic disease, because what these two reveal is the apparent clinical stability only and that may not be the true reflection of stability status of the disease at the cellular level.[21]

Longevity of Stability

Another important indicator is the longevity of stability status of vitiligo—how long would the disease remain stable, after achieving "stability"? When will it start to become unstable again in future? These are hard to predict as there are very few long-term follow-up studies to determine relapse after surgery. It is also known that the disease is extremely variable in behavior.

Table 3: Vitiligo disease activity score (VIDA).

Disease activity	VIDA score
Active in past 6 weeks	+4
Active in past 3 months	+3
Active in past 6 months	+2
Active in past 1 year	+1
Stable for at least 1 year	0
Stable for at least 1 year and spontaneous repigmentation	–1

Induced vs Spontaneous Stability

Stability can be induced by treatment with steroids, PUVA and narrow band phototherapy.[26,27] These treatments may stabilize the disease by promoting apoptosis of the perilesional and circulating melanocyte-specific cytotoxic CD8 cells.[27,28] However, relapse may occur after stopping treatment. There are no clear cut answers as to how long such induced stability would be maintained. A recent study proposed 1 year as the "period of stability of repigmentation" (as opposed to period of inactivity discussed so far)—suggesting that, to qualify as stable, the repigmentated status (not just absence of spread) must be maintained for a period of not less than 1 year.[29]

Cellular Stability

The above factors have focused on clinical stability. It is obvious that, assessment of "cellular" stability is of paramount importance and the cellular parameters should also be taken into consideration, along with the clinical stability. Markers such as CD8 may prove useful in indicating stability of a lesion. Very recently a group of workers while determining the markers of the stability of vitiligo (CD8, CD45RO and FOXP3) has observed that percentage of CD8 and CD45RO lymphocytes in lesional skin biopsy may provide objective indication of lesion or area based stability. They have also observed that a higher percentage of cytotoxic CD8 cells is associated with failure of melanocyte transplantation.[30-32] However, such markers are not available routinely.

The above discussion suggests that the subject is open to debate in several aspects. However, this does not mean that we should refrain from using the surgical option till those unexplored areas are charted and the cellular parameters become available; rather we should continue surgical intervention based on logical application of our clinical knowledge and after proper counseling. Clinical criteria based on different factors such as duration of stability, activity of disease, Koebner's phenomenon and TG should all be the criteria to help us choose a suitable patient for surgery. As in any surgical procedure, situation of a given patient and his/her needs should always be paramount in our decision making.

Disease vs Lesional Stability (General vs Local Stability)

There is no consensus regarding the minimum duration of stability or the relative importance of disease and lesional ostability in selecting patients for vitiligo grafting. A recent publication studied 170 patients into two groups: Group A with lesional stability of >1 year but overall disease stability of only 6–11 months and Group B with overall disease stability of >1 year. Patients underwent either tissue or cellular vitiligo grafting on the selected lesions and the repigmentation achieved was scored from 0 (no repigmentation) to 6 (100% repigmentation). Average repigmentation achieved (on scale of 0 to 6) was 3.8 and 4.04 in Group A and Group B, respectively. In Group A, ≥90% repigmentation was achieved in 36.6% (30/82) patients, while 37.5% (33/88) achieved similar results in Group B. Additionally, 47.6% (39/82) and 53.4% (47/88) of cases achieved partial repigmentation in Group A and Group B, respectively. Statistical analysis revealed no significant differences between the two groups with respect to the repigmentation achieved or adverse effects observed. The study concluded that lesional stability seems to be as relevant as the overall disease stability in selecting patients for surgical intervention in vitiligo.[33]

CASE SELECTION

Surgery is indicated for patients with stable lesions of vitiligo vulgaris, localized or segmental vitiligo lesions, though it may be done for all types of vitiligo (including segmental, generalized and acrofacial types), that do not respond to medical treatment and are stable. A test graft may be considered whenever there is a doubt about the stability, or there is doubtful history. Acral lesions do not respond well to surgery and hence such patients should be counseled properly. Age of the patient is an important consideration, though there is no age limit for surgery. Younger patients respond better to surgery[34,35] but performing surgery in children may need general anesthesia, with its inherent risks and in whom the future course of the disease is extremely variable. Hence, it needs to be emphasized that each case should be considered individually on its merit.

PATIENT COUNSELING AND INFORMATION

Counseling should include detailed information about nature of the disease, the type and rationale of the surgical treatment chosen, expected outcome, need for proper immobilization after surgery and possible complications. Concurrent need for concomitant medical therapy and phototherapy should all be emphasized. It should be stressed that surgical treatment only provides a cosmetic camouflage to the skin, but does not control disease activity; the objective is only cosmetic coverage, not perfect pigmentation. Areas such as lips, eyelids need special consideration in view of their special anatomical features. It is also important to assess psychological outlook and social problems of the patient.

PATIENT EXAMINATION

The stability of the disease should be assessed by a detailed history and examination of lesions. History taking should include questions about occurrence of recent lesions, increase in size of the existing lesions, occurrence of lesions at site of injury and family history. Physical examination should include proper systemic and cutaneous examination to rule out any underlying conditions, presence of keloids, etc.

A detailed consent form describing the procedure and possible complications should be signed by the patient. The consent form should specifically state the limitations of the procedure, possibility of future disease progression and the need for repeated procedures for satisfactory results. Preoperative photography is of vital importance, as in any surgical method of treatment and it also helps in medicolegal situations.

Preoperative Investigations

Routine investigations such as hemoglobin estimation, blood counts, bleeding and clotting time, and blood sugar estimation are adequate in most cases. In elderly patients, electrocardiogram (ECG) may be needed.

CHOICE OF METHOD OF SURGERY

The appropriate surgical method is chosen taking different factors into consideration: area affected, age of patient, patients' attitude and requirements, facility available, expertise of the surgeon and cost of surgery. Each of the methods has its advantages and disadvantages. In general punch grafting is the easiest method, but is also associated with most side effects and least cosmetic acceptance. Suction blister grafting yields outstanding results both at donor and recipient areas, but has the limitation of limited yield of graft. Split thickness graft is quick and yield large grafts, but need surgical skill and the graft may be thicker. Cellular methods are safer, need less donor and hence are associated with more rapid healing, but are more expensive, need more training and specific infrastructure. An overview of different methods is shown in Tables 4 and Table 5 shows the choice of different methods for each area. The techniques are discussed in detail in subsequent chapters.

CONCLUSION

Vitiligo surgery has made major advances in techniques and it is now possible to cover large areas. However, the

Table 4: Overview of surgical techniques in stable vitiligo.

Technique	Indications	Advantages	Disadvantages
Minipunch grafting	Small irregular areas: Acral areas, palms, soles	▪ Simple, easy, inexpensive office procedure	▪ Scarring is frequent at the donor site ▪ Cobblestoning is common. Least cosmetic acceptance ▪ Results are not immediate as it needs follow-up phototherapy and takes 2–3 months for pigment spread
Suction blister grafting	Small areas: Lips, eyelids	▪ No scarring at the donor site ▪ Good cosmetic results, particularly on the lips ▪ Safe and inexpensive technique ▪ Does not require special surgical skills	▪ Time consuming procedure ▪ Yields only small size grafts
Thin split thickness skin grafting	Suitable for large areas	▪ Most commonly used technique ▪ Covers large areas over a short period of time ▪ Pigmentation is uniform ▪ Systemic PUVA therapy is not required routinely ▪ Difficult areas such as eyelids, inner canthus of eyes, areola, nipples and genitals can be treated	▪ Hyperpigmentation and hypertrophy is common, especially on exposed areas and dark-skinned patients ▪ In extensive vitiligo there is a limitation of availability of the donor skin ▪ Needs surgical skill ▪ Donor healing may be delayed
Autologous noncultured epidermal cell suspension	All areas can be treated	▪ Larger areas can be treated at a single session with small donor skin ▪ Repigmentation is uniform	▪ Laboratory facilities are required ▪ Pigmentation takes up to 2–3 months ▪ Expensive technique ▪ Needs special training
Cultured melanocyte grafting	All areas can be treated	▪ The melanocytes can be expanded up to 100 times by culture methods; hence large areas can be treated in a single session	▪ It is an expensive technique requiring a fully equipped tissue culture laboratory with experienced staff ▪ The long-term safety of culture media and carcinogenic potential need further evaluation ▪ Still experimental

Table 5: Summarizes the choice of method for a given area.

Area	Method of choice	Alternative methods	Comment
Face	Suction blister, epidermal cell suspension	Split thickness grafts	Thin graft needed for good results; high degree of cosmesis expected
Lip Eyelids Genitals	Suction blister, epidermal cell suspension	Split thickness grafts Punch grafting	Immobilization is difficult
Other areas such as abdomen, legs	Split thickness grafts epidermal cell suspension	Punch grafts	
Acral areas Palms, soles	Punch grafts		No method yields consistent results Results unsatisfactory

criteria for stability are yet to be defined clearly—perhaps this is because the etiology of vitiligo is yet to be understood fully. More follow-up studies, cellular marker studies are needed to define better criteria.

REFERENCES

1. Behl PN. Homologous thin Thiersch's grafts in treatment of vitiligo. Curr Med Pract. 1964;8:218-21.
2. Falabella R. Epidermal grafting: an original technique and its application in achromic and granulating areas. Arch Dermatol. 1971;104:592-600.
3. Orentriech N, Selmanwitz VJ. Autograft repigmentation of leucoderma. Arch Dermatol. 1972;105:784-6.
4. Falabella R. Repigmentation of leucoderma by minigrafts of normally pigmented, autologous skin. J Dermatol Surg Oncol. 1978:4:916-9.
5. Falabella R. Repigmentation of segmental vitiligo by autologous minigrafting. J Am Acad Dermatol. 1983;9: 514-21.
6. Lerner AB, Halaban R, Klaus SN, et al. Transplantation of human melanocytes. J Invest Dermatol. 1987;89:219-24.
7. Lerner AB. Repopulation of pigmented cells in patients with vitiligo. Arch Dermatol. 1988;124:1701-2.
8. Falabella R, Escobar C, Borrero I. Treatment of refractory and stable vitiligo by transplantation of in vitro cultured epidermal autografts bearing melanocytes. J Am Acad Dermatol. 1992;26:230-6.

9. Skouge JW, Morison WL, Diwan RV, et al. Autografting and PUVA. A combination therapy for vitiligo. J Dermatol Surg Oncol. 1992;18:357-60.
10. Hann SK, Im S, Bong HW, et al. Treatment of stable vitiligo with autologous epidermal grafting and PUVA. J Am Acad Dermatol. 1995;32:943-8.
11. Olsson MJ, Juhlin L. Repigmentation of vitiligo by transplantation of cultured autologous melanocytes. Acta Derm Venereol (Stockh). 1993;73:49-51.
12. Malakar S, Dhar S. Repigmentation of vitiligo patches by transplantation of hair follicles. Int J Dermatol. 1999;38:237-8.
13. Olsson MJ, Juhlin L. Long-term follow-up of leucoderma patients treated with transplants of autologous cultured melanocytes, ultrathin epidermal sheets and basal cell layer suspension. Br J Dermatol. 2002;147:893-904.
14. Lahiri K, Malakar S, Sarma N, et al. Repigmentation of vitiligo with punch grafting and narrow-band UV-B (311 nm) a prospective study. Int J Dermatol. 2006;45:649-55.
15. Njoo MD, Das PK, Bos JD, et al. Association of the Koebner phenomen with disease activity and therapeutic responsiveness in vitiligo vulgaris. Arch Dermatol. 1999;135:407-13.
16. Parsad D, Gupta S. Standard guidelines of care for vitiligo surgery. Indian J Dermatol Venereol Leprol. 2008;74: S37-45.
17. Malakar S, Lahiri K, Malakar RS. How unstable is the concept of stability in surgical repigmentation of vitiligo? Dermatol. 2000;201:182-3.
18. Falabella R. Surgical treatment of vitiligo: why, when and how. J Eur Acad Dermatol Venereol. 2003;17:518-20.
19. Falabella R, Arrunategui A, Barona MI, et al. The minigrafting test for vitiligo: detection of stable lesions for melanocyte transplantation. J Am Acad Dermatol. 1995;32:228-32.
20. Westerhof W, Boersma B. The minigrafting test for vitiligo: detection of stable lesions for melanocyte transplantation. J Am Acad Dermatol. 1995;33:1061.
21. Lahiri K, Malakar S, Banerjee U, et al. Clinico-cellular stability of vitiligo in surgical repigmentation: an unexplored frontier. Dermatol. 2004;209:170-1.
22. Malakar S, Dhar S. Rejection of punch grafts in three cases of herpes labialis induced lip leucoderma, caution and precaution. Dermatol. 1997;195:414.
23. Malakar S, Dhar S. Acyclovir can abort rejection of punch grafts in herpes-simplex induced lip leucoderma. Dermatol. 1999; 199:75.
24. Juhlin L. How unstable is the concept of stability in surgical repigmentation of vitiligo. Dermatol. 2000;201:183.
25. Falabella R, Escobar C, Borrero I. Treatment of refractory and stable vitiligo by transplantation of in vitro cultured epidermal autografts bearing melanocytes. J Am Acad Dermatol. 1992;26:230-6.
26. Lahiri K, Malakar S, Sarma N, et al. Inducing repigmentation by regrafting and phototherapy (311nm) in punch failure cases of lip vitiligo-a pilot study. Indian J Dermatol Venereol Leprol. 2004;70:156-8.
27. JP Ortonne. Vitiligo pathogenesis: What's new? J Eur Acad Dermatol Venereol, volume 17, suppl 3. Barcelona, Spain: 2003;30.
28. van den Wijngaard RM, Aten J, Scheepmaker A, et al. Expression and modulation of apoptosis regulatory molecules in human melanocytes: significance in vitiligo. Br J Dermatol. 2000;143:573-81.
29. Parsad D, Pandhi R, Dogra S, et al. Clinical study of repigmentation patterns with different treatment modalities and their correlation with speed and stability of repigmentation in 352 vitiliginous patches. J Am Acad Dermatol. 2004;50:63-7.
30. Rao A, Gupta S, Dinda AK, Sharma A, Sharma VK, Kumar G, et al. Study of clinical, biochemical and immunological factors determining stability of disease in patients with generalized vitiligo undergoing melanocyte transplantation. Br J Dermatol 2012;166(6):1230-6.
31. Kumar R, Parsad D. Melanocytorrhagy and apoptosis in vitiligo: Connecting jigsaw pieces. Indian J Dermatol Venereol Leprol. 2012;78:19-23.
32. Rao A, Gupta S, Sharma VK. Determinants of success of melanocyte transplantation in vitiligo: role of cytotoxic CD8 Tcells. Pigment Cell Res. 2011;24:833.
33. Majid I, Mysore V, Salim T, Lahiri K, Chatterji M, Khunger N, Talwar S, Sachhidanand S, Barua S. Is lesional stability in vitiligo more important than disease stability for performing surgical interventions? results from a multicentric study. J Cutan Aesthet Surg. 2017;9:13-9.
34. Gupta S, Kumar B. Epidermal grafting in vitiligo: Influence of age, site of lesion, and type of disease on outcome. J Am Acad Dermatol. 2003;49:99-104.
35. Gupta S, Kumar B. Epidermal grafting for vitiligo in adolescents. Pediatr Dermatol. 2002;19:159-62.

Chapter 34

Minigrafting for Vitiligo

Koushik Lahiri

Key Messages

- Minigrafting in vitiligo remains the easiest, fastest and cheapest of all surgical options in vitiligo.
- If deployed properly, it can produce excellent result.
- Stability must be assessed before opting for surgical options in vitiligo.
- Optimal punch sizes are 1, 1.2 and 1.5 mm. Punch sizes more than 1.5 mm are to be avoided.
- Cobblestoning and polka dotting remain the main complication if larger punches are used.
- Phototherapy, after minigrafting evokes encouraging results.

HISTORICAL PERSPECTIVE

Vitiligo is the most significant form of cutaneous achromia which is an illusive, if not enigmatic problem down the ages. In all the ancient civilizations and religions, there is some reference to vitiligo. In the *Rigveda,* it was referred to as '*Kilas*' meaning a white spotted deer. It is interesting to note that as per a Vedic myth the anthropomorphic adoration of the sun, Bhagavantam, developed vitiligo after being gazed upon by his illegitimate son.[1] The disease was mentioned in '*Tarkh- e-Tibbl-e-Iran*' in the period of the *Aushooriyan*, as early as 2200 BC. In 1550 BC, information regarding vitiligo was noted in the Ebers Papyrus.[2] Unfortunately in some of the prominent ancient texts, the disease was confused with leprosy and also other skin diseases like psoriasis. This was referred to as *Swethakushtha* (white leprosy) in the *Atharba Veda* (1400 BC).[3] An accurate description also exists in a collection of Japanese Shinto prayers, Amarakosa, dating from 1200 BC.[4] In the Old Testament, the white spots were also described in Verse 2 of Chapter 13 of Leviticus under the Hebrew word *Zora at* or *Tzaraat/Tzoraath. Tsoraath* was translated using the Greek word "Lepros," which means a scale or scales. Along with this the phonetic resemblance of the word *Tsoraath* (which in Ashkenazi pronunciation would read *tsoraas*) led to the belief that 'leprosy' was psoriasis. In truth, in all likelihood, most cases of biblical 'leprosy' were achromic or hypochromic disorders that would include vitiligo, some cases of psoriasis, cases of pityriasis alba, probably albinism, and also leprosy. The word got translated as 'lepra' in the Greek and English translations of the Bible. Also the theory of vitiligo as a dirty/polluted/contaminated disease was initiated, as the word *Tzaraat* refers to a group of skin diseases, which according to the Old Testament, renders one ritually unclean.[5] The exact word 'Vitiligo' may have been derived from the Latin word *vitium* meaning 'blemish,' or possibly *vitulum* meaning 'small blemish.[5] Another theory is that the Latin derivation is from the white, glistening flesh of calves (vitelius). Others believe that the actual word was first used by Celsus in his tome De Medicina in the first century AD.[4,6,7] References to this disease can also be found in the ancient Koran and Buddhist scripts.[7] The treatment has undergone an enormous evolutionary change from the Vedic days of *Vasuchika* to the most modern transplantation techniques. However, the ultimate goal remains the same, which is, replenishment of lost pigment.

With standard medical treatment options many patients respond. But several patients remain recalcitrant or respond only partially. Any attempt of repigmentation of these resistant patches with conventional medicinal modalities is often unsuccessful and sometimes exasperating, indicating the absence of melanocytes reservoir to induce repigmentation. Under these circumstances, melanocytes repopulation of the achromic areas is not possible unless a new source of pigment cells is placed by surgical methods within the depigmented lesion.[8]

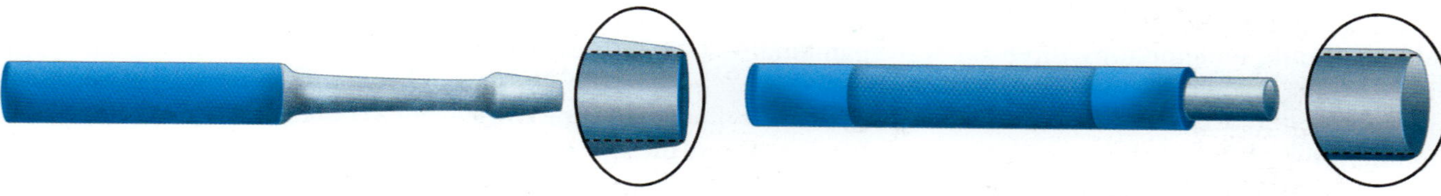

Fig. 1: Keyes punch.

Fig. 2: Loo trephine.

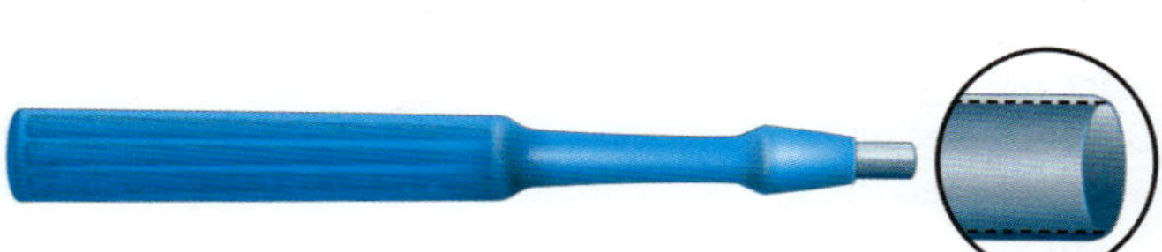

Fig. 3: Disposable punch.

Different corrective surgical methods have evolved during the last four decades. Some of these are: Thin Thiersch's graft (Behl, 1964),[9] epidermal grafting by suction blister (Falabella, 1971),[10] punch grafting (Orenteich, 1972),[11] minipunch grafting (Falabella, 1978, 1983),[12,13] cultured melanocytes grafting (Lerner, 1987, 1988),[14,15] grafting of cultured epidermis (Falabella, 1992),[16] autografting and PUVA (Skouge, 1992 and Hann, 1995)[17,18] transplantation of autologous cultured melanocytes, (Olsson, 1993),[19] single hair transplant (Malakar, Dhar, 1999),[20] ultrathin epidermal sheets and basal cell layer suspension (Olsson, 2002),[21] Minigrafting and NB-UVB (Lahiri, Malakar, 2005).[22]

Among all these mini-punch grafting is the easiest, fastest, least aggressive and minimal expensive method.

THE PUNCH INSTRUMENT

The skin punch or surgical punch is an instrument which is used almost solely by dermatologists. It is interesting to note that originally it was used as a trephine to cut through the skull bone. Its use was documented in abscess removal from tibia as early as in 1852.[23] In 1878 Watson described the use of it in the correction of accidental gunpowder disfigurement.[24] But the importance of cutaneous punch instrument in dermatology was first established by Keyes in 1887.[25]

The Keyes punch (Fig. 1) has been used in dermatology since then for diagnostic purpose. Its rounded sharp cutting end and thick handle make it very much appropriate for small skin biopsies. Because of the thick walls with angled sides above the cutting edge, tissue leans to be pushed away as the punch is made, causing less dermis to be cut through (in diameter) than overlying epidermis. This is also a function of the bevel, which is outside the barrel of the Keye's punch.[26]

To overcome these difficulties other punches have been developed.[27]

The walls of the Loo trephine (Fig. 2) are thinner and less slanted than those of the Keye's punch, making it advantageous to use on depressed scars or minor autotransplants (where a straight vertical incision is needed). This is difficult to do with Keye's punch.

The newer disposable punches (Fig. 3) are excellent for punch biopsies or excisional work on cysts. The razor-sharp edge is a great benefit. The punch is made in a number of different dimensions.

EVOLUTION OF MINIPUNCH GRAFTING

In the history of skin grafting a couple of observations can be mentioned as a preamble to further discussion on punch grafting.

The first documented successful result of experimental skin grafting was described in sheep by Baronio in 1804.[28] But it took another almost one and half century to get the first recorded autograft response of dark-skinned autografts when transplanted to light areas in spotted guniea pigs by Lewin and Peck in 1941.[29]

In 1972 Norman Orentriech first reported autograft repigmentation in human. He treated a black woman with long-standing leucoderma that followed a chemical burn many years back when she was treated with home remedy which included a copper penny dipped in vinegar for presumptive tinea infection on her cheek. Orentriech deployed nine 1 and 2 mm diameter normal skin autografts and observed the 'pigment spread phenomenon'. He reported a maximum of 1 mm pigment spread from both 1 and 2 mm grafts.[11]

In 1976 Labuono and Shatin made a similar observation after transplanting hair bulbs with hair punch grafting within the leucodermic scars of DLE.[30]

Falabella in 1978 reported a novel method of repigmenting leucoderma. With the help of a power driven dermabrasion unit he used dental burrs to create abrasion 2–3 mm in diameter and less than 1 mm in depth and 5 mm apart. In the donor area skin was raised by means of a curved needle, and was snipped off just below it to harvest 1–2 mm size minigrafts. He reported about 3 mm perigraft pigment spread by this technique. Three patients, one with piebaldism, another with chemical leucoderma and a third with post-burn depigmentation were treated by this method.[31] He observed that this superficial split thickness grafts evoked a much better outcome than the full thickness hair punch grafting by Labuono.

In the same article, interestingly, it was concluded that '...true vitiligo is not treatable by transplantation of grafts of normally pigmented, autologous skin.'[31]

Miniature punches of 1.5 mm diameter was used by Falabella while repigmenting three cases of segmental Vitiligo in 1983.[32]

Behl (1985) expressed some reservation while commenting on Falabella's work on minigrafting and claimed better results with thin Thiersch grafting. In a rejoinder Falabella reiterated his faith on miniature punch grafting and countered with his sets of reasons and logics in favor of punch grafting.[33,34]

In the following years Falabella reported success with mini-punch grafting in chemical leucoderma, post-dermabrasion leucoderma and focal and segmental vitiligo.[35-37]

While repigmenting stable leucoderma with autologous minigrafting Falabella made an important observation regarding the relationship between the donor graft area and the area of surgical repigmentation and found that an 1 mm donor graft can originate a pigmented spot 25 times larger than its size.[35]

In 1995 it was Falabella again who combined epidermal grafting and minigrafting in treating vitiligo and piebaldism.[38]

Westerhof in 1994 reported success with punch grafting in stable vitiligo and observed a maximum of 5 mm of pigment spread.[39] In the subsequent year (1995) Boersma stressed on the importance of proper selection of cases before minigrafting.[40]

Various studies point towards the high effectiveness of the procedure.[41-44] An assortment of different evaluation parameters of mini-punch grafting has also evolved over the years.[45-48]

TEST GRAFTING

Before embarking upon any surgical intervention in vitiligo proper assessment of the stability status is of paramount importance.

Clinically, stability can be judged by three simple indicators:

1. History: Lack of progression of old lesions and absence of development of any new lesion within a specified period (6 months to 2 years):
2. Koebner phenomenon (Kp): Absence of a recent Kp either from history (Kp-h) or experimentally induced (Kp-e).
3. Test grafting: On the backdrop of a pervasive incongruity about the minimal period of stability an attempt was made for the first time by Falabella in 1995 to Fathom stability before surgery by introducing minigrafting test. [48]

The objective of this test vowed to serve several purposes:

- Establishing the stability of the depigmenting process
- Determine a means by which patients could be selected
- Identifying patients who may respond to pigment cell transplantation
- To anticipate the response to surgical repair.

In the original suggested procedure a few grafts (1.0–1.2 mm) were placed in the center of the depigmented lesion to be scrutinized. Dressing was done by Micorpore® adhesive tape and kept for a couple of weeks. After removal of the tape the area was exposed to sunlight for 15 minutes daily for a period of 3 months. No treatment was permitted during this test period.

All test sites are visualized under Wood's light. The test was considered positive if unequivocal repigmentation takes place beyond 1 mm from the border of the implanted grafts. On the other hand, if less than 1 mm or no repigmentation was observed the test was considered as negative.

In some of the biggest series this evaluation has been termed as 'test grafting' (TG) and found this to be a more reliable exercise than the unjustified dependence on period of stability alone.[42, 43]

Over the years this 'test' has been vindicated and acknowledged as a powerful tool for detecting stable vitiligo, which anticipates the repigmentation success in vitiligo when surgery becomes a therapeutic option.

PROCEDURE OF MINIGRAFTING (FIGS. 4 TO 6)[31,41-43]

After proper assessment of the stability status and routine physical examination and investigations an informed consent is taken from the patient. The donor and recipient areas are surgically prepared.

1. The instruments required are 1.5 or 1.2 mm punches, small jeweller's or graft holding forceps and small curved tip scissors (Fig. 5).
2. Recipient area is prepared first. 2% lignocaine with or without adrenaline is infiltrated as local anesthetic.
3. To minimize the chance of developing any perigraft halo, the initial recipient chambers are made on or

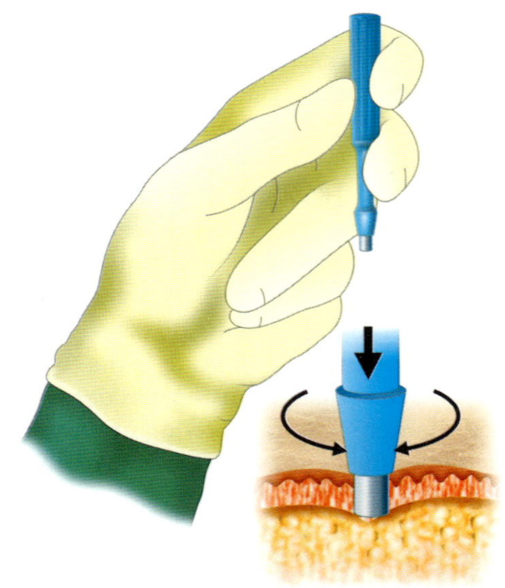

Fig. 4: Correct positioning of the hand while taking grafts with a miniature punch.

very close to the border of the lesion. The punched out chambers are spaced according to the result of test grafting or at a gap of 5–10 mm from each other.

4. The donor area is either upper lateral portion of thigh or gluteal area. Punch impressions are made very close to each other so that from a small area maximum number of grafts can be taken.

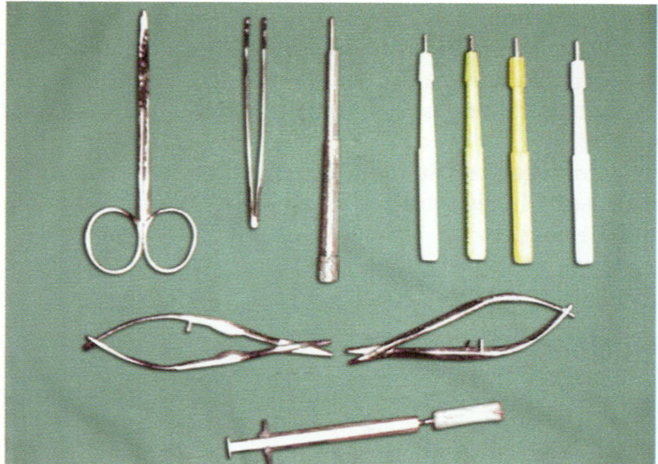

Fig. 5: Instrument needed for minigrafting.

5. Same sized punches are used for both donor and recipient area.
6. The grafts were placed directly from donor (buttock/upper thigh) to the recipient areas. This speeds up the procedure and lessens the chance of infection. Care is taken, so that the graft edges are not folded, the tissue is not crushed or placed upside down. The needle of the syringe or the tip of the scissors is used for proper placement of grafts in the recipient chambers.
7. Hemostasis is achieved by pressing a saline soaked gauze piece over the area.
8. For the recipient area three layers of dressing from inside out were: Paraffin-embedded non-adherent sterile gauze (Jelonet®), sterile Surgipad® and bio-occlusive Micropore® (Figs. 6A to E).
9. For the donor area only Surgipad® and Micropore® are used.
10. The recipient area may be immobilized if necessary. Proper instructions for special areas like lips are necessary. To secure the recipient area these patients are advised to take liquid diet for first 24 hours, preferably with a straw. Patients are allowed normal diet after this period.

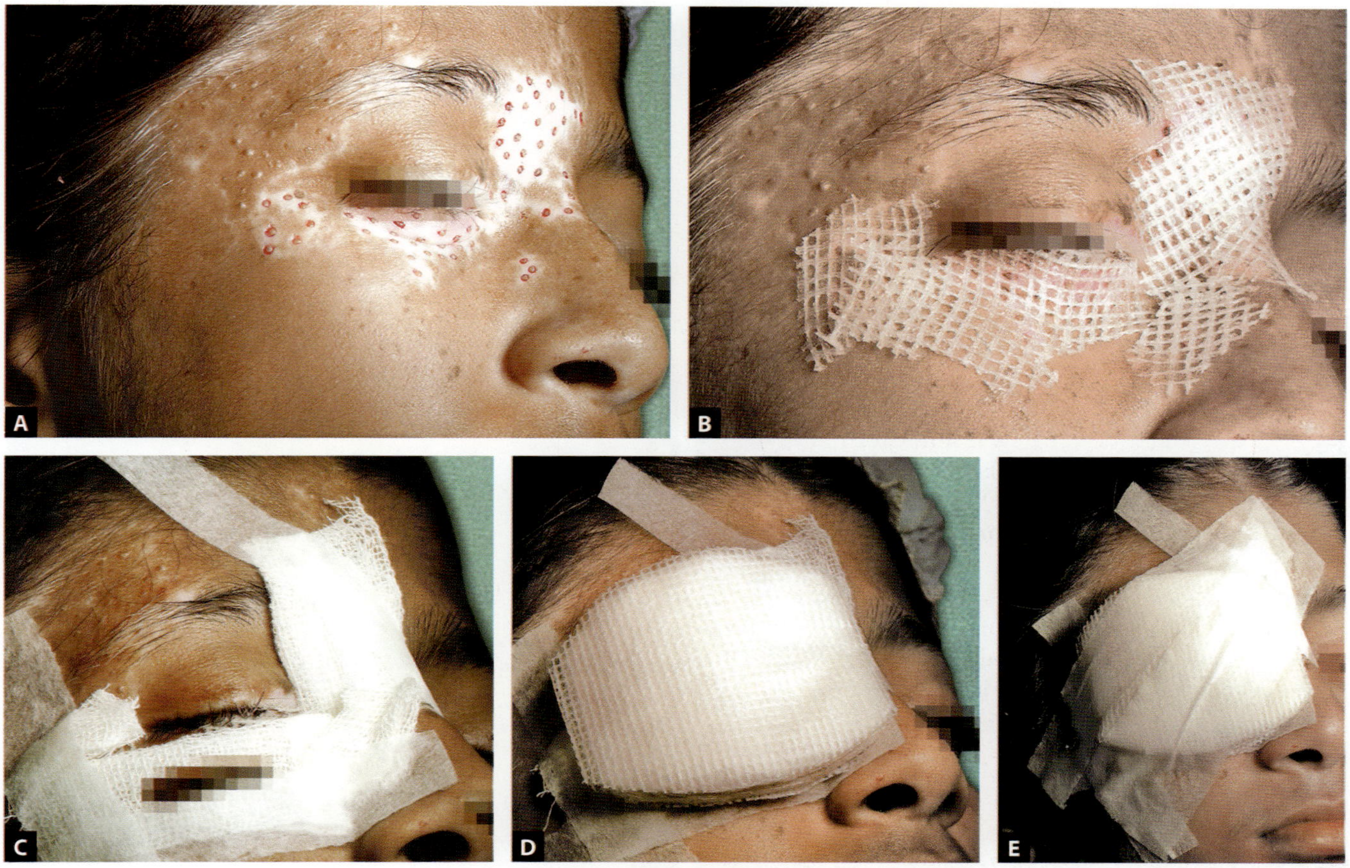

Figs. 6A to E: Three layers of dressing from inside out: Paraffin-embedded nonadherent sterile gauze (Jelonet®), sterile Surgipad® and bio-occlusive Micropore.®

11. Sometimes dressings are opened after 24 hours to look for any dislodgement of grafts, if found any, they are replaced.
12. Finally after 4–7 days the dressings are removed.

FOLLOW UP AND COURSE OF EVENTS

Post-surgically the patients are exposed to PUVA,[17,18]/ PUVASOL (Psoralen plus UVA from Sunlight),[42,43] or NB-UVB[22] or even kept as such in some studies.[29] The patients are followed up fortnightly for initial 2 months and then monthly, up to complete repigmentation is achieved.

In the donor site after healing with secondary intention minimal superficial scarring is expected and acceptable.

Scabs may fall off from the recipient site within 7–14 days. Though in many instances there may not be any scab formation. Perigraft repigmentation is expected to start around 3–4 weeks.[42-44]

The entire depigmented and grafted area is expected to be completely repigmenetd within 3–6 months, based on the area of grafting and body part involved. Minigrafting can be deployed on any part of the body (Figs. 7 to 11).

COMPLICATIONS[41-43]

Complications are seen in PG frequently and are enumerated in Table 1. By proper selection of cases and with proper technique, most of these complications are entirely avoidable. Cobblestoning (Fig. 12) is regarded as the most common of them all.[42,43,49] It was observed that with time it got corrected in most of the cases.[39] In resistant cases, corrective electrofulguration may be needed.[50] It can be avoided by avoiding punches more than 1.5 mm in diameter. On face and lips, it should be even smaller (1.2 or 1 mm). Rejection of grafts is another complication, particularly seen in herpes labialis-induced lip leukoderma.[51-54]

By proper selection of cases most of these complications are entirely avoidable.

Cobble stoning is regarded as the commonest of them all.[42,43,49]

It was observed that with time it got corrected in most of the cases.[42] In resistant cases corrective electrofulguration may be needed.[50]

DISCUSSION AND ANALYTICAL PERSPECTIVE

Surgical correction of vitiligo and other cutaneous achromia has come a long way in last four decades.

But among all other methods, autologous miniature punch grafting has already established its place as the easiest, fastest, least aggressive and of course one of the most effective means of vitiligo therapy.

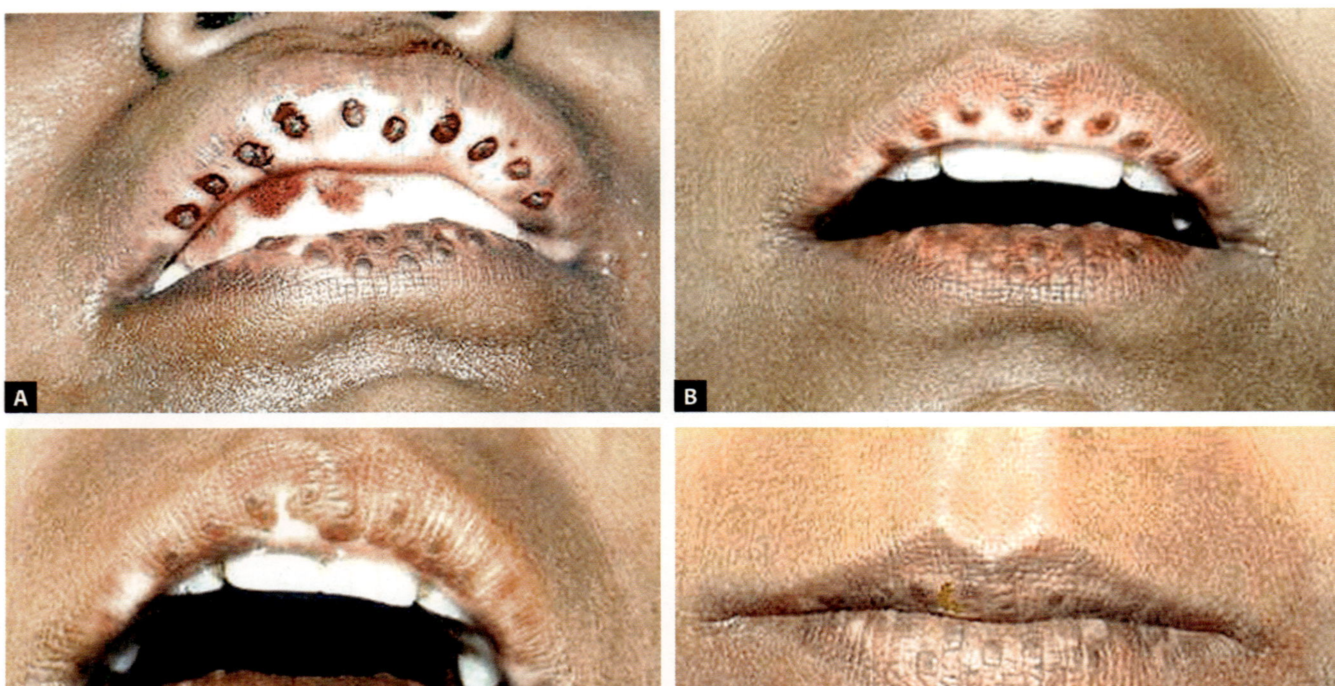

Figs. 7A to D: Minigrafting on lips. Upper lip showing gradual repigmentation. Lower lip showing resolving of cobblestoning.

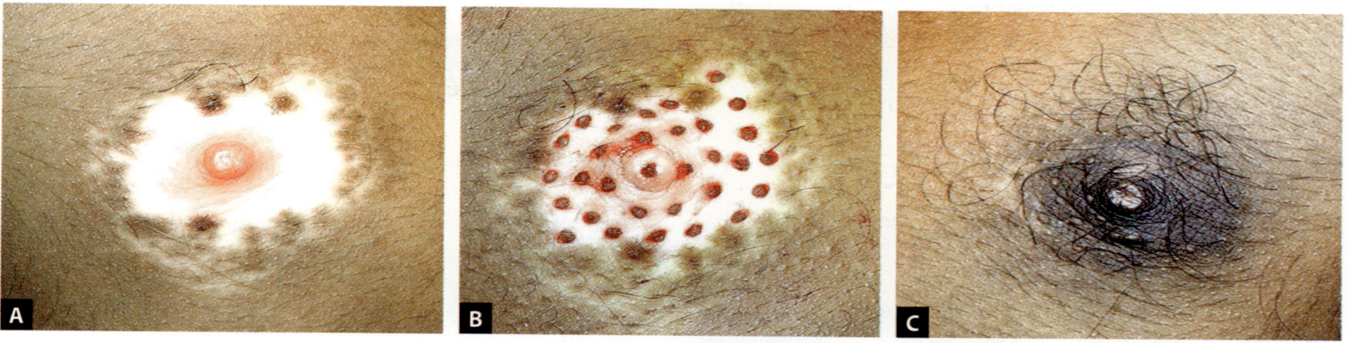

Figs. 8A to C: Minigrafting on male nipple, without any glue or stay suture, showing graft take-up and repigmentation.

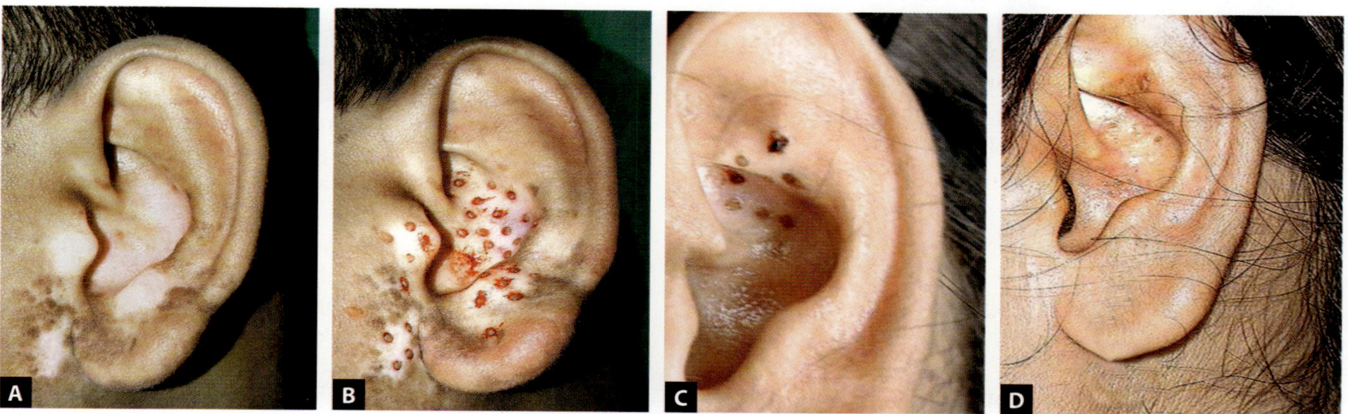

Figs. 9A to D: Minigrafting on inner part of the external ear.

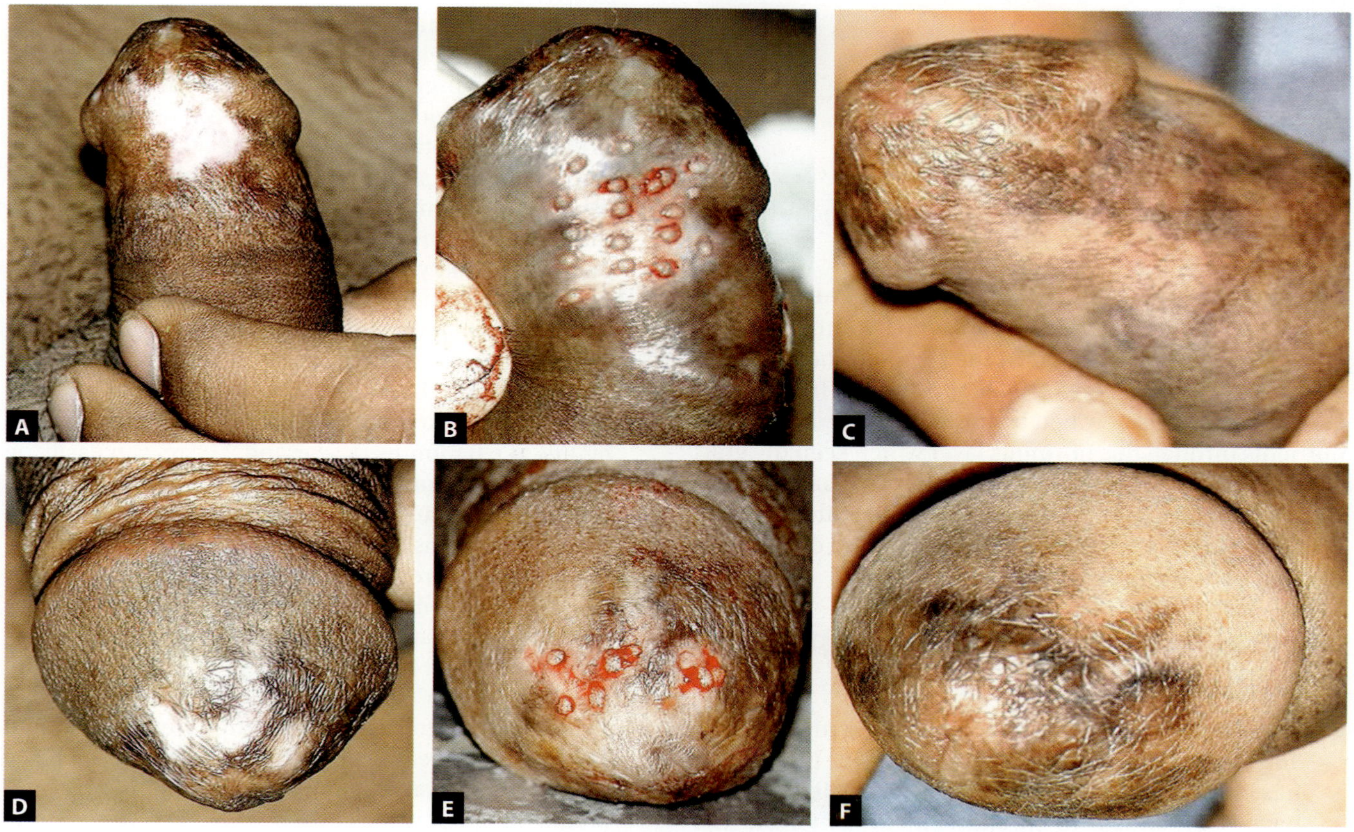

Figs. 10A to F: Minigrafting on ventral and dorsal aspect of glans penis.

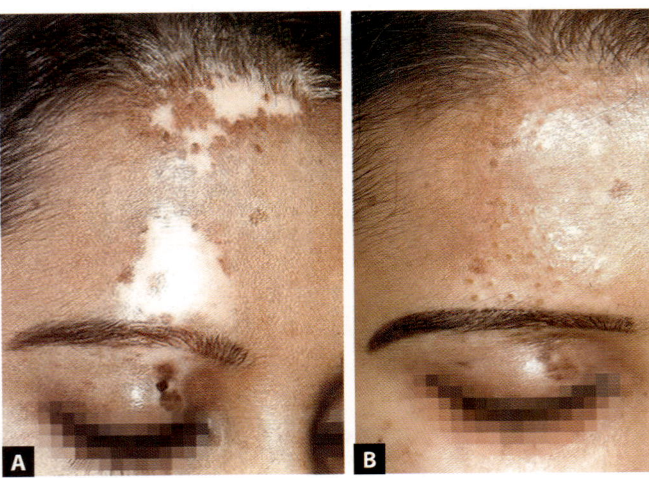

Figs. 11A and B: (A) Segmental vitiligo with leucotrichia; (B) Complete repigmentation with resolving cobblestoning and repigmentation of leucotrichia.

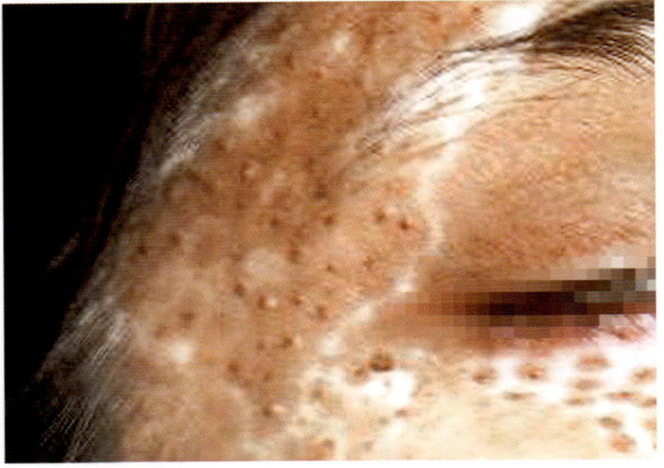

Fig. 12: Cobblestoning and perigraft halo.

When the graft is taken off, the piece of tissue is completely detached from the donor site and then it is placed on the vascular bed in the recipient holes. From this vascular bed it derives its blood supply. Initially the graft adheres to its new bed by fibrin. There is diffusion of nutrients through this fibrinous layer which keep the graft alive initially. Within 2–3 days, capillary linkage occurs with vascularization of the graft. The thinner the graft the denser the capillary network in the superficial dermis and thus earlier is the process of vascularization.[55]

Several Aspects of PG Need Special Consideration

- **Mechanism of pigmentation of grafting procedures**: The mechanism of pigmentation of grafting procedures has been studied in several studies. Melanocytes have been shown to spread centrifugally from the infundibulum of hair follicle to the basal cell layer and

Table 1: Complications of minigrafting.

Recipient site	Donor site
Cobblestoning (Fig. 12)	Keloid
Polka dot	Hypertrophic scar
Variegated appearance and color mismatch	Superficial scar
Static graft (no pigment spread)	Depigmentation/spread of disease
Depigmentation of graft	Contact dermatitis to adhesive tapes
Perigraft halo (Fig. 12)	
Graft dislodgement/rejection	
Hypertrophic scar and keloid formation	

recolonize the epidermis with active and functional melanocytes.[56,57] But the presence of pilosebaceous apparatus within the minigrafts is not at all necessary for the repigmentation process. Because in suction blister grafts only epithelial cells present in the grafts are enough to induce repigmentation.[58] In 1970 Billingham and Silvers have demonstrated the phenomenon of melanocytes migration from graft's edge within the achromic skin to recolonize and replenish the area with functional and active melanocytes.[59]
- **Relapse after grafting:** The major limitation of all grafting techniques is lack of specific criteria for defining stability.[60-65] It is often hard to predict how long the disease will remain stable. Similarly, it is difficult to envisage when it will start to become unstable.[66,67] This fact has made assessment of results difficult. Treatment of relapsed cases is considered difficult. However, repigmentation has been successfully induced in previous graft failure cases under NB-UVB (311 nm) phototherapy.[22] Even after recognizing the significance of stability and after three decades of experience in vitiligo surgery, it is quite ironic to note the little consensus regarding the optimal required period of stability. The complete lack of unanimity can be glaring in some instances (Table 2). In one study the minimal period of stability as a prerequisite for grafting was mentioned to be as little a period as 4 months.[60] While on the other side of the spectrum in another study it was taken as three years.[13,14] Other variable figures like 6 months, 1 year and 2 years can easily be obtained from some other studies as well.[30,31,52]

Even same author has taken different period of stability into consideration in different articles.[16,33]

The curious reverse Koebner's phenomenon after PG; spontaneous repigmentation of distant non-grafted vitiligo patches after PG have been reported.[68-70] It was attributed to possible release of cytokines from grafts.

Size of the grafted lesion varied between 15 and 144 cm² in different studies (Table 3). Like wise the size of the punch instrument differed in different studies (Table 4). But now the consensus being towards using smaller punches likes 1.2 or 1.5 mm. Falabella even

Table. 2: Minimum period of stability in different studies.

Author Ref	Year	Period of stability
Das SS, Pasricha JS[60]	1992	**4 months**
Boersma BR, Westerhof W[38]	1995	**6 months**
Jha AK, Pandey SS, Shukla VK[61]	1992	**1 year**
Savant SS[40]	1992	**2 years**
Falabella R[37]	1995	**2 years**
Falabella R[16]	1992	**3 years**

Table 3: Maximum grafted area in different studies.

Author Ref	Year	Maximum grafted area (cm ^{2})
Jha AK, Pandey SS, Shukla VK[61]	1992	**15**
Das S, Pasricha JS[60]	1992	**80**
Boersma BR, Westerhof W[39]	1995	**96**
Malakar S, Dhar S[43]	1999	**>100**
Falabella R[36]	1988	**110**
Lahiri K, Sengupta SR[42]	1997	**144**

Table. 4: Size of graft in different studies.

Author Ref	Year	Size of punch (diameter in mm)
Das S, Pasricha JS[60]	1992	**4**
Jha AK, Pandey SS, Shukla VK[61]	1992	**3 and 4**
Boersma BR, Westerhof W[39]	1995	**2**
Lahiri K, Sengupta SR[42]	1997	**2**
Malakar S, Dhar S[43]	1999	**2**
Malakar S, Lahiri K[49]	2004	**1.5**
Falabella R[36]	1988	**1.2**
Orentriech N, Selmanwitz VJ[11]	1972	**1 and 2**

Table 5: Appearance of repigmentation time in different studies.

Author Ref	Year	Earliest AOR (in days)
Lahiri K, Malakar S et al[22]	2005	14
Lahiri K, Sengupta SR[42]	1997	14
Malakar S, Dhar S[43]	1999	16
Savant SS[40]	1992	30–45

Table 6: Maximum pigment spread (MPS) in different studies.

Author Ref	Year	MPS (in mm)
Orentriech N, Selmanwitz VJ[11]	1972	**1**
Falabella R[30]	1978	**2-3**
Falabella R[36]	1988	**3-4**
Westerhof W, Boersma M[38]	1994	**5**
Savant SS[40]	1992	**5-15**
Lahiri K, Sengupta SR[42]	1997	**1-10**
Malakar S, Dhar S[43]	1999	
Lahiri K, Malakar S et al.[22]	2005	**12**

recommends 1 mm grafts for facial region and 1.2 mm for other body parts.[63]

In this way the commonest complication of punch grafting can also be avoided. Though the rate of cobblestoning was substantial in most of the study, it was found that with time it got corrected. In resistant cases electrofulguration is helpful.[65]

Repigmentation of leucotrichia with PG and NB-UVB was noticed.[22] The same was also observed and documented before with PUVASOL and PG.[67]

- **Time of appearance of repigmentation:** Another important parameter is the post-graft appearance of repigmentation (AOR) time. It was found to be between 2–6 weeks in different studies (Table 5).

After PG and PUVASOL (psoralen plus ultraviolet A from solar radiation), appearance of repigmentation (AOR) time in different regions varied between 14 and 39 days, with an overall average being approximately 21.6 days as shown in one study.[42] With the deployment of NB-UVB along with PG appearance of repigmentation (AOR) time in different regions varied between 14 and 32 days, with an overall average being approximately 20.6 days.[22]

- **Maximum pigment spread**: Orentriech in his original article (1972) observed that whether 1 or 2 mm grafts were employed, the pigment spread was consistently 1 mm.[11]

Various other results can be found in the literature (Table 6). Falabella while establishing a relationship between donor graft and the area of surgical repigmentation, found that a 1 mm donor graft can repigment an area 25 times larger than the graft it self.[34] In a later study with 1.5 mm grafts and NB-UVB in type IV and V skin type subjects, this value was found to be more than double of that (56.21 times).[22] Previously in one study with PUVA-SOL this relationship was found to be 42 times.[44] Bigger grafts, darker skin types and deployment of NB phototherapy all may have accounted for this high statistical value.

CONCLUSION

Considering all the indicators and parameters, it can be concluded that minigrafting is an easy, inexpensive, effective method of treating stable and recalcitrant vitiligo.[71] The advantages and disadvantages are summarized in Box 1.

ACKNOWLEDGMENTS

Some Figures and Tables used in this chapter have also been used in the following chapter and chapters by me

Box 1: Advantages and disadvantages of minipunch grafting.

Advantages

- Easiest, fastest and least expensive method
- Can be performed anywhere on any site (except angle of the mouth)
- Particularly suitable for areola
- It is perhaps the only suitable method for palm, though results may not be fully satisfactory

Disadvantages

- Side effects are common, particularly cobblestoning
- Phototherapy is always necessary after grafting
- Perfect match may not occur

and my coauthors. With the permission of the concerned editors and publisher, I would like to properly acknowledge the original source:

- Lahiri K, Malakar S, Sarma N, et al. Repigmentation of vitiligo with punch grafting and narrow-band UV-B (311 nm)—a prospective study. Int J Dermatol. 2006;45(6):649- 55.
- Malakar S, Lahiri K. Spontaneous repigmentation in vitiligo: why it is important? Int J Dermatol. 2006;45(4): 478-9.
- Malakar S, Lahiri K. Minigrafting for vitiligo. In: Gupta S, Olsson MJ, Kanwar AJ, Ortonne JP (Eds). Surgical Management of Vitiligo, 1st edITION. Oxford: Blackwell Publishing; 2007. pp. 87-95.
- Lahiri K. Evolution and evaluation of autologous mini-punch grafting in vitiligo. Indian J Dermatol. 2009; 54(2):159-67.

REFERENCES

1. Millington GW, Levell NJ. Vitiligo: the historical curse of depigmentation. Int J Dermatol. 2007;46(9):900-5.
2. Ebbel B. The Papyrus Ebers. Copenhagen. Levin and Muntisgaard; 1937.
3. Whitney MD. Atharvaveda Samhita (Translation and notes). Harvard Oriental series, volume 7, Lannman, Cambridge: Harvard University Press; 1905.
4. Nair BK. Vitiligo—a retrospect. Int J Dermatol. 1978;17(9): 755-7.
5. Freilich AR. Tzaraat—biblical leprosy. J Am Acad Dermatol. 1982;6(1):131-4.
6. Mercurialis H. De morbidis cutaneis et omnibus corporis humani excrementis tractatus. Venezia. Paulus et Antonium Meietos; 1572.
7. Sutton RL. On definition of vitiligo. Arch Dermatol. 1965;91:288.
8. Ortonne JP, Mosher DB, Fitzpatrick TB. Vitiligo and Other Hypomelanoses of Hair and Skin. New York: Plenum Medical; 1983.
9. Behl PN. Homologous thin Thiersch's grafts in treatment of Vitiligo. Curr Med Pract. 1964;8:218-21.
10. Falabella R. Epidermal grafting: an original technique and its application in achromic and granulating areas. Arch Dermatol. 1971;104(6):592-600.
11. Orentriech N, Selmanwitz VJ. Autograft repigmentation of leucoderma. Arch Dermatol. 1972;105(5):734-6.
12. Falabella R. Repigmentation of leukoderma by minigrafts of normally pigmented, autologous skin. J Dermatol Surg Oncol. 1978:4:916-9.
13. Falabella R. Repigmentation of segmental vitiligo by autologous minigrafting. J Am Acad Dermatol. 1983;9: 514- 21.
14. Lerner AB, Halaban R, Klaus SN, et al. Transplantation of human melanocytes. J Invest Dermatol. 1987;89:219-24.
15. Lerner AB. Repopulation of pigmented cells in patients with vitiligo. Arch Dermatol. 1988;124(11):1701-2.
16. Falabella R, Escobar C, Borrero I. Treatment of refractory and stable vitiligo by transplantation of in vitro cultured epidermal autografts bearing melanocytes. J Am Acad Dermatol. 1992;26(2 Pt 1):230-6.
17. Skouge JW, Morison WL, Diwan RV, et al. Autografting and PUVA. A combination therapy for vitiligo. Dermatol Surg Oncol. 1992;18(5):357-60.
18. Hann SK, Im S, Bong HW, et al. Treatment of stable vitiligo with autologous epidermal grafting and PUVA. J Am Acad Dermatol. 1995;32(6):943-8.
19. Olsson MJ, Juhlin L. Repigmentation of vitiligo by transplantation of cultured autologous melanocytes. Acta Derm Venereol (Stockh). 1993;73:49-51.
20. Malakar S, Dhar S. Repigmentation of vitiligo patches by transplantation of hair follicles. Int J Dermatol. 1999;38(3):237-8.
21. Olsson MJ, Juhlin L. Long-term follow-up of leucoderma patients treated with transplants of autologous cultured melanocytes, ultrathin epidermal sheets and basal cell layer suspension. Br J Dermatol. 2002;147(5):893-904.
22. Lahiri K, Malakar S, Sarma N, et al. Repigmentation of vitiligo with punch grafting and narrow-band UV-B (311 nm)—a prospective study. Int J Dermatol. 2006;45(6):649-55.
23. Thompson CJS. The evolution and development of surgical instruments. IV. The trepan. Br J Surg. 1937;25:726.
24. Watson BA. Gunpowder disfigurements. St Luis Med Surg J. 1878;35:145.
25. Keyes EL. The cutaneous punch. J Cutan Geniturin Dis. 1887;5:98.
26. Hagerman D, Wilson H. The skin biopsy punch: evolution and modification. Cutis. 1970;6:1139.
27. Stegman SJ. Commentary: The cutaneous punch. Arch Dermatol. 1982;118:943.
28. Baronio G. Degli innesti animali. Stamperia e Fonderia del genio. Milano; 1804.
29. Lewin ML, Peck SM. Pigment studies in skin grafts on experimental animals. J Invest Dermatol. 1941;4:504.
30. Labuono P, Shatin H. Transplantation of hair bulbs and melanocytes into leucodermic scars. J Dermatol Surg Oncol. 1976;2:53-5.
31. Falabella R. Repigmentation of leucoderma by minigrafts of normally pigmented, autologous skin. J Dermatol Surg Oncol. 1978;4:916-8.
32. Falabella R. Repigmentation of segmental vitiligo by autologous mimigrafting. J Am Acad Dermatol. 1983;9: 514-21.
33. Behl PN. Repigmentation of segmental vitiligo by autologous minigrafting. J Am Acad Dermatol. 1985;12:118-9.
34. Falabella R. Reply. J Am Acad Dermatol. 1985;12:119.
35. Falabella R. Repigmentation of stable leucoderma by autologous minigrafting. J Dermatol Surg Oncol. 1986;12:172-9.
36. Falabella R. Post-dermabrasion leucoderma. J Dermatol Surg Oncol. 1987;13:44-8.
37. Falabella R. Treatment of localized vitiligo by autologous minigrafting. Arch Dermatol. 1988;124:1649-55.

38. Falabella R, Barona M, Escobar, C et al. Surgical combination therapy for vitiligo and piebaldism. Dermatologic Surgery. 1995;21(10):852-7.
39. Westerhof W, Boersma B, et al. Grafting techniques in leucoderma. Book of Abstract. 7th International Congress of Dermatology. New Delhi, India; 1994.
40. Boersma BR, Westerhof W, et al. Repigmentation in vitiligo vulgaris by autologous minigrafting: Results in nineteen patients. J Am Acad Dermatol. 1995;33(6):990-5.
41. Savant SS. Autologous miniature punch grafting in vitiligo. Ind J Dermatol Venereol Leprol. 1992;58:310-4.
42. Malakar S. Punch Grafting. In: A Paul (Ed). An Approach to Dermatosurgery, 1st edition. Calcutta: 1996. pp.44-6.
43. Lahiri K, Sengupta SR. Treatment of stable and recalcitrant depigmented skin conditions by autologous punch grafting. Ind J Dermatol Venereol Leprol. 1997;63:11-4.
44. Malakar S, Dhar S. Treatment of stable and recalcitrant vitiligo by autologous miniature punch grafting: A prospective study of 1,000 patients. Dermatology. 1999;198:133-9.
45. Lahiri K, Sengupta SR. A regionwise comparative study of post-punch graft appearance of repigmentation (AOR) time in cutaneous achromia. Indian J Dermatol. 1998;43(1):13-5.
46. Lahiri K, Sengupta SR. A clinico-microscopic corroboration of surgical repigmentation—a study of 30 cases. IJD. 1998;43(3):99-101.
47. Lahiri K, Sengupta SR. A regionwise comparative study of the extent of post-punch graft surgical repigmentation in cutaneous achromia. Ind J Dermatol Venereol Leprol. 1998;64(4):173-5.
48. Lahiri K, Sengupta SR. Relationship between donor graft area and area of surgical repigmentation. Indian J Dermatol. 1999;44(1)11-4.
49. Falabella R, Arrunategui A, Barona MI, Alzate A. The minigrafting test for vitiligo: Detection of stable lesions for melanocyte transplantation. J Am Acad Dermatol. 1995;32:228-32.
50. Malakar S, Lahiri K. Punch grafting for lip leucoderma. Dermatology. 2004;208(2):125-8.
51. Malakar S, Lahiri K. Electrosurgery in cobblestoning. Indian J Dermatol. 2000;45(1): 46-7.
52. Malakar S, Dhar S. Rejection of punch grafts in three cases of herpes labialis induced lip leucoderma, caution and precaution. Dermatology. 1997;195:414.
53. Malakar S, Dhar S. Acyclovir can abort rejection of punch grafts in herpes-simplex induced lip leucoderma. Dermatology. 1999;199:75.
54. Malakar S, Lahri K. Successful repigmentation of six cases of herpes labialis induced lip leucoderma by micropigmentation. Dermatology. 2001;203:194.
55. Lahiri K, Malakar S. Herpes simplex induced lip leucoderma: revisited. Dermatology. 2004;208:182.
56. Burge S, Rayment R. Free skin grafts. In: Simple Skin Surgery. 1st edition. Bombay. Blackwell Scientific Publications; 1986. pp.71-84.
57. Parrish JA, Fitzpatrick TB, Shea C, et al. Photochemotherapy of vitiligo: use of orally administered psoralen and a high-intensity long-wave ultraviolet light system. Arch Dermatol. 1976;112:1531-4.
58. Ortonne JP, Schmnitt D, Thivolet J, et al. PUVA induced repigmentation of vitiligo, scanning electron microscopy of hair follicles. J Invest Dermatol, 1980;74:40-2.
59. Suvanprakorn P, Dee-Analap S, Pongsomboon CH, et al. Melanocyte autologous grafting for treatment of leukoderma. J Am Acad Dermatol. 1985;13:968-74.
60. Billingham RE, Silvers WK. Studies on the migratory behaviour of melanocytes in guinea pig skin. I. J Exp Med. 1970;131:101-17.
61. Das SS, Pasricha JS. Punch grafting as a treatment for residual lesions in vitiligo. Ind J Dermatol Venereol Leprol. 1992;58:315-9.
62. Jha AK, Pandey SS, Shukla VK. Punch grafting in vitiligo. Ind J Dermatol Venereol Leprol. 1992;58:328-30.
63. Singh KG, Bajaj AK. Autologous miniature skin punch grafting in vitiligo. Ind J Dermatol Venereol Leprol. 1995;61:77-80.
64. Falabella R. Surgical treatment of vitiligo: why, when and how (Editorial). J Eur Acad Dermatol Venereol. 2003;17: 518-20.
65. Malakar S, Lahiri K. Electrosurgery in cobblestoning. Indian J Dermatol. 2000;45(1):46-7.
66. Malakar S, Dhar S. Repigmentation of leukotrichia over vitiligo patches after punch grafting. Indian J Dermatol Venereol Leprol. 1998;64(5):252-3.
67. Malakar S, Lahiri K. How unstable is the concept of stability in surgical repigmentation of vitiligo? Dermatol. 2000;201:182-3.
68. Lahiri K, Malakar S, Banerjee U, et al. Clinico-cellular stability of vitiligo in surgical repigmentation: an unexplored frontier. Dermatology. 2004;209:170-1.
69. Malakar S. Spontaneous repigmentation of vitiligo patches other than the grafted site. Indian J Dermatol. 1997;47(2): 68-70.
70. Malakar S, Dhar S. Spontaneous repigmentation of vitiligo patches distant from the autologous skin graft sites: a remote reverse Koebner's phenomenon? Dermatology. 1998;197(3):274.
71. Malakar S, Lahiri K. Spontaneous repigmentation in vitiligo: why it is important. Int J Dermatol. 2006;45(4):478-9.

Chapter

35

Suction Blister Epidermal Grafting

Shyamanta Barua

Key Messages

- Suction blister epidermal grafting is a simple, easy, safe and inexpensive method in surgical management of vitiligo.
- It arguably yields the best cosmetic results amongst all available methods of tissue grafting employed in vitiligo surgery.
- It is a time consuming procedure and yields only small grafts that can cover limited area(s) of vitiliginous skin in a single session.
- It is useful to treat small, localized patches of vitiligo and is best suitable for eyelids, lips, areolae and face.
- It is not associated with any scarring at either the donor or recipient sites.

INTRODUCTION

Suction blister epidermal grafting (SBEG) is a method of tissue grafting in vitiligo surgery where the pigmented epidermis is harvested from the donor site by prolonged suction at a negative pressure to raise a blister followed by transplantation of the blister roof to the dermabraded or laser ablated vitiliginous recipient site leading to transfer of melanocytes to the underlying dermal surface and resulting in repigmentation of the achromic site.

The suction used in SBEG causes a physiological split at the dermoepidermal junction and results in very thin skin grafts.[1-3] Light and electron microscopic studies have shown that the cleavage in suction blisters takes place between the base of the basal cells and the basal lamina of the basement membrane.[4] These pure epidermal grafts, in the absence of donor dermal tissue, adopt most of the characteristics of the recipient area, thus leading to excellent color match and cosmetic outcome.[2,5,6] Melanocyte transfer from the epidermal grafts to the underlying dermal surface generally occurs within 48–72 hours and complete repigmentation of the achromic recipient site is usually achieved within 3 months.[7]

HISTORICAL ASPECTS

It was Unna[8] in the late 19th century who first observed and documented that dry cupping on intact skin can occasionally produce blisters. In 1950, Blank and Miller[9] achieved the first in vitro separation of epidermis from dermis by the use of suction. The in vivo induction of blister was first reported in 1961 by Slowey and Leider[10] and subsequently by Kiistala and Mustakallio.[11,12] Suction blister technique was first used for transplantation of viable epidermis in achromic lesions by Falabella in 1971.[7] Suvanprakorn et al.[13] reported in 1985 successful repigmentation of lesions of vitiligo by transplantation of epidermis obtained through suction blistering.

Various types of suction apparatus have been used over the years starting from the angiosterrometer,[11] the conventional respiratory or gastrointestinal suction pump,[7] the oil rotatory pump,[14] to the manually operated suction unit.[5] The initial suction blister device consisted of a motor-driven suction pump with cups, vacuum bottle, and a mercury manometer.[15] This heavy, cumbersome and expensive device underwent several modifications aimed at simplifying the apparatus and the procedure.[16-20]

Mukhtar et al.[16] made a very significant modification by using disposable syringes for production of the blister. This made the device very simple but could not measure the negative pressure inside the syringe. This drawback was overcome by Gupta et al.[17] who developed a modified suction blister device. This consisted of a disposable syringe of variable capacity (5, 10, or 20 cc) attached to a three-way tap with a latex rubber tube, a 50 cc syringe for aspiration of air to produce the vacuum, and a manometer to measure the negative pressure. Gupta et al., in a subsequent study,[20] made the manometer superfluous by calculating the column of vacuum or the amount of aspirated air that is necessary for the production of a specific pressure gradient. Kaliyadan et al.[21] substituted the 50 cc syringe with a microdermabrasion device having a vacuum pump to generate negative pressure.

Burm et al.[22] developed a suction device consisting of only two units — a portable suction pump (Medi-Pump, Model 1130D, Tomas Ind., Inc., USA) and cylindrical plastic suction cups containing an independent one-way check valve. A negative pressure cutaneous suction chamber system (NPCSCS, Electronic Diversities, MD, USA) that combines high negative pressure (up to -508 mm Hg) and thermal regulation allowing for rapid induction of blisters was designed by Alexis et al.[23]

PATIENT SELECTION

Proper selection of the patient is the most important factor for achieving a good cosmetic result with any grafting procedure in vitiligo. The age of the patient, the site of vitiligo, keloidal tendency and most importantly, the stability of the disease, are the factors that need consideration.[24]

The minimum duration of stability for vitiligo grafting is still a contentious issue with the recommended duration ranging from 6 months to as long as 4 years in different clinical studies.[25-27] The most accepted consensus is to select a patient with no history of progression of lesions, no new lesions, and no history of a Koebner's phenomenon over at least 1 year before the procedure.[28] Another debatable issue is the relative importance of lesional versus disease stability. A recent multicentric study[29] concluded that lesional stability is as relevant as the overall disease stability in selecting patients for surgical intervention in vitiligo.

The indications and contraindications of SBEG are listed in Box 1.

PROCEDURE

A written informed consent and preoperative photographic documentation of the vitiliginous areas considered for surgery must be made. Premedication with antibiotics may be necessary only in selected cases, especially if large areas are to be grafted. All instruments and equipment (Box 2) required for SBEG must be kept ready in the operating trolley (Fig. 1).

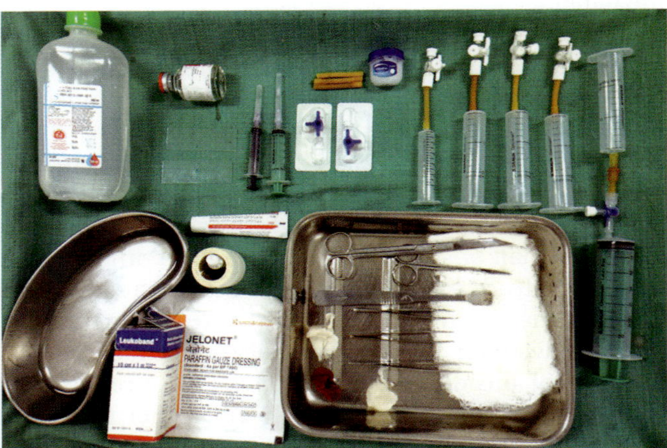

Fig. 1: The SBEG surgical trolley.

Preparation of Donor Site

Falabella,[7] in his original study, had used the inner aspect of the thigh as the site for raising suction blisters. Other preferred donor sites for SBEG include the medial aspect of forearm and arm, the abdomen, buttocks, and the anterolateral aspect of the thigh or leg.[14,17,30-33] As a rule, covered sites such as the gluteal region or the thigh are preferred since there is always a risk, however minimal, of pigmentary changes occuring at the donor site.[34]

The area is surgically prepared by shaving and local cleaning with 10% povidone iodine and spirit. A topical local anesthetic may be applied as the procedure is painful. Alternatively, especially in patients with lower pain threshold, the donor area is infiltrated with 1% xylocaine as a field block.[30,34]

Suction Application and Blister Induction

Blisters may be raised using syringes[17] or suction pump and suction cups[22] or a negative pressure cutaneous suction chamber system.[23] Using syringes to raise blisters is the most commonly employed method.

The plunger of a 20 cc syringe is removed and a three-way connector is attached to its needle end piece through

Box 1: Indications and contraindications of SBEG.[30]

Indications
- Stable vitiligo
- Secondary leukoderma
- Piebaldism

Contraindications
- Active unstable vitiligo
- Infection
- Keloidal tendency

Box 2: Instruments and equipment for SBEG.

- Sterile disposable syringes (5 cc; 10/20 cc; 50cc)
- Three-way connectors and polyvinyl tubing
- Petroleum jelly (@ Vaseline)
- 1% xylocaine vial or topical anesthetic cream
- 0.9% sodium chloride solution
- 10% povidone iodine and spirit swabs
- Dermabrader — manual or electrical
- Iris scissors
- Jeweler's forceps
- Graft spreading rods and spatula
- Sterile glass slides
- Surgical glue (N-butyl 2-cyanoacrylate)
- Surgical dressing material
- Lasers (CO_2 or Erbium:YAG) — optional

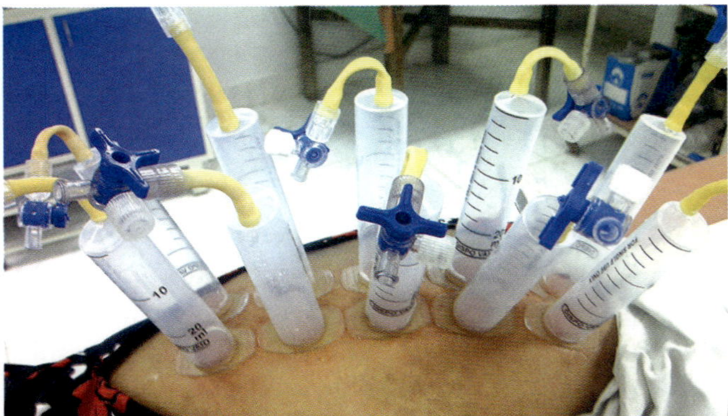

Fig. 2: Multiple 20 cc syringes applied next to each other for suction induced blistering.

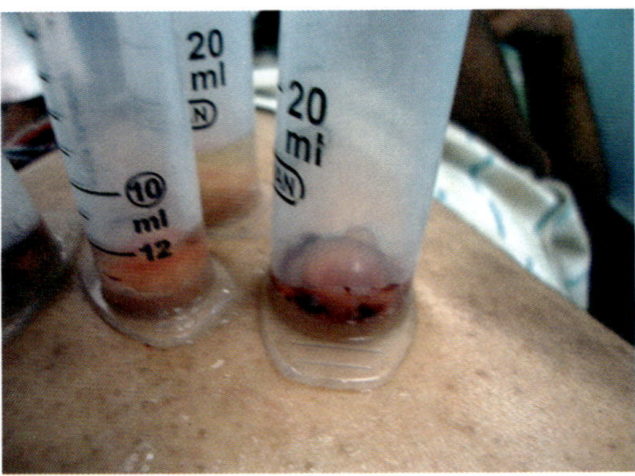

Fig. 3: Appearance of blisters within 20 cc syringes.

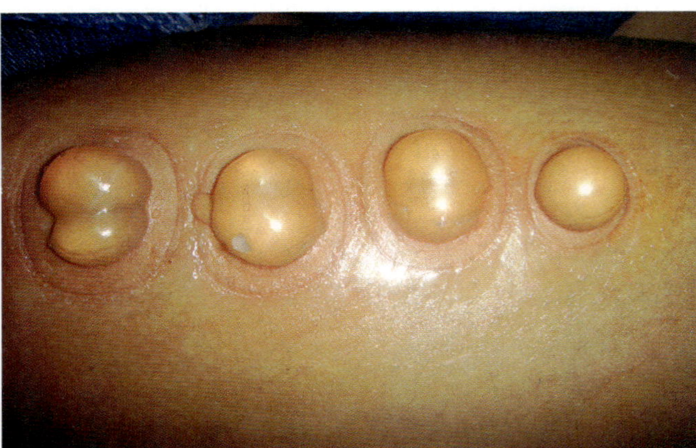

Fig. 4: Formation of unilocular blisters.

polyvinyl tubing, generally cut from IV infusion set. The basal rim of the syringe is coated with petroleum jelly and then applied to the fully stretched donor site. The needle end piece of the 50 cc syringe is then attached to the other adopter of the three-way connector connected to the 20 cc syringe. The three-way connector is unlocked and air is sucked out from the 20 cc syringe by the 50 cc syringe to create negative pressure. The connector is then locked and the aspirated air from the 50 cc syringe is evacuated. Further unlocking of the connector and aspiration of air can be done to increase the negative pressure within the 20 cc syringe.[2,14,15,33]

Once the desired negative pressure is attained, the three-way connector is locked and the 50 cc syringe is disconnected to maintain constant negative pressure within the 20 cc syringe. This pressure generally sucks in 0.5 cm donor skin inside the syringe. Multiple such 20 cc syringes can be applied similarly next to each other as per the area of the recipient site required to be grafted (Fig. 2). Instead of 20 cc syringes, 10 cc syringes can be used if the area to be grafted is minimal. It has, however, been noted that syringes larger than 20 cc take a long time to generate a blister, and those smaller than 10 cc provide blisters that are difficult to handle.[31,34]

Box 3: Factors that determine SBIT.[35]

- Diameter of the suction syringe or cup
- Site of suction blistering
- Age and gender of the patient
- Gradient of negative pressure
- Temperature of suction area
- Pathological variation
- Intradermal injection of saline or anesthetic solution
- Pretreatment with phototherapy or photochemotherapy

Appearance of multiple blisters (Fig. 3) can be seen through the 10 cc or 20 cc syringes, as the case may be. These slowly coalesce to form single or 1–3 unilocular blisters (Fig. 4), large enough to be grafted. This is taken as the end point of suction application when the syringes are disconnected by unlocking the 3-way connector.[15]

The time reported for suction blistering varies widely in different studies from 45 minutes to more than 3 hours[7,14,35,36] Several factors (Box 3) can affect suction blister induction time (SBIT).[35] Syringe-induced blister formation in a given patient is mostly dependent on the anatomic site, the pressure gradient generated, and the length of time the gradient is applied.[17] It was observed that the ideal pressure gradient required to produce suction blisters varied according to age and gender of the patient.[20]

Various measures have been devised to reduce the time required for blister formation. The blistering process can be augmented by applying intracavity positive pressure using intradermal normal saline injection passed through normal skin near the imminent bulla formation site.[37] This is also useful if there is a single small blister inadequate for grafting or if there are multiple small blisters separate from each other. Saline infiltration leads to coalescence of these blisters or even enlarges the size of a single blister that is present.[17,34,35] Even ultraviolet A (UVA) exposure[32] and intraepidermal injection of anesthetic solutions[38] have been reported to shorten the time of blister formation. Other measures include application of heat using infrared lamps, Wood's lamp or even hairdryer.[39]

Preparation of Recipient Site

Once the blisters form at the donor site, the recipient site is prepared surgically and infiltrated with 1% lignocaine as field block. It is necessary to deepithelialize the recipient skin for melanocyte adherence and survival.[40] This can be done with one of the following methods:

Dermabrasion

Controlled mechanical abrasion of the epidermis and a variable segment of the upper dermis can be performed with wire brush, diamond fraise, curette, manual dermabrader, sandpaper, and others.[41] Diamond-impregnated cylindrical fraises are preferred over wire brushes as the latter cause deeper destruction than required for SBEG. Both can be attached to hand-held micromotor controlled by a foot pedal rheostat. The heads are driven at rotational speed between 12,000 and 15,000 rpm to obtain slow, gradual controlled denudation.[42]

Manual dermabraders of appropriate size are more useful for smaller areas or areas with thinner epidermis, such as eyelids. Manual dermabrasion with sterile sandpaper is another alternative. Zaimi et al.[43] recently developed a simple, reliable, inexpensive manual dermabrasion technique performed with a presterilized scratch pad.

Dermabrasion should be stopped on appearance of uniform pinpoint bleeding points to avoid scarring at recipient site. Dermabrasion is best extended for 1–2 mm beyond the border of vitiliginous area.[24]

Suction Blistering

The recipient vitiliginous patch can be denuded by producing suction blisters. The advantage is that only epidermis is removed and there is no risk of scarring. Moreover, the roof of recipient site blister can be used as an autologous biological dressing. The latter retains the moisture, reduces chances of infection, and helps in faster healing.[44]

Cryoblistering

Liquid nitrogen is applied using a large cotton applicator for 5–10 seconds, usually 2–3 days prior to the date of surgery. Blisters will develop within few hours though grafting is performed 48 hours later when edema and inflammation subside.[45] Just before grafting, the depigmented bullous epidermis is unroofed with scissors and wound bed is cleaned. The main concern with cryoblistering is the risk of post-inflammatory hyperpigmentation and hypertrophic scarring.[46]

Laser Ablation

The continuous wave, pulsed, and ultrapulse carbon dioxide laser, and Er:YAG laser can be used to de-epithelialize the recipient site in SBEG. Laser ablation has several advantages over other methods: it is a faster procedure, there is less thermal damage to the perilesional normal skin and de-epithelialization can be done precisely on irregular shapes and surfaces. However, it adds significantly to the overall cost of the procedure.[47,48]

Phototoxic Blistering

The lesions are painted with 0.75% 8-methoxypsoralen and then exposed to 15 J/cm^2 of UVA. Care should be taken to protect the surrounding skin with a physical sunscreen. The procedure is repeated after 4 hours. The lesional blisters develop in about 24 hours. The advantages of phototoxic blistering are that it removes only epidermis, there is little or no bleeding and there is easy demarcation of margins as only depigmented skin blisters.[14,49]

Once the recipient bed is created for the epidermal graft, hemostasis is achieved by pressure and area is kept covered with normal saline soaked gauze(s).[50]

Graft Harvesting

The well-formed unilocular blister is cut all along its border with curved iris scissors (Fig. 5) parallel to the skin surface. Care should be taken to avoid touching the floor of the blister as it causes pain.[34] One edge of a sterile glass slide, smeared with petroleum jelly or antibiotic cream, is kept near the blister (Fig. 6). A pair of fine tipped or Jeweler's forceps is placed beneath the graft. The graft is lifted gently and is everted on the glass slide with the dermal side facing upwards (Fig. 7). This prevents the future chances of graft rejection, due to wrong placement of epidermal side of graft on the dermabraded area.

Anchoring filaments attached to the under surface of the graft along with the coagulum of fibrin and blood are delicately scraped away with flat surface of the spatula. The graft is then spread to its maximum size over the glass slide with the help of Jeweler's forceps and kept moist with normal saline. A fine gauze[51] and acetate sheet,[52] latter commonly known as transparency sheet used in overhead projectors, are other alternatives as graft carrier.

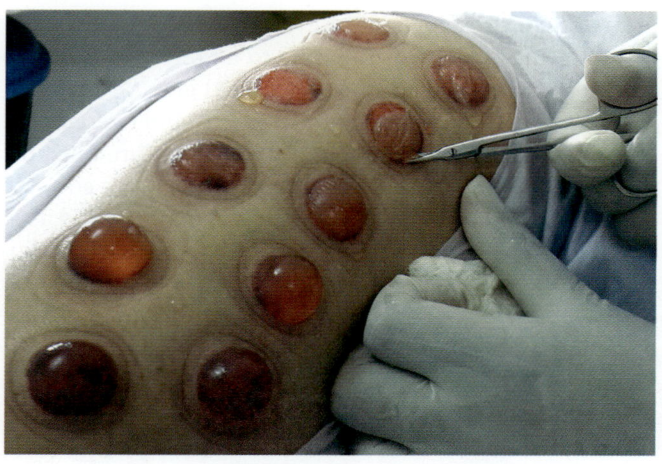

Fig. 5: Curved iris scissors to cut blisters.

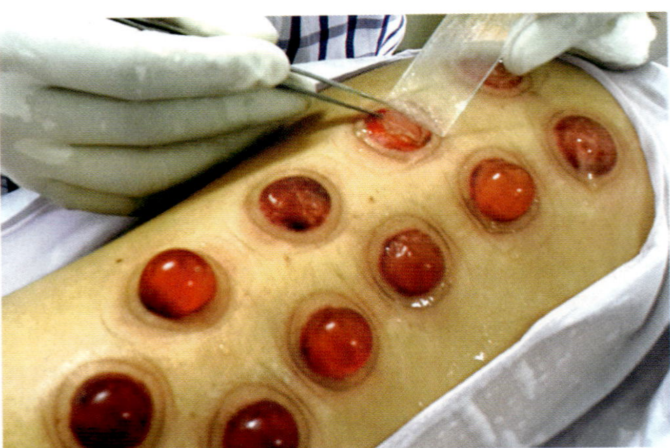

Fig. 6: Vaseline smeared sterile glass slide placed at blister edge to harvest blister graft.

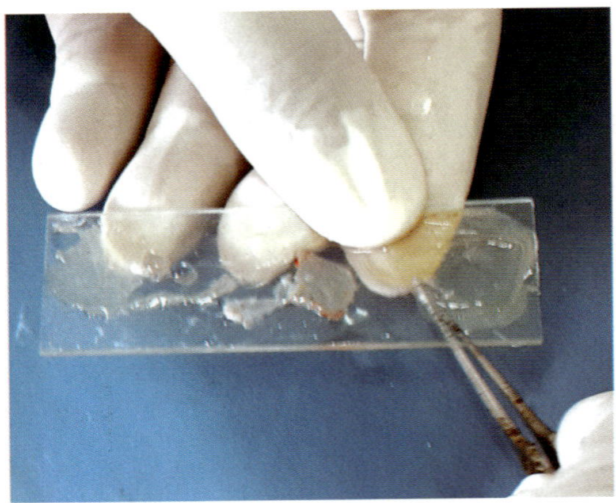

Fig. 7: Blister graft everted on glass slide with dermal side facing upwards.

Graft Transfer

The glass slide with the spread out graft is then inverted over the denuded recipient area in such a manner that it sticks to the underlying dermabraded or laser ablated raw surface. All the grafts are transferred in similar manner and placed next to each other with overlapping of their borders so as not to leave any raw surface uncovered. Special care is taken to erase the curling tendency of the edges, if any, with the help of graft spreading rods. At the periphery, the graft edges should extend 1–2 mm beyond the dermabraded wound edge, thus crossing over to the rim of normal surrounding skin.[15,30]

As blister formation at the donor site is unpredictable, clinicians have to manage with partially formed blisters to cover the recipient area. Moreover, graft placement is difficult in some areas, such as the angle of the mouth. In such circumstances, the paper that sandwiches the sterile petrolatum-soaked gauze can be used to transfer the harvested grafts.[53]

Graft Fixation and Dressing

The graft is pressed firmly over the recipient site with sterile moist gauze to remove any serous exudate underneath the graft; this also helps the graft to adhere to the under surface. Alternatively, drops of surgical glue (N-butyl-2-cyanoacrylate) are applied along the free and overlapped edges of the grafts, especially in lip vitiligo.[3] Care must be taken to wait for 2 minutes for the glue to dry out so as to ensure firm adhesion. Fibrin glue has also been used as a fixative in SBEG.[54]

Postsurgical dressing significantly impact graft survival and thereby affect repigmentation outcomes.[40] The pressure dressing in the recipient area is done with double layer framycetin tulle, moist gauze, followed by sterile gauze and elastocrepe bandage (Fig. 8). The donor area is dressed with framycetin tulle and dry sterile gauze(s). The recipient area can be immobilized, if considered necessary. The patient is given a course of antibiotics and anti-inflammatory drugs for 5–7 days.[30]

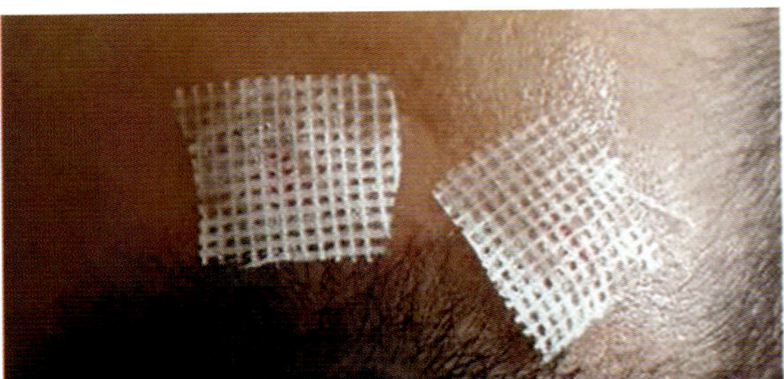

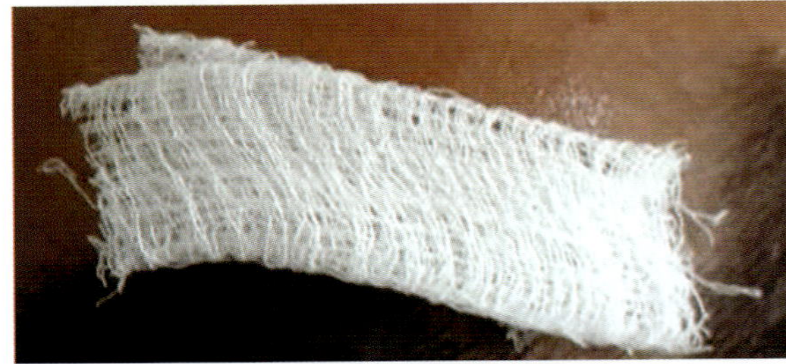

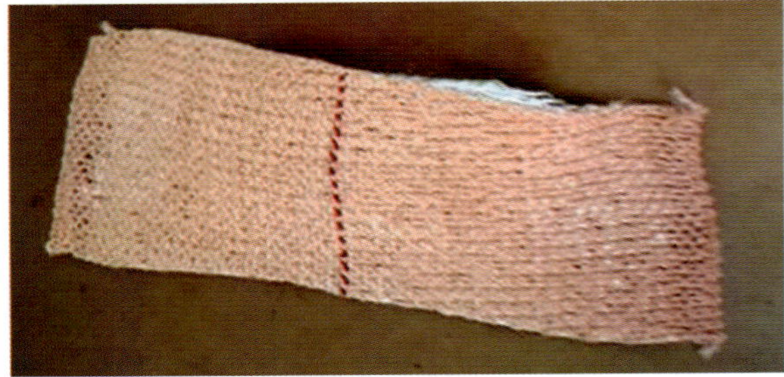

Fig. 8: Layered dressing of recipient site.

Dressing Removal

The dressing in the recipient site is removed after 5–7 days. The adhesive plaster is lifted up from one corner and removed slowly with simultaneous downward pressure on the underlying dressing. The dressing pad is then lifted up with forceps and its base is separated from the gauze slowly with artery forceps with simultaneous downward pressure on the underline gauze.[30] The remaining dressing layers, i.e. the gauze, framycetin tulle are then soaked with normal saline and removed in the same manner, to avoid tearing of the grafts from its bed. Redressing for another 2–3 days is required. Final dressing is removed on the 10th day and the patient advised to bathe regularly. The dressing over the donor site is removed after 24 hours and cleaned daily.[34]

COURSE OF GRAFTS

During the period of contact between grafts and the recipient bed, melanocytes migrate to the depigmented recipient skin resulting in pigmentation.[3] The pigment spreads from the graft to the surrounding area. The melanocyte transfer to the underlying denuded dermal surface takes place within 48–72 hours.[7] The graft either dries off or gets macerated over lips or other mucous membranes by 10–12 days and either comes out or can be peeled off manually leaving behind hyperpigmented and erythematous achromatic areas.

The grafted areas are postoperatively exposed to sunlight directly or treated with psoralen UVA (PUVA) or PUVA solar (PUVASOL) or narrow-band ultraviolet B (NB-UVB) phototherapy.[31] Institution of NB-UVB therapy post-transplantation may stimulate melanocyte activity and spreading and thus, accelerate repigmentation of transplanted vitiliginous areas. Moreover, the immunosuppressive action of NB-UVB may provide protection for melanocytes in proliferation and migration.[55] Complete repigmentation with excellent cosmesis due to uniform color match is observed by 2–3 months.[56]

EFFICACY

SBEG is one of the most effective methods among all transplantation procedures in vitiligo. A meta-analysis showed that 87% of patients who underwent the procedure achieved more than 75% repigmentation. This outcome was similar to that of split thickness grafting (87%), but better than minigrafting (68%) and grafting of noncultured epidermal suspensions (31%).[36] The success rate of SBEG was higher in patients younger than 20 years and in segmental and focal vitiligo (91% achieving >75% repigmentation) than generalized vitiligo (53%, $P<.001$).[57] The meta-analyses, however, failed to demonstrate any statistically significant difference in outcomes on different body areas.

COMPLICATIONS

The complications associated with the procedure are perigraft halo of depigmentation, wrinkling and displacement of the graft and graft rejection. Other rare complications include infection, hematoma and ecchymosis.[24,40]

Box 4: Advantages and limitations of SBEG.

Advantages

- It is a simple, safe and inexpensive procedure
- It offers excellent cosmetic results with no scarring at the donor or recipient sites
- It is useful to treat small, localized patches of vitiligo
- It is the most suitable method for facial vitiligo and for areas like the lips and areolae

Limitations

- It is a time-consuming procedure
- It yields only small grafts that can cover limited area(s) of vitiliginous skin in a single session
- It carries the remote risk of failure of blister induction
- It is not suitable for palms and sole

The advantages and limitations of SBEG are summarized in Box 4.

CONCLUSION

SBEG is perhaps the simplest, although time consuming, tissue grafting method for surgical management of medically recalcitrant but stable vitiligo and other secondary leukodermas. It does not require costly equipment or special surgical skills and small to medium sized vitiliginous areas can easily be treated by this method. As the split is physiological, the graft obtained is very thin and provides excellent cosmetic results especially on mucosae like lips. This method is, however, unsuitable for large areas that require more number of grafts and multiple surgical sessions. It is hoped that future research and innovation will lead to the development of more effective equipment to raise large suction blisters, rapidly and reliably.

REFERENCES

1. Lee DY. The use of suction blisters for recipient site in epidermal grafting: The implications for vitiligo. J Eur Acad Dermatol Venereol. 2009;23:241-2.
2. Gupta S, Jain VK, Saraswat PK. Suction blister epidermal grafting versus punch skin grafting in recalcitrant and stable vitiligo. Dermatol Surg. 1999;25:955-8.
3. Gupta S, Sandhu K, Kanwar A, Kumar B. Melanocyte transfer via epidermal grafts for vitiligo of labial mucosa. Dermatol Surg. 2004;30:45-8.
4. Hunter JAA, McVittie E, Comaish JS. Light and electron microscopic studies of physical injury to the skin. Br J Dermatol. 1974;90:481-90.
5. Kiistala U. Suction blister device for separation of viable epidermis from dermis. J Invest Dermatol. 1968;50:129-37.
6. Lee AY, Jang JH. Autologous epidermal grafting with PUVA-irradiated donor skin for the treatment of vitiligo. Int J Dermatol. 1998;37:551-4.
7. Falabella R. Epidermal grafting: an original technique and its application in achromic and granulating areas. Arch Dermatol. 1971;104:592-600.
8. Unna P. Zur anatomic der blasenbildung an der man-schlichen haut. Vjschr Derm Syph. 1878;5:1-4.

9. Blank H, Miller OG. A method for separating the epidermis from dermis. J Invest Dermatol. 1950;15:9-12.
10. Slowey C, Leider M. Abstract of a preliminary report: the production of bulla by quantitated suction. Arch Dermatol. 1961;83:1029-30.
11. Kiistala U, Mustakallio KK. In-vivo separation of epidermis by production of suction blisters. Lancet. 1964;1:1444-5.
12. Kiistala U, Mustakallio KK. Dermo-epidermal separation with suction: electron microscopic and histo-chemical study of initial events of blistering of human skin. J Invest Dermatol. 1967;48:456-77.
13. Suvanprakorn P, Dee-Ananiap SP, et al. Melanocyte autologous grafting for the treatment of leukoderma. J Am Acad Dermatol. 1985;13:968-74.
14. Koga M. Epidermal grafting using tops of suction blisters in the treatment of vitiligo. Arch Dermatol. 1988;124: 1656-8.
15. Gupta S, Goel A. Suction blister epidermal grafting. In: Gupta S, Olsson MJ, Kanwar AJ, Ortonne JP (Eds). Surgical Management of Vitiligo, 1st edition. Blackwell Publishing Ltd. 2007:96-107.
16. Mukhtar M, Singh S, Shukla VK, Pandey SS. Surgical pearl: suction syringe for epidermal grafting in vitiligo. J Am Acad Dermatol. 1997;37:638-9.
17. Gupta S, Shroff S, Gupta S. Modified technique of suction blistering for epidermal grafting in vitiligo. Int J Dermatol. 1999;38:306-9.
18. Radmanesh M, Ebrahimi A. Double syringe blistering by adding a three-way connector for grafting stable vitiligo patches. J Dermatol Treatment. 2000;11:43-6.
19. Kim HV, Yun SK. Suction device for epidermal grafting in vitiligo: employing a syringe and a manometer to provide an adequate negative pressure. J Dermatol Surg. 2001;26: 702-4.
20. Gupta S, Ajith C, Kanwar AJ, Kumar B. Surgical pearl: standardized suction syringe for epidermal grafting. J Am Acad Dermatol. 2005;52:348-50.
21. Kaliyadan F, Manoj J, Venkatakrishnan S. Using a microdermabrasion machine as a suction blister device. Indian J Dermatol Venereol Leprol. 2008;74:392-3.
22. Burm JS. Simple suction device for autologous epidermal grafting. Plast Reconstr Surg. 2000;106:1225-6.
23. Alexis AF, Wilson DC, Todhunter JA, Stiller MJ. Reassessment of the suction blister model of wound healing: introduction of a new higher pressure device. Int J Dermatol. 1999;38: 613-7.
24. Majid I. Grafting in Vitiligo: How to get better results and how to avoid complication. J Cutan Anesthet Surg. 2013;6:83-9.
25. Juhlin L. How unstable is the concept of stability in surgical repigmentation of vitiligo. Dermatology. 2000;201:183.
26. Lahiri K. Stability in vitiligo: what's that? J Cutan Aesthet Surg. 2009;2:38-40.
27. Lahiri K, Malakar S. The concept of stability of vitiligo: A reappraisal. Indian J Dermatol. 2012;57:83-9.
28. Parsad D, Gupta S. IADVL Dermatosurgery Task Force. Standard guidelines of care for vitiligo surgery. Indian J Dermatol Venereol Leprol. 2008;74:s37-45.
29. Majid I, Mysore V, Salim T, et al. Is lesional stability in vitiligo more important than disease stability for performing surgical interventions? Results from a multicentric study. J Cutan Aesthet Surg. 2016;9:13-9.
30. Savant SS. Skin grafting. In: Savant SS (Ed). Textbook of Dermatosurgery and Cosmetology, 2nd edition. Mumbai: ASCAD; 2005:149-65.
31. Hann SK, Im S, Bong HW, Park YK. Treatment of stable vitiligo with autologous epidermal grafting and PUVA. J Am Acad Dermatol. 1995;32:943-8.
32. Suga Y, Butt KI, Takimoto R, et al. Successful treatment of vitiligo with PUVA pigmented autologous epidermal grafting. Int J Dermatol. 1996;35:518-22.
33. Laxmisha C, Thappa DM. Reliable site for suction blister induction and harvesting. Indian J Dermatol Venereol Leprol. 2005;71:321-4.
34. Khunger N, Kathuria SD, Ramesh V. Tissue grafts in vitiligo surgery: past, present, and future. Indian J Dermatol. 2009; 54:150-8.
35. Gupta S, Kumar B. Suction blister induction time: 15 min or 150 min? Dermatol Surg. 2000;26:754-6.
36. Njoo MD, Westerhof W, Bos JD, Bossuyt MM. A systematic review of autologous transplantation methods in vitiligo. Arch Dermatol. 1998;134:1543-9.
37. Gupta S, Chandrashekar BS, Reddy R, et al. Rapid induction of suction blisters by intra-cavity positive pressure enhancement. Dermatol Surg. 2011;37:843-5.
38. Hanafusa T, Yamaguchi Y, Nakamura M, et al. Establishment of suction blister roof grafting by injection of local anesthesia beneath the epidermis: Less painful and more rapid formation of blisters. J Dermatol Sci. 2008;50: 243-7.
39. Arora S, Kar BK. Reduction of blister formation time in suction blister epidermal grafting in vitiligo patients using a household hair dryer. J Cutan Aesthet Surg. 2016;9: 232-5.
40. Al-Hadidi N, Griffith JL, Al-Jamal MS, Hamzavi I. Role of recipient-site preparation techniques and post-operative wound dressing in the surgical management of vitiligo. J Cutan Aesthet Surg. 2015;8:79-87.
41. Orentreich N, Orentreich DS. Dermabrasion as a complement to dermatology. Clin Plast Surg. 1998;25: 63–80.
42. Baker TM. Dermabrasion as a complement to aesthetic surgery. Clin Plast Surg. 1998;25:81-8.
43. Zaimi I, Romanzi A, Gherardini G. Tricks and tips for manual dermabrasion. Dermatol Surg. 2016;42: 1393-4.
44. Gupta S, Kumar B. Surgical pearl: autologous biological dressing for epidermal grafting in vitiligo and other achromic disorders. J Am Acad Dermatol. 2003;48: 430-1.
45. Falabella R. Repigmentation of leukoderma by autologous epidermal grafting. J Dermatol Surg Oncol. 1984;10: 136-44.
46. Kim HY, Kang KY. Epidermal grafts for treatment of stable and progressive vitiligo. J Am Acad Dermatol. 1999;40: 412-7.
47. Lee DY, Park JH, Choi SC, Lee JH. Comparison of recipient site preparations in epidermal grafting for vitiligo: Suction blister and CO2 laser. J Eur Acad Dermatol Venereol 2009; 23:1448-9.
48. Sachdev M, Krupashankar DS. Suction blister grafting for stable vitiligo using pulsed Er:YAG laser ablation for recipient site. Int J Dermatol. 2000;39:471-3.

49. Albert S, Srinivas CR, Shenoi SD, et al. Phototoxic blister induction in vitiligo surgery. Br J Dermatol. 1999;141:30-1.
50. Savant SS. Suction blister technique. In: Savant SS (Ed). Textbook of Dermatosurgery and Cosmetology, 2nd edition. Mumbai: ASCAD;2005:351-8.
51. Tang WY, De Han J, Lu NZ, et al. Surgical pearl: fine gauze is a useful carrier for epidermal graft in the treatment of vitiligo by means of the suction blister method. J Am Acad Dermatol. 1999;40:247-9.
52. Albert S, Shenoi SD. Acetate sheets in the transfer of epidermal grafts in vitiligo. J Am Acad Dermatol. 2001;44: 719-20.
53. Ashique KT, Srinivas CR. Resizing blister roof grafts for vitiligo surgery. J Am Acad Dermatol. 2014;71:e39-40.
54. Kim H, Kang J, Hwang S, et al. Fibrin glue fixation for suction blister epidermal grafting in two patients with stable vitiligo. Ann Dermatol. 2014;26:751-4.
55. Zhang D, Hong W, Fu L, et al. A randomized controlled study of the effects of different modalities of narrow-band ultraviolet B therapy on the outcome of cultured autologous melanocytes transplantation in treating vitiligo. Dermatol Surg. 2014;40:420-6.
56. Falabella R. Surgical repigmentation of leukoderma. In: Wheeland RG (Ed). Cutaneous Surgery, 1st edition, Philadelphia: WB Saunders Company; 1994;1090-9.
57. Gupta S, Kumar B. Epidermal grafting in vitiligo: influence of age, site of lesion, and type of disease on outcome. J Am Acad Dermatol. 2003;49:99-104.

Chapter 36

Thin Split Thickness Skin Grafting for Vitiligo

Niti Khunger, Rajat Kandhari

Key Messages

- STSG is a simple, cost effective technique requiring a fair amount of surgical skill.
- Harvesting uniformly thick STG, Dermabrasion, Proper graft placement and Immobilization are the limiting steps of STSG.
- Amongst the tissue graft techniques, it covers the large area with yield coverage of 1:1.

INTRODUCTION

Conventional thin split thickness skin grafting (STSG) technique continues to be the most commonly practiced and also the most successful amongst all methods of vitiligo surgery.[1] Although, STSG requires a fair amount of surgical skill, it is a relatively simple and cost effective procedure as compared to melanocyte suspension technique. The ability to cover larger areas in a single sitting, achieving high rates of repigmentation and producing pigmented skin almost immediately after surgery make this a popular technique for the treatment of stable, recalcitrant vitiligo. The technique can be used not only for stable vitiligo, but also for secondary leukoderma (post burns, post herpes infection, contact leukoderma and post discoid lupus erythematosus) and piebaldism.

HISTORY

Haxthausen first transplanted thin split thickness skin grafts from normal to vitiliginous skin in three cases, to study the pathogenesis of the disease.[2] Behl, in 1964, was the first to report the use of thin Thiersch's skin graft to treat vitiligo.[3] The technique involves the free transfer of epidermis containing melanocytes from one donor site to another recipient vitiliginous site.[4] Kahn et al.[5,6] used a modification of this technique where they used ultrathin epidermal sheets or ultrathin split thickness grafts (less than 0.08–0.15 mm) which were obtained with the help of a power dermatome, to successfully repigment large vitiliginous areas. This technique was later employed by Olson and Juhlin[7] to transplant melanocytes to the dermabraded vitiliginous areas.

DEFINITION

Split thickness skin grafting (STSG) involves transfer of epidermis and often a thin uppermost part of superficial dermis to achieve transfer of melanocytes and keratinocytes from donor skin to the dermabraded vitiliginous skin.[8] The thickness of the graft ranges from 0.1 mm to 0.7 mm[9] and different harvesting techniques have been used.[10]

PRINCIPLE OF SPLIT THICKNESS SKIN GRAFTING

There are three biological changes which are observed following skin grafting.[11]

Graft Uptake and Adherence

The first 72 hours after placement of the graft are the most crucial for graft uptake as fibrin bonding occurs during this time. The graft appears pink at this stage. Bleeding, infection and mechanical movement due to improper immobilization of the area can lead to graft failure at this stage. The fibrin bonding is followed by onset of vascular anastomosis and fibrovascular growth. The graft imbibes wound exudate by capillary action through the sponge like structure of the graft dermis and through the dermal blood vessels. This prevents graft desiccation, maintains graft vessel patency and provides nourishment for the graft.

Graft Revascularization

Revascularization of the graft begins at 2–3 days post grafting. This stage involves establishment of direct anastomoses between graft and recipient blood vessels, a process known as inosculation. Insufficient vascular proliferation, development of a thick layer of fibrin or hematoma or seroma can lead to failure of graft uptake in this stage. Hence, a compression bandage is useful to prevent this.

Contracture

Graft contracture can occur either immediately after harvesting the graft or after grafting at the recipient site. This occurs due to contraction of the elastin fibers. Myofibroblasts are said to be responsible for graft contraction. The ability of a graft to resist contraction is related to the thickness of the deep dermal component, as it provides inhibition of the myofibroblast function due to unknown mechanisms.[12] The chances of graft contracture in a thin graft are more as compared to a thicker graft since the deep dermal component is lacking. This can lead to achromic fissures and perigraft halo. Overlapping of graft edges at the recipient site can prevent these complications.

Patient Selection Criteria

This has been dealt with in detail in the chapter on overview of vitiligo and in several previous reviews.[13-21] Specific features are discussed below:

- *Failure of medical treatment:* STSG can be used to cover large vitiliginous areas, as compared to suction blister technique or miniature punch grafting which are used for relatively smaller areas.
- *Site and extent of lesions:* The success rate of this procedure is low in certain sites. The fingers, elbows or other sites prone to movement show considerably lower success rates than other sites

Required Equipment

Dermabraders

Manual (Dr Manekshaw's hand held metallic dermabrader) or electrical (wire brush or diamond fraises).

Skin Grafting Equipment

- For harvesting the graft: Humby's skin grafting knife, Padget's or Davol's dermatome, straight artery forceps with a razor blade or Silver's razor blade holding knife (Figs. 1A and B).
- Graft spreading rods or spatula
- Nontraumatizing ring forceps
- Surgical glue: Cyanoacrylate adhesive (N-butyl 2-cyanoacrylate)
- Other equipment includes: iris scissors, sterile Petri dishes.

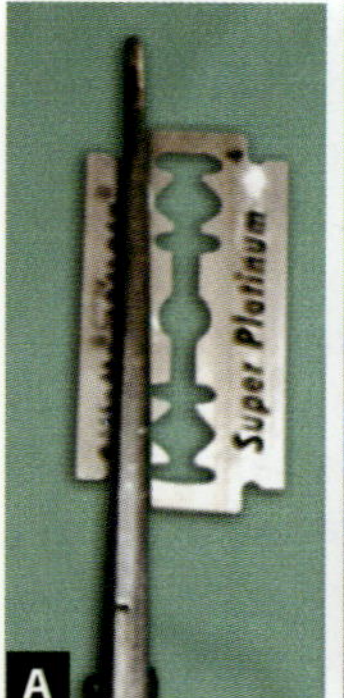

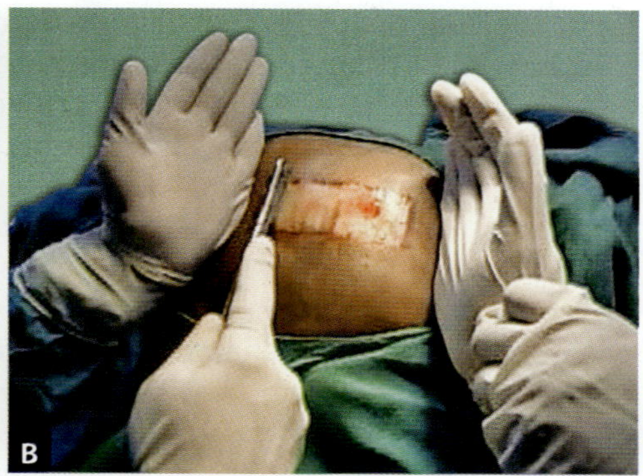

Figs. 1A and B: (A) Stainless steel blade mounted on a straight artery forceps; (B) Harvesting of split skin graft AB.

Technique

Preoperative Preparation

Shaving of the donor and recipient area is important prior to the procedure. In recipient areas where there is thick terminal hair, as the hair grows, it tends to lift up the graft. Hence, plucking the hair with a forceps after giving anesthesia, instead of shaving is said to delay hair growth, thereby preventing the graft from being lifted up.[21,22] As an alternative, chemical depilation of the hair can be carried out.[21]

STSG consists of the following steps:

Harvesting the Graft

Donor Site Preparation and Anesthesia

Harvesting the ideal split thickness graft with uniform thickness requires special surgical skill. The gluteal area is the most preferred site for obtaining a graft for obvious cosmetic reasons, though it is relatively a difficult area to harvest because of the curvature and needs more skill. Alternatively, the anterolateral aspect of the thigh, the arms[5] or the abdomen can be used as a donor site. After appropriate surgical cleansing, the required donor area is calculated and marked with a surgical pen. Topical anesthesia with eutectic mixture of local anesthetics (EMLA) may be sufficient, but in certain cases, anesthesia with lignocaine 2% may be needed.[10] A field block with 1% lignocaine at the edges should be given instead of infiltration anesthesia within the donor area to prevent an uneven surface. This can lead to harvesting a graft of uneven thickness.[23]

Graft Harvesting Technique

The procedure is commenced by an assistant stretching the skin firmly at one end, applying downward and outward traction with the help of the flat of his hand and the surgeon providing outward traction at the other end. This is done to flatten the skin as much as possible and thereby decreasing the drag felt while harvesting the graft. A split thickness graft of uniform thickness is harvested using either a sterile razor blade mounted on a Kocher's forceps (Fig. 1A) or a blade holding instrument. A straight-tip forceps such as Kelly or Rochester-Pean forceps can also be used to hold the razor blade.[10] Alternatively, a hand dermatome, Silver's knife,[24] Humby's knife[25] or a motor driven Zimmer dermatome (Zimmer Inc. Warsaw Ind USA) can also be used. While harvesting the graft, the cutting blade is held parallel to the skin surface and a sliding to-and-fro motion is then employed to cut tangentially throughout the upper dermis. The angle at which the blade is applied controls the depth of the graft (usually at 10–15°) and one should aim at obtaining a thin, translucent uniform graft. Pin point bleeding at the donor site signifies suitable depth of the graft taken. The harvested graft is then transferred to a sterile Petri-dish containing normal saline. Hemostasis is then attained at the donor site with pressure and the area is dressed with a nonadherent dressing.

Donor Area Dressing

Options for dressing the donor site include occlusive dressings (DuoDerm), semiocclusive dressings (Tegaderm),[26] semi-open dressings (Vaseline gauze) and no dressing.[27] The semiocclusive dressings are deemed to be superior as they have the fastest healing rates (average of 9 days to re-epithelialization), lowest subjective pain scores and lowest infection rates (3%).[26] They also have the advantage of being transparent and allowing ongoing inspection of the site. The rate of healing of the donor site is proportional to the number of epithelial appendages remaining and inversely proportional to the thickness of graft harvested.

Recipient Site: Preparation, Graft Placement and Immobilization

Preparation of the recipient site is a critical step to achieve successful repigmentation. The objective is to prepare a uniform denudation of the epidermis at the dermo-epidermal level to allow for plasmatic imbibition in the first 24 to 48 hours, and then vascular ingrowth to provide cellular nutrition to the donor graft, which is crucial for graft survival. There are various techniques that have been described, which include: mechanical dermabrasion using a motor driven diamond fraise or handheld dermabraders, CO_2 and Er:YAG lasers, blister formation by cryotherapy with liquid nitrogen, suction blisters and phototoxic blisters induced by psoralen plus ultraviolet A (PUVA).[28] Mechanical dermabrasion using a motor driven diamond fraise is the most commonly used technique.

Preparation

After appropriate surgical cleansing, the vitiliginous area is first marked with a surgical pen. Anesthesia may be administered using 1% lignocaine, infiltrated into four quadrants, deep dermal and subcutaneous, covering the vitiliginous area and the surrounding 4–5 cm of normal perilesional skin. Alternatively, topical anesthetic cream is applied under occlusion 2–3 hours before the procedure is sufficient in most cases.[29] For larger areas, a nerve block or general anesthesia is usually required.

Dermabrasion

The vitiliginous area (Fig. 2A) is then abraded with the help of an electric high speed dermabrader with a diamond fraise end piece. Dermabrasion must be done evenly all over the depigmented area and 2–3 mm of the perilesional normal skin, in order to prevent the development of a perigraft halo postoperatively. Dermabrasion is done till punctuate papillary bleeding is seen, which is the level of the dermoepidermal junction at the level of the papillary dermis (Fig. 2B). A manual metallic dermabrader may be used by beginners as it provides better depth control. Alternatively, an Er:YAG laser or an ultrapulse CO_2 laser can be used, particularly for critical anatomical sites. The ultrapulse CO_2 is considered better since it has the ability to achieve an epidermal-dermal split with a single pass and also achieves better hemostasis, as compared to the Er:YAG laser.[30]

Placement of Graft

Once the recipient area is abraded, the graft is transferred onto the dermabraded recipient skin, taking care to place the dermal surface facing down. The graft may be placed over a sterile glass slide with the dermal side up. Two to three punctures with a 24G needle to make tiny holes in the graft can be made in order to prevent serum accumulation under the graft. The slide is then everted on the recipient area so that the dermal side faces down. Ideally, the graft should be little larger than the recipient site, and should extend 3–5 mm beyond the edges of the abraded area. The edges of the graft should be evened out with the help of a spatula. This helps in preventing curling of the graft and thereby preventing a beaded border appearance. Once the graft has been placed one must ensure that no air, blood, serum or debris from the dermabraded area is trapped underneath the graft.

Immobilization

Proper immobilization of the graft is of utmost importance, and failure to do so may result in wrinkling and beading of the graft resulting in a relative decrease in the size of the graft. Collection of serum under the graft and poor immobilization are the two main factors for failure of graft uptake.

Various methods such as surgical adhesive, octyl-2-cyanoacrylate with a pressure dressing, the composite film and graft unit (FGU),[31] flexible collodion[3] and sprays such as Opsite spray (Smith and Nephew, United Kingdom)[32] have been tried in order to prevent the above mentioned complications. The octyl-2-cyanoacrylate adhesive is excellent to secure the graft and in addition

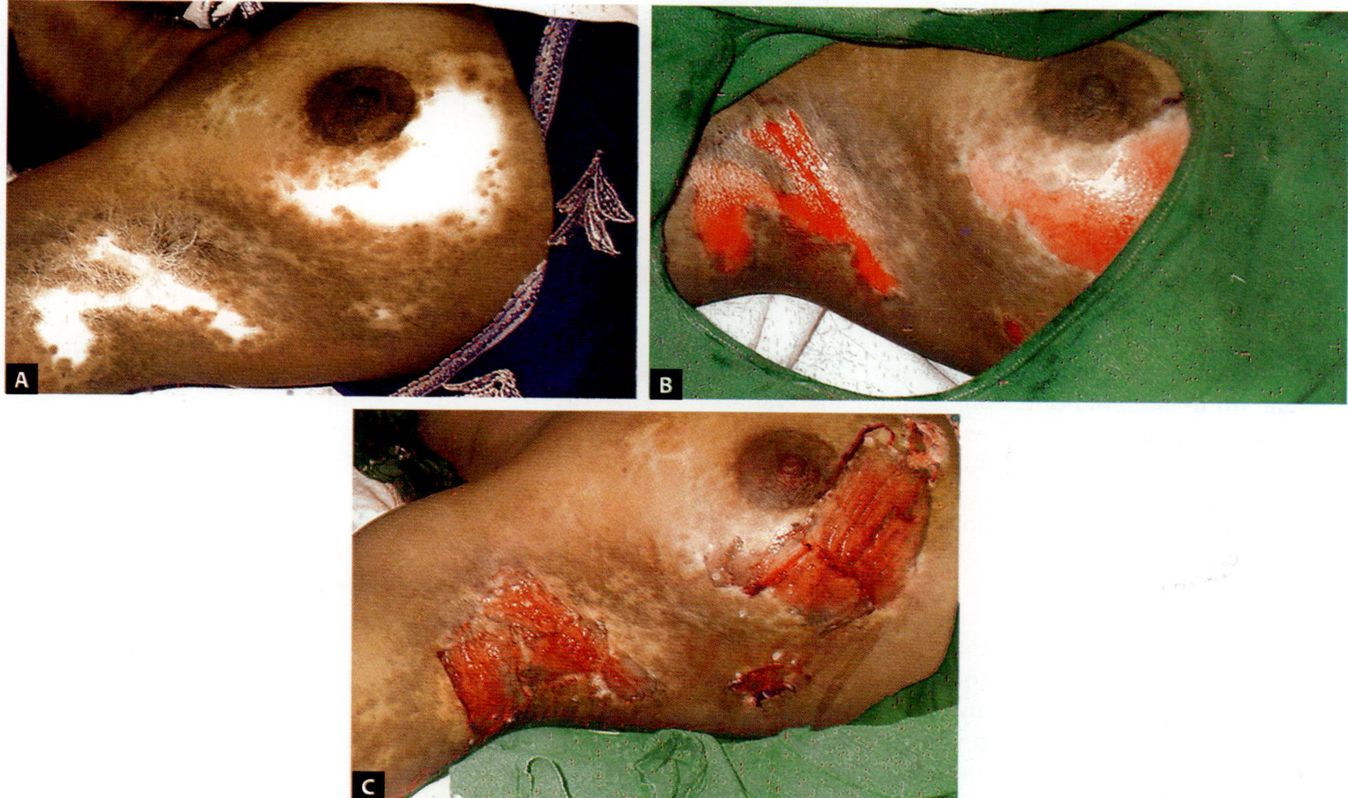

Figs. 2A to C: (A) Lesion before dermabrasion; (B) Dermabraded recipient area; (C) Graft fixed with surgical glue.

also exhibits antimicrobial properties against *Staphylococci, Pseudomonas,* and *Escherichia coli.*[33] It is best applied at the edges of the graft in an interrupted manner (Fig. 2C). In a study of 50 patients of stable, recalcitrant vitiligo, treated with STSG of over 180 lesions, cyanoacrylate adhesive was effective in immobilizing the grafts especially over the mobile areas.[34] The composite FGU consists of a semipermeable thin film (Tegaderm) and the harvested thin graft, wherein the film is placed over the graft and slightly beyond it. The adhesive nature of the film prevents beading or curling of the graft. A pressure dressing may be given with an elastocrepe bandage to avoid hematoma or seroma formation.

Postoperative Care

The patient is counseled regarding strict immobilization of the site where the graft is placed. Antibiotics are administered for a week. The first dressing change is done preferably after 24 hours, to check for formation of any seroma or hematoma underneath the graft. Drainage of the seroma or hematoma is done by making a small incision over the collection and expressing the underlying contents. One should not attempt to express the fluid out from the edge of the graft as this may disrupt the adherence of the whole graft. In case of a flexible collodion dressing windows of 0.5 cm diameter are made with the help of acetone to observe for seroma, blood or air.[16]

Dressing is subsequently changed after 1 week by which time the graft is usually taken up and healing is complete. When removing the dressing, one can moisten it with saline to reduce adherence to the graft. The dressing may then be carefully removed to prevent lifting the graft-off of the underlying wound bed. Donor site dressing is also changed after 1 week.

Expected Outcomes

The systematic reviews by Njoo et al.[35] on autologous transplantation methods show that the highest mean success rates are achieved by STSG, which range from 87% to 91%. Agrawal et al.[36] treated 32 sites in 21 patients with stable refractory vitiligo using this technique. They reported 100% repigmentation in 68% of the patches and 90–95% repigmentation in the remaining patches. It took an average.[6] 3 months to achieve close to a full color match.

Compared to other techniques split-thickness grafting appears to be better than control, suction blister, or combined split-thickness or suction grafts.[37] Compared to blister grafting, the STSG can cover a larger surface area. Ozdemir et al.[38] demonstrated a higher percent of repigmentation with the STSG technique than the suction blister grafting in a single patient. As compared to mini punch grafting the STSG technique produces far more cosmetically superior results and matching over larger areas. Repigmentation is greater in patients treated with photochemotherapy plus split thickness skin graft versus punch grafts.[39]

Complications

Complications may occur either at recipient site or donor site.

At the Recipient Site

These include the following:

- Graft rejection
- Seroma or hematoma formation: The most common cause of graft rejection is accumulation of air bubbles, serum (seroma) or blood (hematoma) underneath the graft surface. They prevent adherence of the graft to the underlying wound bed, thereby depleting the graft of the required nutrition. Meshing the graft can be considered as an effective way of preventing seroma formation.[40] Movement or shifting of the graft is also a cause of graft rejection as it results in disrupting the attachment of the graft to the recipient site. One must counsel the patient regarding immobilization, especially if the graft is placed on a joint. Longitudinal strips of grafts arranged parallel to the skin creases can be used at these sites.[8] Another common cause of failure of graft uptake is due to technical error wherein the graft is placed upside down, with the epidermal surface of the graft in contact with the dermal surface of the wound bed. Trauma to the graft or excessive stretching of the graft may also result in partial failure of graft uptake. A recipient site having poor vascularity or surface contamination can also result in graft failure.
- Textural abnormalities: Failure to even out the edges of the graft results in "curling" or "branching", resulting in peripheral beading at the graft edge or a "stuck on tire patch" appearance.
- Hyperpigmentation: This is a relatively common complication, especially in dark skinned individuals and takes a long time to resolve (Fig. 3).[41] This can be treated with topical retinoids or chemical peeling (personal observation) or with laser resurfacing, or at times, with superficial dermabrasion.
- Perigraft halo: Peripheral depigmentation or achromic fissures at the graft edge occurs primarily due to graft contraction (Fig. 3). The graft should ideally extend 3–5 mm beyond the abraded area to avoid this complication. They can be treated with topical or systemic psoralens or NB-UVB.[23] Al-Mutairi et al.[42] have used excimer laser (308 nm) after grafting to minimize the chances of developing perigraft halo or achromic fissures.[26]
- Hypertrophy: Thick grafts usually are the cause of hypertrophy. This usually subsides spontaneously in 3–4 months. Topical retinoids or topical midpotent corticosteroids can be used to treat this complication.[23]
- Milia: Formation of milia is common on the face and neck, which is due to remnants of epidermis following dermabrasion (Figs. 4A to C). They resolve spontaneously or can be expressed out.
- Secondary infection: If proper aseptic precautions are maintained, secondary infection is relatively uncommon complication of this procedure.[43]

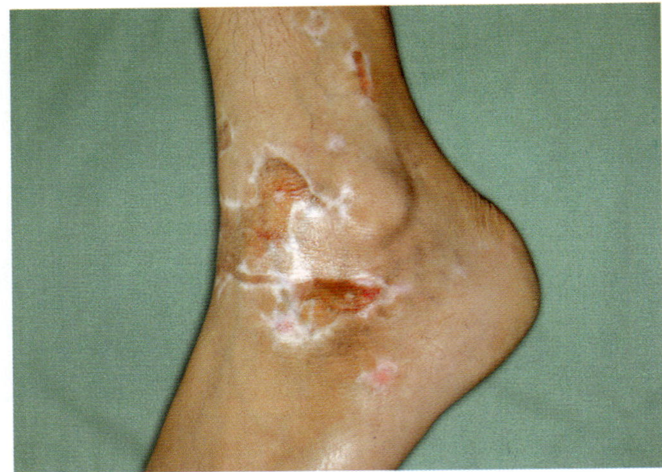

Fig. 3: Split skin graft showing hyperpigmentation and perigraft halo.

- Reactivation of vitiligo: This may occur at the graft site or the perigraft area.

Complications at the Donor Site

These include the following:

- Post-inflammatory hyperpigmentation: This is common in darker skins and can persist even up to 1 year.
- Scarring: Superficial scarring can occur at the donor site, especially when thick grafts have been harvested.
- Recurrence or koebnerization: Occurrence of vitiligo at the donor site.

Advantages and Disadvantages of STSG

Advantages and disadvantages of STSG are shown in Box 1.

Technique Modifications at Special Sites

Certain areas such as eyelids, lips, acral areas and genital area are difficult areas to graft. Successful results can be attained by managing difficult to treat sites with modifications in the original technique.

Eyelids: The thinnest graft should be selected for the eyelid area. Eye shields may be used by beginners during dermabrasion for protection. Strict immobilization is required for the first 72 hours, and this can be achieved by cyanoacrylate adhesive and pressure bandage (Figs. 4A to C).

Lips: Although, the suction blister technique is considered a good option for small areas on the lip, the split thickness graft gives optimal results for slightly larger areas. Care should be taken to secure the graft with cyanoacrylate adhesive first along the mucosal side and then straightening out the graft onto the surrounding normal skin.

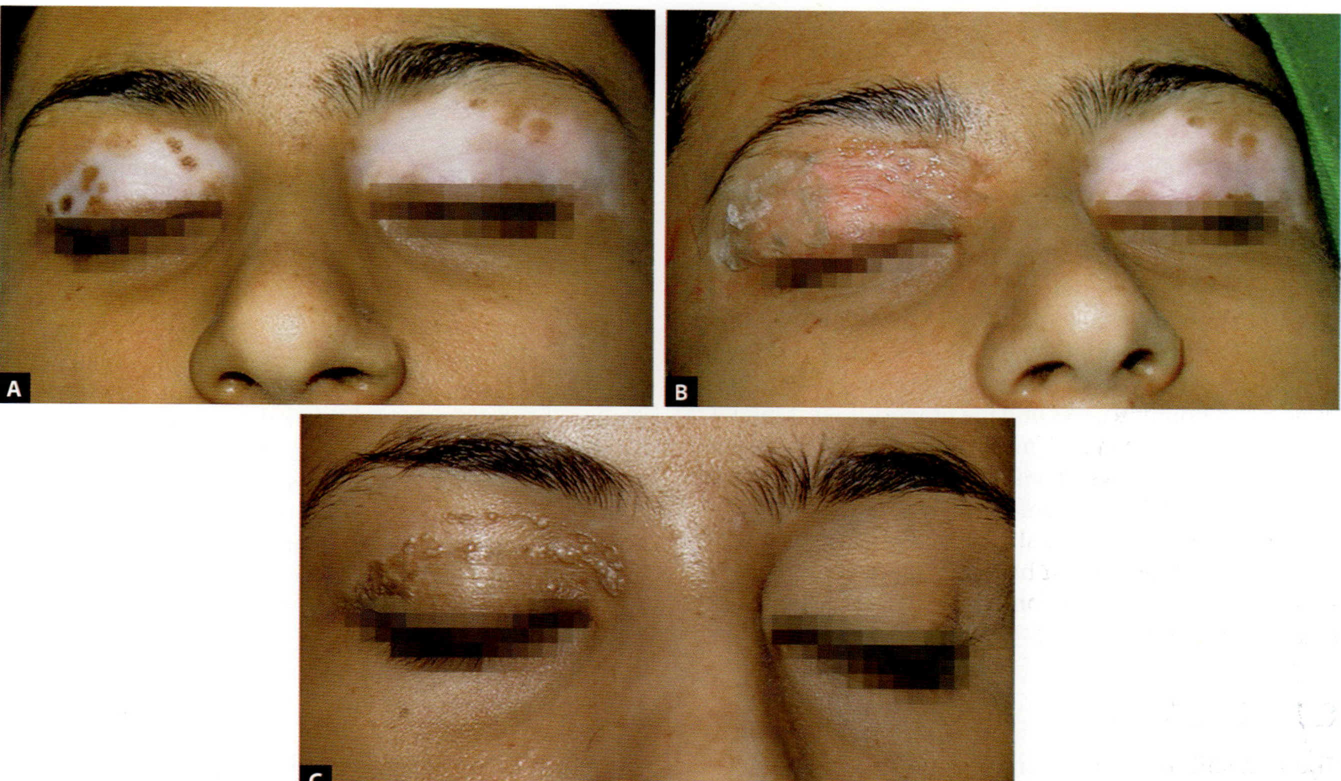

Figs. 4A to C: (A) Vitiligo lesions on eyelids; (B) Vitiligo lesion after grafting on right eyelid; (C) Excellent results, but with milia on right eyelid.

Box 1: Advantages and disadvantages of split thickness skin grafting

Advantages of thin split thickness skin grafting

- Large areas can be covered in a single sitting, resulting in quick results over a short period of time
- Grafted areas appear skin colored immediately after the operation
- Excellent cosmetic matching over large areas
- Uniform pigmentation—no "cobblestoning" as compared to miniature punch grafing[39]
- Relatively simple and cost effective procedure. No reagents, laboratory facilities or elaborate equipment is required, as compared to noncultured or cultured melanocyte suspensions
- Repigmentation of leukotrichia is possible with this technique[44,45]
- Difficult areas such as eyelids, inner canthus of eyes, areola and nipples can be treated with relatively successful outcomes
- Procedure is less time consuming as compared to punch grafting, suction blister grafting and melanocyte suspension methods

Disadvantages

- Hyperpigmentation is common, especially in dark skinned individuals and particularly on the exposed areas
- Superficial scarring may occur at the donor site
- Multiple sittings may be required when large areas need to be covered
- Surgical skill is required to take adequate sized, thin grafts. However, the use of electric dermatomes has made it simpler to harvest uniform thin grafts
- Tips, palms, soles and mucous membranes are difficult to graft by this method. Inherent differences occur in the histology of the oral mucosa and skin, and any procedure involving partial-thickness grafts from keratinized skin may lead to mismatch in texture and disfigurement.[46] Scarring and contracture at the recipient area in addition to the donor site morbidity is a common phenomenon when split thickness grafts are applied in the oral mucosa to cover the full-thickness defects[47,48]
- Furthermore, there is a risk of malignant transformation in such keratinized grafts applied in the oral mucosa[49]
- The STSG technique provides a yield of 1:1 ratio,[50] although a modification of the technique called the "flip- top" graft may be used; wherein 3–5 mm thinly shaved dermoepidermal fragments are inserted under very thin flaps raised on the recipient site. Repigmentation occurs by coalescence of pigment spread arising from multiple grafts within a few months after grafting[51]

Alternately, the graft may be secured by 5-0 Prolene(R) sutures at the edges, to prevent graft displacement. It is preferable to admit the patient and give intravenous fluids and nil orally for the first 24 hours. A semisolid or liquid diet through a straw is advised till the dressing is removed. Sutures and dressing are removed in a week.[28]

Acral areas: The presence of a thicker epidermis, leading to inadequate dermabrasion and inability to prepare a good vascular bed, makes the acral sites one of the toughest sites to treat with this technique. These sites are also more prone to friction and trauma, making koebnerization a common phenomenon.[52] Thin split thickness grafting may be used for dorsal sites, and immobilization is essential, by splinting the fingers. The dorsa of fingers and periungual areas take up mini punch grafts better than STSGs, wherein graft contracture and rejection are major limitations.

Genital areas: Conventional surgical therapies such as mini-punch grafts or ultrathin split-thickness grafts from keratinized skin are not suitable for the nonkeratinized mucosa of the glans penis because this may lead to gross mismatch in texture and color.[53] History of genital herpes must be taken before attempting a surgery at these sites, as it can be a potential reason for failure of the surgical procedure. Long-term prophylaxis with acyclovir should be given in proven and doubtful cases and the prognosis is explained.[21] Autologous, noncultured melanocyte- keratinocyte cell transplantation is considered as the preferred and effective surgical option for management of genital vitiligo.[54,55]

The above discussion shows that a surgeon dealing with vitiligo surgery must have adequate expertise of all various methods as often combination treatments give the best results[56] (Figs. 5A and B).

CONCLUSION

The thin split thickness skin graft technique is effective, simple to learn, gives rapid results, provides good cosmesis and can be used to treat large as well as "difficult to treat" areas. Furthermore, it is a cost effective procedure which does not require elaborate settings. The above mentioned reasons make it one of the most popular surgical modalities used for treating stable vitiligo. However the newer modalities of cellular transplants, which have been simplified and have better textural results are the preferred modalities particularly for larger areas, whereas split thickness grafting techniques are preferred if immediate results are required.

Treatment Pearls

1. Acquire training—mastering split thickness skin grafting requires a certain amount of skill, training and practice—preferably learn the technique, observe and assist closely before attempting a solo procedure.
2. "Practice makes perfect": For beginners practice taking small but ultrathin grafts of uniform thickness which is devoid of dermal tissue as this is the key to good cosmesis and an appropriate color match. Slowly graduate to taking larger grafts and attempting larger areas. There are various ways of harvesting the graft, choose one you are most comfortable with.
3. Dermabrade the skin 1–2 mm beyond the margins of the vitiligo lesion and place the grafts beyond the dermabraded margins to minimize the chances of perigraft halo formation.
4. Proper immobilization is essential after grafting to ensure satisfactory results.
5. Use ring blocks at the donor site to ensures a smooth surface for graft placement. Infiltration anesthesia at the donor area may lead to an irregular surface.
6. Use NBUVB, PUVA, or excimer laser if there is a delay in the onset of repigmentation—practice caution as overuse of psoralens may lead to hyperpigmentation.
7. Counsel your patient well, regarding the advantages and disadvantages.

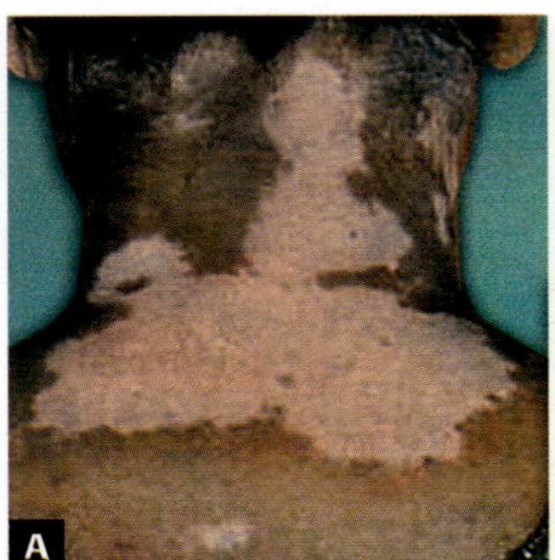

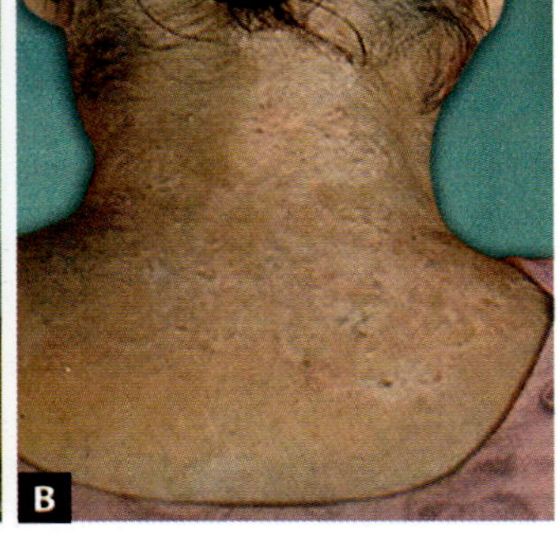

Figs. 5A and B: (A) Vitiligo patch on upper back and neck; (B) Excellent result after split thickness grafting.

REFERENCES

1. Mulekar SV, Isedeh P. Surgical interventions for vitiligo: an evidence-based review. Br J Dermatol. 2013;169:57-66.
2. Falabella R. History and chronology of development of surgical therapies for vitiligo. In: Gupta S, Olsson MS, Kanwar AJ, Ortonne JP (Eds). Surgical management of vitiligo, 1st edition. Massachusetts, USA: Blackwell Publishing; 2007:41-8.
3. Behl PN. Treatment of vitiligo with homologous thin Thiersch's skin grafts. Curr Med Pract. 1964;8:218-21.
4. Skouge JW. Split thickness skin grafting. In: Skouge JW, Gerkin RL (Eds). Skin Grafting, 1st edition. New York:Churchill Livingstone Inc; 1991;5-45.
5. Kahn AM, Cohen MJ. Vitiligo: Treatment by dermabrasion and epithelial sheet grafting. J Am Acad Dermatol. 1995;33; 646-8.
6. Kahn AM, Cohen MJ. Repigmentation in vitiligo patients. Melanocyte transfer via ultra-thin grafts. Dermatol Surg.1998;24(3):365-7.
7. Olsson MJ, Juhlin L. Epidermal sheet grafts for repigmentation of vitiligo and piebaldism, with a review of surgical techniques. Acta Derm Venereol. 1997;77:463-6.
8. Sameem F, Sultan SJ, Ahmad QM. Split thickness skin grafting in patients with stable vitiligo. J Cutan Aesthet Surg. 2011;4:38-40.
9. Khunger N. Vitiligo surgery. In: Robinson JK (ed.). Surgery of the skin: procedural dermatology. 2nd edition. UK: Elsevier Health Sciences; 2010. pp. 683-92.
10. Foroozan M, Pouaha J, Truchetet F. Simple method for harvesting split-thickness skin grafts. Dermatol Surg. 2010;36:1743-5.
11. Khunger N. Thin split-thickness skin grafts for vitiligo. In: Gupta S (Ed). In surgical management of vitiligo. Blackwell Publishing Ltd; 2007;108-14.
12. Rudolph R. Inhibition of myofibroblasts by skin grafts. Plast Reconstr Surg. 1979;63(4):473-80.
13. Kim HY, Kang KY. Epidermal grafts for treatment of stable and progressive vitiligo. J Am Acad Dermatol. 1999;41:412-7.
14. Mutalik S, Ginzburg A. Surgical management of stable vitiligo: a review with personal experience. Dermatol Surg. 2000;26:248-54.

15. Boersma BR, Westerhof W, Bos JD. Repigmentation in vitiligo vulgaris by autologous minigrafting: result in nineteen patients. J Am Acad Dermatol. 1995;33:990-5.
16. Kim HU, Yun SK. Suction device for epidermal grafting in vitiligo: employing a syringe and manometer to provide an adequate negative pressure. Dermatol Surg. 2000;26:702-4.
17. Hann SK, Im S, Bong HW, et al. Treatment of stable vitiligo with autologous epidermal grafting and PUVA. J Am Acad Dermatol. 1995;32:943-8.
18. Falabella R, Escobar C, Borrero I. Treatment of refractory and stable vitiligo by transplantation of in vitro cultured epidermal autografts bearing melanocytes. J Am Acad Dermatol. 1992;26:230-6.
19. Parsad D, Gupta S. IADVL Dermatosurgery Task Force. Standard guidelines of care for vitiligo surgery. Indian J Dermatol Venereol Leprol. 2008;74:S37-45.
20. Falabella R, Arrunategui A, Barona MI, et al. The minigrafting test for vitiligo: detection of stable lesions for melanocyte transplantation. J Am Acad Dermatol. 1995;32:228-32.
21. Khunger N. Vitiligo Surgery. In: Khunger N, Sachdev M (Eds). Practical manual of cosmetic dermatology and surgery, 1st edition. India: Mehta Publishers; 2010.
22. Van Geel N, Ongenae K, de Mil M, et al. Modified technique of autologous noncultured epidermal cell transplantation for repigmenting vitiligo: a pilot study. Dermatol Surg. 2001;27:873-6.
23. Khunger N, Kathuria SD, Ramesh V. Tissue grafts in vitiligo surgery- past, present and future. Indian J Dermatol. 2009:54(2):150-8.
24. Ozdemir M, Centikale O, Wolf R, et al. Comparison of two surgical approaches for treating vitiligo: a preliminary study. Int J Dermatol. 2002;41(3):135-8.
25. McGregor IA, McGregor AD. Fundamental techniques of plastic surgery, 9th edition. Edinburg: Churchill Livingstone; 1995;35-9.
26. Terrill PJ, Goh RC, Bailey MJ. Split-thickness skin graft donor sites: a comparative study of two absorbent dressings. J Wound Care. 2007;16(10):433-8.
27. Kilinc H, Sensoz O, Ozdemir R, et al. Which dressing for split-thickness skin graft donor sites? Ann Plast Surg. 2001;46(4):409-14.
28. Al-Hadidi N, Griffith JL, Al-Jamal MS, Hamzavi I. Role of Recipient-site Preparation Techniques and Post-operative Wound Dressing in the Surgical Management of Vitiligo. J Cutan Aesthet Surg. 2015;8:79-87.
29. Juhlin L, Olsson MJ. Optimal application times of eutectic mixtures of local anesthetics (EMLA) cream before dermabrasion of vitiliginous skin. Eur J Dermatol. 1995;5:365-70.
30. Oh CK, Cha JH, Lim LY, et al. Treatment of vitiligo with suction epidermal grafting by the use of an ultrapulse CO_2 laser with a computerized pattern generator. Dermatol Surg. 2001;27(6):565-8.
31. Malakar S, Malakar RS. Surgical pearl: composite film and graft unit for the recipient area dressing after split-thickness skin grafting in vitiligo. J Am Acad Dermatol. 2001;44:856-7.
32. Mysore V. Punch grafting in vitiligo. Gulf J Dermatol. 2000;7:27-31.
33. Toriumi DM, O'Grody K, Desai D, et al. Use of octyl-2-cyanoacrylate for skin closure in facial plastic surgery. Plast Reconstr Surg. 1998;102(6):2209-19.
34. Khunger N, Lahiri K, Mysore V. Surgical treatment of vitiligo. In: Robinson JK, Hanke W, Siegel DM, Fratila A (Eds). Surgery of the Skin, 2nd Edition. Elsevier Inc. USA; 2010;683-93.
35. Njoo MD, Westerhof W, Bos JD, et al. A systematic review of autologous transplantation methods in vitiligo. Arch Dermatol. 1998;134:1543-9.
36. Agrawal K, Agrawal A. Vitiligo: repigmentation with dermabrasion and thin split-thickness skin graft. Dermatol Surg. 1995;21:295-300.
37. Whitton ME, Ashcroft DM, Gonzalez U. Therapeutic interventions for vitiligo. J Am Acad Dermatol. 2008;59(4):713-7.
38. Ozdemir M, Cetinkale O, Wolf R, et al. Comparison of two surgical approaches for treating vitiligo: a preliminary study. Int J Dermatol. 2002;41(3):135-8.
39. Khandpur S, Sharma VK, Manchanda Y. Comparison of minipunch grafting versus split-skin grafting in chronic stable vitiligo. Dermatol Surg. 2005;31:436-41.
40. Acikel C, Ulkur E, Celikoz B. Carbon dioxide laser resurfacing and thin skin grafting in the treatment of "stable and recalcitrant" vitiligo. Plast Reconstr Surg. 2003;111:1291-8.
41. Khunger N. Recent advances in the surgical treatment of vitiligo. In: Ghosh S (Ed). Recent advances in dermatology, volume 2. India: Jaypee Medical Publishers (P) Ltd; 2007;319-40.
42. Al-Mutairi N, Manchanda Y, Al-Doukhi A, et al. Long-term results of split-skin grafting in combination with excimer laser for stable vitiligo. Dermatol Surg. 2010;36(4):499-505.
43. Behl PN, Azad O, Kak R, et al. Autologous thin Thierschs grafts in vitiligo: experience of 8000 cases 50000 grafts (1959-98) with modified technique in 198 cases in the year 1997-98. Indian J Derm Venereol Leprol. 1999;65(3):117-21.
44. Agrawal K, Agrawal A. Vitiligo: surgical repigmentation of leukotrichia. Dermatol Surg. 1995;21(8):711-5.
45. Bose SK. Is there any treatment of leukotrichia in stable vitiligo? J Dermatol. 1997;24(9):615-7.
46. Gupta S, Sandhu K, Kanwar A, et al. Melanocyte transfer via epidermal grafts for vitiligo of labial mucosa. Dermatol Surg. 2004;30(1):45-8.
47. Rhee PH, Friedman CD, Ridge JA, et al. The use of processed allograft dermal matrix for intraoral resurfacing: an alternative to split-thickness skin grafts. Arch Otolaryngol Head Neck Surg. 1998;124(11):1201-4.
48. Mitchell R. The use of collagen in oral surgery. Ann Acad Med Singapore. 1986;15(3):355-60.
49. Sa'do B, Nakamura N, Higuchi Y, et al. Squamous cell carcinoma of the oral cavity derived from a skin graft: a case report. Head Neck. 1994;16(1):79-82.
50. Falabella R. Surgical approaches for stable vitiligo. Dermatol Surg. 2005;31(10):1277-84.
51. McGovern TW, Bolognia J, Leffell DJ. Flip-top pigment transplantation: a novel transplantation procedure for the treatment of depigmentation. Arch Dermatol. 1999;135(11):1305-7.
52. Mutalik S. Surgical management of acral vitiligo. In: Gupta S (Ed). Surgical management of vitiligo. Blackwell Publishing Ltd; 2007;225-8.
53. Gupta S. Commentary on: genital vitiligo treated by autologous, noncultured melanocyte-keratinocyte cell transplant. Derm Surg 2005;31:1740.
54. Mulekar SV, Al Issa A, Al Eisa A, Asaad M. Genital vitiligo treated by autologous, noncultured melanocyte-keratinocyte cell transplantation. Dermatol Surg. 2005;31:1737-40.
55. Mulekar SV, Al Issa A, Al Eisa A. Treatment of vitiligo on difficult-to-treat sites using autologous noncultured cellular grafting. Dermatol Surg. 2009;35(1):66-71.
56. Pahwa M, Gupta S, Khunger N. Multi modal single step vitiligo surgery(MMSSVS): A novel approach. Dermatol Surg. 2010;36(10):1627-31.

Chapter

37A

Epidermal Noncultured Cell Suspension in Vitiligo

Munish Paul

Key Messages

- Tissue grafts have the limitation of smaller area coverage
- Cellular grafts need a small size of donor, which can then be used to cover a large vitiligo area
- The vital steps in epidermal noncultured suspension include donor harvesting, trypsinization to separate the cells, antitrypsinization to remove excess trypsin, centrifugation to make a suspension of cells
- The donor recipient area coverage is in the ratio 1:8–1:10
- It is suitable for all areas
- Limitations include higher cost, need for trained staff and a longer learning curve.

INTRODUCTION

As discussed in earlier Chapters, medical treatments are not successful in all cases of vitiligo.[1-3] Tissue grafts have the limitations that large amount of donor skin is needed as there is no cell expansion in these methods.[4,5] Hence, transplantation of autologous cultured and noncultured melanocytes which involve cell suspension without culture or keratinocyte/melanocyte co-cultures[6-10] are gaining popularity. Transplantation of noncultured melanocytes/keratinocytes suspension has the advantage that cell culture is not needed and that skin harvesting from the donor area, cell separation and application of melanocytes can all be undertaken in a single 3 hour procedure.

Indications, contraindications, case selection, preoperative investigations have all been dealt with in earlier chapters. This Chapter will deal therefore only with specific details of the procedure.

PROCEDURE

- Harvesting a skin graft
- Trypsinization and cell separation
- Dermabrasion of the recipient (vitiligo) site
- Transfer and fixing of melanocyte rich cell suspension.

Accompanying Box 1 and Figures 1 to 8 demonstrate these steps.

Harvesting of Skin Graft

The lateral aspect of the gluteal region is selected as the donor area. Care should be taken to ensure that the donor area has no vitiligo patches. The area of split thickness donor skin taken is one-tenth of the recipient area while dealing with large confluent patches. In cases having multiple scattered small patches, larger donor skin is taken, approximately one-fifth of the recipient area. Under aseptic precautions, a very superficial sample is harvested using a shaving blade held in straight Kocher's forceps. The donor area is dressed with liquid paraffin dressing (Fairlee™) and a sterile gauze pad.

Cell Separation Technique (Box 1)

This is the most important step and consists of three steps; trypsinization, removal of excess trypsin by antitrypsin and centrifugation to obtain a cell suspension.

1. *Trypsinization*: The cell separation is done ideally under aseptic precautions in a laminar flow bench kept in the operation theatre. If laminar flow bench is not available, the sterile environment of the theater is adequate. The skin sample harvested is transferred to a Petri dish containing 5 mL of the 0.2% w/v trypsin solution, epidermal side facing upwards, and incubated for 45 min at 37°C.

Box 1: Steps in obtaining epidermal noncultured cell suspension (Figs. 1 to 8)

- Step 1: A split thickness thin graft is harvested under local/topical anesthesia
- Step 2: Graft is placed in a Petri dish containing 5 mL of 0.2% trypsin + 0.8% ethylenediaminetetraacetic acid (EDTA) solution
- Step 3: Graft is soaked completely in the solution and spread out with epidermal surface facing upwards
- Step 4: Incubated in an incubator at 37° for 45 minutes to 2 hours
- Step 5: Trypsin solution is neutralized by 5 mL of 0.5% trypsin inhibitor
- Step 6: Dermis is teased out from the epidermis and discarded
- Step 7: The cells are separated from the epidermis and transferred to a test tube
- Step 8: The test tube with epidermal cells is centrifuged for 5 minutes to obtain a pellet rich in cells
- Step 9: The pellet is resuspended in phosphate-buffered saline (PBS)/ Dulbecco's modified Eagle's medium (DMEM) and transferred to 1 mL tuberculin syringe, ready for application onto the recipient area

2. *Removal of excess trypsin*: After incubation for 45 minutes-2 hours, the action of trypsin is neutralized with trypsin inhibitor (Life Technologies, USA). The epidermis is separated from the dermis and transferred to a test tube containing 2 mL of DMEM: Nutrient mixture F-12 (DMEM/F-12) medium (Life Technologies) and vortex-mixed for 15 seconds. The epidermis is further broken into smaller pieces in a Petri dish and washed with the DMEM/F-12 medium and finally transferred to a test tube containing the DMEM/F-12 medium.
3. *Centrifugation*: The test tube is then centrifuged for 6 minutes. The supernatant is discarded and the pellet at the bottom is suspended in a 1 mL insulin syringe. The final volume prepared varies from 0.2–0.5 mL depending on the size of the graft taken and the area to be treated.

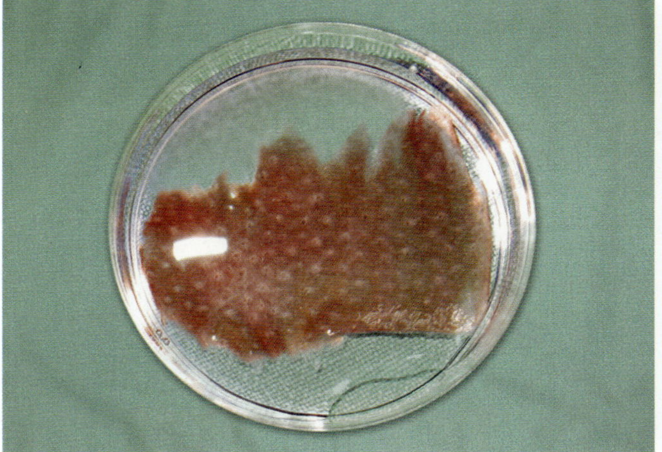

Fig. 1: In the first step a very thin skin graft is taken from the thigh and incubated at 37° with trypsin enzyme for 45 minutes to induce separation of the various layers of the skin. The size of donor area required is only 1/10 of the vitiligo area to be operated.

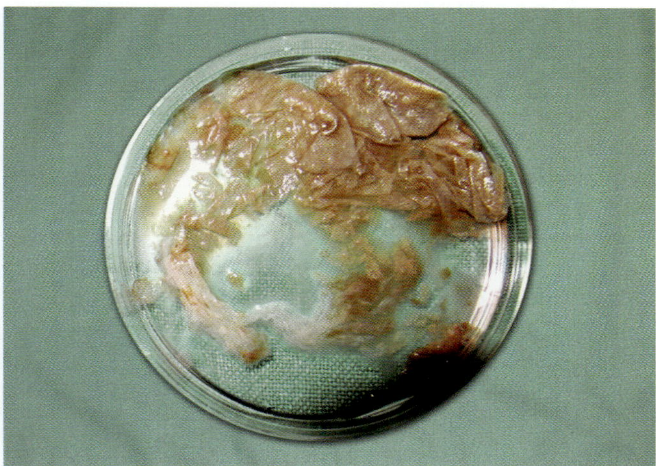

Fig. 2: The trypsin enzyme dissolves the various layers of skin so that the epidermis (upper layer), dermis (middle layer) are separated and skin is now in a liquid state.

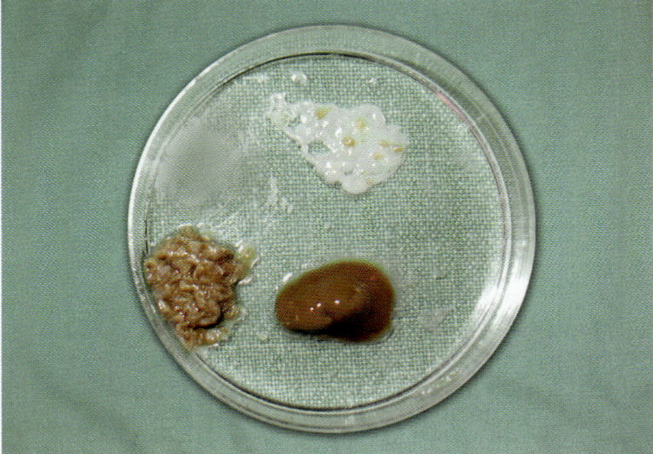

Fig. 3: All the layers of skin have separated: White is dermis, light brown fraction is upper epidermis and dark brown is melanocyte rich cell suspension.

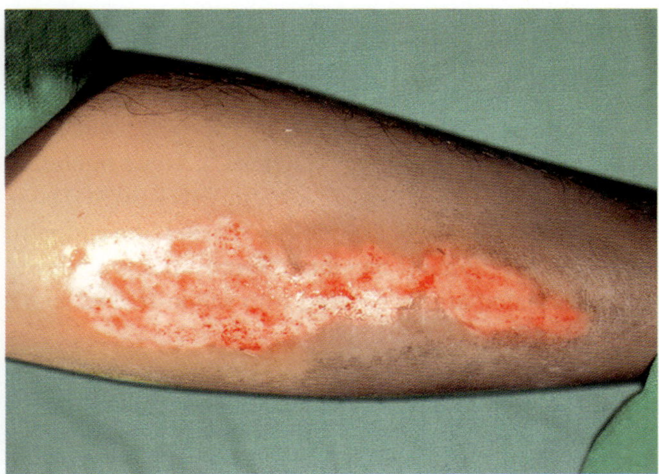

Fig. 4: The skin of the vitiligo area to be treated is removed very superficially with a erbium yag laser or diamond burrs.

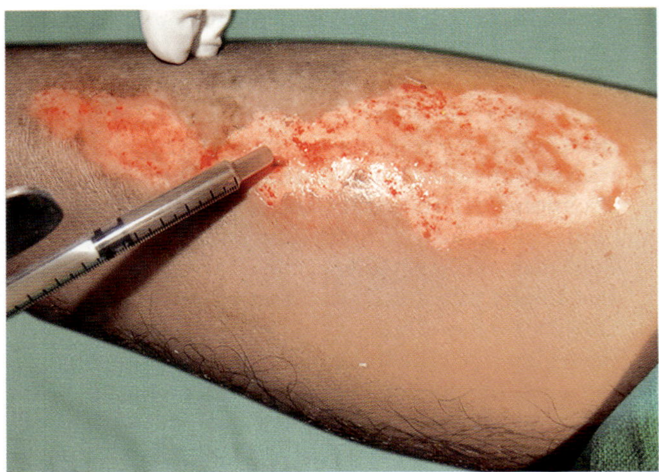

Fig. 5: The melanocyte rich cell suspension (pigment cells) is applied on the laser ablated area uniformly.

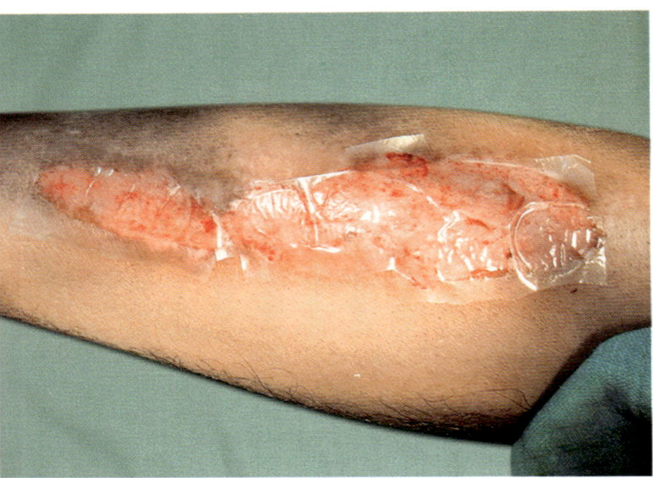

Fig. 6: Collagen dressings are applied on the transplanted cells to ensure that they get fixed completely on the area to be operated.

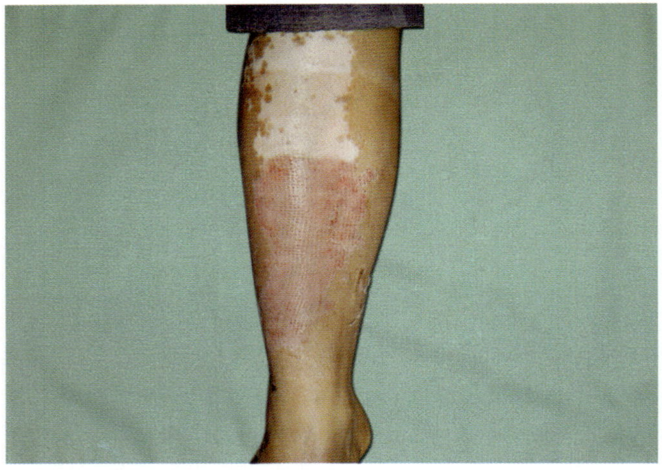

Fig. 7: The operated area heals completely in 7 days and looks pink in color. At this stage, concealer makeup can be used and patient can resume normal bath and activity.

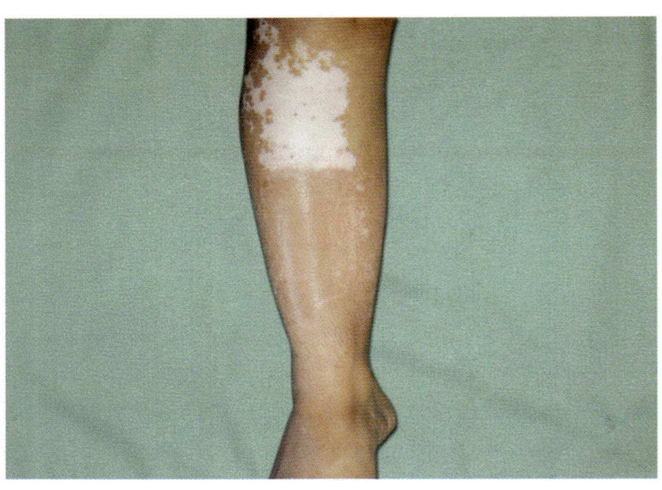

Fig. 8: The operated area has completely achieved pigmentation in 3 months and there is good color and texture matching.

Dermabrasion of the Recipient Site

The recipient site is abraded with a dermabrader fitted with a diamond fraise wheel (Delasco™). While operating close to the eyelid margins, an erbium:YAG (Er:YAG) laser is used with a fluence of 1,000 mJ, 1–2 passes. The endpoint of ablation is pinpoint bleeding. Hemostasis is achieved and the ablated area is covered with saline-soaked gauze pieces.

Transplantation Technique

The cell suspension is spread evenly on the dermabraded area with 1 mL insulin syringe and covered with collagen dressing (Collomedica laboratories) to hold the cells applied. This is covered with liquid paraffin dressing and gauze pieces. Patients are instructed to lie still in the same position for at least 1 hour to ensure cell fixation and then shifted to a room and further instructed to avoid excessive movements of the treated area for at least 6 hours.

POSTPROCEDURE INSTRUCTIONS

All patients are instructed to take complete rest and avoid all vigorous physical activities. Patients are prescribed oral antibacterial agents for 5 days and nonsteroidal anti-inflammatory drugs (NSAIDs) for 3 days. The dressings are removed after 1 week in most cases. Patients are asked to follow-up at weeks 1 and 3 and then at 3 month intervals. Patients are instructed not to scrub the area. Patients are permitted to use make-up on the treated area 10 days after the removal of dressings.

ONSET OF PIGMENTATION

The onset of pigmentation usually occurs in 3–6 weeks and it can take 3–6 months for the patches to achieve significant pigmentation. Psoralen ultraviolet A (PUVA) with sunlight or phototherapy can be initiated after 3 weeks. Vitiligo patches which do not recover even after 6 months will need to be transplanted again. Figures 9 to 12 show before and after photographs in different areas-hands, neck and scalp. Box 2 shows the advantages and disadvantages of non-cultured epidermal cell suspension (NCECS) technique.

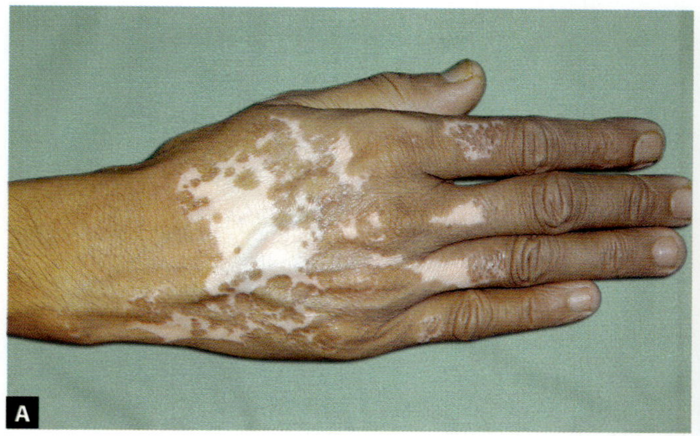

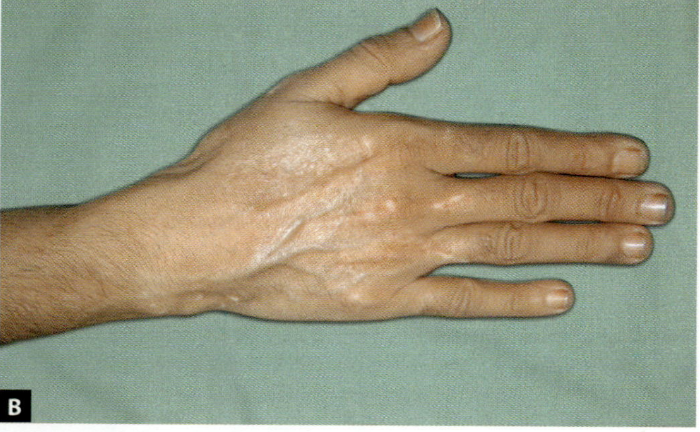

Figs. 9A and B: Vitiligo hand (A) Pretreatment; (B) Post cell transfer.

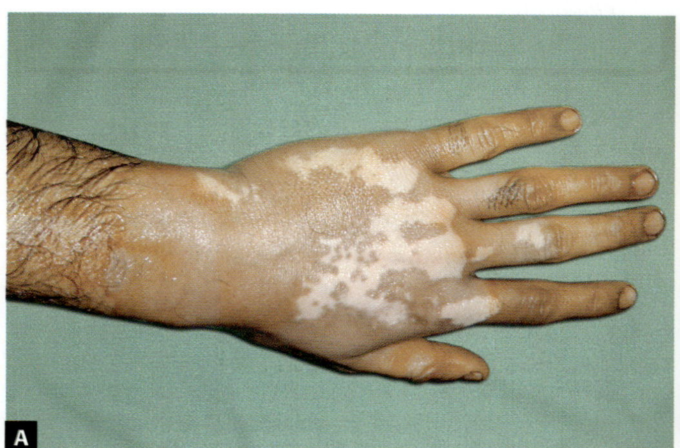

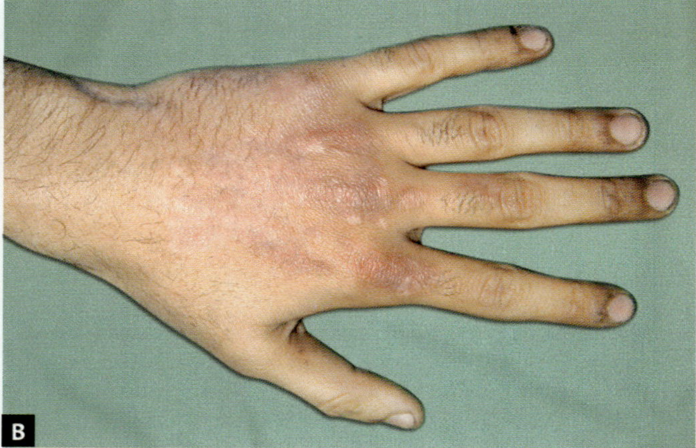

Figs. 10A and B: Vitiligo hand (A) Pretreatment; (B) Post cell transfer.

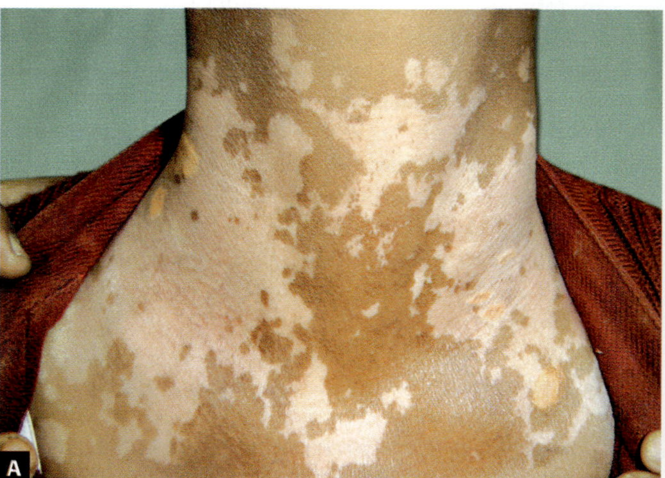

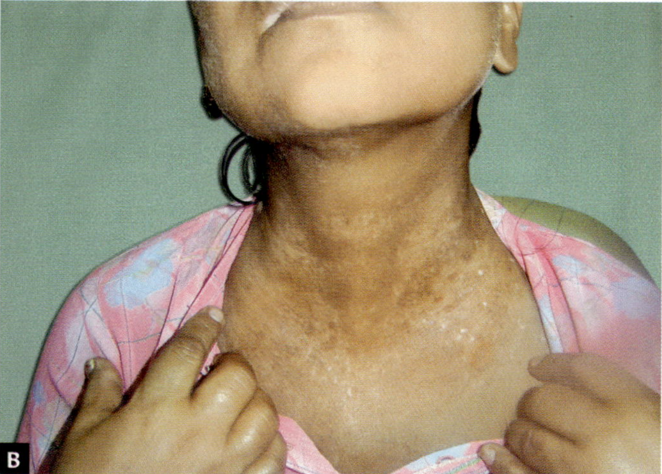

Figs. 11A and B: Vitiligo neck (A) Before treatment; (B) Post cell transfer.

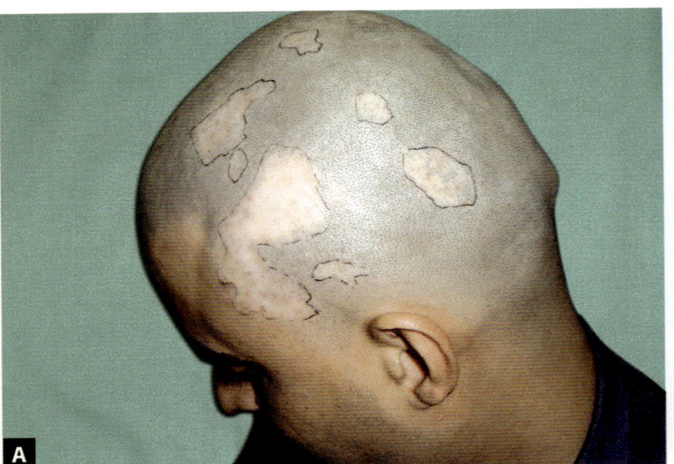

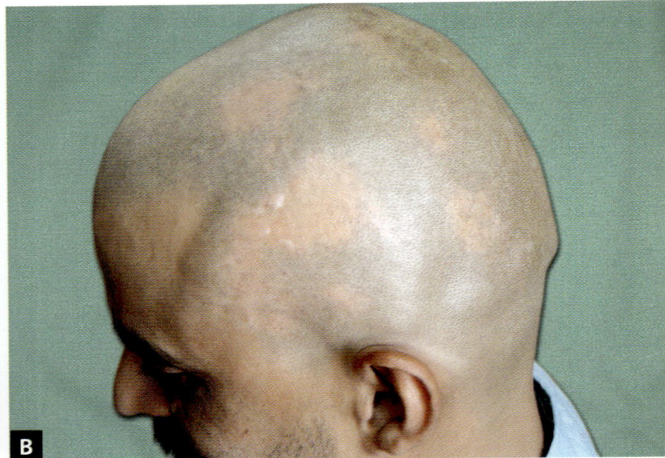

Figs. 12A and B: Vitiligo scalp: (A) Pretreatment; (B) Post cell transfer.

Box 2: Advantages and disadvantages of the procedure

Advantages

- Donor recipient ratio 1:10, i.e. with just 10 cm^2 of donor size a vitiligo patch of 100 cm^2 can be treated
- Excellent texture and color matching
- No stuck-on look (as seen in split thickness grafting) or cobblestoning (as with punch grafting)
- Large areas can be treated in a single session
- Patient can use cosmetic camouflage as early as 10 days postoperatively

Disadvantages

- Complex procedure as compared to simple punch or split thickness grafting
- Longer training and supervision required to perfect the procedure
- Variables such as trypsin strength, media used, temperature and time of incubation, centrifugation can alter results
- More expensive

Modifications of the Procedure

Noncultured epidermal cell suspension (NCECS) has only 4 basic steps, i.e. harvesting the graft, cell separation, resurfacing the vitiligo area and transferring the cell suspension and stabilizing it. Various authors have reported modifications which can be incorporated while performing this procedure:

- *Making the cell suspension more viscous and uniform:*[11] The suspension obtained is often too watery and runs off. Nanny van Geel et al.[11] reported the use of hyaluronic acid to the final pellet, in the ratio reported the use of Hyaluronic acid addition to the final pellet in the ratio of 1:1, this increases the viscosity and prevents runaway of the final cell suspension.
- *Cold trypsinization:* Yvon Gauthier et al.[9] described a two-step technique; recipient area is prepared by inducing cryoblisters with liquid nitrogen and then the melanocyte keratinocyte suspension is injected into the blisters. The donor area used is the skin of the scalp which is incubated in 0.25% trypsin for 18 hours at 4°. This is referred to as cold trypsinization and avoids centrifugation.
- *Cryopreservation of cell suspension*
- *Using suction blister roofs as donor skin*[13]
- *Use of timed surgery for removing epidermis in epidermis.*[14]

These are described in more detail in the next Chapter.

- Four compartment method of NCES:[15] Four compartment(FC) method, a simplified and cost-effective method of noncultured epidermal cell suspension for the treatment of vitiligo. A split-thickness graft is taken using a shaving blade held by long straight artery forceps. The skin graft is then transferred to the FC Petri dish in compartment 1 which contains 0.25% trypsin and 0.02% EDTA solution and is incubated at 37 °C for 1 hour. After 1 hour, the trypsinized graft is washed sequentially to remove trypsin in phosphate-buffered saline (PBS) in compartments 2 and 3. Then the graft is shifted to compartment 4. In this compartment, the dermis is separated from the epidermis using sterile forceps, and cells are dislodged gently from the basement membrane and suspended in PBS. This suspension of epidermal cells, comprising a mixture of keratinocytes and melanocytes, is used for transplantation over the dermabraded area of the patient.

This technique makes the NCECS process cost-effective and simple enough to be performed in the clinic without laboratory equipment. The following items are required in the FC method: a Petri dish with four compartments, forceps, PBS, trypsin solution and a sterile syringe.

Advantages of the FC Method

- No need for the following items: Trypsin inhibitor, pipettes, autoclaved tips, centrifuge tube and centrifuge machine
- There is no need for centrifugation; overnight cold trypsinization at 4°C in an ordinary refrigerator is performed

- PBS washing is used to remove trypsin and hence there is no need to use any trypsin inhibitor
- Pipette and tips are replaced by syringes.

- *In vivo preparation of NCES:*[16] In this process, cell separation and harvesting is performed inside sterile blisters induced by suction on the patient's thigh. This technique is simple, inexpensive, and requires minimal processing and handling of the tissue outside the body.
  Procedure:
  - Suction blisters are raised on the lateral aspect of the patient's upper thigh
  - With a 24-G hypodermic needle, the blister fluid is aspirated and 1 mL of 0.25% trypsin-0.002% EDTA solution is introduced into the blister cavity, body heat acts as an incubator at a temperature of around 37.8C
  - Within 45 minutes, epidermal melanocytes and basal keratinocytes, which are in contact with the trypsin-EDTA solution, detach to form a cellular suspension inside the blister cavity. This suspension is aspirated and transferred to a sterile Petri dish following which the dermal side of blisters are scrapped to release basal layer cells into the suspension. The suspension is then transplanted onto dermabraded vitiligo patches (Figs. 13A to F).

  Advantages
  - It does not require specialized training or laboratory equipment
  - There is no lag period between harvesting and transplantation
  - There is minimal handling of tissue outside the body, thus reducing risk of contamination
  - The blister cavity provides a closed system, essentially creating a mini-laboratory in the patient's own skin
  - This procedure is suitable for dermatologists in smaller centers where conventional cellular transplantation cannot be performed because of lack of infrastructure.
- *Using hair as donor*: This is described in detail in the next Chapter

8. *Modifications of NCES while operating on the acral areas*
   Acral vitiligo is the most difficult variety of vitiligo to manage. The reason for failure is that acral areas are difficult to operate; dermabrasion is difficult to perform and retention of the cell suspension is also difficult. The procedure of NCES has to be modified to improve the chances of take up of the melanocytes and subsequent results and a few pearls are described in Table 1.

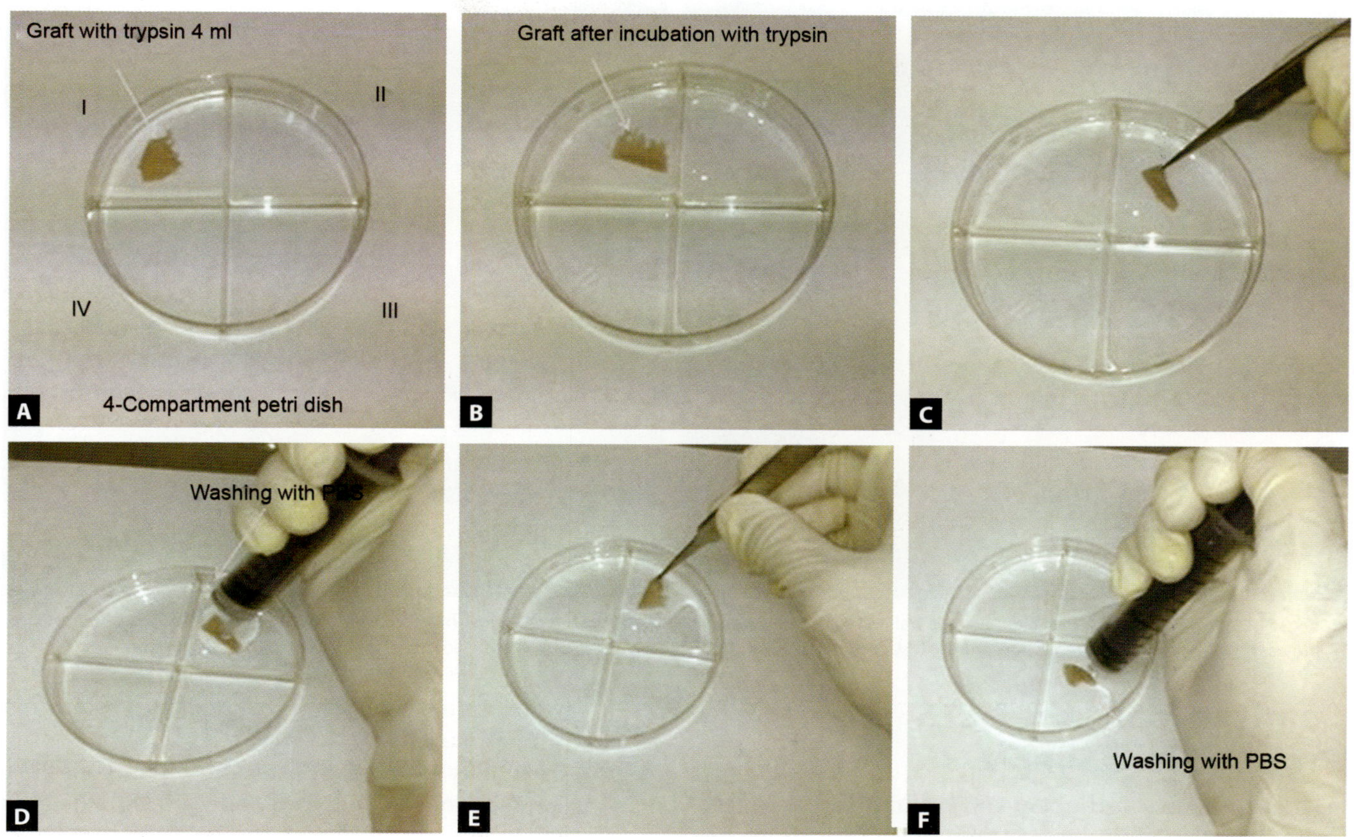

Figs. 13A to F: (A) trypsin added to skin graft (B) skin graft in trypsin after incubation (C-F) Washing with PBS to remove trypsin in compartments II and III.

Table 1: Modifications of the procedure for specific acral areas.

Site	Recipient site preparation	Retaining the cellular grafts
Eyes	▪ Dermabrasion (DA) ▪ Use cylindrical burrs ▪ Stabilize well, use a corneal shield to provide base for dermabrasion	▪ For small areas, use only collagen and leave it open ▪ For larger area (full eyelid): apply collagen>> paraffin>> guaze>> pad>> close eye for 7 days
Finger tips	▪ Deeper dermabrasion	▪ Dress each finger individually and then the whole hand
Lips	▪ Use infiltration ▪ Put a gauze inside mouth to make the lips taut ▪ Use CO_2 laser or erbium YAG Laser	▪ Collagen>> Paraffin>> suture with 4-0 prolene
Penis/ Scrotum	▪ Pear-shaped burr for dermabrasion ▪ Pinch skin around to make it taught ▪ Use CO_2 laser or erbium YAG laser	▪ Cut collagen in small pieces and sprinkle ▪ Admit patient ▪ Put in urinary catheter ▪ Use drugs to reduce erection

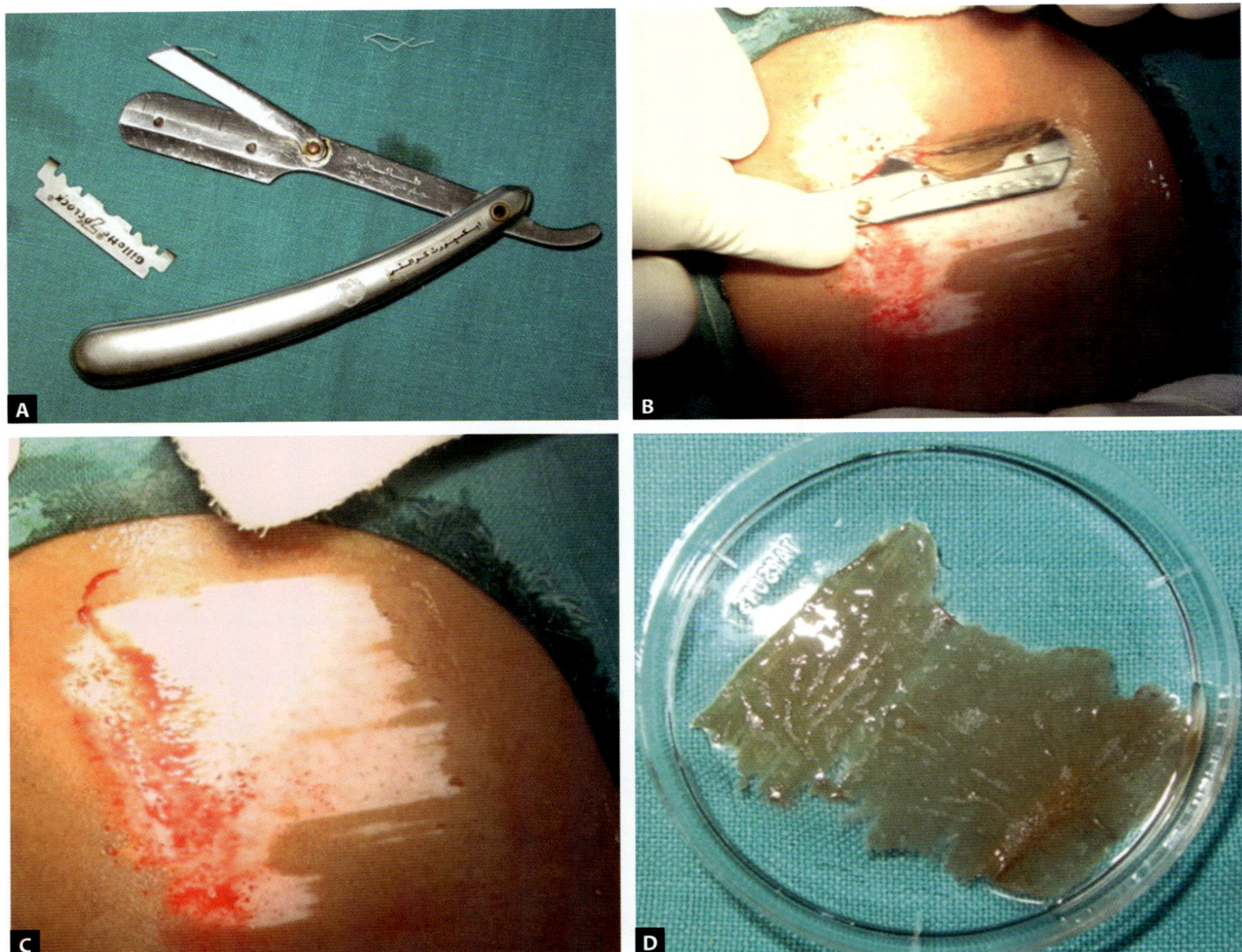

Figs. 14A to D: (A) Ustra : A simple device to harvest grafts (B) Ultra thin graft being harvested with the USTRA (C) Pinpoint Bleed at the donor area shows that the graft harvested is very thin and superficial (D) Graft harvested with USTRA, graft is floating, not curled up denoting minimum dermis.

Pearls to Make the NCES Process More Simple

- Using a simple instrument-USTRA to harvest skin grafts.
  - The first and foremost step in NCES is to harvest an ultrathin graft, because if the graft is thick, i.e. with dermis it cannot be separated by trypsinzation (Figs. 14A to D).
  - The ability to cut a split-thickness skin graft free-handedly needs long experience. Several devices have been improvized to simplify this task. However, the size and elaborate arrangements of

dermatomes often preclude their use. The various options available are Humby's skin grafting knife, Silver's skin grafting knife, Dermatomes: Davol's, Padgets

- Most dermatosurgeons are comfortable using a blade in straight artery forceps
- The author has been using USTRA which is commonly used shaving handle for harvesting ultra thin grafts. Normal shaving blade can be inserted in this and no complicated adjustments are required.

- Suction blister roofs can be used as donor skin
- Laminar air flow is not mandatory to conduct cell separation; Use of a laminar air flow has been conventionally recommended for carrying out the cell separation procedure, but this adds to the cost of treatment. However, if the cell separation is carried out in a sterile OT, there is no requirement of laminar air flow
- Incubator is not mandatory; Ideally incubation should be done at 37° in an incubator but even if it's done in the open with room temperature of 25–35°, cell separation cell separation can be achieved.
- Cutting down the incubation time of the graft in tryspin EDTA solution:Recommended incubation time is 45 mins at 37°. If the grafts harvested are ultra-thin, the incubation time can be cut down to just 30 mins (instead of 45 mins) in hot trypsinization method at 37°.
- Avoiding trypsin inhibitor: Anti-trypsin solution is the most expensive chemical in the NCES process. However, DMEM F 12 media, patients own serum or PBS can be used to neutralize trypsin.
- Using Pixel collagen to hold the cells: Retaining the cell suspension in some areas like the eyelid, scrotal skin, penile skin, areola, perianal area skin is a challenge because the skin tends to be mobile and expansile. By cutting the collagen sheet into very small pieces, graft take is enhanced, as the multiple small pieces adhere better and are more mobile with the skin stretching. We have coined the term Pixel collagen for this step i.e. cutting the dry collagen sheet in small pixel pieces and applying them.

CONCLUSION

NCES method has established itself as an effective and safe method of treating vitiligo and has replaced split skin grafting in many centers. The several modifications introduced over the last few years have enhanced its utility.

REFERENCES

1. Pasricha JS, Khaitan BK. Oral mini pulse therapy with betamethasone in vitiligo patients having extensive or fast spreading disease. Int J Dermatol. 1993;32:753-7.
2. An appraisal of narrow band (TL-01) UVB phototherapy. Br J Dermatol. 1997;137:327-30.
3. Moshar DB, Pathak MA, Fitzpatrick TB. Photochemotherapy for vitiligo: an approach to diagnosis and management in phototherapy in dermatology. New York: Mosby Yearbook; 1993;114-6.
4. Falabella R. Treatment of localized vitiligo by autologous minigrafting. Arch Dermatol. 1988;124:1649-55.
5. Savant SS. Autologous miniature punch skin grafting in stable vitiligo. Indian J Dermatol Venereol Leprol. 1992;58:310-4.
6. Lerner AB, Halaban R, Klaus SN, et al. Transplantation of human melanocytes. J Invest Dermatol. 1987;89:219-24.
7. Olsson MJ, Juhlin L. Repigmentation of vitiligo by transplantation of cultured autologous melanocytes. Acta Derm Venereol. 1993;73:49-51.
8. Olsson MJ, Juhlin L. Leucoderma treated by transplantation of basal cell layer enriched suspension. BR J Dermatol. 1998;138:644-8.
9. Gauthier Y, Surleve-Bazeille J. Autologous grafting with non-cultured malanocytes: a simplified method for treatment of depigmented lesions. J Am Acad Deramatol. 1992;26:191-4.
10. Mulekar SV. Melanocyte-keratinocyte cell transplantation for stable vitiligo. Int J Dermatol. 2003;42:132-6.
11. Van Geel N1, Ongenae K, De Mil M, Naeyaert JM. Modified technique of autologous non cultured epidermal cell transplantation for repigmenting vitiligo: a Pilot study. Dematol Surgery. 2001;27:873-6.
12. Olsson MJ, Moellmann G, Lerner AB, et al. Vitiligo: repigmentation with cultured melanocytes after cryostorage. Acta Derm Venereol. 1994;74:226-8.
13. Chen FY, Chang JS, Yang PY, et al. Transplantation of cultured autologous pure melanocytes after laser abrasion for the treatment of segmental vitiligo. J Dermatol. 2000;27:434-9.
14. Guerra L, Capurro S, Melchi F, et al. Treatment of "stable" vitiligo by timedsurgery and transplantation of cultured epidermal autografts. Arch Dermatol. 2000;136:1380-9.
15. Kumar R1, Parsad D, Singh C, Yadav S. Four compartment method: a simplified and cost-effective method of noncultured epidermal cell suspension for the treatment of vitiligo. Br J Dermatol. 2014 Mar;170(3):581-5. doi: 10.1111/bjd.12725.
16. Gupta S1, Sahni K2, Tembhre MK2, Mathur S3, Sharma VK2. A novel point-of-care in vivo technique for preparation of epidermal cell suspension for transplantation in vitiligo. J Am Acad Dermatol. 2015 Feb;72(2):e65-6. doi: 10.1016/j.jaad.2014.10.042.

Chapter

37B

Vitiligo Surgery: Mega Sessions

Munish Paul

Key Messages

- Local anesthesia permits to operate only small areas in one session, because of issues of pain, apprehension and xylocaine toxicity.
- Extensive areas: Gega sessions (>400 cm^2), Mega Sessions (150–400 cm^2) can be performed comfortably and safely under general anesthesia.
- General anesthesia requires OT equipped with anesthesia equipment, cardiac monitors, life saving equipment's and trained staff to handle emergencies.
- Non-culture epidermal suspension (NCECS) technique scores over other vitiligo grafting techniques because of the excellent donor recipient ratio, i.e. 1: 10.
- Pain para and postoperative, blood loss, are important issues while doing large areas in one session.
- The percentage and extent of repigmentation of the mega and gega session is similar to that of regular sessions.

INTRODUCTION

Surgical management of stable vitiligo[1] has evolved and come a long way. More and more dermatologists are now apt at various vitiligo and other surgeries. Most dermatologists either work from their own clinics or centers or perform various procedures in a minor theater, doing most procedures under local anesthesia. Most vitiligo surgeries are done for small areas, usually of size 50-100 sq. cm. This chapter focuses on surgical management of extensive vitiligo and offers tips for performing such surgeries.

A patient of stable vitiligo may have a large area to be operated and may not have time for multiple sessions such as those coming from a foreign country, or those with a marriage in the offing. Currently there are no definite guidelines as to how much maximum area can be operated in a single session. We take up cases with larger areas 150 to 400 cm^2 for such mega sessions (Table 1).

Table 1: Terminology used while doing NCECS over large areas.

Terminology	*Area to be operated in cm^2*
Regular NCECS session	Up to 150 cm^2
Mega sessions	150–400 cm^2
Gega sessions	Area > 400 cm^2

CASE SELECTION

1. Only patients having disease stability for 1 year are taken up for surgery.
   Stability is taken up on these criteria:
   - No new patches since one year
   - No extension of existing patches since one year
   - No loss of pigmentation in patches which had achieved repigmentation since one year
   - No vitiligo patches at the site of injury i.e. koebenerization since one year.
2. General anesthesia (GA) should be preferred in these cases:
   - Extensive area, i.e. 150 cm^2 and above
   - Young/apprehensive patient having extensive area
   - Patient is medically fit and doesn't have major comorbidities which may pose as a contraindication for GA.
3. Site, area, selection:
   - Ideally only one side of the body should be operated, i.e. we should try to avoid doing both hand/both feet-both eyes in one go. Bandaging both hands or feet for a week at a stretch can be quite disabling for the patient
   - Since turning or changing a patients position under GA is difficult and compromises sterility, patches to be operated in extensive cases need to

be planned in way that no/minimum change of position is required. Example; areas over the chest and abdomen can be done in one session, lesions over the back need a separate session.
- All areas should be photographed, measured and marked before the GA is induced so that no patches are missed out
- Total recipient area should be calculated so that donor area to be harvested is more precise.

Anesthesia: Safe upper limit of local anesthetic xylocaine (2%) without adrenaline is 4.5 mg/kg (up to 300 mg) and with epinephrine 7 mg/kg (up to 500 mg). This implies that in safe limits only a small amount of xylocaine can be injected and thus a small area can be operated at one time. Regional blocks can be used but they again require training and expertise to be really effective. Local anesthesia cannot be used in small children and apprehensive adults. The main limitation is pain and its effective management intraoperation and postoperation. Hence transplantation for extensive areas will require general anesthesia and local anesthesia is not suitable while operating on large areas.

The use of GA (general anesthesia) makes the process simpler as the issues of pain relief is taken care of and the surgeon as well as the patient, both are equally comfortable. The setting is thus conducive for taking up extensive cases in single session.

Operation theater set up: It is imperative to have a complete OT set up which is equipped with anesthesia equipment, cardiac monitors, lifesaving equipment's. The staff should be trained to handle emergencies. An anesthetist has to be present throughout the procedure till the patient is completely out of anesthesia; admission facilities are required for short stay to monitor the patient post operatively for 6–8 hrs.

PREOPERATIVE COUNSELING AND INFORMED CONSENT[2]

The surgical process starts with a detailed history of the patient pertaining to vitiligo and general health and associated diseases esp. in regards to the use of general anesthesia

It's important to always remember that general anesthesia requires meticulous planning right from the patient evaluation, OT set up, Anesthesia drugs, equipment, gases, emergency drugs, trained staff and vigilant pre- and postoperative care. Even if the duration of anesthesia is short, the risks and complications can be similar to a long case and if they occur can be very unforgiving.

A detailed consent form elaborating the procedure and possible complications, risks should be signed by the patient and a witness. The consent form should specifically cover the limitations, risks of the NCES procedure as well as that of the general anesthesia.

Preoperative laboratory studies include complete hemogram including platelet counts, bleeding and clotting time (or prothrombin and activated partial thromboplastin time), thyroid profile, LFT, KFT, serum electrolytes, chest X ray PA view, ECG in adults. Screening for antibodies for hepatitis B, C and HIV is recommended.

The type of anesthesia used is to be decided on a case to case basis depending on the site, extent of the area, age of the patient, comorbidities. Most cases can be managed with just IV sedation with drugs combination like ketamine, midazolam, propofol. Intubation is not required in most of the cases of NCES and the cocktails of anesthesia drugs used by an experienced anesthetist can make the whole process go smooth.

DURATION OF ANESTHESIA

The duration of anesthesia required is usually short as it is required only for the painful steps of the procedure:

a. Analgesia is required at the time of harvesting of skin graft which on an average needs only 2–5 mins.
b. Secondly, analgesia is needed during dermabrasion that varies from 20–30 mins depending on the area to be covered.

   Once the skin grafts are harvested, they are trypsinized immediately while the dermabrasion is being carried out. The cell separation process, dressings etc requires no further anesthesia and patient need not be under anesthesia at that point of time.
c. Lastly, the application of dry collagen sheets on the dermabraded skin also produces stinging and burning sensation, which warrants a second "shot" of anesthesia cocktail in some patients.

DONOR-RECIPIENT RATIO

This is the second and most important consideration while taking up large vitiligo areas for surgery. Vitiligo is a cosmetic problem and if in the process of repigmenting the vitiligo patch ends up scarring the donor area, the purpose of the procedure is lost.

NCECS has the advantage that with a small skin graft from the donor area, a large recipient vitiligo area can be treated. The commonest donor recipient ratio being used is 1: 10, i.e. if we harvest a skin graft of 3 cm × 3 cm, i.e. 9 cm^2; we can almost treat 90 cm^2 of vitiligo area. A smaller graft implies minimum scar over the donor area.

Other tissue grafting methods are not suitable for large areas for the following reasons:

Punch grafting[3,4] (tissue graft) is the easiest and least expensive method, but it is time consuming, seldom produces even uniform repigmentation. In minipunch grafting, the donor recipient ratio is 1: 3, i.e. a punch can only spread the pigment three times its size. Hence it is not suitable for large areas.

In suction blister grafting[5] the donor recipient ratio is 1:1 and although the cosmetic results are good, there is limitation in raising blisters. Hence blister grafting is suitable only in small areas.

Ultrathin epidermal sheet grafting can treat larger areas (up to 200 cm^2) (Figs. 1 to 3) but requires skill and experience to take such large grafts. Ultrathin split thickness grafting[6] involves harvesting of large sheets of skin; the donor recipient ratio is 1:1 or at times even 1.5: 1- because if the graft harvested is relatively thick it has to be discarded as only the thinnest graft would give a better cosmetic result. Hence a large area is at a risk of donor skin scarring and disfigurement, depigmentation at the donor site. The graft on the recipient site can have a stuck on appearance and in many cases hyperpigmentation, perigraft halo, milia formation are encountered. The overall cosmetic result is not very cosmetically appealing (Figs. 4 and 5).

CULTURED METHODS

Culture methods[7] have a definite edge in that they provide an unlimited number of cells for transplantation, i.e. 100 fold. However, culture methods require extensive labs,

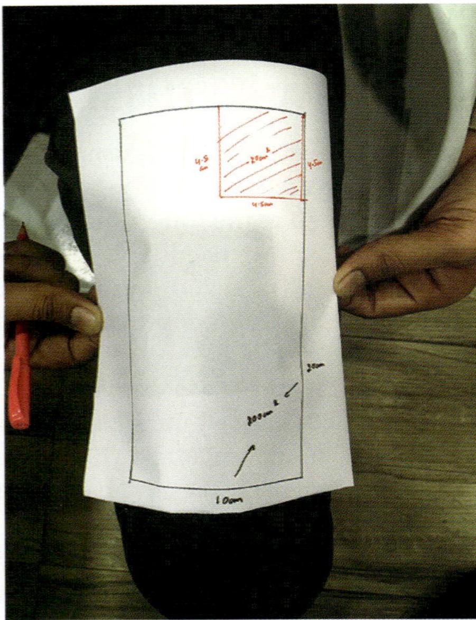

Fig. 1: Donor area calculation to cover 200 cm^2 of vitiligo area. If a split thickness graft is to be harvested 10 × 20 cm^2, i.e. 200 cm^2, if NCES is planned then 1/10 area, i.e. 4.5 × 4.5 cm, i.e. 20.25 cm^2, if is needed.

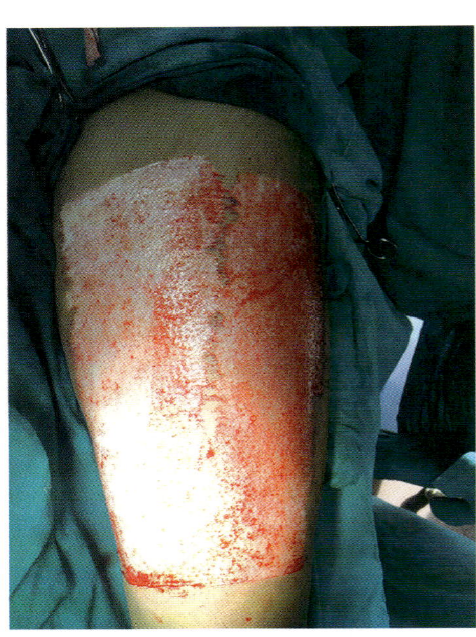

Fig. 2: 200 cm^2 of split thickness graft harvested.

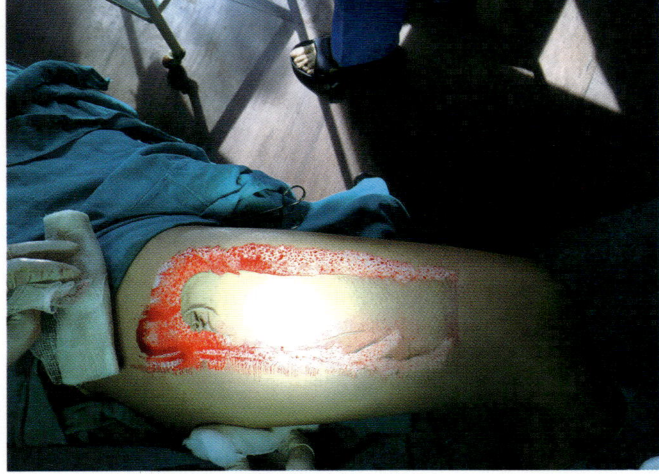

Fig. 3: Large graft harvested, pinpoint to continuous bleed seen on the donor bed suggestive of a level of papillary to reticular dermis.

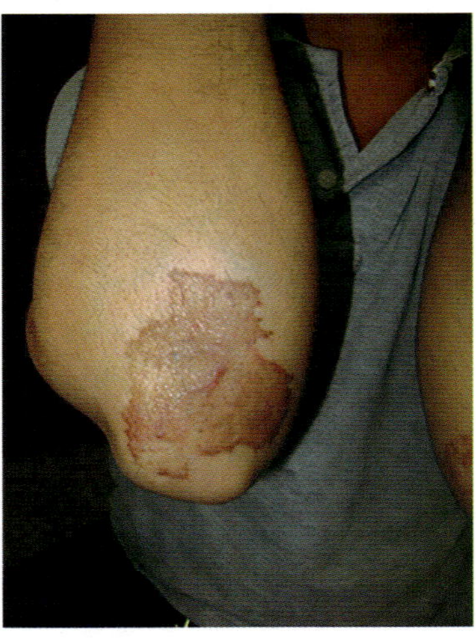

Fig. 4: Limitation of STG: Stuck on appearance, milia formation, hypertrophic margins, perigraft halo.

equipment and trained personnel and hence the cost of procedure goes up make it unaffordable for most patients. There are also concerns of contamination, bacterial/ fungal overgrowths.

Hence the NCECS is the ideally suited for vitiligo surgery of extensive areas. However, punch grafting may be preferred if the dermatosurgeon is not trained for NCECS or split skin grafting. Split skin ultrathin grafts may be preferred by a surgeon who has the expertise for taking large grafts, if facilities do not exist for NCECS.

PROCEDURE DETAILS: SPECIAL ISSUES WHILE DOING LARGE AREA (> 200 CM^2)

Preparation of the NCECS[8,9] has already been covered in details in the previous chapter and hence only relevant steps are described here.

DONOR AREA CALCULATION

Preoperatively, all recipient areas are marked and photographed. Calculation of the area that needs to be operated is done (Fig. 1, table1). Fig 2 to 9 show different steps of donor harvesting. The process of NCECS is the same as has been described in previous chapters.

RECIPIENT AREA PREPARATION IN NCECS/STG (FIGS. 10 TO 15)

While doing large areas, dermabrasion with diamond burrs and with micromotor is preferred since its fast and large areas (200–500 cm^2) can be done in just 20–30 mins.

While dermabrading an even level of dermabrasion up to the papillary dermis should be achieved–this is evident by fine pinpoint bleeding. At times there can be at times some skip zones, because of the clouding the operating field by the oozing blood. These are areas of inadequate level of dermabrasion should be watched for closely. After the entire area has been dermabraded, adequate hemostasis is achieved with saline soaked gauzes for 10 mins and a relook is taken. The areas not showing pinpoint bleed are further dermabraded to create an even surface. This avoids skip zones in the repigmentation.

While doing margins it is important to go 5 mm into the normal skin, this reduces the incidence of perigraft achromic fissures.

SPECIAL CARE WITH EXTENSIVE PUNCH GRAFTING

While doing extensive punching it is better to have at least two dermatologists operating at the same time so that one person can harvest the grafts from the thigh and the other can prepare the recipient wells. The surgeon preparing the recipient site keeps a count of the number of punches required which is conveyed to the harvesting surgeon. The recipient sites in PG tend to bleed more and should be covered with moist saline gauzes to achieve hemostasis. Excessive bleeding clouds the field which can lead to certain areas being left out it is advised that the placement of grafts is started only after the entire recipient area is prepared and bleeding controlled.

After placing the punches in the wells area is covered with paraffin dressing, gauze, pad and bandage.

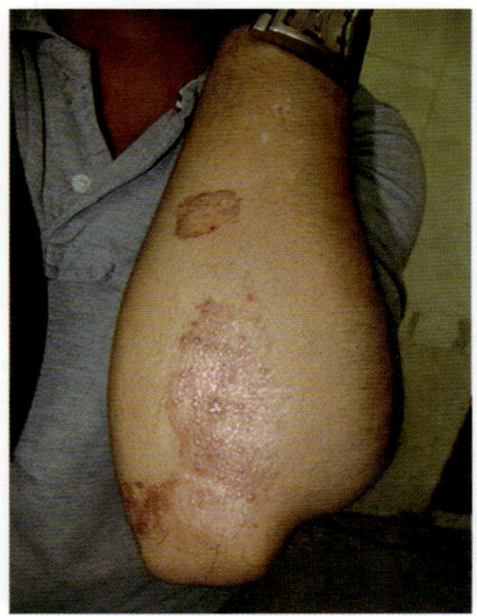

Fig. 5: Limitation of STG: Hyperpigmentation and stuck on appearance.

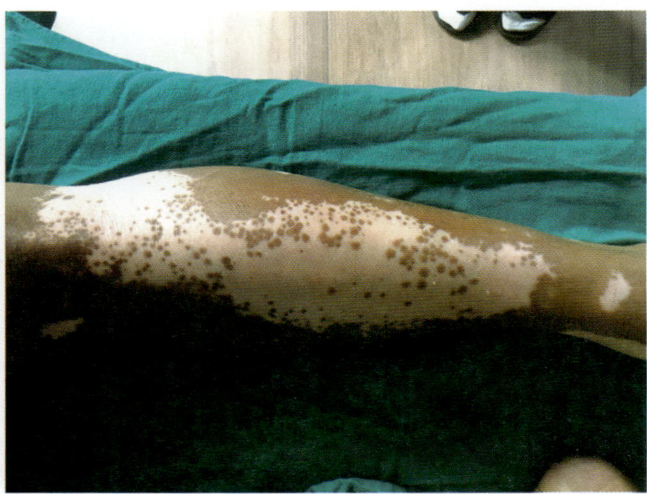

Fig. 6: Extensive vitiligo patch over the shin approx 250 cm^2.

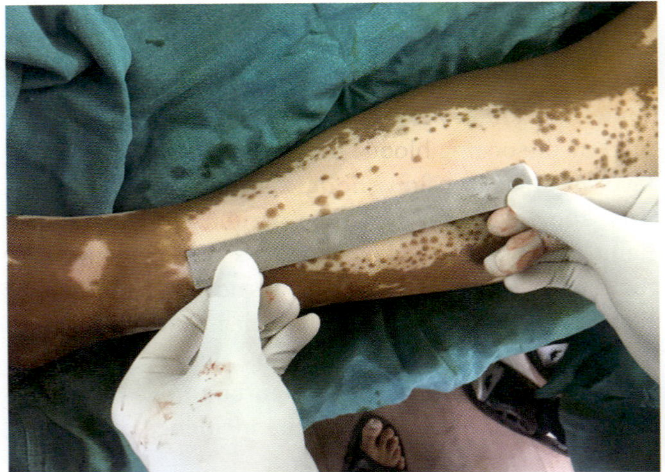

Fig. 7: Area calculation presurgical over the recipient area.

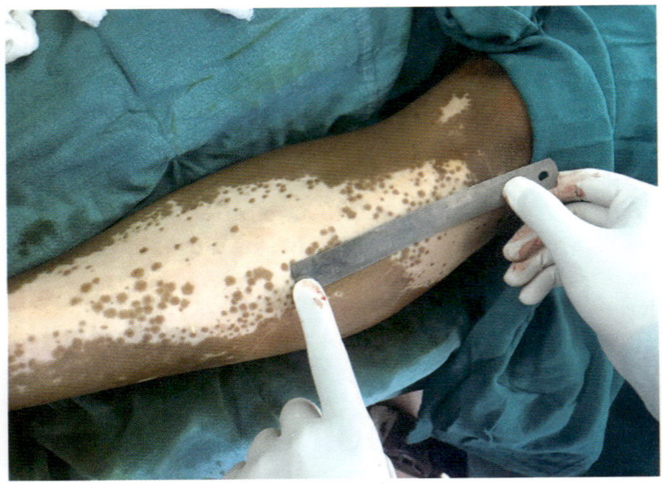

Fig. 8: Area calculation presurgical over the recipient area.

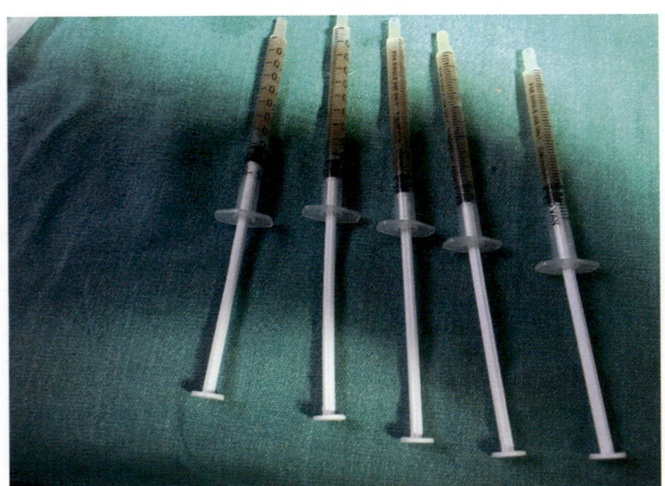

Fig. 9: 4.5 mL of cell suspension for the 250 cm^2 area.

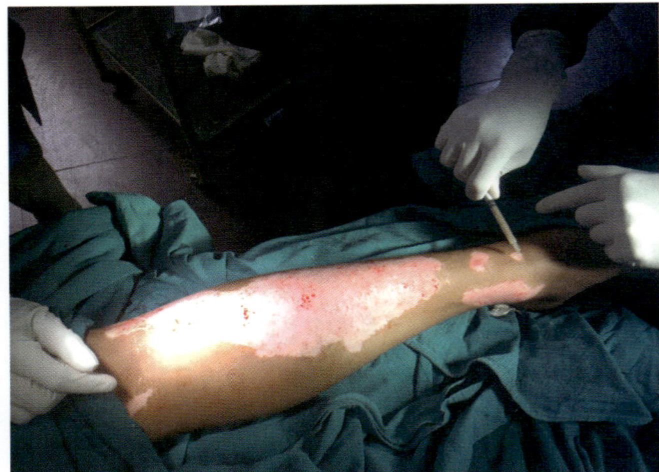

Fig. 10: Uniform spread of the cell suspension over the derma braded area.

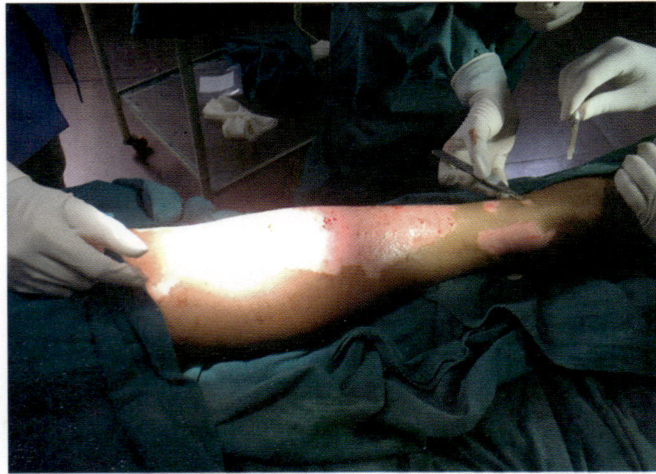

Fig. 11: Collagen dressing to hold the cell suspension in place.

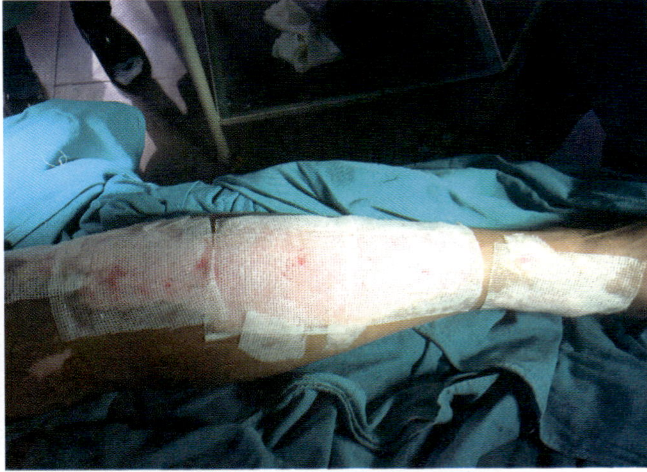

Fig. 12: Single layer of collagen dressing as the second layer of dressing.

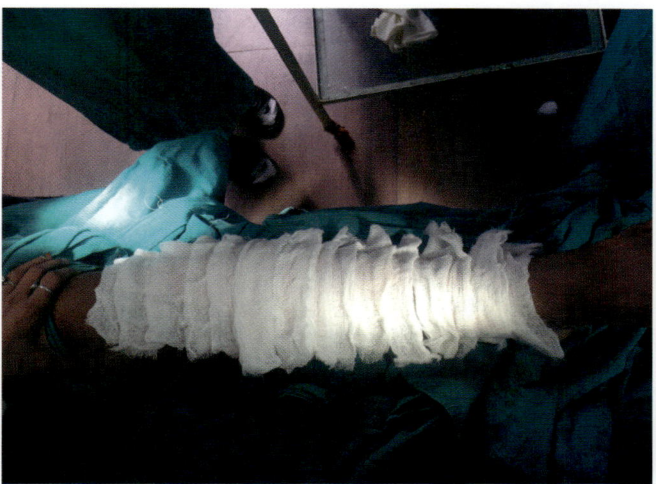

Fig. 13: Dry gauze as the third layer of dressing.

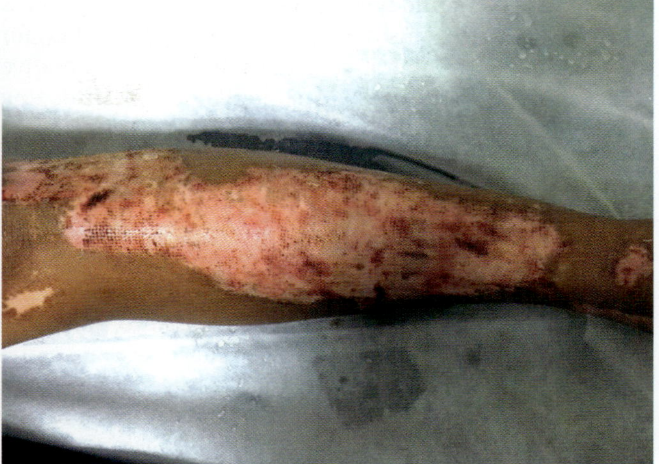

Fig. 14: Complete epithelialization and healing at day 7.

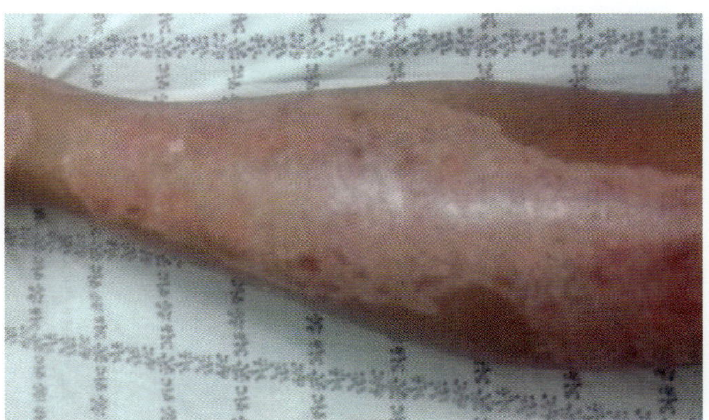

Fig. 15: Early pigmentation at 8 weeks.

SPECIAL CARE WITH SPLIT THICKNESS GRAFTS

Since a large sheet of ultrathin skin is required it requires considerable experience and expertise. The thigh has to stretched tightly by an assistant one side while the surgeon gives traction with his free hand. A slightly larger graft has to be harvested because if the graft is too thick at places it doesn't give good cosmetic appearance.

After harvesting, the thigh is tightly wrapped with an adrenaline-soaked bandage to achieve hemostasis and left for at least 15–20 mins the dressing over the donor area is done after ensuring there is no bleeding, with guaze rolls.

The graft harvested can be given slits with a 15 no scalpel blade (to create a mesh) this allows space for the fluids to ooze out and prevents blood collection and graft upliftment. If a mechanical masher is available it can expand the graft to cover a larger area.

The grafts are then laid out on the dermabraded vitiligo area and are secured on the edges with stay sutures given

Table 2: Rough estimate for deciding the donor-recipient ratio.

Recipient areas	Donor-recipient ratio
Single confluent patch	1:10
Few scattered large patches	1: 8
Multiple small patches	1:5

with 5-0 prolene. This is then covered with paraffin dressing and dressed.

Immobilization of the recipient area is very important lest the graft can get dislodged—some surgeons even prefer to give a Plaster of Paris cast or splints to immobilize the area.

PAIN MANAGEMENT

Adequate care of the postoperative pain since is essential since large amount of skin has been derma braded In most of our patients we have found an IM or IV Diclofenac 2 mL, i.e. 80 mg injection is adequate to keep the patient comfortable. Few patients would need an additional dose of pentazocine, Phenergan.

FLUID AND ELECTROLYTE MANAGEMENT

NCECS is a surgery with little blood loss because the level of dermabrasion is only up to the papillary dermis. There is not much bleeding and even in extensive areas, i.e. 400 cm^2 the amount of blood loss is less than 20 mL. Since a small donor area is required and the grafts are ultra-thin there is not much of a blood loss from the donor site as well.

In harvesting extensive sheets of skin as in split thickness grafting there is more blood loss. In punch grafting also there is more blood loss since the punches are up to the mid dermis there is considerably more bleeding at both the donor and recipient areas.

The patient should be kept well hydrated with IV fluids since most GA patients need to be Nil per Oral (NPO) for almost 8 hours preoperative and 4-6 hours postoperative and also since a large area is operated there can be oozing postoperative.

RESULTS (FIG. 16 TO 24)

The percentage and extent of repigmentation of the mega and gega session is similar to that of regular sessions The onset of pigmentation color and texture matching is no different in these large area surgeries, even the retention of pigmentation and relapse rates were similar to the surgeries of limited area We did not observe any koebnerization being induced, i.e. the disease becoming unstable immediately after the procedure. Hence larger areas per session can be taken up, to reduce the total number of procedures a patient has to go through to repigment a certain amount of area.

CONCLUSION

Taking up mega or gega sessions of NCECS is safe and effective. Doing large areas in a single session is the best way to manage a patient having extensive vitiligo in minimum sessions. However case selection has to be done carefully and after thorough counseling. The process requires planning and dedicated team of dermatologists, anesthetist, OT nursing staff technicians, and post nursing care to make the procedure safe and comfortable for the patient.

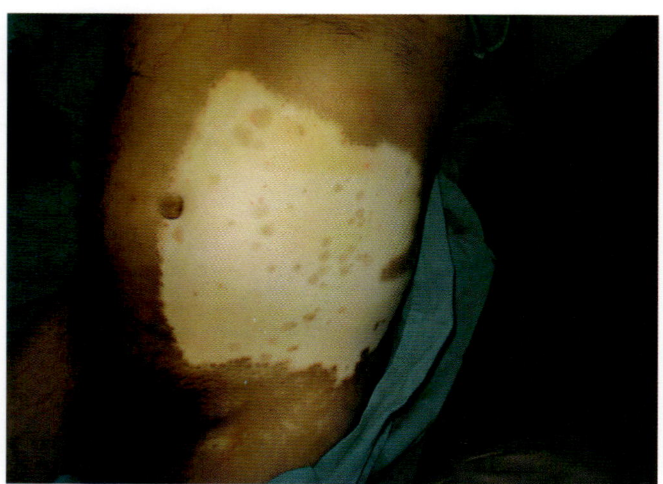

Fig. 16: Extensive vitiligo area (350 cm^2): Segmental variety.

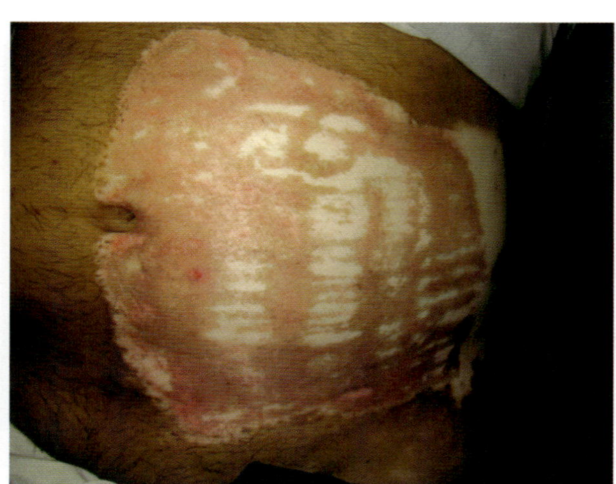

Fig. 17: At 3 weeks postoperation, entire area epithelized, area appears erythematous, and some skip zones visible indicating a more superficial level of dermabrasion in those areas.

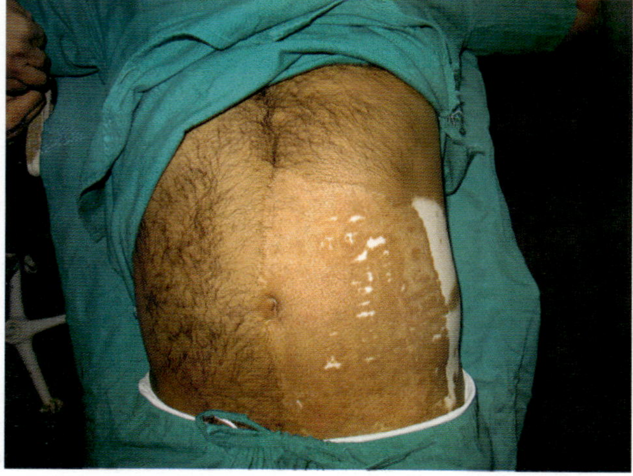

Fig. 18: 6 months postoperation entire area repigmented including the skip zones.

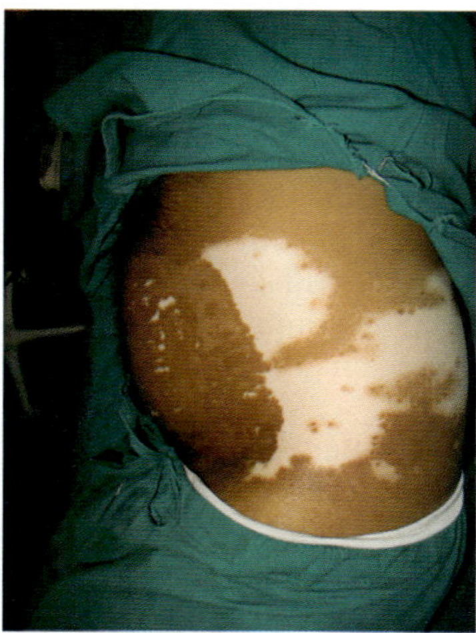

Fig. 19: 2nd session of cell transplant in the same patient.

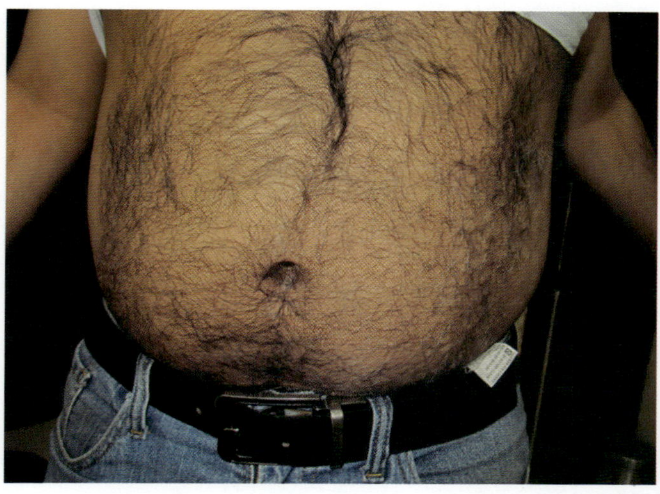

Fig. 20: Entire area repigmented well with, leukotrichia also replaced by pigmented hair.

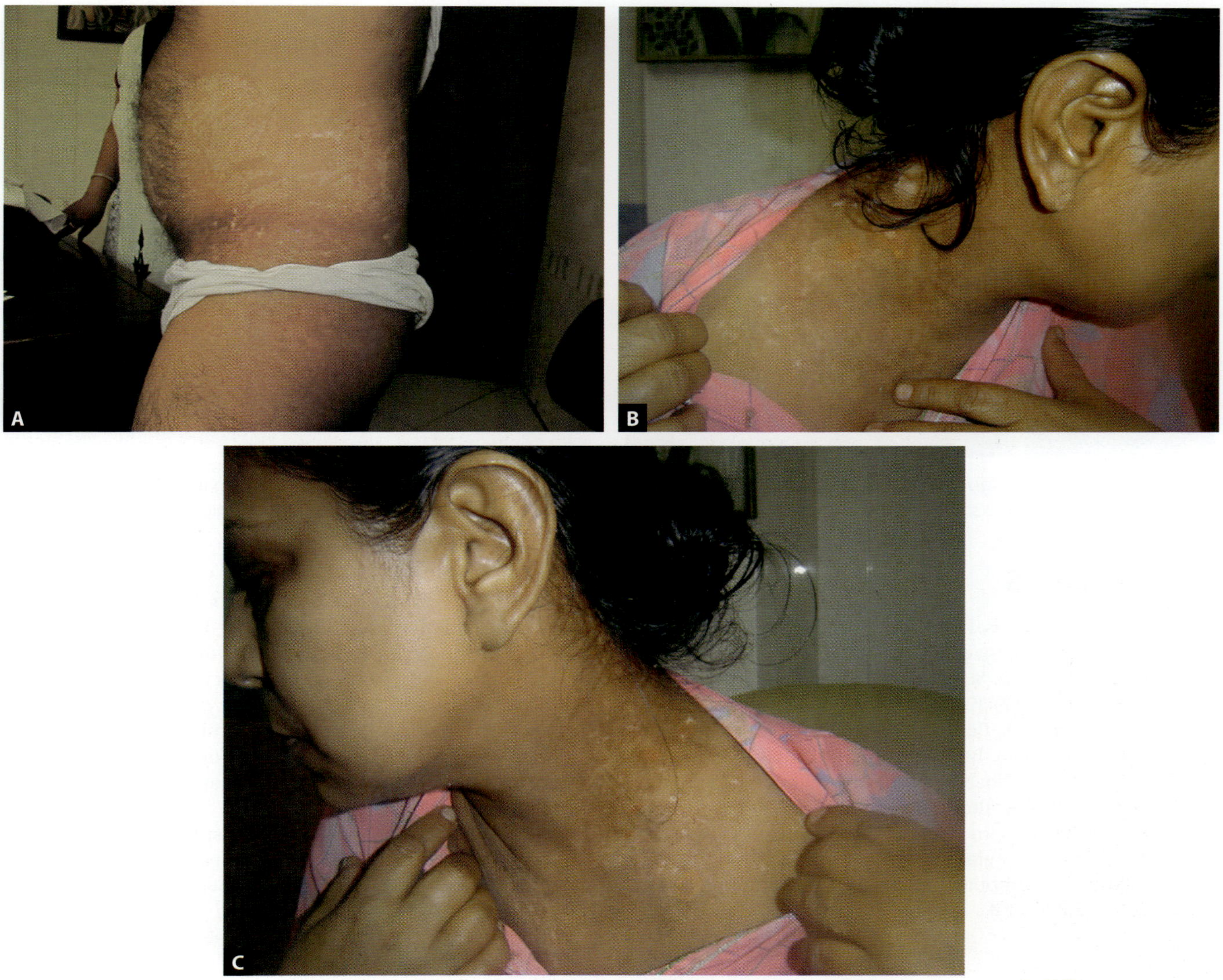

Figs. 21A to C: Good texture and colour matching in the entire area.

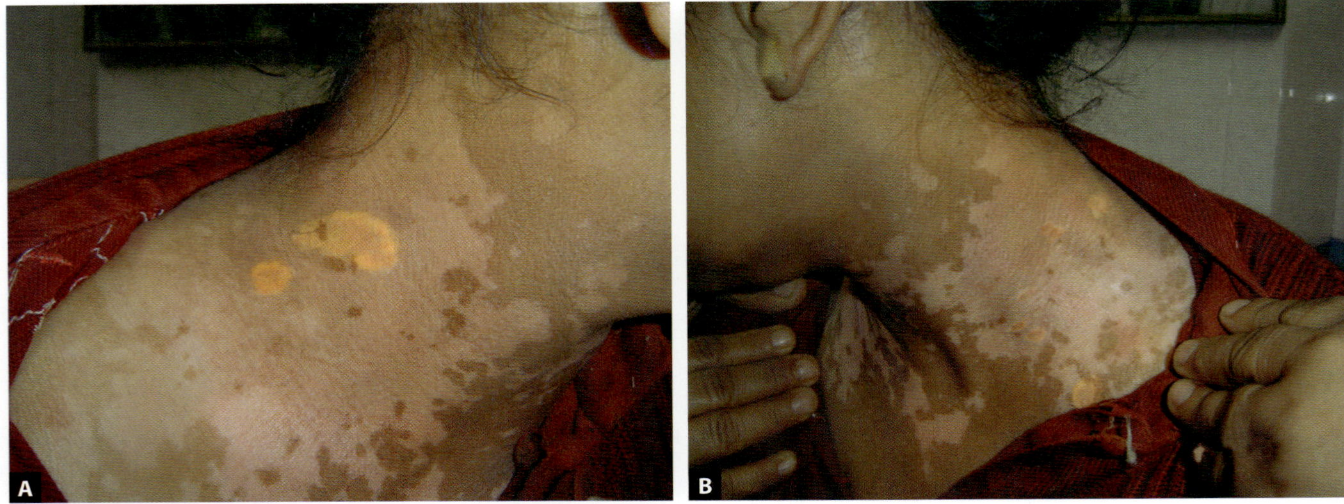

Figs. 22A and B: NCECS over neck, chest, and a previously tattooed area.

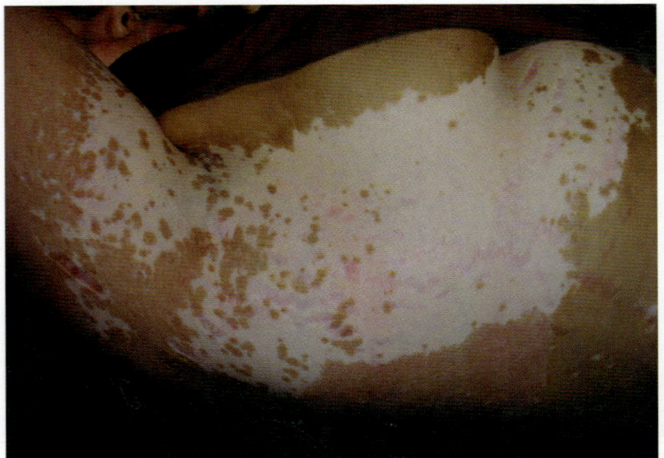

Fig. 23: Extensive vitiligo > 400 cm^2 over the trunk, few areas showing stretch marks because of long-term steroid use.

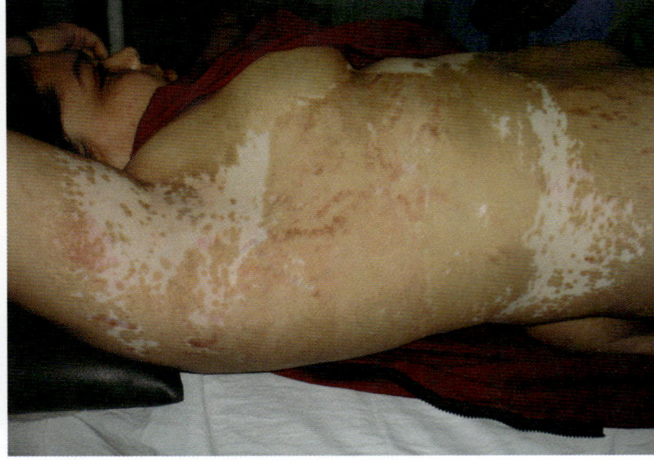

Fig. 24: Good texture and color matching in the entire area, even the stretch marks showing repigmentation.

REFERENCES

1. Manchanda K, Bansal M, Pandey SS. Surgical management of vitiligo—An approach to the patient. NJDVL. 2013;11(1):6.
2. Parsad D, Gupta S. Standard guidelines of care for vitiligo surgery. 2008;74(7):37-45.
3. Taieb A, Alomar A, Böhm M, et al. Guidelines for the management of vitiligo. Br J Dermatol. 2013;168(1):5-19.
4. Van Geel N, Ongenae K, Naetert JM. Surgical techniques for vitiligo. Review dermatology. 2001; 202:162-6.
5. Oh CK, Cha JH, Lim LY, et al. Treatment of vitiligo with suction epidermal grafting by the use of an ultrapulse CO_2 laser with a computerised pattern generator. Dermatol Surg. 2001;27:563-8.
6. Khunger N. Thin split thickness skin grafts for vitiligo in surgical management of vitiligo. Gupta S et al. (Eds). Blackwell Publishing Ltd. 2007:108-14.
7. Olsson MJ, Juhlin L. Repigmentation of vitiligo by transplantation of cultured melanocytes. Acta Dermatol Venereol (Stock). 1993;73:49-51.
8. Munish Paul. Autologous non-cultured basal cell-enriched epidermal cell suspension transplantation in vitiligo: Indian experience. J Cutan Aesthet Surg. 2011; 4(1): 23-28.
9. Mulekar SV. Long term follow-up study of segmental and focal vitiligo treated by autologous non-cultured melanocyte-keratinocyte cell transplantation. Arch Dermatol. 2004:1211-15.

Chapter 38

Noncultured Extracted Hair Follicle Outer Root Sheath Cell Suspension

Savita Yadav, Sanjay Singh, Somesh Gupta

Key Messages

- Noncultured Extracted Hair Follicle Outer Root Sheath Cell Suspension (NCHF-ORF-CS) also called follicular cell suspension is a recently described surgical method of repigmentation in vitiligo.
- Procedure is technically minimally demanding and can be completed on the same day.
- Major advantage is lack of visible scarring at donor site.
- Large areas can be treated with suspension prepared from small number of hair follicles.
- Technique is in its initial phase of development and may require further standardization.

INTRODUCTION

Vitiligo is an acquired autoimmune pigmentary disorder with a worldwide prevalence and significant burden in Indian subcontinent. Both medical and surgical modalities have been tried in management of vitiligo. There are no uniform guidelines or recommendations available for surgical management. Clinical stability of disease for a period of more than a year remains a preempt requirement for patients undergoing surgical interventions, which includes: No new lesion, nonprogression of existing lesions, spontaneous repigmentation, absence of koebnerization, and positive minigraft test.[1] Surgical therapies have been found to be useful in segmental vitiligo, nonsegmental vitiligo resistant to medical therapies and stable for at least 1–2 years.[2] Various surgical procedures like minigrafts, hair follicle transplantation, split thickness grafts, suction blister grafts, noncultured epidermal cell suspension (NCES), and cultured autologous melanocytes transplantation have been used. The basic principle of above mentioned surgical modalities is transfer of melanocytes from uninvolved skin to the stable vitiligo lesion. This leads to rapid repopulation of melanocytes by proliferation and migration leading to repigmentation of depigmented skin.[3] Autologous noncultured hair follicle outer root sheath cell suspension (NCHF-ORS-CS), also known as hair follicular cell suspension (FCS) is a recently described surgical modality for the management of vitiligo.

The major advantage of cell suspension (either cultured or noncultured) over conventional methods is treatment of larger affected area by use of small donor area and better color and texture match with the surrounding skin. Culture techniques are time consuming, technically demanding, expensive, and also require trained personnel with sophisticated culture laboratory facilities. The use of various growth factors and additives in the culture medium [e.g. 12-O-tetradecanoylphorbol 13-acetate (TPA)] raises concern about the safety of this procedure. In contrast, noncultured cell suspension techniques like NCES and NCHF-ORS-CS obviate the need of these additives, can be used to treat large vitiliginous areas (eight- to ten-fold size of donor skin), technically less demanding and the procedure can be completed in few hours on an outpatient basis.

AUTOLOGOUS NONCULTURED HAIR FOLLICLE OUTER ROOT SHEATH CELL SUSPENSION/FOLLICULAR CELL SUSPENSION

Basic Concepts

The maintenance of the melanocytes in epidermis as well as hair follicle is dependent on melanocyte stem cells (MelSCs), a quiescent cell population that is located in the bulge region of the hair follicle and acts as a melanocyte reservoir. These stem cells can migrate into the epidermis and give rise to differentiated pigment-producing melanocytes. Under normal circumstances, these melanocytes remain inactive but become active to produce melanin when stimulated by ultraviolet radiation, wound, or dermabrasion.[2,4]

Repigmentation of vitiligo depends on three possible sources of melanocytes: (1) from the hair follicle where stem cells are found, (2) from the normal skin at margins, and (3) unaffected melanocytes within depigmented areas.[5] This leads to four clinical patterns of repigmentation: (1) follicular, (2) marginal, (3) diffuse, and (4) combined, of which follicular pattern is the most common.[3]

Cui et al. in their study observed dopa-positive melanocytes (active) in the epidermis of normal skin while dopa-negative melanocytes (inactive) were seen in the ORS of normal hair follicles, which serve as a melanocyte reservoir. In vitiligo patients, the dopa-positive melanocytes in the epidermis were completely absent, whereas the dopa-negative melanocytes present in ORS of hair follicles were unaffected. Treatment leads to stimulation of the inactive melanocytes present in the middle and/or lower parts of the ORS resulting in their proliferation and migration upward along the surface of the ORS to the adjacent epidermis. Continued radial migration of the melanocytes leads to appearance of perifollicular repigmentation in vitiligo lesions. The melanocytes undergo continuous maturation and become active during their upward migration. In conclusion, these inactive melanocytes in ORS function as reservoir and are a potential source for repigmentation of vitiligo lesions. These observations signify the very important role of hair follicle in repigmentation of vitiligo lesions.[6]

Meyer et al. studied normal human scalp hair follicles by using immunohistochemistry and quantitative histomorphometry. They found bulge region as relatively immunoprivileged area of human skin and this leads to protection of the hair follicle epithelial stem cell reservoir from autoaggressive immune attacks.[7] MelSCs reside in the bulge region that might be responsible for their protection from damage by immune cells, which possibly explains the persistence of pigmented hairs in vitiligo lesions in most of the cases.

Theoretical Advantages of Follicular Cell Suspension over Epidermal Cell Suspension

Hair follicle melanocytes differ from epidermal melanocytes in various ways (Table 1). Epidermal and follicular melanins are independent units and this fact is strongly approved by presence of white hair on highly pigmented skin.[8] The follicular melanin unit consists of one melanocyte to five keratinocytes in the hair bulb and 1:1 in the basal layer of the hair bulb, while in epidermal melanin unit, there is one melanocyte for every 36 keratinocytes. One of the most striking difference between the two melanocytes subpopulations is that the hair bulb melanocytes are cyclically active during anagen phase, whereas epidermal melanogenesis is a continuous process.[9] Furthermore, even small number of hair melanocytes can produce sufficient melanin to pigment up to 1.5 m of the hair shaft. Because of these properties, the hair appears to be better source of melanocytes than epidermis for cell suspension techniques. The FCS has many other advantages besides the unique characteristics of hair follicle melanocytes. FCS requires few hair follicles, which means less volume of tissue in comparison with NCES. There is intact interfollicular area after follicular extraction by using 1 mm punch. This leads to earlier and better wound healing at donor site compared to conventional shave biopsy technique in NCES, where continuous sheet of epidermis is taken from thigh. Follicular unit extraction (FUE) wound heals by minimal scarring. Furthermore, these scars are located over hairy sites and practically invisible leading to cosmetically very acceptable donor site to the patients, while with NCES technique there is a risk (though low) of keloid or hypertrophic scar formation over the donor site with its associated cosmetic disfigurement. The technique of preparation of FCS is relatively simple, when compared

Table 1: Comparison of follicular and epidermal melanin units.

	Follicular melanin unit	*Epidermal melanin unit*
Activity	Cyclical activity, tightly coupled to hair growth cycle	Continuously active
Ratio with keratinocytes	1:1–1:5	1:36
Size	Larger, have more longer and extensive dendrites	Smaller, less dendritic
Melanosomes	Larger	Smaller (2–4 times smaller)
Melanin granules	Minimally degraded in hair cortex	Completely degraded in the differentiating keratinocytes
Golgi apparatus and rough endoplasmic reticulum	More developed	Less developed
Susceptibility to immune destruction	Relatively less due to their immunologically privileged location (the bulge area)	More
Aging	More influenced by aging (hair graying)	Less influenced by aging

to NCES as it does not require separation of the epidermis from dermis and manual breaking of epidermal samples into small pieces.

Procedure of Follicular Cell Suspension (Fig. 1)

Step 1: Follicular Unit Extraction

Occipital scalp is the preferred donor site by most of cutaneous surgeons. Few hairs are delineated in this area and trimmed to a length of approximately 2 mm. Anagen hairs are preferred for extraction as they have more number of active melanocytes. Field block anesthesia using 2% lignocaine with adrenaline is given encircling the delineated donor area. With the help of 1 mm punch (manual or motorized), intact hair follicles are extracted. This is a very critical step as hair follicles should be taken in toto to avoid transaction of hair follicles. Then the hair follicle is gently extracted using a hair follicle holding forceps. Depending on the area to be transplanted, approximately, 50–100 pigmented follicles are extracted. On an average, 15–25 hair follicles are sufficient to repigment approximately 20 cm^2 area.[2] The intact hair follicles are collected in normal saline and transferred immediately to the laboratory. The donor area is dressed using mupirocin ointment and sterile cotton pads.

Step 2: Preparation of Cell Suspension

The extracted hair follicles are washed three times under aseptic conditions with phosphate-buffered saline (PBS) containing various antibiotic and antifungal agents such as penicillin, streptomycin, kanamycin, and amphotericin B. The extracted hair follicles are incubated in test tubes with 0.25% trypsin and 0.05% ethylenediaminetetraacetic acid (EDTA) at 37°C for 30 minutes, to prepare the single cell suspension.[3] Within 15–20 minutes of first incubation, the cells from the ORS start separating from each other. After 30 minutes of incubation, the hair follicles are gently stroked with a forceps to separate the loosened up cells and hair follicles are then transferred to the second test tube for further incubation for 30 minutes. At this point, we add trypsin inhibitor to the first test tube to arrest continued digestion of the loosened cells, which have remained behind in the first test tube. The same procedure is repeated in the second and the third test tubes. Only thin keratinous shafts are left behind at the end of three such cycles. Finally, the contents of all three test tubes are collected in a single test tube and single cell suspension is prepared by filtering with 70 µm cell strainer. The final cell pellet is obtained by centrifuging the combined cell suspension at 1,000 rpm for 5 minutes. The cell pellet thus obtained is resuspended in small amount (0.25 mL or 0.5 mL, depending on the size of recipient area) of PBS or

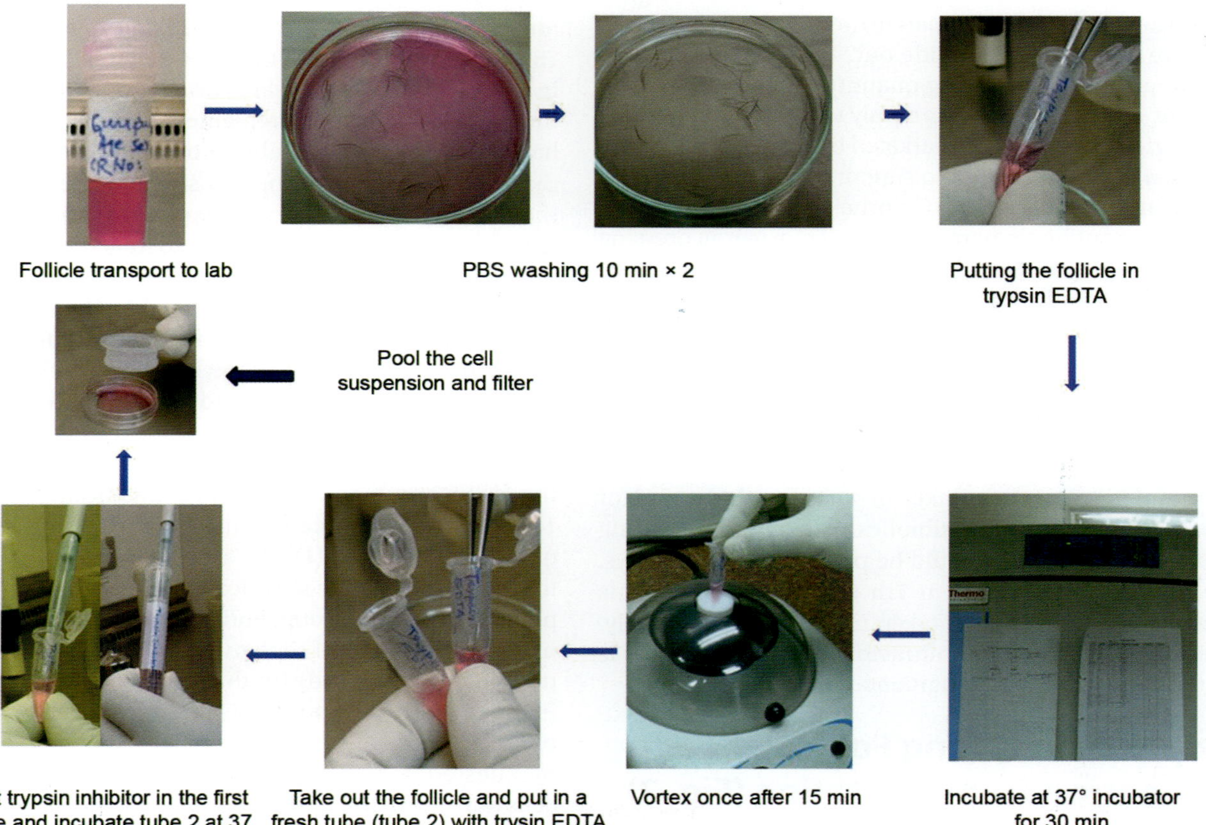

Fig. 1: Steps of preparation of extracted hair follicular outer root sheath cell suspension.

Dulbecco's modified Eagle›s medium (DMEM). The whole laboratory process usually takes around 2–3 hours.

The trypsin used can be either porcine or bovine source derived or recombinant trypsin. Trypsin from porcine or bovine source has a risk of zoonotic disease transmission such as transmission of endogenous retroviruses. Manira et al. compared effects of animal-derived trypsin and recombinant trypsin on human skin cell culture expansion and found similar results in both groups in terms of cell yield and expression of specific cellular markers.[10]

Step 3: Transplantation

Under strict aseptic measures, the recipient site is cleaned and draped. Local anesthesia with 2% lignocaine is given to the area to be treated. Most of cutaneous surgeons avoid using adrenaline with lignocaine as it leads to vasoconstriction that might result in poor graft intake or complete failure. In addition, it masks the bleeding, which may result in deeper dermabrasion. Recipient site is abraded with manual or motorized dermabrader until tiny bleeding points appear which suggest dermoepidermal junction. Further dermabrasion should not be carried out as it might lead to scarring. Five millimeter of normal-looking skin beyond the margin of vitiliginous skin is also abraded to avoid the halo phenomenon.

Cell suspension is aspirated using a spatula or pipette, and the suspension is evenly spread over the recipient site followed by application of five-layered dressing composed of collagen sheet, antibiotic-containing paraffin gauze, surgical cotton gauze/pad, thin transparent dressing film, and elastic adhesive bandage from inside out. There are no specific existent guidelines regarding quantity of suspension to be used per unit area. Most commonly used collagen sheet is of fish origin. In India, it is marketed by name of NeuSkin-F (Chennai). It is considered to support epidermal cells and to help in their migration.[11] Chlorhexidine is preferred as antibiotic in antibiotic-paraffin gauze. Transparent dressing film (Tegaderm) and elastic adhesive bandage (Dynaplast) are used to stabilize the graft. The patient should be kept under observation for at least for 1–2 hours after procedure.

Postoperative Care

Restriction of movement of recipient site, keeping area clean and dry, minimizing local manipulation are important measures to be taken in postoperative period for at least 7 days. Systemic antibiotics preferentially covering *Staphylococcus aureus* should be prescribed for 5–7 days. The dressing is removed at 7th day follow-up. At this time, the recipient site has taken up the graft adequately. Topical/oral psoralen plus ultraviolet A (PUVA) therapy is started to induce rapid repigmentation at recipient site.

Response following Follicular Cell Suspension Transplantation (Fig. 2)

There is significant scarcity of literature regarding response following FCS transplantation. Only few studies have assessed the results of this technique till date. Vanscheidt et al. in their study on five patients of stable vitiligo used autologous ORS cell suspension prepared by using trypsin on plucked anagen scalp hair follicles. Erbium-doped yttrium aluminum garnet (Er-YAG) laser was used for dermabrasion at recipient site. Post re-epithelialization, lesions were treated with narrow-band ultraviolet-B 2–3 times weekly. Authors found almost complete (>90%) repigmentation in three out of five patients with vitiligo, around 50% repigmentation in one patient and less than 10% repigmentation in the other.[12] Mohanty et al. in their prospective study on 14 patients of stable vitiligo (at least for 3 months) used extracted FCS and found more than 75% repigmentation in 9 out of 14 patients. Three patients in study had less than 1 year of disease stability and none of them had more than 75% repigmentation, while 11 patients had at least 1 year of stability of which 9 showed more than 75% repigmentation. This study further emphasizes the concept of stability of 1 year before undergoing any vitiligo surgery. Authors used 15–25 follicular units, which provided 25,000–50,000 cells that were sufficient to treat up to 25 cm^2 area.[13] Similarly, Shah et al. in their study on 25 patients of stable vitiligo noticed excellent repigmentation (90–100%) in 60% cases with FCS technique.[14] A randomized comparative study on 30 patients with 47 vitiligo lesions have compared FCS with NCES. There was excellent repigmentation (90–100%) in 83.3% of lesions in the NCES group and 65.2% of lesions in the FCS group. There was a significant improvement in dermatology quality-of-life index (DLQI) score in both but patients in the NCES group were significantly more satisfied than the patients in the FCS group. Both group showed similar color match and pattern of repigmentation.[15] Kumar et al. in a preliminary pilot study on three human subjects noticed FUE as a better method of follicle harvesting than follicular plucking (FP). Authors found partial loss of stem cell niche manifested as low mean percentage of CD200 positive cells during FP. The average cell yield per follicle was 2,500 and 250 by the FUE and FP method, respectively, which showed significant statistical difference.[16]

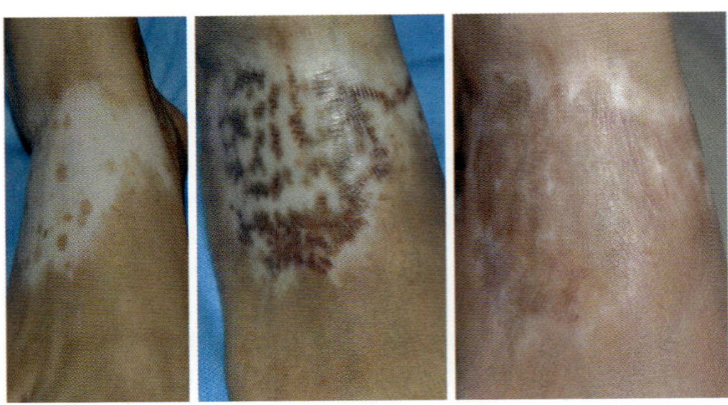

Fig. 2: Vitiligo patch before surgery, 3 weeks after hair follicular outer root sheath cell suspension transplantation with pigmentation resembling peri-follicular pigmentation, and 6 months post transplantation with 90% repigmentation.

Furthermore, Vinay et al. in a study on 30 patients of stable vitiligo analyzed factors affecting the repigmentation in patients treated with FCS. Marked repigmentation (>75%) was seen in 21 out of 60 (35%) lesions while 10 out of 21 lesions showed excellent repigmentation (>90%). Authors have concluded that the number of melanocytes and hair follicle stem cells transplanted, and absence of dermal inflammation were important determinants of optimal repigmentation.[17]

CONCLUSION

Follicular cell suspension is a new addition to various options in vitiligo surgery. It is a novel, less invasive, cosmetically acceptable technique, which requires less expertise. Efficacy of this procedure is now established by few studies. However, a study with a larger sample size will be required to further explore the efficacy of this procedure. Furthermore, head-to-head comparative trials are needed to compare the efficacy of FCS and NCES. Overall, FCS technique is an addition to the armamentarium for management of stable vitiligo.

REFERENCES

1. Mulekar SV. Surgical management of vitiligo. Expert Rev Dermatol. 2014;229-39. [online] Available from http://www.tandfonline.com/doi/abs/10.1586/edm.10.9. [Accessed February, 2017].
2. Kumar A, Mohanty S, Sahni K, et al. Extracted hair follicle outer root sheath cell suspension for pigment cell restoration in vitiligo. J Cutan Aesthetic Surg. 2013;6:121-5.
3. Sawatkar GU, Vinay K, Dogra S, et al. Follicular cell suspension: a new surgical modality for the treatment of vitiligo. Pigment Int. 2015;2:4.
4. Goldstein NB, Koster MI, Hoaglin LG, et al. Narrow-band ultraviolet B treatment for human vitiligo is associated with proliferation, migration, and differentiation of melanocyte precursors. J Invest Dermatol. 2015;135:2068-76.
5. Falabella R. Vitiligo and the melanocyte reservoir. Indian J Dermatol. 2009;54:313-8.
6. Cui J, Shen LY, Wang GC. Role of hair follicles in the repigmentation of vitiligo. J Invest Dermatol. 1991;97:410-6.
7. Meyer KC, Klatte JE, Dinh HV, et al. Evidence that the bulge region is a site of relative immune privilege in human hair follicles. Br J Dermatol. 2008;159:1077-85.
8. D'Mello SA, Finlay GJ, Baguley BC, et al. Signaling pathways in melanogenesis. Int J Mol Sci. 2016;17:pii: E1144.
9. Tobin DJ, Slominski A, Botchkarev V, et al. The fate of hair follicle melanocytes during the hair growth cycle. J Investig Dermatol Symp Proc. 1999;4:323-32.
10. Manira M, Khairul Anuar K, Seet WT, et al. Comparison of the effects between animal-derived trypsin and recombinant trypsin on human skin cells proliferation, gene, and protein expression. Cell Tissue Bank. 2014;15:41-9.
11. Scharffetter-Kochanek K, Klein CE, Heinen G, et al. Migration of a human keratinocyte cell line (HACAT) to interstitial collagen type I is mediated by the alpha 2 beta 1-integrin receptor. J Invest Dermatol. 1992;98:3-11.
12. Vanscheidt W, Hunziker T. Repigmentation by outer-root-sheath-derived melanocytes: proof of concept in vitiligo and leucoderma. Dermatol Basel Switz. 2009;218:342-3.
13. Mohanty S, Kumar A, Dhawan J, et al. Noncultured extracted hair follicle outer root sheath cell suspension for transplantation in vitiligo. Br J Dermatol. 2011;164:1241-6.
14. Shah AN, Marfatia RK, Saikia SS. A study of noncultured extracted hair follicle outer root sheath cell suspension for transplantation in vitiligo. Int J Trichol. 2016;8:67-72.
15. Singh C, Parsad D, Kanwar AJ, et al. Comparison between autologous noncultured extracted hair follicle outer root sheath cell suspension and autologous noncultured epidermal cell suspension in the treatment of stable vitiligo: a randomized study. Br J Dermatol. 2013;169:287-93.
16. Kumar A, Gupta S, Mohanty S, et al. Stem cell niche is partially lost during follicular plucking: a preliminary pilot study. Int J Trichol. 2013;5:97-100.
17. Vinay K, Dogra S, Parsad D, et al. Clinical and treatment characteristics determining therapeutic outcome in patients undergoing autologous non-cultured outer root sheath hair follicle cell suspension for treatment of stable vitiligo. J Eur Acad Dermatol Venereol. 2015;29:31-7.

Chapter 39

Cultured Melanocyte Transplantation

Kanika Sahni, Davinder Parsad

Key Messages

- Cultured cellular graft represents a major advance in vitiligo surgery as it has a donor to recipient area of around 1:100 and hence a very small donor graft is adequate to cover a very large area.
- The other major advantage of this technique is it contains the possibility to cryopreserve these cells in cell banks and reculture them whenever these are needed for transplantation in future.
- However, the lack of complete standardization, relatively inadequate data, the need for expensive laboratory equipment and technical knowledge of cell culture limit the use of this modality to a few centers only at present and the technique still needs to evolve before it can find widespread practical application.

INTRODUCTION

The ideal surgical treatment modality for vitiligo should be effective in all cases, rapid, cheap, easy to perform, safe, and cheap. None of the currently available modalities provides all the above advantages. Tissue grafts possess several limitations such as inability to cover large areas in a single sitting and non-uniform repigmentation and textural change (esp. punch grafting and split thickness skin grafting). Cultured melanocyte grafting have overcome these problems, as they are able to cover large areas with uniform pigmentation, from small grafts in less number of sittings, hence contributing to greater patient comfort, with less textural changes of donor skin. The other major advantage of these techniques is the possibility to cryo-preserve these cells in cell-banks and reculture them whenever these are needed for transplantation in future. Hence, cellular graft represents a major advance in vitiligo surgery. However, the lack of complete standardization, relatively inadequate data, the need for expensive laboratory equipment and technical knowledge of cell culture limit the use of this modality to a few centers only at present and the technique still needs to evolve before it can find widespread practical application.

Cultured melanocyte suspensions are of two types: Pure melanocyte cell suspension and coculture with keratinocytes. The latter are more manageable and make it easier to treat many large achromic patches at the same time. In addition, these cocultures allow melanocytes to grow in more physiologic conditions: The maintenance of an optimal numerical relationship with the keratinocytes provides a more suitable environment for their development, possibly owing to the release of growth factors essential for their functions.

Background and History

The first clinical use of cultured epidermis was reported in the 1980s to treat burns[1] and later extended to the treatment of many other disorders including vitiligo. The idea of obtaining a large population of melanocytes from small samples of normally pigmented skin by growing them in the laboratory thus seemed attractive and plausible. However, initial attempts at culturing melanocytes were unsuccessful because of the slow multiplication rate and the overgrowth of other more rapidly multiplying cells like keratinocytes and fibroblasts. The first successful culture of melanocytes was from tissue obtained from metastatic melanoma patients, but at that time, attempts to culture them from normal skin or non-metastatic melanoma failed. The first break came in 1980 when Eisenger and Marko[2] were able to successfully culture melanocytes from newborn foreskins and adult skin by the addition of phorbol-12-myristate-13-acetate (PMA) and cholera toxin. The technique was further refined by the addition of isobutylmethylxanthine (IBMX) and human placental extract. Cholera toxin and IBMX served to keep intracellular levels of cAMP high. The placental extract was believed to be a source of basic fibroblast growth factor (bFGF) while at a concentration of 10 ng/mL, PMA was found to be toxic to human keratinocytes but not melanocytes; and in fact was found to promote the attachment and proliferation of melanocytes. They observed that PMA at 10 ng/mL had a toxic effect mainly on keratinocytes, whereas 10 nM cholera toxin inhibit growth of fibroblasts. In 1984; Gilchrest et al.[3] reported the selective cultivation and long term maintenance in culture, of human melanocytes from newborn and adult epidermis, which they were able to serially passage up to 6 times.

The next breakthrough occurred in 1987 with the first report of the use of cultured melanocytes to pigment leukodermas, when Lerner et al. successfully treated a patient of piebaldism by injecting cultured melanocytes into suction blisters prepared at the depigmented site. This opened new avenues in the field of the application of tissue cultures for treatment of cutaneous depigmenting disorders.The procedure included obtaining a thin skin graft (from roofs of suction-induced blisters) which was enzymatically dissociated to provide a suspension which was later cultured in vitro in a medium containing 12-O-tertadecanoyl-phorbol-13-acetate (TPA), newborn calf serum and cholera toxin to yield a growth of melanocytes after 1 month of incubation. Initial cultivation which yielded growth of melanocytes mixed with fibroblasts was later supplemented with 100 µg/mL geneticin to eliminate fibroblasts and yield pure melanocyte cultures.

However, reports on mutagenicity of phorbol esters later led to their exclusion from media and it had to be later replaced by bFGF.[4]

In the last few decades, the procedure has undergone several modifications. Donor skin has variously been obtained using biopsy (punch biopsy/split thickness skin graft/full thickness skin grafts) or suction/cryo-induced blisters. Several methods have been used to prepare the recipient site including dermabrasion, suction/cryo-induced blisters, or lasers (Er:YAG or CO_2). Recently, the use of hyaluronic acid sheets[5] and amniotic membrane[6] as scaffolds for cultured melanocytes has been reported to be successful.

Patient Selection

The technique of cultured autologous melanocytes can be used for repigmentation of skin in all types of vitiligo and piebaldism. Case selection should be done carefully, as discussed in earlier chapters, as per existing guidelines.[7,8] Apart from the general recommendations for vitiligo surgery, cultured autologous melanocyte transplantation is particularly useful for patients with large achromic patches. However, it must be explained to patients that involvement of large body surface area by vitiligo is in itself a poor prognostic factor for repigmentation by both medical and surgical means. In addition, acrofacial vitiligo, especially involvement of tips of fingers and toes, may have a poorer response to cultured melanocyte grafting compared to lesions on other sites. In a large study of the use of the procedure in 105 achromic lesions, the authors reported poor results in the treatment of extremity lesions and those in periorificial areas. The average percentages of repigmentation of extremities and periorificial sites were 8% and 35% respectively compared to 88–96% repigmentation of all other body sites.[9]

Technique

The ideal donor recipient (DR) ratio is not yet accurately defined. Interestingly, in a recent study Hong et al,[10] found no significant differences in repigmentation after cultured melanocyte transplantation based on donor-recipient ratio. They divided 102 patients undergoing transplantation of cultured pure melanocytes into two groups, (1) a low DR ratio group, with DR ratio ≤1 : 10 (mean 1 : 8, 35 cases) and (2) a high DR ratio group with DR ratio >1:10 (mean 1:27, 67 cases) and found results to be comparable between the two groups. They concluded that although cultured autologous melanocyte transplantation is an expensive and complicated procedure, it provides the highest DR ratios (>1:10 and up to 1:60).

The following steps are involved in melanocyte culture:

- Technique of culture
- Preparation
- Donor site
- Recipient site
- Dressing and follow-up.

TECHNIQUE OF CULTURE

- **Collection of the samples:** The skin biopsies are obtained from the normally pigmented skin for transplantation, and if necessary, additionally from lesional or perilesional skin for experimental purposes. Various methods have been used to obtain skin samples from donor site, including punch grafts, split thickness skin grafts, full thickness skin grafts and roofs of suction blisters. However, it is our personal experience that for transplantation purposes the ideal graft is a split thickness skin graft comprising of epidermis and superficial part of dermis. It provides a good yield of melanocytes and does not leave behind any scarring. A 4 × 4 cm size graft is usually obtained from the upper thigh or gluteal area under lignocaine infiltration and/or topical eutectic mixture of local anesthetics (EMLA) anesthesia, with proper aseptic precautions. The graft is collected in phosphate buffer saline (PBS) with antibiotics (50-U/mL penicillin and 0.05 mg/mL streptomycin), in a sterile container (labelled with patient details) and immediately transported to the laboratory on ice. If the lag period is more than 4 hours, then the graft is placed in complete M2 melanocyte

Flowchart 1: Technique for melanocyte culture.

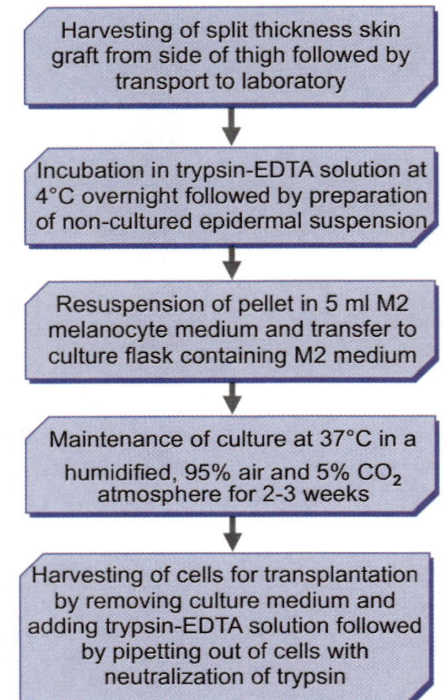

medium (PromoCell, Heidelberg, Cat. No. C-24300) and kept at 8°C. The donor area is dressed with sterile nonadherent chlorhexidine gauze (Bactigras, TJ Smith & Nephew Ltd., Hull, U.K.) followed by a sterile surgical pad that is kept in place with a sterile transparent occlusive dressing (Tegaderm O, 3M Healthcare, St. Paul, MN).

b. **Processing of the graft** (Flowchart 1): In the laboratory, the grafts are trimmed with sharp scissors to remove all fat and the deeper dermis. They are then transferred to a petridish with trypsin-EDTA (0.25% trypsin and 0.02% EDTA) and the sample is turned back and forth with the help of jeweler's forceps to ensure that it comes in complete contact with the solution. The grafts are placed with the epidermal side facing upwards, and then cut into pieces of about 5 × 5 mm. This is followed by incubation at 4°C overnight. On the next day, the trypsin/EDTA solution is removed and trypsin activity is terminated by adding 3 mL (15°C) of 0.5 mg/mL trypsin inhibitor (Sigma, St Louis, MO, USA) in PBS.

The trypsin inhibitor is then pipetted out and PBS or M2 melanocyte medium is added and the epidermis is separated from the dermis using sterile forceps. The tissue is then pipetted well so as to separate cells of the dermoepidermal junction from the tissue and the solid waste of tissue is removed. The PBS containing cells is then centrifuged at 1,000 rpm for 5 minutes to obtain a pellet. The supernatant and the floating fragments are removed and the pellet is resuspended in 5 mL M2 melanocyte medium and transferred to a 75 or 150 cm^2 culture flask containing M2 medium and placed flat to prevent cells from adhering to the sides of flask. The empty centrifuge tube is rinsed twice with M2 medium, which is also transferred to the culture flask, to ensure that all cells are collected (Figs. 1A and B).

The cell number is adjusted to 2.5 × 10^4 cells per cm^2. Care is taken to avoid media containing phorbol esters when the culture is being done for transplantation purposes. The culture is maintained at 37°C in a humidified, 95% air and 5% CO_2 atmosphere. The medium is to be changed at 3–4 days intervals and the cells should be examined daily microscopically to look for contamination or infection and also to look for outgrowth of cells. When confluence occurs, the cells are split by trypsin treatment for 5 minutes at room temperature and subcultured. Cell viability may be assessed by trypan blue exclusion assay, which is based on uptake of trypan blue dye by nonviable cells as a result of disintegration of the cellular membrane.

If a 100% pure melanocyte culture is needed for research purpose, 45 µg/mL geniticin (G418; 45 µg/mL) can be added to the medium for 3 days, starting from the 10th day of the culture. Genticin selectively suppress the fibroblasts. To eliminate keratinocytes, the level of Ca^{2+} levels may be elevated to 1.6 mM for 2 days, since high Ca levels are toxic to keratinocytes but not melanocytes.

However, for therapeutic purposes these interventions are not necessary since they do not interfere with melanocyte growth to a sufficient degree. In fact, few remaining keratinocytes may in fact aid in the growth and differentiation of melanocytes. Usually, between 10 × 10^6 to 50 × 10^6 cells are obtained at the end of 2 weeks at which stage, the cells are ready for transplantation.

To harvest the cells for transplantation, after removing culture medium from the flask, a small amount of trypsin/EDTA solution is added and the flask is shaken slightly to allow the solution to come in contact with all the cells. The cells are hence incubated for 5 minutes and then the flask is tilted to check whether the cells have detached sufficiently. The suspension is then pipetted out, the trypsin is neutralized with trypsin inhibitor which is then pipetted out and the solution centrifuged at 1,000 rpm for 5 minutes and the pellet resuspended in M2 medium and transplanted onto the recipient site.

SURGICAL TECHNIQUES

Patient preparation, donor area and recipient area and follow-up have been discussed in earlier chapters and are essentially similar to what is followed for tissue grafts. Application of the cultured cell suspension is similar to what has been discussed in noncultured epidermal cell suspension.

The patient is asked to give rest to the operated area and to limit mobility at the site. First follow-up visit is at 7 days when the dressing at both donor and recipient sites is

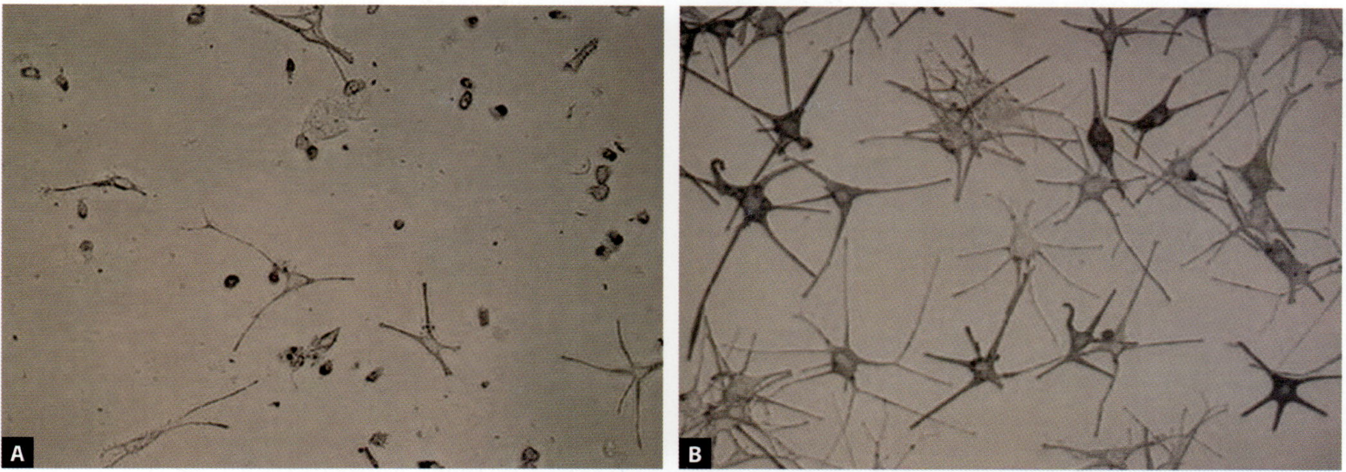

Figs. 1A and B: Cultured melanocytes after 5 and 15 days respectively.

removed. Both the sites are expected to be re-epithelialized by then and appear pink in color. Over the next 2–4 weeks small brown spots of pigment start appearing on the pink area and by 16–24 weeks maximal repigmentation is expected. Patients may be advised to undergo phototherapy in the postoperative period (NBUVB/PUVA/PUV Asol) or simply asked to expose the area to sunlight for 10–15 minutes daily.

Cryopreservation

In order to allow cultured melanocytes to be preserved for prolonged periods, the cells may be lifted into suspension by trypsinization and centrifuged to form a pellet as above. The pellet is to be then resuspended in cryoprotectant, which is a solution consisting of 8% dimethyl sulfoxide (DMSO) in undiluted newborn calf serum (or a commercially available cryoprotectant). Usually 1 mL of cryoprotectant is to be used for each 10 million cells and the suspension is transferred to cryotube which is kept on ice for 10 minutes and then placed in a freezer and frozen at a temperature of –70°C to –85°C.

Whenever needed, these cells can be thawed by placing in a 37°C water bath, after which the suspension is transferred to a test tube containing culture medium. This is centrifuged at 1,000 rpm for 5 minutes and pellet is resuspended in culture medium or PBS for transplantation. About 70% of cells retain viability after 1 year.

MODIFICATIONS AND NEW DEVELOPMENTS

- **12, 13-dibutyrate (PDBu) for melanocyte culture:** A study has attempted to compare the efficacy of another phorbol ester, Phorbol 12, 13-dibutyrate (PDBu) in melanocyte culture because of its less hydrophobic nature compared to phorbol 12-myristate 13-acetate (PMA). In PDBu, melanocytes acquired proliferative status and bipolar morphology quicker with less survival of keratinocytes. PDBu has also been found to have a higher proliferative induction capacity than PMA and melanocytes survived longer in PDBu compared to PMA.[11]
- **Amniotic membrane as a scaffold for melanocyte transplantation:** In a pilot study on four patients, Redondo et al.[6] replated cultured epidermal melanocytes onto the basement membrane (BM) side of amniotic membrane at a density of 5 – 25 × 10^3 cell/cm^2 after which they allowed the melanocytes to grow for another 3–4 days. Following this, they mounted these amniotic membranes on sterile vaseline gauze following which the amniotic membranes were placed on the dermabraded recipient site with the BM side down. They were able to achieve excellent repigmentation in all patients and observed repigmentation of the marginal area also, which is found to persist as a halo of depigmentation following other surgical procedures in some patients.

  They hypothesized that AMs are an easily available substrate which offer anti-inflammatory and antimicrobial properties with lack of antigenicity which facilitates the re-epithelialization of skin and reduces scarring.
- **Hyaluronic acid micropore sheets as scaffold:**[5] Another modification is the use of hyaluronic acid micropore sheet as a scaffold for culture of melanocytes. Andreassi et al. transferred cultured melanocytes and keratinocytes from suspension onto a 10 × 10 cm sized sheet of hyaluronic acid fixed on the bottom of a dish of same shape and size. The cells were allowed to proliferate and form a keratinizing stratified epithelium that reproduces the structure of epidermis. This sheet was then transferred to dermabraded recipient sites and repopulation of the areas occurred via passage of cells through the micropores. In their experience on 85 patients treated in the course of 7 years, they observed

more or less intense repigmentation in most of the treated lesions.

- **Preparation of recipient site:** A number of methods have been used for dermabrasion of the recipient site which have been described in earlier chapters. The new ones are use of Er:YAG laser,[12] CO_2 laser and recently Timed surgery. Timed surgery is a programmed diathermosurgery device which allows precise control of all operational parameters (electric power, appropriate shape of the output waveform, emission time, dimension of the electrode). Guerra et al.[9] used the above device for denudation of epidermis by coagulating it at 1 W using the dull portion of a 0.2 mm electrode bent at an angle, so as to allow the electrode to skim over the skin surface. The coagulated epidermis was then gently removed with the same electrode, but without electric power.

RESULTS

There has been a recent study comparing the results of cultured melanocyte (CM) transplantation with non cultured epidermal suspension (NCES) transplantation and it was found that excellent response was seen in 62.17% cases with the NCES technique and in 52% with the CM technique. Thus though results were comparable, CM offers the potential for significant expansion of donor-recipient ratio from 1:10 to 1:100.[13] Another similar study found better repigmentation followed CM transplantation as compared to NCES transplantation in vitiligo.[14] Bao et al. compared blister grafting with NCES and CM transplantation and found BG inferior to both CM and NCES while both the cellular techniques were not significantly different.[15] There have been two recent reports that highlighted the repigmentation of leukotrichia after CM transplantation.[16,17]

CONCLUSION

Cultured melanocyte transplantation is a promising technique for the management of resistant stable vitiligo with a special advantage of being able to cover large areas with small grafts. However, it requires technical expertise and expensive laboratory set-up and hence has not gained widespread popularity. In the hands of experienced personnel, it has the potential to give satisfactory and gratifying results.

REFERENCES

1. O'Connor NE, Mulliken JB, Banks-Schlegel S, et al. Grafting of burns with cultured epithelium prepared from autologous epidermal cells. Lancet. 1981;1:75-8.
2. Eisinger M, Marko O. Selective proliferation of normal human melanocytes in vitro in the presence of phorbol ester and cholera toxin. Proc Natl Acad Sci U S A. 1982;79:2018-22.
3. Gilchrest BA, Vrabel MA, Flynn E, Szabo G. Selective cultivation of human melanocytes from newborn and adult epidermis. J Invest Dermatol. 1984; 83:370-6.
4. Löntz W, Olsson MJ, Moellmann G, Lerner AB. Pigment cell transplantation for treatment of vitiligo: a progress report. J Am Acad Dermatol. 1994;30:591-7.
5. Andreassi L, Pianigiani E, Andreassi A, et al. A new model of epidermal culture for the surgical treatment of vitiligo. Int J Dermatol. 1998;37:595-8.
6. Redondo P, Gimondo de Azcarate A, Marquar L, GarcGa-Guzman M, Andreu E, Prosper F. Amniotic membrane as a scaffold for melanocyte transplantation in patients with stable vitiligo. Dermatol Res Pract. 2011; 2011: 532139.
7. Prasad D, Gupta S; IDVAL Dermatosurgery Taskforce. Standard guidelines of care for vitiligo surgery. Indian J Dermatol Venereol Leprol. 2008 Jan;74 Suppl:S37-45.
8. Falabella R, Arrunategui A, Barona MI, Alzate A. The minigrafting test for vitiligo: detection of stable lesions for melanocyte transplantation. J Am Acad Dermatol. 1995;32:228-32.
9. Guerra L, Capurro S, Melchi F, Primavera G, Bondanza S, Cancedda R, et al. Treatment of 'stable vetiligo by timedsurgery and transplantation of cultured epidesmal autografts. Arch Dermatol. 2000;136:1380-9.
10. Hong WS, Hu DN, Qian GP, McCormick SA, Xu AE. Ratio of size of recipient and donor areas in treatment of vitiligo by autologous cultured melanocyte transplantation. Br J Dermatol. 2011;165(3):520-5.
11. Padma D, Bhat KM. A comparison between Phorbol 12 Myristate 13 Acetate and Phorbol 12, 13 Dibutyrate in Human Melanocyte Culture. J Clin Diagn Res. 2016;10(1):GC01-4.
12. Kaufmann R, Greiner D, Kippenberger S, Bernd A. Grafting of in vitro cultured melanocytes onto laser-ablated lesions in vetiligo. Acta Derm Venereol. 1998;78(2):136-8.
13. Verma R, Grewal RS, Chatterjee M, Pragasam V, Vasudevan B, Mitra D. A comparative study of efficacy of cultured versus non cultured melanocyte transfer in the management of stable vitiligo. Med J Armed Forces India. 2014;70(1): 26-31.
14. Verma G, Varkhande SR, Kar HK, Rani R. Evaluation of repigmentation with cultured melanocyte transplantation (CMT) compared with non-cultured epidermal cell transplantation in vitiligo at 12th week reveals better repigmentation with CMT. J Invest Dermatol. 2015;135(10):2533-5.
15. Bao H, Hong W, Fu L, Wei X, Qian G, Xu A. Blister roof grafting, cultured melanocytes transplantation and non-cultured epidermal cell suspension transplantation in treating stable vitiligo: a mutual self-control study. J Dermatolog Treat. 2015;26(6):571-4.
16. Yao L, Zhong SX, Hu DN, Guo JW, Li SS, Xie XL, et al. Repigmentation of leukotrichia in vitiligo with transplantation of cultured autologous melanocytes. Int J Dermatol. 2014;53(8):1016-8.
17. Wu XG, Xu AE. Successful treatment of vitiligo on the scalp of a 9-year-old girl using autologous cultured Pure melanocyte transplantation. Pediatr Dermatol. 2017;34(1):e22-e23.

Chapter 40

Phototherapy with Grafting Procedures in Vitiligo

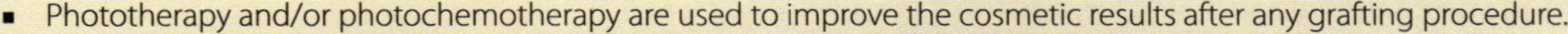

Imran Majid

Key Messages

- Phototherapy and/or photochemotherapy are used to improve the cosmetic results after any grafting procedure.
- Among the different phototherapeutic procedures used, NBUVB is currently most favored.
- Excimer laser and targeted phototherapy are the most recent additions to the phototherapy armamentarium for this purpose.

INTRODUCTION

The idea behind performing a grafting procedure in resistant vitiligo is to donate viable melanocytes to the recipient lesion. These melanocytes are donated in the form of tissue or cellular components, known as tissue and cellular grafting procedures respectively. After the grafting procedure the donated melanocytes can be stimulated by using topical or oral drugs or different forms of phototherapy to hasten and increase the chances of repigmentation. The idea behind using phototherapy after the surgical procedure is to stimulate and/or cause a proliferation of the donated melanocytes at the recipient site. Phototherapy and photochemotherapy have been used as supplemental therapies in all forms of tissue and cellular grafting procedures like miniature punch grafting (MPG), suction blister grafting (SBG), split-thickness (STSG) and ultra-thin skin grafting (UTSG) as well as in different cellular grafting techniques.

PUVA AND PUVASOL

Psoralens with UVA (PUVA) or with sun exposure (PUVAsol) have been very commonly used in combination with miniature punch grafting.[1-6] The main idea behind using this supplemental therapy is to enhance the pigment spread after miniature punch grafting. Most of the clinical studies on MPG have found this adjuvant therapy to be beneficial in their patients. In one clinical study, PUVAsol has been compared with topical corticosteroids as post-procedure therapy in MPG.[7] The study found both the therapies to be almost equally effective in enhancing the repigmentation after the surgical procedure.

PUVA and PUVAsol therapy has also been used with split-thickness skin grafting (STSG) and also with SBG with good results.[8,9] Even pre-irradiation of donor skin with UVA has been seen to increase the number of available melanocytes for the recipient area after STSG.[10]

In general, the photochemotherapy is started either immediately after the removal of dressings or one to two weeks after that and then continued for a period of two to six months or till complete repigmentation is achieved. The protocol followed is usually similar to that followed in other vitiligo patients with twice to thrice-weekly exposures. The dosages used as well as any dose enhancements are also similarly followed.

Adverse effects can occur especially with the use of topical PUVAsol and the patients can develop phototoxicity if over-exposure occurs. Hyperpigmentation of the grafted area can also be seen. All the usual precautions needed in photochemotherapy need to be followed and all the contraindications have to be excluded before starting the photochemotherapy regimen.

NARROWBAND UVB

Narrowband UVB (NBUVB) enjoys the status of being the most effective monotherapy in generalized vitiligo at present. It has now been experimentally proven that this treatment causes proliferation and migration of melanocytes from the outer root sheath of the hair follicles in vitiligo.[11] This beneficial property of Narrowband UVB is taken advantage of in vitiligo grafting. NBUVB is used after the procedure to enhance the repigmentation and to cause a better cosmetic match.

The post-procedure use of NBUVB has been described in almost all the tissue grafting procedures like MPG, SBG, UTSG and STSG.[12-15] One clinical study on punch-grafting failure cases found excellent results when the same areas, which had not pigmented earlier, were re-grafted under NBUVB cover.[13]

In cases with UTSG, NBUVB is supposed to cause a better and early onset of repigmentation. It is also claimed to minimize the chances of achromic fissures or perigraft halo of depigmentation in this type of tissue grafting (Figs. 1A and B). Clinical studies have reported excellent repigmentation with a good color match when UTSG was supplemented with NBUVB exposure.[14]

In addition to tissue grafting procedures, NBUVB has been used in cellular grafting as well. There are reports of combined use of NBUVB with basal cell suspension technique as well as with epidermal cell cultures.[15,16]

As in the case of PUVA, Narrowband UVB is started within about two to three weeks after the grafting procedure and the exposure is given twice or thrice a week. The exposure is limited to the grafted area only in usual cases and the dose increments are given as in other cases of vitiligo. The phototherapy regimen is followed till complete repigmentation of the grafted area is achieved. In cases showing partial repigmentation only at the end of three to four months with no further spread of pigment with NBUVB exposures, the phototherapy regimen is usually stopped.

TARGETED PHOTOTHERAPY

Targeted phototherapy is the most recent addition to phototherapy armamentarium and it specifically 'targets' the lesional skin only while the rest of the skin remains unexposed. As a result, the uninvolved skin remains protected and the lesional skin can be exposed to higher energies to achieve a rapid therapeutic effect. Additionally, adverse effects of whole body irradiation are also avoided.

Different targeted phototherapy devices have been used in vitiligo till date and these include the XeCl excimer laser, excimer lamp and targeted UVB devices delivering either broadband UVB (BBUVB) or NBUVB light. All these devices are useful therapeutic modalities in vitiligo and thus can prove helpful when used in the postoperative period after vitiligo grafting. However, only excimer laser has been reported in combination with tissue and cellular grafting procedures in vitiligo till date in the world literature.

EXCIMER LASER

This laser system has also been used in patients undergoing split-thickness skin grafting and the results obtained have been reported as excellent in 100% patients at the end of one-year of follow up.[17] In a comparison study excimer laser has been found to be equally efficacious as NBUVB when used postoperatively in cases with MPG.[18] However, patients needed a much lower cumulative dose of phototherapy when excimer laser was used.

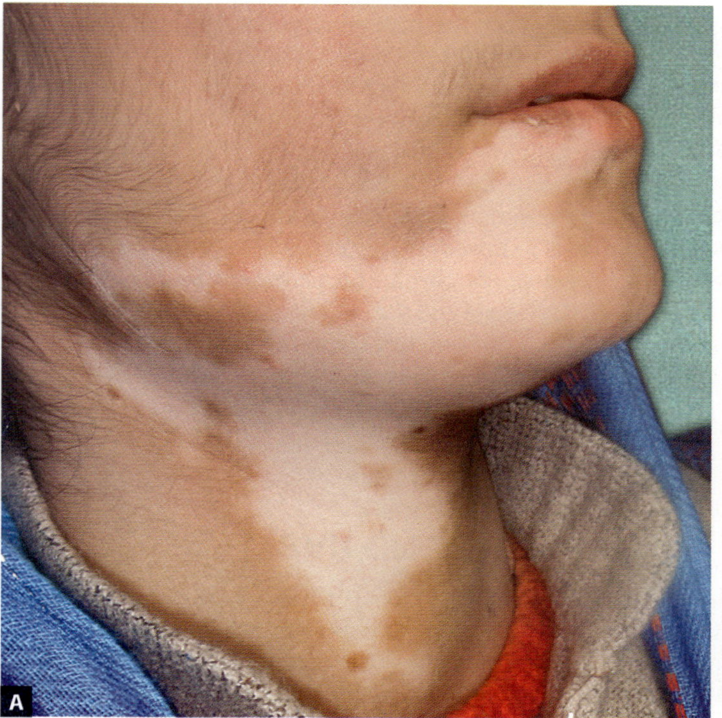

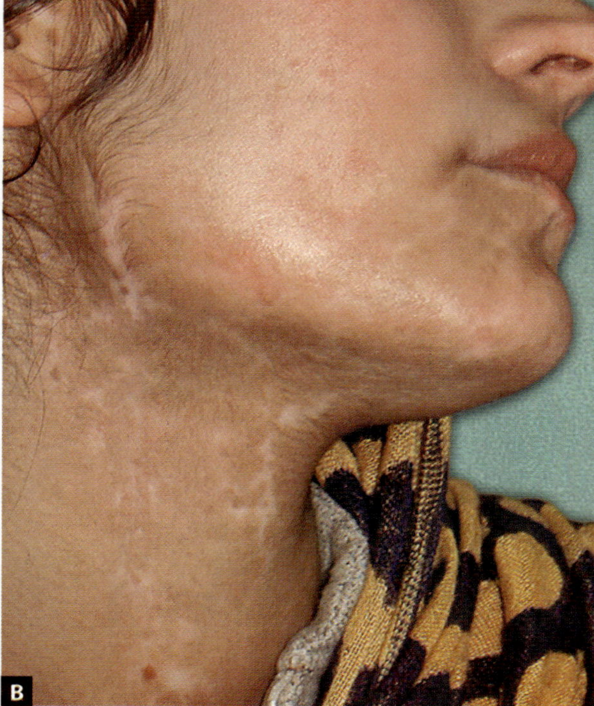

Figs. 1A and B: (A) Segmental vitiligo on neck; (B) Post-treatment picture after ultrathin skin grafting and NBUVB.

SUMMARY

Phototherapy in the form of NBUVB and excimer lasers or photochemotherapy with PUVA and PUVAsol can be used as supplemental therapies to improve the cosmetic results achieved in both cellular as well as tissue grafting techniques in vitiligo (Box 1).

Box 1: Tips for phototherapy after vitiligo grafting.

- Using any form of phototherapy after a surgical procedure improves the cosmetic outcome
- The type of phototherapy to be used depends on the availability of equipment, the cost factor involved and the type of patient to be treated
- Narrowband UVB (NBUVB) scores over PUVA and PUVASOL as it is safer and does not need any postexposure safety precautions for the eyes
- Phototherapy needs to be started within 1–2 weeks after the removal of dressing for maximum stimulation of donated melanocytes
- In general, the phototherapy regimen is continued till a satisfactory outcome is achieved or till there is no further improvement observed at the grafted site
- The phototherapy protocol to be followed as well as any precautions and contraindications are the same as when the phototherapy regimen is used alone
- Targeted phototherapy has the advantages of being safer and yielding quicker results

REFERENCES

1. Lahiri K, Sengupta SR. Treatment of stable and recalcitrant depigmented skin conditions by autologous punch grafting. Indian J Dermatol Venereol Leprol. 1997;63:11-14.
2. Malakar S, Dhar S. Treatment of stable and recalcitrant vitiligo by autologous mimiature punch grafting: A prospective study of 1,000 patients. Dermatology. 1999;198: 133-9.
3. Bonafe JL, Lassere J, Chavoin JP, et al. Pigmenation induced in vitiligo by normal skin grafts and PUVA stimulation: a preliminary study. Dermatologica. 1983;166:113-6.
4. Skouge JW, Morison WL, Diwan RV, Rotter S. Autografting and PUVA: A combination therapy for vitiligo. Dermatol Surg Oncol. 1992;18:357-60.
5. Hann SK, Im S, Bong HW, Park YK. Treatment of stable vitiligo with autologous epidermal grafting and PUVA. J Am Acad Dermatol. 1995;32:943-8.
6. Savant SS. Autologous miniature punch grafting in stable vitiligo. Ind J Dermatol Venereol Leprol. 1992;58:310-4.
7. Barman KD, Khaitan BK, Verma KK. A comparative study of punch grafting followed by topical corticosteroid versus punch grafting followed by PUVA therapy in stable vitiligo. Dermatol Surg. 2004;30:49-53.
8. Hann SK, Im S, Bong HW, Park YK. Treatment of stable vitiligo with autologous epidermal grafting and PUVA. J Am Acad Dermatol. 1995;32:943-8.
9. Awad SS, Raof HA, El-Din WH, El-Domyati M. Epithelial grafting for vitiligo requires ultraviolet a phototherapy to increase success rate. J Cosm Dermatol 2007;6:119-24.
10. Lee AY, Jang JH. Autologous grafting with PUVA-irradiated donor skin for the treatment of vitiligo. Int J Dermatol. 1998;37:551-4.
11. Wu C-S, Yu C-L, Wu C-S, et al. Narrowband ultraviolet-B stimulates proliferation and migration of cultured melanocytes. Exp Dermatol. 2004;13:755-63.
12. Lahiri K, Malakar S, Sarma N, Banerjee U. Repigmentation of vitiligo with punch grafting and narrow-band UV-B (311 nm) a prospective study. Int J Dermatol. 2005;45: 649-55.
13. Lahiri K, Malakar S. Inducing repigmentation by regrafting and phototherapy (311 nm) in punch failure cases of lip vitiligo: A pilot study. Indian J Dermato Venereol Leprol. 2004;70:156-8.
14. Majid I, Imran S. Ultrathin split-thickness skin grafting followed by narrowband UVB therapy for stable vitiligo: An effective and cosmetically satisfying treatment option. Indian J Dermatol, Venereol Leprol. 2012;78(2):159.
15. Mysore V, Salim T. cellular grafts in management of leukoderma. Indian J Dermatol. 2009;54:142-9.
16. Elisa P, Massimiliano R, Andrea A, et al. Autologous epidermal cultures and narrowband Ultraviolet B in the surgical treatment of vitiligo. Dermatol Surg. 2010;31: 155-9.
17. Al-Mutairi N, Manchanda Y, Al-Doukhi A, Al-Haddad A. Long-term results of split-skin grafting in combination with excimer laser for stable vitiligo. Dermatol Surg. 2010;36:499-505.
18. Linthorst Homan MW, Spuls Pl, Nieuweboer-Krobotova L, et al. A randomized comparison of excimer laser versus narrow-band ultraviolet B phototherapy after punch grafting in stable vitiligo patients. J Eur Acad Dermatol Venereol. 2012;26(6):690-5.

Chapter

41

Vitiligo: Other Modalities of Treatment

Dilip Kachhawa

Key Messages 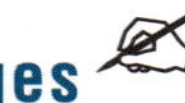

- Many minor and simple surgical procedures have been practiced for small and stable patches of vitiligo.
- Tattooing, despite its multitude of disadvantages, may be useful in some special situations especially for difficult areas like angle of the mouth, areola and nipple.
- Surgical excision with primary closure can be done for a patch over the mucosal surface and places where a small linear scar is acceptable.
- Other miscellaneous techniques such as epidermal cell transfer technique (Jodhpur technique), Follicular Unit Extraction Transplant, mesh grafting are newer surgical approaches.

INTRODUCTION

Apart from the hitherto described standard methods of grafting, several minor techniques have been described by several authors in the previous chapters. These, though not widely used, do have their role in selected cases and are described below.

MICROPIGMENTATION/TATTOOING

Micropigmentation involves implanting small particles (mostly iron oxide pigment) into the middle layer of dermis similar to a tattoo. The procedure is sometimes called 'permanent cosmetics.'

It is a therapeutic modality in which inert, artificial pigments in various combinations to match the patients skin color are introduced into the mid-dermis level of the lesion.[1] Micropigmentation is a useful procedure for the cosmetic camouflage of vitiliginous patches especially involving mucosal and mucocutaneous areas particularly in brown or black skinned races like Asians and Africans (Figs. 1A to D).[2] Tattooing as the treatment of vitiligo has been performed for the following indications:

- In a situation which needs urgent pigment correction of the depigmented patch.
- In special sites like angles of the mouth where graft retention is poor.

Various tattoo pigments include:

- White: Titanium dioxide
- Red: Cinnabar, Mercuric sulfate
- Black: Iron oxide
- Yellow: Cadmium sulfate
- Camel yellow: Iron oxide
- Light brown: Iron oxide
- Dark brown-: Iron oxide.

All tattoo pigments must be autoclaved before use.

Procedure

The procedure includes an informed consent, cleaning with normal saline followed by tumescent anesthesia with injection 2% of xylocaine. Tattoo pigments are mixed in a desired proportion, depending on the site and to get an appropriate color match. Actual micropigmentation is done with number 10 pony sewing needle after appropriate sterilization in a cidex solution. Alternatively, a motorized tattoo instrument can also be used. Micropigmentation is done until the color matches the surrounding skin.Pressure is given with gauze for about 2 min to stop bleeding if any. After the procedure, the area is cleaned with saline. Immediate side-effects such as bleeding and hematoma are noted in some studies.[3]

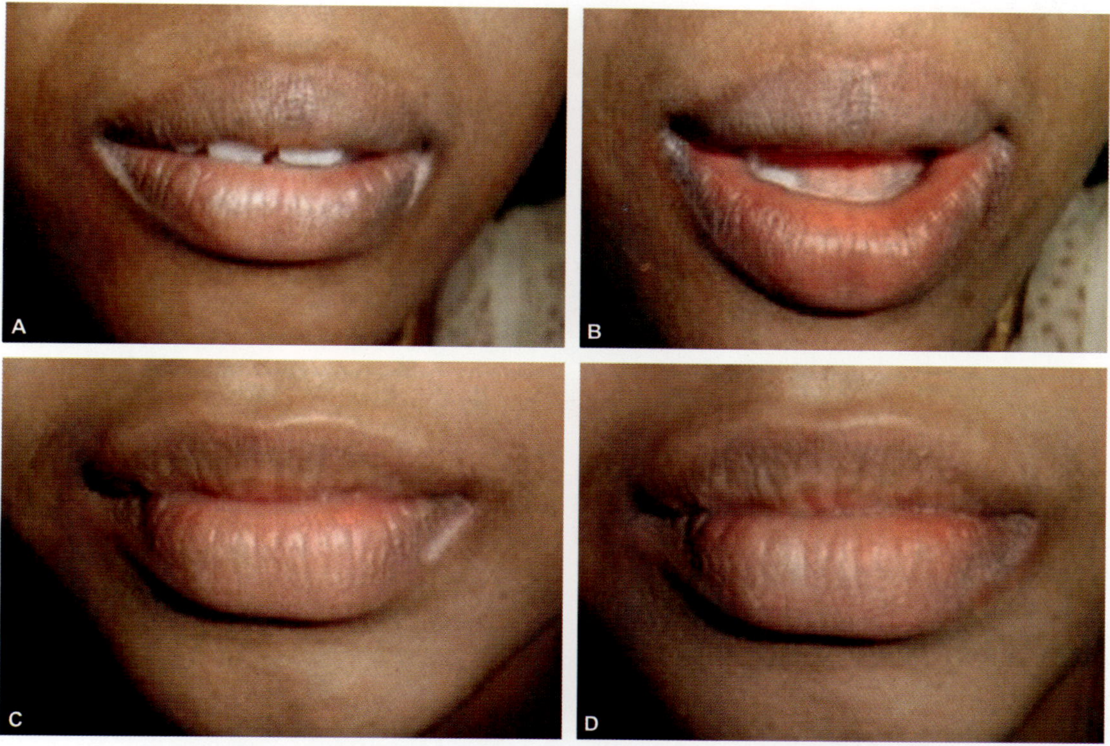

Figs. 1A to D: Vitiligo of lateral lower lip before and after micropigmentation.
Courtesy: Journal of Cutaneous and Asthetic Surgery (JCAS).

Advantages and Disadvantages of Micropigmentation

Micropigmentation can:

- Help blend the color of vitiligo to more closely match that of surrounding skin.
- Breaks up the texture of the vitiligo skin by softening and flattening it.

However, there are several disadvantages of the technique, which precludes the routine use of the technique; these include blackening due to oxidation,[4] photosensitization to cadmium sulfate, bleaching of pigment (i.e. unsightly and inappropriate look of implanted pigment with time), fading of pigment over a period of time, which is unacceptable to the patient. Greenish discoloration due to Tyndall effect may also be seen. Such pigment mismatch keeps changing over a period of time and further poses serious difficulty for correction with other surgical modalities of treatment. Reaction to tattoos can include allergic hypersensitivity: granulomatous, lichenoid and pseudolymphomatous types. The reactions are seen to be more common with red, yellow, green and blue pigments and are very uncommon with the more commonly used black and brown tattoos.

What to expect after the procedure:

- Swelling in the treated area which resolves spontaneously or with ice pack application.
- Improved appearance in treated area within a few days.
- Full healing of treated area in four to six weeks.

SURGICAL REMOVAL OF THE DEPIGMENTED AREAS

Surgical removal followed by primary closure of a small depigmented patch of vitiligo has been practiced in situations of urgency to get rid of the lesion, if the lesion is small, as most grafting methods need few weeks for the repigmentation to occur. This modality can be a useful surgical treatment option as long as the lesion is amenable for surgical excision and closure with a good resultant scar which is acceptable to the patient. The most common site for such treatment is ideally a small patch of vitiligo over the lip and mucosal areas, since the retention of cellular grafts over the mucosal surfaces is poor.[5,6]

THERAPEUTIC WOUNDING

Superficial wounding of epidermis as a therapeutic modality has been practiced for small and stable patches of vitiligo.[7] In this procedure, dermabrasion or wounding by other means is performed without subsequent grafting procedure. This technique is suited for hairy areas and induces repigmentation of the lesion by altering epidermal cytokines milieu which stimulates inactive melanocytes present in the outer root sheath of hairs. The melanocytes which appear in the epidermis 8–10 days after dermabrasion are two to three times larger than normal melanocytes with a hypertrophic cellular body, elongated dendrites and intense 3,4-dihydroxyphenylalanine (DOPA) oxidase activity.[8] Wounding can be performed by various modalities such as manual or motor dermabrasion, laser ablation by CO_2[8] and Er:YAG lasers,[9] cryosurgery,[10] needling,[11] spot chemical peeling with 88% phenol[12] solution, trichloroacetic acid 30–50% or 5% 5-Flurouracil.[13] This modality is not a suitable treatment for places such as mucosa, and palms and soles where the hair follicles are absent.

EPIDERMAL CELL TRANSFER TECHNIQUE (JODHPUR TECHNIQUE)

Dilip Kachhawa[14] has described a unique method in which donor area is dermabraded and the dermabraded material consisting of epidermis and dermis is collected and applied directly on to the dermabraded recipient area. Lateral area of thigh is selected as donor area needed for collecting grafting material which is approximately one-third of recipient area.

The procedure consists of three steps:

1. The donor and recipient site (Fig. 2A) is anesthetized under proper aseptic conditions.
2. An antibiotic ointment (2% mupirocin ointment) is then applied over the donor site. The purpose of ointment is to collect the epidermal material during subsequent dermabrasion. Dermabrasion is performed by using manual dermabrader or motorized microdermabrader gently at slower rpm (approx. 5000 rpm) rolling the fraise continuously till pinpoint bleeding points are visible. At this juncture, dermabrasion is stopped and the epidermal material entangled in the ointment is collected with the help of a spatula or graft spreader. A paste-like material is thus obtained containing ointment, melanocytes and keratinocytes.
4. Procedure at recipient site: This site is prepared in the same way as for split thickness grafting (STG) by dermabrasion upto the level of upper dermis. The paste like epidermal cell material obtained above is spread on this dermabraded recipient site as a thin film (Fig. 2B). Above this grafted material collagen dressing is

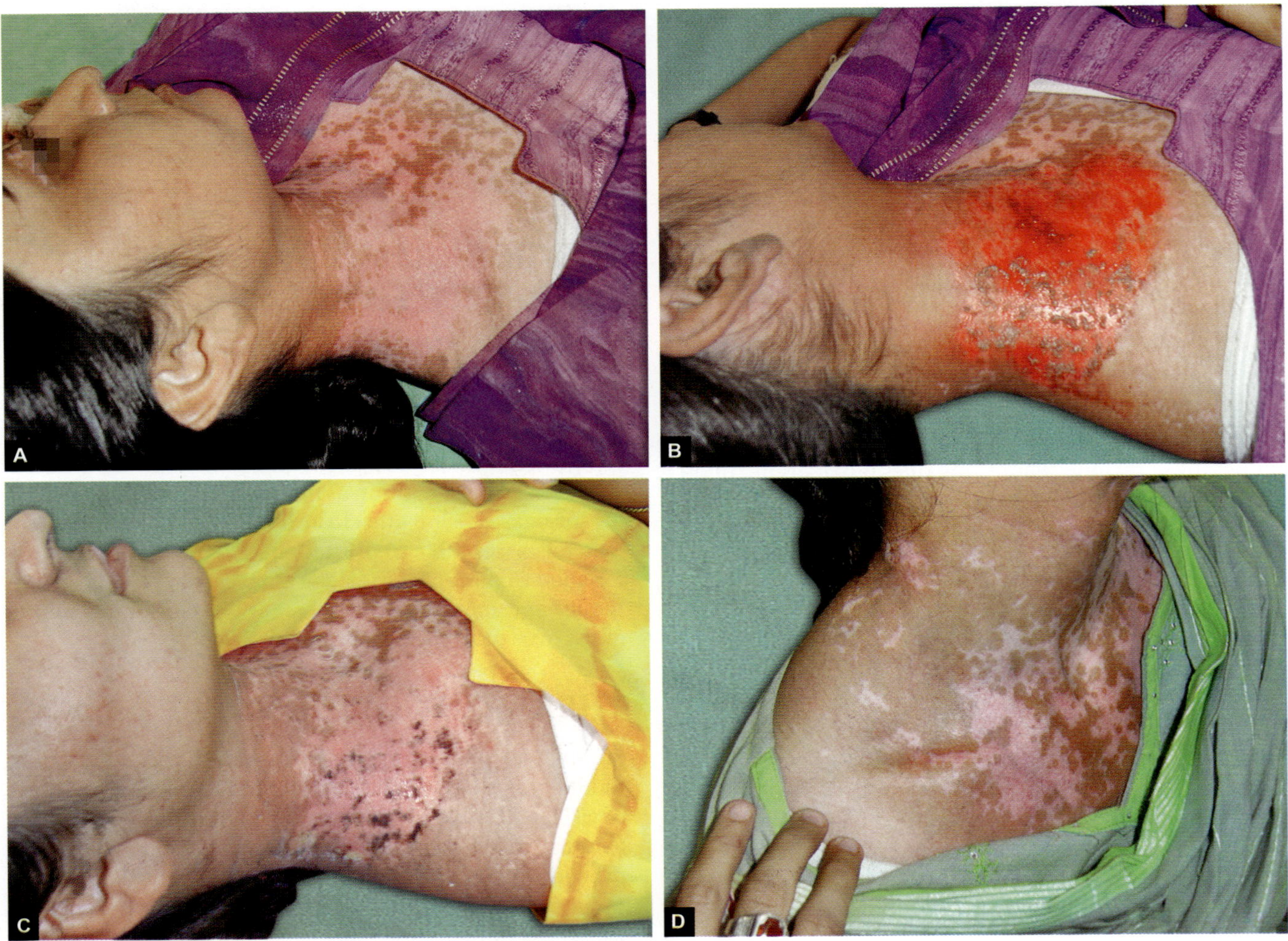

Figs. 2A to D: (A) Before surgery; (B) Just after grafting with paste-like material containing melanocytes and keratinocytes; (C) After 1 week of grafting, grafted material is seen as black eschar; (D) After 20 weeks pigmentation seen over grafted sites.

done followed by placement of three layered ointment soaked sterile gauge and left for 7 days, after which it is removed and a blackish eschar is seen, which falls off on its own in the next 3–5 days (Fig. 2C). PUVAsol therapy is started after 14–21 days. Repigmentation is observed after4–6 weeks of the procedure and significant pigmentation occurs by 16–20 weeks (Fig. 2D).

This method has advantages such as simplicity, lack of skill needed for grafting and no requirement for any special grafting equipment.

FOLLICULAR UNIT EXTRACTION TRANSPLANT

Follicular unit grafting[15] is another new technique that can be employed for stable vitiligo lesions. After giving tumescent anesthesia (lignocaine with 1:100,000 adrenaline diluted in the ratio of 1:10 with normal saline), the donor follicles are extracted using micropunches [follicular unit extraction (FUE) technique]. The donor area chosen is the occipital or postauricular region of the scalp as per the patient's requirement, i.e. the number of hair required, the characteristics of the hair at the recipient site, etc (Figs. 3A and B). The hair follicles are then transplanted intact as follicular units. After infiltrative anesthesia at the recipient site, transplantation is done using 18-G needle to create slits in the recipient area and the hair follicle is gently inserted using a jeweller's forceps. Topical corticosteroid and tacrolimus or topical PUVAsol therapy are given to enhance repigmentation after a few weeks.

Extraction of individual follicular units from occipital area, chest, back, beard, etc., not only avoids scarring and can be usefully employed even in the surgically difficult sites such as non-glabrous skin, eyelash or angle of the mouth (Figs. 4A and B). This technique is also devoid of complications such as cobblestoning, hypertrophic scar, and postoperative hyperpigmentation which may be seen with other grafting procedures. However, using this

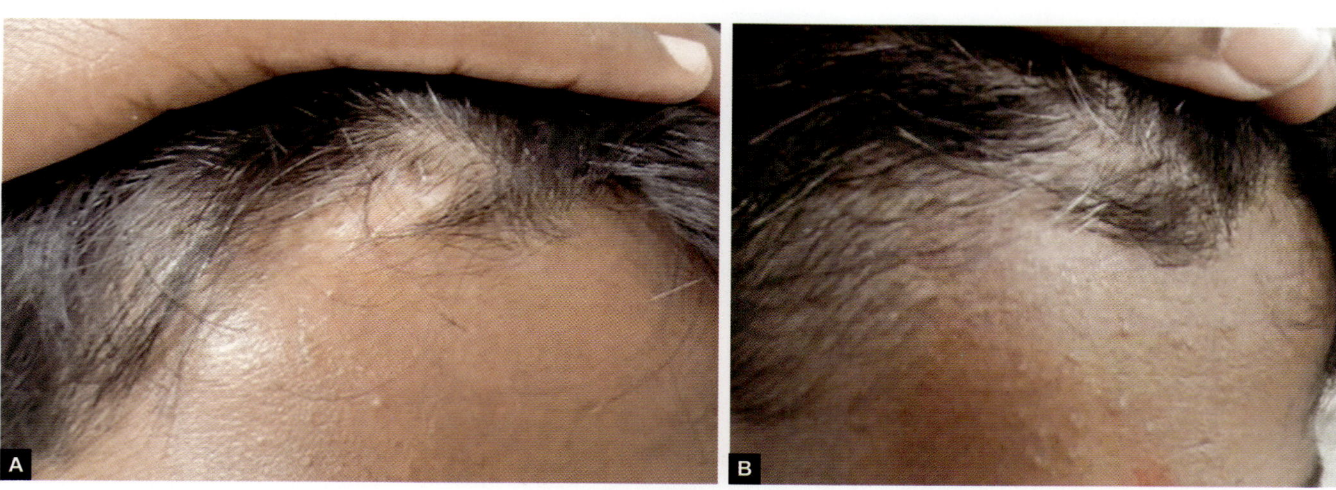

Figs. 3A and B: (A) Vitiligo lesion over scalp-before the procedure; (B) Six months after the procedure; improvement in vitiligo and leukotrichia with excellent color match.

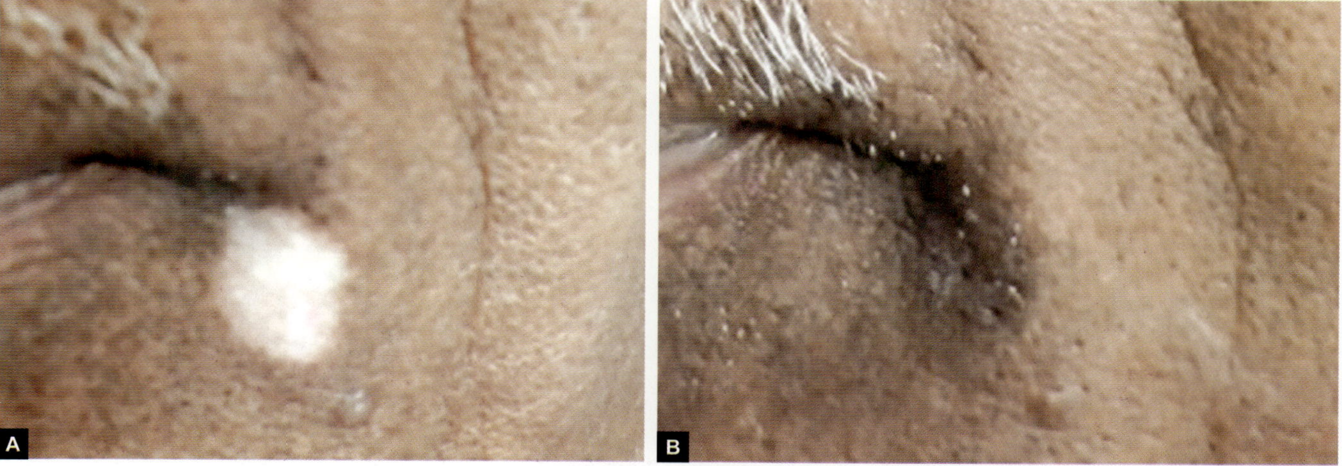

Figs. 4A and B: (A) Vitiligo lesion over the moustache before the procedure; (B) 2 months after the procedure.

technique it is difficult to treat medium to large lesions and glabrous areas. Also, vitiliginous skin heals slowly with this method because the grafted melanocytes require a long time to spread.

SMASH GRAFTING

It is a modification of split thickness grafting (STG). In this technique, STG is cut in very small pieces and a paste like material is prepared and used as a graft on pre-dermabraded recipient site. Advantages of this technique are—(1) thick graft can be used, (2) uniform pigmentation seen, (3) avoids stuck on appearance of graft.[16,1]

CONCLUSION

Surgical methods are the modalitiy of choice for stable recalcitrant vitiligo patches. Newer cell based or tissue based techniques provide a good color match along with repigmentation. Hence, patient satisfaction can be achieved by employing these novel methods of repigmentation.

PEARLS

- The pigmentation of micropigmentation tends to fade over time, requiring a periodic touch-up.
- Therapeutic wounding is suitable only for hairy areas.
- Jodhpur technique is a simple, economical and effective technique for treatment of stable vitiligo patches.
- FUE transplant is devoid of any cosmetic side-effects, but the results are slow to appear.

REFERENCES

1. Savant SS. Tattooing. In: Savant SS (Ed). Textbook of Dermatosurgery and Cosmetology, 2nd edition. Mumbai: ASCAD;2005;337-44.
2. Thami GP. Micropigmentation. In: Gupta S, Olsson MJ, Kanwar AJ, Ortonne JP (Eds). Surgical Management of Vitiligo, 1st edition. Oxford: Blackwell publishing; 2006;249-53.
3. Francis A, Criton S, Shojan A, Philip R. Micropigmentation in vitiligo of lateral lower lip. J Cutan Aesthet Surg. 2013; 6(4):236–7.
4. Garg G, Thami GP. Micropigmentation: tattooing for medical purposes. Dermatol Surg. 2005;31:928-31.
5. Gupta DK. Excision with primary closure. Microskin grafting for vitiligo, 1st edition. New York: Springer; 2009;11-4.
6. Sacchidanand S, Purohit V, Sujaya SN. Surgical excision and primary closure for the treatment of lip vitiligo J Cutan Aesthet Surg. 2011; 4(3):216-7.
7. Savant SS. Therapeutic spot and regional dermabrasion in stable vitiligo. Indian J Dermatol Venereol Leprol. 1996;62: 139-45.
8. Staricco RGJ. The melanocytes and the hair follicle. J Invest Dermatol. 1960;35:185-94.
9. Savant SS. Therapeutic wounding. In: Savant SS (Ed). Textbook of Dermatosurgery and Cosmetology, 2nd edition. Mumbai: ASCAD; 2005;370-7.
10. Savant SS. Cryosurgery with liquid nitrogen in stable vitiligo. Indian J Dermatol Venereol Leprol. 1999;65:246-7.
11. Ahmad TJ, Rashid T, Rani Z. Needling: An adjunct to narrowband ultraviolet B therapy in localized fixed vitiligo. J Pak Assoc Derma. 2008;18:149-53.
12. Savant SS, Shenoy S. Chemical peeling with phenol: For the treatment of stable vitiligo and alopecia areata. Indian J Dermatol Venereol Leprol. 1999;65:93-8.
13. Gauthier Y, Anbar T, Lepreux S, Cario-André M, Benzekri L. Possible mechanisms by which topical 5-fluorouracil and dermabrasion could induce pigment spread in vitiligo skin: An experimental study ISRN Dermatol. 2013:852497.
14. Kachhawa D, Kalla G. Keratinocyte-melanocyte graft technique followed by PUVA therapy for stable vitiligo. Indian J Dermatol Venereol Leprol. 2008;74:622-4.
15. Sacchidanand S, Thakur P, Purohit V, Sujaya SN. Follicular unit extraction as a therapeutic option for Vitiligo. J Cutan Aesthet Surg. 2013;6:229-31.
16. Krishnan A, Kar S Smashed skin grafting or smash grafting —a novel method of vitiligo surgery. Int J Dermatol. 2012;51 (10):1242-7.

Chapter

42

Innovations and Pearls in the Surgical Management of Vitiligo

KT Ashique, Feroze Kaliyadan

Key Messages

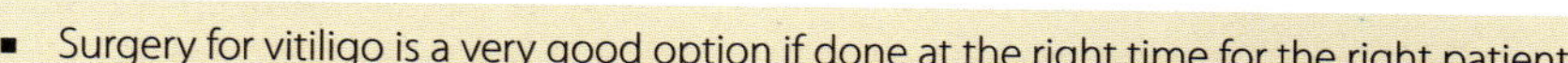

- Surgery for vitiligo is a very good option if done at the right time for the right patient.
- There are various methods, viz. Punch grafting, Suction blister grafting, Cellular grafting.
- Innovations and improvisations have made the procedures versatile.
- Things have been simplified to a great extent that vitiligo surgeries can be undertaken even in poor resource settings.

"There is a way to do it better. Find it".

—*THOMAS ALVA EDISON*

INTRODUCTION

Moving forward in any field is impossible without innovations.[1] A lot of new techniques and modifications have happened in the recent times in the surgical management of vitiligo. A few salient works from published literature are reviewed here. They are all pointers towards new dimension in research in vitiligo surgery. The most common methods used in the surgical treatment of vitiligo include: punch grafting, suction blister grafting, autologous melanocyte-keratinocyte suspension transfer. Cultured melanocyte transplantation, though effective, is limited by the need for extensive laboratory support and a tedious process. Simple techniques like using phenol over the depigmented lesions to induce pigmentation have been described.[2] This chapter describes some practical tips and pearls which can be used in improving the outcome of surgical treatment in vitiligo.

SUCTION BLISTER EPIDERMAL GRAFT

Suction blister epidermal grafting, being very easy and less demanding in terms of expertise and expenditure, is widely carried out as an office-based procedure. To overcome the limitation of shortage of graft to cover the recipient area especially when there is lesser than expected number of blister formed, Ashique et al. found a simple technique to split the graft into fragments and each fragment can be placed easily at the recipient area with utmost ease.[3] The advantage of this technique is zero investment in terms of money and since the graft is placed on a paper, it is easy for the surgeon to place them even at difficult areas like the angle of the mouth, lips below the eyes, etc. (Figs. 1A to D).

Different techniques have been suggested for simplifying the process and to increase the speed of blister formations for suction blister grafting. Gupta et al. described an apparatus consisting of a cylindrical funnel connected with a three-way tap, and suction was given by a 50 mL syringe for producing suction blisters.[4] Kaliyadan described use of a microdermabrasion machine for producing suction blisters.[5] Various methods have been used to speed up the blister formation including application of ultraviolet (UV) light, infrared light, liquid nitrogen and injection of local anesthetic or saline into the donor site.[6-9]

Some pearls have also been suggested for transfer of the suction blister graft-like using the gloved finger or the hypodermic needle.[10,11]

RECIPIENT SITE PREPARATION

Another very simple and low cost technique which makes vitiligo surgery even more simplified. Gupta et al. in their study found that a hypodermic needle could be used for dermabrasion of the recipient site while preparing the

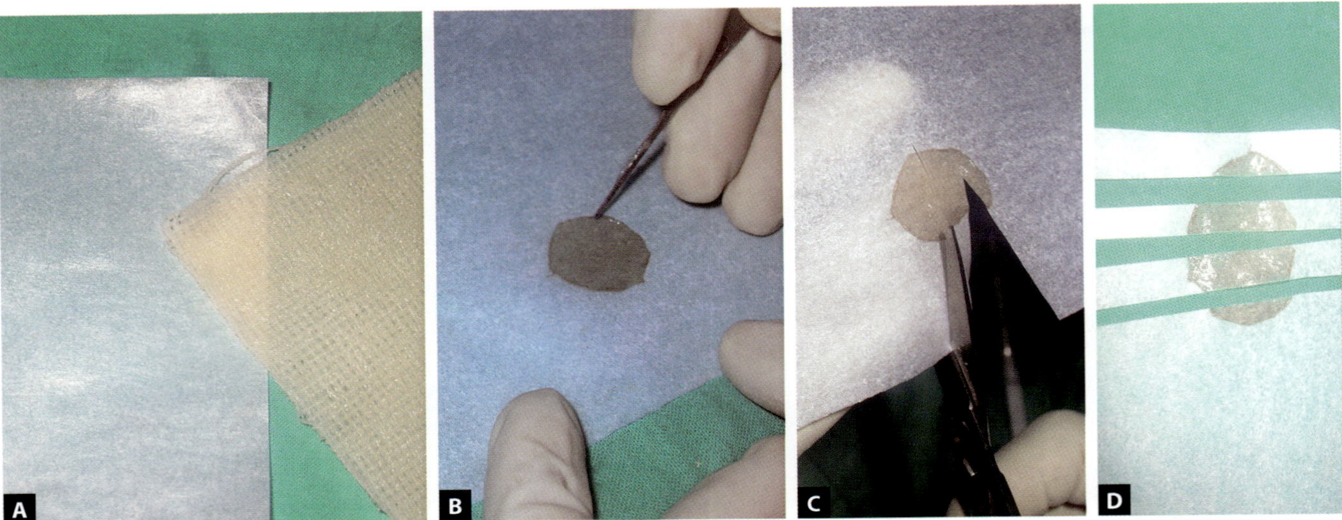

Figs. 1A to D: (A) The oil paper that comes sandwiching the jelonet dressing; (B) The blister roof harvested and placed on the paper; (C) The graft easily cut with the paper; and (D) The split grafts ready for placement at the recipient end.

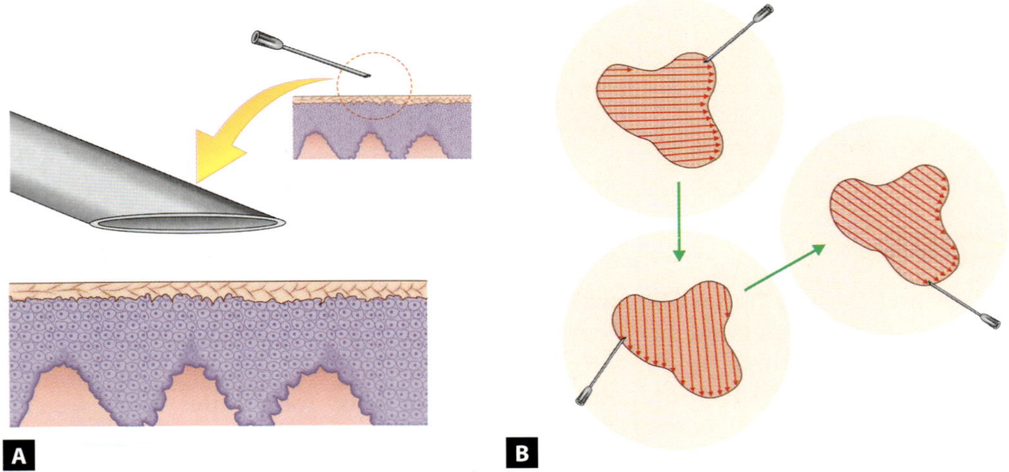

Figs. 2A and B: (A) Dermabrasion of the recipient site for vitiligo surgery with the beveled end of the needle held at 45° to the skin surface; and (B) The direction of motion of the strokes one after the other till pinpoint bleeding is attained.
Source: Dr Sanjeev Gupta, MD, DNB. Professor and HOD, Department of Dermatology and Venereology, Maharishi Markandeshwar Institute of Medical Sciences and Research, Mullana, Haryana.

area for placing the graft or suspension.[12] A 20 or 22 gauge needle is held with the thumb and index finger and with the beveled end in contact with the skin surface, multiple longitudinal, transverse and oblique stokes were made till pinpoint bleeding was noticed (Figs. 2A and B). The technique bypasses the need for motorized dermabrader in small patches and the procedure becomes more accessible to the surgeons in the resource poor setting. The technique is also useful in repair of perilesional depigmentation after surgery.

While motor dermabrasion is the most commonly used method, some options to speed up the process include using radiofrequency ablation and ablative lasers.[13,14] Suction blister production for preparation of the recipient site has also been described.[15]

EPIDERMAL CELL SUSPENSION

Gupta et al. described a very novel and interesting technique of preparation of cell suspension on the patient's body itself and the technique help to do away with the bulky centrifuge for incubation.[16] The normal body temperature of the patient works as the ideal temperature for cell separation. The technique involves creating blisters on the patient body as in suction blister grafting, aspirating the fluid and injecting with the cavity with trypsin-ethylenediaminetetraacetic acid (EDTA) solution and left for 45 minutes. This becomes a biological incubation in body temperature and then the fluid is again aspirated and kept in a petridish. The roof of the blister is also excised and scrapped off the basal layer. The entire suspension is

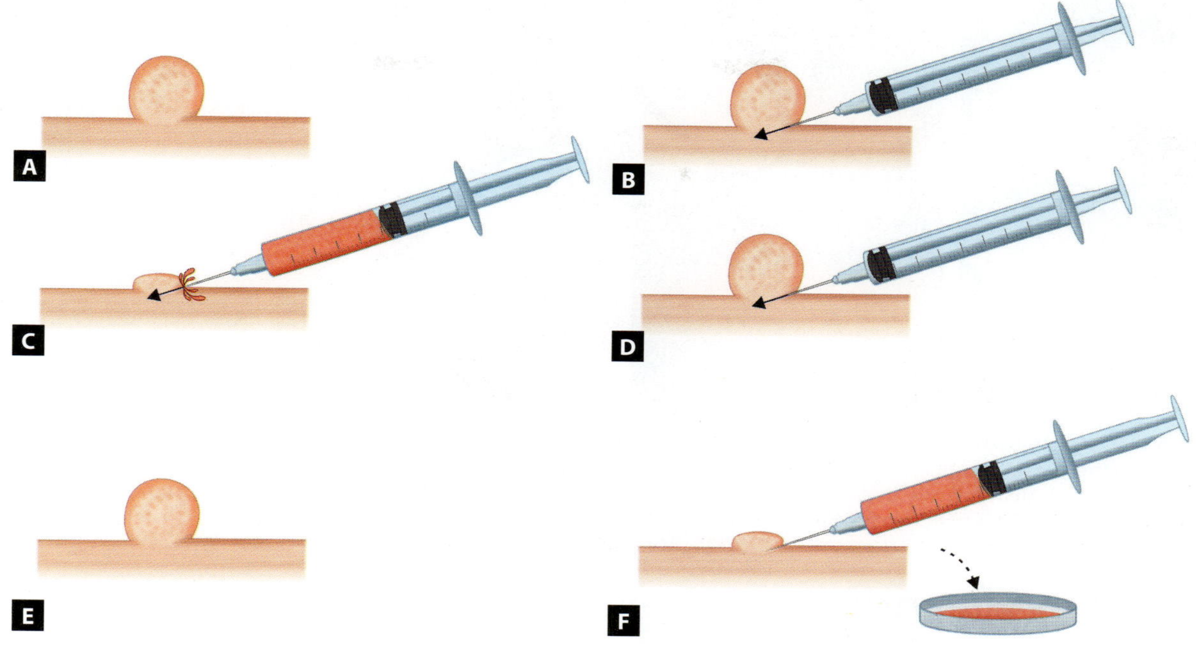

Figs. 3A to F: (A) Full-formed blister produced by suction; (B) The blister cavity is approached from the side with a syringe dermally (C) Aspiration of the blister fluid from the blister and leaving the blister roof intact (D) Injection of recombinant trypsin-EDTA into the intact blister cavity (E) Blister being used a autologous apparatus for incubation in body temparature (F) Incubated Cell suspension thus formed is aspirated and transferred to petridish.
(EDTA: Ethylene diamine tetra acetic acid).

used for transplantation on the prepared recipient area. The procedure hence makes cellular grafting easier even in low resource settings where infrastructure is a limitation (Figs. 3A to F).

Gauthier et al. also described a technique of injecting the epidermal cell suspension into a suction blister raised on the recipient site.[17]

Another tip for melanocyte suspension is to use that instead of trypsin inhibitor the grafts can be washed by Dulbecco's modified eagle medium (DMEM) or any other suitable medium. This cuts down the cost of the procedure to a great extent as the most expensive reagent in the whole procedure is the trypsin inhibitor only. Even patient's own serum can be used as an alternate to DMEM medium with equally good results. This, or using hyaluronic acid, also helps to increase the viscosity of the suspension.[18-20]

Gupta et al., a technique to harvest epidermal brushings from the donor site as a source for non-cultured melanocyte transfer in vitiligo surgery.[21] Manual dermabraders were used to abrade the skin. The first brushings which predominantly constituted the horny layer was discarded and subsequent brushings were used for trypsinizing-like the conventional cellular grafting procedure (Figs. 4A and B). The pellet was made into a suspension with phosphate buffered saline and applied to the recipient area and dressings given. The biggest advantage of this procedure was the complete absence of scarring at the donor area and repeated harvesting was possible from the site. The learning curve for skin harvesting with knife being more the chances of scarring at the donor site after the procedure are high. This can be completely avoided by this technique of donor harvesting as it does not require much expertise.

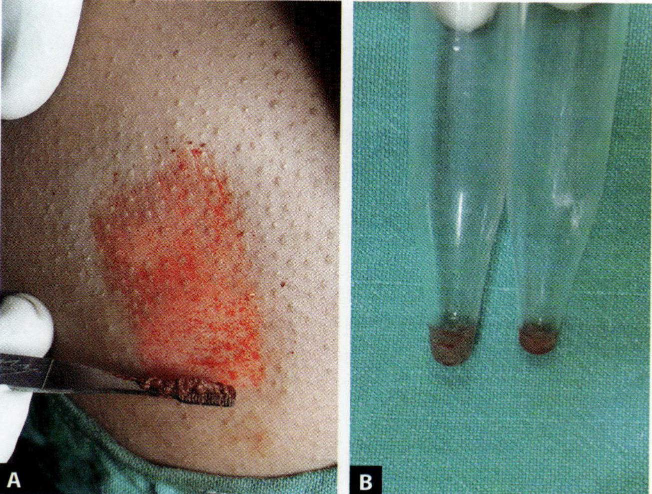

Figs. 4A and B: (A) Brushing from the skin taken with manual dermabrasion; and (B) Basal layer transferred to test tube for trypsinizing and further steps of cellular grafting.

Source: Dr Sanjeev Gupta, MD, DNB. Professor and HOD, Department of Dermatology and Venereology, Maharishi Markandeshwar Institute of Medical Sciences and Research, Mullana, Haryana.

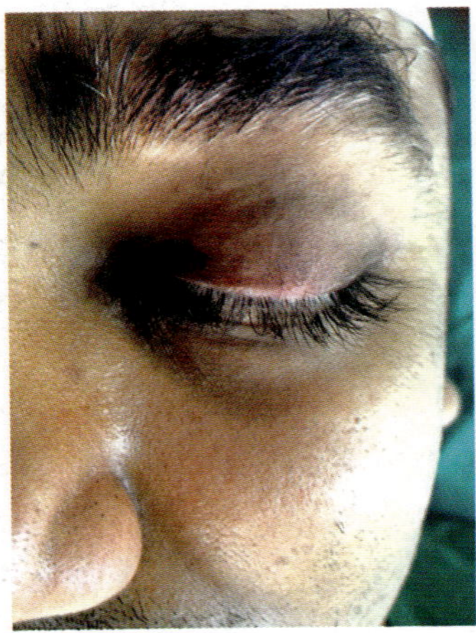
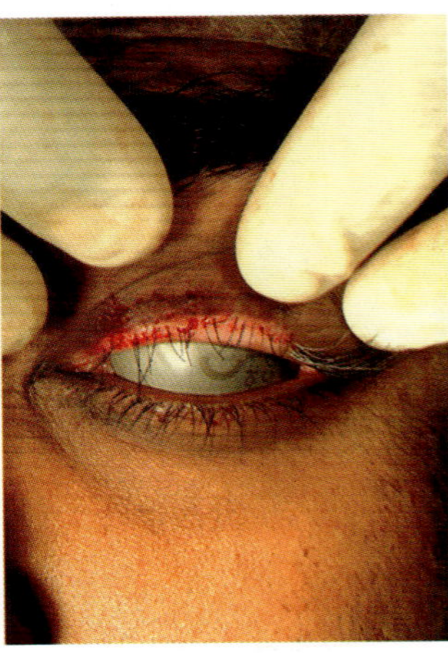

Fig. 5: Follicular unit transfer done as a treatment option for vitiligo involving the eye lid margin.
Source: Dr Kumaresan M MD, Professor, Department of Dermatology, PSG Institute of Medical Sciences and Research, Coimbatore, Tamil Nadu.

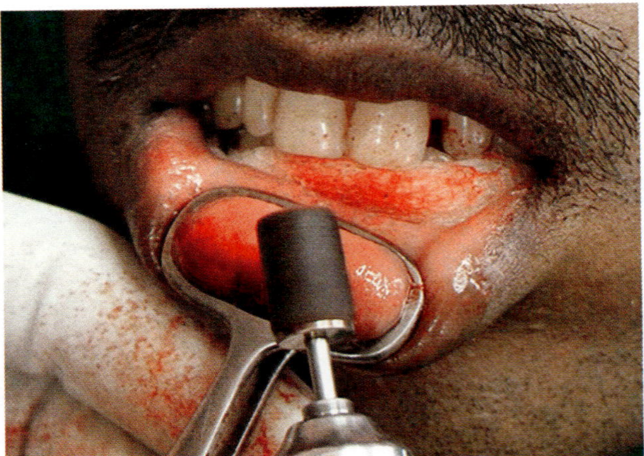

Fig. 6: Modified chalazion clamp with bigger ring in place as the lower lip is being dermabraded with a motorized dermabrader. The clamp also makes handling the lip easy during the dermabrasion.

NEEDLING OR MICRONEEDLING

Malik et al. in their study found excellent repigmentation (70–80%) in patients with large patches of stable vitiligo with this technique.[22] Under topical anesthesia with 1% lidocaine cream, patient underwent microneedling with dermoroller for about 15–20 minutes. The end point was fine pinpoint bleeding and then a 1% tacrolimus ointment was applied. The procedure was repeated approximately 7 to 8 times over a period of 3 months. The advantage of this procedure is the cost-effectiveness due to less infrastructure and the procedure can be carried out as an office-based procedure to treat large patches.

Zawar et al. attempted needling technique to treat stable vitiligo on the leg.[23] The procedure involved anesthetizing the area with topical lidocaine and under all aseptic precautions, a 20 gauge needle was inserted at 45° to the surface and innumerable punctures were made to produce pinpoint bleeding. The procedure was repeated three times 2 weeks apart. The procedure is very cheap and can be carried out in any setting with utmost ease.

HAIR FOLLICLE TRANSPLANT

Some authors have reported good results with follicular transplant in the case of vitiligo (Fig. 5).[24,25] Non-cultured extracted hair follicle outer root sheath cell suspension has also been used in the treatment of vitiligo with the advantage that the yield of melanocytes is more.[26]

CHALAZION CLAMP REVISITED

The chalazion clamp has found a lot of application in dermatologic surgery in the present form. During lip surgery like dermabrasion of the lips for preparing the recipient area is cumbersome for two reasons. First the slipperiness of the lip when contact with the saliva and the blood and second the vascularity and bleeding which makes dermabrasion a bit difficult in addition. The smaller size of the ring has been a limitation and this was overcome by a modification as devised by Ashique et al.[27] The larger ring in the modified chalazion clamp (25 × 10 mm) makes the instrument more versatile by allowing more space within the ring for dermabrasion. The clamp in place acts as a handle to maneuver the lip during procedures at ease (Fig. 6).

CONCLUSION

Surgical management of vitiligo has been a remarkable breakthrough and innovations have been happening in all the procedures undertaken. There are scopes for further research and improvisations at various levels of the procedures.

REFERENCES

1. Srinivas CR. Innovations in dermatology. Indian J Dermatol Venereol Leprol. 2016;82(6):641-4.
2. Mysore V. Use of phenol to induce pigmentation in vitiligo. J Cosmet Dermatol. 2002;1(2):99-100.
3. Ashique KT, Srinivas CR. Resizing blister roof grafts for vitiligo surgery. J Am Acad Dermatol. 2014;71(2):e39-40.
4. Gupta S, Shroff S, Gupta S. Modified technique of suction blistering for epidermal grafting in vitiligo. Int J Dermatol. 1999;38(4):306-9.
5. Kaliyadan F, Manoj J, Venkitakrishnan S. Using a microdermabrasion machine as a suction blister device. Indian J Dermatol Venereol Leprol. 2008;74(4):392-3.
6. Kaliyadan F, Venkitakrishnan S, Manoj J. Use of a wood's lamp as a ultraviolet light source to improve the speed and quality of suction blister harvesting. Indian J Dermatol Venereol Leprol. 2010;76(4):429-31.
7. Laxmisha C, Babu A, Mohan Thappa D. Letter: infrared lamps for faster suction blister induction. Dermatol Surg. 2006;32(8):1111-2.

8. Hanafusa T, Yamaguchi Y, Nakamura M, et al. Establishment of suction blister roof grafting by injection of local anesthesia beneath the epidermis: less painful and more rapid formation of blisters. J Dermatol Sci. 2008;50(3):243-7.
9. Gupta S, Kumar B. Suction blister induction time: 15 minutes or 150 minutes? Dermatol Surg. 2000;26(8):754-6.
10. Laxmisha C, Thappa DM. Surgical Pearl: gloved finger as a transport platform for epidermal graft of suction blister. J Am Acad Dermatol. 2007;57(5 Suppl):S118-9.
11. Laxmisha C, Thappa DM. Surgical pearl: Use of hypodermic needle to transfer minigrafts. J Am Acad Dermatol. 2006; 54(4):707.
12. Gupta S, Gupta S, Kumar A. The hypodermic needle as a dermabrading device for recipient area preparation for skin grafting in vitiligo. J Am Acad Dermatol. 2015;72(4): e105-6.
13. Kaliyadan F. Using the ball-shaped attachment of a radiofrequency ablation device for preparation of recipient site in vitiligo surgery. Indian J Dermatol. 2011;56(4): 459-60.
14. Komen L, Vrijman C, Wietze van der Veen JP, et al. Observations on CO_2 laser preparation of recipient site for noncultured cell suspension transplantation in vitiligo. J Cutan Aesthet Surg. 2016;9(2):133-5.
15. Lee DY, Park JH, Choi SC, et al. Comparison of recipient site preparations in epidermal grafting for vitiligo: suction blister and CO_2 laser. J Eur Acad Dermatol Venereol. 2009;23:1448-9.
16. Gupta S, Sahni K, Tembhre MK, et al. A novel point-of-care in vivo technique for preparation of epidermal cell suspension for transplantation in vitiligo. J Am Acad Dermatol. 2015;72(2):e65-6.
17. Gauthier Y, Surleve-Bazeille JE. Autologous grafting with noncultured melanocytes: a simplified method for treatment of depigmented lesions. J Am Acad Dermatol. 1992;26(2 Pt 1):191-4.
18. Mulekar SV. Long-term follow-up study of segmental and focal vitiligo treated by autologous, noncultured melanocyte-keratinocyte cell transplantation. Arch Dermatol. 2004;140(10):1211-5.
19. Majid I. Grafting in Vitiligo: How to Get Better Results and How to Avoid Complications. J Cutan Aesthet Surg. 2013;6(2):83-9.
20. van Geel N, Ongenae K, De Mil M, et al. Modified technique of autologous noncultured epidermal cell transplantation for repigmenting vitiligo: a pilot study. Dermatol Surg. 2001;27(10):873-6.
21. Gupta S, Kumar A, Mahendra A, et al. A minimally invasive, scarless technique of donor tissue harvesting for noncultured epidermal cell suspension transplantation in vitiligo. J Am Acad Dermatol. 2015;73(6):e213-5.
22. Malik N, Singh Y, Goyal T. A simple office-based procedure for patients with extensive vitiligo. J Am Acad Dermatol. 2016;75(5):e195-7.
23. Zawar VP, Karad GM. Needling in unresponsive stable vitiligo. J Am Acad Dermatol. 2016;75(5):e199-e200.
24. Kumaresan M. Single-hair follicular unit transplant for stable vitiligo. J Cutan Aesthet Surg. 2011;4(1):41-3.
25. Thakur P, Sacchidanand S, Nataraj HV, et al. A Study of Hair Follicular Transplantation as a Treatment Option for Vitiligo. J Cutan Aesthet Surg. 2015;8(4):211-7.
26. Shah AN, Marfatia RK, Saikia SS. A Study of Noncultured Extracted Hair Follicle Outer Root Sheath Cell Suspension for Transplantation in Vitiligo. Int J Trichology. 2016;8 (2):67-72.
27. Ashique KT, Kaliyadan F. Reinventing the Chalazion clamp: Modification of the instrument for the procedural dermatologist. J Am Acad Dermatol. 2016;75(5):e193-4.

Chapter 43

Surgical Management of Non-vitiligo Leukoderma: An Update (A Review)

Sanjeev Mulekar, Madhulika Mhatre

Key Messages 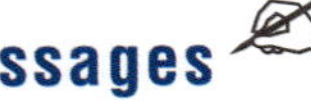

- Non-vitiligo leukodermas form an important spectrum of hypopigmented disorders.
- Conditions include piebaldism, nevus depigmentosus, Halo nevus, post-burn leukoderma, post-discoid lupus erythematosus (DLE) depigmentation, post-laser leukoderma, post-dermabrasion leukoderma.
- Piebaldism and post-burn leukoderma respond to various surgical transplantation methods consistently.
- Nevus depigmentatosus may recur post-surgery.
- Halo nevus shows consistent results.

INTRODUCTION

Leukoderma and hypopigmentation are generic terms used to designate disorders characterized by lightening of skin due to reduced epidermal melanin. Hypomelanosis is a more specific term that denotes absence or reduction of melanin in the skin, while amelanosis indicates total absence of melanin. The term depigmentation refers to the total loss of skin color.[1]

Leukodermas may be genetic or acquired. Among the genetic hypomelanotic disorders, vitiligo is by far the most common leukoderma encountered in the clinical practice: piebaldism and nevus depigmentosus are also commonly seen. Postinflammatory leukodermas may result from many inflammatory dermatoses such as burns, discoid lupus erythematosus (DLE), and treatment with laser and dermabrasion. Halo nevus is a specific type of leukoderma that occurs around a melanocyte nevus. These are not genetically determined, but can be considered as experiments of nature that demonstrate that there are mechanisms in humans that can selectively damage pigment cells.[2]

Leukodermas are most striking of all human disease phenotypes due to their characteristic stark patches of white skin, exposing patients to cosmetic embarrassment and social stigma in many societies. However, many of them with absolute stability do not respond to the conventional conservative therapies such as psoralen-ultraviolet A (PUVA) or narrowband UVB (NB-UVB). Therefore, surgical therapies need to be considered. While there are many published reports on surgical treatment for vitiligo, there is paucity of data on surgical treatment modalities for other hypopigmented disorders.

In this chapter, we review published studies on surgical management of non-vitiligo leukoderma. Pubmed search of all published English literature was conducted by using keywords: leukoderma, piebaldism, nevus depigmentosus, halo nevus, post-discoid depigmentation, and post-burn leukoderma. Level of evidence was graded on a five-point scale as follows:[3] (I) at least one properly designed randomized controlled trial; (II-1) well-designed controlled trial without randomization; (II-2) well-designed cohort or case-control analytic study, preferably more than one center or research group; (II-3) multiple time series with or without intervention or dramatic results from uncontrolled studies; and (III) clinical experience, descriptive studies, or reports of expert committees.

SURGICAL TREATMENT MODALITIES

- Tissue grafting
  - split-thickness tissue grafting
  - punch grafting
  - suction blister roof grafting.

  Pieces of pigmented skin are used to transfer melanocytes from normal pigmented parts of a patient's body to hypomelanotic or achromic areas. A dermatome is used to obtain a split-thickness thin graft in the first technique. Punch grafting uses a punch tool to harvest the skin sample. In suction-blister grafting the roof of an induced blister is the source of melanocytes.

- Cellular grafting: Epidermal cells are extracted from a skin sample and transplanted as a suspension. Cellular grafting can be accomplished either by in vitro culture of melanocytes and/or keratinocytes or by noncultured cell suspension.

INDICATIONS

- Piebaldism
- Nevus depigmentosus
- Halo nevus
- Post-burn leukoderma
- Post-DLE leukoderma
- Post-laser leukoderma
- Post-dermabrasion leukoderma

Piebaldism (Figs. 1A and B)

It is an autosomal dominant genetic skin disease characterized by a white forelock and large vitiligo like amelanotic macules, generally located on the forehead, ventral and lateral chest and abdomen, mid-upper arms to wrists and mid-thighs to mid-calves.[4] Melanocytes are either absent or greatly reduced in piebald lesions, although islands of hyperpigmentation may occur within leukodermic patches.[5] It does not respond to medical therapy.[4] Several surgical methods, such as minigrafts, epidermal grafts and split-thickness skin grafts have been used to treat piebaldism successfully.[6-9] Repigmentation of achromic areas of piebaldism has also been reported with noncultured epidermal cellular grafting[10] and pure melanocyte and epidermal cultured techniques which has an advantage of treating large surface areas with smaller skin biopsy sample.[11-14] *However, the value of this data is limited by the low number of patients and/or by the small size of treated lesions.* Only one study by Guerra et al. reported treatment of very large areas without any scarring by epidermal culture (Table 1).

Table 1: Piebaldism.

Method	*Study*	*Patients*	*Repigmentation*	*Type of study*	*Level of evidence*	*Reference*
Cultured autologous	Lerner AB	1	Excellent	Case report		Jm Invest Dermatol 1987[11]
Cultured autologous	Kumagai N	1	Normal			Annals of Plastic Surgery 1997[13]
Split-thickness graft	Njoo MD	12	95% to 100%			BJD 1998[8]
Cultures Autologous	Guerra L	6	95%			BJD 2004[14]
Punch grafts	Selmanowitz VJ					Cutis 1979[6]
Epidermal sheet grafts	Olsson, Juhlin					Acta derm venereol 1997[7]
Cultured and noncultured autologous melanocytes, autologous ultrathin epidermal sheets	Olsson, Juhlin			Retrospective questionnaire study	III	BJD 2002[9]
Noncultured cellular	Van Geel et al.	3	Mean 85–90%			BJD 2010[10]
Cultured epidermis + minigrafting	Falabella	1	100%			Dermatol Surg 1995[12]

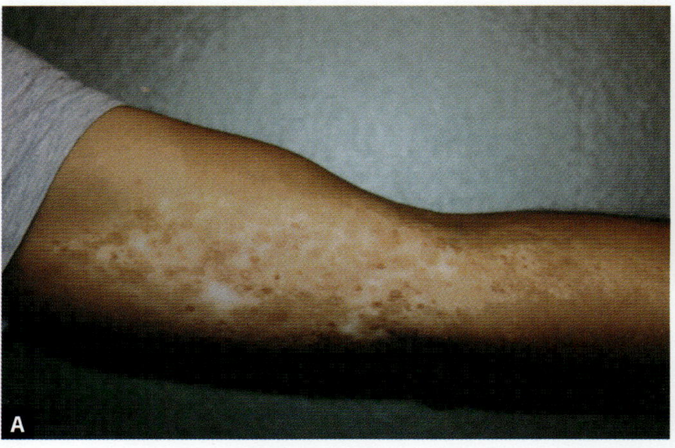

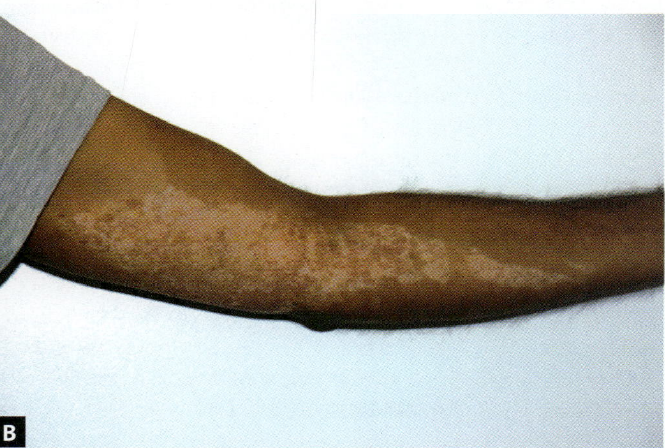

Figs. 1A and B: (A) Piebaldism pretreatment; (B) Piebaldism posttreatment. Please note color mismatch.

Nevus Depigmentosus (Figs. 2A and B)

Nevus depigmentosus is a congenital, nonprogressive cutaneous hypomelanosis, which can present as a circumscribed irregular, oval or round macule or as a unilateral band or streak with a block-like configuration or arranged along Blaschko's lines.[15] The lesions are hypomelanotic and remain unchanged throughout life although they may enlarge proportionately with the growing child. Different therapeutic attempts have been made to achieve repigmentation of nevus, such as epidermal grafting, noncultured melanocyte-keratinocyte suspension and cultured epidermis-bearing melanocytes.[10,16-21] All authors except Olsson have reported successful repigmentation varying from 80% to 100%. Long-term outcome has been monitored over a period of 2.5 years with sustained repigmentation by Raskovic,[21] but Kim DY reported recurrence of nevus 8 years after successful repigmentation.[17] Mulekar et al.[20] in a prospective uncontrolled study observed 80–100% uneven repigmentation in 2, and 100% good quality repigmentation in 1 out of 6 patients treated with noncultured melanocyte transplantation, while 2 failed to repigment. Based on the available evidence *it can be concluded that though repigmentation of nevus depigmentosus is possible by grafting techniques, the results are inconsistent and recurrence is possible* (Table 2).

Halo Nevus (Figs. 3A and B)

Halo nevus is a pigmented nevus surrounded by ring of depigmentation that may progress to spontaneous disappearance of the nevus.[22] The cause of the halo is difficult to explain solely by cellular or humoral mechanism and could be attributed to a product released from damaged nevus cells or a cytokine produced by the inflammatory cells.[2] The treatment of halo nevus is

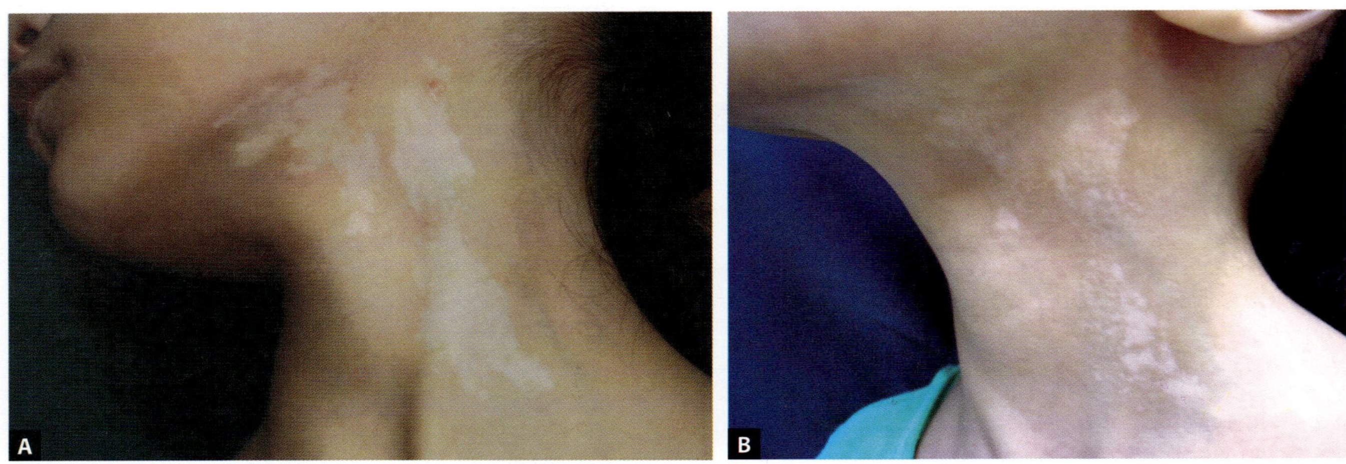

Figs. 2A and B: (A) Nevus depigmentosus pretreatment; (B) Nevus depigmentosus posttreatment. Please note incomplete repigmentation.

Table 2: Nevus depigmentosus.

Method	*Study*	*Patients*	*Repigmentation*	*Type of study*	*Level of evidence*	*Reference*
Epidermal graft	Gupta S, Goel A	1	Good- in grafted area	Single case report	III	Dermatol Surg 2005[16]
Epidermal graft	Kim DY ParkYK Hann SK	1	Good-after 8 years recurred	Single case report	III	JAAD 2008[17]
Cultured epidermis	Raskovic D et al.	1	Complete	Single case report	III	JAAD 2006[21]
Noncultured epidermis	Gauthier Y et al.	1	80%		III	JAAD 1992[18]
Noncultured epidermis	Olsson M, Juhlin L	1	0%		III	BJD 1998[19]
Noncultured epidermis	Mulekar et al.	5	Poor result- 2 patients 80–100% - 3 patients			JCAS 2011[20]
Noncultured epidermal cellular grafting	van Geel et al	1	78%			BJD 2010[10]

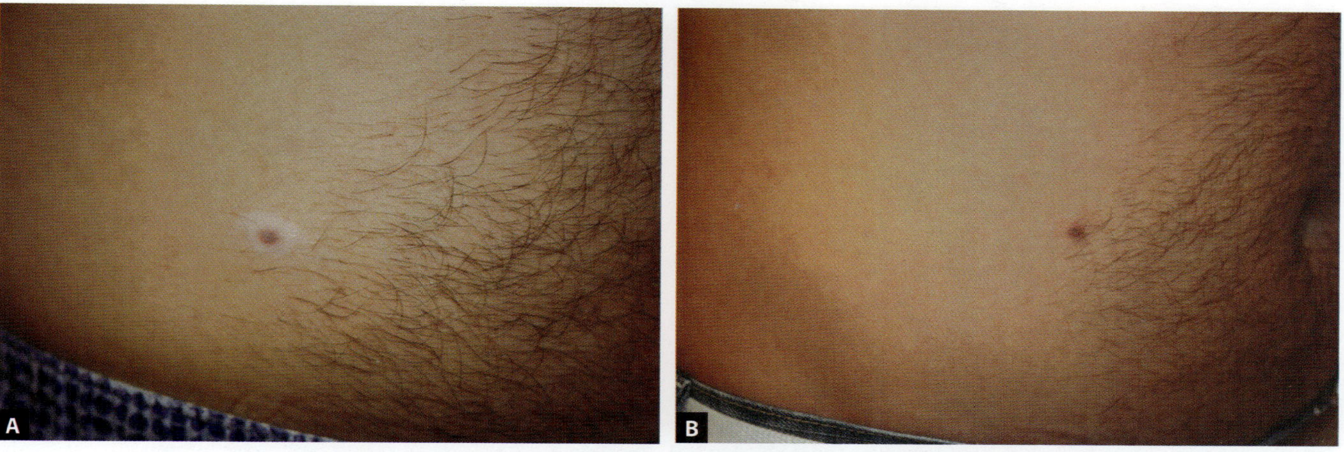

Figs. 3A and B: (A) Halo nevus pretreatment; (B) Halo nevus posttreatment.

Table 3: Halo nevus.

Method	Study	Patients	Repigmentation	Type of study	Level of evidence	Reference
Noncultured epidermal cellular grafting	van Geel et al.	11	91%		III	BJD 2010[10]
Cultured and noncultured autologous melanocytes, autologous ultrathin epidermal sheets	Olsson, Juhlin	2 1	65–95% 22–64%	Retrospective questionnaire study	III	BJD 2002[9]

controversial because it is suspected but unproven that it may result from nevus cells that are atypical or may undergo malignant transformation. Recommendations range from observation requiring no therapy to excision biopsy.[2] PubMed search revealed only two studies which reported long-term results of different surgical therapies. Van Geel et al. reported 11 patients of halo nevi treated with noncultured epidermal cellular grafting with a mean repigmentation of 91% and 90% of patients achieving a repigmentation of greater-than or equal to 75%. A diffuse hypopigmented color mismatch was more frequently observed. In some exceptional cases peripheral white ring was also present.[10] Olsson and Juhlin reported three cases of halo nevi each treated by transplantation of cultured autologous melanocytes, autologous ultrathin epidermal sheets and autologous basal cell layer suspension, respectively.[9] Two patients who received cellular grafting showed 65–95% repigmentation and one who was grafted with ultrathin epidermal sheet showed 22–64% repigmentation of the trunk and the neck. We have experienced consistent repigmentation with very good color matching of most halo nevi treated in patients with skin type three to five (Table 3).

Post-burn Leukoderma (Figs. 4A and B)

It usually results when deeper burns heal with secondary intention. It is characterized by chalk white depigmented lesions of variable size and shape with disappearance of melanocytes which appears at the site of the burn injury and remains unchanged subsequently. The exact mechanism of developing leukoderma following burn injuries is not known. Medical therapies are not known to be effective in the treatment of post-burn leukoderma. Tissue grafting methods reported to treat post-burn leukoderma are chip skin grafting, epidermal grafting, and thin skin grafting. There are three prospective uncontrolled studies and two case report series. Kahn and Cohen reported excellent graft take in 29 out of 30 operative procedures performed on 21 patients with depigmentation following burn injuries. Color match was rated excellent in 34% (n=10) of the procedures and good in 62% (n=19). The follow-up period varied from 2 weeks to 94 months with an average of 17 months. Among the adverse effect most patients developed milia following the procedure.[23] Acikel et al. treated 13 patients with thin split-thickness grafting with a follow-up period 1 to 12 months (average 8 months). The surface area of the treated leukoderma sites range from 0.5–3% of total body surface area. The skin graft taken was 100% in 12 patients while one graft was lost due to hematoma. The color match was rated excellent in five of the procedures (38.5%), good in six (46%), and fair in two (15%).[24] Three patients of post-burn gas leukoderma treated with epidermal grafts showed 100% repigmentation with good color matching. The follow-up period was 6–14 months. The size of the lesions treated is not mentioned.[25] In another series three patients treated with minigrafting with adequate repigmentation. Cobblestone appearance was seen in one of them.[26] Falabella described for the first

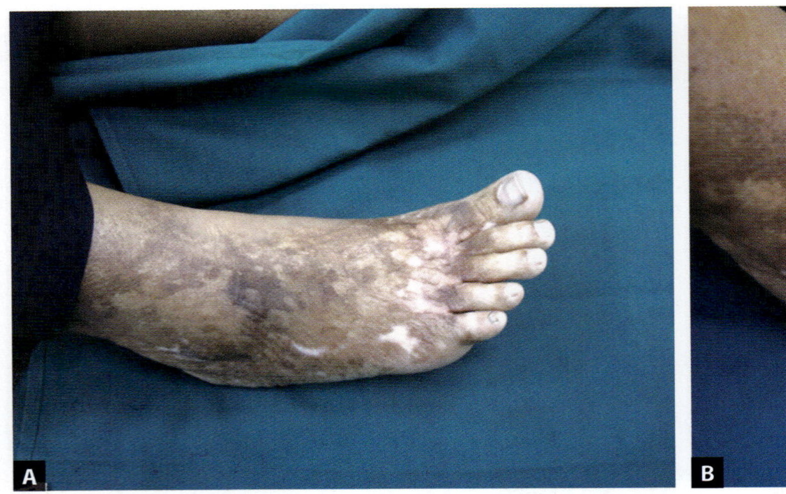
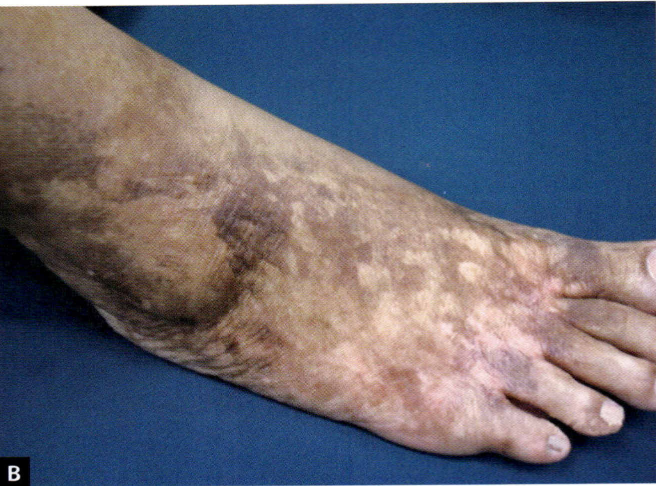

Figs. 4A and B: (A) Post-burn leukoderma pretreatment; (B) Post-burn leukoderma posttreatment.

Table 4: Post-burn leukoderma.

Method	Study	Patients	Repigmentation	Type of study	Level of evidence	Reference
Dermabrasion + Chip skin graft	Harashina T				Evidence unavailable	Br J Plast Surg 1985
Dermabrasion + thin skin graft	Onur erol O				Evidence unavailable	Plast Reconstr Surg 1990
Thin skin graft	Kahn AM	20	Good, excellent	Prospective uncontrolled		Burns 1996[23]
Thin minigraft	Fuji M	3	Excellent	Case report		Dermatol Surg 2007[26]
Epidermal graft	Falabella R	4		Case report		Arch Dermatol 1971[27]
Autologous graft	Suvanprakorn P	3	Good	Prospective uncontrolled study		JAAD 1985[25]
CO_2 laser + dermabrasion + thin skin graft	Acikel C	13	Excellent	Prospective uncontrolled		Plast Reconstr Surg 2000[24]
Noncultured epidermis	Mulekar et al.	10	Excellent			Burns 2011[28]

time epidermal grafting in three patients with post-burn leukoderma with 100% take of the grafts.[27] Mulekar et al. reported for the first time good to excellent repigmentation in post-burn leukoderma with noncultured melanocyte-keratinocyte transplantation[28] (Table 4).

Post-discoid Lupus Erythematosus Leukoderma

Long-standing lesions of DLE may heal with depigmented scars and are very difficult to induce repigmentation by conventional methods such as use of topical steroids and topical or systemic photosensitizes. In addition, histopathologically, DLE lesions destroy areas deep to the hair follicles in the skin thus destroying the main reservoir for melanocytes. Epidermal grafts by suction blister which is well-known to improve recalcitrant vitiligo was used to treat four patients of post-discoid depigmentation with repigmentation of more 100% of the grafted area due to the peripheral spread of the pigment.[29] Use of noncultured melanocyte-keratinocyte suspension is another modality to treat post-DLE depigmentation[30] (Table 5).

Post-laser Leukoderma (Figs. 5A and B)

Various lasers are used in the treatment of melasma, tattoo removal, telangiectasia, etc. This may result in loss of pigment and is usually restricted to the area of treatment. We treated one patient of depigmented macules on face resulted by treatment of telangiectasia with V-beam laser with noncultured melanocyte-keratinocyte transplantation. Olsson reported his experience of treating leukoderma caused by laser. However, these reports are anecdotal and in the form of personal experience.[31]

Table 5: Post-discoid lupus erythematosus.

Method	Study	Patients	Repigmentation	Type of study	Level of evidence	Reference
Epidermal graft	Gupta S	1	75%	Case		Dermatology 2001[29]
Noncultured MKTP	Mulekar et al.	1	98%	Case		Dermatol Surg 2008[30]

Abbreviations: MKTP, melanocyte-keratinocyte transplantation

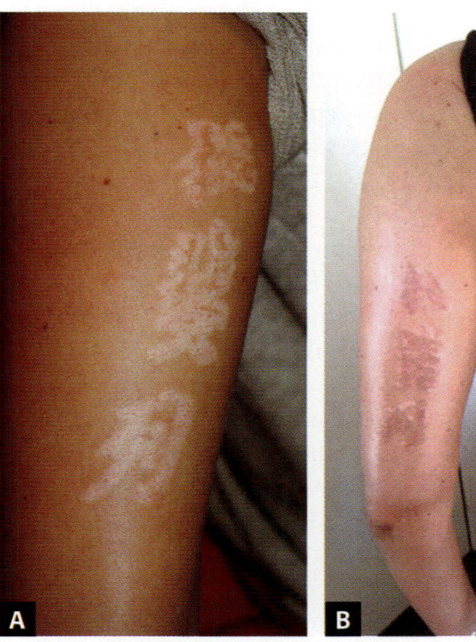

Figs. 5A and B: (A) Post-laser leukoderma pretreatment; (B) Post-laser leukoderma posttreatment. Please note initial hyperpigmentation.

Post-dermabrasion Leukoderma

Mechanical dermabrasion using diamond fraize wheels was commonly practiced by plastic surgeons for facial resurfacing. There is only a single report by Flabella of treatment of post-dermabrasion leukoderma which may be a rare complication.[32]

DISCUSSION

Non-vitiligo leukoderma makes an important spectrum of hypopigmented disorders most of them are responsive to surgical intervention. However, there seems to be lack of awareness among patients and physicians about the possible ways of intervention. This has led to lack of sufficient literature supporting the therapeutic options.

Among the conditions discussed earlier, piebaldism and post-burn leukoderma respond to various surgical transplantation methods consistently. Therefore, these conditions may be recommended to be treated by surgical transplantation methods. Hypopigmentation observed in halo nevus shows repigmentation when treated with cell suspension transplantation. Patients with halo nevi are psychologically disturbed due to their cosmetic appearance resembling the headlights of a car as described by one, especially after tanning in summer in European continent, and due to its resemblance to vitiligo in the South and Middle East Asia. Initial reports of successful repigmentation should be followed up with long-term observation to assess the potential recurrence and development of atypical melanocytes. No untoward effects have been reported by any of the investigators till date.

Nevus depigmentosus is a matter of concern for both the patient and physician. Though, positive results have been reported by many, the quality of repigmentation remains an area of uncertainty, and recurrence possible. More studies are indicated to find the mechanism of melanosome distribution in nevoid lesion. We advise caution and in depth discussion with patient and his or her parents before exercising the surgical intervention.

Hypothetically, postinflammatory depigmentation should respond well to surgical transplantation unless associated with underlining autoimmune cause. Laser procedures are on the rise, especially for tattoo removal, treatment of telangiectasia and hypopigmentation due to laser are likely to increase in near future. Awareness of potential of surgical transplantation methods will increase the reports of such cases.

Questions may be raised about the lack of controlled studies to prove the efficacy of the surgical methods in these disorders. However, studies by Prof Lerner[11] and van Geel[33] support the efficacy of cellular suspension against a placebo in a case of piebaldism and vitiligo patients, respectively. The efficacy of cellular transplantation seems to be beyond doubt at least in those conditions associated with complete loss or absence of melanocytes.

SUMMARY

Non-vitiligo leukodermas form an important spectrum of hypopigmented disorders; treatment with surgical modalities should be better studied in the management of these patients.

REFERENCES

1. Ortonne JP. Vitiligo and other disorders of hypopigmentation. C 66 In: Bolognia J, Jorizzo JL, Rapini RP (Eds). Dermatology. London UK: Mosby Publisher; 2003. pp. 947-73
2. Brochez L, Boone B, Naeyaert JM. Hypomelanoses associated with melanocytic neoplasia. In: Nordlund JJ,

Boissy RE, Hearing VJ, King RA, Oetting WS, Ortonne JP (Eds). The Pigmentary System, 2nd edition. Oxford UK: Blackwell Publishing Ltd; 2006. pp.705-24

3. Harris RP, Helfand M, Woolf SH, et al. Current methods of the US Preventive Service Task Force: a review of the process. Am J Prev Med. 2001;20(3 suppl):21-35.
4. Mosher DB, Fitzpatrick TB, Ortonne JP, et al. Hypomelanoses and hypermelanoses. In: Freedberg IM, Eisen AZ, Wolf K et al. (Eds) Dermatology in General Medicine, 5th edition. New York: McGraw-Hill; 1999. pp. 961.
5. Spritz RA. Piebaldism, Waardenberg syndrome, and related disorders of melanocyte development. Semin Cutan Med Surg. 1997;16:15-23.
6. Selmanowitz VJ. Pigmentary correction of piebaldism by autografts. II. Pathomechanisms and pigment spread in piebaldism. Cutis. 1979;24:66-73.
7. Olsson MJ, Juhlin L. Epidermal sheet grafts for repigmentation of vitiligo and piebaldism, with a review of surgical techniques. Acta Derm Venereol (stock) 1997; 77:463-6.
8. Njoo MD, Nieuweboer-krobotova L, Westerhof W. repigmentation of leucodermic defects in piebaldism by dermabrasion and thin split-thickness skin grafting in combination with minigrafting. Br J Dermatol. 1998;139: 829-33.
9. Olsson, Juhlin L. Long-term follow-up of leukoderma patients treated with transplants of autologous cultured melanocytes, ultrathin epidermal sheets, and basal cell layer suspension. Br J Dermatol. 2002;147:893-904.
10. van Geel N, Wallaeys E, Goh BK, et al. Long term results of non cultured cellular epidermal grafting in vitiligo, halo nevi, piebaldism and nevus depigmentosus. Br J Dermatol. 2010;163:1186-93.
11. Lerner AB, Halaban R, Klaus S, et al. Transplantation of human melanocytes. J Invest Dermatol. 1987;89:219-24.
12. Falabella R, Barona MI, Escobar C, et al. Surgical combination therapy for vitiligo and piebaldism. Dermatol Surg. 1995;21:852-7.
13. Kumagai N, Uchikoshi T. Treatment of extensive hypomelanosis with autologous cultured epithelium. Am Plast Surg. 1997;39:68-73.
14. Guerra L, Primavera G, Raskovic D, et al. Permanent repigmentation of piebaldism by erbium:YAG laser and autologous cultured epidermis. Br J Dermatol. 2004;150: 715-21.
15. Lernia VD. Segmental nevus depigmentosus: analysis of 120 patients. Pediatr Dermatol. 1999;16:349-53.
16. Gupta S, Goel A. Letter to the editor: nevus depigmentosus needs transplant of epidermal sheets. Dermatol Surg. 2005; 31:1746-7.
17. Kim DY, Park YK, Hann SK. Recurrence of nevus depigmentosus after an autologous epidermal graft. J Am Acad Dermatol. 2008;58:527-8.
18. Gauthier Y, Surleve-Bazeille JE. Autologous grafting with noncultured melanocytes: A simplified method for treatment of depigmented lesions. J Am Acad Dermatol. 1992;26:191-4.
19. Olsson MJ, Juhlin L. Leucoderma treated by transplantation of a basal cell layer enriched suspension. Br J Dermatol. 1998;138:644-8.
20. Mulekar SV, Al Issa A, Al Eisa A. Nevus depigmentosus: treated by melanocyte-keratinocyte transplantation with review of the literature. J Cutan Aesthet Surg. 2011;4:29-32.
21. Raskovic D, Bondanza S, Gobello T, et al. Autologous in vitro reconstituted epidermis in the treatment of a large nevus depigmentosus. J Am Acad Dermatol. 2006;54(Suppl):S238-40.
22. Wayte DM, Helwig EB. Halo nevi. Cancer. 1968;22:69-90.
23. Kahn AM. Cohen MJ. Treatment for depigmentation following burn injuries. Burns. 1996:22(7);552-4.
24. Acikel C. Ulkur E, Guler MM. Treatment of burn scar depigmentation by carbon dioxide laser-assisted dermabrasion and thin skin grafting. Plast Reconstr Surg. 2000;105:(6)1973-8.
25. Suvanprakorn P, Dee-Ananlap S, Pongsomboon C, Klaus S. Melanocyte autologous grafting for treatment of leukoderma. J Am Acad Dermatol. 1985:13;968-74.
26. Fuji M, Terashi H, Hashikawa K, et al. Thin minigrafting technique for post burn leukoderma. Dermatol Surg. 2007;33:1368-73.
27. Falabella R. Epidermal grafting an original technique and its application in achromic and granulating areas. Arch Derm. 1971;104:592-600.
28. Mulekar SV, Al Issa A, Al Eisa A. Treatment of post burn leucoderma with non-cultured melanocyte-keratinocyte transplantation. Burns. 2011;37:448-52.
29. Gupta S. Epidermal grafting for depigmentation due to discoid lupus erythematosus. Dermatology. 2001;202: 320-3.
30. Mulekar SV, Ghwish B, Al Issa A, et al. Melanocyte-keratinocyte transplantation for postdiscoid lupus erythematosus depigmentation. Dermatol Surg. 2008;34:261-3.
31. Olsson MJ. Surgical treatments of leukodermas other than vitiligo vulgaris. In: Gupta S, Olsson MJ, Kanwar AJ, Ortonne JP (Eds). Surgical Management of Vitiligo. Oxford, UK: Blackwell Publishing; 2007. pp. 238-45.
32. Falabella R. Repigmentation of stable leukoderma. J Dermatol Surg Oncol. 1987;13:44-8.
33. van Geel N, Ongenae K, De Mil M, et al. Double-blind placebo-controlled study of autologous transplanted epidermal cell suspensions for repigmenting vitiligo. Arch Dermatol. 2004;140:1203-8.

Chapter

44

Complications of Vitiligo Surgery

Niti Khunger, Alka Goel

Key Messages

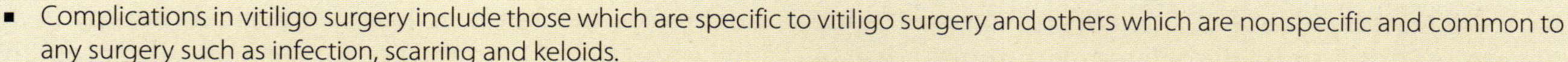

- Complications in vitiligo surgery include those which are specific to vitiligo surgery and others which are nonspecific and common to any surgery such as infection, scarring and keloids.
- Specific complications include failure of complete pigmentation due to poor choice of patient (unstable disease), poor choice or execution of technique.
- Punch grafting is associated with the highest number of side effects. Cellular grafts are associated with least incidence of side effects. Since criteria for case selection (stability) are inadequately defined, relapse is a possibility in all cases and this needs to emphasized during counseling.

INTRODUCTION

Complications in vitiligo surgery include those which are specific to the technique and those which are common to any surgery (Table 1). Some complications are common to any surgery such as reactions to anesthetic agents, infections, keloid formation, etc. To avoid these complications, the surgery should be performed in an operation theater setting, with all aseptic precautions to avoid infection. Presence of infection will not only lead to graft failure, but can also lead to scarring. Bleeding and oozing from the donor site can occur, particularly over a large area. A pressure dressing, with layers of gauze pad and adhesive bandage will minimize this side effect.

Table 1: General complications of vitiligo surgery.

Non-specific	*Specific to vitiligo surgery*
• Reaction to anesthetic agents	• Inadequate graft material
• Pain	• Failure of graft uptake
• Bleeding	• Failure of pigmentation
• Infection	• Partial repigmentation
• Scarring	• Cosmetic mismatch
• Keloids	• Relapse of disease with reversal of pigmentation

Specific Complications

Specific complications can occur in the donor as well as the recipient area and are discussed here. Some complications occur in relation to improper case selection, poor choice of method or poor technique, which are common to all vitiligo surgeries. Such complications are shown in Box 1. Inadequate graft material less than required in the recipient area is more common with ultrathin grafts that contract after harvesting, such as with suction blister technique and ultrathin split thickness grafts. To avoid this the donor area should be at least 5-10% more than the recipient area. Failure of graft uptake can occur due to inadequate immobilization over mobile areas and over joints, lips, eyelids, or collection of serous fluid under the graft. This is more common with thin split thickness skin grafts and suction blister grafts. Strict immobilization by the use of splints over mobile areas and pressure dressings

Box 1: Tips to achieve good results and avoid complications.[41]

- Avoid
- Procedures in patients with a keloid diathesis
- Patients with unstable, active vitiligo
- Thick dermoepidermal grafts with knife or dermatome
- Punch grafts larger than 1.2 mm (1.0 mm ideal for facial areas)
- Extensive areas without planning full treatment
- Manipulation of recipient sites with excessively invasive methods

will minimize this complication. In very thin grafts, it may be difficult to distinguish the epidermal and dermal side. There will be failure of graft uptake if the epidermal side is put face down. To avoid this a sterile slide can be pressed on the donor graft after harvesting and everted so that the dermal side faces upwards. Cosmetic disfigurement and color mismatch of graft are common with tissue grafts and infrequent with cellular grafts. Hence, they are now the preferred method of treatment. Relapse of disease with depigmentation of the graft can occur in spite of correct technique, due to reactivation of vitiligo. A stable case with no signs of active disease should be taken up for surgery. A recent report suggests that lesional stability is more important than disease stability. However activity of vitiligo is unpredictable and this should be clearly explained to the patient before the surgery. The details of stability of the disease are discussed in the previous chapter.

Complications related to a specific technique may occur in both the recipient and donor areas and are enumerated in Table 2. In general, cellular grafts appear to have the least incidence of side effects, whereas tissue grafts are reported to be associated with more adverse effects. The maximum number of adverse events are seen when mini punch grafting (MPG) and thin split-thickness skin grafting[1] (Table 2). These complications are discussed below.

Color Mismatch (Hyperpigmentation and Hypopigmentation)

Repigmentation may not occur in the same manner in all patients. A slight degree of hyperpigmentation is frequently observed with all methods, and especially in darker skin types, Fitzpatrick phototype IV–VI[2]. A possible role of arachidonic acid metabolites has been suggested due to higher levels of tyrosinase and immunoreactive b-locus protein found when pigment cells were in vitro cultured for 2 days with prostaglandin D2, leukotriene B4, C4, D4, E4, thromboxane B2 and 12-hydroxyeicosatetraenoic acid.[3] Prostaglandin E2 has also been thought to have a similar role.[4] Some patients have a tendency for hyperpigmentation, which may be determined by examining areas of recent superficial skin trauma. Such patients should be counseled regarding the risk of hyperpigmentation at the donor and recipient site. This hyperpigmentation may persist for years (Figs. 1A and B). It is difficult to manage due to possible risk of reactivation of the disease, associated with hypopigmenting agents. Sunscreens should be advocated on the exposed areas once repigmentation has occurred. Topical steroids like fluticasone proprionate or mometasone furoate may be used. Topical tretinoin 0.025% and salicylic acid peels have been found to be beneficial in persistent cases (personal observation). Hypopigmentation is more common with non-cultured melanocyte cell suspensions, if concentration of melanocytes in the suspension is not adequate. It may also occur due to reactivation of vitiligo. This can be managed with PUVA therapy, narrowband UVB (NBUVB)[5] or the excimer lamp or laser,[6] if topical therapy is not successful (Fig. 2). Nowadays, for cosmetically acceptable

Table 2: Complications observed at recipient and donor area in transplantation procedures.

Recipient area	Donor area
Hyperpigmentation	Hyperpigmentation
Perigraft halo- or hypopigmented borders	Hypopigmentation
Cobblestone appearance	Scarring
Contact dermatitis to topical medication	Koebner's phenomenon
Milia/inclusion cysts	Infection
Thick margins/stuck-on appearance	Hypertrophic scar/keloid formation
Variegated appearance	
Infection	
Scarring	

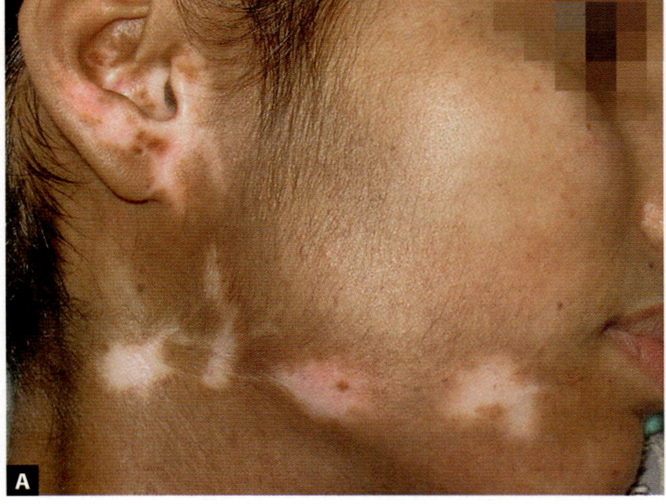

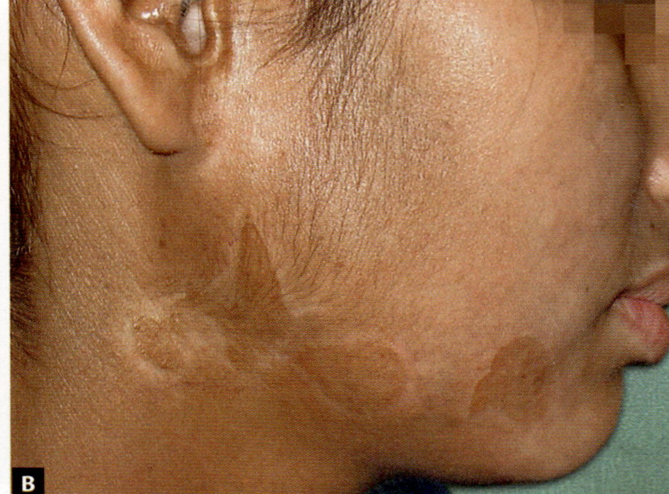

Figs. 1A and B: Persistent hyperpigmentation on the face after split skin grafting.

repigmentation at recipient site newer techniques like CO_2 laser and Er:YAG laser are being utilized to prepare the recipient site.[7]

Perigraft Halo and Achromic Fissures

Perigraft halo is a rim of depigmentation that remains at the outer edge of grafted vitiligo lesion while achromic fissures are areas of depigmentation between the grafts (Figs. 3A and B). They are caused by the combined effect of initial contracture of the graft when it is harvested and contraction of the dermal elastin fibers occurring at the recipient site.[7] Immunological reactions at the periphery of the recipient area may also be responsible. Pigment spread may also not be complete, particularly in tissue grafts leading to perigraft halo. This complication may be prevented by overlapping of graft edges at the recipient site and applying the graft 1–2 mm beyond the depigmented area.[7] Proper postoperative dressing and splinting and prolonged application of pressure will also prevent contracture. Postoperative PUVA therapy or NBUVB therapy is usually corrective.

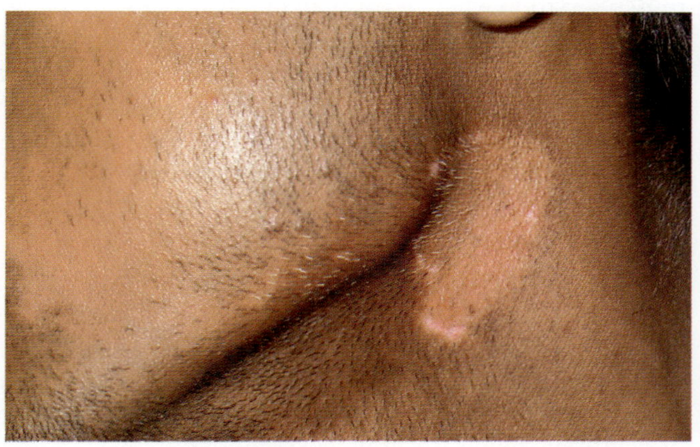

Fig. 2: Hypopigmentation following grafting.

Cobblestoning (Raised Grafts) and Sunken Pits (Sunken Grafts)

Cobblestone appearance at the recipient site is one of the most common and distressing complication seen with minipunch grafting[3,8,9] (Fig. 4). Various studies have reported cobblestone appearance in 22–47% of the patients.[8-11] This occurs when large punches are used to obtain donor grafts or when punch recipient sites are not deep enough leading to variable protrusions. Cobblestoning may be prevented by using punches of smaller size (ideally 1–1.5 mm),[12] using thinner grafts, trimming excess dermis if any from the bottom of grafts,[8,10] and punching the recipient pits 1 mm deeper than the size of the donor grafts.[11] The recommended sizes of biopsy punch to be used for mini punch grafting are 1.0 mm for facial areas and 1.2 mm at other sites, particularly in young patients.[12] Preventing overcrowding by keeping the grafts at least 5 mm apart from each other also reduces this complication.[13] Silicone gel sheets may be used to prevent or minimize the chances of cobblestoning.[14] It has been observed that with time cobblestoning gets corrected in most of the cases.[15] In resistant cases, corrective electrofulguration may be needed.[15,16] Sinking pit or sunken graft is seen when the minigrafts used are not smaller than the punched hole sizes.[8] To avoid sunken grafts, appropriate thickness grafts should be chosen.

Graft Hypertrophy

This complication is seen when the donor grafts are thick (Fig. 5). They usually resolve spontaneously over a period of 3-4 months. Topical steroids and topical retinoids may be used if it is persistent.

Scarring at Donor Site

Some degree of scarring is inevitable while harvesting punch grafts and split thickness grafts. Scarring at the donor site is not seen with suction blister grafting as the

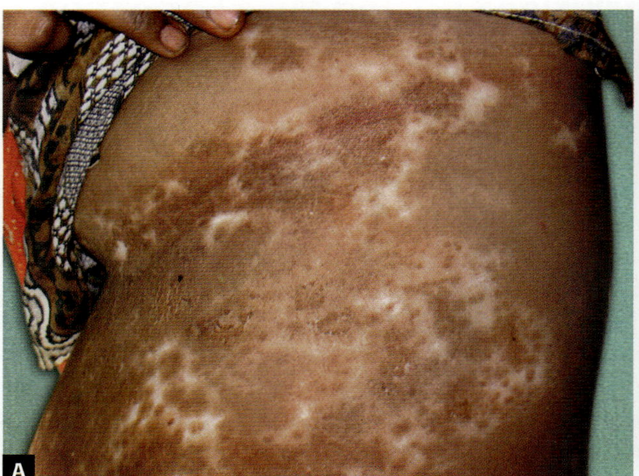

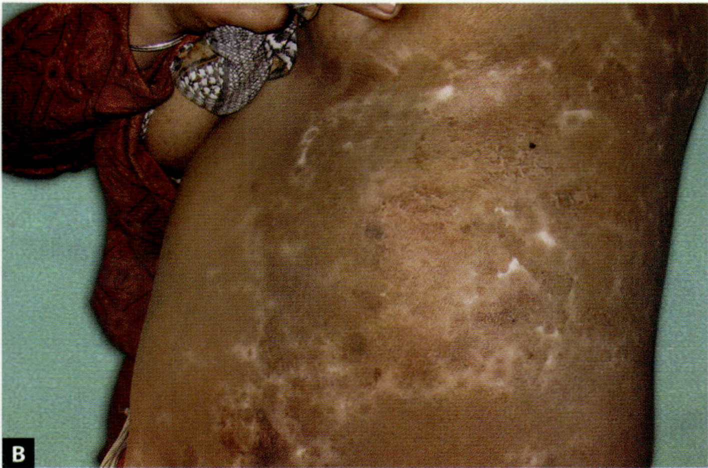

Figs. 3A and B: Perigraft halo with achromic fissures, gradually improving with phototherapy.

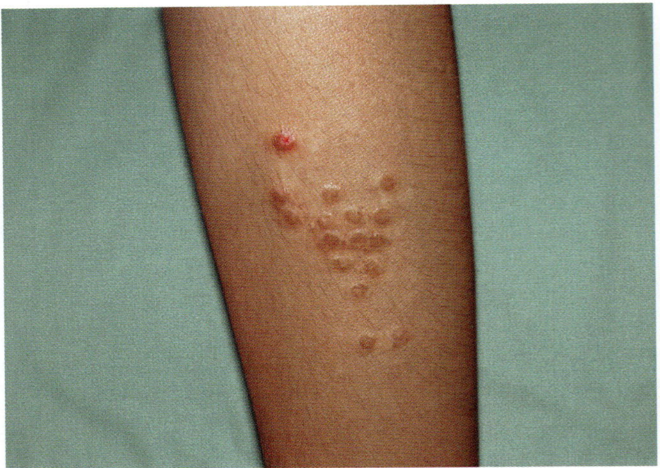

Fig. 4: Persistent cobblestoning in a punch grafting.

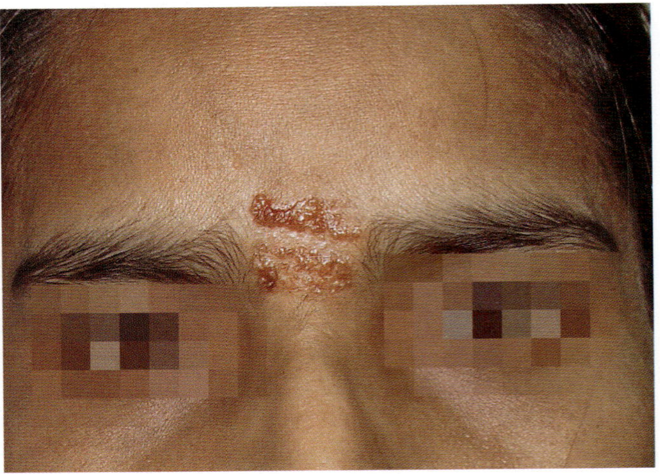

Fig. 5: Graft hypertrophy along with milia formation.

grafts are purely epidermal. Hence, donor site should be selected with care such as the unexposed area (gluteal region). Scarring on thigh is more visible and hence should be avoided. To avoid scarring in punch grafting, the donor punches should be very superficial and smaller than 2 mm. Scarring following graft can be prevented by taking very thin dermo-epidermal grafts of preferably 0.1–0.3 mm thickness with a suitable dermatome.[2] Plain knives or surgical blades are not preferred for shaving large grafts as they do not provide regular and even graft thickness. Surgical skill is acquired with experience and harvesting thin grafts without scarring leads to good cosmetic results, with the added advantage of being able to reuse the same donor site, if required. Dermatomes are ideal for harvesting large thin grafts of even thickness.

Hypertrophic Scars or Keloids

Hypertrophic scars, thick grafts and grafted areas with uneven surfaces may be seen with all the procedures. Hypertrophic scars can also develop at the donor site due to the inability to regulate the depth while attempting to obtain ultrathin grafts or with punch grafts. The risk is high in dark skin individuals with a tendency to keloid formation. Hence, before performing the procedure, old scars should be carefully examined. The motor-driven diamond fraise or wire-brush used for dermabrasion at recipient sites might lead to formation of hypertrophic scar if dermabrasion is done deeply.[13] Hypertrophic scarring, if it occurs, subsides spontaneously over 3–4 months in most cases. Topical retinoids may be used to hasten the response.[7] Individuals prone to keloids should be evaluated and surgery should preferably be avoided. Suction blister grafting or cellular techniques are better options in such patients, if vitiligo surgery is an absolute necessity. Punch grafting or split-thickness grafting should not be performed in such patients. Appropriate evaluation of old scars, accidental or surgical, should be done and if doubts still persist, a minigrafting test area should be done before the definitive procedure.[17]

Curling of Borders with Beaded Appearance of the Periphery of Grafts

It is usually seen in mesh grafting and flip-top pigment transplantation when grafts with inappropriate thickness are taken. Curling of borders can be prevented by stretching the grafts and smoothening out the edges after placement of the grafts. Postoperative pressure and splinting is also helpful. Once beading has occurred, the 'beads' can be snipped off with the scissors or can be lightly dermabraded.

Thick Margins or Stuck-on Tyre Appearance

These occur due to thick grafts. This usually subsides spontaneously over a period of 3–4 months as development of scar tissue below the graft will smooth out the graft, but may persist for longer periods.

Inclusion Cyst and Milia Formation

Milia are small epithelial cysts seen commonly in the first 6 months following split-thickness grafting (Fig. 5). They develop due to persistence of remnant of epithelial cells following dermabrasion or due to occlusion of sweat ducts where the outflow is blocked in combination with rapid proliferation of epithelial cells at the end of sweat ducts.[18] It is a temporary phenomenon, commonly seen over the face and neck following split thickness grafts and not seen with surgical techniques using cellular grafts. Untreated milia resolve spontaneously after sometime and do not recur or they can be expressed out with a sterile needle. The incidence of milia formation can be reduced by uniform and even dermabrasion and thorough cleaning of the dermabraded recipient site before application of the graft.[7]

Graft Rejection or Failure of Graft Uptake

Bleeding below the graft with hematoma formation, infection or excessive movement, with shifting of grafts and upside down placement of graft can lead to graft rejection.[7]

This can be minimized by:

- Placing the graft on the recipient patches after the bleeding is controlled.
- Postoperative immobilization by securing the graft by proper pressure dressings and use of splints over mobile areas.
- Prophylactic antibiotics.

Failure of graft uptake is more common in the acral areas, particularly fingers and toes. Adequate immobilization with splints and adequate deep level of dermabrasion may minimize the risk of graft failure. Overall, thin split-thickness graft has the highest success rate as compared to other methods.

Variegated Appearance

Depending on the technique used, the final results of repigmented areas may vary from patient to patient. The graft may initially appear variegated but later, they lighten up and the border merges so as to match the surrounding skin color in most patients, except a few who may have permanent hyperpigmentation. For successful repigmentation, preparation of recipient site is important and newer techniques may be helpful in it.[19]

Infection

Infection is a very infrequent complication observed in available literature. Prevention of infection is important and appropriate aseptic precautions should be taken while performing transplant procedures.[20]

Koebner's Phenomenon

Reactivation of vitiligo at the donor or recipient site or appearance of new lesions may occur in unstable cases or if the disease becomes reactive after a period of stability. This can be minimized with proper selection of stable vitiligo patients.[21]

Individual Transplant Procedures and their Complications

Table 3 summarizes the side effects seen in each type of grafting technique.

Tissue Grafts

Tissue grafts in general have more complications than cellular grafts.

Mini Punch Grafts

Minigrafting has perhaps the highest complication rate amongst all grafting methods. Cobblestone appearance, variegated appearance and color mismatch, perigraft halo, graft dislodgment/rejection, static graft (no pigment spread), depigmentation of graft, hypertrophic scar and keloid formation are the main complications seen at recipient site. Superficial scarring, Koebner's phenomenon and hypertrophic scar formation may be seen at donor site.[6,11,12]

Suction Blisters Epidermal Grafts

Suction blister epidermal grafting (SBEG) is generally a safe technique. Perigraft halo of depigmentation, wrinkling and displacement of the graft and graft rejection are usually the main complications seen. Temporary hyperpigmentation at donor and recipient site, Koebner's phenomenon, and keloid formation has also been observed in a few studies.[12,22-24] Higher suction pressure if used to raise blisters, may cause rupture of epidermis and hemorrhagic blisters.[10] Liquid nitrogen, if used excessively, can result in severe inflammation causing hypertrophic scarring and postinflammatory hyperpigmentation. It can also cause cryodamage of peripheral melanocytes resulting in a hypopigmented rim around the recipient site.[20] The chance of scarring at the donor site is minimal because the dermis remains intact.

Thin Split-thickness Skin Grafts

Complications in this technique are usually operator dependent. Scarring at the donor site can occur in inexperienced hands. Recipient area may show complications, such as stuck-on appearance , perigraft halo, curling of the graft with beaded appearance, displacement of the grafts, cosmetically mismatched pigmentation, and milia formation.

Hair Follicular Grafts

Hair follicle grafting has been performed by a few authors to treat small patches in hair-bearing areas and has been found useful in treating lesions with leukotrichia.[25-27] Previously hair follicles were harvested by small strip grafting of hair-bearing scalp from the occipital area followed by separation of single hairs which are then transplanted into vitiligo patches 5–10 mm apart. Currently, follicular unit extraction(FUE) is the method of choice for harvesting hair follicles. Hair follicles are harvested from the occipital are using 0.9 or 0.1 mm metallic punches mounted on a micromotor. Though no major complications were seen in the available studies, this method has several limitations. Hair dissection is a tedious, time-consuming and delicate procedure and needs proper training. It is difficult to treat large vitiligo lesions because of the limited number of donor hairs and vitiliginous skin heals slowly because the grafted melanocytes require a long time to spread.[26] Besides it can only be used in hair bearing areas.

Table 3: Nature of adverse events in transplantation procedures.

		n=76	*SBEG*	*MPG*	*NCES*	*CM*	*CE*	*HFG*
			n=441	*n*=1295	*n*=318	*n*=259	*n*=170	*n*=21
Recipient area	Hyperpigmentation	2	53	312	3		1	
	Hypopigmented borders	4	1	5	20			
	Cobblestoning			397				
	Contact dermatitis due to topical medications		6	3				
	Inclusion cysts	20						
	Thick margins/stuck on appearance	9						
	Variegated appearance		7	244				
	Infection	2	9	3	1			
	Scarring			19			2	
	All adverse events	37	76	983	24		3	
Donor area	Hyperpigmentation	1	131					
	Scarring	30		60				
	Koebner's phenomenon		4	3		3		
	Infection			1				
	All adverse events	31	135	64		3		

Source: Gupta et al.[1]
Abbreviations: SBEG, Suction blister epidermal grafts; MPG, Mini punch grafting; NCES, Noncultured epidermal cell suspension; CM, Cultured melanocytes; CE, Cultured epithelial graft; HFG, Hair follicle graft.

Cellular Grafts

Cellular grafts generally have lesser incidence of side effects.

Autologous Noncultured Epidermal Cell Suspension

Reported adverse effects on recipient and donor areas are in general, minimal as compared to tissue grafts. Mild textural changes at the donor site, cosmetic mismatch at recipient site, either hypo- or hyperpigmentation at the recipient site are common complaints. Hyperpigmentation or hypopigmentation and hypopigmented halo at the edge of the graft may be seen.[28-32] These can be minimized by taking appropriate concentration of melanocytes in the suspension.

Hair Follicle Melanocyte Cell Suspension

Melanocyte cell suspension obtained from the outer root sheath of the hair follicle is a recently described technique in vitiligo surgery.[33-35] It is based on the principle that the outer root sheath and bulge area of the hair follicle is a reservoir of inactive melanocytes (melanocyte stem cells), which when activated produce melanin pigment and are responsible for perifollicular repigmentation seen clinically in a repigmenting patch of vitiligo. In this technique, hair follicles are extracted by follicular unit extraction (FUE) using a one mm biopsy punch from the occipital area, trypsinized for 90 minutes in an incubator and the melanocytes are suspended in DMEM medium similar to epidermal cell suspension method.[35] They are then transplanted to the recipient vitiliginous sites prepared after dermabrasion. In the study by Shah et al.[34] excellent repigmentation (90–100%) was achieved in 60% of patients. No side effects were observed in the donor site. In the recipient site hyperpigmentation was observed in 75% of patients, which reduced after few months in a few patients. Pruritis (25%), xerosis (10%) and infection were transient side effects. Hyperpigmentation and color mismatch were also observed by Donaparthi and Chopra.[35] In their comparative study, the results were also inferior when compared to epidermal cell suspension. Clearly there is a need to further standardize this procedure to obtain uniform excellent results.

Transplantation of Cultured Autologous Melanocytes

This procedure treats larger areas successfully without the need for additional phototherapy and is associated with minimal complications at the donor/recipient site.[36-38] However, cultured epidermis is difficult to handle and manipulation affects cell vitality. Mutagenicity and possible risk of cancer have also been cited as potential risks. One of the additives, TPA, also known as 12-otetradecanoylphorbol-13-acetate, is a selective growth accelerator of the melanocytes. Since this is a tumor promoter, concerns about its long-term safety have been expressed. The recent availability of TPA free and serum-free media is a possible solution to this problem. Beta fibroblast growth factor (ß-FGF)[30,31] has also been used as a substitute and is believed to provide satisfactory result.

Autologous Cultured Epithelial Graft (CEG)

There has been limited data on these methods and only few center perform these techniques.[32-36] The fact that melanocytes can be cultured together with keratinocytes makes this technique useful in vitiligo patients refractory to all other known therapies.[36] No major complications have been reported in various studies but this technique is expensive, requires sophisticated laboratory and trained personnel.[32-36] It may be the therapy of future when simplified and becomes cost-effective.

Review of Literature

A systematic review of autologous transplantation methods[37,38] showed the highest rate of success (87%) with suction blister and, while the average success rates for other methods varied from 13–53%. The maximum incidence of adverse effects were seen with tissue grafts mainly punch grafting, i.e. cobblestone appearance on the recipient site (27%) and scar formation on the donor sites (40%), followed by split thickness grafting and suction blister epidermal grafting. Cellular grafting was associated with the lowest number of adverse effects. In the recipient site, cobblestone appearance was the predominant complication in punch grafts, whereas hyperpigmentation and thickening of grafts were common in suction blister epidermal grafts and split thickness skin grafts (STSGs). In the donor site, superficial scarring and hypopigmentation are the common findings in punch grafts, whereas hyperpigmentation is the main problem in SBEG and to minimize complications and increase chances of success, certain modifications of the technique can be done at different sites (Box 1).[39,40]

CONCLUSION

To conclude, with the advancement in the techniques and horizontal spread of training, surgical therapies are more frequently practiced especially in Asian countries. Serious postoperative complications arising from dermatologic surgery are uncommon. Not every patient with vitiligo is a good candidate for surgical repigmentation and the key for success is an appropriate selection of patients, since there are specific criteria that must be fulfilled for vitiligo surgery.[16,17,42] Proper patient counseling about the nature of the disease and the surgery, limitations of the procedure and whether more procedures will be needed for optimal outcome should be done. Patient should be counseled for all possible therapeutic options and should be given liberty to choose from the available modalities. Many complications may be prevented by preoperative evaluation, sound surgical technique and careful follow-up care.[43]

REFERENCES

1. Gupta S, Narang T, Olsson MJ, et al. Surgical management of vitiligo and other leukodermas: evidence-based practice guidelines. In: Gupta S, Olson MJ, Kanwar AJ, et al. (Eds). Surgical Management of Vitiligo. Oxford, UK: Blackwell Publishing Ltd; 2007;69-79.
2. Falabella R. Surgical approaches for stable vitiligo. Dermatol Surg. 2005;31:1277-84.
3. Falabella R. Treatment of localized vitiligo by autologous minigrafting. Arch Dermatol. 1988;124:1649-55.
4. Tomita Y, Iwamoto M, Masuda T, et al. Stimulatory effect of 381 prostaglandin E2 on the configuration of normal human melanocytes in-vitro. J Invest Dermatol. 1987;89:299-301.
5. Lahiri K, Malakar S, Sarma N, Banerjee U. Repigmentation of vitiligo with punch grafting and narrow-band UV-B (311 nm): A prospective study. Int J Dermatol 2005;45:649-55.
6. Linthorst Homan MW, Spuls PI, Nieuweboer-Krobotova L, de Korte J, Sprangers MA, Bos JD, et al. A randomized comparison of excimer laser versus narrow-band ultraviolet B phototherapy after punch grafting in stable vitiligo patients. J Eur Acad Dermatol Venereol 2012;26:690-5.
7. Khunger N. Thin split-thickness skin grafts for vitiligo. In: Gupta S, et al. (Eds). Surgical management of vitiligo. Blackwell Publishing Ltd; 2007;108-14.
8. Savant SS. Autologous miniature punch skin grafting in stable vitiligo. Ind J Dermatol Venereol Leprol. 1992;58: 310-4.
9. Malakar S, Dhar S. Treatment of stable and recalcitrant vitiligo by autologous miniature punch grafting: a prospective study of 1000 patients. Dermatology. 1999;198: 133-9.
10. Mutalik S, Ginzburg A. Surgical management of stable vitiligo: a review with personal experience. Dermatol Surg. 2000;26:248-54.
11. Boersma BR, Westerhof W, Bos JD. Repigmentation in vitiligo vulgaris by autologous minigrafting: Results in nineteen patients. J Am Acad Dermatol. 1995;33:990-5.
12. Falabella R. Surgical therapies for vitiligo and other leukodermas, part 1: minigrafting and suction epidermal grafting. Dermatologic Ther. 2001;14:7-14.
13. Mulekar S. Surgical management of vitiligo. Expert Rev Dermatol. 2010;5:229-39.
14. Agarwal US, Jain D, Gulati R, Bhargava P, Mathur NK. Silicone gel sheet dressings for prevention of post-minigraft cobblestoning in vitiligo. Dermatol Surg 1999;25:102-4.
15. Lahiri K, Sengupta SR. Treatment of stable and recalcitrant depigmented skin conditions by autologous punch grafting. Indian J Dermatol Venereol. 1997;63:11-4.
16. Malakar S, Lahiri K. Electrosurgery in cobblestoning. Indian J Dermatol. 2000;45:46-7.
17. Falabella R, Arrunategui A, Barona MI, et al. The minigrafting test for vitiligo: detection of stable lesions for melanocyte transplantion. J Am Acad Dermatol. 1995;32:228-32.
18. Olson MJ. In Treatment of leukoderma by transplantation of ultrathin epidermal sheets. In: Gupta S, et al (Eds). Surgical management of vitiligo. Blackwell Publishing Ltd; 2007;11523.
19. Majid I. Grafting in vitiligo: How to get better results and how to avoid complications. J Cutan Aesthet Surg. 2013;6: 83-89.
20. Falabella R. Surgical therapies for vitiligo. Clin Dermatol. 1997;15:927-39.

21. Parsad D, Gupta S. Standard guidelines of care for vitiligo surgery. Indian J Dermatol Venereol Leprol. 2008;74: S3745.
22. Mutalik S, Ginzberg A. Surgical management of stable vitiligo: A review with personal experience. Dermatologic Surgery. 2000;26:248-54.
23. Gupta S, Kumar B. Epidermal grafting in vitiligo: Influence of age, site of lesion, and type of disease on outcome. J Am Acad Dermatol. 2003;49:99-104.
24. Hann SK, Im S, Bong HW, et al. Treatment of stable vitiligo with autologous epidermal grafts and PUVA. J Am Acad Dermatol. 1995;32:943-8.
25. Na GY, Seo SK, Choi SK. Single hair grafting for the treatment of vitiligo. J Am Acad Dermatol. 1998;38:580-4.
26. Malakar S, Dhar S. Repigmentation of vitiligo patches by transplantation of hair follicles. Int J Dermatol. 1999;38: 237-8.
27. Kumaresan M. Single-hair follicular unit transplant for vitiligo. J Cutan Aesthet Surg. 2011;4:41-3.
28. Gauthier Y, Surleve-Bazeille JE. Autologous grafting with noncultured melanocytes: A simplified method for treatment of depigmented lesions. J Am Acad Dermatol. 1992;26:191-4.
29. Olsson MJ, Juhlin L. Leucoderma treated by transplantation of basal cell layer enriched suspension. Br J Dermatol. 1998;138:644-8.
30. van Geel N, Wallaeys E, Goh BK, et al. Long-term results of non cultured epidermal cellular grafting in vitiligo, halo nevi, piebaldism and nevus depigmentosus. Br J Dermatol. 2010;163:1186-93.
31. Mulekar SV. Long-term follow-up study of 142 patients with vitiligo vulgaris treated by autologous non-cultured melanocyte-Keratinocyte cell transplantation. Int J Dermatol. 2005:44:841-5.
32. Van Geel N, Goh BK, Wallaeys E, et al. A review of non-cultured epidermal cellular grafting in vitiligo. J Cutan Aesthet Surg. 2011;4:17-22.
33. Kumar A, Mohanty S, Sahni K, Kumar R, Gupta S. Extracted Hair Follicle Outer Root Sheath Cell Suspension for Pigment Cell Restoration in Vitiligo. J Cutan Aesthet Surg. 2013;6:121-25.
34. Shah AN, Marfatia RK, Saikia SS. A study of noncultured extracted hair follicle outer root sheath cell suspension for transplantation in vitiligo. Int J Trichol 2016;8:67-72
35. Donaparthi N, Chopra A. Comparative Study of Efficacy of Epidermal Melanocyte Transfer Versus Hair Follicular Melanocyte Transfer in Stable Vitiligo. Ind J of Dermatol. 2016;6:640-644.
36. Chen YF, Yang PY, Hu DN, et al. Treatment of vitiligo by transplantation of cultured pure melanocytes suspension: Analysis of 120 cases. J Am Acad Dermatol. 2004;51:68-74.
37. Redondo P, del Olmo J, Garcia-Guzman M, et al. Repigmentation of vitiligo by transplantation of autologous melanocyte cells cultured on amniotic membrane. Br J Dermatol. 2008;158:1168-71.
38. Czajkowski R, Placek W, Drewa T, et al. Autologous cultured melanocytes in vitiligo treatment. Dermatol Surg. 2007;33:1027-36.
39. Falabella R, Escobar C, Borrero I. Transplantation of in vitro-cultured epidermis bearing melanocytes for repigmenting vitiligo. J Am Acad Dermatol. 1989;21:257-64.
40. Falabella R, Escobar C, Borrero I. Treatment of refractory and stable vitiligo by transplantation of in vitro cultured epidermal autografts bearing melanocytes. J Am Acad Dermatol. 1992;26:230
41. Jha AK, Pandey AS, Gulati AK, et al. Inoculation of a cultured autologous epidermal suspension containing melanocytes in vitiligo. Arch Dermatol. 1993;129:785-6.
42. Njoo MD, Westerhof W, Bos JD, et al. A systematic review of autologous transplantation methods in vitiligo. Arch Dermatol.1998;134:1543-9.
43. Kaufmann R, Greiner D, Kippenberger S, et al. Grafting of in vitro cultured melanocytes onto laser-ablated lesions in vitiligo. Acta Derm Venereol. 1998;78:136-8.

Chapter

45

Overview of Acne Scarring

Anil Abraham

Key Messages 

- Acne scarring causes significant psychic trauma, maladjustment between parent and children, general insecurity and feelings of inferiority.
- Acne scars are classified as atrophic and hypertrophic. Atrophic scars are in turn classified as rolling, icepick and box scars.
- Treatment has to be tailored as per the type of scar in the patient and hence is variable.
- Quantitative grading systems are useful for assessing severity and plan treatment modalities.

"And wrath has left its scar—that fire of hell has left its frightful scar upon my soul."

INTRODUCTION

There is no single disease which causes more psychic trauma, maladjustment between parent and children, general insecurity, feelings of inferiority and greater sums of psychic suffering than does acne vulgaris.[1]

Acne vulgaris is a common skin disorder known to occur in up to 80% of people between 11 years and 30 years of age and 5% of older adults but is now being recognized as a chronic disease with devastating sequelae.[2-4] Modern therapy ensures that a considerable proportion of all patients can be offered effective treatment of their disease, but the morbidity is not restricted solely to the lesions of acne and sequelae too have their serious consequences.

EPIDEMIOLOGY

There is limited epidemiologic data available on the prevalence of acne scarring.[5] Scarring was recorded in 14% of women and 11% of men among 749 patients aged 25 and 58 years.[3] Western authors have reported scarring associated in 30–95% of patients of acne vulgaris.[6,7] The prevalence data from Varanasi reported acne in 50.6% of adolescent boys and 38.13% of girls.[8] Adityan and Thappa observed scarring and hyperpigmentation in 39.5% and 24.6% of patients respectively.[9] They also supported the relatively high incidence of scarring as observed by Western authors in patients with longer duration of the disease hence stressing the need for early treatment.[9,10] Majority of the scars occurred on the face with truncal involvement seen more commonly in males.[11] Atrophic scarring appears to be the most common subtype although there is a lack of good epidemiologic data on relative prevalence rates of different types of scarring.[12]

PSYCHOSOCIAL IMPACT OF ACNE SCARRING

Scars are an indelible reminder of possible dreaded outcome of acne. One of the most common stigmata of acne is the scars which can play havoc with the social functioning of the patient leading to severe psychologic depression.[13] Acne scarring patients are reported to have greater levels of stress and anxiety than other medical conditions.[14] Social withdrawal has been reported among individuals with acne scars. The problem is compounded by the fact that there is no predictive tool to identify patients at risk of scarring from the severity of acne. The condition of acne which is easily dismissed as self-limiting is estimated to reduce the quality of life (QOL) as great as that with epilepsy, asthma, diabetes or arthritis.[15] Treatment of the acne scars is often the first request of the patient in consultation even before the treatment of acne lesions. Limited treatment options for acne scars leave prevention as the best remedy for scar prone patients.[7]

Indians appear to accept acne more readily and its impact on QOL in Indian population is of lower magnitude.

PATHOGENESIS OF ACNE SCARRING

Injury to the normal skin initiates a cascade of wound healing events which are: (1) inflammation, (2) granulation tissue formation, and (3) matrix remodeling. Acne scars result from an aberrant response to wound healing at various stages:

Inflammation

The process of inflammation in acne is unique in being localized to the pilosebaceous follicles and in the role of the local milieu in initiating the cascade. Proliferation of *Propionibacterium* acnes leads to stimulation of the innate immune response and activation of both the classical and alternate complement pathway leading to inflammation.[16,17] Potential modulation at this step can go a long way in preventing scarring. The ultimate appearance of a scar correlates to the extent and depth of inflammation. When the preceding inflammation extends significantly into the dermis, resulting degradation of the dermal matrix is much more extensive hence a greater potential for scarring.[12]

Initial vasoconstriction for hemostasis is followed by vasodilatation and erythema. Melanogenesis is also stimulated at this step. This step is important for development of post-acne erythema and hyperpigmentation.[18] Holland et al. assessed the differences in the cell mediated immune responses between acne prone and not prone patients. The authors concluded that the specific immune response was initially small and ineffective with small number of CD4+ T cells majority of which were skin homing cells followed by massive influx of macrophages and skin homing cells with angiogenesis in resolving lesions.[19] Hence, the inflammatory reaction at the pilosebaceous gland is stronger and has a longer duration in patients with scars, but is slow to develop hence justifying the need to treat early inflammation to prevent acne scarring.

Granulation Tissue Formation

The new skin composition in a normal wound is dominated by type III collagen, with a small percentage (20%) of type I collagen. There is a shift in the balance of collagen type in mature scars to be similar to that of unwounded skin, with approximately 80% of type I collagen.[18]

Matrix Remodeling

Matrix metalloproteinases (MMPs) are extracellular matrix (ECM) degrading enzymes that interact and form a lytic cascade for remodeling of the ECM. Activation of NF-kB and activator protein-1 (AP-1) leads to upregulation of MMPs like MMP-1, MMP-8, MMP-9 and MMP-13.

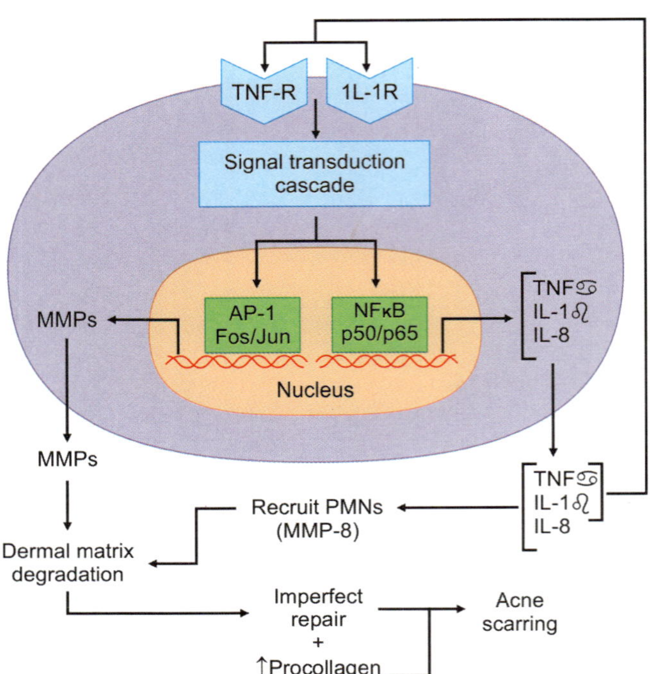

Fig. 1: A hypothetical model of pathophysiology of inflammatory acne and dermal damage leading to scarring.

(*Source:* Kang S, Cho S, Chung JH, et al. Inflammation and extracellular matrix degradation mediated by activated transcription factors nuclear factor-kappaB and activator protein-1 in inflammatory acne lesions in vivo. Am J Pathol. 2005;166:1691-9.)

Each of these are involved in degradation of collagen. Prolonged cycles of upregulation of MMPs and subsequent procollagen synthesis are prolonged in acne scar prone patients.[20] An imbalance in the ratio of MMPs to tissue inhibitors of MMPs results in the development of atrophic or hypertrophic scars (Fig. 1).[19] For example, higher levels of MMP-2 and lower levels of MMP–9 are found in hypertrophic and keloid scars causing lack and/or late apoptotic death of myofibroblasts hence prolonging the fibrogenesis.

CLASSIFICATION

The guiding principle of scar subtype classification must be done with therapeutic options in mind.

Acne scars can be broadly categorized as either a result of increased or lack of tissue formation or damage of tissue (hypertrophic and atrophic respectively).

Atrophic Acne Scars

Atrophic acne scars are more common than hypertrophic scars with a ratio of 3:1. Atrophic scars can be broadly classified into three types (Fig. 2).

Ice Pick Scars

Ice pick scars are narrow in diameter (<2 mm), deep, sharply marginated epithelial tracts that extend vertically

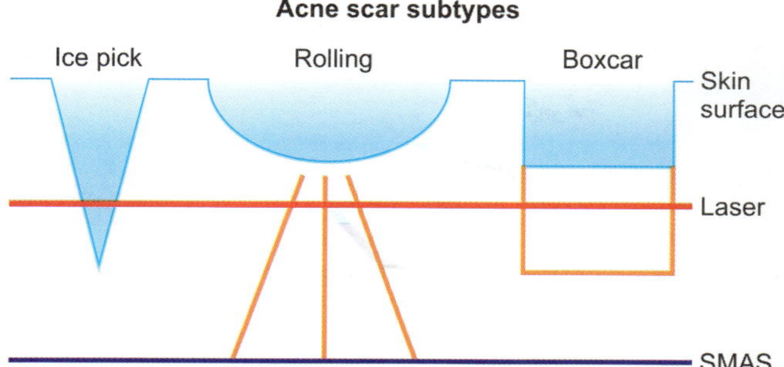

Fig. 2: A novel classification system: three basic scar types—icepick, rolling and boxcar (superficial and deep). Yellow reference line denotes depth of ablation and resurfacing capability of the CO_2 laser. Green line represents superficial musculoaponeurotic system to which fibrous bands adhere, creating rolling scars.
(*Source*: Jacob CI, Dover JS, Kaminer MS. Acne scarring: a classification system and review of treatment options. J Am Acad Dermatol. 2001;45:109-17)

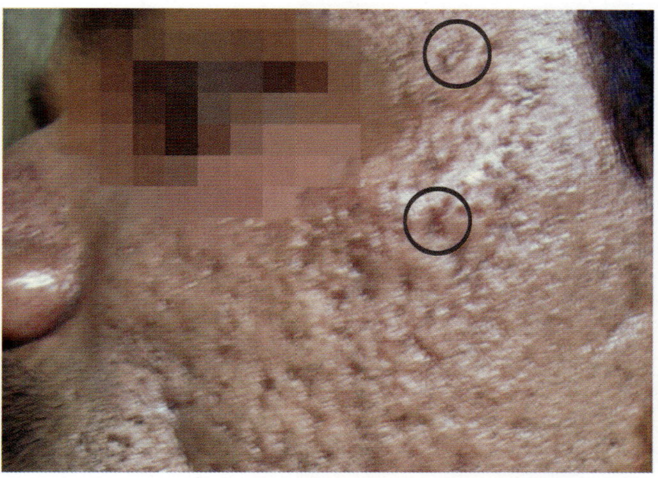

Fig. 4: Rolling scars with undulating appearance.

to the deep dermis or subcutaneous tissue.[9] The opening is usually wider than the deeper infundibulum as the scar tapers from the surface to its deepest apex, hence forming a V shape (Fig. 3).

Rolling Scars

Rolling scars are poorly demarcated depressions of the skin with vertical extension limited to the depth corresponding to epidermal thickness. They occur from dermal tethering of otherwise relatively normal-appearing skin and are usually wider than 4–5 mm. Abnormal fibrous anchoring of the dermis to the subcutis leads to superficial shadowing and a rolling or undulating appearance to the overlying skin (Fig. 4).

Boxcar Scars

Boxcar or U-shaped scars are uniform, round or oval scars with well-established vertical edges that reach a depth

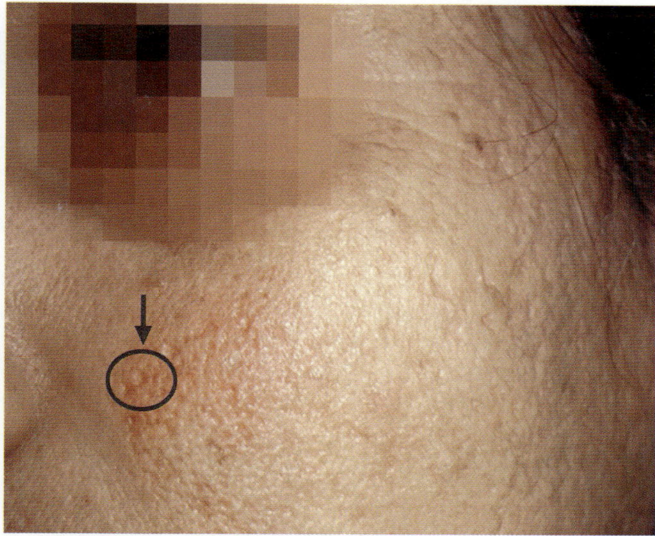

Fig. 3: Arrow highlights icepick type of scarring.

corresponding to the superficial or deep dermis and are usually wider at the surface. They may be shallow (0.1–0.5 mm) or deep (0.5 mm) and are most often 1.5–4.0 mm in diameter (Fig. 5). With atrophic scars, the icepick type represents 60–70% of total scars, the boxcar 20–30% and rolling scars 15–25%.[12]

Hypertrophic Scars

Hypertrophic and keloidal scars are associated with excess collagen deposition and decreased collagenase activity.

Hypertrophic scars are typically pink, raised and firm with thick hyalinized collagen bundles that remain within the borders of the original site of injury.

In contrast, keloids form as reddish-purple papules and nodules that proliferate beyond the borders of the original wound; histologically, they are characterized by thick bundles of hyalinized acellular collagen arranged in whorls. Hypertrophic acne scars and acne-associated keloids occur predominantly on the torso (upper and mid aspect of back, sternum and clavicular areas, shoulders and deltoids, and occasionally over the jaw angles).

GRADES OF ACNE SCARRING

Goodman and Baron devised a qualitative scarring grading system that is simple and universally applicable except in severe cases where different patterns are simultaneously present in a patient (Table 1).[21]

A quantitative grading system developed by the same authors was found to be reasonably accurate and reproducible with good inter investigator reliability based on counting (1–10, 11–20, >20) of scar type (atrophic, macular, boxcar, hypertrophic and keloidal) and severity (mild, moderate and severe). Points are assigned to each respective category and totaled from 0 to a maximum of 84.[9] This system assigns fewer points to macular and mild

Table 1: Qualitative scarring grading system.

Grade of post-acne scarring	*Level of disease*	*Clinical features*
1	Macular	These scars can be erythematous, hyper or hypopigmented flat marks
2	Mild	Mild atrophy or hypertrophy scars that may not be obvious at social distances of 50 cm or greater and may be covered adequately by make-up or the normal shadow of shaved beard hair in men or normal body hair if extrafacial
3	Moderate	Moderate atrophic or hypertrophic scarring that is obvious at social distances of 50 cm or greater and is not covered easily by make-up or the normal shadow of shaved beard hair in men or body hair if extrafacial, but is still able to be flattened by manual stretching of the skin (if atrophic)
4	Severe	Severe atrophic or hypertrophic scarring that is evident at social distances greater than 50 cm and is not covered easily by make-up or the normal shadow of shaved beard hair in men or body hair if extrafacial and is not able to be flattened by manual stretching of the skin

Source: Goodman GJ, Baron JA. Postacne scarring: a qualitative global scarring grading system. Dermatol Surg. 2006;32:1458-66

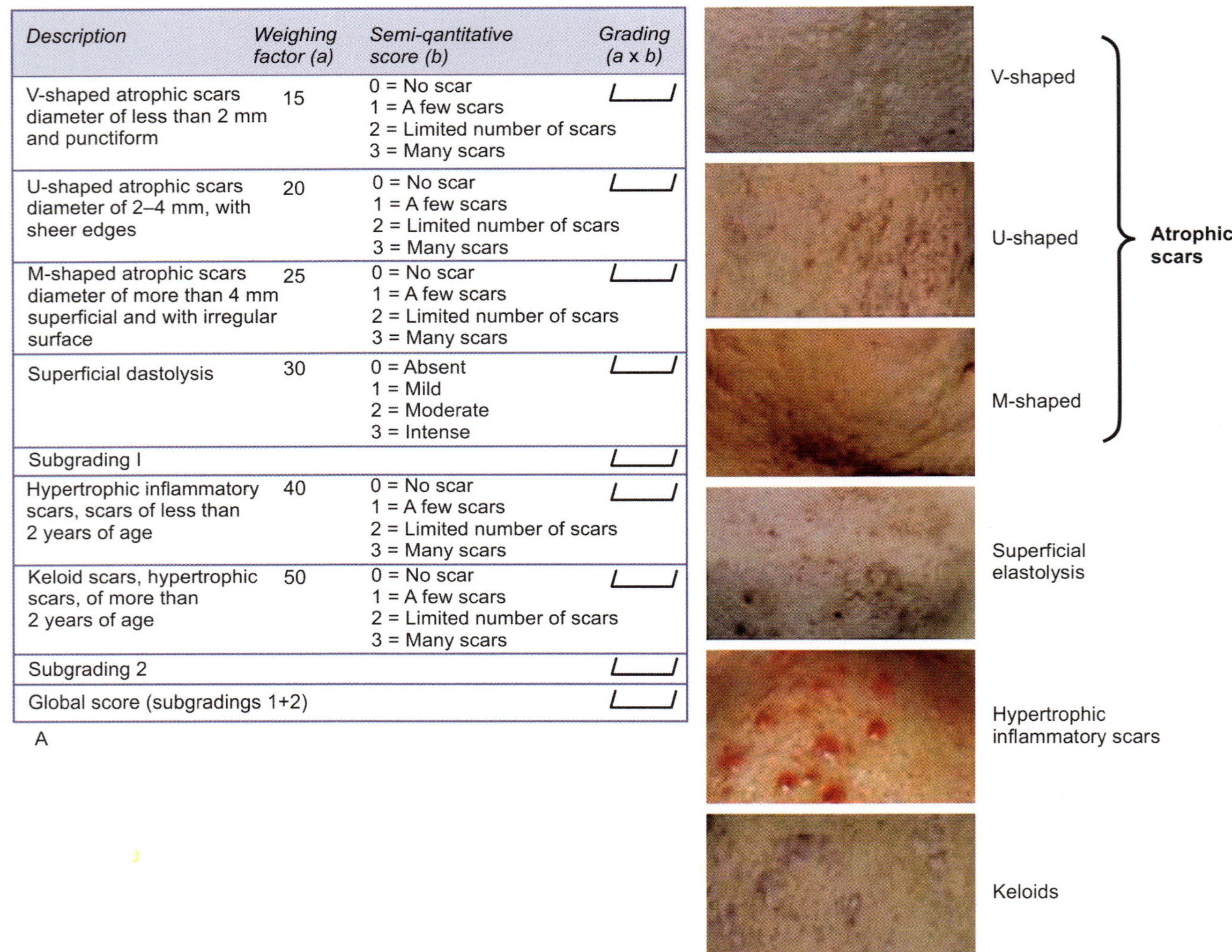

Description	*Weighing factor (a)*	*Semi-qantitative score (b)*	*Grading (a x b)*
V-shaped atrophic scars diameter of less than 2 mm and punctiform	15	0 = No scar 1 = A few scars 2 = Limited number of scars 3 = Many scars	
U-shaped atrophic scars diameter of 2–4 mm, with sheer edges	20	0 = No scar 1 = A few scars 2 = Limited number of scars 3 = Many scars	
M-shaped atrophic scars diameter of more than 4 mm superficial and with irregular surface	25	0 = No scar 1 = A few scars 2 = Limited number of scars 3 = Many scars	
Superficial dastolysis	30	0 = Absent 1 = Mild 2 = Moderate 3 = Intense	
Subgrading I			
Hypertrophic inflammatory scars, scars of less than 2 years of age	40	0 = No scar 1 = A few scars 2 = Limited number of scars 3 = Many scars	
Keloid scars, hypertrophic scars, of more than 2 years of age	50	0 = No scar 1 = A few scars 2 = Limited number of scars 3 = Many scars	
Subgrading 2			
Global score (subgradings 1+2)			

Fig. 5: The ECCA grading scale.

Source: Dreno B, Khammari A, Orain N, et al. ECCA grading scale: an original validated acne scar grading scale for clinical practice in dermatology. Dermatology. 2007;214:46-51.)

atrophic scars than to moderate and severe atrophic scars (macular or mildly atrophic: 1 point; moderately atrophic: 2 points; punched out or linear-troughed severe scars: 3 points; hyperplastic papular scars: 4 points).

The ECCA (***Echelle d'Evaluation clinique des Cicatrices d'acné***) for facial acne scarring is another quantitative scale designed with the aim of standardizing discussion on scar treatment and it is based on the sum of individual types of scars and their numerical extent (Fig. 5). Scar types considered to be more visibly disfiguring were weighted more heavily. Specific scar types and their associated weighting factors were the following:

- Atrophic scars with diameter less than 2 mm: 15
- U-shaped atrophic scars with a diameter of 2–4 mm: 20
- M-shaped atrophic scars with diameter greater than 4 mm: 25
- Superficial elastolysis: 30
- Hypertrophic scars with a less than 2-year duration: 40
- Hypertrophic scars of greater than 2-year duration: 50

A semiquantitative assessment of the number of each of these scar types was then determined with a four-point scale, in which:

- 0 indicates no scars
- 1 indicates less than 5 scars
- 2 indicates between 5 and 20 scars
- 3 indicates more than 20 scars.

With this method, the relative extent of scarring for each scar type was calculated. The total score can vary from 0 to 540. The potential advantages of this system include independent accounting of specific scar types, thereby providing for separate atrophic and hypertrophic subscores in addition to total scores. Potential shortcomings include restriction to facial involvement, time intensity and undetermined clinical relevance of score ranges.[21] Objective evaluation of the scars is necessary for standardization in discussion, treatment and research. Grading devices focusing on 3-dimensional grid-based mapping of lesions and molded skin replicas have been devised for comparison examination.[22]

However, these are not as applicable in practical, daily use by the average physician.

PREVENTION OF SCARRING

The occurrence of scarring is hard to predict. At present, the best method of preventing or limiting scarring is to treat acne early to minimize the extent and duration of inflammation. Patients seeking treatment of acne should be educated that scarring is permanent sequelae that can occur and that it is more likely with long-term inflammation. In addition, the importance of adherence with treatment to minimize the potential for scarring should be emphasized.[23]

REFERENCES

1. Sultzberger MB, Zaidems SH. Psychogenic factors in dermatological disorders. Med Clin North Am. 1948;32:669-85.
2. Kraning KK, Odland GF. Prevalence, morbidity, and cost of dermatological diseases. J Invest Dermatol. 1979;73: 395-401.
3. Goulden V, Stables GI, Cunliffe WJ. Prevalence of facial acne in adults. J Am Acad Dermatol. 1999;41:577-80.
4. Niemeier V, Kupfer J, Demmelbauer-Ebner M, et al. Coping with acne vulgaris: evaluation of the chronic skin disorder questionnaire in patients with acne. Dermatology. 1998;196:108-15.
5. Cunliffe W. Clinical features of acne. In: Cunliffe WC (Ed). Acne, 1st edition. Chicago: Martin Dunitz-Year Book; 1989; 20-32.
6. Goodman GJ. Management of post-acne scarring: what are the options for treatment? Am J Clin Dermatol. 2000;1:3-17.
7. Cunliffe WJ. The sebaceous gland and acne–40 years on. Dermatology. 1998;196:9-15.
8. Pandey SS. Epidemiology of acne vulgaris (thesis Abstract VII). Indian J Dermatol. 1983;28:109-10.
9. Adityan B, Thappa DM. Profile of acne vulgaris–A hospital-based study from South India. Indian J Dermatol Venereol Leprol. 2009;75:272-8.
10. Kane A, Niang SO, Diagne AC, et al. Epidemiological, clinical, and therapeutic features of acne in Dakar, Senegal. Int J Dermatol. 2007;46:36-8.
11. Layton AM, Henderson CA, Cunliffe WJ. A clinical evaluation of acne scarring and its incidence. Clin Exp Dermatol. 1994;19:303-8.
12. Jacob CI, Dover JS, Kaminer MS. Acne scarring: a classification system and review of treatment options. J Am Acad Dermatol. 2001;45:109-17.
13. Koo JY, Smith LL. Psychologic aspects of acne. Pediatr Dermatol. 1991;8:185-8.
14. Cunliffe WJ, Gould DJ. Prevalence of facial acne vulgaris in late adolescence and in adults. Br Med J. 1979;1:1109-11.
15. Mallon EM, Newton JN, Klassen A. The quality of life in acne: a comparison with general medical conditions using genetic questionnaires. Br J Dermatol. 1999;140:672-6.
16. Farrar MD, Ingham E. Acne: inflammation. Clin Dermatol. 2004;22:380-4.
17. Webster GF, Leyden JJ, Nilsson UR. Complement activation in acne vulgaris: consumption of complement by comedones. Infect Immune. 1979;26:183-6.
18. Farraum CL, Arpey CJ. Normal cutaneous wound healing: clinical correlation with cellular and molecular events. Dermatol Surg. 2005;31:674-86.
19. Holland DB, Jeremy AH, Roberts SG, et al. Inflammation in acne scarring: a comparison of the response in lesions from patients prone and not prone to scar. Br J Dermatol. 2004;150:72-81.
20. Kang S, Cho S, Chung J, et al. Inflammation and extracellular matrix degradation mediated by activated transcription factors nuclear factor-kB and activator protein-1 in inflammatory acne lesions in vivo. Am J Pathol. 2005; 166:1691-9.
21. Goodman G, Baron JA. Post acne scarring: a qualitative global scarring grading system. Dermatol Surg. 2006;32: 1458-66.
22. Friedman PM, Skover GR, Payonk G, et al. 3D in-vivo optical skin imaging for topographical quantitative assessment of non-ablative laser technology. Dermatol Surg. 2002;28:199-204.
23. Dreno B, Khammari A, Orain N, et al. ECCA grading scale: an original validated acne scar grading scale for clinical practice in dermatology. Dermatol. 2007;214:46-51.

Chapter

46

Surgical Management of Acne Scars

T Salim, Ragini Ghiya

Key Messages

- Acne scarring requires a combination approach; each type of scar may need a different treatment
- A combination of resurfacing techniques, scar revisions, subcision, punch elevation or excision may be needed
- Trichloroacetic acid (TCA) CROSS is a technique advocated for ice pick scars
- Subscission is recommended for boat-shaped scars
- Dermal grafts are useful to fill up depression and are a replacement for fillers.

INTRODUCTION

The previous Chapter has dealt with an overview of acne scars, their classification and pathophysiology. This Chapter deals with surgical management of acne scars.

Numerous invasive, semi-invasive and noninvasive techniques have been used to remove, replace or raise acne scars, and in turn resurface the cutaneous surface and reduce shadows. The currently available treatments for acne scarring includes:[1,2]

- Aesthetic approach: Chemical peels, microdermabrasion, dermal fillers
- Surgical approach: Punch techniques, subcision, dermal grafting, fat transfer, implantation of autologous collagen, and cultured and expanded autologous fibroblasts, focal treatment with trichloroacetic acid (TCA), and microneedling, dermabrasion, scar revision and cryoslush
- Laser resurfacing including ablative, nonablative and fractional resurfacing.

The treatments vary in severity and efficacy (Fig. 1). Treatment options like ablative laser resurfacing or mechanical dermabrasion offer significant improvement in facial scars, but are invariably associated with considerable morbidity and downtime.[2] On the other hand, treatments like microdermabrasion, superficial peels and nonablative laser resurfacing are associated with a minimal or no downtime, but do not show the same level of therapeutic efficacy.[3,4] This Chapter will focus on different surgical techniques for acne scar revision, while laser resurfacing is dealt with in the next Chapter. Other techniques such as scar revisions, chemical peels, microdermabrasion, etc. have been dealt with in different Chapters. This Chapter will therefore only briefly mention relevant features of these techniques. For details, the reader is referred to individual chapters.

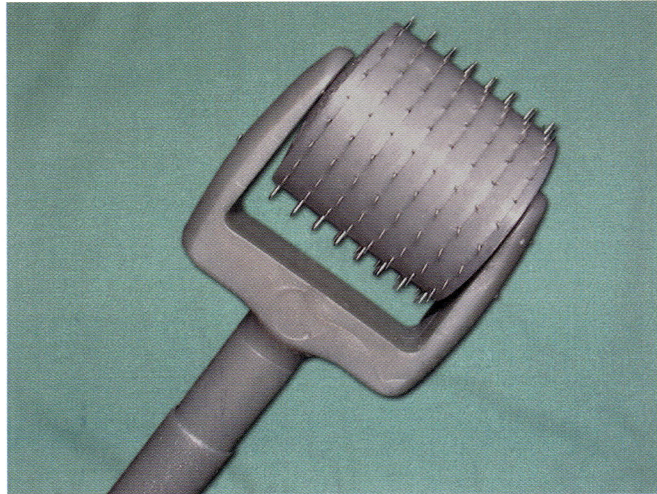

Fig. 1: Microneedling instrument.

The specific surgical techniques for management of post-acne scarring include:

- Microneedling
- Subcision
- Punch techniques

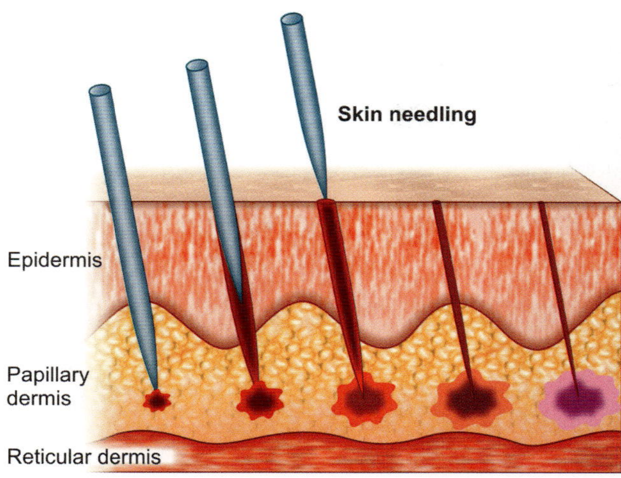

Fig. 2: Microneedling principle.

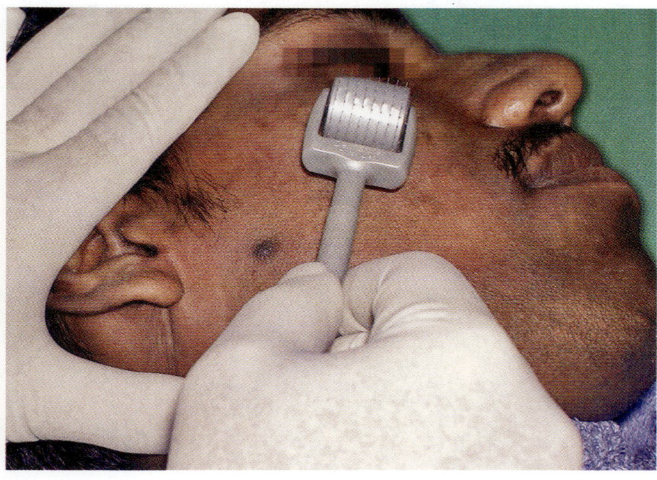

Fig. 3: Microneedling procedure.

- Trichloroacetic acid chemical reconstruction of skin scars (TCA CROSS)
- Dermal grafting.

MICRONEEDLING

Microneedling[5-12] [skin needling therapy, dermaroller therapy or collagen induction therapy (CIT)] has been dealt with in a separate Chapter and only relevant and specific points are discussed here. It is a relatively new technique with efficacy and safety in the management of atrophic acne scars.

The dermaroller used to treat acne scars is a hand held device with drum-shaped roller studded with 192 fine microneedles of 0.1 mm diameter in eight rows (Fig. 1). The device is available in needle length ranging from 0.5 to 2 mm. Dermaroller with 1.5 mm needle length is commonly used in acne scar therapy. Deeper atrophic scar may require 2 mm instrument. There are also motorized dermastamps and homecare dermastamps available for percutaneous collagen induction. Motorized dermastamps are needle cartridges attached to a motor device similar to a mesogun having a to-and-fro movement inducing pricks. The speed and depth of the needling can be adjusted according to the scars.

Indications

- This technique works best on acne scars of Grade 3 and Grade 4
- It is recommended for the rolling acne scars and boxcar scars.

Contraindications

- Active herpes labialis
- Keloidal tendency
- Patients on isotretinoin therapy within the preceding 6 months
- Bleeding disorders.

Procedure

The procedure is carried out under topical anesthesia. Patient is prepared in a similar manner to a surgical procedure. The facial skin is disinfected and anesthetized using a thick application of topical anesthetic cream (eutectic mixture of prilocaine and lignocaine). This is left for 30–45 minutes.

The treatment is then carried out by rolling the needling tool over the areas affected by acne scars, four times in four different directions: horizontally, vertically, and diagonally right and left. This ensured an even pricking pattern, resulting in about 250–300 pricks/cm^2. It has been shown that rolling with a dermaroller (192 needles, 200 μm length and 70 μm diameter) (Fig. 1) over an area for 15 times will result in approximately 250 holes/cm^2.

The microneedles penetrate through the epidermis but do not remove it; the epidermis is only punctured and heals rapidly. As the needles are set in a roller, every needle initially penetrates at an angle and then goes deeper as the roller turns. Finally, the needle is extracted at a converse angle, therefore curving the tracts and reflecting the path of the needle as it rolls into and then out of the skin for about 1.5–2 mm into the dermis[8] (Fig. 2). The epidermis, and particularly the stratum corneum, remains intact except for the minute holes, which are about four cells in diameter.

Endpoint for each treatment is the presence of uniform bleeding points over the scarred area. In patients with deep-seated scarring, the skin is stretched in a perpendicular direction to the dermaroller movement so that the base of the scars could also be reached (Fig. 3).

Postprocedure Care

Immediately after the procedure, the area is mildly swollen, with superficial bruising. After the initial bleeding stops within a few minutes, there is a serous ooze, which stops within the first few hours after the operation. Treated area is cleaned with sterile saline solution to remove the

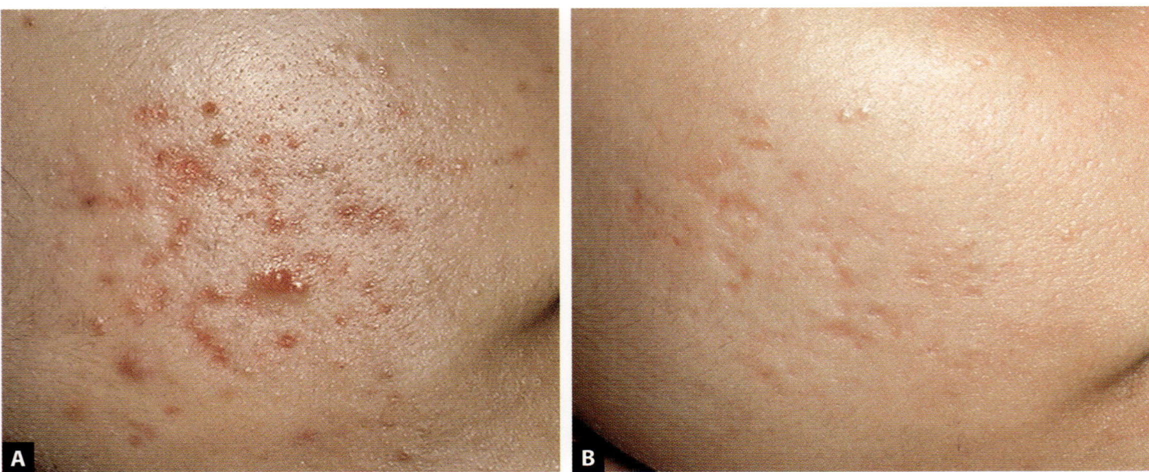

Figs. 4A and B: (A) Dermaroller before; and (B) after 6 months.

Table 1: Advantages and disadvantages of different surgical modalities of acne scar correction.

Modality	*Advantages*	*Disadvantages*
Chemical peeling	Noninvasive, minimal downtime	Less effective, needs multiple sessions
Microdermabrasion	Noninvasive, minimal downtime	Less effective, needs multiple sessions
TCA CROSS	Noninvasive, minimal downtime Ideal for ice pick scars	Risk of postinflammatory hyper or hypopigmentation in Indian skin
Microneedling	Easy, safe. Can be combined with topical drug delivery or topical platelet rich plasma application for better results	Full result may take 8–12 months as collagen deposition occurs slowly
Subscision	Effective for all kind of depressed scars	Downtime, needs proper training on part of dermatologist
Punch techniques	Effective for box scars, large ice pick scars	Should be combined with laser resurfacing few weeks later, downtime, needs proper training on part of dermatologist
Fillers Fat transfer	Effective for all kind of depressed soft scars	Should be preceded by subscision in most cases, costly (except fat transfer), needs to be followed by laser or chemical peel for skin texture correction
Cryoslush	Noninvasive, minimal downtime	Effective only in superficial scars
Scar revision	Effective for linear scars	Needs proper training for operating dermatologist
Lasers	Noninvasive, minimal downtime	Good for superficial scars only. Has to be preceded by punch techniques or subcision for deep scars

serous ooze and bleed. Patient may require oral analgesics if the treatment is done with needle size greater than 2 mm. The edema and erythema subsides in few hours. As the epidermis is not abraded, there is no need for photoprotection as a postprocedure care.

A total number of treatment sessions required is three to four, repeated at 4–8 weeks interval.[8]

Outcome

In accordance with the literature, the full result may take 8–12 months of treatment, as the deposition of new collagen takes place slowly (Figs. 4A and B). Improvement in acne scar continues even after 6 months after the last dermaroller therapy. As shown by Fernandes and Signorini,[8] microneedling has undisputable advantages compared with conventional methods (Table 1). The most important is that the epidermis remains intact because it is not damaged, eliminating most of the risks and negative side effects of chemical peeling or laser resurfacing.[13]

Many studies have confirmed the effectiveness of microneedling in acne scars. G Fabbrocini et al. confirmed that dermaroller therapy was highly effective in treatment of rolling acne scars.[8] A recent Indian study by Majid I, found that, in 21 patients with Grade 3 scarring treated with microneedling, an excellent response was noted in 16 patients (reduction to Grade 1 or less). Overall, 26 out of the total of 36 patients (72.2%) showed an excellent response to dermaroller treatment while 6 others achieved a good response (16.7%).[14] This technique can be employed in darker skin types without the fear of inducing postinflammatory hyperpigmentation. Relative advantages and disadvantages are mentioned in Table 2.

Table 2: Microneedling in acne scars—advantages and disadvantages.

Advantages	*Disadvantages*
▪ Can be done in all types of skin ▪ It can be done with topical anesthesia ▪ Skin becomes thicker ▪ The healing phase is short ▪ Cost-effective ▪ It can be done on people who have had laser resurfacing or those with very thin skin ▪ Reduces telangiectasias along with acne scars ▪ Simple technique. Easy to master ▪ Minimal chances for postinflammatory hyper and hypopigmentation	▪ Overaggressive needling may cause scarring ▪ Mild treatment—it takes a longer time to see the result than with laser resurfacing ▪ Multiple sessions required ▪ Unsightly swelling and bruising while using deeper needles (>2 mm)

Practical Tips

- Select patients with Grade 2 and 3 acne scars
- Counsel the patient about the gradual improvement of scars and need of multiple sessions
- Use good quality instruments to avoid complications
- Combine other techniques for faster and improved results.

SUBCISION

Subcision or subcutaneous incisionless surgery is a surgical intervention used to treat a variety of skin depressions including atrophic acne scars, depressed scars and wrinkles for years.[6,15] This procedure acts by releasing the subcutaneous fibrotic strands that pull down the overlying tissue in a rolling scar.

History

In 1957, Spangler reported use of Bowmen's iris needle to cut the fibrous strands beneath the deeply depressed facial scar.[16] The same technique was later described by David Orentreinch and Norman Orentreinch under "subcutaneous incisionless surgery" in 1995 with use of a tribeveled hypodermic needle.[6]

Principle

The mechanisms of scar improvement in subcision are:

- Releasing fibrotic strands underlying scars
- Organization of blood in the induced dermal pocket
- Connective tissue formation in the area.[6]

Thus, the depressed scar is lifted by the releasing action of the procedure as well as from connective tissue that forms in the course of normal wound healing (Figs. 5A and B).

Indications

- This is the first scar revision technique to be performed in any case of pitted acne scars before taking up for other procedures
- Rolling acne scars—particularly scars that improve with stretching the skin.

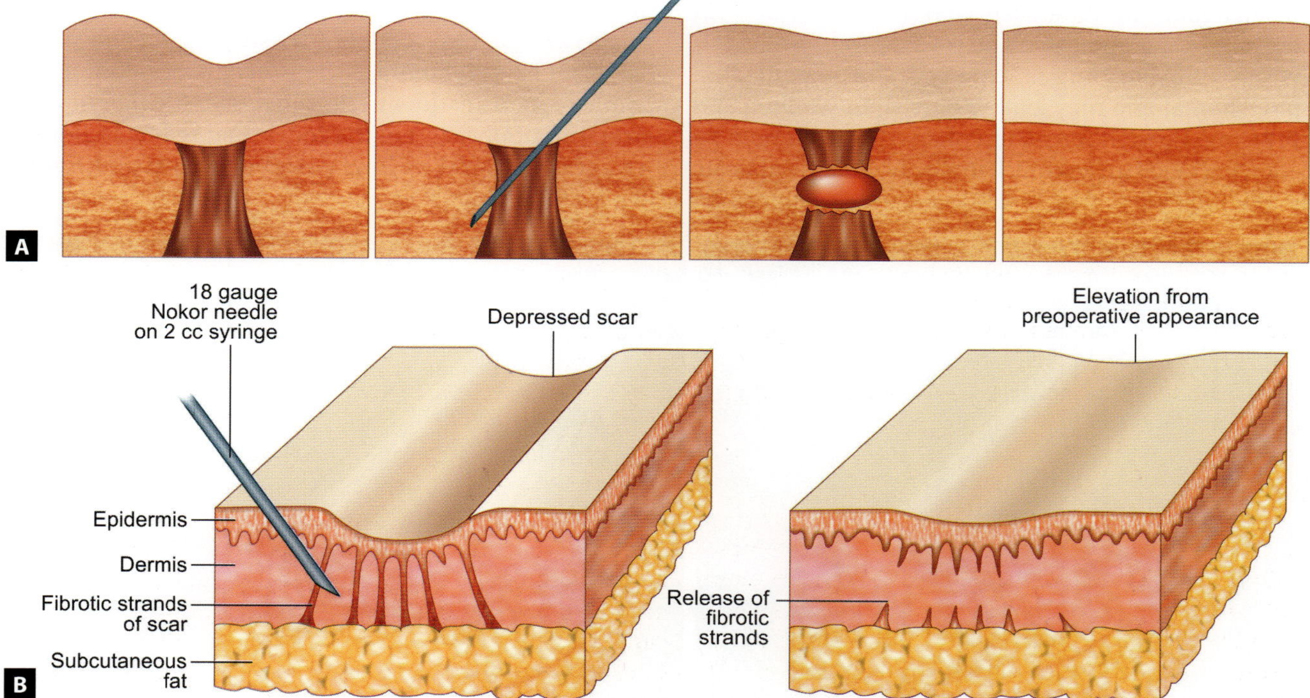

Figs. 5A and B: Subcision principle.

Treatment Procedure

The scarred area is marked and subcutaneous anesthesia (lidocaine 1% with epinephrine 1:100,000) given . The best needle to perform subcision is 18 gauge, 1.5 inch Nokor Admix needle. In the absence of Nokor needle injection needles ranging from 16 gauge to 23 gauge can be used. The needle is inserted with blade facing upward, at the periphery of the scarred area. Afterward, it is turned so that the tip is in a horizontal orientation (parallel to skin surface—side to side) just below dermal-subcutaneous junction plane and gently swept across the site. A snapping sound is heard as the bands are broken. In addition, a gentle piston like (to-and-fro) motion has been used to advance needle through fibrous band to release them. Procedure is done in two directions in each scarred area. For maximal pressure release of the fibrotic strands, it is better to approach larger scars from multiple puncture sites. The needle can be fixed on a 2 cc syringe so that the syringe works as a handle (Figs. 6A and B). Firm pressure should be applied postoperatively for at least 5 minutes to achieve hemostasis. Treatment can be repeated at an interval of 6 weeks for up to two to three successive treatments.

Complications

Bleeding, hematoma, hypertrophic scaring and scar recurrence are complications. Some degree of swelling is invariable and patient needs to be counseled. Bluish discoloration and swelling persists for 5–7 days.

Practical Tips

- When treating multiple scars with subcision, start with the most dependent area and work upward.
- While mild bleeding is expected and beneficial, a large hematoma may lead to persistent swelling and bruising. Prevent formation of a large hematoma by allowing blood to flow out, if undue bleeding is noticed.
- Subcision can be combined with suction. Doing repeated suction by microdermabrasion device, of the subcised scars, may prevent redepression by induction of repeated hemorrhage in dermal pocket, delay in healing and more new connective tissue formation at the scar area. Aalami Harandi et al. followed a subcision suction method by starting suction sessions on the 3rd day after subcision and continuing every other day for 2 weeks. There was significant and persistent improvement in short time, without considerable complication.[17]
- Subcision can be combined with subdermal implants. Balighi et al. treated acne scars with subcision and implantation of absorbable plain catgut pieces passed through the insertion puncture of the needle. However, the subdermal catgut implant led to no significant superior results in the above mentioned study.[18] Autologous fat or dermal tissue can be used as subdermal implants.[19] The use of these implants may cause an inflammatory response leading to fibrous tissue formation in the subcised area and theoretically improve the result of subcision.
- Subcision can be combined with most other acne scar treatments. Superior results can be achieved by combination therapy.[20]

Bilevel Subcision

The author combined subcision at two different levels in the same session with promising results. Instead of combining 2 different techniques, a bilevel subcision is done at two different planes so as to break the fibrotic bands of individual scars and induce neocollagenesis at a deeper level. Apart from improvement of scars, this technique also reduces the skin sagging and induce excellent skin tightening. The procedure is done under tumescent anesthesia thereby protecting all vital structures. Subcision of the individual scars are done at a superficial level as in classical subcison and further

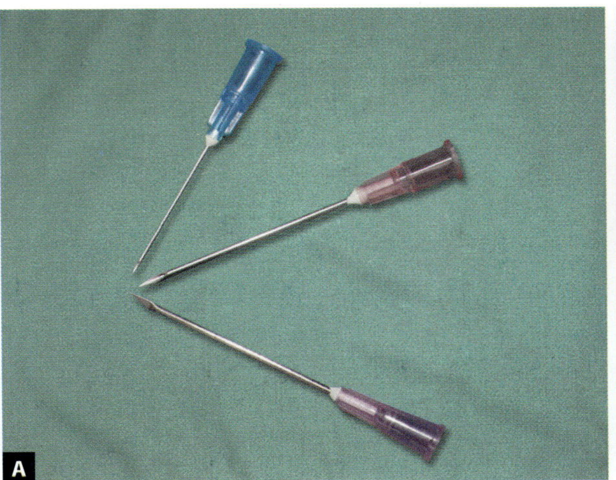

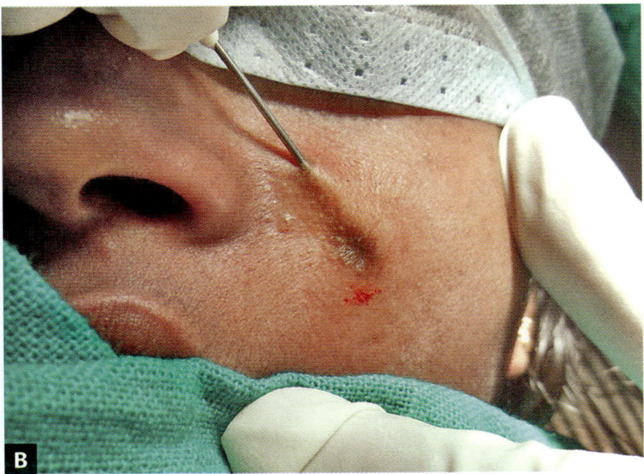

Figs. 6A and B: (A) Nokor needles; and (B) Subcision.

a deeper full plane subcision is done at upper subcuticular level. This can be performed, preferably using a blunt cannula or even a nokor needle. Figures 7A to D show the principle of bilevel subcision.

One side of the face can be treated by approaching through 3 points for deep subcision (Figs. 8 and 9). Each scar can be individually subcised at a superficial level. There is edema and feeling of tightness during the first one week. It takes 7 to 10 days for the swelling to subside. Scars become better over the next few months and maximum effects are seen at the end of a year along with overall facial tightening and pore reduction.

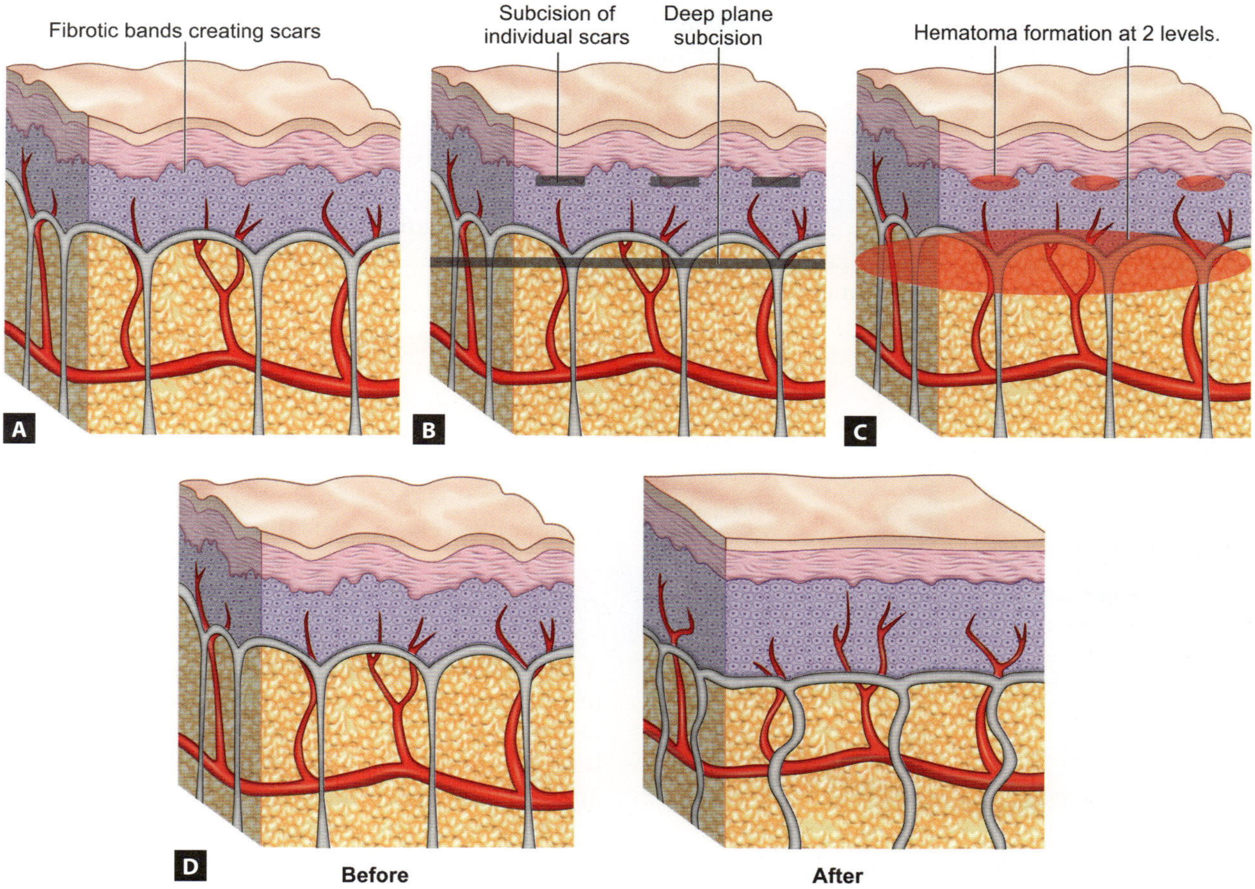

Figs. 7A to D: (A) Schematic representation of scar; (B) Sites of bilevel subcision. Just below individual scars and deeper plane; (C) Hematoma formation; (D) Before and after bilevel subcision.

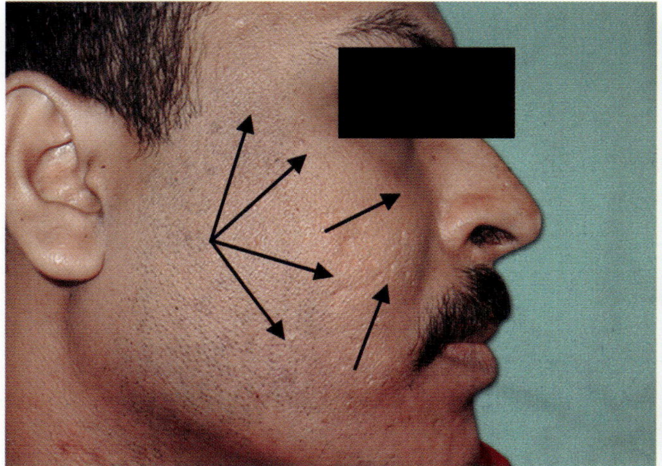

Fig. 8: Three points of entry for deeper subcision. Fanning movement can cover major area over the face.

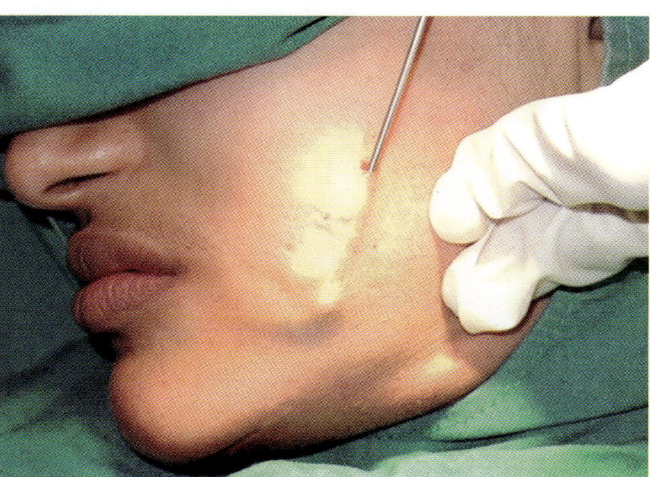

Fig. 9: Deep subcision using a cannula.

PUNCH TECHNIQUES

All punch techniques remove a pitted scar with a small rim of normal tissue. There are some scars which are circular, are small, punched out in appearance and have normal or altered texture of skin. Examples of such scars include acne scars with white atrophic bases or sharply punched out "ice pick" scars. Punch techniques can be of use in the management of these scars. The punch techniques include: punch excision, punch flotation or punch elevation and punch replacement grafting.

Punch Excision

Indication

Punch excision is recommended for ice pick scars and deep boxcar scars less than 3.5 mm diameter (Fig. 10).

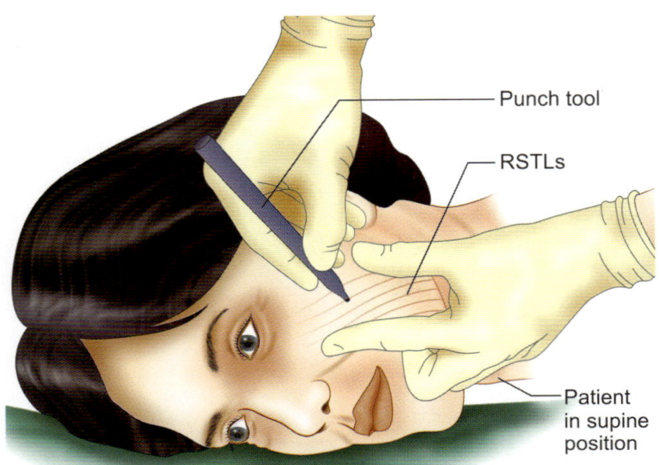

Fig. 10: Punch excision—schematic illustration. Note use of nondominant hand to apply outward traction perpendicular to facial relaxed skin tension lines. The punch tool is placed perpendicular to the skin and used with a quick rotating motion to remove the scar.

Procedure

This is done under local anesthesia. Scars are excised with a 1.5, 2, 2.5 or 3 mm biopsy punch as per size of the scar (Figs. 11A and B). By placing outward traction on the punch site at the time of excision, the circular wound is changed into an ellipse. To ensure that the ellipse runs parallel to the relaxed skin tension lines, the outward traction should be applied perpendicular to the skin lines. The scar tissue is removed and the wound sutured with one to three interrupted sutures using 6-0 nylon or prolene. If the punch excision is 2.5 mm or greater, a 6-0 vicryl (ethicon) subcutaneous suture can be placed prior to epidermal closure. This absorbable deep suture helps to promote wound edge eversion and facilitates proper healing (Figs. 12A and B).

Punch Flotation

Indications

Punch flotation works best for wide (>3 mm) boxcar acne scars that do not have significant color or textural irregularities (Figs. 13A to D).

Procedure

A punch that is exactly sized to match the inner diameter of the crateriform scar is selected for treatment. The punch is performed using a quick, rotating motion. This releases the bound-down scar. The plug is elevated with forceps and carefully freed from the underlying tissue. The plug is then elevated and positioned to lie slightly higher than the surrounding skin. The elevated punch can be secured in position by applying cyanoacrylate tissue adhesive and further closing with wound closure tapes like Steri-Strips (3M Corp.)

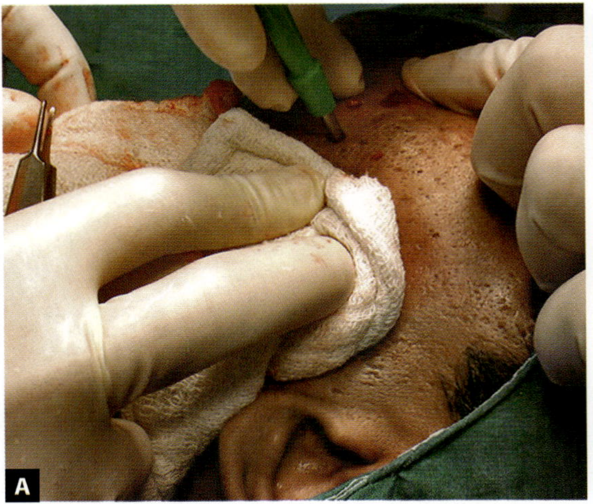

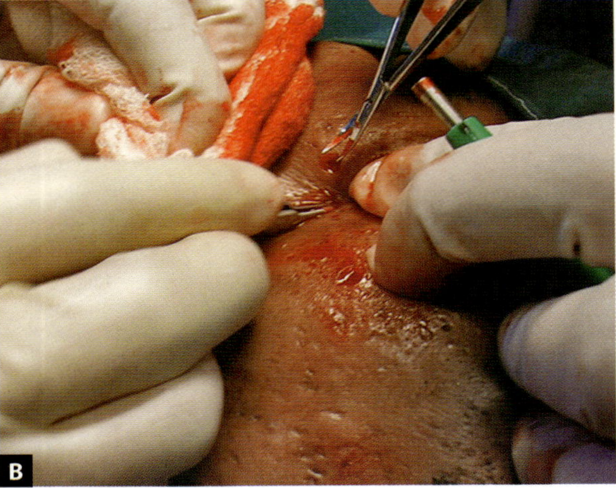

Figs. 11A and B: Punch excision and closure.

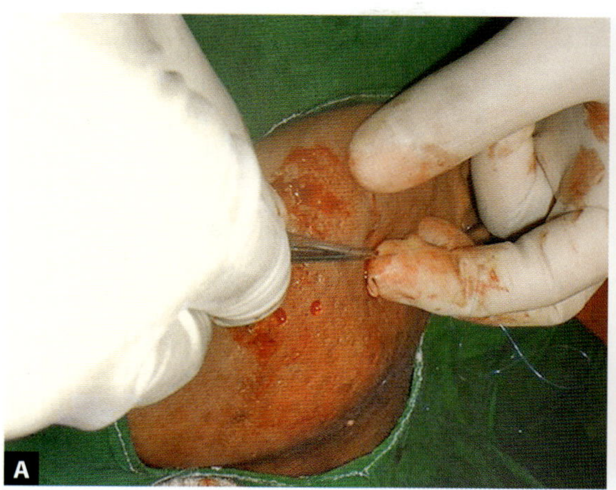
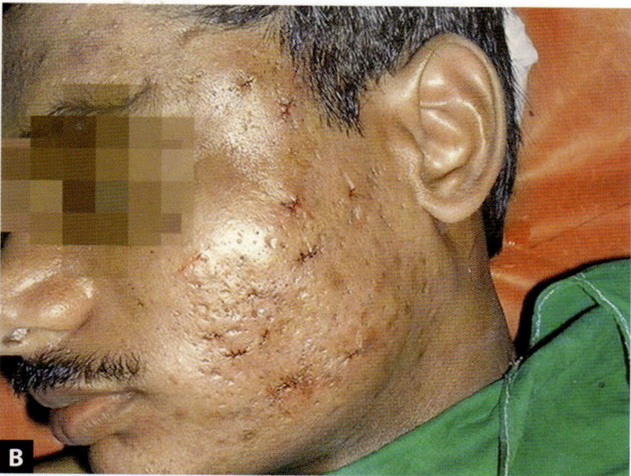

Figs. 12A and B: Punch excision and closure.

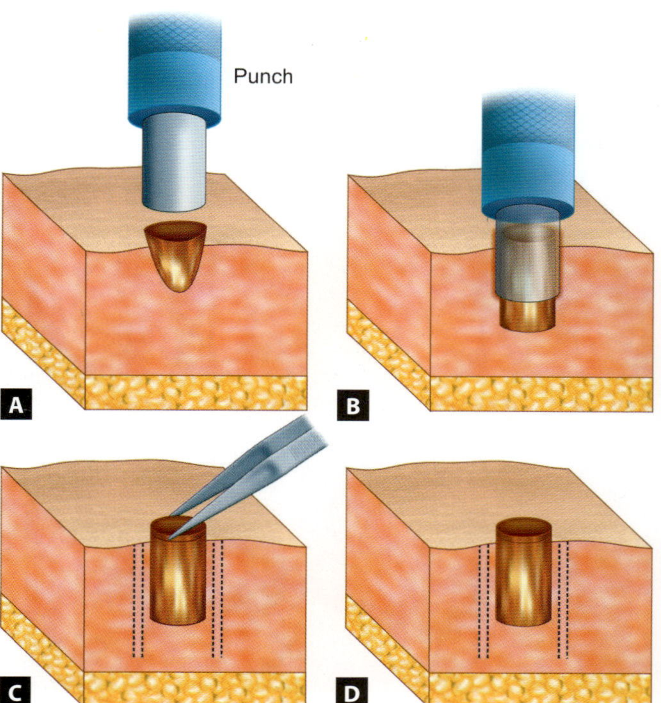

Figs. 13A to D: Punch flotation—schematic.

Punch Replacement Grafting

Indications

This procedure is utilized for deep, irregular pits and tethered boxcar scars with altered skin texture.

Procedure

The technique is similar to that of a punch flotation, but replaces the plug with a donor plug instead of elevating the original defect. The scar plug is removed and a graft plug of tissue obtained from the postauricular area or inner arm transferred to the plug site. The donor punch graft should be 0.5 mm larger than the punch used to excise the scar. Grafts can be secured into place by cyanoacrylate tissue adhesive and wound closure tapes.

Limitations of Punch Techniques

Punch replacement and punch flotation techniques are more successful for scars located on less mobile regions of the face such as the malar area and the forehead and less successful in perioral sites. Complications that may be observed include poor graft take, graft extrusion, and graft visibility. Poor color and textural mismatch are also frequently observed. Multiple procedures may be needed. Since the advent of lasers, these procedures are performed less frequently.

Practical Tips

- Punch techniques have to be combined with other scar revision modalities for effective management of acne scars.
- Punch techniques followed by resurfacing 4–8 weeks later improves the scar significantly.[20,21] Several studies have suggested that if resurfacing is performed in this postoperative period, the healing takes on almost a fetal type, with distribution of the extracellular matrix glycoprotein, integrin subunits in the epidermis[22] and dermal collagen fibers becoming unidirectional parallel to the epidermal surface after dermabrasion.
- Dermabrasion after excision, but before closure, improves the subsequent scar appearance.[23]
- Recently, simultaneous resurfacing with a CO_2 laser and punch excision[24] has been advocated.

CHEMICAL RECONSTRUCTION OF SKIN SCARS

Chemical reconstruction of skin scars (CROSS) is a technique using high strength trichloroacetic acid (TCA) focally on the atrophic acne scars to induce collagenization and cosmetic improvement. Lee and colleagues reported the use of high concentration (65% and 100%) trichloroacetic acid (TCA) applied locally to atrophic acne scars. The authors labeled this technique CROSS.[25]

Trichloroacetic acid is a versatile peeling agent because the peel depth varies according to its concentration.[26] It is also self-neutralizing and not absorbed in the systemic circulation; hence, high concentrations can be safely used without risk of systemic absorption.

Principle

Application of the caustic agent TCA causes precipitation of proteins, coagulative necrosis of cells in the epidermis, and necrosis of collagen in the papillary to upper reticular dermis.[27] There is an increase in dermal volume as a result of an increase in collagen production, glycosaminoglycan, and elastin fragmentation and reorganization of dermal collagen. The dermal remodeling continues for several months. During the remodeling phase, type III collagen is gradually replaced by type I collagen. The fibroblasts are oriented parallel to the epidermis which leads to improvement of scars.[27,28]

Indications

TCA CROSS is indicated for ice pick scars. In fact, it is the best treatment for this otherwise difficult to treat scar. Since, the ice pick scars are deep, destruction of the floor and wall of the pits followed by dermal remodeling leads to gradual improvement.

Procedure

The scars are marked with a surgical marking pen (Figs. 14A to D). The face is cleaned with spirit and degreased with acetone. The procedure is carried out with the patient sitting comfortably as lying down can cause effacement of appearance of the scars. The skin is stretched, and 100% TCA is focally applied with a wooden toothpick pressing firmly up to the bottom of the depressed area of atrophic scar taking care to avoid spillage to the surrounding skin. The skin is monitored carefully and kept stretched until a frosted appearance is seen. Frosting is a result of coagulation of epidermal and dermal proteins and is generally seen in 10–15 seconds. The patient is asked to wash the face after the procedure. Photoprotection is recommended. TCA CROSS can be repeated at 4-week intervals for a total of three treatments.[26,29]

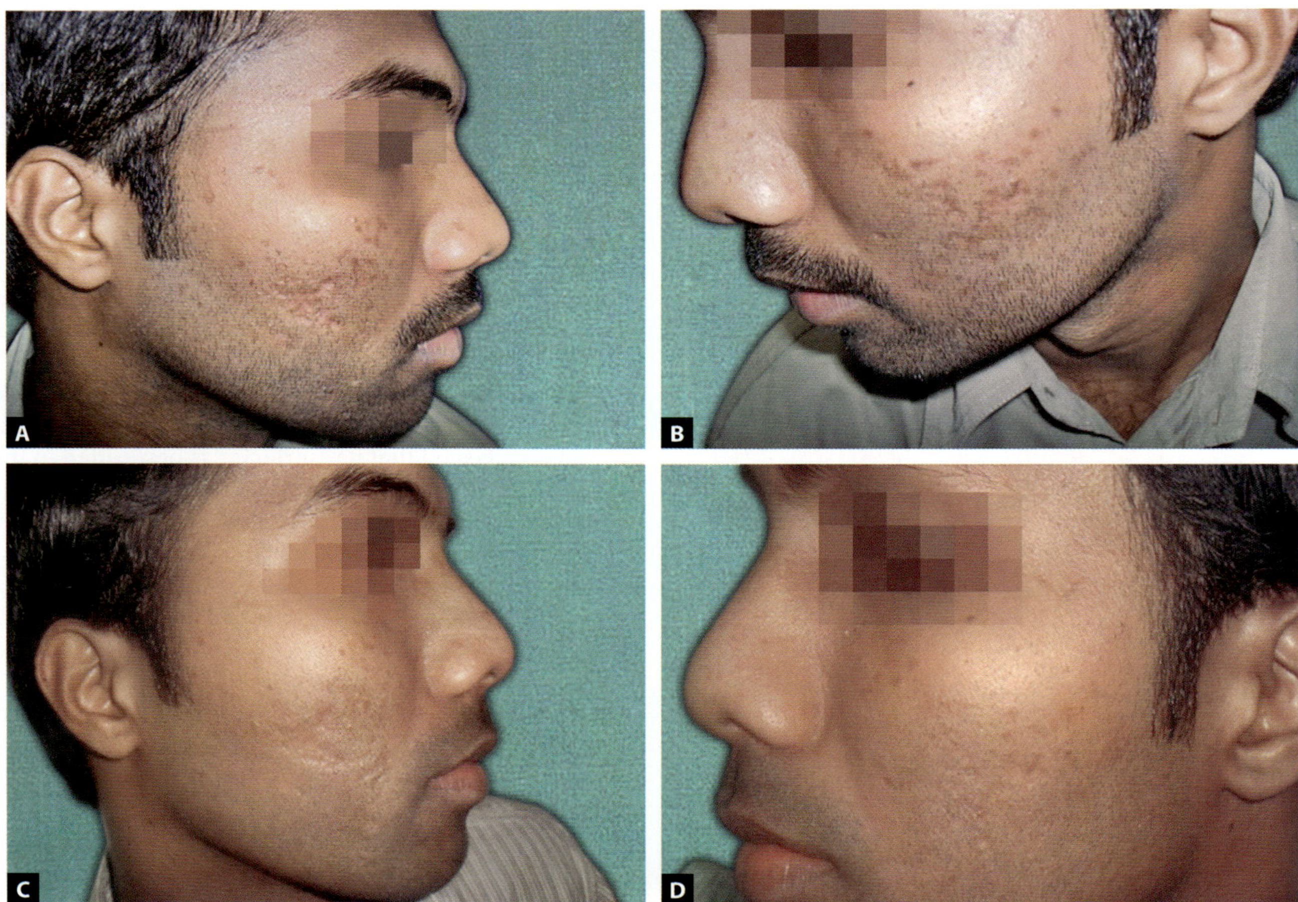

Figs. 14A to D: TCA CROSS: (A and C) Before; (B and D) After.
Courtesy: BS Chandrashekar.

Complications

Transient postinflammatory hyperpigmentation and hypopigmentation are the reported complications of TCA CROSS.[26]

Concentration of TCA ranged from 50% to 100% in various studies.[25,26,29,30] None of the studies have reported any significant side effects even after applying 100% TCA on type V skin.[26] However, the results were better with increased concentration.

In a split face study comparing TCA CROSS 100% applied twice at 12-week interval with a 1,550 nm Er:Glass fractional laser applied thrice at 6-week interval, the CROSS technique was reported to be superior for ice pick scars.[30]

Practical Tips

- Priming the skin with hydroquinone and tretinoin cream for 2 weeks before the procedure helps in reducing the incidence of postinflammatory hyperpigmentation that is expected after using high concentrations of TCA in dark skins
- Photoprotection should be strictly followed in all patients on TCA CROSS
- Care should be taken to avoid spillage of TCA to normal skin
- Application of TCA should be limited to the ice pick scars and care should be taken not to apply the agent to rim of the opening of the pit.

DERMAL GRAFTING[31-33]

Dermal grafts has been reported to be effective as a filler material for treating depressed scars. This technique builds on previous subcision and consists of placing dermal grafts into precise pockets under the skin. A dermal graft is a skin graft from which epidermis and subcutaneous fat have been removed.

Dermis can be used for filling up the defects in a cost effective way. Dermal grafts have shown long-term survival in various published data and are almost permanent. Survival rates of dermal grafts are much higher than fat transplants.

Advantages of Using Dermal Graft

- Not susceptible to infection
- Can be accurately tailored for a variety of defects
- Creates a permanent spacer between overlying skin and underlying fibrous band of tissue
- Readily available material
- Easy to perform.

Procedure

Two different techniques of dermal grafting using the conventional technique and enzymatic separation are discussed below.

Conventional Technique

Procedure is done under local anesthesia (Figs. 15 and 16).

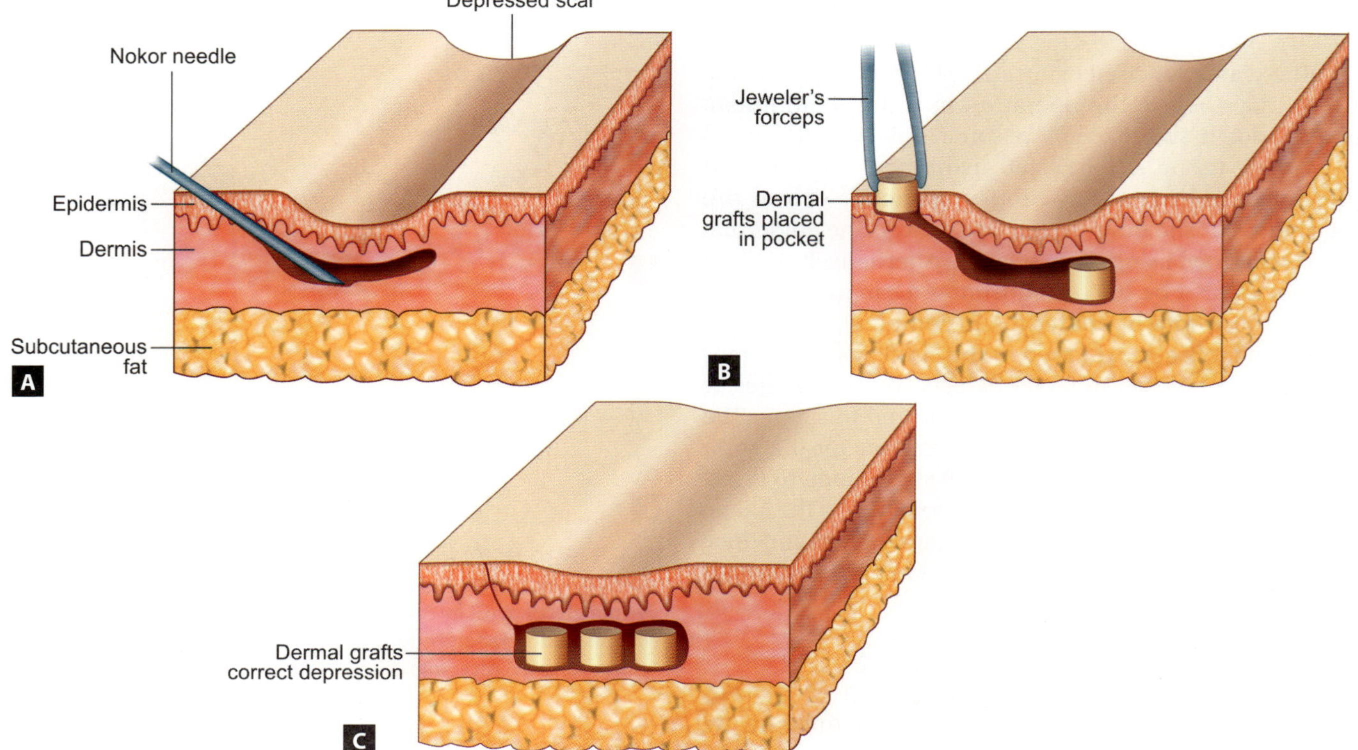

Figs. 15A to C: Dermal grafting conventional technique principle.

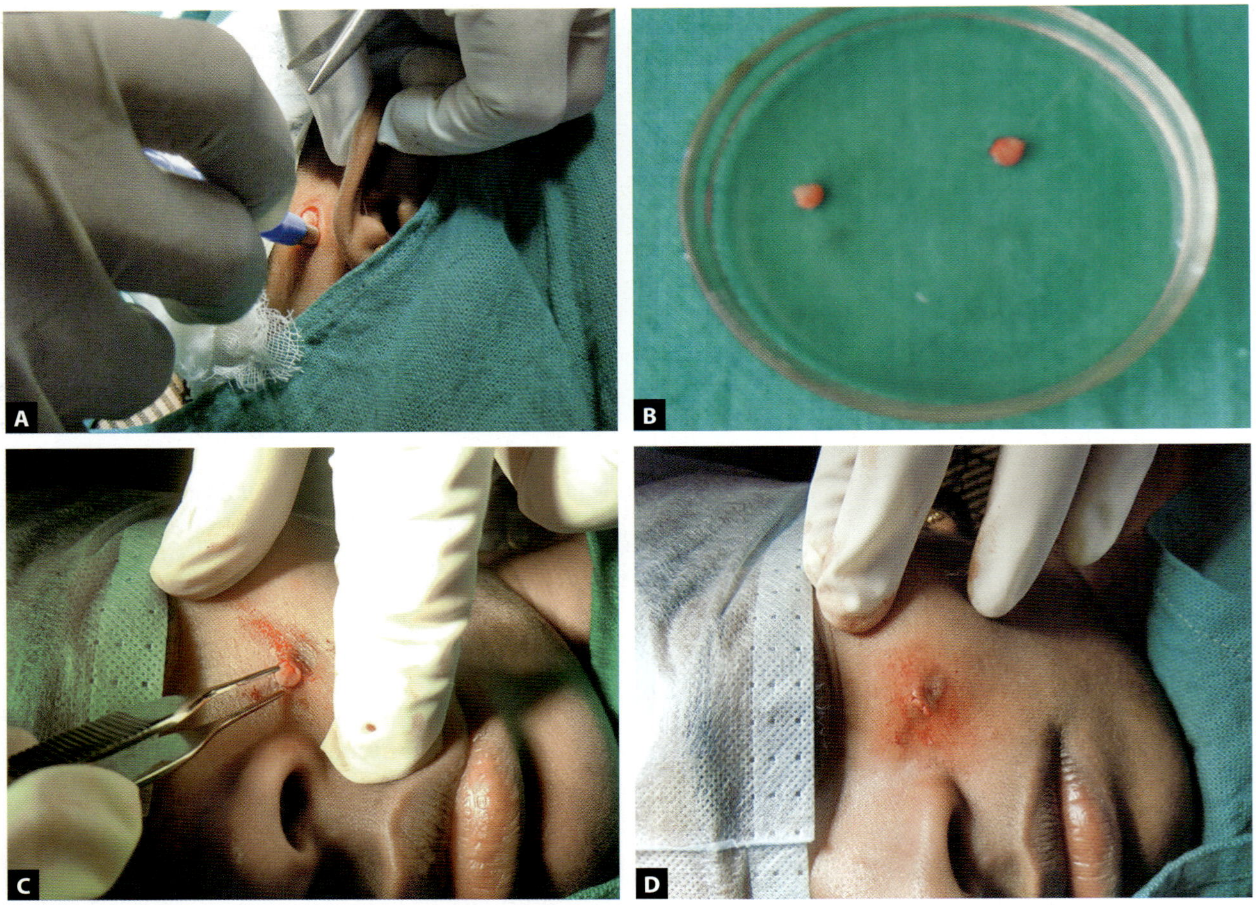

Figs. 16A to D: (A) Dermal grafting—conventional harvesting donor graft; (B) Dermal grafting—conventional donor graft with epidermis removed; (C) Dermal grafting—conventional placement of donor graft in the scar; and (D) Dermal grafting—conventional graft in place after closure.

The scar is subcised using a 18 gauge or Nokor needle 10–14 days before the operation in order to stimulate granulation tissue and achieve some initial correction.

Donor tissue is harvested using any conventional dermatomes or using biopsy punches from the postauricular site down to the fascia level. The epidermal part is trimmed using a fine scissors. Alternatively, dermal tissue can also be harvested from a dermabraded area where the whole of epidermis is completely removed. Excess of fat is also trimmed in the similar way. Dermo-fat graft can be used in larger defects. These punches or long narrow strip of dermis is transferred to saline. The defective area is tunneled to create a space for the graft; as per the size of the defect. A small slit is made to insert the grafts. The grafts are trimmed according to the shape of the defect. The graft is inserted using a forceps and once complete correction has occurred, the slit is sutured with prolene.

Enzymatic Technique

This is a technique of dermal grafting developed by the author (Figs. 17A to D). The technique uses trypsin to make the firm dermal tissue soft and moldable.

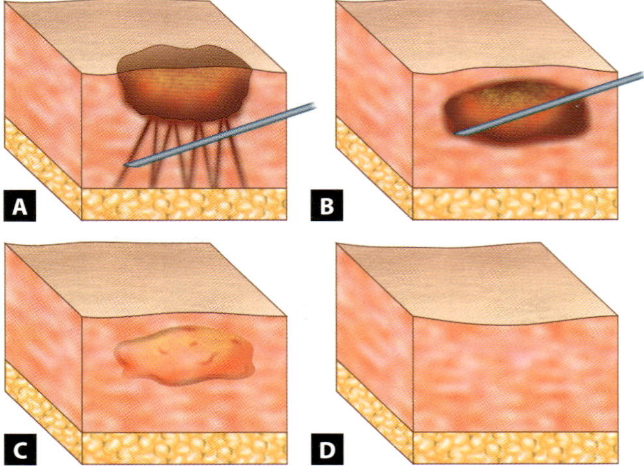

Figs. 17A to D: (A) Initial subscision prior to enzymatic dermal grafting; (B) Creation of a dermal pocket prior to enzymatic dermal grafting; (C) Injection of dermal suspension obtained from enzymatic dermal grafting with a wide bore needle or directly by syringe; and (D) After injection of suspension.

Full thickness skin graft is harvested as in case of conventional technique. This is then transferred into a

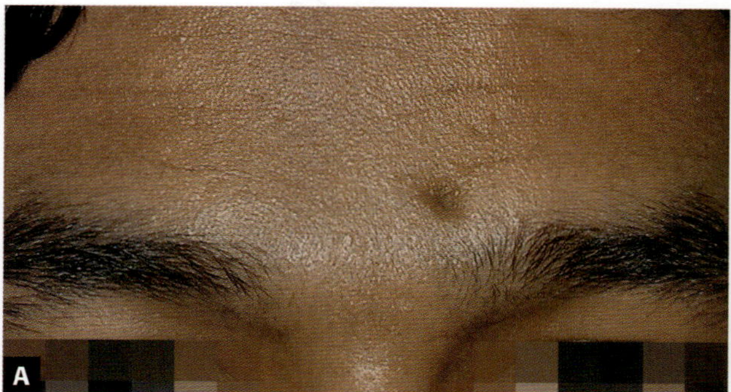

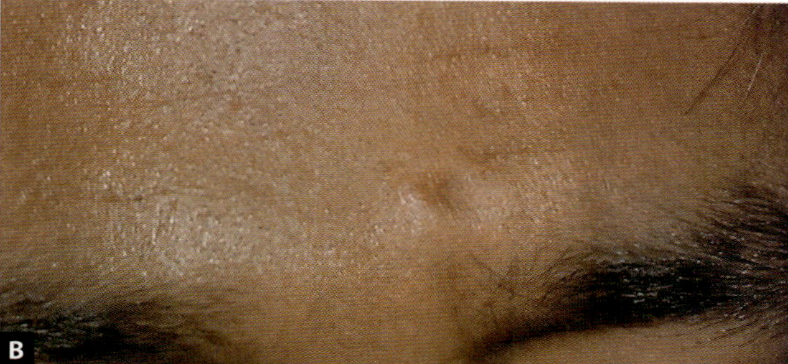

Figs. 18A and B: Dermal grafting—enzymatic separation before and after 3 months.

petridish containing 0.25% of trypsin in EDTA solution. This is incubated at 37° C for 75 minutes. After incubation, the tissue is transferred to phosphate buffered saline and the epidermis is manually separated.

The dermal tissue separated by enzymatic technique is soft, flexible and easily moldable in comparison with the firm dermal tissue harvested by the conventional technique. This is filled into the defect as in case of conventional technique. Or it can be transferred into 1 cc syringe and pushed into the defect. Area can be molded by external manipulation. The slit made for inserting the material is then sutured. Result achieved can be gratifying (Figs. 18A and B).

Practical Tips

- Epidermis should be removed entirely. Any epidermal tissue left along with the dermal graft can induce cyst formation
- Great care should be taken while handling the dermal tissue. Any contamination can lead to infection and rejection of the graft.

OTHER MODALITIES FOR TREATMENT OF ACNE SCAR

In addition to the above methods, there are a number of other methods which have been described individually in different chapters. Relevant points of these techniques are mentioned here briefly.

Chemical Peeling

As is well-known superficial peels are useful for superficial acne scars only. Peeling agents that can be used for acne scars are salicylic acid (20–30%), TCA (10%, 15% and 25%), glycolic acid (25–35%) and Jessner's peel. TCA (35%) can cause medium depth peeling and hence can be used for deeper scars, but should be used with great caution in Indian skin due to high chances of postinflammatory pigmentation. Salicylic acid (20–30%) is the peeling agent of choice in active acne and it can be used for superficial acne scars, particularly in those with seborrheic skin. Glycolic acid is effective peeling agent even at low concentrations but there is great patient variability in terms of reactivity and efficacy. Details of each peel are dealt with in separate chapters on chemical peels.

Microdermabrasion

It has become popular because of the ease of its technique, safety and low cost. Microdermabrasion is mainly indicated for the treatment of superficial acne scars and is ineffective for deeper scars. The patient must be adequately counseled regarding the limitations of the procedure, the need for multiple sittings, and expected outcome and complications. The key to effective microdermabrasion is stretching the skin under tension for effective abrasion and achieving a vacuum to aspirate the epidermal debris and used crystals. Treatment is repeated weekly until the desired result is obtained. Microdermabrasion is a safe procedure particularly in darker skin and requires no downtime.

Soft Tissue Augmentation (Fillers)

The popularity of soft tissue augmentation with dermal fillers and autologous fat implantation is increasing because of minimal downtime, immediate results and availability of an array of newer agents. It is mainly indicated for the treatment of soft atrophic acne scars with loss of dermal tissue. Dermal fillers placed under the scars, elevate them and bring the surface of the scars in level with the surface of surrounding skin. It may be combined with lasers or other modality to improve skin textural abnormalities. It may be preceded by subcision or microneedling to break the fibrous septa preventing scars to raise to the surface after filler injection.

Many preparations can be used for this including hyaluronic acid fillers, autologous fat, etc. Fillers working by fibroplasia like poly-L-lactic acid (PLLA, Sculptra) and calcium hydroxyapatite (CaHA, Radiesse) have attracted attention in recent years because of their longer correction duration due to their collagen stimulating effect. Liquid injectable silicone, one of the permanent filler, is also being used for correction of acne scars giving long-term correction.

However, their high cost and temporary duration of result is a disadvantage.

Scar Revisions

In selected cases, when scarring is linear and extensive, scar revision techniques such as Z, M and Y plasty may be useful. These need to be performed by a dermatosurgeon properly trained in performing these procedures. Details of the procedures are given in the section on "Scar Revision".

Cryotherapy

Cryoslush and cryopeel are used for the treatment of nodulocystic acne, inflammatory papule and pustule. In the cryoslush method (Figs. 19A and B), solid CO_2 is crushed and a few drops of acetone are added to make a paste. This paste is rapidly applied to the lesions with a gauze ball for 2–10 seconds. Superficial peeling is achieved due to epidermal necrosis, which causes desquamation of comedones, resolution of inflammatory papules, pustules, nodules and cysts. In the cryopeel method, a spray of liquid nitrogen is used for 2–3 seconds, instead of a CO_2 slush. However, pigmentary changes are commonly observed, particularly in darker-skinned patients and so this procedure should be used carefully only after proper counseling of the patient. Persistent erythema and scarring may also occur.

CONCLUSION

The treatment of postacne scars is a multimodality approach and any single modality usually does not bring satisfactory correction. Each modality has its advantages and disadvantages (Table 1). The main goal of treatment is to achieve maximal improvement rather than perfection in most of the cases. The surgical procedures (punch excision, punch elevation and subcision) can be combined in one treatment session, if necessary, for different scar types. Most patients who have had punch excision or elevation should undergo laser resurfacing few months later for further textural refinement. Laser skin resurfacing can be used after subcision, but is not always necessary. Laser skin resurfacing alone is not as effective for rolling scars because it does not release the fibrous tethers. Patients must be reminded that collagen remodeling can take several months to occur, and maximum benefit from resurfacing or microneedling may not be evident until that time. Dermal fillers can be combined with any procedure for elevation of scar depressions. Many complications can be prevented by thorough preoperative evaluation, sound surgical technique and careful follow-up care. Good patient rapport and effective communication with patients are invaluable.

There are multiple surgical options that can be tailored to each individual's needs, tolerance and goals along with the physician's assessments, skills and expectations. The right procedure has to be combined in the right sequence to achieve the best result.

This Chapter deals with only some of the surgical methods in acne scar revision. For information on lasers and other adjunctive therapies, please refer appropriate sections.

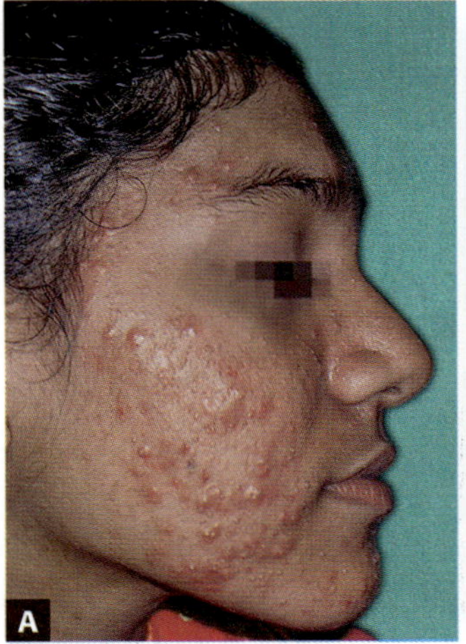

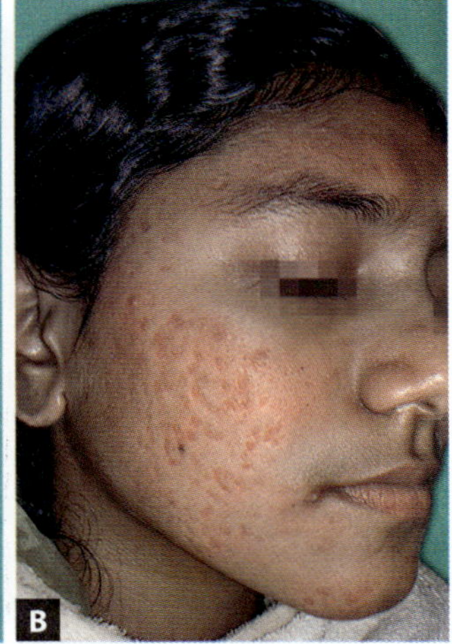

Figs. 19A and B: Cryoslush (A) before and (B) after in active acne.
Courtesy: BS Chandrashekar.

Tips and Pearls

- Subcision is an underutilized technique, but yields excellent results in trained hands
- Chemical peeling and microdermabrasion (MDA) gives limited improvement and needs multiple sessions
- The main goal of treatment is to achieve maximal improvement rather than perfection in most of the cases
- Punch excision techniques should be followed by resurfacing to achieve optimum results
- Dermal fillers can be combined with any other treatment modality
- Multiple treatments combined in a rational way can help bring satisfactory improvement rather than any single modality used alone

REFERENCES

1. Jacob CI, Dover JS, Kaminer MS. Acne scarring: a classification system and review of treatment options. J Am Acad Dermatol. 2001;45:109-17.
2. Alster TS. Cutaneous resurfacing with CO_2 and erbium: YAG lasers: Preoperative, intraoperative and postoperative considerations. Plast Reconstr Surg. 1999;103:619-32.
3. Ang P, Barlow RJ. Non-ablative laser resurfacing: a systematic review of the literature. Clin Exp Dermatol. 2002;27:630-5.
4. Shim EK, Barnette D, Hughes K, et al. Microdermabrasion: a clinical and histopathologic study. Dermatol Surg. 2001;27:524-30.
5. Fernandes D. Minimally invasive percutaneous collagen induction. Oral Maxillofac Surg Clin North Am. 2005;17:51-63.
6. Orentreich DS, Orentreich N. Subcutaneous incisionless (subcision) surgery for the correction of depressed scars and wrinkles. Dermatol Surg. 1995;21:543-9.

7. Camirand A, Doucet J. Needle dermabrasion. Aesthetic Plast Surg. 1997;21:48-51.
8. Fabbrocini G, Fardella N, Monfrecola A, et al. Acne scarring treatment using skin needling. Clin Exp Dermatol. 2009;34: 874-9.
9. Rawlins JM, Lam WL, Karoo RO, et al. Quantifying collagen type in mature burn scars: A novel approach using histology and digital image analysis. J Burn Care Res. 2006;27: 60-5.
10. Ferguson MW, O'Kane S. Scar-free healing: From embryonic mechanisms to adult therapeutic intervention. Philos Trans R Soc Lond B Biol Sci. 2004;359:839-50.
11. Bandyopadhyay B, Fan J, Guan S, et al. A "traffic control" role for TGFbeta3: Orchestrating dermal and epidermal cell motility during wound healing. J Cell Biol. 2006;172: 1093-105.
12. Aust MC, Fernandes D, Kolokythas P, et al. Percutaneous collagen induction therapy. An alternative treatment for scars, wrinkles and skin laxity. Plast Reconstr Surg. 2008;121: 1421-9.
13. Fernandes D, Signorini M. Combating photoaging with percutaneous collagen induction. Clin Dermatol. 2008;26: 192-9.
14. Majid I. Microneedling therapy in atrophic facial scars: an objective assessment. J Cutan Aesthet Surg. 2009;2:26-30.
15. Goodman GJ. Therapeutic undermining of scars (subcision). Australas J Dermatol. 2001;42:114-7.
16. Spangler AS. New treatment for pitted scars. AMA Arch Dermatol. 1957;76:708-11.
17. Aalami HS, Balighi K, Lajevardi V, et al. Subcision-suction method: a new successful combination therapy in treatment of atrophic acne scars and other depressed scars. J Eur Acad Dermatol Venereol. 2011;25:92-9.
18. Balighi K, Robati RM, Moslehi H, et al. Subcision in acne scar with and without subdermal implant: a clinical trial. J Eur Acad Dermatol Venereol. 2008;22:707-11.
19. Pinski KS, Coleman WP. Microlipoinjection and autologous collagen. Dermatol Clin. 1995;13:339-51.
20. Katz BE, Oca AG. A controlled study of the effectiveness of spot dermabrasion ('scarabrasion') on the appearance of surgical scars. J Am Acad Dermatol. 1991;24:462-6.
21. Yarborough JM Jr. Ablation of facial scars by programmed dermabrasion. J Dermatol Surg Oncol. 1988;14:292-4.
22. Harmon CB, Zelickson BD, Roenigk RK, et al. Dermabrasive scar revision: immunohistochemical and ultrastructural evaluation. Dermatol Surg. 1995;21:503-8.
23. Caver CV. Versatile dermabrasion. J Dermatol Surg Oncol. 1980;6:665-7.
24. Gravelink JM, White VR. Concurrent use of laser skin resurfacing and punch excision in the treatment of facial acne scarring. Dermatol Surg. 1998;24:527-30.
25. Lee JB, Chung WG, Kwahck H, et al. Focal treatment of acne scars with trichloroacetic acid: chemical reconstruction of skin scars method. Dermatol Surg. 2002;28:1017-21.
26. Khunger N, Bhardwaj D, Khunger M. Evaluation of CROSS technique with 100% TCA in the management of ice pick acne scars in darker skin types. Journal of Cosmetic Dermatology. 2011;10:51-7.
27. Yug A, Lane JE, Howard MS, et al. Histologic study of depressed acne scars treated with serial high-concentration (95%) trichloroacetic acid. Dermatol Surg. 2006;32: 985-90.
28. Brodland DG, Cullimore KC, Roenigk RK, et al. Depths of chemicoexcision induced by various concentrations and application techniques of trichloracetic acid in a porcine model. J Dermatol Surg Oncol. 1989;15:967-71.
29. Fabbrocini G, Cacciapuoti S, Fardella N, et al. CROSS technique: chemical reconstruction of skin scars method. Dermatol Therapy. 2008;21:S29-32.
30. Kim HJ, Kim TG, Kwon YS, et al. Comparison of a 1,550 nm erbium: glass fractional laser and a chemical reconstruction of skin scars (CROSS) Method in the treatment of acne scars: A simultaneous split-face trial. Lasers Surg Med. 2009;41:545-9.
31. Arndt KA. Scar revision. Procedures in cosmetic dermatology. Elsevier. 2006;45-66.
32. Besecker B, Hart CG. A new treatment option for acne scars: allograft dermis. Dermatology nursing / Dermatology Nurses Association. 1999;11:111-4.
33. Burres SA. Recollagenation of acne scars. Dermatologic Surgery. 1996;22:364-7.

Chapter

47

Acne Scars: Treatment with Lasers

Imran Majid

Key Messages

- Lasers, particularly fractional lasers, are an integral part of the management of acne scars.
- Both fractional ablative and nonablative lasers are useful.
- Ablative fractional lasers score over nonablative lasers in terms of efficacy of scar amelioration. However, the former are associated with significant downtime.
- Among the different morphological types of acne scars, rolling and superficial boxcar scars respond the best to laser resurfacing treatment.
- In severe types of scarring, lasers have to be combined with other antiscar modalities for optimum results.

INTRODUCTION

Post-acne scarring is one of the most feared and long-lasting complications of inflammatory acne.[1] The condition is associated with a lot of psychological trauma as the involved site is most often the face. There is a long list of treatment options available for amelioration of post-acne scars but the outcome from any of these treatment options is still far from being ideal. Lasers are among the most recent additions to this list of therapeutic options. A number of laser and light devices are currently used in managing acne scars and these devices will be discussed in this chapter. What needs to be remembered, however, is that majority of patients with acne scars have more than one morphological types and grades of scars and this warrants the use of multiple treatment options to reach a satisfactory level of improvement.

INDICATIONS OF LASER TREATMENT IN ACNE SCARS

Laser treatment for acne scars can be considered in any patient in whom the scars are causing a significant psychological impact. In general patients with Grade 2 to Grade 4 scars by the Goodman and Baron grading system are thought to be the ideal candidates for laser treatment.[2] While patients with Grade 1 scars can be managed by simpler scar amelioration techniques like peels with or without topical retinoids or even microdermabrasion techniques, laser resurfacing can be used in such cases if the psychological impact is really high in an individual patient.[2,3] Patients with the most severe, Grade 4 scars are the most difficult to treat and generally do not show a considerable improvement after any single treatment option. These patients have to be treated with a cocktail of multiple treatment options like surgical techniques, fillers, subcisions and laser resurfacing.

Lasers are indicated in the treatment of all the different morphological types of acne scars. However, the response to laser resurfacing varies among these morphological variants. Among the different morphological types of acne scars, rolling and superficial boxcar scars respond the best to laser resurfacing treatment.[4,5] Pitted scars and especially deeper boxcar scars usually respond less satisfactorily to laser resurfacing than the above mentioned scar types. In such cases laser resurfacing needs to be combined with surgical procedures like punch excision or punch floatation or with TCA CROSS technique to improve the therapeutic results.[4-6]

LASERS USED FOR ACNE SCARS

Lasers used in the treatment of post-acne scars can be broadly divided into two main groups—ablative and non-ablative lasers. This classification is simply done on the basis of whether the laser leads to an ablative injury to the epidermis/dermis or not during the treatment process.

Ablative Lasers

Ablative lasers, as the term denotes, cause an injury or ablation of the epidermis and a part of the dermis with resultant collagen deposition as a part of the healing response. This collagen deposition in the dermis along with a renewal of the epidermal layer is responsible for amelioration of post-acne atrophic scars as well as any pigment dyschromias.

The two main ablative lasers used for acne scars are the CO_2 and erbium lasers. The CO_2 laser emits light at the 10,600 nm wavelength and is the more ablative of the two. It causes vaporization of the epidermis and the papillary dermis to a depth of about 50–150 μm.[7] The depth of this vaporization depends largely on the energy level that is used. In addition to this vaporizing effect there is an additional thermal injury extending up to another 20–40 μm zone around the vaporization zone.[8] The erbium yttrium aluminum garnet (Er:YAG) laser, on the other hand, emits light in the 2,940 nm wavelength and the depth of ablation with this laser is less than that achieved with CO_2 laser. In addition it causes minimal surrounding thermal damage of about 5–15 μm.[8] The depth of ablation can be increased by increasing number of laser passes (stacking) and similarly the extent of surrounding thermal damage can be increased by increasing the laser pulse duration (Variable pulse). see chapter on Er:YAG laser for more details.

As a rule, ablative lasers are the most effective in treatment of post-acne scars but the high incidence of adverse effects limits their use. These adverse effects include a prolonged erythema and exfoliation of the skin, post-treatment hyper- and hypopigmentation and even the risk of scarring and secondary infections. Another disadvantage of these ablative lasers is the prolonged downtime associated with their use.

Nonablative Lasers

While ablative procedures result in removal of entire epidermis and parts of dermis and cause a dramatic and impressive reduction in scar severity, their side effect profile is equally serious especially in dark skinned races.[8,9] This is where the nonablative lasers score as they can also reduce acne scarring without significant downtime. However, the efficacy of these lasers is considered to be less as compared with the ablative lasers. The underlying principle of laser remodeling by nonablative lasers is induction of controlled injury to the dermal collagen without any damage to the epidermis. This controlled injury leads to a healing response with dermal collagen remodeling. This causes a tightening effect on the skin with resultant improvement in the appearance of the scars.[8,9]

The nonablative lasers used for treatment of acne scars can be divided into two groups:

1. *Infrared lasers:* These include 1,450 nm diode laser, 1,064 nm Q-switched Nd:YAG laser, 1,320 nm Nd:YAG laser and 1,540 nm Er:glass laser.
2. *Visible light lasers:* This list includes the commonly used intense pulsed light (IPL), pulsed dye lasers, light emitting diodes, broadband light sources, etc.

Among the above two groups infrared lasers are the ones that have been used and studied more commonly than the other group. Treatment with nonablative lasers can provide modest improvement scores in acne scar management. Typically the treatment comprises of multiple sessions at 3–4 week intervals and the overall score is presumed to improve with more number of sessions. The first nonablative laser that was used for treatment of acne scars was the 1,450 nm diode laser. This laser provides an additional advantage of treating active acne in addition to the acne scars through its effect on sebaceous glands.[10] Another laser device in the infrared range that has been used in the management of post-acne scars is the 1,320 nm Nd:YAG laser.[11] This laser system has been compared with the 1450 nm diode laser and the comparison study showed both the lasers to be effective and safe with relatively better efficacy from the latter.[12] A combination of serial TCA peels and 1,450 nm diode laser treatments has also been assessed in a study with a small sample size and the combination has been shown to be more effective than laser treatment alone.[13]

FRACTIONAL PHOTOTHERMOLYSIS

Fractional photothermolysis is a relatively new concept in laser rejuvenation wherein the laser system, instead of causing a photoinjury to the whole skin, produces longitudinal arrays of microscopic thermal injury to specific depths in the dermis. These longitudinal thermal wounds are known as microscopic treatment zones (MTZs) and they are separated from each other by normal, non-injured skin. The term "fractional" is in fact derived from this fact only that only a fraction of the whole skin is treated rather than the whole skin surface. This "fractionated treatment" minimizes the chances of any serious adverse effects to the skin and also shortens the downtime after treatment. The technology provides a fine balance between the undesirable side effects of ablative lasers and the limited efficacy of nonablative ones. Fractional photothermolysis was initially used for the treatment of photoaging[14] but the technology is now used in many more indications especially post-acne scarring.

In fractional photothermolysis, the skipped non-injured part of the skin provides the source of keratinocytes that migrate into the laser-treated injured areas.[15] This phenomenon of kertinocyte migration is seen within the first 24 hours after treatment. After migration into the treatment zone the donated keratinocytes facilitate the removal of necrotic debris from the skin in the form of denatured dermal tissue, melanin and other constituents.[15,16] This necrotic debris is known by the name of 'microscopic epidermal necrotic debris' (MENDs). Elimination of this microscopic debris (MENDs) is followed by laying-down of new collagen in the dermis and a resultant anti-scarring and anti-aging effect.

Fractional photothermolysis is also divided into the ablative and nonablative platforms depending upon the wavelength of the laser used and the effects of the laser on the skin. In the treatment of acne scars both the ablative and nonablative fractional lasers have been used. Fractional photothermolysis is summarized in Box 1.

Nonablative Fractional Resurfacing for Acne Scars

Fractional lasers with wavelengths in the range of 1,410–1,550 nm are the ones referred to as nonablative fractional lasers. These lasers cause columns of coagulative change in the dermis without injuring the epidermis. As the stratum corneum remains intact the healing is fairly rapid without any sequalae. Among the nonablative fractional lasers, the one that has been the most commonly used till date is the 1,550 nm erbium doped fiber laser known as Fraxel laser (Reliant technologies, USA). Most of the studies on this laser device have reported improvements in the scar appearance in the range of 50% or even up to 75% after multiple sessions at monthly intervals.[17-19] The erbium-doped fiber laser has even been used in patients with darker skin with good results.[20,21] The most important advantage of nonablative lasers is that there is no significant downtime after treatment with these devices. This is of significant practical benefit as many patients are not ready to accept downtime over many days after any treatment for acne scars (Table 1).

Box 1: Summary of fractional lasers.

- Fractional lasers are the most commonly used lasers for acne scars at present
- Fractional lasers treat only a small fraction or part of the skin by causing longitudinal columns of injury known as microscopic treatment zones (MTZs)
- Two main categories of fractional lasers are used: Nonablative and ablative fractional lasers
- Nonablative lasers are associated with minimal downtime and are considered safer than ablative lasers
- Ablative fractional lasers are claimed to be more efficacious than nonablative lasers

ABLATIVE FRACTIONAL LASER RESURFACING

Ablative fractional lasers have been designed to deliver the best of both worlds by applying ablative laser technology in a fractionated pattern that provides the efficacy of ablative laser treatment but minimizes the side effect profile to a considerable degree. Fractional ablative lasers cause a direct vaporizing effect on the epidermis and some part of the dermis in a microscopic columnar pattern. In addition there is a zone of coagulation of variable thickness around these columns. The depth and diameter of these columns depends upon the laser device used as well as the energy and pulse width used during the procedure (Figs. 1A to C).

Table 1: Some studies on nonablative lasers in acne scars.

Laser used	*Study type*	*Results*
1,560 Erbium; Mosaic[6]	Prospective split face study on comparison between laser and CROSS technique in 20 patients	Laser gave better results in rolling scars while ice pick scars showed similar results with both
1,560 Erbium glass, Fraxel SR[18]	Prospective study in 29 patients	16% patients achieved >75% improvement while 62% showed 50–75% improvement
1,560 Erbium[32]	Prospective study in 53 cases	50–75% improvement in 90% patients after 3 sessions
1,540 Erbium, Starlux[33]	Prospective split face study	About 50% patients shoed moderate improvement

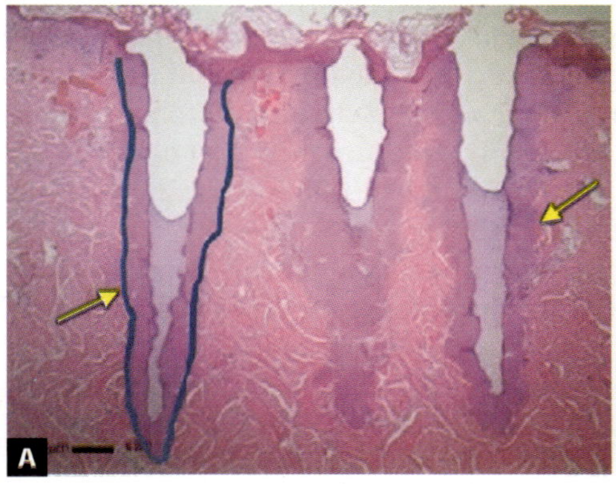

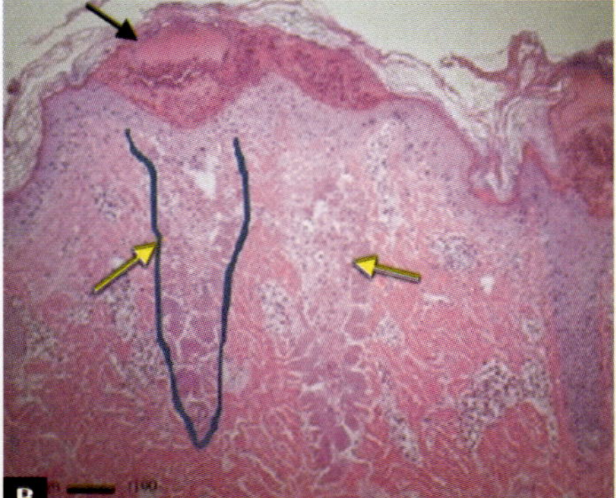

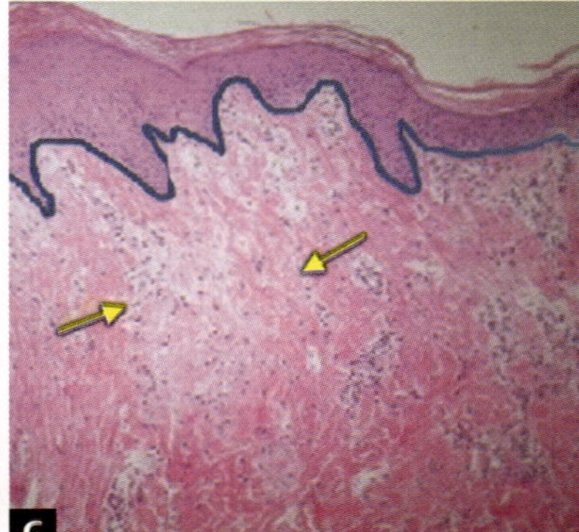

Figs. 1A to C: Histological pictures showing the longitudinal ablation and healing response with fractional CO_2 laser: (A) Immediately after; (B) Post 2 Days; (C) Post 14 days.
(*Courtesy:* Lutronics Corp)

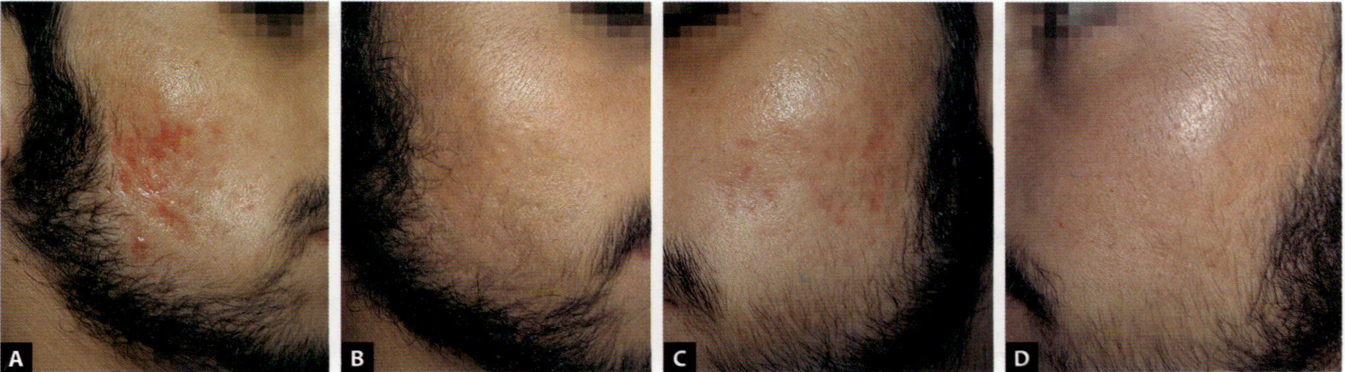

Figs. 2A to D: Predominantly rolling scars showing excellent improvement after fractional CO_2 laser resurfacing.

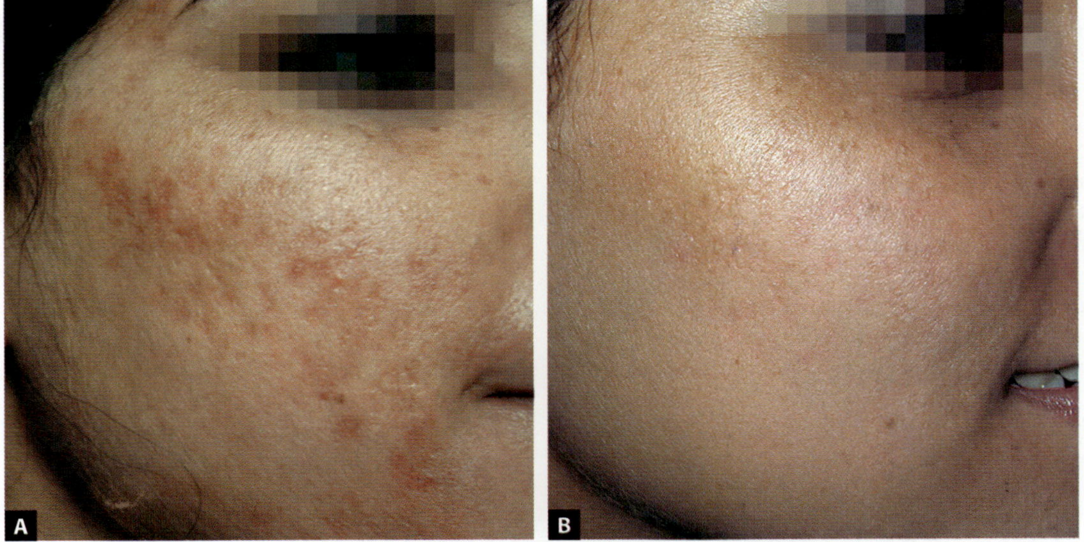

Figs. 3A and B: Early scars show better results after fractional CO_2 laser resurfacing.

Table 2: Some studies on ablative fractional lasers in acne scars.

Laser used	*Study design*	*Results*
Fractional CO_2, Ultrapulse[20]	Prospective study in 20 cases	50% patients showed >50% improvement
Fractional CO_2 Fraxel[24]	Prospective study in 16 cases	43–79.9% improvement on clinician's assessment
Fractional CO_2 Cynosure[34]	Prospective study in 15 cases	Good to excellent improvement reported by 79% patients
Erbium YAG, Pixel[35]	Prospective study in 26 patients	Mean improvement of 79% in all patients treated with 5 treatments 3 weeks apart
Fractional CO_2 Ellipse[23]	Prospective study in 13 cases	85% patients achieved 25-50% improvement
Fractional CO_2 Qray FRX[25]	Prospective study in 60 cases	Excellent improvement in 43.3% cases and good results in 25%. Rolling and superficial boxcar scars responded better and pits responded the least

The use of fractional ablative lasers in acne scars has seen an increasing trend over the last few years. The level of scar improvement achieved with these lasers has been claimed to be more than with nonablative lasers (Figs. 2 and 3). These lasers have been used in almost all races and skin types with good to excellent efficacy and a favorable adverse effect profile.

Two ablative fractional laser devices are reported to be useful in acne scars—fractional CO_2 laser and fractional Er:YAG laser (Table 2).

FRACTIONAL CO_2 LASER IN ACNE SCARS

Among all ablative and nonablative fractional lasers the one that has been the most commonly used and reported successful is the fractional CO_2 laser. A number of clinical studies have confirmed the efficacy of this laser system in acne scars.[22-25] The range of improvement reported with fractional CO_2 laser has varied from one study to another. This is mainly because of non-uniform means of assessment of treatment response. There is still a lack of reproducible objective means of assessing therapeutic response in acne scars.

STEPS OF FRACTIONAL LASER TREATMENT FOR ACNE SCARS

The procedure is done usually under the effect of topical anesthesia under occlusion. An eutectic mixture of prilocaine/tetracaine and lignocaine is commonly used and kept for 45 minutes to 1 hour.

A smoke evacuator should be available and needs to be used as it removes the viral particles along with the smoke.

A proper fluence and density settings are then selected according to the scar type and severity. Deeper scars need higher fluencies as the depth of penetration of the laser beam is directly proportional to it. It is important to treat the shoulder or margins of scars to achieve a good therapeutic benefit.

A topical non-comedogenic antibiotic cream is advised in the postoperative period. Patients with a history of herpes simplex need to be given antiviral prophylaxis 1-day prior and 5 days after the procedure. Patients are advised to avoid sun exposure after the procedure to minimize the chances of post-inflammatory hyperpigmentation. It is important to counsel the patients about the downtime. Patients do experience erythema and crusting for few days after the procedure and this may limit their social activities for these days.

COMPLICATIONS OF LASER TREATMENT FOR ACNE SCARS

Adverse effects that are reported most commonly with ablative fractional lasers are erythema and crusting that can remain for 4–7 days after treatment session. In addition patients may suffer from post-inflammatory hyperpigmentation, flaking and dryness of the skin, pruritus, bronzing of skin and aggravation of active acne.[23,24]

Among all these complications mentioned the one that is the most important in colored or darker skin is post-inflammatory hyperpigmentation and even depigmentation. To avoid this complication it is important to use lower fluences and lower MTZ densities and to avoid overlapping of laser passes over the skin. It is equally important to avoid any post-treatment sun exposure and to use sunscreens properly in the postprocedure period.

In addition, if the laser is not used cautiously and judiciously, it can also lead to prolonged erythema and edema, purpura especially if the patient is taking non-steroidal anti-inflammatory drug (NSAIDs), aggravation of scarring, painful crusting and permanent scarring and hypopigmentation (Box 2).[26,27]

Box 2: Adverse effects of fractional laser resurfacing.

- Erythema and crusting
- Post-inflammatory hyperpigmentation
- Acne flare up
- Pruritus
- Bronzing of skin
- Severe adverse effects include purpura, prolonged erythema, aggravation of scarring and hypopigmentation

COMBINATION TREATMENTS WITH LASERS IN ACNE SCARS

Fractional lasers resurfacing can be combined with other procedures to cause a synergistic effect in treating acne scars. The most popular combination treatments are TCA CROSS, medium depth peels and surgical procedures like subcision, punch elevation and punch floatation. Combination with TCA CROSS can tackle coexistent pitted scars which respond less to fractional laser treatment. Similarly subcision can be used prior to fractional laser resurfacing with significant benefit. Subcision is used to decrease the depth of deep rolling or boxcar scars and this makes them more amenable to treatment with fractional lasers.

Another popular combination treatment nowadays is platelet-rich plasma. There are few reports of successful combined use of fractional laser resurfacing with autologous platelet-rich plasma. Lastly, fractional laser treatment can be combined with autologous fat grafting or with hyaluronic acid filler injections.[28-31]

CONCLUSION

Lasers have found a permanent place in the treatment of facial acne scars. Among the nonsurgical modalities they are perhaps the most efficacious in causing scar amelioration. Among the different lasers available for this indication, fractional lasers are the ones that are the most favored as of now. However, before using any of these lasers, it is imperative to know the right laser and the right parameters for an individual patient. Using the wrong setting or the incorrect laser can harm and even disfigure the patient.

REFERENCES

1. Orentreich D, Orentreich N. Acne scar revision update. Dermatol Clin. 1987;5:359-68.
2. Goodman GJ, Baron JA. The management of post-acne scarring. Dermatol Surg. 2007;33:1175-88.
3. Goodman GJ. Management of post-acne scarring: what are the options for treatment? Am J Clin Dermatol. 2000;1:3-17.
4. Rivera AE. Acne scarring: A review and current treatment modalities. J Am Acad Dermatol. 2008;59:659-76.
5. Goel A, Krupashankar DS, Aurangabadkar S, et al. Fractional lasers in dermatology—Current status and

recommendations. Indian J Dermatol Venereol Leprol. 2011;77:369-79.
6. Kim HJ, Kim TG, Kwon YS, et al. Comparison of a 1,550 nm Erbium: Glass fractional laser and a chemical reconstruction of skin scars (CROSS) method in the treatment of acne scars: a simultaneous split-face trial. Lasers Surg Med. 2009;41:545-9.
7. Tanzi EL, Alster TS. Laser treatment of scars. Skin Therapy Lett. 2004;9:4-7.
8. Tanzi EL, Alster TS. Treatment of atrophic facial acne scars with a dual-mode Er:YAG laser. Dermatol Surg. 2002;28: 551-5.
9. Alster T, Zaulyanov L. Laser scar revision: a review. Dermatol Surg. 2007;33:131-40.
10. Paithankar DY, Ross EV, Saleh BA, et al. Acne treatment with a 1,450 nm wavelength and cryogen spray cooling. Lasers Surg Med. 2002;31:106-14.
11. Rogachefsky AS, Hussain M, Goldberg DJ. Atrophic and a mixed pattern of acne scars improved with a 1,320-nm Nd:YAG laser. Dermatol Surg. 2003;29:904-8.
12. Tanzi EL, Alster TS. Comparison of a 1,450-nm diode laser and a 1320-nm Nd:YAG laser in the treatment of atrophic facial scars: a prospective clinial and histologic study. Dermatol Surg. 2004;30:152-7.
13. Carniol PJ, Vynatheya J, Carniol E. Evaluation of acne scar treatment with a 1,450-nm midinfrared laser and 30% trichloroacetic acid peels. Arc Facial Plast Surg. 2005;7:251-5.
14. Manstein D, Herron GS, Sink RK, Tanner H, Anderson RR. Fractional photothermolysis: a new concept for cutaneous remodeling using microscopic patterns of thermal injury. Lasers Surg Med. 2004;34:426-38.
15. Khan MH, Sink RK, Manstein D, et al. Intradermally focused infrared laser pulses: thermal effects at defined tissue depths. Lasers Surg Med. 2005;36:270-80.
16. Manstein D, Herron GS, Sink RK, et al. Fractional photothermolysis: a new concept for cutaneous remodeling using microscopic patterns of thermal injury. Lasers Surg Med. 2004;34:426-38.
17. Alster TS, Tanzi EL, Lazarus M. The use of fractional laser photothermolysis for the treatment of atrophic scars. Dermatol Surg. 2007;33:295-9.
18. Chrastil B, Glaich AS, Goldberg LH, Friedman PM. Second-generation 1,550-nm fractional photothermolysis for the treatment of acne scars. Dermatol Surg. 2008;34:1327-32.
19. Rahman Z, Tanner H, Jiang K. Treatment of atrophic scars with the 1,550 nm erbium-fiber fractional laser. Lasers Surg Med. 2006;38:24.
20. Hu S, Chen MC, Lee MC, Yang LC, Keoprasom N. Fractional resurfacing for the treatment of atrophic facial acne scars in Asian skin. Dermatol Surg. 2009;35:826-32.
21. Mahmoud BH, Srivastava D, Janiga JJ, et al. Safety and efficacy of erbium-doped yttrium aluminun garnet fractionated laser for treatment of acne scars in type IV to VI skin. Dermatol Surg. 2010;36:602-9.
22. Cho SB, Lee SJ, Kang JM, et al. The efficacy and safety of 10,600-nm carbon dioxide fractional laser for acne scars in Asian patients. Dermatol Surg. 2009;35:1955-61.
23. Manuskiatti W, Triwongwaranat D, Varothai S, et al. Efficacy and safety of a carbon-dioxide ablative fractional resurfacing device for treatment of atrophic acne scars in Asians. J Am Acad Dermatol. 2010;63:247-83.
24. Chapas AM, Brightman L, Sukal S, et al. Successful treatment of acneiform scarring with CO_2 ablative fractional resurfacing. Lasers Surg Med. 2008;40:381-6.
25. Majid I, Imran S. Fractional CO_2 laser resurfacing as monotherapy in the treatment of atrophic facial acne scars. J Cutan Aesthet Surg. 2014;7(2):87.
26. Fife DJ, Zachary CB. Delayed pinpoint purpura after fractionated carbon dioxide treatment in a patient taking ibuprofen in the postoperative period. Dermatol Surg. 2009;35:553.
27. Metelista AI, Alster TS. Fractionated laser resurfacing treatment complications: a review. Dermatol Surg. 2010;36:299-306.
28. Zhu JT, Xuan M, Zhang YN, et al. The efficacy of autologous platelet-rich plasma combined with erbium fractional laser therapy for facial acne scars or acne. Molecular Medicine Reports. 2013;8(1):233-7.
29. Faghihi G, Keyvan S, Asilian A, et al. Efficacy of autologous platelet-rich plasma combined with fractional ablative carbon dioxide resurfacing laser in treatment of facial atrophic acne scars: A split-face randomized clinical trial. Indian J Dermatol Venereol Leprol. 2016;82(2):162.
30. Nofal E, Helmy A, Nofal A, et al. Platelet-rich plasma versus CROSS technique with 100% trichloroacetic acid versus combined skin needling and platelet rich plasma in the treatment of atrophic acne scars: a comparative study. Dermatologic Surgery. 2014;40(8):864-73.
31. Gawdat HI, Hegazy RA, Fawzy MM, Fathy M. Autologous platelet rich plasma: topical versus intradermal after fractional ablative carbon dioxide laser treatment of atrophic acne scars. Dermatologic Surgery. 2014;40(2): 152-61.
32. Alster TS, Tanzi EL, Lazarus E. The use of fractional laser photothermolysis for the treatment of atrophic scars. Dermatol Surg. 2007;33:295-9.
33. Hedelund L, Moreau KER, Boyer D, et al. Fractional nonablative laser resurfacing for atrophic acne scars. A renomized controlled trial with blinded response evaluation. Lasers Med Sci. 2010;25:749-54.
34. Katz B. Efficacy of a new fractional CO_2 laser in the treatment of photodamage and acne scarring. Dermatol Ther. 2010;23:403-06.
35. Deng H, Yuan D, Yan C, et al. A 2940-nm fractional photothermolysis laser in the treatment of acne scarring: a pilot study in China. J Drugs Dermatol. 2009;8:978-80.

Chapter

48

Approach to Management of Post-acne Scars

BS Chandrashekar, Mysore Venkataram

Key Messages 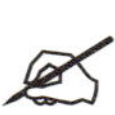

- Combination of different treatments are needed for management of different types of acne scars.
- Fractional lasers represent a major advance in the management of acne scars.
- Scarring and delayed wound healing was described earlier in patients undergoing laser procedures when on isotretinoin, but now there are studies suggesting the contrary.
- Postinflammatory hyperpigmentation remains the biggest challenge faced during interventions for acne scar and proper counselling is important.
- Newer technologies like Microneedling Radiofrequency and Tixel® have shown promising results in the management of acne scars.

INTRODUCTION

The management techniques of post-acne scars have greatly improved with introduction of new treatments such as fractional lasers. It is now possible to manage even severe scars, with far better results than ever possible before, with minimal side effects and healing time. Added to this, early management with isotretinoin has resulted in better medical management for prevention of scars. This has led to greater patient satisfaction, but also enhanced expectations. The previous three Chapters have dealt with different aspects of acne scar surgery—including classification and pathophysiology, different surgical techniques and lasers. This Chapter deals with a summary of approach to management of acne scars. The reader is also referred to the guidelines of care for acne scars by the taskforce on dermatosurgery, Indian Association of Dermatologists, Venereologists and Leprologists.[1]

PRETREATMENT CONSIDERATIONS

It is important to understand that the management of acne scars is time-consuming and any improvement seen occurs gradually. A combination of medical and surgical approaches is needed, with frequent visits to the clinic, over several months. Further, as in any treatments on the face, adverse effects are not acceptable to patients and leads to patient dissatisfaction. It is therefore important to establish an open, free communication and good rapport with patients, to gain their trust and confidence.

Counselling should include frank and free discussion of all aspects of the treatments such as time taken, number of sessions, outcomes expected, post-treatment course and care, downtime and discomfort, pre and post-treatment conditioning regimens. An effort should be made to understand patients' expectations, pain threshold and work schedules. Informed consent is mandatory and so are pre and post-treatment photographs. Often the improvement is gradual, and patients may express disappointment at the lack of improvements. Photographs are of great help in such cases. It is important for the patients to have realistic expectations as in all aesthetic treatments, particularly in management of scars. Patients have to be counselled that despite recent advances, severe scarring remains a difficult challenge to manage.

Examination of skin should include an assessment of scars, type, extent, tendency for pigmentation and keloid formation. Table 1 shows the summary of techniques for different grades of post-acne scarring. Table 2 summarizes the treatment for each type of scar (Fig. 1).

Flowcharts 1 to 3 summarizes a stepwise approach to management of different types of scars.

Table 1: Summary of treatment modalities for different grades of post-acne scarring.

Grades of post-acne scarring	*Level of disease*	*Treatment modalities*
1	Macular ▪ Erythematous ▪ Hyperpigmented ▪ Hypopigmented	 IPL, vascular lasers Hydroquinone, topical retinoids, azelaic, kojic acids, microdermabrasion,[2] salicylic acid and glycolic peels[3,4] Spot dermabrasion, epidermal—melanocyte cell suspension
2	Mild	Microdermabrasion, chemical peels, microneedling, nonablative lasers
3	Moderate	▪ Subcision ▪ Scar revisions ▪ Medium depth peels ▪ TCA CROSS[5] ▪ Fractional lasers—Erbium: YAG, CO_2, Erbium glass ▪ Intralesional steroid/cytotoxic therapy for hypertrophic scars[6]
4	Severe	▪ Combination of all the above treatments ▪ Fat injections ▪ Dermabrasion ▪ Ablative lasers ▪ Microneedling radio frequency ▪ Tixel®

Note: that the recommendations in the table are not absolute and variations can exist dependingon the preference of the physician and needs of the patient (IPL: Intense pulsed laser; TCA CROSS: Chemical reconstruction of skin scars using trichloroacetic acid).

Table 2: Summary of treatment procedures for different types of scars.

Type of scar	*Treatment options*	*Comment*
Erythematous macule	IPL, vascular lasers	Often persists for a long time
Hyperpigmented macule	Hydroquinone, topical retinoids, azelaic, kojic acids, salicylic acid (Fig. 2) and glycolic peels, microdermabrasion (Fig. 3)	Determine tendency for pigmentation before choosing treatment option. Prior priming with depigmenting agents is necessary
Hypopigmented macule	Spot dermabrasion, epidermal—melanocyte cell suspension	Not common in Indian skin
Ice pick scars	TCA CROSS (<1.5 mm) (Fig. 4) excision and suturing (> 1.5 mm) fractional lasers	TCA CROSS is the preferred treatment of choice; counsel about mild postinflammatory pigmentation
Punched out round scars (Boxcar scars)	Round scars—punch techniques—elevation if overlying skin is normal; excision and suturing/grafting if abnormal Irregular scars—fractional lasers, scar revisions	Proper patient counseling is important Fractional lasers can provide modest improvement
Boat-shaped, rolling scars	Subcision, dermaroller fractional lasers (Fig. 5)	Subcision is an underused technique—yields satisfactory results if done properly
Depressed scars	Fillers, dermal graft, fat injection dermaroller (Fig. 6)	In selected cases only
Hypertrophic scars	Silicone sheets, intralesional injections of steroids, radiofrequency debulking (Fig. 7), ablative lasers, dermabrasion	Multiple sessions needed; postoperative pigmentation and scarring are frequent
Scars aggravated by muscle action	Botulinum toxin	

(IPL: Intense pulsed laser; TCA CROSS: Chemical reconstruction of skin scars using trichloroacetic acid).

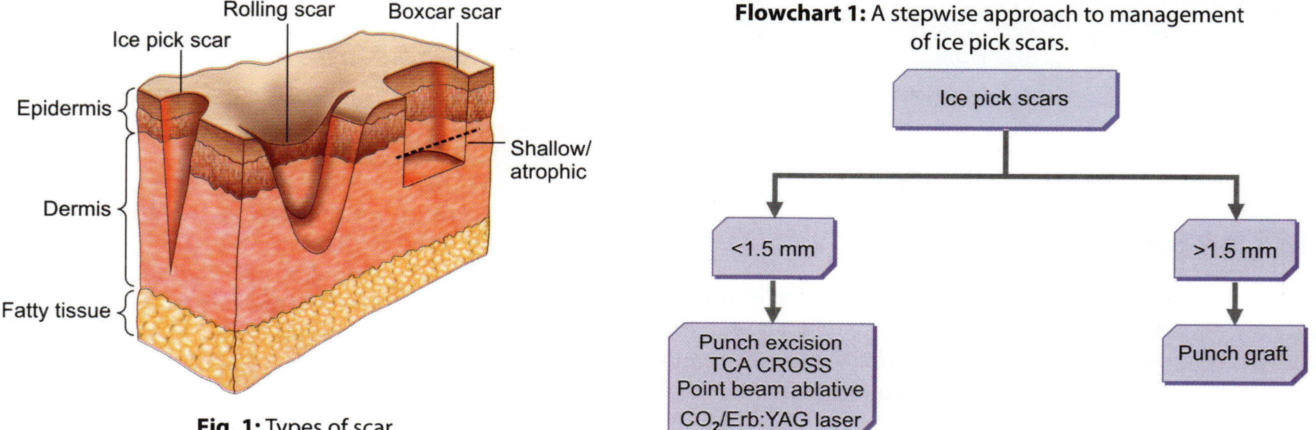

Fig. 1: Types of scar.

Flowchart 1: A stepwise approach to management of ice pick scars.

Flowchart 2: A stepwise approach to management of boxcar scars.

Flowchart 3: A stepwise approach to management of shallow/ atrophic and valley scars.

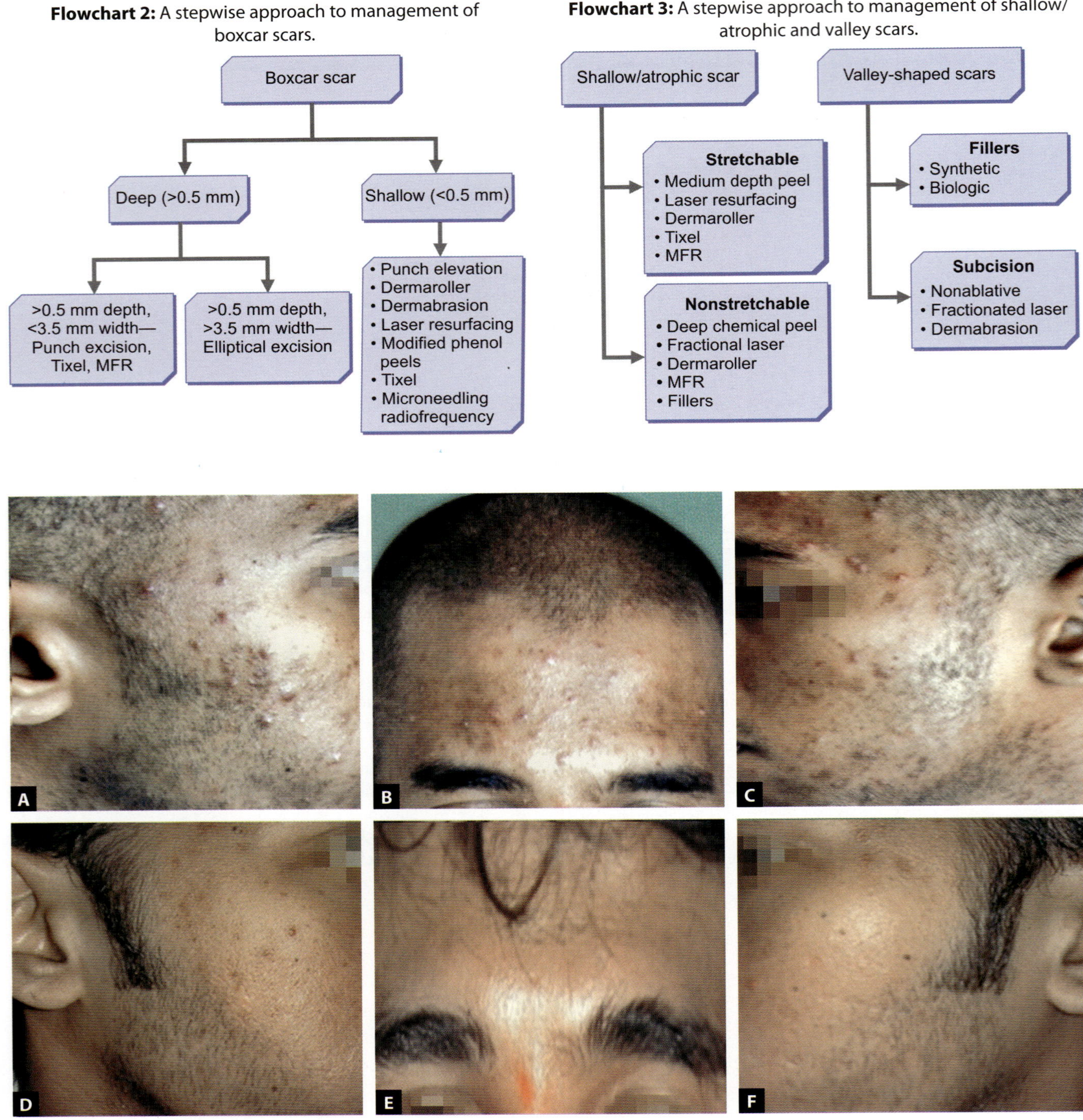

Figs. 2A to F: Hyperpigmented scars treated with retinoic acid and glycolic acid.

ISOTRETINOIN AND ACNE SCAR MANAGEMENT

It is an established fact that the advent of isotretinoin has greatly enhanced the management of acne vulgaris, even the most severe variants. However, the subject of use of different resurfacing techniques in patients treated with the drug has remained a matter of debate. It is generally agreed that care should be exercised in patients with a history of recent isotretinoin use as the drug may lead to delay in healing and atypical scar formation. A 6–12-month waiting period following discontinuation of isotretinoin has been recommended before performing resurfacing procedures.[7] This recommendation is based on earlier reports of keloid formation and atypical scar formation after use of dermabrasion and argon lasers, which are invasive and ablative procedures.[8-11] However, several

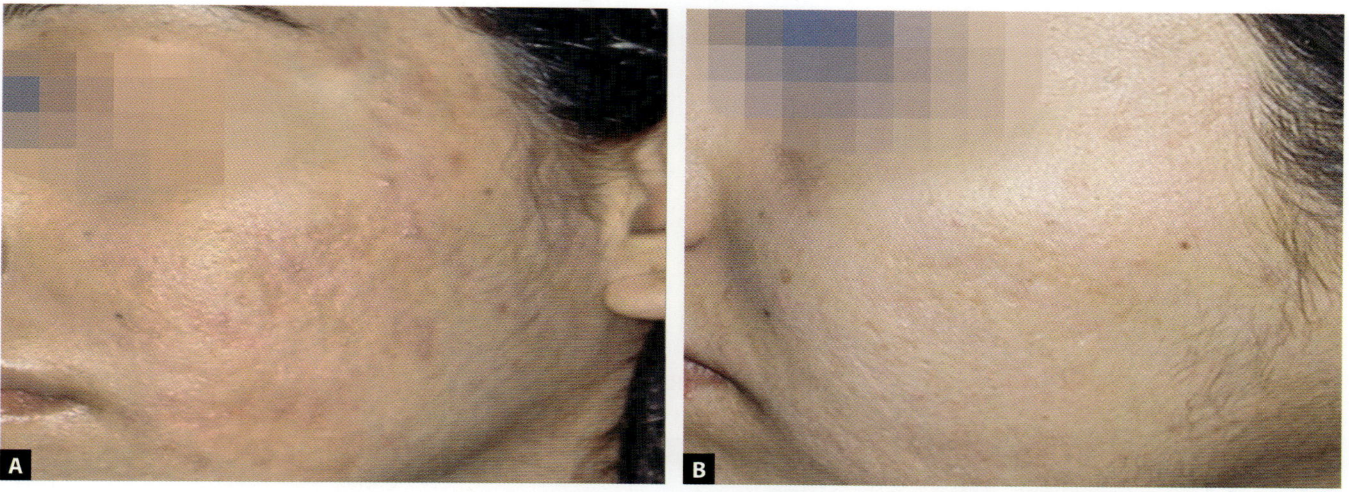

Figs. 3A and B: Microdermabrasion for mild scarring; (A) before and (B) after.

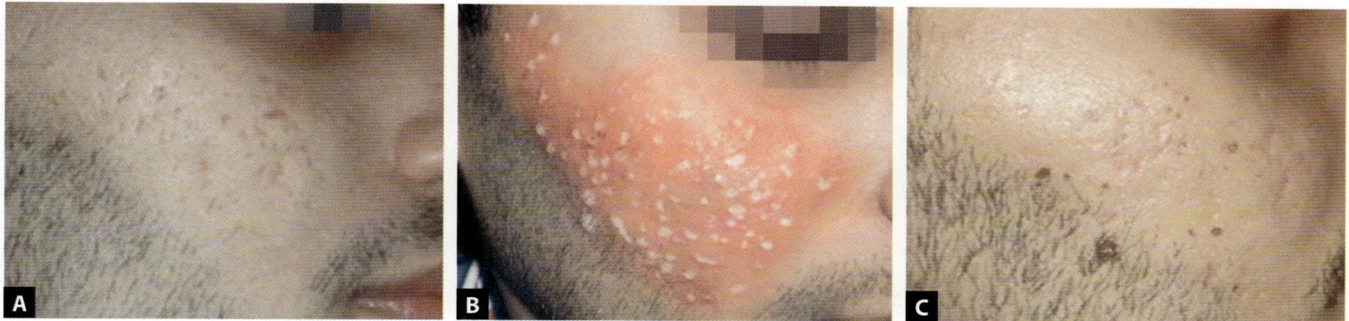

Figs. 4A to C: TCA CROSS for ice pick scars, (A) before, (B) immediately after TCA CROSS and (C) final results.

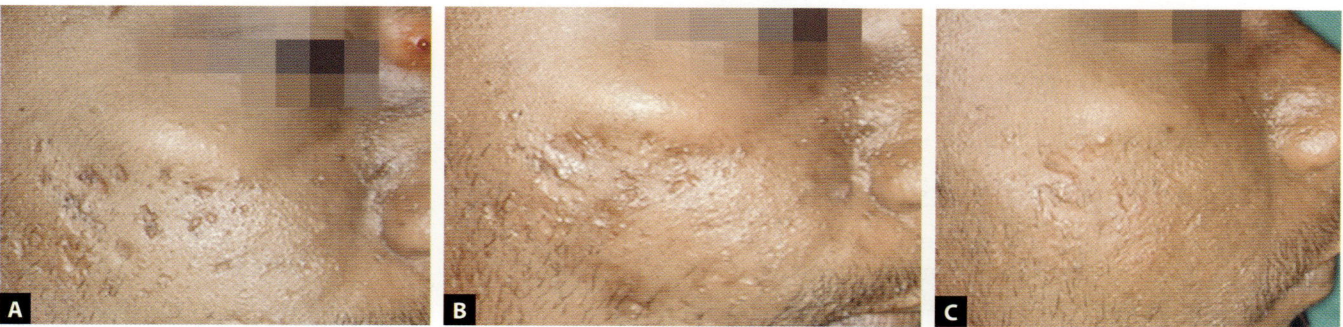

Figs. 5A to C: Fractional Erbium:YAG laser—six sessions; before and after.

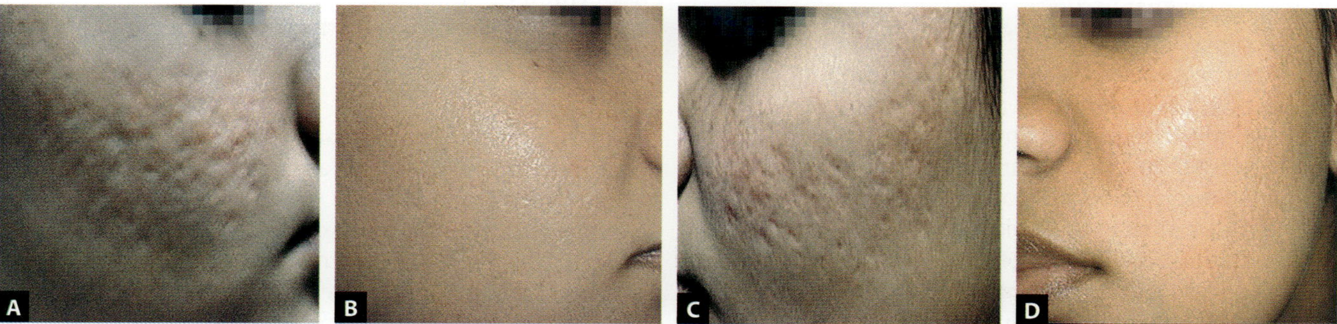

Figs. 6A to D: Microneedling for boxcar scars before (A and C) and after treatment (B and D).

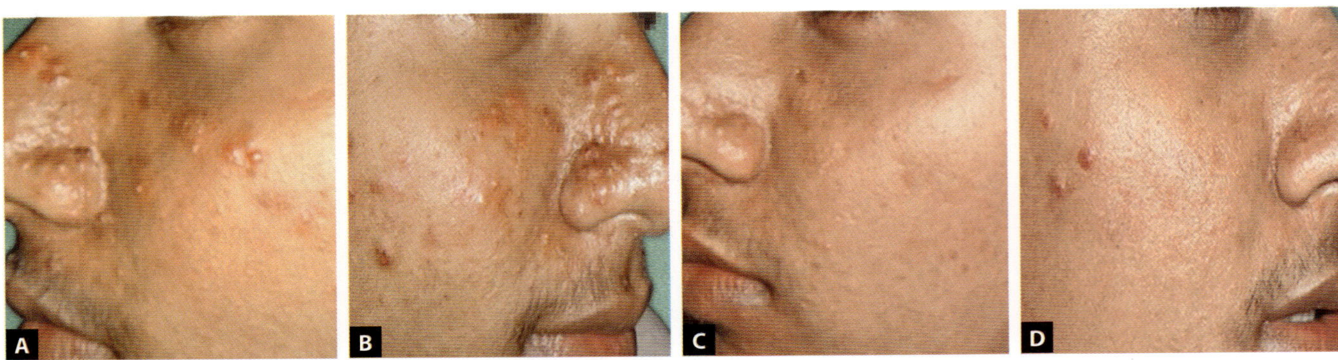

Figs. 7A to D: Radio debulking.

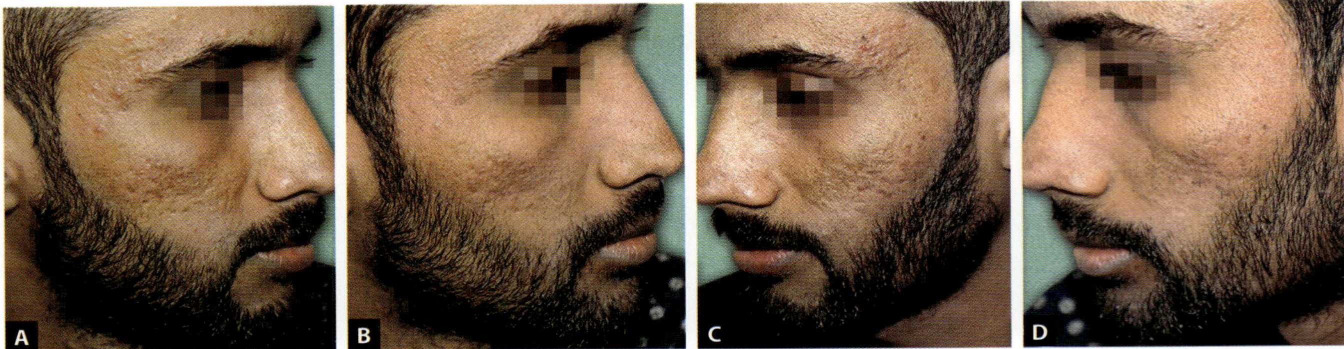

Figs. 8A to D: Boxscars and rolling scars treated with microneedling radiofrequency.

recent publications have documented the safety of different procedures such as laser hair removal and dermabrasion in patients recently treated with isotretinoin.[12-19] This subject has been dealt with in greater detail in the Chapter on safety of procedures in patients on isotretinoin.

NEWER TECHNOLOGIES IN ACNE SCAR MANAGEMENT

Microneedling Radiofrequency

Microneedling radiofrequency system is a novel fractional resurfacing technique for the treatment of acne scars (Figs. 8A to D). It creates controlled thermal damage in the dermis and stimulates wound-healing response thus initiating a collagen remodeling process by using thermal production from tissue impedance and subsequent heat diffusion to deeper tissue.

The procedure is repeated 4 to 6 times with an interval of 6 weeks between each session, since the time for collagen remodeling lasts around 4–6 weeks. The treatment regimens can be changed depending on the scar type. Needle depths range from 0.5 mm to 3.5 mm, and is modified depending on the anatomical site and pass number. Power levels are adjusted according to the needle depth and site. Exposure times range from 10 ms to 1000 ms.

The advantages of fractional radiofrequency include, less epidermal disruption by only 5%, compared with 10–70% of that of fractional ablative laser systems,[20] faster healing process, lesser incidence of postinflammatory hyperpigmentation in darker skin tones, minimal downtime and control over the depth of treatment.[21]

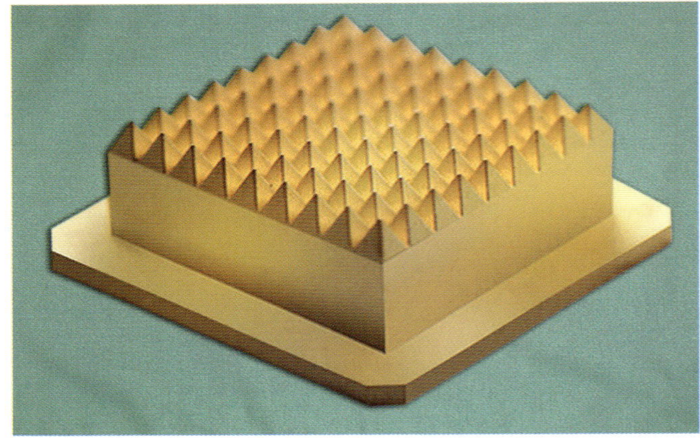

Fig. 9: Tixel® tip.

Tixel®

Tixel® is a nonlaser fractional treatment device based on thermomechanical ablation technology similar in effectiveness to fractional CO_2 laser treatment. The energy is emitted through a matrix of 81 tiny pyramid-shaped pins (Fig. 9) made of biocompatible materials covering a treatment area of 1 cm², heated to a temperature of 400°C.[22] During treatment, the pins are introduced to the surface of the skin at a precisely controlled speed, after which the

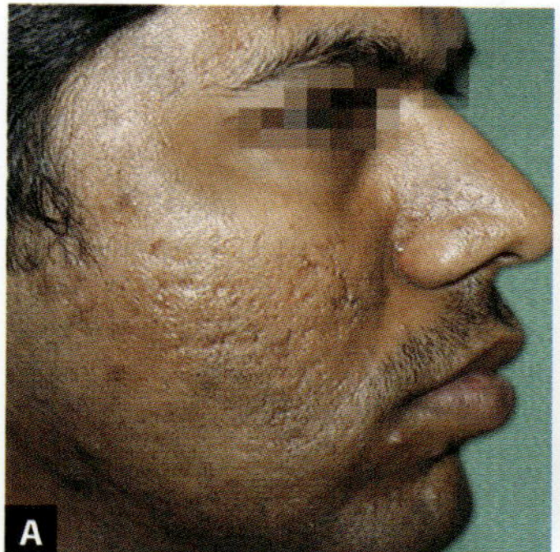

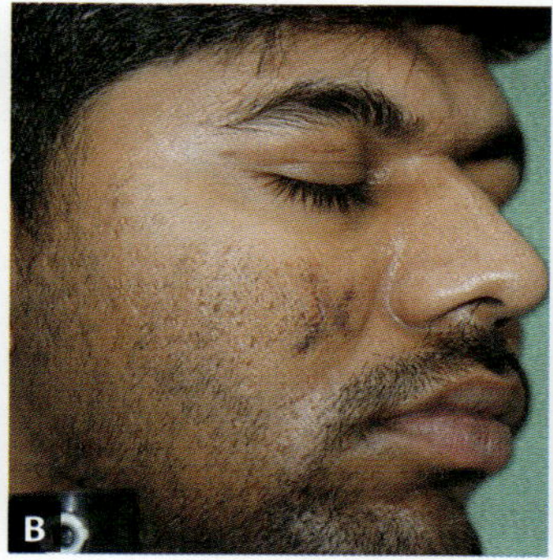

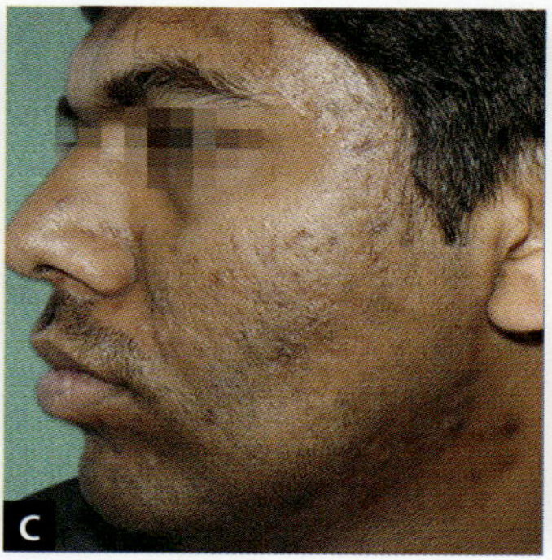

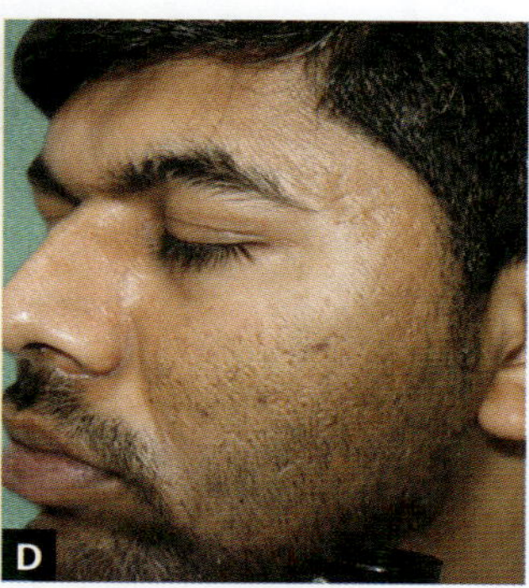

Figs. 10A to C: Acne scars treated with Tixel®.

thermal energy stored in the pins is rapidly transferred upon brief contact with the skin. The ensuing evaporation of water from the skin occurs instantaneously, resulting in the formation of tiny craters in the treatment zone.

The parameters for treatment are changed according to the severity of acne scars (Fig. 10). Treatment sessions are spaced 1 month apart, and 3–5 sessions are advised. The extent of thermal damage is closely related to the pulse duration and the type of tip. Longer pulses create a larger crater diameter and deeper thermal damage while shorter pulses create permeable channels for transdermal transfer of drugs. Exposure time (pulse duration) ranges from 5 to 18 milliseconds. Pulse protrusion is the distance that the pyramid's distal section extends beyond the distance gauge surface and it ranges from 100 to 700 μm with a micropore width of 170 μm.

In contrast to thermal damage created by CO_2 lasers, histopathologic studies have shown that Tixel® has extremely high control over the diameter and depth of craters, which are as deep as CO_2, but narrower. There is less charring and crusting, safe to use with darker skin tones, lesser pain without anesthesia or cooling, absence of fumes during the procedure and less downtime and post care.

SUMMARY

The patient's quest for the treatment of acne scars begins even before the treatment of acne. With the ever evolving research, better technologies with greater safety profile are getting developed. Till the ideal technology for acne scars is perfected, the treatment has to be tailored for each patient according to their type of scars.

REFERENCES

1. Khunger N. Standard guidelines of care for acne surgery. IJDVL. 2008;74:S28-36.
2. Alkhawam L, Alam M. Dermabrasion and microdermabrasion. Facial Plast Surg. 2009;25:301-10.
3. Landau M. Chemical peels. ClinDermatol. 2008;26:200-8.
4. Fabbrocini G, De Padova MP, Tosti A. Chemical peels: what's new and what isn't new but still works well. Facial Plast Surg. 2009;25:329-36.
5. Fabbrocini G, Cacciapuoti S, Fardella N, et al. CROSS technique: chemical reconstruction of skin scars method. DermatolTher. 2008;21:S29-S32.
6. Manuskiatti W, Wanitphakdeedecha R, Fitzpatrick RE. Effect of pulse width of a 595-nm flashlamp-pumped pulsed dyelaser on the treatment response of keloidal and hypertrophicsternotomy scars. Dermatol Surg. 2007;33:152-61.
7. Rivera AE. Acne scarring: A review and current treatment modalities. J Am Acad Dermatol. 2008;59:659-76.
8. Dogan G. Possible isotretinoin-induced keloids in a patient with Behçet's disease. Clin Exp Dermatol. 2006;31:535-7.
9. Rubenstein R, Roenigk HH Jr, Stegman SJ, et al. A typical keloids after dermabrasion of patients taking isotretinoin. J Am Acad Dermatol. 1986;15:280-5.
10. Katz BE, Mac Farlane DF. Atypical facial scarring after isotretinoin therapy in a patient with previous dermabrasion. J Am Acad Dermatol. 1994;30:852-3.
11. Peteiro C, Toribio J. Keloid formation induced by isotretinoin therapy. Int J Dermatol. 1999;38:228-9.
12. Cassano N, Arpaia N, Vena GA. Diode laser hair removal andisotretinoin therapy. Dermatol Surg. 2005;31:380-1.
13. Khatri KA, Garcia V. Light-assisted hair removal in patients undergoing isotretinoin therapy. Dermatol Surg. 2006;32:875-7.
14. Khatri KA. Diode laser hair removal in patients undergoing isotretinoin therapy. Dermatol Surg. 2004;30:1205-7.
15. Khatri KA. The safety of long-pulsed Nd:YAG laser hair removal in skin types III-V patients during concomitanti sotretinoin therapy. J Cosmet Laser Ther. 2009;11:56-60.
16. Roenigk HH Jr, Pinski JB, Robinson JK, et al. Acne, retinoids,and dermabrasion. J Dermatol Surg Oncol. 1985;11:396-8.
17. Bagatin E, Guadanhim LR, Yarak S, et al. Dermabrasion for acne scars during treatment with oral isotretinoin. Dermatol Surg. 2010;36:483-9.
18. Chandrashekar BS, Varsha DV, Vasanth V, et al. Safety of performing invasive acne scar treatment and laser hair removal in patients on oral isotretinoin: a retrospective study of 110 patients. Int J Dermatol. 2014;53:1281-5. doi:10.1111/ijd.12544
19. Mahadevappa OH, et al. Surgical outcome in patients taking concomitant or recent intake of oral isotretinoin:A multicentric study-ISO-AIMS study. Journal of Cutaneous and Aesthetic Surgery. 2016;9(2):106-14.
20. Hruza G, Taub AF, Collier SL, Mulholland SR. Skin rejuvenation and wrinkle reduction using a fractional radiofrequency system. J Drugs Dermatol. 2009;8(3):259-65.
21. Chandrashekar BS, Sriram R, Mysore R, et al. Evaluation of microneedling fractional radiofrequency device for treatment of acne scars. J Cutan Aesthet Surg. 2014;7(2):93-7.
22. Elman M, Fournier N, Barnéon G, et al. Fractional treatment of aging skin with Tixel, a clinical and histological evaluation. J Cosmet Laser Ther. 2016;18(1):31-7.

Chapter 49

Mohs Micrographic Surgery

Nicholas Collier,
Venura Samarasinghe, Vishal Madan

Key Messages

- The Mohs micrographic surgery (MMS) procedure allows histological verification of tumor clearance prior to wound closure. This treatment offers unsurpassed cure rates along with maximal conservation of adjacent healthy skin, thus reducing morbidity and mortality.
- MMS is a specialized procedure, to treat selected cutaneous tumors.
- MMS is most commonly used in the treatment of basal cell carcinomas on the face, squamous cell carcinoma. It is also used to treat squamous cell carcinoma, lentigo maligna and a number of rare aggressive cutaneous tumor types.
- Limitations of use of MMS include the time and cost of the surgeon and technician and the cost of specialized equipment such as the cryostat.

INTRODUCTION

Conventional surgery involves excision of a tumor with a preselected wide margin of normal skin and then processing of the pathology specimen in vertical sections at 2–4 mm intervals, akin to a 'bread loaf' series of sections through the tumor. Less than 1% of the tumor margin is examined in this method of sampling and thus there is a possibility of the tumor being present at sites not sectioned during processing. Histopathology reports from this method of sectioning will commonly state that 'the tumor *appears* excised from the levels viewed'.

MMS is a specialized method of skin cancer removal allowing unparalleled clearance rates and maximal preservation of healthy skin. The initial stage involves the removal of the tumor with a narrow margin of clinically normal skin. This layer of skin is marked to allow orientation, flattened, frozen and sectioned horizontally to ensure visualization of the complete peripheral and deep margins. Intraoperative microscopic examination is performed with areas of residual tumor carefully marked and layers of skin adjacent to the involved margins removed. This process continues until complete tumor clearance is assured.

Thus, MMS offers a higher cure rate than standard surgery for skin cancer treatment, reducing the morbidity and mortality from future recurrence, and simultaneously allowing maximal conservation of adjacent healthy skin. This is especially important when managing reconstructions in the cosmetically and functionally sensitive sites of the face.

HISTORY

In the mid-1930s, when working as a cancer research assistant during medical school, Frederick Mohs observed that injection of 20% solution of zinc chloride induced in situ tissue fixation, preserving the cells for microscopic examination. From this finding, Mohs developed a process of fixing tissue using zinc chloride in vivo and excising the tumor in horizontal layers under microscopic control until complete clearance had been achieved.[1]

The new technique, called chemosurgery, was first reported by Mohs in 1941.[2] The main complication of chemosurgery was the use of zinc chloride as the in vivo tumor fixative as it caused significant pain and tissue irritation. From 1953, zinc chloride fixation was replaced by the production of fresh frozen tissue sections for the microscopic examination. This allowed multiple stages to be completed in a single day and averted tissue irritation to permit immediate repair of the wound.

In 1969, using his technique, Mohs reported 66 basal cell carcinomas (BCC) and 4 squamous cell carcinomas (SCC) with 100% 5-year cure rate.[3] In 1974, Tromovitch and

Stegman presented a further series of patients managed to further acclaim.[4,5] Subsequently, the technique was renamed Mohs micrographic surgery (MMS) and has become the treatment of choice in high risk, large, contiguous skin tumors especially over critical anatomical sites of the head and neck.

INDICATIONS

MMS has been widely reported to provide greater cure rates in multiple cutaneous tumors in comparison to all other treatment modalities. In general, large tumors critical site tumors requiring greatest tissue conservation, locally aggressive tumors and recurrent tumors are best treated by MMS.

Table 1 provides a list of some cutaneous malignancies managed by MMS.[6-8] Some of the more common indications for MMS are discussed in further detail.

BASAL CELL CARCINOMA

Basal cell carcinoma is the most common skin cancer worldwide and also the most common indication for MMS. The main sub-types of BCC are nodular, superficial and infiltrative.[9] Rarer subtypes include cystic, morphoeic and basosquamous. Subtypes may co-exist, forming a mixed pattern and having pigmented variants. The histopathological findings are dependent on the subtype but are characterized by palisading basaloid cells connected to the epidermis with retraction artefact on hematoxylin and eosin staining. High-risk BCCs are optimally treated by MMS. Features compatible with high-risk BCC are listed in Table 2.[10] Rowe et al. published a review of all BCC studies published since 1947.[11] The group found a recurrence rate of 10.1% at 5 year follow-up for standard excision (SE) compared to 1% for MMS at 5-year follow-up. Results were even more striking for recurrent BCC (rBCC). MMS provides recurrence rates of 5.6% at 5 years for rBCC in comparison to 17.4% at 5 years for SE.[11]

Table 1: Cutaneous tumors treated with Mohs surgery.

Basal cell carcinoma	***Squamous cell carcinoma***
Dermatofibrosarcoma protuberans	Leiomyosarcoma
Microcystic adnexal carcinoma	Atypical fibroxanthoma
Extramammary Paget's disease	Melanoma
Sebaceous carcinoma	Adenoid cystic carcinoma
Bowen's disease	

Table 2: High-risk BCC.

Large size >2 cm	***Recurrent BCC***
Morphoeic or micronodular subtype	Perineural/perivascular invasion
H-zone of face	

Malhotra et al. performed a retrospective analysis for periocular BCC utilizing data from the Australian Mohs database. Of 1,295 patients treated with MMS, 5-year recurrence rates were found to be 0% for primary tumors and 7.8% for rBCC.[12] Treatment of periorbital BCC is particularly important as recurrences may be associated with orbital invasion and if extensive, may even require orbital exenteration.

A Dutch randomized clinical trial comparing MMS and surgical excision (SE) for the treatment of facial BCCs demonstrated a trend towards lower recurrence rates of SE (4.1%) in comparison to MMS (2.1%) for primary facial BCC at 5 year follow-up ($p = 0.23$).[13] The 10 year-follow-up results were published in 2014.[14] Recurrence rates for primary and recurrent BCC treated by MMS and surgical excision were 4.4% vs 12.2% ($p = 0.1$) for primary lesions and 3.9% vs 13.5% ($p = 0.02$) for recurrent lesions. It was noted that a substantial number of primary (56%) and recurrent (14%) BCCs were found to recur more than 5 years after treatment.

Squamous Cell Carcinoma

Squamous cell carcinoma usually present as enlarging red or skin-colored keratotic, papules, nodules or plaques, which may be ulcerated, tender and bleeding. Cutaneous SCC most often develops over chronically, actinically damaged skin on the head, neck and other photoexposed sites.

The typical histological findings are malignant keratinocytes invading into the dermis and are described in further detail in various dermatopathology books. Mortality from SCC occurs predominantly within a high-risk subgroup of patients. This high-risk subgroup can be identified from factors listed in Table 3.[15]

For primary cutaneous SCC, a retrospective review of all studies found MMS to provide an overall cure rate of 97% at 5 years. When the data were further analyzed, the following cure rates of MMS compared to SE were found respectively: 96.9% versus 89.1% (lip), 94.7% versus 81.3% (ear), 74.8% versus 59.3% (size over 2 cm), 67.4% versus 46.4% (poorly differentiated histologic subtype) and 90% versus 77.7% (recurrent SCC).[16]

Leibovitch et al. undertook a prospective study of 5- year survival rates for 1,263 patients treated with MMS for cutaneous SCC from 1993 to 2002. 5-year cure rates were 97.4% in patients presenting with primary SCC and 94.1% for patients presenting with recurrent SCC.[17] For organ transplant recipients, subclinical invasion of SCC can

Table 3: Factors indicating high-risk SCC.

Tumor size over 2 cm	***Tumor depth >4 mm***
Moderate, poorly differentiated SCC	Ear, lip, hand, genital anatomic location
Perineural or perivascular invasion	Recurrent SCC
SCC arising from scars or chronic ulcers	SCC arising in immunosuppressed patients

occur up to 6 mm wide of the macroscopic tumor margins and often the SCC is biologically more aggressive.[18] MMS would be indicated in these high-risk patients.

Dermatofibrosarcoma Protuberans

Dermatofibrosarcoma protuberans (DFSP) is a slow-growing cutaneous fibrohistiocytic malignancy. Extensive subclinical invasion often occurs, contributing to the high recurrence rates after standard excision. DFSP usually presents as an asymptomatic purplish-red nodule or plaque. Areas of induration, telangiectasia or atrophy may be present. Approximately 10% of DFSP transform into a high-grade sarcoma variant. Histological examination shows monomorphic spindle-shaped cells forming a cartwheel arrangement. The deeply-invading tumor cells create a honeycomb appearance and stain positive for CD34 and negative for factor XHIa.[19]

Paradisi et al. carried out a retrospective review of all published reports of DFSP treated with MMS versus standard excision. The pooled data for MMS revealed that out of 463 patients, 6 tumors recurred [1.3%, confidence interval (Cl) 4.4%–28.1%] compared with 288 recurrences from 1,394 patients treated with SE (20.7%, 95% Cl 18.6%–22.9%). DFSP treated with SE were 16 times more likely to recur than those treated with MMS.[20]

A recent large single center retrospective review of 158 patients with dermatofibrosarcoma treated by MMS (67) and wide local excision (91) demonstrated substantially lower recurrence rates with MMS (30.8% vs 3.0% $p < 0.001$). Additionally, the mean defects were smaller with MMS (10.7 cm vs 8.8 cm p = 0.004).[21]

Microcystic Adnexal Carcinoma

Microcystic adnexal carcinoma (MAC) is a locally aggressive cutaneous malignancy with follicular and sweat gland differentiation. MAC presents as a smooth skin-colored or yellowish slow-growing indurated plaque or cystic nodule usually located on the central face. Clinical differential diagnoses include benign adnexal tumors (e.g. trichoepithelioma, trichoadenoma, syringoma), morphoeic BCC and SCC. Histological examination reveals the presence of islands of cells forming pilar and gland-like structures, with keratin cysts and a desmoplastic stroma. Perineural and muscular invasion help to differentiate MAC from syringomas histologically. Immunohistochemistry with carcinoembryonic antigen (CEA), epithelial membrane antigen (EMA) and cytokeratin may help with histological diagnosis.[22]

A retrospective review of 44 patients with MAC was performed using data in the Australian Mohs database over a 9-year period. Perineural invasion occurred in 18% of the cases and 32% of the cases were recurrences from other treatment modalities. The 5-year cure rates with MMS were found to be 5%.[23] In comparison, SE had a reported recurrence rate of at least 30%. Defects managed by MMS have clinical margins four times larger than predicted, highlighting the invasive nature of the neoplasm and importance of microscopic margin control.[24]

Leiomyosarcoma

Primary LMS is a rare mesenchymal malignancy arising from smooth muscle and occurs in cutaneous and subcutaneous forms. The cutaneous type develops from hair follicle arrector pili muscles and the subcutaneous type from the smooth muscles of the blood vessel vasculature. Secondary LMS arise from visceral metastasis. LMSs typically present as red or light brown nodules which may ulcerate. Histology classically shows dermal spindle-shaped cells with blunt-ended nuclei, and are actin and vimentin positive.[25]

Standard excision has a reported recurrence rate of 30–45%. Humphreys et al reviewed 15 cases of LMS treated with MMS in the literature and found the overall recurrence rate to be 13%.[26] Subsequently, Starling and Coldiron reported a further 11 patients treated over a 16- year period by MMS. The average defect size was 15.0cm^2 and recurrence rates were 0% at 4.5 years.[27]

Atypical Fibroxanthoma

Atypical fibroxanthoma (AFX) is a fibrohistiocytic tumor usually developing over sun-exposed areas in elderly men and presents as a rapidly enlarging pink, red or brown nodule, often with ulceration. Histological examination reveals atypical spindle cells and epithelioid fibrohistiocytic cells, often with multinucleated giant cells. Immunohistochemistry is positive for actin and vimentin. These features may be indistinct from those of undifferentiated pleomorphic sarcoma (UPS) and some authors believe AFX to be a superficial variant of UPS.[28]

Ang et al. reviewed 88 cases of AFX treated at the Mayo clinic over a 24-year period. 23 cases were treated with standard excision and 59 cases were treated with MMS. Recurrence rates for SE were 8.7% with median follow-up of 8.7 years in comparison to 0% for MMS at median follow-up of 4.5 years.[29]

Porocarcinoma

Porocarcinomas are malignant tumors which develop from the eccrine duct and acrosyringium. They are estimated to account for between 1 in 10,000 and 1 in 20,000 cutaneous cancers.[30] Porocarcinomas present as firm, erythematous to violaceous nodules, usually less than 2 cm in diameter. They can develop from an existing poroma or arise de novo. Whilst they can affect a wide age range, they predominately affect patients between 60 to 80 years of age.[31] Lesions occur most commonly on the lower leg but unlike poromas, are not common on the acral skin.[32]

Wide local excision was historically the treatment of choice, however recurrence rates affected approximately

20%, with distant metastases in 10% and mortality rates of 5–10%.[33,34] A recent review from the Mayo clinic included 9 cases with a mean follow-up period of 3.3 years, and demonstrating no recurrence or disease-related mortality.[35]

Extramammary Paget's Disease

Primary cutaneous extramammary Paget's disease (EMPD) is an adenocarcinoma originating most likely from apocrine glands or epidermal stem cells. Secondary EMPD is associated with an underlying adnexal carcinoma or a regional visceral carcinoma, usually rectum, bladder, urethra, cervix, prostate or vulva. Clinical presentation is of scaly or macerated plaques, with indistinct margins most commonly over genital skin. Histology shows Paget cells which are large round cells with big nucleoli. EMPD cells have high mucopolysaccharide levels, staining positive for periodic acid-Schiff and Alcian blue at pH 2.5.[36]

Lee et al. reviewed 35 Korean patients with EMPD over a 10-year period. Recurrence rates at mean 5.3-year follow-up were 36.4% with SE in comparison with 18.2% for MMS.[37]

Hendi et al. performed a literature review for recurrence rates after MMS in comparison to other modalities. Results showed a 5-year cure rate of 80% with MMS for primary EMPD and 56% for recurrent EMPD in comparison to other treatment modalities with a 33–60% 5 year cure rate. The group recommended that if SE is performed, 5 cm wide margins would be required to clear 97% of all tumors.[38]

Lentigo Maligna Melanoma

Melanoma usually presents as a changing pigmented lesion, which, dependent on Breslow thickness, is associated with a substantial risk of local, regional and distant metastasis. Subtypes include superficial spreading, nodular, lentigo maligna melanoma (LMM) and acral lentiginous melanoma. Histopathology is characterized by invasive melanocytes, and may pose a significant diagnostic challenge for a pathologist.[39-41] SE involves 5 mm clinical margins of normal skin for LM, and 10 mm margins for thin melanoma of less than 1.0 mm Breslow thickness. The adequacy of 5 mm margins to consistently achieve clearance of insitu melanoma has been questioned.[42]

Zitelli et al. reported on 625 consecutive patients diagnosed with melanoma of the head and neck region. Margins of 9 mm were required to remove 98.5% of insitu lesions, whilst 12 mm margins removed 96.6% of melanomas of Breslow thickness 2.01–4.00. Patients had a mean follow-up of 4.8 years. 5-year survival results compared favorably with matched results from standard wide local excision. The authors argued for wider than standard margins of 9 mm for insitu disease and melanoma less than 1 mm Breslow, but narrower margins of 12 mm for lesions with a Breslow thickness between 1 mm and 4 mm.[43]

Thus, in areas where tissue needs to be conserved such as the head and neck region, MMS may be advantageous for LMM.[43,44] However, the use of MMS for melanoma has been contentious due to both the inferior quality of slides produced with frozen section in comparison to traditional paraffin embedded sections, and also to the difficulty in differentiating malignant melanocytes from atypical melanocytes in photodamaged skin. With the improvement in immunohistochemistry techniques on frozen sections for melanoma and reduction in turnaround time to produce the sections, MMS may become more widely utilized in melanoma treatment. Further randomized controlled trials are required comparing SE to MMS.

MOHS SUITE (SURGICAL FACILITY)

The Mohs suite is best designed with the surgical theater in close proximity to the Mohs laboratory containing the cryostat machine (used to produce the frozen sections) and the office where the microscope is situated. This will facilitate transportation of the tissue between the locations and allow optimal communication between the Mohs surgeon and histotechnician.

Equipment required for the cryostat include surgical blade, specimen button or chuck, antiroll brush, forceps, inking dyes to mark tissue margins, optimal cutting temperature (OCT) medium for embedding, mounting medium, tissue fixing solutions, tissue stains, slides, cover slips, chemical disposal area, wash basin and eye wash station. The laboratory requires adequate ventilation to remove chemical fumes from the staining process and most laboratories have a backup cryostat in case of malfunction of the primary machine.

DEVELOPING TECHNIQUES

MMS techniques have been in continuous development for many decades and the excellent outcomes and degree of skill required set a high bar for the introduction of changes in the technique. The technique is, however, both time-consuming and associated with high costs compared with standard surgery. Therefore improvements are constantly being sought and noninvasive methods for in vivo determination of tumor margins developed. The goal of these approaches is to save time and cost while maintaining efficacy; the more important developing ones are discussed below.

Confocal Microscopy

Confocal microscopy is capable of providing images of a quality sufficient to be considered as a potential alternative to the traditional histopathology approaches used in MMS. This has potential advantages as the histological quality of the frozen sections normally used in MMS is inferior than that of traditional histopathology based on formalin fixation and paraffin embedded sections. This quality sacrifice is being traded off for increased speed and a similar trade-off might be attainable using confocal microscopy.

The technique enables collection of images at different skin depths (down to the penetration limit) and these images are then manipulated by software to create the desired image output. The confocal microscope uses point illumination and only takes images at one depth level at a time. It is this which gives it an optical resolution that is much better than with the usual wide-field microscopes, this improved resolution being particularly marked in the depth direction. By focusing in a specific focal plane, the image is freed from interference from adjacent planes, both above and below. This increased optical resolution and contrast is achieved by eliminating all light reflected from other than the focal point. This is accomplished by adding a small pinhole before the detector, in the confocal plane, hence the name. As the pinhole produces an ellipsoid of much greater length than width, there is an intrinsically lower axial resolution. Thus, the horizontal images can achieve a resolution of 1.25 μm axially, but only 5 μm laterally this, however, is sufficient to observe cellular morphology.

In order to maximize the detection depth in the skin, near-infrared light (830 nm) is used. This is produced by a laser diode, thereby achieving good resolution down to at least 200 μm. In practice, images are produced *en face*, horizontal and parallel to the skin and are visually sectioned to resemble the histopathology specimen in MMS.[45]

As only a small point inside the tissue is in focus at any one time, it is necessary to scan the resultant images and recreate composite images using a computer. This allows for the composite images to be manipulated. Two forms of output have proved particularly useful; these are the stack mode and the mosaic mode. In the stack mode, the skin is viewed at consecutive levels from the epidermis down to the papillary dermis, at which point the resolution begins to deteriorate. In the mosaic mode, a composite image is made (stitched together) from the individual images, the resulting mosaics displaying large areas of tissue at the low magnification needed for MMS.[46]

Reflectance Confocal Microscopy

This seems to be the best of the newer techniques for lateral margin detection, allowing identification of tumor characteristics at the cellular level.[47]

In reflectance confocal microscopy (RCM) no staining is required. The images are gray scale and the reflectivity of the tissue determines the contrast.

In detecting BCC tumor during MMS, RCM has been shown to have a sensitivity of 96.6% and a specificity of 89.2%, with a positive predictive value of 93.0% and a negative predictive value of 94.7%.[48]

Fluorescence Confocal Microscopy

Fluorescence confocal microscopes have been shown to have application to the MMS technique in the examination of ex vivo tissue.[46,48] Ex vivo fluorescence confocal microscopy (FCM) can be used for real-time imaging of tissue arising directly from MMS excisions. There are differences and similarities between RCM and FCM.

In contrast with RCM, where no staining is used, FCM does use stains as contrast agents. For example, a common technique used in FCM is staining with acridine orange, which by specifically staining the nuclei increases the contrast of nucleated cells, and hence these show up clearly in contrast to the weak fluorescence arising from the dermis.[46] This offers an advantage over RCM, as in RCM, the dermis reflects brightly, hindering observation.

As with RCM, FCM produces high-resolution individual images which are manipulated by software to produce mosaics; the images are said to be "stitched together". Again the images are thin optical sections but, in the case of FCM, the individual images are larger, typically 750 μm × 750 μm and these are stitched together to give wide field-of-view mosaics, typically 12 mm × 12 mm, which show large areas of tissue at low magnification which is the desirable output for MMS. In FCM this image collection and manipulation takes less than three minutes, thereby enabling real-time pathology.[46]

MMS predominately treats BCCs. Up to 1% of BCCs, termed locally advanced BCCs, are clinically determined as non-amenable to curative surgery or radiotherapy.[49] BCCs develop through inappropriate activation of the hedgehog pathway. Newly-approved hedgehog pathway inhibitors (vismodegib and sonidegib) are available and both have been shown to substantially shrink tumors in 40–50% of patients. Their long-term use is often limited by resistance and tumors often recur. Adverse effects frequently include muscle cramps, alopecia and dysgeusia.[50] An area of current research involves their neoadjuvant use to shrink the tumor, thereby enabling surgery and potentially limiting functional or cosmetic impairment from surgery.

A crucial question is whether the tumor shrinkage occurs coherently, without residual islands of BCC being left behind. For excision to be effective, clear margins are essential, and for this, shrinkage induced by hedgehog inhibitors would need to occur evenly without leaving BCC cells behind in the vacated areas. It is not yet clear how much of a problem this will prove to be, but this aspect is receiving attention.[51-55]

An investigator-initiated open-label clinical trial of vismodegib as a neoadjuvant to surgery was conducted with 15 patients with high-risk BCC; 11 of these completed the trial, and 4 patients could not complete more than 3 months due to the adverse effects from vismodegib.[53]

This trial showed that 2 to 6 months of vismodegib treatment produced a 27% reduction of the surgical defect area from baseline.[52] These 11 patients had 13 BCCs selected as targets for excision, mainly of the infiltrative

BCC subtype. It was found that vismodegib treatment needed to last for a minimum of 3 months in order to produce a significant reduction in BCC size.[53]

MOHS MICROGRAPHIC SURGERY TECHNIQUE

Performing successful MMS is dependent on the production and interpretation of high-quality frozen horizontal (en face) sections. The procedure involves different steps as shown in the accompanying Box 1. If residual tumor is present on microscopic examination, the involved microscopic margins are identified on the defect utilizing the Mohs map and further Mohs layers are removed precisely from the areas of residual tumor. The process is repeated until the entire tumor has been removed.

Step 1: Preoperative Assessment

MMS is a lengthy procedure and may not be suitable for all patients, for example those with dementia. It is important to offer a choice of treatment modalities to patients, with discussion of the benefits and disadvantages of each treatment and to allow patients to make informed decisions.

A routine preoperative assessment will include a review of current and past medical problems, medications, herbal treatments, smoking and alcohol consumption, and discussion of the risks of surgery. Anticoagulants should not be stopped prior to the operation, due to increased risk of postoperative venous thromboembolism.[56] Patients are requested to stop smoking to aid local tissue perfusion and stop alcohol consumption and relevant herbal treatments (e.g. garlic, ginger, gingko) to reduce hemorrhagic complications. Patients should be provided with written information on the procedure.

Large tumors may require preoperative imaging to assess for muscle or bony invasion. If the defect is likely to be large, preoperative liaison with the relevant plastic, oculoplastic, ear-nose-throat or maxillofacial surgeon may be necessary to coordinate the complex repair post-MMS.

Box 1: Steps of Mohs micrographic surgery.

1. Preoperative screening
2. Removing of the first Mohs layer
3. Accurate paper mapping of the removed tissue in relation to the defect created
4. Inking of margins for orientation
5. Tissue grossing (flattening), embedding, cutting of tissue sections (cryotomy)
6. Fixing of the cut sections, staining
7. Interpretation of the slides produced
8. Repetition of steps 2–7 if residual tumor is present

Step 2: Excision of First Mohs Layer and Mapping of the Tumor

Prior to infiltration of local anesthesia (LA), the clinical margins of the tumor must be marked in addition to important skin tension lines and anatomic subunits using a skin marker pen. A premixed solution of 1% lignocaine and epinephrine (1 in 200,000) as local anesthetic is typically used for injection. Marcaine may be injected additionally or in combination to provide anesthesia of longer duration.

Prior to excising the first Mohs layer, curettage is used for initial tumor debulking (Fig. 1). In addition to debulking of the tumor, reports have suggested that the curettage can be used to precisely remove subclinical extension of tumor by palpation of abnormal tissue, thereby reducing the number of Mohs stages required. However, other studies have shown that wider curettage may unnecessarily remove extra normal tissue and result in a larger Mohs defect.[57]

Following debulking of the tumor, the margin of the first Mohs layer is scored with a 1–2 mm narrow width of epidermis. Perpendicular marking nicks are made through the scored peripheral margin onto the surrounding skin for future orientation. Typically, nicks are made at 12 o'clock, 6 o'clock and 9 o'clock positions. The blade is then classically held at a 45° angle to the skin, incision is made upto the subcutaneous tissue maintaining the angle, and then the tumor is removed in a horizontal deep plane to provide a 'saucer' shaped layer of tissue (Fig. 2). 'Saucerization' facilitates flattening of the tissue and allows the entire peripheral and deep margin to be examined in one plane. It is important to ensure that the complete margin of epidermis is present and the incision has not incised through the curetted tissue. Radiofrequency ablation or hyfrecator is used to cauterize any bleeding points after removal of the first layer and the surgical area is bandaged and patient asked to wait in the waiting hall until the results of first layer are microscopically interpreted.

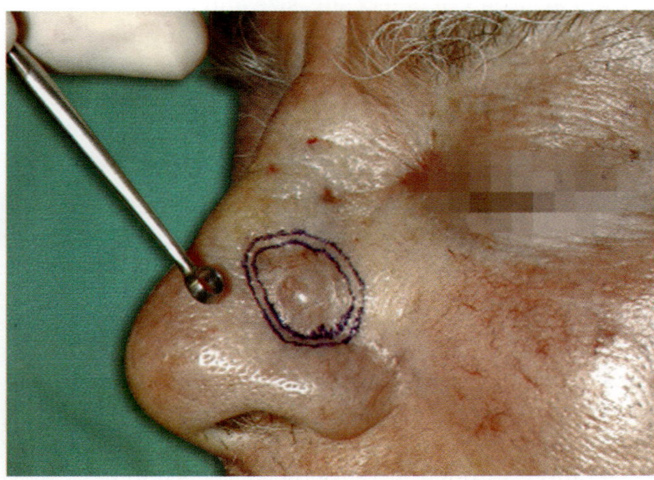

Fig. 1: Curetting or debulking the tumor.

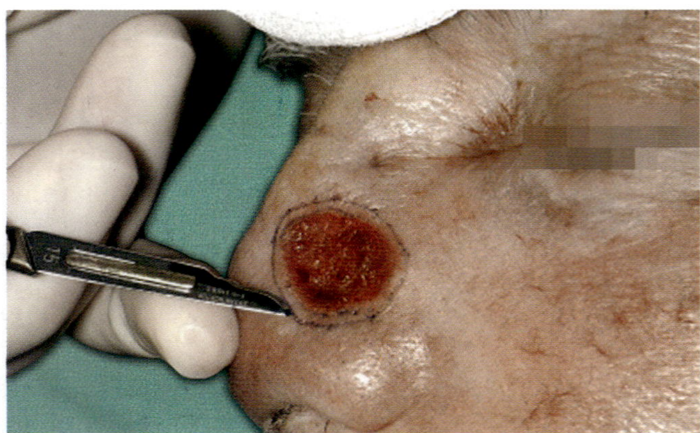

Fig. 2: Incising the Mohs layer at 45° angle.

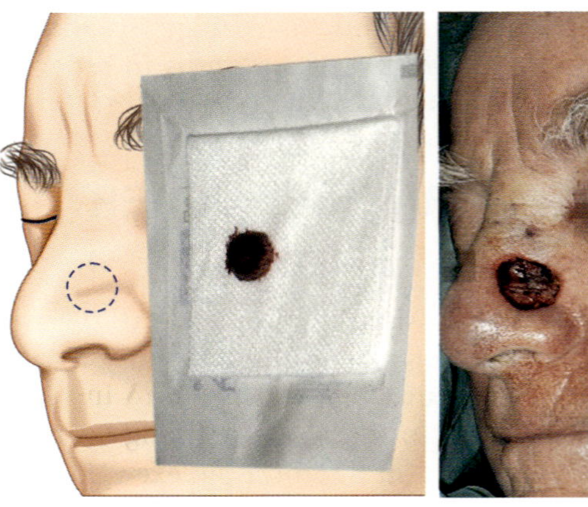

Fig. 3: Mohs template design.

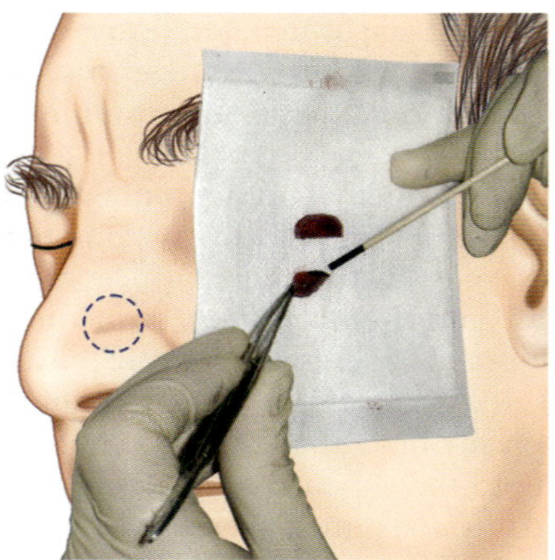

Fig. 4: Color coding the sections.

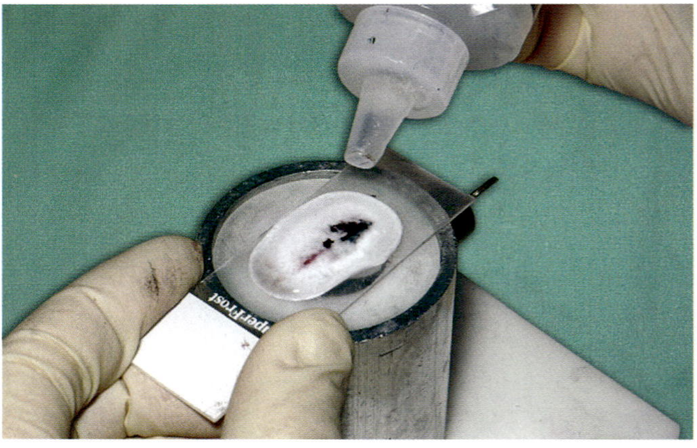

Fig. 5: Embedding medium (e.g. OCT compound) is applied around the periphery of the tissue.

The excised tissue is placed on a square of gauze. A hand-drawn Mohs map of the wound is created to represent the in vivo wound with marking nicks (Fig. 3). Large specimens may require division for placement onto a glass slide. Each subdivision must be numbered and marked on the Mohs map. Digital photographs may be used in place of hand-drawn maps and printed to provide greater accuracy of defect site, size and orientation.

The tissue margins are marked using ink and the corresponding site and color drawn onto the Mohs map. One color is standard on a superior or medial edge, another color at the inferior or lateral edge (Fig. 4). The same color coordination should be used for all Mohs stages and procedures to reduce errors of orientation.

Step 3: Tissue Grossing, Embedding and Sectioning

The tissue is placed on a slide and carefully checked to ensure that the entire margins are flat and in contact with the slide surface. The edges can be maneuvered flat using cotton tip applicators or forceps. Relaxation incisions may be required through the superficial surface to help gross (flatten) the specimen.

Next, an embedding medium (e.g. optimal cutting temperature compound) is applied around the periphery of the tissue and the entire block is frozen in the cryostat freeze bar (Fig. 5). The freezing process should occur quickly to avoid the formation of ice crystal and subsequent tissue artefact.

The frozen block is then placed, deep margin face up, on a chuck using further OCT medium for adherence and the entire button mounted on the cryostat stage ready for sectioning. Alternative techniques of embedding include using a heat extractor, embedding machine or isopentane histobath.

The frozen tissue block is next sectioned in the microtome. The block should be carefully sectioned until a complete skin edge is obtained, which can be checked for by the histotechnician using a microscope prior to proceeding to fixation. If a complete margin is not present, deeper cuts are required.

Step 4: Tissue Fixation and Staining

The section is placed on a positively charged slide to improve adherence. Two or three sections may be placed simultaneously on one slide. The tissue is then fixed, most commonly using either 10% neutral buffered formalin, alcoholic formalin, alcohol, or acetone. Once the tissue has been fixed, the next step is staining of the tissue.

Hematoxylin and eosin is the most frequently used tissue stain. Toluidine blue may be used in BCC to highlight mucopolysaccharides surrounding islands of tumor. Once the tissue is stained, excess dye is cleared using xylene substitutes.

Increasingly, immunohistochemical staining is also performed on the frozen sections. These include cytokeratin stains for BCC and SCC, Ber-EP4 for BCC, CD34 for DFSP and HMB-45, and Mel-5, S-100 and Melan-A for melanoma.[58]

Cytokeratin staining for BCC in MMS is a useful adjunct in morphologically complex cases where there is a dense inflammatory infiltrate surrounding suspicious cells that can hinder identification of scanty tumor cells which are difficult to determine with hematoxylin and eosin or toluidine blue staining. A recent study demonstrated pancytokeratins AE1/AE3 to be a highly effective stain for BCC in MMS and showed consistent staining, both in terms of intensity of staining and sensitivity of greater than 99%.[59]

Finally, a coverslip is placed over the section using a coverslip adhesive and the slide is ready to be reviewed by the Mohs surgeon.

Step 5: Interpreting the Frozen Section

Examination of the Mohs frozen section allows review of the entire peripheral and deep margin for residual tumor (Fig. 6). If residual tumor is present, further Mohs layers are required. The site of the residual tumor is marked onto the Mohs map and then reflected onto the in vivo defect on the patient. The patient is brought back to the operative room and utilizing the orientation nicks made onto the skin in step 3, the residual tumor site is marked and further Mohs layers taken. A 1–2 mm margin of normal skin is taken from both peripheral and deep involved margins for future orientation and the entire process repeated until all of the tumor has been removed. The wound can then be repaired to provide optimum cosmetic and functional result. The choice of wound repair is dependent on the anatomical site, the quality of the adjacent tissue and individual patient characteristics. The ideal repair for one patient will not necessarily be the best repair for another patient. Commonly used modalities of wound repair include secondary intention healing, skin grafting and utilisation of local skin flaps, which can be performed on the same or next day.

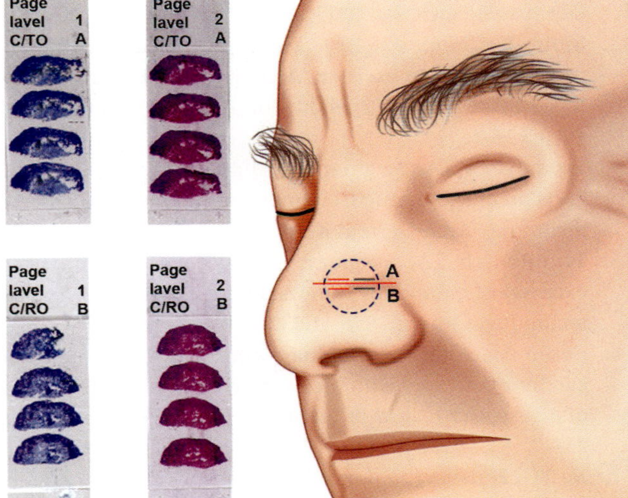

Fig. 6: Sections are ready to be read by the Mohs surgeon.

SLOW MOHS MICROGRAPHIC SURGERY

The classical technique for MMS described above has also been modified to use traditional formalin fixation and paraffin embedded sections to still ensure 100% margin control. This method is known as slow Mohs and each stage takes 24–48 hours. The advantage is a higher quality of histological sections than standard Mohs frozen sections, especially useful for melanoma which may be difficult to interpret on frozen sections.

A large series of 750 BCCs treated with slow Mohs found a cure rate of 97.8% for primary tumors and 95.3% for recurrent tumors at 5-year follow-up.[60] Slides were read jointly by the Mohs surgeon and dermatopathologist. The primary disadvantage of slow Mohs is the 1–2 days turnaround time for the production of the paraffin embedded slides. This necessitates several patient visits, but is a viable option when traditional MMS is not feasible. Slow Mohs has also been reported for use with SCC with equivalent cure rates and can be used with any tumor type.[61]

Cost-effectiveness of Mohs Micrographic Surgery

MMS is more expensive than conventional surgery; the main expenses of MMS arise from the labor costs of the Mohs surgeon, nurses, assistants, histotechnicians and receptionists and increased length of time taken to perform MMS in contrast to standard surgery.

A study by Smeets et al. and Essers et al. found MMS to be significantly more expensive than SE for primary and recurrent BCC, and independent of the BCC subtype or anatomical site.[13,62] However, Bialy et al. found MMS to be cost comparable to SE when tumor recurrence rates post-procedure, thus necessitating further procedures were was accounted for.[63] Cook and Zitelli described 400 consecutive tumors and also showed that the cost of MMS to have equivalency to SE.[64]

Table 4: List of potential errors in technique.

Step	Error	Adverse consequence
Step 2 Excision	Incision angle over 45°	Difficulty flattening specimen into one plane
	Incising through curetted area when taking Mohs layer	Complete peripheral margin will not be available for assessment
Step 2 Mapping	Inaccuracy of drawing Mohs map	Incorrect orientation
	Too much ink used	Ink spill onto other margins confusing orientation
Step 3 Grossing	Edges not unrolled during grossing	Tangential sections
Step 3 Embedding	Slow freeze during embedding	Ice formation in tissue sample causing artifact
Step 3 Sectioning	Sections curl on anti-roll plate	Misalignment of anti-roll plate, or cold blade
	Torn sections	Dull blade or blade contains nicks
	Thin and thick sections	Loose chuck or blade holder
	Foreign tissue on blade from a previous procedure	Introduction of foreign tissue (floater) into section
Step 4 Tissue fixation	Tissue in fixing medium for insufficient time	Inadequate dehydration of tissue resulting in reduced quality of staining
Step 4 Tissue staining	Foreign tissue in staining medium from a previous procedure	Introduction of foreign tissue into section (floater)
	Incorrect labeling of slides	Errors of tumor mapping
Step 5 Interpreting frozen section	Misinterpretation of benign histology for malignant and vice versa	Errors of false negative or false positive margins
	Inflammation masking underlying tumor cells	Errors of false negative margins
	Misinterpretation of perineural invasion	Errors of false negative margins

POTENTIAL ERRORS AND LIMITATIONS OF MOHS MICROGRAPHIC SURGERY

Errors can occur at all steps along the process of performing MMS. Table 4 highlights potential areas of difficulty to be aware of in the procedure and Box 2 summarizes some of the common limitations of MMS.

CONCLUSION

Surgical treatment of skin tumors can have a significant impact on the quality of life for a patient. MMS provides the highest cure rates, utilizing margin control whilst sparing the maximum amount of healthy tissue.

This allows for optimum functional and cosmetic repair. MMS should be the treatment of choice for high-risk skin tumors in critical anatomical sites on the head and neck. MMS is a technical procedure requiring specialized training for 1–2 years before independent practice is commenced. A Mohs surgeon in Australia performs on an average 200–300 cases per year; in the USA the number of cases is on average 1000.[65] India has a lower incidence of skin cancer and it should be mandatory that dermatologists in India performing MMS have followed a suitable training program, and subsequently completed a minimum number of MMS cases per year to ensure that the highest standards of the MMS technique is maintained.

Box 2: Limitations of Mohs micrographic surgery.

- Time-consuming process
- Quality of frozen sections inferior to standard paraffin embedded sections for histological interpretation
- Dedicated histotechnician required for preparation of frozen sections
- Tumors which grow in a noncontiguous manner may be associated with falsely negative margins

REFERENCES

1. Wood LD, Ammirati CT. An overview of Mohs micrographic surgery for the treatment of basal cell carcinoma. Dermatologic clinics. 2011;29(2):153-60.
2. Mohs F. Chemosurgery: a microscopically controlled method of cancer excision. Arch Surg. 1941;42:279-95.
3. Mohs FE. Cancer of eyelids. Bull Am Coll Chemosurgery. 1970;3:10-1.
4. Tromovitch TA, Stegman SJ. Microscopically controlled excision of skin tumors: chemosurgery (Mohs): fresh tissue technique. Arch Dermatol. 1974;110:231-2.
5. Tromovitch TA, Stegman SJ. Microscopie-controlled excision of cutaneous tumors: chemosurgery, fresh tissue technique. Cancer. 1978;41:653-8.
6. Berlin AL, Amin SP, Goldberg DJ. Extraocular sebaceous carcinoma treated with Mohs micrographic surgery: report of a case and review of literature. Dermatol Surg. 2008;34: 254-7.
7. Xu YG, Hinshaw M, Longley BJ, et al. Cutaneous adenoid cystic carcinoma with perineural invasion treated by mohs micrographic surgery-a case report with literature review. J Oncol. 2010;2010:469049.

8. Leibovitch I, Huilgol SC, Selva D, et al. Cutaneous squamous carcinoma in situ (Bowen's disease): treatment with Mohs micrographic surgery. J Am Acad Dermatol. 2005;52:997-1002.
9. Arits AH, Mosterd K, Essers BA, et al. Photodynamic therapy versus topical imiquimod versus topical fluorouracil for treatment of superficial basal-cell carcinoma: a single blind, non-inferiority, randomised controlled trial. Lancet Oncol. 2013;14:647-54.
10. Samarasinghe V, Madan V, Lear JT. Focus on Basal cell carcinoma. J Skin Cancer. 2011;2011:328615.
11. Rowe DE, Carroll RJ, Day CL Jr. Long-term recurrence rates in previously untreated (primary) basal cell carcinoma: implications for patient follow-up. J Dermatol Surg Oncol. 1989;15:315-28.
12. Malhotra R, Huilgol SC, Huynh NT, et al. The Australian Mohs database, part II: periocular basal cell carcinoma outcome at 5-year follow-up. Ophthalmology. 2004;111: 631-6.
13. Smeets NW, Krekels GA, Ostertag JU, et al. Surgical excision vs Mohs' micrographic surgery for basal-cell carcinoma of the face: randomised controlled trial. Lancet. 2004;364: 1766-72.
14. van Loo E, Mosterd K, Krekels GA, et al. Surgical excision versus Mohs' micrographic surgery for basal cell carcinoma of the face: A randomised clinical trial with 10 year follow-up. Eur J Cancer. 2014;50:3011-20.
15. Samarasinghe V, Madan V, Lear JT. Management of high-risk squamous cell carcinoma of the skin. Expert Rev Anticancer Ther. 2011;11:763-9.
16. Rowe DE, Carroll RJ, Day CL Jr. Prognostic factors for local recurrence, metastasis, and survival rates in squamous cell carcinoma of the skin, ear, and lip. Implications for treatment modality selection. J Am Acad Dermatol. 1992; 26:976-90.
17. Leibovitch I, Huilgol SC, Selva D, et al. Cutaneous squamous cell carcinoma treated with Mohs micrographic surgery in Australia I. Experience over 10 years. J Am Acad Dermatol. 2005;53:253-60.
18. Brodland DG, Zitelli JA. Surgical margins for excision of primary cutaneous squamous cell carcinoma. J Am Acad Dermatol. 1992;27:241-8.
19. Angouridakis N, Kafas P, Jerjes W, et al. Dermatofibrosarcoma protuberans with fibrosarcomatous transformation of the head and neck. Head Neck Oncol. 2011;3:5.
20. Paradisi A, Abeni D, Rusciani A, et al. Dermatofibrosarcoma protuberans: wide local excision vs. Mohs micrographic surgery. Cancer Treat Rev. 2008;34:728-36.
21. Lowe GC, Onajin O, Baum CL, et al. A Comparison of Mohs Micrographic Surgery and Wide Local Excision for Treatment of Dermatofibrosarcoma Protuberans With Long-Term Follow-up: The Mayo Clinic Experience. Dermatol Surg. 2016.
22. Wetter R, Goldstein GD. Microcystic adnexal carcinoma: a diagnostic and therapeutic challenge. Dermatol Ther. 2008; 21:452-8.
23. Leibovitch I, Huilgol SC, Selva D, et al. Microcystic adnexal carcinoma: treatment with Mohs micrographic surgery. J Am Acad Dermatol. 2005;52:295-300.
24. Chiller K, Passaro D, Scheuller M, et al. Microcystic adnexal carcinoma: forty-eight cases, their treatment, and their outcome. Arch Dermatol. 2000;136:1355-9.
25. Annest NM, Grekin SJ, Stone MS, et al. Cutaneous leiomyosarcoma: a tumor of the head and neck. Dermatol Surg. 2007;33:628-33.
26. Humphreys TR, Finkelstein DH, Lee JB. Superficial leiomyosarcoma treated with Mohs micrographic surgery. Dermatol Surg. 2004;30:108-12.
27. Starling J, 3rd, Coldiron BM. Mohs micrographic surgery for the treatment of cutaneous leiomyosarcoma. J Am Acad Dermatol. 2011;64:1119-22.
28. Iorizzo LJ, 3rd, Brown MD. Atypical fibroxanthoma: a review of the literature. Dermatol Surg. 2011;37:146-57.
29. Ang GC, Roenigk RK, Otley CC, et al. More than 2 decades of treating atypical fibroxanthoma at mayo clinic: what have we learned from 91 patients? Dermatol Surg. 2009;35: 765-72.
30. Wick MR, Goellner JR, Wolfe JT, 3rd, et al. Adnexal carcinomas of the skin. I. Eccrine carcinomas. Cancer. 1985; 56:1147-62.
31. Robson A, Greene J, Ansari N, et al. Eccrine porocarcinoma (malignant eccrine poroma): a clinicopathologic study of 69 cases. Am J Surg Pathol. 2001;25:710-20.
32. Riera-Leal L, Guevara-Gutierrez E, Barrientos-Garcia JG, et al. Eccrine porocarcinoma: epidemiologic and histopathologic characteristics. Int J Dermatol. 2015;54: 580-6.
33. Song SS, Wu Lee W, Hamman MS, et al. Mohs micrographic surgery for eccrine porocarcinoma: an update and review of the literature. Dermatol Surg. 2015;41:301-6.
34. Skowron F, Poulhalon N, Balme B, et al. [Primary eccrine porocarcinoma: a clinicopathological study of 50 cases]. Ann Dermatol Venereol. 2014;141:258-64.
35. Tolkachjov SN, Hocker TL, Camilleri MJ, et al. Treatment of Porocarcinoma With Mohs Micrographic Surgery: The Mayo Clinic Experience. Dermatol Surg. 2016;42:745-50.
36. Lam C, Funaro D. Extramammary Paget's disease: Summary of current knowledge. Dermatol Clin. 2010;28:807-26.
37. Lee KY, Roh MR, Chung WG, et al. Comparison of Mohs micrographic surgery and wide excision for extramammary Paget's Disease: Korean experience. Dermatol Surg. 2009; 35:34-40.
38. Hendi A, Brodland DG, Zitelli JA. Extramammary Paget's disease: surgical treatment with Mohs micrographic surgery. J Am Acad Dermatol. 2004;51:767-73.
39. Higgins HW, 2nd, Lee KC, Galan A, et al. Melanoma in situ: Part II. Histopathology, treatment, and clinical management. J Am Acad Dermatol. 2015;73:193-203; quiz -4.
40. King R. Lentiginous melanoma. Arch Pathol Lab Med. 2011; 135:337-41.
41. Kallini JR, Jain SK, Khachemoune A. Lentigo maligna: review of salient characteristics and management. Am J Clin Dermatol. 2013;14:473-80.
42. Felton S, Taylor RS, Srivastava D. Excision Margins for Melanoma In Situ on the Head and Neck. Dermatol Surg. 2016;42:327-34.
43. Bricca GM, Brodland DG, Ren D, et al. Cutaneous head and neck melanoma treated with Mohs micrographic surgery. J Am Acad Dermatol. 2005;52:92-100.
44. Stigall LE, Brodland DG, Zitelli JA. The use of Mohs micrographic surgery (MMS) for melanoma in situ (MIS) of the trunk and proximal extremities. J Am Acad Dermatol. 2016;75:1015-21.

45. Que SK, Fraga-Braghiroli N, Grant-Kels JM, et al. Through the looking glass: Basics and principles of reflectance confocal microscopy. J Am Acad Dermatol. 2015;73:276-84.
46. Bennassar A, Vilata A, Puig S, et al. Ex vivo fluorescence confocal microscopy for fast evaluation of tumor margins during Mohs surgery. Br J Dermatol. 2014;170:360-5.
47. Venturini M, Gualdi G, Zanca A, et al. A new approach for presurgical margin assessment by reflectance confocal microscopy of basal cell carcinoma. Br J Dermatol. 2016; 174:380-5.
48. Gareau DS, Karen JK, Dusza SW, et al. Sensitivity and specificity for detecting basal cell carcinomas in Mohs excisions with confocal fluorescence mosaicing microscopy. J Biomed Opt. 2009;14:034012.
49. Dreier J, Dummer R, Felderer L, et al. Emerging drugs and combination strategies for basal cell carcinoma. Expert Opin Emerg Drugs. 2014;19:353-65.
50. Sekulic A, Von Hoff D. Hedgehog Pathway Inhibition. Cell, 2016;164:831.
51. Wolfe CM, Green WH, Cognetta AB Jr, et al. Basal cell carcinoma rebound after cessation of vismodegib in a nevoid basal cell carcinoma syndrome patient. Dermatol Surg. 2012;38:1863-6.
52. Ally MS, Aasi S, Wysong A, et al. An investigator-initiated open-label clinical trial of vismodegib as a neoadjuvant to surgery for high-risk basal cell carcinoma. Journal of the American Academy of Dermatology. 2014;71(5):904-11.
53. Ally MS, Aasi S, Wysong A, et al. An investigator-initiated open-label clinical trial of vismodegib as a neoadjuvant to surgery for high-risk basal cell carcinoma. J Am Acad Dermatol. 2014;71:904-11.
54. Alcalay J, Tauber G, Fenig E, et al. Vismodegib as a neoadjuvant treatment to Mohs surgery for aggressive basal cell carcinoma. J Drugs Dermatol. 2015;14:219-23.
55. Sofen H, Gross KG, Goldberg LH, et al. A phase II, multicenter, open-label, 3-cohort trial evaluating the efficacy and safety of vismodegib in operable basal cell carcinoma. J Am Acad Dermatol. 2015; 73: 99-105 e1.
56. Stables G, Lawrence CM. Management of patients taking anticoagulant, aspirin, non-steroidal anti-inflammatory and other anti-platelet drugs undergoing dermatological surgery. Clin Exp Dermatol. 2002; 27: 432-5.
57. Guardiano RA, Grande DJ. A direct comparison of visual inspection, curettage, and epiluminescence microscopy in determining tumor extent before the initial margins are determined for Mohs micrographic surgery. Dermatol Surg. 2010;36:1240-4.
58. El Tal AK, Abrou AE, Stiff MA, et al. Immunostaining in Mohs micrographic surgery: a review. Dermatol Surg. 2010; 36:275-90.
59. Orchard GE, Wojcik K, Shams F, et al. Pan-cytokeratin markers for rapid frozen section immunocytochemistry from head and facial Mohs cases of basal cell carcinoma: a comparison and evaluation to determine the marker of choice. Br J Biomed Sci. 2015;72:61-6.
60. Lawrence CM, Haniffa M, Dahl MG. Formalin-fixed tissue Mohs surgery (slow Mohs) for basal cell carcinoma: 5-year follow-up data. Br J Dermatol. 2009;160:573-80.
61. Turner RJ, Leonard N, Malcolm AJ, et al. A retrospective study of outcome of Mohs' micrographic surgery for cutaneous squamous cell carcinoma using formalin fixed sections. Br J Dermatol. 2000;142:752-7.
62. Essers BA, Dirksen CD, Nieman FH et al. Cost-effectiveness of Mohs Micrographic Surgery vs Surgical Excision for Basal Cell Carcinoma of the Face. Arch Dermatol. 2006;142: 187-94.
63. Bialy TL, Whalen J, Veledar E, et al. Mohs micrographic surgery vs traditional surgical excision: a cost comparison analysis. Arch Dermatol. 2004;140:736-42.
64. Cook J, Zitelli JA. Mohs micrographic surgery: a cost analysis. J Am Acad Dermatol. 1998;39:698-703.
65. Rutherford T, Elliott T, Vinciullo C. Mohs surgery in Australia: a survey of work practices. Australas J Dermatol. 2011;52:98-103.

Chapter

50

Melanoma

Nicholas Collier, Firas Al-Niami, Vishal Madan

Key Messages

- Melanoma is the most serious form of skin cancer, accounting for the majority of skin cancer deaths, and has a rising worldwide incidence.
- Surgical treatment of melanoma can be curative in early stages, and early recognition and management is therefore essential.
- Superficial spreading melanoma is the commonest subtype worldwide; however, in Asian skin where melanoma is much less common the acral subtype is most frequently found.
- The prognosis of melanoma varies widely and depends on several factors, including the depth of the tumor, sentinel-node status, presence of ulceration and dermal mitotic rate.
- Treatment of advanced melanoma has seen recent striking advances, notably in immune checkpoint inhibitors and molecular targeted therapies.

INTRODUCTION AND HISTORY

Melanoma derives from the Greek words *melas* and *oma* meaning black tumor. The earliest description of melanoma is attributed to Hippocrates in the 5th century.[1] It was however in 1838 that the term melanoma was first proposed by Carswell.[2] By the mid-twentieth century, the disease had been described as melanosarcoma, melanocarcinoma and nevocarcinoma. It is now well-understood that melanoma is a neoplastic disease of the melanocytes, cells that arise from the neural crest. During early gestation, melanocytes migrate from the neural crest to the skin, mucous membranes, uveal tract and meninges. The overwhelming majority of melanoma occurs in the skin and depends on the presence of melanocytes and not necessarily the process of melanogenesis, as seen for example in the amelanotic variant in albinos who lack melanogenesis. Other variants such as mucosal and uveal melanoma will not be discussed in this chapter.

The terms melanoma and malignant melanoma describe the same disease and are therefore interchangeable. The latter term is however redundant as all cases of melanoma are malignant. Melanoma is a disease that can be associated with a high mortality and therefore timely recognition and management of the disease is essential to reduce this risk.

EPIDEMIOLOGY

Melanoma is an important public health problem and, although having been addressed by sustained sun protection initiatives and early detection interventions, its worldwide incidence continues to increase. Evidence of increasing melanoma incidence in Caucasian populations over recent decades is shown by most epidemiological studies; this is presumed to be related to changes in sun exposure and recreational behavior.[3] In the United States for example, the incidence of melanoma increased from 4.2 per 100,000 in the period 1969-1971, to 21.8 per 100,000 for the period 2009 to 2013.[4,5] Worldwide however, the highest yearly incidence was reported in New Zealand, with 77.7 cases per 100,000.[6] Racial differences have been shown to exist for melanoma subtypes in the US population.[7] Despite the fact that among all variants of skin cancer melanoma represents less than 10% of the cases, at least two-thirds of the skin cancer associated deaths are attributed to melanoma. However, it is much less common in Indian skin.

In Germany, a nationwide screening program for those aged ≥35 years commenced in 2008 and, out of approximately half a million persons screened, 0.3% were diagnosed with melanoma. The results suggest that this screening was not associated with significant changes in incidence.[8]

ETIOLOGY

The principal function of melanocytes is the production of photoprotective melanin pigments. Melanocytes are generally only intermittently mitotic as melanin production does not require high cell turnover.[9] Exposure to ultraviolet (UV) rays has been linked to the development of melanoma and is the only well-established environmental factor.[10] Intermittent exposures to UV, and in particular when associated with sunburns, greatly increase the risk for the development of the disease. In particular, sunburns acquired during childhood and early adolescence carries the greatest risk.[11] This highlights the fact that it is not only the UV exposure that contributes to the induction of melanoma, but also the duration, pattern and age of exposure. The current explanation for the role of UV in the pathogenesis of melanoma is related to the increased cell turnover of the melanocytes following UV radiation in order to produce photoprotective melanin. This proliferative response requires a delicate balance between negative and positive cell cycle regulatory signals. Any alteration in these signals can result in uncontrolled cell division, which is the hallmark of malignancy.

There is abundant evidence now that the skin phenotypes at greatest risk for melanoma are those with skin types I and II.[12] People with freckles, red or blonde hair, increased number of nevi, and those with a family history of melanoma carry a greater risk. The ability to acquire a tan appears to be protective. The incidence of melanoma in people with skin type IV is much lower than skin types I and II.[13] The issue of sunbeds in relation to melanoma has been a topic of intense discussion. There is evidence to support the role of sunbed use in the development of melanoma and this has been shown in several studies.[14,15] Similar to the exposure to solar UV radiation, sunbed use during early adulthood appears to be associated with a higher risk for the development of melanoma.[16]

Genetics plays a role in the pathogenesis of melanoma in a subset of patients. Several genes have been implicated that confer a higher susceptibility to melanoma in high-risk families.[17,18] There are as yet unidentified melanoma susceptibility genes. Genes which code for cyclin-dependent kinase inhibitor 2A *(CDKN2A)*, also known as p16 and MTS, and cyclin-dependent kinase 4 *(CDK4)* are associated with an increased risk of melanoma.[19,20] Both *CDKN2A* and *CDK4* play a critical role in the regulation of the cell cycle. Mutations of these genes can trigger uncontrolled melanocyte proliferation and differentiation, leading to the development of melanoma.

Of these genes, *CDKN2A* is currently the major melanoma susceptibility gene, accounting for approximately 20–40% of hereditary melanoma or approximately 0.2–2% of all melanomas.[21] An increased risk for pancreatic cancer with *CDKN2A* has also been established in some families and therefore carriers of this mutation should be warned about this risk. Currently, testing for *CDKN2A* is available and is usually considered if the patient has a greater than 10% pretest probability of carrying the mutation. In addition to the presence of melanoma, these include: two or more family members with melanoma, family member with multiple primary melanomas, family history of melanoma and pancreatic cancer, first-degree relative with a proven *CDKN2A* mutation carrier and lastly any individual with multiple primary melanomas regardless of the family history. Individuals in whom *CDKN2A* or the other two genes is found require aggressive management with intensive regular surveillance, with strong emphasis on regular self-examination. Melanoma patients who fall into this so-called "familial" category due to the presence of either of these genes are at 30–70 fold higher risk of developing melanoma than the general population and therefore represent a very high-risk group.[22]

In summary, multiple factors play a role in the pathogenesis of melanoma, with UV being the main environmental one. Carrying a germline mutation in *CDKN2A* is associated with the greatest risk, followed by a strong family history of melanoma, then the presence of atypical nevus syndrome and finally phenotypic characteristics indicative of sun sensitivity such as red hair, multiple freckles and the tendency for sunburns.

CLINICAL VARIANTS OF PRIMARY CUTANEOUS MELANOMA

The features classically observed in a developing melanoma include changes in color, shape, size and border. History is important as often patients notice a change in an existing nevus. In approximately 75% of cases of cases however, melanoma may arise de novo from background of normal skin with only 25% thought to develop in a cutaneous melanocytic nevus. The "ABCD" diagnostic system is a simple and helpful tool in evaluating cutaneous pigmented lesions:

A = Asymmetry
B = Border irregularity
C = Color variation
D = Diameter greater than 6 mm.

Asymmetry means asymmetry of pattern or shape. The border of most melanomas becomes irregular as a result of uneven growth within the lesion.

Irregularity of pigment is of importance and the presence of varying shades of pigmentation may be a clue for melanoma. Multiple colors and color variation may be observed in melanoma. In melanoma cancerous cells can spread throughout the dermis, into the subcutis and upwards through pagetoid spread into the epidermis.

The blue and gray colors seen can be explained by the Tyndall effect where shorter wavelength blue light is more widely reflected and scattered than longer wavelength red light.[23] When melanin is present in the deeper subcutis it appears blue, due to more blue light being reflected back. In melanoma, unlike benign nevi, melanoma cells can travel to the epidermis though pagetoid spread giving rise to dark brown and black colors. Whitish areas within a melanoma may indicate "regression" where histologically, lymphocytes can be seen replacing the tumor with fibrous stroma, clinically producing a pale scar-like area.[24]

The diameter of the lesion exceeding 6 mm is not particularly diagnostic as many benign lesions may be over 6 mm. However, melanomas developing in dysplastic nevi are usually 6 mm or more in diameter and an increase in the size of a nevus may be indicative of malignant transformation.

The overwhelming majority of cutaneous melanomas fall into the following clinicopathological subsets: superficial spreading melanoma (SSM), nodular melanoma (NM), lentigo maligna melanoma (LMM) and acral lentiginous melanoma (ALM). In some cases, neither the clinical presentation nor the histological appearances permit classification of the melanoma, in which the tumor is designated as indeterminate. It is important to note that some melanomas may lack pigment and thus these are often misdiagnosed. These are referred to as "amelanotic melanomas" and can belong to any of the aforementioned subtypes.

Melanoma in situ and lentigo maligna (LM) are both confined to the epidermis and will be dealt with only briefly-in this chapter.

Superficial Spreading Melanoma

Superficial spreading melanoma is the most common subtype of melanoma among white populations accounting for approximately 70% of all cases.[25] This clinical variant of melanoma can occur on both sun-exposed and non-sun-exposed surfaces and tends to show a predilection for the lower legs in women and upper back in men; areas prone to intermittent, rather than chronic, sun exposure. Clinically, the lesions tend to have irregular borders with variable shades and degrees of pigmentation (Fig. 1). Clinical signs of regression include notching, an area of central hypopigmentation, or an asymmetrical halo of hypopigmentation.

Nodular Melanoma

This is the subtype with the most aggressive potential. The most frequently affected sites are the head, neck and limbs.

Typically, this presents with a rapidly growing nodule that often arises de novo (Fig. 2). The surface may appear smooth or ulcerated. It is common for this subtype to have a uniform color which may be black, blue or gray. At the time of clinical detection, the tumor has usually invaded deeply into the dermis, accounting for the worse prognosis in this subtype.[26]

Lentigo Maligna Melanoma

LMM represents about 10% of melanomas among Caucasians and is rarely seen in Asian and black skin.[25] It is the invasive form of the precursor lesion LM, the latter being an in situ type of melanoma occurring on sun-damaged skin. LMM typically occurs on the head and neck of elderly people. Clinically, this often presents as a tan or brown macule or patch, often speckled with minute brown or black flecks, with irregular borders and often with varying shades of pigmentation (Fig. 3). Regression may present as notching or scalloping of the borders, with or without the presence of white or gray shades within the lesion. It is estimated that the lifetime risk of LM progressing to LMM is around 5%.[27]

Acral Lentiginous Melanoma

ALM is the least common subtype of melanoma among skin types I and II but is the most common among skin types V and VI.[25,28-30] This variant occurs on the palms or soles; areas with comparatively minimal exposure to UV radiation. The sole of the foot is the most common site for this tumor which may initially appear as a "dirty patch". Some authors

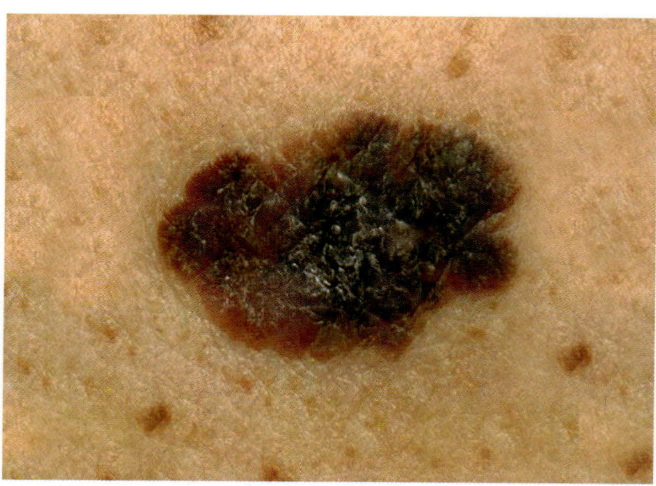

Fig. 1: Superficial spreading melanoma.

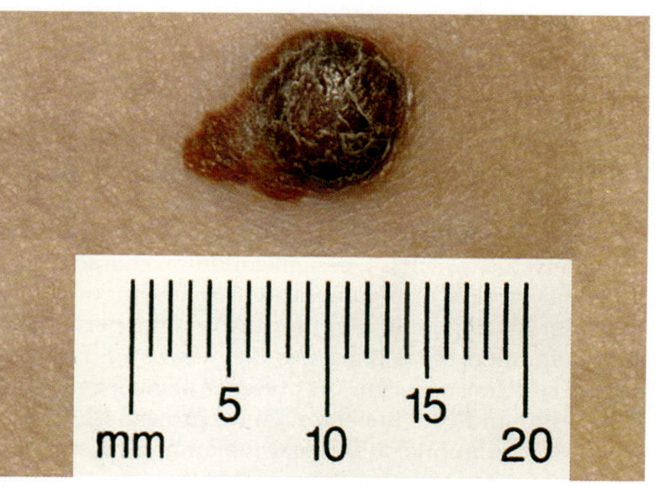

Fig. 2: Nodular melanoma.

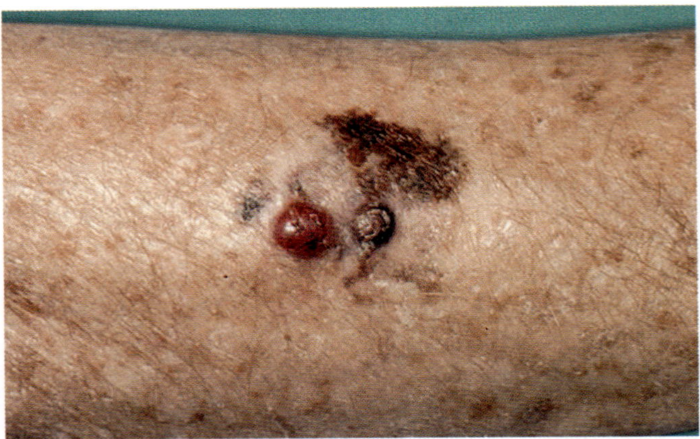

Fig. 3: Lentigo maligna melanoma.

proposed to use the term "acral" melanoma to include a subset of these tumors which display histological features more in keeping with SSM rather than a lentiginous pattern such as LM. This subtype of melanoma often has greater depth of penetration at the time of diagnosis than its superficial clinical appearance, as an irregular flat area of diffuse pigmentation, may suggest. The colors may form a mosaic of tan, dark brown, and black. The border is often irregular and ill-defined. As the tumor advances, its borders become highly irregular and notched.

Dermoscopy is a clinically useful tool aiding differentiation between benign and malignant acral pigmented lesions. At acral sites pigmented lesions can be seen with a parallel pattern of pigmentation. There are two main types of parallel pigmentation. In benign lesions, the pigment is commonly seen in a parallel furrow pattern where the pigment lines are often narrow. Conversely a parallel ridge pattern where the pigment lines are broad with narrower non-pigmented lines is a cause for concern, and suggestive of an ALM.

A less common but distinctive variant of ALM is subungual melanoma. The great toe and thumb are the sites most commonly affected, accounting for over three-quarters of the cases.[31] Similar to ALM on the palms and soles, this variant is more common among Asians and Blacks compared to Caucasians.[32]

Subungual melanoma may be first evident as a split nail, a swelling of part of the nail bed, an ulcerated area, or as a longitudinal black or brown streak in the nail bed, often associated with nail dystrophy. The latter is an important clue to alert the dermatologist of the possibility of this diagnosis, as nail dystrophy is not a feature of longitudinal melanonychia, which is a benign condition characterized by linear streaks of pigmentation. Involvement of the brown or black pigment on the surrounding periungual area is an important sign in this diagnosis and has been termed Hutchinson's sign. The presence of this sign should be taken to indicate melanoma until proven otherwise. Cases of amelanotic subungual melanoma resembling paronychia or traumatic subungual hematomas may pose a particular diagnostic challenge.

HISTOPATHOLOGY

The histopathological features of melanoma can at times be challenging and require considerable expertise. This is largely due to the fact that no single histological criterion definitely separates benign from malignant melanocytic lesions. Criteria for the diagnosis of melanoma include assessment of both architectural and cytological features. Histological features that are more often present in melanoma than in benign nevi, include: asymmetry, ulceration, cytological atypia, pagetoid spread in the epidermis, lack of maturation and dermal mitoses. Architectural characteristics include: an increased number of atypical melanocytes (singly or in nests), lateral extension of atypical melanocytes along the dermoepidermal junction, loss of maturation (normally the nuclei of the melanocytes appear smaller as they descend deeper into the dermis, referred to as maturation), extension of melanocytes along the epithelia of adnexal structures, variation in size and shape of nests of atypical melanocytes, and asymmetry of the overall lesion.

Cytological criteria include: large nuclei with prominent nucleoli, irregular shape of the nuclei, variable hyperchromatism, pleomorphism, and the presence of mitotic figures (their absence however does not rule out melanoma).

The growth and spread of melanoma has been described as occurring in an initial horizontal growth phase or radial growth phase, in which the melanoma is primarily confined to the epidermis, followed by a vertical growth phase, in which the melanoma acquires the ability to invade deeper into the dermis. Pagetoid spread is defined as the presence of atypical melanocytes, singly or in nests, above the basal layer and can be a clue to the diagnosis of melanoma.

It is important to note that, although in many cases the diagnosis of melanoma can be established on hematoxylin and eosin-stained sections, the use of immunohistochemistry can be valuable in certain cases where doubt exists. This technique uses the expression of certain melanocytic markers or melanoma-associated antigens. These markers include S100, MART-I (also called Melan-A), Tyrosinase, NKIC3, HMB-45 (also known as gp100) and MUM-1. Whilst these markers can help identify melanocytes and subsequently a possible diagnosis of melanoma, it is important to note that some markers, S100 as an example, are sensitive but not specific to melanocytes.[33]

STAGING AND MICROSTAGING OF MELANOMA

The staging of neoplasia, including melanoma, is a system which aims to describe the extent of the disease and typically includes three major areas of the disease; (a) localized to the primary site; (b) the presence of regional lymph node metastasis without evident distant metastases; and (c) the presence of distant metastasis.[34]

Staging systems are of clinical value as they categorize patients into groups whose prognosis and treatment differ significantly from one another.

The definitions of clinical versus pathologic staging depend upon whether the regional lymph nodes are staged by clinical/radiographic imaging or by pathological evaluation. In cases where no histology (other than that of the primary melanoma), either through (sentinel) lymph node biopsy or lymphadenectomy, of the node is performed, the staging then is termed "clinical". Acquiring pathological nodal or visceral histology as parameters for the pathological staging gives far greater accuracy in defining distinctive prognostic subgroups, in comparison to clinical staging alone.

Stages I and II require histopathological features of the primary tumor, whereas pathological stages III and IV require histopathological examinations of the involved lymph nodes and distant metastases. Certain specific histopathological features of melanoma impact on the overall prognosis and these are considered in the following paragraphs:

Breslow Thickness

Breslow thickness (BT) was first introduced by Breslow in 1970.[35] It is a method of measuring the tumor thickness in millimeters from the top of the granular layer to the deepest tumor cell. This is the strongest prognostic variable for melanoma in the primary lesion.[36] Current staging, based on the American Joint Committee on Cancer (AJCC), divides BT to those of less than or equal to 1.0 mm, between 1.01–2.0 mm, between 2.01–4.0 mm and more than 4.0 mm.

In a useful scheme based on Breslow's work, "low-risk" patients are those with tumors less than 0.76 mm in greatest thickness.[35] Patients with tumors having BT ranging between 0.76–1.50 mm in greatest thickness may be designated as "low intermediate risk", whereas the tumors between 1.5–3.99 mm BT are designated as "high intermediate risk", the tumors thicker than 4 mm are at very high-risk for local recurrence(s) as well as metastases.[35,37]

Ulceration

Ulceration of the primary melanoma is associated with an unfavorable survival prognosis. In a population-based study, the survival rate dropped from 91.6% in the non-ulcerated group to 66.2% in the ulcerated group.[38] It is important to note that ulceration in this context implies full thickness loss of the epidermis with reactive changes which include a fibrinous exudate and attenuation or acanthosis of the adjacent epidermis. These features help distinguish true ulceration from epidermal erosions that may represent a biopsy or preparation artefact.

Mitotic Rate Count

Mitotic rate count was introduced in the year 2008 in revised AJCC melanoma guidelines and is considered to be a powerful predictor of survival, particularly in thin tumors, along with BT, sentinel lymph node involvement, and age.[39,40]

The recommended approach is to find an area deemed to be a "hot spot" and then count the mitoses in that field and finally extend this to adjacent fields until an area corresponding to 1 mm² is assessed. If no "hot spot" can be found and mitoses are sparse and randomly scattered throughout the lesion, then a representative mitosis is chosen and, beginning with that field, the count is then extended to adjacent fields until an area corresponding to 1 mm² is assessed. The count is then expressed as the number of mitoses per mm². In the 7th AJCC melanoma staging guidelines, the presence of a single mitotic figure upgrades the tumor from stage la to lb.

Regression

Regression is most often confined to the radial growth phase, and is likely to occur as a consequence of lesional cell destruction by cytotoxic T cells. In most cases however, the disappearance is not complete and is paradoxical. Some studies have shown that the presence of partial regression may correlate to poorer prognosis and increased risk for metastasis.[41]

Tumor-Infiltrating Lymphocytes

Tumor-infiltrating lymphocytes constitute the host inflammatory response to melanoma and this is a diagnostically important microscopic feature; however it remains unclear as to whether this is associated with a prognostic outcome.[42] This reaction pattern can either be brisk (a dense band of lymphocytes among tumor cells across the entire base, or throughout the tumor), non-brisk, or absent.

Tumor (Micro) Satellites

Tumor (micro) satellites are discrete foci of tumor in the connective tissue (separated by at least 0.3 mm of normal collagen), discontinuous from the main tumor, and are considered to most likely represent locoregional metastases.[43] The presence of this microscopic feature in the primary tumor upgrades the staging to at least stage III (in the absence of distant metastasis which would define stage IV). Their presence is therefore of prognostic importance and is associated with a worse outcome.

DIAGNOSTIC METHODS IN MELANOMA

Early diagnosis of melanoma is essential in decreasing morbidity and mortality and therefore any suspicion of melanoma should be dealt with promptly. Clinical examination carried out visually by a trained dermatologist only leads to the correct diagnosis in around two-thirds of the cases. Accuracy can be further increased by the use of aids such as serial photography, dermoscopy, and confocal microscopy.[44] Histopathological diagnoses remains the "gold standard" in confirming or ruling out melanoma and should be used for all suspicious nevi. The accepted recommendations are to excise the entire suspected nevus with a 2 mm margin for initial histological assessment.[45-47] Punch biopsies should be avoided due to the risk of sampling error. Incisional biopsies may be performed in selected cases of LM and in suspicious areas of giant congenital nevi, but this requires an expert opinion and assessment to avoid misdiagnosis. The author has performed a study of the biopsy techniques and outcomes in LM, and found that those who underwent punch biopsies had a high percentage of sampling error, cases where the correct diagnosis was shown to be LMM upon excision followed by excisional biopsy.[48] None of the larger incisional biopsies showed any sampling error, findings that further demonstrate the risk of sampling error and misdiagnosis in punch biopsies of pigmented lesions. Once the diagnosis of melanoma has been confirmed histologically following excisional biopsy, further wide excision should take place, with the margins required depending (largely) on the BT of the primary tumor.

PROGNOSIS

The prognosis of a patient with melanoma is largely dependent on the stage at the time of diagnosis (Table 1). As stated previously, early detection is essential in melanoma and the prognosis for thin melanomas with no locoregional metastasis is generally good. The local recurrence (as defined by any recurrence within 2 cm of the excisional surgical scar of a primary melanoma) rate is estimated to be approximately 4%; this percentage being greater in either thicker or ulcerated tumors or where the location of the primary melanoma is on the head or neck. This recurrence concept differs from that of a "second primary melanoma" which occurs in 3--4% in patients with a primary melanoma. The risk of local recurrence is however greatly increased in patients with the atypical nevus syndrome, multiple primaries, or the presence of a germline mutation.

Table 1: Approximate melanoma 5- and 10-year survival rates.

	*5-year survival**	*10-year survival**
Stage IA	97%	95%
Stage IB	92%	86%
Stage IIA	81%	67%
Stage IIB	70%	57%
Stage IIC	53%	40%
Stage IIIA	78%	68%
Stage IIIB	59%	43%
Stage IIIC	40%	24%
Stage IV	15–20%	10–15%

**Adapted from* Balch et al[49]

Stage III melanoma patients are a heterogeneous group with respect to both their risk of distant metastases and their melanoma-specific mortality. The 5-year survival rates range from 82%, for patients with non-ulcerated melanomas, who had a single clinically occult nodal metastasis, to 29%, for patients with ulcerated primary melanomas and greater than 4 nodal macrometastases (Table 2).[50] Major prognostic factors in this group are the number of metastatic lymph nodes and the tumor burden. Tumor burden is likely to be lower where the nodal metastases are clinically occult (as detected by sentinel or elective lymph node dissection) than where they are clinically palpable. The prognosis in stage IV melanoma is generally very poor and the major prognostic factor is the site of distant metastases, with a poorer prognosis for visceral than for non-visceral (e.g. skin and distant lymph nodes) metastases, however the newer systemic therapies have improved these prognoses.[49]

SURGICAL MANAGEMENT

Surgical excision is the treatment of choice for the primary cutaneous lesions of melanoma and should result in a high cure rate if performed at an early stage. It is the only currently available firmly established curative treatment in melanoma. Elliptical excision of the lesion with primary closure should be performed. The fundamental issue is the removal of an appropriate margin of normal skin to minimize the important complication of tumor persistence and recurrence. Lack of adequate surgical margins can result in local recurrence, due to the persistence of malignant cells from the primary lesion, or as a result of microscopic satellites that exist beyond the margins of excision. The depth of the therapeutic excision has conventionally been to the muscle fascia or deeper, to reduce risk of local recurrence.

Lateral surgical excision margins for melanoma depend on the BT and are based on numerous multicentered trials.[51-57] Evidence from currently-available data show increased overall survival in favor of wide excision and this should therefore be implemented in all cases of melanoma following the initial excision of the lesion with narrow (usually 2 mm) margins.[58]

Current practice is to excise melanoma in situ and LM with at least 5 mm margin.[47] This is, however, not supported by evidence through randomized clinical trials but is more a consensus of experts in the field.

Table 2: Five-year survival rates for patients with stage III disease stratified by number of metastatic nodes, primary tumor ulceration, and nodal tumor burden.

Primary tumor ulceration	*Number of nodal micrometastases*			*Number of nodal macrometastases*		
	1	*2–3*	*≥4*	*1*	*2–3*	*≥4*
Absent	82%	73%	38%	52%	47%	45%
Present	57%	54%	34%	49%	38%	29%

Adapted from Balch et al.[50]

In cases of melanoma with a BT of up to 1 mm, a 1 cm margin is required and this is supported by data from three randomized controlled trials.[51] In melanoma cases with a BT between 1.01–2.00 mm, four randomized controlled trials have taken place;[51-54] however, only one trial compared 1 cm margin against a larger margin and therefore not enough evidence exists on the long-term outcome of 1 cm versus 2 cm but the general consensus from the available data (other trials compared 2 cm vs. greater margins) is that a 2 cm margin is preferable if technically possible.

In melanomas with a BT between 2.01–4.00 mm, the current evidence stems from two trials comparing 2 cm versus 4 cm margins and 1 cm versus 3 cm margins.[52-56] Results from the latter trial showed significantly higher rates of locoregional recurrences in patients treated with 1 cm margins, with subsequent reduction in melanoma-specific survival. The data from the trial comparing 2 cm versus 4 cm margins showed no difference in local recurrence, and therefore the overall consensus is that, from this group of patients, a minimum of 2 cm margin is required, although 3 cm margins are equally appropriate.[55-60]

In melanomas greater than 4 mm, the risk of local recurrence and distant metastasis is estimated to be more than 50% and therefore adequate surgical excision is required to minimize this risk. Currently, there is only one trial in this group comparing 1 cm against 3 cm margins with the results showing a significant increase in local recurrence in the 1 cm group.[56] As there are no data available to support margins less than 3 cm being as effective, the available evidence can only suggests a margin of 3 cm in this group.

Sentinel Lymph Node Biopsy

Melanoma predominately metastasises via the lymphatic system with patients developing nodal metastases.

Historically, treatment involved wide local excision and elective lymph node dissection (ELND), where regional lymph nodes were removed. Subsequent studies, however, demonstrated no survival benefit from ELND, in comparison with observation and subsequent lymph node dissection for clinically apparent disease.[61-63]

Thin melanomas are less likely to metastasise via the lymphatic system, while many thick melanomas have already developed distant metastases. This risk of lymph node involvement in thin melanomas is generally accepted to be below 5%, and this is particularly true for those of BT <0.75 mm without a high mitotic rate or ulceration.[64-66] Overall the rate of nodal metastasis in melanoma is approximately 20%, rising to 40% in thick melanomas.[67]

Clinical examination and, to a lesser degree, ultrasonography, are poorly sensitive tools to detect early nodal involvement. There was need for a sensitive tool to select the minority of patients with nodal involvement who would benefit from lymphadenectomy and avoid the cost and complications of the procedure in the remainder.

The technique of lymphatic mapping and sentinel lymph node biopsy was first proposed in the 1980s as a procedure for identifying patients with clinical stage I and II melanoma who have microscopic disease, who would benefit from lymphadenectomy.[68] The rationale for this approach is the concept that different regions in the skin have specific patterns of lymphatic drainage to the regional lymph nodes and that, for a given region of the skin, there is at least one specific lymph node that is the "sentinel" node among the regional lymph nodes to which cutaneous afferent lymphatic vessels drain first. The sentinel node is the most likely first site of metastasis and therefore, if this is negative histologically (i.e. free from melanoma deposits), then the remaining lymph nodes in the basin are unlikely to contain metastatic disease.

Locating the sentinel node is achieved through injection of radiolabeled colloids and blue dyes. These can be used singly or preferably in conjunction. Injection is into the dermis at the site of the primary melanoma. Uptake is detected either visually or with a gamma probe, and the affected node (or nodes) removed for histological examination. In 1992, a seminal paper was published demonstrating this procedure to be an accurate means of assessing the presence or absence of microscopic nodal disease with a false-negative rate of less than 1%.[69]

The goals of sentinel node biopsy include accurate staging, enhanced disease-free survival and improved survival. It is intended to identify patients with clinically node-negative disease who in fact have microscopic metastases. The procedure is also intended to identify patients with pathologically node-negative disease for whom additional treatment may not be indicated.[66,69,70]

To date, the effect of sentinel lymph node biopsy and complete lymph node dissection on survival remains controversial. The landmark Multicenter Selective Lymphadenectomy Trial I (MSLT I) was the first and largest randomized trial, to date, to evaluate the potential survival benefit of this procedure.[71] This multinational trial recruited over 2000 patients who were followed for 10 years, with the final report published in 2014.[67]

MSLT I examined whether SNLB with immediate completion lymphadenectomy (CLD) if positive provided better outcomes than observation and CLD when nodal disease was clinically detected. This study confirmed SLNB to be the most powerful prognostic factor for disease recurrence (HR 2.64) and death from melanoma (HR 2.40). In patients with intermediate-thickness melanoma (BT 1.2–3.5 mm) the 10-year survival rates were 62.1% for those with positive nodes and 85.1% for those with tumor-free nodes (p <0.001).[67]

The disease-specific survival rate is defined as the percentage of people in a study or treatment group who have not died from a specific disease, but not other causes, in a defined period of time. MSLT I demonstrated that the 10-year disease-specific survival rate was not significantly different between the biopsy and observation arms in both intermediate thickness (81.4% vs 78.3%, p = 0.18) and thick melanomas (58.9% vs 64.4%, $p = 0.56$). Within the subgroup of patients who had nodal metastases, latent analysis was, somewhat controversially, performed. This post-hoc analysis reported an increased 10-year melanoma-specific survival with SLNB (62.1 vs 41.5 $p = 0.006$); no difference was found with thick melanomas (BT >3.5 mm). The issue of whether sentinel lymph node biopsy provides a survival benefit to certain subgroups of patients remains a matter of continuous debate, which, given the size and cost of this study may not be answered for some time. Complication rates were not given in the final report; however, a recent systematic review reported overall complication rates from SLNB as 11.3%. Common complications included seroma (5.1%), infection (2.9%), lymphedema (1.3%), hematoma (0.5%) and nerve injury (0.3%).[72]

MSLT I also demonstrated an increased disease-free survival in the SLNB arm in both intermediate and thick melanomas. Survival rates in patients who developed locoregional recurrence following a negative biopsy were similar to those in the observation arm.

The rates of lymphedema appear lower, in patients receiving "early" CLD following positive SLN, than in patients treated with "late" CLD following observation and clinical recurrence (20.4% vs 12.4% $p = 0.04$). Late CLD was also associated with a greater number of positive nodes and a longer length of hospitalization, but there was no difference in acute morbidity.[73]

Current thinking and practice, largely based from the MSLT I trial and other studies, is that sentinel lymph node biopsy should be offered to patients with BT of 0.76–4.0mm.[49,66,74-77] The procedure is therefore primarily intended to be used as a prognostic tool for staging the patient.

Primary tumors with BT greater than 4 mm have a very high percentage of distant metastases with around a quarter demonstrating direct distant metastases not involving the draining lymph node basin.[78] SLNB is unlikely to be of benefit in this subgroup of patients.

Details of the required margins as well as considerations for SLNB can be found in Table 3.

A further trial MSLT, II is due to complete in 2022. This involves patients who have all had positive SLNB. The study seeks to assess whether there is additional benefit to immediate CLD in comparison with observation and CLD for clinically recurrent disease, as most patients will only present with micrometastases in the sentinel nodes.[79]

Table 3: Recommended excision margins and SLNB.

Breslow thickness	Recommended surgical excision margins	Sentinel lymph node biopsy
Less than 1 mm	1 cm	Not recommended*
1–2 mm	2 cm	Recommended
2–4 mm	2 cm	Recommended
Greater than 4 mm	At least 2 cm (3 cm if surgically possible)	Not recommended

*Consider sentinel lymph node biopsy if Breslow thickness is greater or equal to 0.76 mm and ulceration or mitotic figures are present.

MEDICAL MANAGEMENT OF ADVANCED MELANOMA

Melanoma with dissemination to distant sites and visceral organs (stage IV) was, with the exception of rare cases of surgery for oligometastatic disease, almost invariably incurable, with a median survival time of 9 months.[49]

Adjuvant medical management is indicated in both intermediate and high-risk melanoma (stages IIb and III) and in particular where lymph node micrometastases or metastases are found. Stage IV melanoma normally requires medical management.

Less than a decade ago medical treatments in melanoma were restricted to non-targeted treatments including cytotoxic chemotherapy, radiotherapy and cytokine immunotherapy. Huge efforts in both clinical and scientific research have, since 2011, begun to result in new therapies that can alter the course of the disease.[78,80,81]

Melanoma shows a high degree of biological diversity with activating mutations having been demonstrated as arising from many genes including *BRAF*, *NRAS*, *KIT*, *GNAQ*, and *GNA11*. Where the systemic therapy is targeted on the tumor cells rather than the immune cells, this makes it appropriate to identify the presence of relevant mutations before commencing targeted therapies.[82]

In order to understand these diverse therapeutic options, which continue to evolve, it is important to understand the various pathways involved in the initiation and proliferation of the cancer. Immunotherapy acts on the ability of the host immune system to destroy cancer cells. It is a term that encompasses a spectrum of therapeutic approaches that range from nonspecific immune stimulation to precisely targeted modalities.

These newly approved therapies, for the treatment of advanced and metastatic melanoma, fall into two main categories: targeted molecular therapies which inhibit tumor pathways, and checkpoint inhibitor immunotherapies.[83] These new therapies represent a significant improvement. In a minority of patients, and particularly with the immunotherapies, they can lead to durable response. Further progress may require a deeper understanding of the mechanisms of resistance, particularly to the targeted molecular therapies.[83-85]

When pembrolizumab was approved in September 2014, the FDA announcement included the observations that it was "the sixth new melanoma treatment approved since 2011, a result of promising advances in melanoma research" and "Many of these treatments have different mechanisms of action and bring new options to patients with melanoma".

Systemic Therapy

Prior to the advent of targeted and immune therapies for advanced melanoma, the standard systemic treatment was limited to chemotherapy, and, in selected patients, the cytokine interleukin-2; the only other approved systemic treatment in this era was interferon-α.[86] This limited choice of inadequate treatments had persisted for many years. Dacarbazine was the benchmark standard systematic therapy, in spite of it never having been shown to be superior to the best supportive care in a randomized control trial.[86] Significant improvements in therapy for metastatic melanoma have been made recently, but these treatments, like their precursors, are associated with significant adverse events, and managing these incurs substantial costs.[87]

Cytotoxic Chemotherapy

The treatment of metastatic melanoma by standard chemotherapy to target neoplastic cells has been widely used for many years and trialed in melanoma patients, with overall poor results. In the light of recent successes using targeted and immune therapies for advanced melanoma, it is now reasonable to question whether chemotherapy still represents a valid treatment option.[86]

Dacarbazine

From its approval in 1976, dacarbazine (DTIC) remained for 22 years the only first-line treatment for advanced melanoma, even though it showed only a 10–20% of overall response rate in phase I and II trials and showed no clear overall survival (OS) benefits.[88] Although improved results in combination with immune checkpoint inhibitors have been shown in trials, dacarbazine has been shown to be inferior in head-to-head trials with newer therapies and its place in the armamentarium against melanoma is increasingly to be questioned.[86,89]

Other Chemotherapy Regimens

Trials of multidrug chemotherapy-based combinations showed themselves to be more toxic than single-agent dacarbazine, without improving overall survival. A common chemotherapy regimen previously used in metastatic melanoma combines cisplatin, vinblastine, and dacarbazine (CVD) but has shown no significant improvement compared with dacarbazine. Other studied combinations include carboplatin and paclitaxel, but no clear improvement has yet been shown.

Albumin-bound paclitaxel, nab-paclitaxel, has shown some promise with a recently-reported phase III trial. This trial demonstrated improved progression-free survival in comparison with dacarbazine, but no statistically significant difference in overall survival. Side effects of neuropathy and neutropenia were more common with nab-paclitaxel, and thrombocytopenia more frequent with dacarbazine.[89]

Cytokine Immunotherapy

Cytokines are released by immune cells, keratinocytes, and melanoma cells and can diminish or augment various immune responses. They nonspecifically stimulate or repress the immune system and increase the effectiveness of the host's natural ability to prevent tumor progression and overcome tumor-derived immunosuppression.

Interferon

The original approved treatment in the setting of adjuvant therapy, that is surgically resected primary melanoma with resection of lymph nodes if positive, was interferon-α indicated for high-risk group melanoma patients (stages IIb and III)[90,91]

Only modest overall activity of adjuvant interferon (INF) therapy was seen in 25 years of trials.[92] However, melanoma patients have experienced durable therapeutic benefits with immunotherapy and high-dose interferon alfa-2b (INF-α2b) for one year and pegylated (PEG) INF-α2b for five years have been approved as adjuvant therapies.[93]

In 2011, PEG INF-α2b was approved for adjuvant use in melanoma patients who had metastases in lymph nodes (stage III melanoma) and were within twelve weeks of surgical resection of the primary melanoma. This was based on a trial which showed a marginally significant improvement in relapse-free survival with treatment, compared with the observation arm. There was however no difference in overall or distant metastasis-free survival, and the treatment was associated with serious adverse effects; patients with ulcerated melanoma and lower disease burden had the greatest benefit.[92]

Interleukin-2

Interleukin-2 (IL-2), discovered in 1976, is an immune-modulating glycoprotein produced by T lymphocytes. IL-2 stimulates T cell proliferation, inducing activation of cytotoxic T lymphocytes and NK cells.[42] Systemic IL-2 has been FDA-approved for the treatment of metastatic melanoma since 1998, but its response rates have been low (10–15%) at the cost of high morbidity.[94]

Checkpoint Inhibitors (Immunostimulatory Monoclonal Antibodies)

What is the mechanism of action of checkpoint inhibitors? Simply put, T cells can destroy some melanoma cells but other melanoma cells can evolve mechanisms to protect themselves from T cells. One method of doing this is to adopt one of the mechanisms by which host cells protect themselves from attack by host T cells. The cells do this by using checkpoints to stop the T cells from attacking. Immune checkpoints are molecules in the immune system which either increase a signal (co-stimulatory molecules) or decrease a signal. Many cancers, including melanoma, protect themselves by decreasing the signal which would otherwise activate T cell responses. It was realized that if these checkpoint molecules, which are expressed by tumor cells and which thereby decrease the immune system's attack on the tumor, could be blockaded, then the immune system would be freed to attack the tumor. Advanced melanoma was chosen as a test for these new blockading drugs, known as checkpoint inhibitors, for several reasons including that skin cancers are intrinsically more accessible and therefore easier to study and also that melanomas often show regression as lighter markings within the melanoma where the immune system has successfully attacked the melanoma. This approach was shown to work in advanced melanoma and is being studied for use in other cancers. The earliest successful drugs were ipilimumab and pembrolizumab which blockaded different checkpoints, namely CTLA-4 and PD-1 and these are explained in more detail below. Checkpoint inhibitor therapy is proceeding apace, with programmed cell death (PD)-1 protein (and its ligands) inhibitors adding to, and improving upon, the breakthrough with ipilimumab, an anti-CTLA-4 antibody. Combinations of the two checkpoint inhibitor types, CTLA-4 and PD-1, show synergistic or additive effects.

Immunotherapy has changed the treatment of metastatic melanoma and improved patient outcomes. Ipilimumab, an inhibitor of cytotoxic T lymphocyte antigen-4 (CTLA-4), was the first approved (in 2011) immune checkpoint inhibitor and demonstrated improved survival in advanced melanoma. More recently, other immune checkpoint inhibitors, including the programmed death-1 (PD-1) inhibitors pembrolizumab and nivolumab (both approved in 2014), have demonstrated efficacy in locally advanced unresectable and metastatic melanoma.[95]

CTLA-4 Checkpoint Inhibitors

Immune checkpoint inhibitors target lymphocytes (T cells) rather than cancer cells, and evoke an anti-tumor immune reaction. Since the activated lymphocytes recognize various tumor-associated antigens, including a mutated antigen, immune checkpoint inhibitors exhibit continuous long-term effectiveness, despite the generation of genetic mutations in cancer cells. Activated and regulatory T cells express the surface protein CTLA-4, which negatively regulates T cell function when it binds to B7 proteins on antigen presenting cells. This effectively induces tolerance, and this binding is with greater affinity than with its alternative, CD28, which is also expressed on the T cell and which, when bound to the B7, positively regulates the T cell. CTLA-4 is upregulated in malignancy thereby sparing the tumor cells expressing it from T cell responses. The aim of blockading the CTLA-4 is to break this mechanism of immune tolerance to the tumor cells and to allow activation of the T cells allowing a prolonged tumor-specific attack. As well as this desirable effect, the breaking of tolerance can also affect antigens on normal host tissues leading to side-effects, for example, the gastrointestinal tract or the endocrine glands or dermatological toxicities, the latter usually being the first to occur.[96] Various autoimmune phenomena have also been observed in patients treated with this drug, most notably vitiligo.

Ipilimumab is a fully human, IgG1 monoclonal antagonist antibody to CTLA-4. Being a CTLA-4 antibody, ipilimumab can act to potentiate an antitumor T cell response by blocking the CTLA-4 on the T cell. This allows the antigen-presenting cell to achieve co-stimulatory binding to CD28 which CTLA-4, if not blocked by ipilimumab, would prevent.[96] In systemic therapies for metastatic melanoma, ipilimumab was the first to be shown to improve outcome survival.[97,98] Survival data, from a pooled analysis of trials, showed ipilimumab to have a response rate similar to chemotherapy (10–15%) but these responses were more durable with ipilimumab, with 20% of patients surviving beyond 5 years.[86,99] A phase III trial showed that, with completely resected high-risk stage III melanoma, recurrence-free survival was significantly improved with adjuvant ipilimumab, but the risk-benefit ratio requires further assessment.[100] Indeed the immune-related adverse events associated with ipilimumab stem from its effect on T cell function, and its side-effect profile, which differs considerably from both chemotherapies and molecular-targeted therapies, requires particular attention and early recognition.[96]

PD-1 Checkpoint Inhibitors

The programmed cell death (PD-1) receptor is a receptor on the surface of T cells which binds to a ligand (PD-L1 or PD-L2) on the surface of normal cells, acting as a checkpoint, thus protecting the normal cells from being attacked by the T cells. Again, as the tumor cells can also express PD-L1 or PD-L2, and thereby avoid a T cell response, which would lead to their destruction. Blockading PD-1 or its ligands stops this checkpoint from frustrating the T cell response, and allows the T cell to be activated and proceed with a response, which eliminates the tumor. Both nivolumab and pembrolizumab are anti-PD-1 monoclonal antibodies, which act, as checkpoint inhibitors in the treatment of melanoma, by blocking the signals which would have otherwise prevented activated T cells from attacking the melanoma cells.

In a phase III study, among previously untreated patients who had metastatic melanoma but had no *BRAF* mutation (and hence would not be candidates for *BRAF* inhibitor therapy—see below), nivolumab was shown to be associated with significant improvements, in both overall and progression-free survival, compared with dacarbazine.[101]

Pembrolizumab targets the PD-1 receptor, thereby blockading a protective mechanism on the cancer cells allowing the immune system to be activated to destroy them. It was approved in 2014 as the first anti-PD1 drug and is intended for use following treatment with ipilimumab, or after treatment with ipilimumab and a *BRAF* inhibitor (see below), in advanced melanoma patients who carry a *BRAF* mutation.

Targeted Molecular Therapies

These novel therapies have emerged as a result of our better understanding of the molecular biology of melanoma and the pathways that are involved in its pathogenesis, a process that leads to distinct deregulation of the cell cycle growth and division.

An important pathway in melanoma is the mitogen-activated protein kinase (MAPK) pathway, also known as the extracellular signal-regulated kinase (ERK) pathway. Activation of MAPK through the RAS-RAF-MEK signaling pathway leads to activation and proliferation of cells.[80] Targeted therapies are aimed at interrupting this signaling pathway leading to its inhibition.

Activating mutations in the serine-threonine kinase *B-RAF (BRAF)* are found in 50% of advanced melanoma patients. These mutations result in constitutive activation of the mitogen-activated protein kinase (MAPK) pathway.[102,103] There has been a rapid expansion of targeted (as well as immune) therapies for melanoma following the discovery of the *BRAF* V600E mutation in approximately 50% of melanoma patients, and the clarification of its role in melanoma pathophysiology. These *BRAF* V600 mutant patients can potentially benefit from mitogen-activated protein kinase (MAPK) pathway inhibitor therapy. The range of such treatments has rapidly expanded. Selective *BRAF* inhibitors including vemurafenib (approved in 2011), dabrafenib (approved in 2013); and MEK inhibitor trametinib (approved in 2013), have extended the potential of molecular targeted therapy for advanced melanoma, demonstrating a significant increase in overall survival rate and long-term benefits in multiple large clinical trials. Furthermore, several new agents and novel therapies are currently under phase III clinical trials with the possibility of approval in the near future.

These new treatments have been heralded as the start of a golden era in oncology and are providing significant survival improvements. In the meantime, new challenges for clinicians have also started to emerge.[88] Certainly, inhibition of the mutated *BRAF* pathway is having a large impact on the management of metastatic melanoma patients, but challenges remain, such as how to combine them with other treatments, and how to sequence the different treatment modalities.[104] Other challenges are those of increasing the numbers of complete responders, delaying the development of resistance, minimising adverse effects, and doing all this at a bearable price. Increasingly the genetic profiles of the patient's tumor will allow clinicians to select treatments with optimum efficacy and toxicities, with the eventual aim of turning metastatic melanoma into a chronic condition, with survival duration measured in years rather than months.[104] It must be borne in mind however, that these targeted molecular therapies for melanoma have inhibited disease progression, but have not been shown to markedly improve melanoma survival; they do however contribute to the increased understanding of melanoma development and progression and are a hopeful step along the road to disease control by therapy.[105]

Dermatological side effects are extremely common with *BRAF* and *MEK* inhibitors, commonly involving the epidermis and adnexal structures. Side effects are somewhat similar to germline mutations in RAS, and therefore these medications have been termed "RASopathic".[106] Frequent non-dermatological side effects include arthralgia, diarrhea and fatigue.

Approximately 20% of patients treated with vemurafenib develop SCC.[107] The initiating event in SCC formation is commonly RAS mutation, preferentially HRAS.[108] It has been reported that *BRAF* inhibition induces the development of SCC, through paradoxical activation of MAPK in keratinocytes with pre-existing RAS mutations.[107]

MEK inhibitors are not associated with SCC and combination of *BRAF* and MEK inhibitors interestingly seem to reduce the common cutaneous side effects.

Other common dermatological reactions include maculopapular and follicular generalized exanthames, alopecia, keratosis pilaris and hyperkeratosis. Photosensitivity is observed in approximately half of patients taking vemurafenib and appears specific to this medication, being rarely found in association with dabrafenib.[109,110] Papulopustular reactions have been reported with MEK inhibitors, typically 2–6 weeks following commencement.[111]

BRAF Inhibitors

Vemurafenib, a tyrosine kinase inhibitor of V600 mutated *BRAF*, was the first molecular targeted therapy to be approved (in 2011) for advanced melanoma. Vemurafenib is a powerful inhibitor of mutated *BRAF*. Vemurafenib is used to treat patients shown by mutational analysis to have V600 mutated *BRAF*, and showed a 50% response rate and a significant decrease in the relative risk of death, compared with dacarbazine (hazard ratio 0.37).[96,112] Vemurafenib is a powerful inhibitor of mutated *BRAF*.

Dabrafenib is a reversible, ATP-competitive inhibitor that selectively inhibits BRAF kinase, with an almost identical overall response rate and progression-free survival benefit to that seen with vemurafenib.[113,114] A phase III trial showed that patients treated with dabrafenib had significantly improved progression-free survival compared with dacarbazine.[110]

MEK Inhibitors

BRAF is a constituent of the MAP kinase (MAPK) signal-transduction pathway. Activating mutations are found in about half of all melanomas. The most common *BRAF* mutation is the V600E and the second most common is the V600K. Together these two mutations account for 95% of the *BRAF* mutations found. Activated *BRAF* phosphorylates and activates mitogen-activated protein kinase (MEK) proteins (MEK1 and MEK2) which then activate downstream MAP kinases which control tumor proliferation and survival.[115]

Trametinib, a MEK inhibitor, in a phase III trial, showed increased rates of progression-free and overall survival in patients with *BRAF*-mutated (V600E or V600K) metastatic melanoma, compared with chemotherapy.[115,116]

For *BRAF* V600 metastatic melanoma patients, combined treatment with *BRAF* and MEK inhibitors increased progression-free survival and objective response rate compared to monotherapy with *BRAF* inhibitors alone, and is now considered the standard of care treatment for these patients.[117]

Although this combination is seen to prevent the MAPK reactivation which can occur with monotherapy with *BRAF* inhibitors, these responses are not durable and further combinations with immunotherapy based on PD-1 blockade are being pursued.[117] A recent phase II trial of a dabrafenib-trametinib combination treatment, for *BRAF* inhibitor-refractory metastatic melanoma, showed no benefit, probably due to failure to inhibit the MAPK pathway, but it did show circulating *BRAF* V600 to be a promising early biomarker of clinical response.[118]

Cobimetinib was approved in November 2015 for the treatment of patients with unresectable or metastatic melanoma with a *BRAF* V600E or V600K mutation, in combination with vemurafenib. This approval was based on the demonstration of improved progression-free survival and overall survival in a phase III trial of patients with previously untreated, *BRAF* V600 mutation-positive, unresectable or metastatic melanoma.[119] Cobimetinib is not indicated for treatment of patients with wild-type *BRAF* melanoma. The most serious risks in patients receiving cobimetinib were new primary malignancies, hemorrhage, cardiomyopathy, severe dermatologic reactions, serous retinopathy and retinal vein occlusion, hepatotoxicity, rhabdomyolysis, and severe photosensitivity reactions.

KIT Inhibitors

The tyrosine kinase c-KIT (KIT) is necessary for melanocyte survival, and mutations in this gene are found in around one-third of mucosal and acral melanomas. KIT has also been shown to be frequently mutated or amplified in mucosal and chronically sun-damaged skin (CSD) melanomas. Mutant KIT signaling occurs in only 5–7% of melanomas overall, therefore this is much less than the approximately 50% *BRAF* V600 melanoma mutation frequency. KIT acts as an oncogene, driving melanoma cell proliferation, progression and migration through complex downstream signalling cascades.[82,120] A phase II trial of imatinib concluded that melanomas that arise on mucosal, acral, or CSD skin should be assessed for *KIT* mutations, but not if *KIT* is amplified only.[82]

INTRALESIONAL THERAPY

Oncolytic Virus Therapy

In addition to systemically delivered immunotherapies, intralesional therapies, such as talimogene laherparepvec (T-VEC), play an important role in the treatment of locoregionally advanced and metastatic melanoma.[95] This is a new immunotherapy using native or attenuated viruses to both destroy melanoma cells selectively, and also induce a systemic anti-tumor immune response. In addition to T-VEC, there are a number of other similar oncolytic viruses in clinical development, for example the Coxsackie virus A21.[121]

T-VEC represents a novel potential therapy for patients with metastatic melanoma. Responses in uninjected lesions provide validation of T-VEC-induced systemic immunotherapeutic effects against melanoma.[122,123]

T-VEC is the first oncolytic virus approved (October 2015), in the therapy of melanoma patients with injectable but non-resectable lesions in the skin and lymph nodes.[124] This provides a new treatment option and is potentially of use, especially for patients with limited disease. It is the first oncolytic virus to show a therapeutic benefit and has been approved following a phase III study in which it was well-tolerated and showed both a higher durable response rate (objective response lasting continuously for ≥6 months), and a longer median overall survival, particularly in untreated patients or those with stage IIIB, IIIC, or IVM1a disease.[125]

T-VEC is an oncolytic HSV-1 virus with deletion of its ICP47 gene, which enables antigen presentation and virus proliferation in melanoma cells. Its immune response is enhanced by replacing the genetic sequence for its neurovirulence factor ICP34.5, by that of the GM-CSF cytokine. It is designed to selectively replicate in tumors, infecting and destroying tumor cells, and additionally inducing immune responses against the tumor.

Intralesional therapy for metastatic melanoma has some advantages over systemic therapy as it allows for delivery of an increased concentration of the agent and reduced systemic exposure, thereby increasing local efficacy and limiting toxicity. This can also operate as an autologous vaccine to induce systemic immunity as the tumor contains the tumor antigens.[126] Until now, in spite of many attempts, few agents progressed to phase III trials. More recently, following the introduction of T-VEC, intralesional therapy is again being pursued due to its relatively good local response rates and tolerable adverse event profile. This may represent a treatment option in selected patients with unresectable, locally-advanced or metastatic melanoma.[126]

Vaccinations

The underlying principle is to use melanoma-associated antigens to stimulate the immune system, either by producing tumor-specific antibodies, or by stimulating effector T cells. Common melanoma-associated antigens are tyrosinase, glycoprotein 100 (gp100) and melanoma antigen recognized by T cells-1 (MART-1). Trials conducted with the use of vaccination using gp100 showed disappointing results.[127]

Stimulating an immune response against melanoma by the use of vaccines remains a challenge. A recent (December 2015) phase III trial involving peptide vaccination showed no significant improvement in relapse-free or overall survival in patients with high-risk resected melanoma.[128]

A study of the long-term outcomes of helper peptide vaccination for metastatic melanoma showed the vaccine (6 MHP) was associated with improved overall survival, but this would require confirmation by a randomized prospective trial.[129] The 6 MHP vaccine is a multipeptide vaccine, designed to induce helper T cells against melanocytic antigens, which has been shown to induce specific Th1-dominant $CD4^+$ T cell responses.

Based on the hypothesis that combining a melanoma vaccine with interleukin-2, an immune activating agent could improve efficacy, a trial was carried out comparing the peptide vaccine gp100 plus interleukin-2 with interleukin-2 alone.[130] The gp100 peptide vaccine showed improved progression-free survival and response rates in melanoma patients treated with high-dose interleukin-2.[130] There are indications that older patients mount immune responses to these vaccines with comparable survival outcomes to younger patients.[131]

Adoptive Cell Transfer

Melanomas express specific antigens that elicit T cell responses and this has encouraged the pursuit of both vaccine-based and adoptive T cell immunotherapy studies. Adoptive cell transfer in the context of melanoma is the concept of isolating peripheral T lymphocytes or tumor-infiltrating lymphocytes with reactivity toward tumor antigens, activating and expanding these cells, and reintroducing them into affected patients. Early trials had limited success, with the reinjected lymphocytes disappearing quickly from the peripheral circulation. Currently the use of adoptive cell transfer is limited to clinical trials. It has shown early signs of potential efficacy in a selected group of patients but no routine clinical treatments are yet available.

Isolated Limb Perfusion and Infusion

Isolated limb perfusion (ILP) is a treatment for regional metastatic melanoma by which higher doses of anticancer drugs (usually chemotherapy) can be used than would be tolerable systemically, often by a factor of 10 times higher. The chemotherapy agents are delivered only to the circulation of the limb involved. There is morbidity associated with ILP, with a limb loss rate of approximately 1% reported.[132] This technique, and the related, but simpler and minimally invasive, isolated limb infusion technique (ILI), have been used in selected patients with stage III unresectable melanoma. These are therapies for regional metastatic melanoma with prevalent intransit disease and are associated with high costs and long hospital stays. Successful randomized clinical trials, comparing ILP/ILI with alternative treatments, are not yet available.[133,134] A recent retrospective review of 203 patients with intransit melanoma found ILP to offer an improved overall response (80% vs 53% $p < 0.001$) but this did not translate into improved progression free survival nor overall survival.[135]

RADIOTHERAPY

Radiotherapy uses beams of high-energy *X*-rays, or sub-atomic particles, to damage DNA and thereby destroy quickly-dividing cancer cells.

The main indication for the use of radiotherapy in melanoma is for palliation.[136] Spread of melanoma to sites such as the brain and bones can cause pain, which can often be alleviated by radiotherapy.[137] A review of American patients with metastatic melanoma found 45% received radiation treatment.[133]

Radiation may be delivered to an entire organ, such as the brain, in several low doses or fractions. Alternatively high doses of targeted stereotactic radiation can be used to localized metastatic growths. General side effects of radiation therapy include skin irritation and fatigue, which often improve a few weeks following treatment. Specific local effects such as lymphedema, mucositis or dysphagia may occur.

Adjuvant radiotherapy for node-positive, stage 3 melanoma patients has been found to not improve overall survival.[138,139]

Radiotherapy can be performed when surgery is contraindicated. A recent literature review studied the use of radiotherapy as a primary treatment for LM in 537 patients with a median follow up period of 3 years. Recurrence occurred in 5% of patients with progression to LMM occurring in 1.4% of patients.[140]

Uncontrolled studies have reported improved local control following adjuvant radiotherapy.[141] Risk of complications and recurrence rates differ, dependent on the anatomic location of the nodal basin involved.[142] Complications include lymphedema and radiation dermatitis. A recent randomized trial demonstrated reduced risk of lymph node relapse (HR0.56, $p = 0.04$) but no difference in relapse-free survival or overall survival.[143]

Preclinical and clinical studies involving radiotherapy combined with treatments, particularly immunotherapy, show potential promise.[144,145]

CONCLUSION

- Melanoma represents around 10% of the cases of skin cancer, however at least two-thirds of skin cancer-associated deaths are attributed to melanoma.
- Ultraviolet (UV) radiation exposure is the main environmental risk factor for melanoma. Other risk factors include germline mutation in *CDKN2A*, a strong family history of melanoma, presence of atypical nevus syndrome and phenotypic characteristics such as red hair, multiple freckles and the tendency for sunburns.

- Superficial spreading, nodular, ALM and LMM are the clinical subtypes of melanoma and they can present with amelanotic variants.
- Histopathological features impacting the prognosis of melanoma include BT, mitotic rate count and the presence of ulceration, regression, tumor infiltrating lymphocytes or and tumor (micro) satellites.
- Surgical excision is the treatment of choice for the primary cutaneous melanoma and often curative in early melanoma.
- Sentinel lymph node status is the most powerful prognostic factor, however the procedure has not clearly demonstrated a survival advantage.
- Licensed checkpoint inhibitors and targeted molecular therapies represent a paradigm shift in the management of advanced melanoma, with checkpoint inhibitors leading to a lasting response in a minority of patients.
- Further treatments and combination treatments offer the hope of providing a substantial improvement to the prognosis of those with advanced melanoma.

REFERENCES

1. Urteaga O, Pack GT. On the antiquity of melanoma. Cancer 1966;19:607-10.
2. Carswell R. Pathological Anatomy: Illustrations of the Elementary Forms of Disease: Longman, Orme, Brown, Green and Longman. 1838.
3. Nikolaou V, Stratigos AJ. Emerging trends in the epidemiology of melanoma. Br J Dermatol. 2014;170:11-9.
4. Howlader N, Noone AM, Krapcho M, Miller D, Bishop K, Altekruse SF, et al (Eds). SEER Cancer Statistics Review, 1975-2013, National Cancer Institute. Bethesda, MD, http://seer.cancer.gov/csr/1975_2013/, based on November 2015 SEER data submission, posted to the SEER web site, April 2016.
5. Marks R. Epidemiology of melanoma. Clin Exp Dermatol. 2000;25:459-63.
6. Jones WO, Harman CR, Ng AK, et al. Incidence of malignant melanoma in Auckland, New Zealand: highest rates in the world. World J Surg. 1999;23:732-5.
7. Wang Y, Zhao Y, Ma S. Racial differences in six major subtypes of melanoma: descriptive epidemiology. BMC Cancer. 2016;16:691.
8. Trautmann F, Meier F, Seidler A, et al. Effects of the German skin cancer screening programme on melanoma incidence and indicators of disease severity. Br J Dermatol. 2016.
9. Youn J, Lee A, Lee Y. The effect of ultraviolet irradiation on epidermal melanocytes and the influence of sunscreen: A histochemical and ultrastructural study. Seoul J Med. 1990;31:253-62.
10. Viola MV, Houghton A, Munster EW. Solar cycles and malignant melanoma. Med Hypotheses, 1979;5:153-60.
11. Green A, Siskind V, Bain C, et al. Sunburn and malignant melanoma. Br J Cancer. 1985;51:393-7.
12. Bliss JM, Ford D, Swerdlow AJ, et al. Risk of cutaneous melanoma associated with pigmentation characteristics and freckling: systematic overview of 10 case-control studies. The International Melanoma Analysis Group (IMAGE). Int J Cancer. 1995;62:367-76.
13. Parkin M, Muir CS, Whelan SL, et al. Cancer Incidence in Five Continents, Vol. 6. Lyon: IARC; 1992.
14. Hery C, Tryggvadottir L, Sigurdsson T, et al. A melanoma epidemic in Iceland: possible influence of sunbed use. Am J Epidemiol. 2010;172:762-7.
15. International Agency for Research on Cancer Working Group on artificial ultraviolet l, skin c. The association of use of sunbeds with cutaneous malignant melanoma and other skin cancers: A systematic review. Int J Cancer. 2007; 120:1116-22.
16. Cust AE, Armstrong BK, Goumas C, et al. Sunbed use during adolescence and early adulthood is associated with increased risk of early-onset melanoma. Int J Cancer. 2011; 128:2425-35.
17. Stratigos AJ, Yang G, Dimisianos R, et al. Germline CDKN2A mutations among Greek patients with early-onset and multiple primary cutaneous melanoma. J Invest Dermatol. 2006;126:399-401.
18. Millikan RC, Hummer A, Begg C, et al. Polymorphisms in nucleotide excision repair genes and risk of multiple primary melanoma: the Genes Environment and Melanoma Study. Carcinogenesis. 2006;27:610-8.
19. Tucker MA, Goldstein AM. Melanoma etiology: where are we? Oncogene. 2003;22:3042-52.
20. Hayward NK. Genetics of melanoma predisposition. Oncogene. 2003;22:3053-62.
21. Goldstein AM, Tucker MA. Screening for CDKN2A mutations in hereditary melanoma. J Natl Cancer Inst. 1997;89:676-8.
22. Goldstein AM, Tucker MA. Genetic epidemiology of familial melanoma. Dermatol Clin. 1995;13:605-12.
23. Weismann K, Lorentzen HF. Dermoscopic color perspective. Arch Dermatol. 2006;142:1250.
24. Naveh HP, Rao UN, Butterfield LH. Melanoma-associated leukoderma-immunology in black and white? Pigment Cell Melanoma Res. 2013;26:796-804.
25. Clark WH Jr., Elder DE, Van Horn M. The biologic forms of malignant melanoma. Hum Pathol. 1986;17:443-50.
26. Baumel B, Eisner LS. Diagnosis and treatment of headache in the elderly. Med Clin North Am. 1991;75:661-75.
27. McKenna JK, Florell SR, Goldman GD, et al. Lentigo maligna/lentigo maligna melanoma: current state of diagnosis and treatment. Dermatol Surg. 2006;32:493-504.
28. Cormier JN, Xing Y, Ding M, et al. Ethnic differences among patients with cutaneous melanoma. Arch Intern Med. 2006; 166:1907-14.
29. Krementz ET, Sutherland CM, Carter RD, et al. Malignant melanoma in the American Black. Ann Surg. 1976;183: 533-42.
30. Madankumar R, Gumaste PV, Martires K, et al. Acral melanocytic lesions in the United States: Prevalence, awareness, and dermoscopic patterns in skin-of-color and non-Hispanic white patients. J Am Acad Dermatol. 2016;74: 724-30.
31. Milton GW, Shaw HM, McCarthy WH. Subungual malignant melanoma: a disease entity separate from other forms of cutaneous melanoma. Australas J Dermatol. 1985;26:61-4.
32. Jimbow K, Takahashi H, Miura S, et al. Biological behavior and natural course of acral malignant melanoma. Clinical and histologic features and prognosis of palmoplantar, subungual, and other acral malignant melanomas. Am J Dermatopathol. 1984;6:43-53.

33. Orchard G. Evaluation of melanocytic neoplasms: application of a pan-melanoma antibody cocktail. Br J Biomed Sci. 2002;59:196-202.
34. Beahrs OH, Myers MH, American Joint Committee on Cancer. Manual for Staging of Cancer, 2nd edition. Philadelphia: Lippincott. 1983:117-22.
35. Breslow A. Thickness, cross-sectional areas and depth of invasion in the prognosis of cutaneous melanoma. Ann Surg. 1970;172:902-8.
36. Ronan SG, Han MC, Das Gupta TK. Histologic prognostic indicators in cutaneous malignant melanoma. Semin Oncol. 1988;15:558-65.
37. Day CL Jr., Lew RA, Mihm MC Jr., et al. The natural break points for primary-tumor thickness in clinical Stage I melanoma. N Engl J Med. 1981;305:1155.
38. Barnhill RL, Fine JA, Roush GC, et al. Predicting five-year outcome for patients with cutaneous melanoma in a population-based study. Cancer. 1996;78:427-32.
39. Gimotty PA, Elder DE, Fraker DL, et al. Identification of high-risk patients among those diagnosed with thin cutaneous melanomas. J Clin Oncol. 2007;25:1129-34.
40. Francken AB, Shaw HM, Thompson JF, et al. The prognostic importance of tumor mitotic rate confirmed in 1317 patients with primary cutaneous melanoma and long follow-up. Ann Surg Oncol. 2004;11:426-33.
41. Clark WH Jr., Elder DE, Guerry Dt, et al. Model predicting survival in stage I melanoma based on tumor progression. J Natl Cancer Inst. 1989;81:1893-904.
42. Gimotty PA, Guerry D, Ming ME, et al. Thin primary cutaneous malignant melanoma: a prognostic tree for 10-year metastasis is more accurate than American Joint Committee on Cancer staging. J Clin Oncol. 2004;22: 3668-76.
43. Harrist TJ, Rigel DS, Day CL Jr., et al. "Microscopic satellites" are more highly associated with regional lymph node metastases than is primary melanoma thickness. Cancer. 1984;53:2183-7.
44. Feit NE, Dusza SW, Marghoob AA. Melanomas detected with the aid of total cutaneous photography. Br J Dermatol. 2004;150:706-14.
45. Lederman JS, Sober AJ. Does biopsy type influence survival in clinical stage I cutaneous melanoma? J Am Acad Dermatol. 1985;13:983-7.
46. Lees VC, Briggs JC. Effect of initial biopsy procedure on prognosis in Stage 1 invasive cutaneous malignant melanoma: review of 1086 patients. Br J Surg. 1991;78: 1108-10.
47. Marsden JR, Newton-Bishop JA, Burrows L, et al. Revised UK guidelines for the management of cutaneous melanoma 2010. Br J Dermatol. 2010;163:238-56.
48. Al-Niaimi F, Jury CS, McLaughlin S, et al. Review of management and outcome in 65 patients with lentigo maligna. Br J Dermatol. 2009;160:211-3.
49. Balch CM, Gershenwald JE, Soong SJ, et al. Final version of 2009 AJCC melanoma staging and classification. J Clin Oncol. 2009;27:6199-206.
50. Balch CM, Gershenwald JE, Soong SJ, et al. Multivariate analysis of prognostic factors among 2,313 patients with stage III melanoma: comparison of nodal micrometastases versus macrometastases. J Clin Oncol. 2010;28:2452-9.
51. Veronesi U, Cascinelli N, Adamus J, et al. Thin stage I primary cutaneous malignant melanoma. Comparison of excision with margins of 1 or 3 cm. N Engl J Med. 1988;318: 1159-62.
52. Balch CM, Urist MM, Karakousis CP, et al. Efficacy of 2-cm surgical margins for intermediate-thickness melanomas (1 to 4 mm). Results of a multi-institutional randomized surgical trial. Ann Surg. 1993;218:262-7; discussion 7-9.
53. Cohn-Cedermark G, Rutqvist LE, Andersson R, et al. Long term results of a randomized study by the Swedish Melanoma Study Group on 2-cm versus 5-cm resection margins for patients with cutaneous melanoma with a tumor thickness of 0.8-2.0 mm. Cancer. 2000;89:1495-501.
54. Khayat D, Rixe O, Martin G, et al. Surgical margins in cutaneous melanoma (2 cm versus 5 cm for lesions measuring less than 2.1-mm thick). Cancer. 2003;97:1941-6.
55. Balch CM, Soong SJ, Smith T, et al. Long-term results of a prospective surgical trial comparing 2 cm vs. 4 cm excision margins for 740 patients with 1-4 mm melanomas. Ann Surg Oncol. 2001;8:101-8.
56. Thomas JM, Newton-Bishop J, A'Hern R, et al. Excision margins in high-risk malignant melanoma. N Engl J Med. 2004;350:757-66.
57. NIH Consensus conference. Diagnosis and treatment of early melanoma. JAMA. 1992;268:1314-9.
58. Sladden MJ, Balch C, Barzilai DA, et al. Surgical excision margins for primary cutaneous melanoma. Cochrane Database Syst Rev 2009: CD004835.
59. Veronesi U, Cascinelli N. Narrow excision (1-cm margin). A safe procedure for thin cutaneous melanoma. Arch Surg. 1991;126:438-41.
60. Balch CM, Soong SJ. Smith T, et al. Long-term results of a prospective trial comparing 2 cm vs. 4 cm excision margins for 740 patients with 1-4 mm melanomas. Ann Surg Oncol. 2001:8:101-8.
61. Cascinelli N, Morabito A, Santinami M, et al. Immediate or delayed dissection of regional nodes in patients with melanoma of the trunk: a randomised trial. WHO Melanoma Programme. Lancet. 1998;351:793-6.
62. Balch CM, Soong S, Ross MI, et al. Long-term results of a multi-institutional randomized trial comparing prognostic factors and surgical results for intermediate thickness melanomas (1.0 to 4.0 mm). Intergroup Melanoma Surgical Trial. Ann Surg Oncol, 2000;7:87-97.
63. Sim FH, Taylor WF, Pritchard DJ, et al. Lymphadenectomy in the management of stage I malignant melanoma: a prospective randomized study. Mayo Clin Proc. 1986;61: 697-705.
64. Wong SL, Brady MS, Busam KJ, et al. Results of sentinel lymph node biopsy in patients with thin melanoma. Ann Surg Oncol. 2006;13:302-9.
65. Puleo CA, Messina JL, Riker AI, et al. Sentinel node biopsy for thin melanomas: which patients should be considered? Cancer Control. 2005;12:230-5.
66. Andtbacka RH, Gershenwald JE. Role of sentinel lymph node biopsy in patients with thin melanoma. J Natl Compr Canc Netw. 2009;7:308-17.
67. Morton DL, Thompson JF, Cochran AJ, et al. Final trial report of sentinel-node biopsy versus nodal observation in melanoma. N Engl J Med. 2014;370:599-609.
68. Gershenwald JE, Ross MI. Sentinel-lymph-node biopsy for cutaneous melanoma. N Engl J Med, 2011;364:1738-45.
69. Morton DL, Wen DR, Wong JH, et al. Technical details of intraoperative lymphatic mapping for early stage melanoma. Arch Surg. 1992;127:392-9.
70. Gannon CJ, Rousseau DL Jr., Ross MI, et al. Accuracy of lymphatic mapping and sentinel lymph node biopsy after previous wide local excision in patients with primary melanoma. Cancer. 2006;107:2647-52.

71. Morton DL, Thompson JF, Cochran AJ, et al. Sentinel-node biopsy or nodal observation in melanoma. N Engl J Med. 2006;355:1307-17.
72. Moody JA, Ali RF, Carbone AC, et al. Complications of sentinel lymph node biopsy for melanoma—A systematic review of the literature. Eur J Surg Oncol. 2016.
73. Faries MB, Thompson JF, Cochran A, et al. The impact on morbidity and length of stay of early versus delayed complete lymphadenectomy in melanoma: results of the Multicenter Selective Lymphadenectomy Trial (I). Ann Surg Oncol. 2010;17:3324-9.
74. Warycha MA, Zakrzewski J, Ni Q, et al. Meta-analysis of sentinel lymph node positivity in thin melanoma (<or=1 mm). Cancer. 2009;115:869-79.
75. Karakousis GC, Gimotty PA, Botbyl JD, et al. Predictors of regional nodal disease in patients with thin melanomas. Ann Surg Oncol. 2006;13:533-41.
76. Kalady MF, White RR, Johnson JL, et al. Thin melanomas: predictive lethal characteristics from a 30-year clinical experience. Ann Surg. 2003;238:528-35; discussion 35-7.
77. Ranieri JM, Wagner JD, Wenck S, et al. The prognostic importance of sentinel lymph node biopsy in thin melanoma. Ann Surg Oncol. 2006;13:927-32.
78. Eggermont AM. Advances in systemic treatment of melanoma. Ann Oncol. 2010;21(7):vii339-44.
79. Morton DL. Overview and update of the phase III Multicenter Selective Lymphadenectomy Trials (MSLT-I and MSLT-II) in melanoma. Clin Exp Metastasis. 2012;29: 699-706.
80. Kudchadkar R. Novel targeted therapies for the treatment of metastatic melanoma. Ochsner J. 2010;10:117-24.
81. Ibrahim SF, Sambandan D, Ratner D. Immunotherapy for cutaneous malignancy. Dermatol Surg. 2011;37:1377-93.
82. Hodi FS, Corless CL, Giobbie-Hurder A, et al. Imatinib for melanomas harboring mutationally activated or amplified KIT arising on mucosal, acral, and chronically sun-damaged skin. J Clin Oncol. 2013;31:3182-90.
83. Franklin C, Livingstone E, Roesch A, et al. Immunotherapy in melanoma: Recent advances and future directions. Eur J Surg Oncol. 2016.
84. Ndoye A, Weeraratna AT. Autophagy—An emerging target for melanoma therapy. F1000Res. 2016;5.
85. Ratterman M, Hallmeyer S, Richards J. Sequencing of New and Old Therapies for Metastatic Melanoma. Curr Treat Options Oncol. 2016;17:52.
86. Carlino MS, Long GV. Is chemotherapy still an option in the treatment of melanoma? Ann Oncol. 2015;26:2203-4.
87. Bilir SP, Ma Q, Zhao Z, et al. Economic burden of toxicities associated with treating metastatic melanoma in the United States. Am Health Drug Benefits. 2016;9:203-13.
88. Zhu Z, Liu W, Gotlieb V. The rapidly evolving therapies for advanced melanoma—Towards immunotherapy, molecular targeted therapy, and beyond. Crit Rev Oncol Hematol. 2016;99:91-9.
89. Maio M, Grob JJ, Aamdal S, et al. Five-year survival rates for treatment-naive patients with advanced melanoma who received ipilimumab plus dacarbazine in a phase III trial. J Clin Oncol. 2015;33:1191-6.
90. Eggermont AM, Suciu S, MacKie R, et al. Post-surgery adjuvant therapy with intermediate doses of interferon alfa 2b versus observation in patients with stage IIb/III melanoma (EORTC 18952): randomised controlled trial. Lancet. 2005;366:1189-96.
91. Wheatley K, Ives N, Hancock B, et al. Does adjuvant interferon-alpha for high-risk melanoma provide a worthwhile benefit? A meta-analysis of the randomised trials. Cancer Treat Rev. 2003;29:241-52.
92. Eggermont AM, Suciu S, Testori A, et al. Long-term results of the randomized phase III trial EORTC 18991 of adjuvant therapy with pegylated interferon alfa-2b versus observation in resected stage III melanoma. J Clin Oncol. 2012;30: 3810-8.
93. Tarhini AA, Kirkwood JM. How much of a good thing? What duration for interferon alfa-2b adjuvant therapy? J Clin Oncol. 2012;30:3773-6.
94. Eklund JW, Kuzel TM. A review of recent findings involving interleukin-2-based cancer therapy. Curr Opin Oncol. 2004; 16:542-6.
95. Luu C, Khushalani NI, Zager JS. Intralesional and systemic immunotherapy for metastatic melanoma. Expert Opin Biol Ther. 2016:1-9.
96. Fecher LA, Agarwala SS, Hodi FS, et al. Ipilimumab and its toxicities: a multidisciplinary approach. Oncologist. 2013; 18:733-43.
97. Robert C, Thomas L, Bondarenko I, et al. Ipilimumab plus dacarbazine for previously untreated metastatic melanoma. N Engl J Med. 2011;364:2517-26.
98. Hodi FS, O'Day SJ, McDermott DF, et al. Improved survival with ipilimumab in patients with metastatic melanoma. N Engl J Med. 2010;363:711-23.
99. Schadendorf D, Hodi FS, Robert C, et al. Pooled analysis of long-term survival data from phase II and phase III trials of ipilimumab in unresectable or metastatic melanoma. J Clin Oncol. 2015;33:1889-94.
100. Eggermont AM, Chiarion-Sileni V, Grob JJ, et al. Adjuvant ipilimumab versus placebo after complete resection of high-risk stage III melanoma (EORTC 18071): a randomised, double-blind, phase 3 trial. Lancet Oncol. 2015;16:522-30.
101. Robert C, Long GV, Brady B, et al. Nivolumab in previously untreated melanoma without *BRAF* mutation. N Engl J Med. 2015;372:320-30.
102. Davies H, Bignell GR, Cox C, et al. Mutations of the *BRAF* gene in human cancer. Nature. 2002;417:949-54.
103. Curtin JA, Fridlyand J, Kageshita T, et al. Distinct sets of genetic alterations in melanoma. N Engl J Med. 2005;353: 2135-47.
104. Marples M. Commentary: *BRAF* inhibitors for metastatic melanoma. Br J Dermatol. 2013;168:471-3.
105. van Akkooi AC, Nijsten T. A costly revolution for a subgroup of patients with metastatic melanoma. Br J Dermatol. 2013; 168:467-70; discussion 70-1.
106. Rinderknecht JD, Goldinger SM, Rozati S, et al. RASopathic skin eruptions during vemurafenib therapy. PLoS One. 2013;8:e58721.
107. Welsh SJ, Corrie PG. Management of *BRAF* and MEK inhibitor toxicities in patients with metastatic melanoma. Ther Adv Med Oncol. 2015;7:122-36.
108. Su F, Viros A, Milagre C, et al. RAS mutations in cutaneous squamous-cell carcinomas in patients treated with *BRAF* inhibitors. N Engl J Med. 2012;366:207-15.
109. Dummer R, Rinderknecht J, Goldinger SM. Ultraviolet A and photosensitivity during vemurafenib therapy. N Engl J Med. 2012;366:480-1.
110. Hauschild A, Grob JJ, Demidov LV, et al. Dabrafenib in BRAF-mutated metastatic melanoma: a multicentre, open-label, phase 3 randomised controlled trial. Lancet. 2012; 380:358-65.

111. Vaubel J, Livingstone E, Schadendorf D, et al. Retarded low-dose doxycycline for EGFR or MEK inhibitor-induced papulopustular rash. J Eur Acad Dermatol Venereol. 2014; 28:1685-9.
112. Chapman PB, Hauschild A, Robert C, et al. Improved survival with vemurafenib in melanoma with *BRAF* V600E mutation. N Engl J Med. 2011;364:2507-16.
113. Hauschild A. Response to a costly revolution for a subgroup of patients with metastatic melanoma. Br J Dermatol. 2013; 168:470-1; discussion 70-1.
114. Cebollero A, Puertolas T, Pajares I, et al. Comparative safety of *BRAF* and MEK inhibitors (vemurafenib, dabrafenib and trametinib) in first-line therapy for *BRAF*-mutated metastatic melanoma. Mol Clin Oncol. 2016;5:458-62.
115. Flaherty KT, Robert C, Hersey P, et al. Improved survival with MEK inhibition in BRAF-mutated melanoma. N Engl J Med. 2012;367:107-14.
116. Latimer NR, Bell H, Abrams KR, et al. Adjusting for treatment switching in the METRIC study shows further improved overall survival with trametinib compared with chemotherapy. Cancer Med. 2016;5:806-15.
117. Homet Moreno B, Mok S, Comin-Anduix B, et al. Combined treatment with dabrafenib and trametinib with immune-stimulating antibodies for *BRAF* mutant melanoma. Oncoimmunology. 2016;5:e1052212.
118. Chen G, McQuade JL, Panka DJ, et al. Clinical, molecular, and immune analysis of dabrafenib-trametinib combination treatment for BRAF inhibitor-refractory metastatic melanoma: A phase 2 clinical trial. JAMA Oncol. 2016;2:1056-64.
119. Larkin J, Ascierto PA, Dreno B, et al. Combined vemurafenib and cobimetinib in BRAF-mutated melanoma. N Engl J Med. 2014;371:1867-76.
120. Posch C, Moslehi H, Sanlorenzo M, et al. Pharmacological inhibitors of c-KIT block mutant c-KIT mediated migration of melanocytes and melanoma cells in vitro and in vivo. Oncotarget. 2016.
121. Dharmadhikari N, Mehnert JM, Kaufman HL. Oncolytic virus immunotherapy for melanoma. Curr Treat Options Oncol. 2015;16:326.
122. Andtbacka RH, Ross M, Puzanov I, et al. Patterns of clinical response with talimogene laherparepvec (T-VEC) in patients with melanoma treated in the OPTiM phase III clinical trial. Ann Surg Oncol. 2016;23:4169-77.
123. Kaufman HL, Amatruda T, Reid T, et al. Systemic versus local responses in melanoma patients treated with talimogene laherparepvec from a multi-institutional phase II study. J Immunother Cancer. 2016;4:12.
124. Pol J, Kroemer G, Galluzzi L. First oncolytic virus approved for melanoma immunotherapy. Oncoimmunology. 2016;5: e1115641.
125. Andtbacka RH, Kaufman HL, Collichio F, et al. Talimogene laherparepvec improves durable response rate in patients with advanced melanoma. J Clin Oncol. 2015;33:2780-8.
126. Sloot S, Rashid OM, Sarnaik AA, et al. Developments in Intralesional therapy for metastatic melanoma. Cancer Control. 2016;23:12-20.
127. Schwartzentruber DJ, Lawson D, Richards J, et al. A phase III multi-institutional randomized study of immunization with the gplOO: 209-217(210M) peptide followed by high-dose IL- 2 compared with high-dose IL-2 alone in patients with metastatic melanoma. J Clin Oncol. 2009;27:18s (suppl; abstr CRA9011).
128. Lawson DH, Lee S, Zhao F, et al. Randomized, placebo-controlled, phase III trial of yeast-derived granulocyte-macrophage colony-stimulating factor (GM-CSF) versus peptide vaccination versus GM-CSF plus peptide vaccination versus placebo in patients with no evidence of disease after complete surgical resection of locally advanced and/ or stage IV melanoma: A trial of the Eastern Cooperative Oncology Group-American College of Radiology Imaging Network Cancer Research Group (E4697). J Clin Oncol. 2015;33:4066-76.
129. Hu Y, Kim H, Blackwell CM, et al. Long-term outcomes of helper peptide vaccination for metastatic melanoma. Ann Surg. 2015;262:456-64; discussion 62-4.
130. Schwartzentruber DJ, Lawson DH, Richards JM, et al. gp100 peptide vaccine and interleukin-2 in patients with advanced melanoma. N Engl J Med. 2011;364:2119-27.
131. Ramirez AG, Wages NA, Hu Y, et al. Defining the effects of age and gender on immune response and outcomes to melanoma vaccination: a retrospective analysis of a single-institution clinical trials' experience. Cancer Immunol Immunother. 2015;64:1531-9.
132. Boesch CE, Meyer T, Waschke L, et al. Long-term outcome of hyperthermic isolated limb perfusion (HILP) in the treatment of locoregionally metastasised malignant melanoma of the extremities. Int J Hyperthermia. 2010;26: 16-20.
133. Ma Q, Zhao Z, Barber BL, et al. Use patterns and costs of isolated limb perfusion and infusion in the treatment of regional metastatic melanoma: A retrospective database analysis. Adv Ther. 2016;33:282-9.
134. Kroon HM. Treatment of locally advanced melanoma by isolated limb infusion with cytotoxic drugs. J Skin Cancer. 2011;2011:106573.
135. Dossett LA, Ben-Shabat I, Olofsson Bagge R, et al. Clinical response and regional toxicity following isolated limb infusion compared with isolated limb perfusion for in-transit melanoma. Ann Surg Oncol. 2016;23:2330-5.
136. Seegenschmiedt MH, Keilholz L, Altendorf-Hofmann A, et al. Palliative radiotherapy for recurrent and metastatic malignant melanoma: prognostic factors for tumor response and long-term outcome: a 20-year experience. Int J Radiat Oncol Biol Phys. 1999;44:607-18.
137. Huguenin PU, Kieser S, Glanzmann C, et al. Radiotherapy for metastatic carcinomas of the kidney or melanomas: an analysis using palliative end points. Int J Radiat Oncol Biol Phys. 1998;41:401-5.
138. Danish HH, Patel KR, Switchenko JM, et al. The influence of postoperative lymph node radiation therapy on overall survival of patients with stage III melanoma, a National Cancer Database analysis. Melanoma Res. 2016;26:595-603.
139. Henderson MA, Burmeister BH, Ainslie J, et al. Adjuvant lymph-node field radiotherapy versus observation only in patients with melanoma at high risk of further lymph-node field relapse after lymphadenectomy (ANZMTG 01.02/ TROG 02.01): 6-year follow-up of a phase 3, randomised controlled trial. Lancet Oncol. 2015;16:1049-60.
140. Fogarty GB, Hong A, Scolyer RA, et al. Radiotherapy for lentigo maligna: a literature review and recommendations for treatment. Br J Dermatol. 2014;170:52-8.

141. Burmeister BH, Mark Smithers B, Burmeister E, et al. A prospective phase II study of adjuvant postoperative radiation therapy following nodal surgery in malignant melanoma-Trans Tasman Radiation Oncology Group (TROG) Study 96.06. Radiother Oncol. 2006;81:136-42.
142. Guadagnolo BA, Zagars GK. Adjuvant radiation therapy for high-risk nodal metastases from cutaneous melanoma. Lancet Oncol. 2009;10:409-16.
143. Burmeister BH, Henderson MA, Ainslie J, et al. Adjuvant radiotherapy versus observation alone for patients at risk of lymph-node field relapse after therapeutic lymphadenectomy for melanoma: a randomised trial. Lancet Oncol. 2012;13:589-97.
144. Hiniker SM, Reddy SA, Maecker HT, et al. A prospective clinical trial combining radiation therapy with systemic immunotherapy in metastatic melanoma. Int J Radiat Oncol Biol Phys. 2016;96:578-88.
145. Barker CA, Postow MA. Combinations of radiation therapy and immunotherapy for melanoma: a review of clinical outcomes. Int J Radiat Oncol Biol Phys. 2014;88:986-97.

Chapter 51

Varicose Veins: An Overview

S Sacchidanand, BS Shivaswamy, Aniketh Venkataram

Key Messages

- Varicose veins are common problems associated with several cutaneous manifestations and may present to a dermatosurgeon.
- Use of Doppler has largely replaced the clinical tests that were used earlier for diagnosis of venous insufficiency.
- Various treatment options exist including compression therapy, sclerotherapy, surgical and endovenous treatments.
- Choice of treatment is based on the trade-off between their advantages and long-term recurrence rates.

VENOUS ANATOMY

The first accurate and nearly complete description of the peripheral venous system was given by Vesalius in De Humanis Corporis Fabrica. The veins of the lower limb can be divided into superficial and deep veins, with the deep muscle fascia being the line of demarcation between the two. The superficial compartment consists of all tissue between the skin and the deep muscle fascia and the deep compartment all the tissue between the fascia and the bones. The saphenous compartment is a sub-compartment of the superficial compartment enclosed between the saphenous fascia and the deep muscle fascia. Communicating veins connect veins in the same compartment whereas perforator veins connect superficial and deep veins.

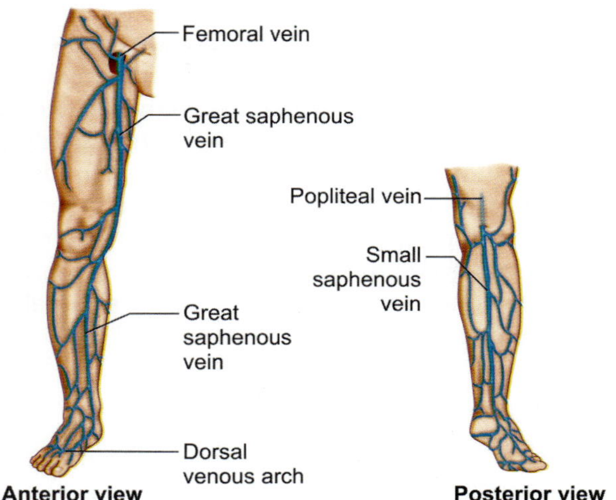

Fig. 1: Anatomy of the greater and lesser saphenous system.

Superficial Veins

The dorsal venous arch of the foot is continuous with the great saphenous vein (GSV) medially and the small saphenous vein (SSV) laterally (Fig. 1). Small superficial veins drain the skin and subcutaneous tissue and form bigger tributaries which eventually drain into the saphenous veins. The GSV, in association with the saphenous nerve ascends anterior to the medial malleolus and then behind the medial aspect of the knee.[1] Proximally it ascends up the medial aspect of the thigh and empties into the common femoral vein at the saphenofemoral junction (SFJ), 2.5 cm below and lateral to the pubic tubercle. Important tributaries of the GSV include the posterior and anterior accessory great saphenous veins which drain just below the knee. Three tributaries, namely the superficial circumflex iliac, superficial epigastric and the superficial external pudendal drain just before the SFJ.

The small saphenous vein begins at the lateral end of the dorsal venous arch and ascends posterior to the lateral malleolus in the subcutaneous fat.[2] It pierces the deep fascia and runs between the two heads of the gastrocnemius muscle before emptying into the popliteal vein. The saphenopopliteal junction (SPJ) is highly variable and rarely the SSV may drain directly into the femoral vein or the GSV. The inter saphenous vein (of Giacomini)

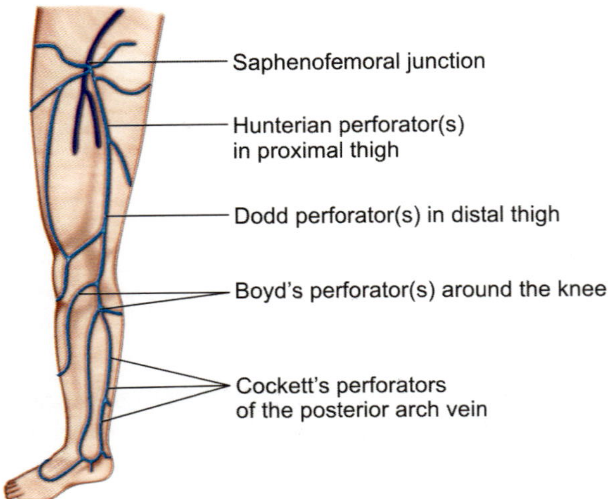

Fig. 2: Perforator system of the lower limb.

is a communication between the GSV and the SSV in the posteromedial aspect of the thigh.

Deep Veins

The Plantar venous arch drains into the medial and lateral plantar veins which continue as the posterior tibial veins. The dorsalis pedis veins on the dorsum of the foot continue as the anterior tibial veins at the ankle. The anterior and posterior tibial veins as well as the peroneal veins accompany their respective arteries and drain into the popliteal veins. The venous sinuses of the calf muscles are drained by the soleal and gastrocnemius veins into the popliteal vein. The popliteal vein continues in the adductor canal as the femoral vein. The deep femoral vein (profunda femoris) drains into the femoral vein to form the common femoral vein, which becomes the external iliac vein after crossing the inguinal ligament.

Perforator Veins

There may be as many as 150 perforators veins in the lower limbs, of which few are clinically important (Fig. 2). These include

a. The foot perforators,
b. Ankle perforators,
c. In the calf, the posterior tibial perforators (of Cockett) connect the posterior accessory GSV to the posterior tibial veins, while the paratibial perforators connect the GSV to the posterior tibial veins,
d. Boyd's perforator is located just below the knee, and
e. Dodd's and Hunter's perforators are located in the thigh.

VENOUS PATHOPHYSIOLOGY

The venous system has the greatest capacitance in the vascular tree. In the supine position, the pressure in the veins of the lower limb is similar to that in other parts of the body. However on standing a dramatic change occurs, the pressure is equal to that of a column of blood from the heart to the foot which is around 100 mm Hg.

The peripheral muscle pumps play a major role in venous return to the heart. The soleal sinuses and plantar veins are drained during walking, when the muscle compression forces blood from the superficial to the deep venous system, and thereon to the proximal vasculature. This outflow from the superficial veins is balanced by inflow with the mean pressure dropping by nearly two-thirds to 30 mm Hg. This reduction in superficial venous pressure is dependent on patent deep veins, perforators and superficial veins with competent valves. Failure of any of these elements can lead to ambulatory venous hypertension.

Venous insufficiency is generally described as primary and chronic venous insufficiency.

Primary venous insufficiency (PVI)—Injury to vein walls and valves, primarily by inflammation leads to elongation and dilatation of the veins secondary to ambulatory venous hypertension which results in the physical manifestations. The first manifestations are telangiectasias in the epidermis and dermis, followed by dilation of the reticular plexus. Progression leads to still deeper varicose veins. The common factor of all these are tortuous walls and dysfunctional valves.

Chronic venous insufficiency (CVI)—This is manifested as skin changes of hyperpigmentation, ulceration and lipodermatosclerosis. The prior theories to explain CVI included the stasis theory and the fibrin cuff-hypoxia theory, both of which have been disproved by studies. The commonly accepted premise now if of leukocyte activation. Leukocytes are trapped in the venous microcirculation secondary to venous hypertension, where they get activated. This leads to the release of various cytokines and growth factors, of which transforming growth factor-beta (TGF-β) appears to be highly significant. Extracellular matrix remodeling ensues with diminished fibroblast function resulting in the clinical manifestations of CVI.

RISK FACTORS

- Heredity—Several studies have suggested a genetic predisposition to the development of varicose veins. This might be related to abnormalities in the *FOXC2* gene.
- Age—Incidence increases with age.
- Sex—Higher prevalence is seen in women, probably related to pregnancy.
- Pregnancy—Hormonal factors are responsible. Varicose veins are generally seen in the first trimester and are thought to be the effect of progesterone on venous dilatation and valvular insufficiency.
- Other factors—Various other risk factors have been postulated including western diet, obesity, straining during micturition and western style toilets have been

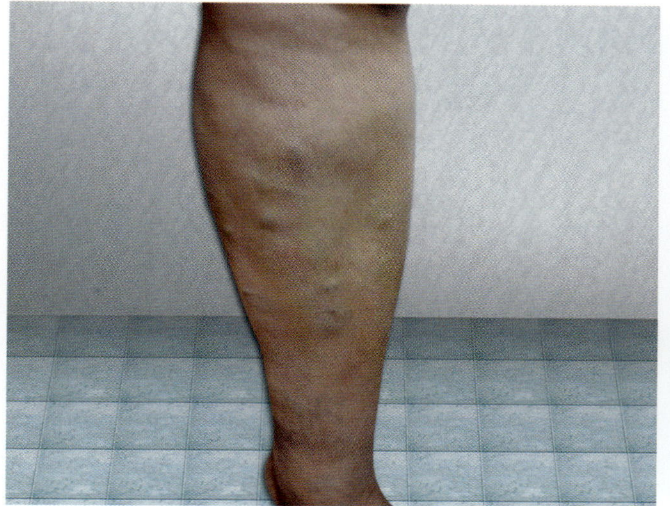

Fig. 3: Tortuous swellings of lower limb veins.

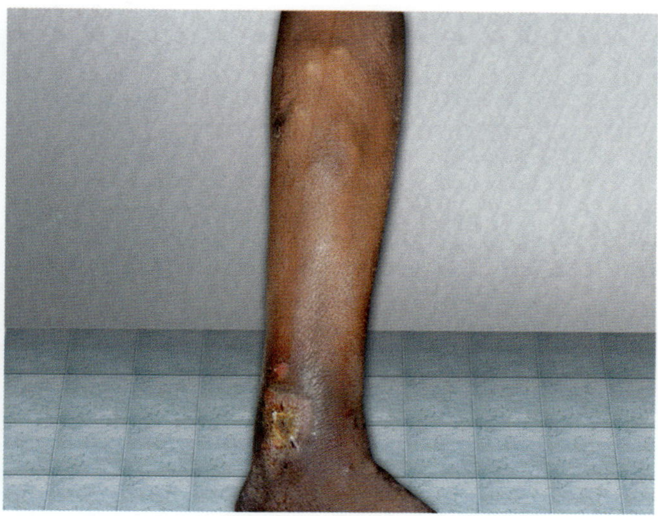

Fig. 4: Venous ulceration over medial malleolus.

suggested with equivocal evidence. Occupations which involve prolonged periods of standing also appear to carry a risk of varicose veins.[3]

CLINICAL FEATURES

- Tortuous swelling of veins of lower limb (Fig. 3)
- Aching and heaviness of the lower limbs, particularly towards the end of the day
- Ankle swelling
- Itching
- Bleeding
- Thrombophlebitis
- Eczema
- Pigmentation
- Ulceration (Fig. 4)
- Exacerbation of symptoms during early days of menstrual cycle.

EXAMINATION

A careful clinical examination can provide the practitioner with an accurate analysis of the venous status of the limb. Several clinical tests are described, many of which have lost their significance with the advent of newer imaging modalities, in particular the hand-held Doppler.

Inspection

The limb should be examined for

- Telangiectasis, reticular veins and varicose veins—including their site and extent
- Pigmentation
- Eczema
- Ulceration
- Swelling

Clinical Tests

- Brodie-Trendelenburg test—the limb is elevated and milked proximally, then a tourniquet tied just below the SFJ and the patient asked to stand quickly.
  - Part 1—the tourniquet is released, rapid filling from above indicates SFJ incompetence.
  - Part 2—the tourniquet is not released, slow filling from below upwards indicates perforator incompetence.
  - This test helps to identify the presence of both junctional as well as perforator incompetence, when both parts of it are performed.
- Tourniquet test—In supine position, the limb is raised and the veins milked proximally to empty them. Multiple tourniquets are tied on either side of suspected incompetent perforators. Then the patient is asked to stand up, and venous filling is observed. Based on which segments between tourniquets are filled, the presence of incompetent perforators are identified.
- Fegan's test—in standing position, bulges in the vein are marked. In supine position, after milking the veins palpate the marked areas. If cresentic gaps are felt, it marks the gaps in the deep fascia where perforators are present and signifies perforator incompetency where perforators are present.
- Schwartz test—In standing position, one hand is placed on the SFJ and the other hand is used to lightly tap on a distal portion of the GSV. Presence of an impulse indicates valvular insufficiency between these two segments.

CLASSIFICATION

The accepted classification at present is the Clinical-Etiological-Anatomical-Pathophysiological (CEAP) (Box 1) classification devised by the ad hoc committee of the American Venous forum in 1994. The revision of

Box 1: CEAP classification.

Clinical	
C0	No visible or palpable signs of venous disease
C1	Telangiectasias (up to 1 mm), reticular veins (1–3 mm)
C2	Varicose veins (0.3 mm)
C3	Edema without skin changes
C4	Skin changes due to venous disease (pigmentation, eczema, lipodermatosclerosis)
C5	Skin changes with healed ulceration
C6	Skin changes with active ulceration
Etiological	
Ec	Congenital (since birth)
Ep	Primary (of undetermined cause)
Es	Secondary (known cause such as thrombotic, traumatic etc)
En	No venous cause identified
Anatomical	
As	Superficial veins
Ad	Deep veins
Ap	Perforator veins
An	No venous location identified
Pathophysiological	
Pr	Reflux
Po	Obstruction
Pro	Reflux and obstruction
Pn	No venous pathology identified

the CEAP is an ongoing process. The clinical part of the classification alone is generally used, while the other components of the classification are generally used for academic purposes. But usage of the entire system provides a thorough assessment of the disease process.

INVESTIGATIONS

The advent of the Doppler technology has transformed the diagnosis of varicose veins, and today any evaluation of a venous insufficiency patient without a Doppler study is considered grossly inadequate (Fig. 5).

Standard Doppler

A Doppler probe emits a sound when blood flows past the probe and records the reflected sound. A uniphasic flow indicates blood flowing in one direction, whereas a biphasic flow indicates blood flowing in reverse direction, indicative of a reflux. This principle is commonly used in a hand-held device, often by the operating surgeon himself to identify sites of reflux and plan the mode of treatment. With distal augmentation of flow by squeezing the calf muscles, normal deep breathing and the Valsalva maneuver, the location of reflux, either junctional or valve can be identified.

Duplex Doppler

This technology combines a B-mode ultrasound (7–8 MHz) with a standard Doppler (3MHz). The B-mode

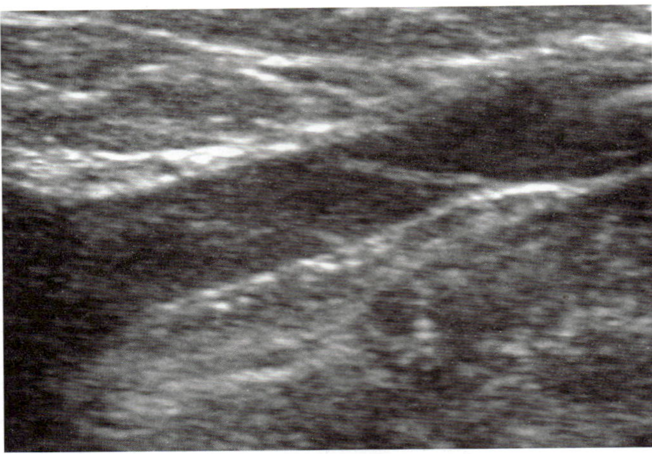

Fig. 5: Doppler scan of great saphenous vein.

ultrasound provides a background gray scale image, on which the Doppler flow image is superimposed to precisely determine the site of reflux.[4] The patient should always be examined in standing position as minor reflux can be missed in supine position. Distal augmentation methods are used to provide a complete picture. Studies have shown the addition of a duplex evaluation greatly increases the accuracy of preoperative assessment and avoids incorrect choice of surgery.[5]

Other investigation methods which are not usually performed include—

1. Plethysmography—This is based on the principle of air displacement. It consists of an air chamber that surrounds the limb from knee to ankle. A reading is taken after the veins are emptied and the patient is made to stand up. The filling of the veins is expressed in millimetres per second.
2. Varicography—in this method, contrast material is injected directly in the superficial varices and then detailed mapping is performed.

These methods have largely been replaced by the Doppler scan.

MANAGEMENT

The ideal management of varicose veins is one that abolishes incompetence, prevents complications, improves cosmesis, and at the same time be associated with low morbidity, short recovery, low recurrence and be cost effective. There exist a wide variety of treatment options which balance these requirements in different proportions (Box 2).[6]

Pharmacological Therapy

Several classes of drugs have been suggested to have venoprotective effects, but most of them lack FDA approval.

a. The most common class of drugs are flavanoids derived from plant glycosides. Studies have shown they subjectively improve symptoms such as pain, night cramps and restless legs. The precise mechanism is

Box 2: Overview of treatment options.

1. Pharmacological therapy
2. Compression therapy
3. Sclerotherapy
4. External lasers
5. Endovenous treatments
   a. Radiofrequency ablation (RFA)
   b. Endovenous laser treatment (EVLT)
   c. Nonthermal ablation
6. Surgical methods
   a. Saphenofemoral ligation
   b. LSV stripping
   c. Phlebectomies
   d. Subfascial ligation of perforators
7. Other methods
   a. Subfascial endoscopic perforator surgery
   b. Ambulatory Conservative Hemodynamic Management (ACHM or CHIVA)
   c. Transilluminated powered phlebectomy
   d. Cryosurgery.

unknown but it is suggested that they reduce venous reflux and inhibit leukocyte activation and migration, leading to beneficial effects in ulcer healing.[7]

b. Calcium dobesilate is another drug that is used to treat symptoms and edema of CVI. It is said to decrease the capillary hyperpermeability thereby reducing edema. However recent studies have failed to demonstrate its superiority as compared to placebo.[8]
c. Pentoxifylline is thought to reduce adhesiveness of white blood cells and decrease oxygen free radicals. Its efficacy in treatment of venous ulcers in conjunction with compression has been demonstrated by several studies.[9]
d. Prostaglandins E1 and F reduce leukocyte activation, and inhibit platelet aggregation. They are found in horse chestnut seed extract used as a traditional medicine.

Compression Therapy

Compression stocking should be considered for CEAP classes 2 to 6. The objective is to provide external graded compression of the limb to counteract venous hypertension. During walking these compression devices provide a compression of up to 80 mm Hg peaks which help to intermittently overcome the venous reflux, which in turn reduces the ambulatory venous hypertension. It also counteracts the forces that favour capillary leakage and help to reduce edema.

Different types of compression devices are available which include stockings, paste boots, layered bandaging and adjustable compression. Patients must be educated about the importance of compliance in order to maximize the beneficial effects of compression. Compression therapy should be used with care in patients with significant arterial insufficiency. Also systemic conditions which affect wound healing and edema such as diabetes mellitus, malnutrition should be addressed simultaneously.

Several reviews have demonstrated the beneficial effects of compression therapy.[10] One meta-analysis suggested the use of 10–20 mm Hg compression as ideal as lower pressures were ineffective and higher pressures provided no added benefit.[11]

Sclerotherapy

Sclerotherapy is defined as the introduction of a chemical into the lumen of a vein to induce endothelial damage that results in thrombosis, subsequent fibrosis and occlusion. It is a very versatile option and has been used to treat a wide range of vein diameters. A number of sclerosing agents have been used including hypertonic saline, sodium tetradecyl sulfate, polidocanol, sodium morrhuate, etc.

For smaller veins, liquid sclerotherapy may be used. Foam sclerotherapy involves the agitation of air into the agent so as to increase the surface area of contact while reducing the volume of solution injected. The common complications of this procedure include hyperpigmentation, pain and urticaria. Rarely cutaneous necrosis, DVT, pulmonary embolism and inadvertent arterial injection are seen.

Sclerotherapy will be dealt with in a separate chapter.

External Lasers

Lasers have been used to treat leg telangiectasias and reticular veins. They have several theoretical advantages over sclerotherapy including reduced pigmentation, matting and allergenic effects. Lasers of various wavelengths are used to selectively treat blood vessels by taking advantage of difference in absorption between different components of the blood vessel. It is important to first treat feeder veins before treating telangiectasias to avoid recurrence. Some of the most common lasers used include CO_2 laser, pulsed dye, KTP, diode. But the most common one is the 1064 nm ND:YAG laser. Lasers have also been used in combination with sclerotherapy to reduce the dosage and side effect profile of both.

Lasers will be dealt with in detail in a separate chapter.

Endovenous Techniques

Radiofrequency Ablation

In this technique, radiofrequency energy is used to produce heat when in contact with the vessel wall which causes endothelial damage, wall contraction and thrombus formation. This leads to fibrosis and constriction of the vein lumen which eventually leads to occlusion.[12] This procedure can be performed under general, regional or most recently tumescent local anesthesia.

Procedure: A duplex scan is performed preoperatively to mark the skin over the vein including the highest point of reflux. Local anesthetic is injected at the selected access site and access obtained. A guidewire is passed into the vein over which the appropriate size of the radiofrequency

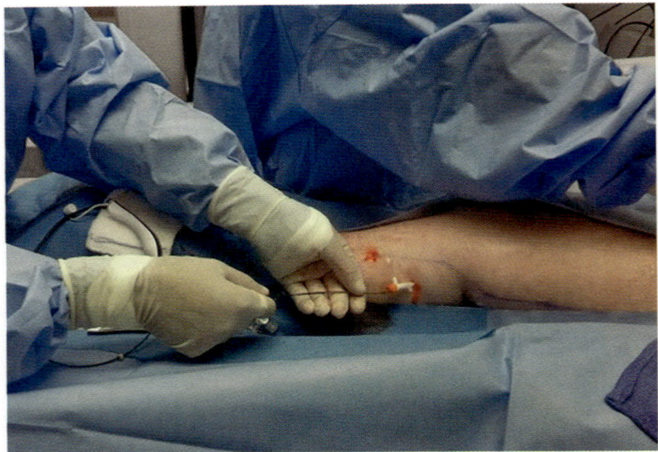

Fig. 6: Radiofrequency catheter advanced over guidewire.

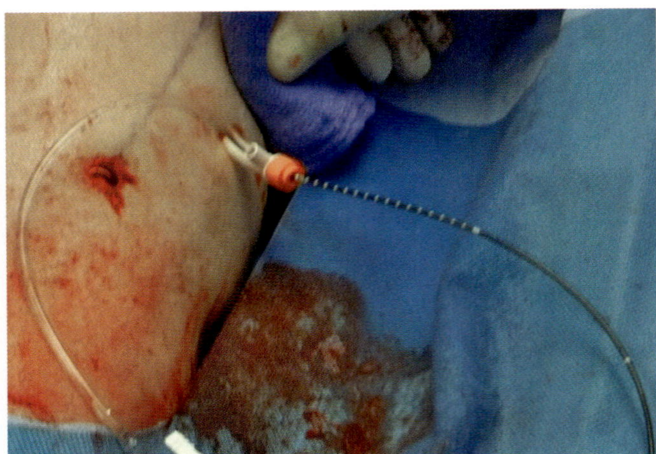

Fig. 7: Catheter sequentially moved to cover entire vein.

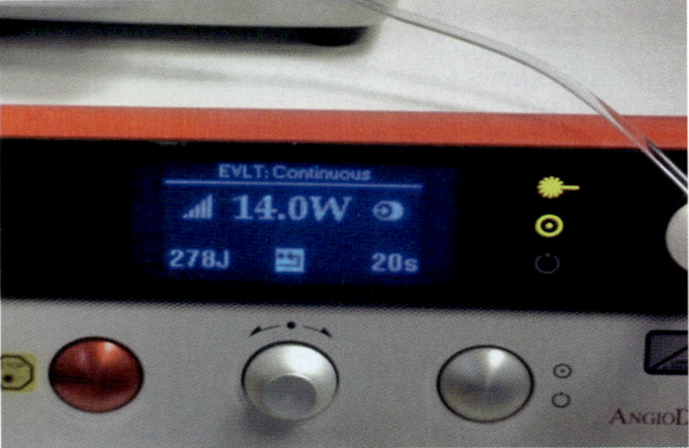

Fig. 8: Endovenous laser generator.

catheter is inserted and advanced to the predetermined site of treatment (Fig. 6). After correct placement of the catheter is confirmed, perivenous tumescent anesthesia is injected which also serves to compress the vein around the catheter and protect surrounding tissues from heat damage. Once the anesthetic is injected, the generator is turned on and a fixed segment of the vein is heated to a predetermined temperature (generally 120°C). After completion of a segment, the catheter is sequentially moved, and successive segments of fixed lengths treated till the entire diseased vein is treated (Fig. 7). If required, a particular segment such as near the SFJ or a large perforator can be ablated twice before proceeding to the next segment. After treatment, a duplex scan is performed to assess reflux and occlusion. Postoperative compression for a week is recommended.

Potential complications include vessel perforation, thrombosis, phlebitis, infection, nerve injury, skin burns. However studies indicate the incidence of these to be low.[12]

One multicenter trial showed 85% of LSV occluded at 2 years, with others showing 88–100%.[13] In comparison with surgery, a study showed an occlusion rate of 95% for RFA versus 100% for surgery on day of procedure, but the time taken to resume daily activities was significantly lower for RFA.[14] A prospective RCT comparing the two for recurrent varices showed no difference in occlusion but significantly fewer complications and operating time for radiofrequency.[15]

Endovenous Laser Ablation

Endovenous laser ablation (EVLA) is very similar to RFA, except for the catheter used and the energy used. Here a bare tipped catheter is used to deliver laser energy that forms steam bubbles in the lumen which causes an inflammatory reaction leading to thrombosis, occlusion and fibrosis.[16]

Numerous frequencies have been used ranging from 810 to 1470 nm (Fig. 8). Research has shown that all laser wavelengths are equally effective but lower wavelengths are associated with more pain and bruising.

***Procedure*:** A duplex scan is performed and the sources of venous reflux are marked on the surface. Venous access is obtained and the microsheath inserted. The distance to the SFJ from the access site is measured and the guide-wire passed through the same distance (Fig. 9). The microsheath is replaced with a long sheath, and the laser fiber is advanced through the sheath. The aiming beam is turned on to identify the fiber tip under the skin (Fig. 10). The position of the tip is confirmed with ultrasound and tumescent anesthesia administered as with RFA.

The next step in the procedure has several variations related to pullback time and amount of energy delivered. Initially pulsed mode of pullback was preferred and time was used to measure pullback. Later it was found that the amount of energy delivered correlated better with treatment efficacy.[17] Currently continuous pullback is used while observing the real time energy monitor to gauge speed of pullback. 50 to 80 J/cm is the average treatment

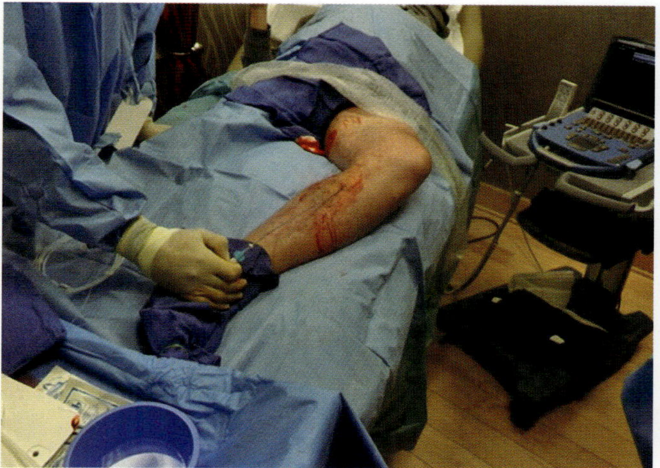

Fig. 9: Laser fiber advanced over guidewire.

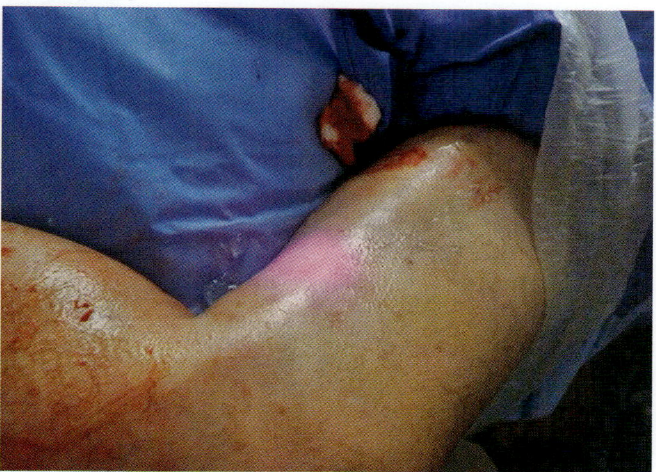

Fig. 10: Fiber tip visible below skin.

energy recommended. After the procedure, patients are advised compression therapy for a minimum of one week.

Ecchymoses and pain are frequently reported side effects of endovenous laser ablation. Nerve injury, skin burns, deep vein thrombosis and pulmonary embolism occur rarely. An exceptional complication is a material or device that by accident remains inside the body after the procedure.[18]

A success rate of 100% one week after EVLT is reported in most studies. Although success rate decreases with time, it remains at least 90%. In a prospective study, 93% of 499 GSV remained occluded 2 years after therapy.[19] Another study comparing EVLT with surgery found lesser neovascularization rates two years after treatment in the EVLT arm.[20] A retrospective study suggested that RFA and EVLT were equally effective, but three DVT were reported after EVLT.[21]

Nonthermal Ablation

The above mentioned techniques require tumescent anesthesia, which has the disadvantage of needing multiple puncture sites. Also to avoid lidocaine toxicity multiple sessions might be needed. To overcome this, nonthermal nontumescent techniques have been developed. However these techniques are still new and long-term results are awaited.

i. Mechanochemical venous ablation (MOCA)—This is a hybrid system which uses a rotating tip with injection of sclerosant. The rotating tip causes intimal abrasion inducing venospasm which is combined with the sclerosant. Closure rates at 8 months are as high as 96.7%.[22]
ii. Cyanoacrylate glue (CAG) closure—Under USG guidance, a catheter is introduced to the site of incompetence. CAG is then injected in combination with external mechanical compression.[23]

Surgical Methods

Surgery should be individualized for the patient, with a combination of SFJ ligation, stripping and stab phlebectomy performed as based on the patient's venous status.

Saphenofemoral Ligation

The GSV can be approached through an oblique incision 1 cm above and parallel to the groin crease. Preoperative duplex marking of the SFJ greatly simplifies the process. After splitting the subcutaneous tissue, the main saphenous trunk is identified and followed to its termination. There are six main tributaries around the SFJ, each of which should be identified and divided to avoid recurrence. These are the inferior epigastric, superficial circumflex iliac, superficial external pudendal, deep external pudendal, and the medial and lateral accessory saphenous veins.

The number and location of these tributaries vary greatly and hence the femoral vein should be dissected above and below the confluence, and the saphenous vein dissected caudally for 10 cm to avoid missing any tributary. Double ligation is generally performed, and if stripping is not being performed, 5 to 10 cm of GSV should be resected (Fig. 11). Care should be taken to avoid leaving a long stump.

GSV Stripping

The SFJ ligation is generally performed in combination with GSV stripping as it markedly reduces recurrence rates.[24] Any incompetent accessory saphenous veins should also be addressed during the surgery, as unresected accessory saphenous veins are probably the main cause of recurrence after surgery. While spinal anesthesia was generally used previously, recently tumescent anesthesia has also been used to perform this procedure in an outpatient setting.

After flush SFJ ligation, a transverse venotomy is performed in the GSV. The stripper is inserted from above and passed distally (Fig. 12). The stripper is passed distally from above to avoid the stripper from passing into a deep vein through an incompetent tributary. Generally metallic

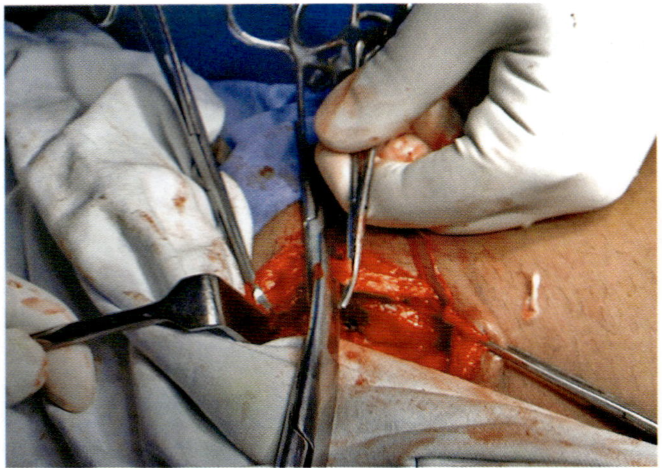

Fig. 11: Saphenofemoral junction ligation.

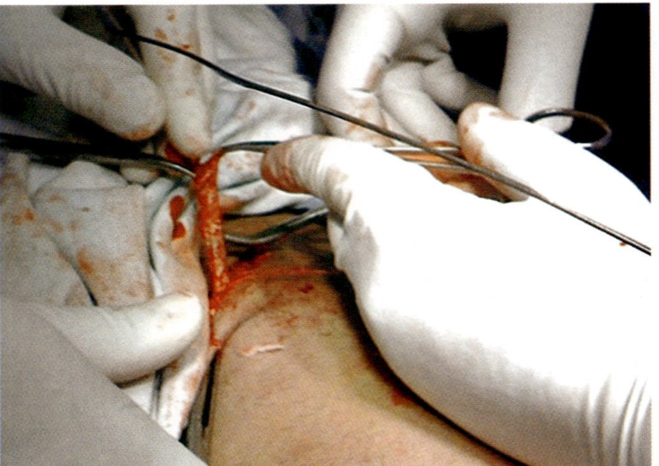

Fig. 12: Venous stripper passed into GSV.

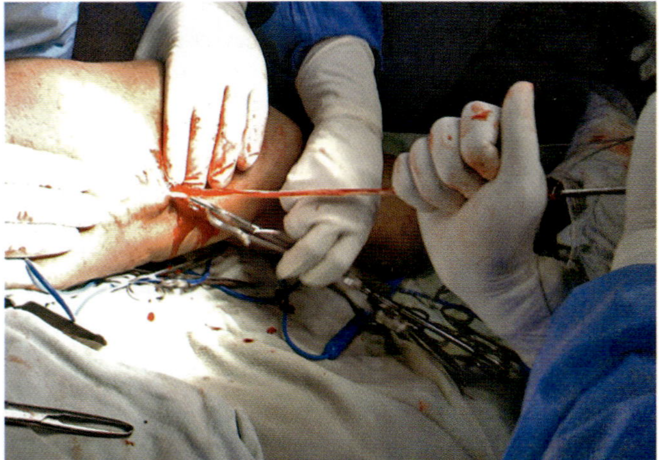

Fig. 13: Greater saphenous vein being stripped from above downwards.

or disposable plastic strippers are used. The stripper head is palpated through the skin as it is passed below. At the desired level, a small transverse incision made over the head through the skin and vein and the head is removed. The vein is fixed to the stripper head with a ligature. The vein is then stripped from above downwards and compression bandage immediately applied (Fig. 13). Stripping from above downwards avoids damage to the saphenous nerve. A larger head size recovers the entire vein and tributaries while a smaller head reduces bruising.

A variation of this technique is the invagination stripper where the stripper head is attached to the luminal surface of then vein and the vein intussuscepts onto itself. This reduces bruising but may lead to incomplete stripping if the vein tears.

Phlebectomies

The SFJ ligation and stripping remove the source of reflux, however leftover superficial varicosities may drain through alternate pathways and may be symptomatic as well as cosmetically problematic. Previously these were removed through large incision, but refinement in technique has allowed for their removal through millimeter sized incisions. This technique is well suited to local anesthesia.

The patient is made to stand erect and the veins to be removed are marked. The limb is prepped and subcutaneous injection of the local anesthetic is done along the length of the vein to be vein to be removed, while care is taken not to inject intravenously.

A stab incision up to 3 mm is made at the most prominent part of the vein using a number 11 blade. The main instrument used is the phlebectomy hook which consists of a hook at one end and a fine spatula at the other end. The spatula end is inserted through the stab into the subcutaneous fascia and used to free the vein from its tissue connections, as far as possible on either side of the incision.

The hook is then inserted at right angles to the vein and the vein is teased out of the incision like a loop. Clamps are applied to either end of the loop and the vein is divided in between. Both ends of the vein are steadily twisted out of the incision with one hand while the other hand is used to apply pressure to the subcutaneous vein to facilitate the process. As much of the vein as possible is pulled out. Occasionally a perforator might avulse causing venous bleeding. In such an instance, continuous pressure for 5–10 minutes usually controls the bleeding.

Postoperatively, the wounds are cleaned and closed with steri-strips (sutures are generally not required or preferred as they lead to a poor cosmetic result). Adhesive wrap is applied to the leg with a thigh high compression stocking. The patient is followed up at a week and three weeks.

Subfascial Ligation of Perforators

This procedure was described with variations by Linton, Cockett and Dodd. It consists of making an incision on the medial aspect of the lower leg till the medial malleolus through the fascia. All perforating veins in the subfascial compartment on the medial and dorsal side are identified, ligated with nonabsorbable sutures and divided.

This procedure did not gain much popularity as it was associated with recurrence and frequent wound complications.

Results

Most studies have shown a significant improvement in quality of life after stripping.[25] In comparison to endovenous ablation, most studies have shown an early postoperative advantage for EVA, but disease specific scores were comparable after time.[26] The earlier return to normal activities in the EVA arm was found to confer advantages.[27]

Other Methods

Subcutaneous Endoscopic Perforator Surgery (SEPS)

SEPS uses endoscopy instruments to ligate incompetent perforators through small incisions. It is highly favored for advanced CVI in view of its minimally invasive nature and safety profile.

The limb is exsanguinated, elevated and then a thigh tourniquet is placed. A small longitudinal incision is made 100 mm distal to tibial tuberosity, and fascia incised after dissecting subcutaneous tissue. A 10 mm port is introduced through which the camera is inserted. A 5 mm port is inserted about 5 mm distal to the first one. Carbon dioxide is insufflated in the subcutaneous tissue and dissection performed. All visualized perforators are interrupted using harmonic scalpel, electrocautery or metallic clips. On completion the ports are removed, the CO_2 expressed and tourniquet removed. Local anesthetic is injected to reduce postoperative pain.

Complications include DVT, thrombophlebitis and neuralgia.[28] The long-term follow-up results of the endoscopic division of perforating veins are comparable with those of the open division of perforating veins.[29]

Ambulatory Conservative Hemodynamic Management (ACHM)

ACHM may be defined as a 'physiological surgery' technique which involves identification (duplex doppler) and ligation of points of deep to superficial reflux rather than ablative surgery. The aim of ACHM is not only to preserve the GSV for use as a future vascular graft, but also to maintain its drainage eliminating reflux points with change of compartments.

Studies so far have been conflicting. One prospective study concluded that the interruption of GSV reflux by this procedure is only temporary.[30] Another RCT comparing CHIVA with stripping concluded that recurrence rates were higher in the stripping arm.[31] Due to the complexity of this technique and doubts about its efficacy it has not been widely adopt.

Transilluminated Powered Phlebectomy

This has been proposed as a quicker and more reliable method for varicose vein avulsion. In this procedure, an endoscopic dissector with a rotating blade and suction is used to hydrodissect the subcutaneous tissue and resect the veins. This is done with the aid of a transilluminator. Using transilluminated powered phlebectomy, multiple and large incisions could be reduced. A perfect cosmetic outcome might be reached.[32] One RCT comparing this procedure with stab phlebectomies concluded that TIPP had the advantage of fewer incisions but was associated with more extensive bruising and prolonged pain.[33]

Cryosurgery

This includes cryosclerosis and cryostripping. These are methods of treating LSV reflux in conjunction with SFJ ligation where the vein is frozen in situ using liquid nitrogen. Complications include hematoma formation and nerve damage. One RCT comparing it to RFA concluded there was no significant difference in late outcome though patients favoured RFA in view of less postoperative pain.[34]

CONCLUSION

Numerous treatment options exist for the management of this common yet non-life-threatening condition. Surgery remains the most common mode of treatment used. Yet in the quest for a less invasive procedure several treatment options are emerging. The trade-off between their obvious advantages and long-term recurrence rates will determine their role in management. In view of multiple options being available, the patients decision may be the final say.

REFERENCES

1. Caggiati A, Bergan JJ. The Saphenous vein: derivation of its name and its relevant anatomy. J Vasc Surg. 2002;35(1): 172-5.
2. Schweighofer G, Mühlberger D, Brenner E. The anatomy of the small Saphenous vein: fascial and neural relations, saphenofemoral junction, and valves. J Vasc Surg. 2010;51(4):982-9.
3. Carpentier PH, Marieq HR, Biro C, et al. Prevalence, risk factors, and clinical patterns of chronic venous disorders of lower limbs: A population-based study in France. J Vasc Surg. 2004;40:650-9.
4. Jutley RS, Cadle I, Cross KS. Preoperative assessment of primary varicose veins: A duplex study of venous incompetence. Eur J Vasc Endovasc Surg. 2001;21(4):370-3.
5. Singh S, Lees TA, Donlon M, et al. Improving the preoperative assessment of varicose veins. Br J Surg. 1997;84(6):801-2.

6. Beale RJ, Gough MJ. Treatment options for primary varicose veins—A review. Eur J Vasc Endovasc Surg. 2005;30:83-95.
7. Shoab SS, Porter J, Scurr JH, Coleridge-Smith PD. Endothelial activation response to oral micronised flavonoid therapy in patients with chronic venous disease—a prospective study. Eur J Vasc Endovasc Surg. 1999;17(4):313-8.
8. Martínez-Zapata MJ, Moreno RM, Gich I, et al. A Randomized, double-blind multicentre clinical trial comparing the efficacy of calcium dobesilate with placebo in the treatment of chronic venous disease. Eur J Vasc Endovasc Surg. 2008;35(3):358-65.
9. Jull AB, Arroll B, Parag V, Waters J. Pentoxifylline for treating venous leg ulcers. Cochrane Database Syst Rev. 2012 Dec 12;12:CD001733. doi: 10.1002/14651858.CD001733.pub3.
10. O'Meara S, Cullum NA, Nelson EA. Compression for venous leg ulcers. Cochrane Database of Systematic Reviews 2009, Issue 1. Art. No.: CD000265. DOI: 10.1002/14651858. CD000265.pub2.
11. Amsler F, Blättler W. Compression therapy for occupational leg symptoms and chronic venous disorders - a meta-analysis of randomised controlled trials. Eur J Vasc Endovasc Surg. 2008;35(3):366-72.
12. Proebstle M, Vago B, Alm J, et al. Treatment of the incompetent great Saphenous vein by endovenous radiofrequency powered segmental thermal ablation: First clinical experience. J Vasc Surg. 2008;47(1):151-6.
13. Merchant RF, DePalma RG, Kabnick LS. Endovascular obliteration of Saphenous reflux: A multicenter study. J Vasc Surg. 2002;35(6):1190-6.
14. Lurie F, Creton D, Eklof B, et al. Prospective randomized study of endovenous radiofrequency obliteration (closure procedure) versus ligation and stripping in a selected patient population (EVOLVeS Study). J Vasc Surg. 2003;38(2): 207-14.
15. Hinchliffe RJ, Ubhi J, Beech A, et al. A prospective randomised controlled trial of VNUS closure versus surgery for the treatment of recurrent long saphenous varicose veins. Eur J Vasc Endovasc Surg. 2006;31(2):212-8.
16. Proebstle TM, Lehr HA, Kargl A, et al. Endovenous treatment of the greater Saphenous vein with a 940-nm diode laser: Thrombotic occlusion after endoluminal thermal damage by laser-generated steam bubbles. J Vasc Surg. 2002; 35(4):729-36.
17. Timperman PE. Prospective evaluation of higher energy great Saphenous vein endovenous laser treatment. J Vasc Interv Radiol. 2005;16(6):791-4.
18. Van den B, Neumann RR, de Roos M, Nijsten KP. Endovenous laser ablation-induced complications: review of the literature and new cases. Dermatologic Surgery. 2009;35(8):1206-14.
19. Min RJ, Khilnani N, Zimmet SE. Endovenous laser treatment of saphenous vein reflux: long-term results. J Vasc Interv Radiol. 2003;14(8):991-6.
20. Theivacumar NS, Darwood R, Gough MJ. Neovascularisation and recurrence 2 years after varicose vein treatment for sapheno-femoral and great saphenous vein reflux: A comparison of surgery and endovenous laser ablation. Eur J Vasc Endovasc Surg. 2009;38(2):203-7.
21. Puggioni A, Kalra M, Carmo M, et al. Endovenous laser therapy and radiofrequency ablation of the great Saphenous vein: analysis of early efficacy and complications. J Vasc Surg. 2005;42(3):488-93.
22. Bootun R, Lane TR, Dharmarajah B, et al. Intra-procedural pain score in a randomised controlled trial comparing mechanochemical ablation to radiofrequency ablation: The Multicentre Venefit™ versus ClariVein® for varicose veins trial. Phlebology 2016;31(1):61-5.
23. Morrison N, Gibson K, McEnroe S, et al. Randomized trial comparing cyanoacrylate embolization and radiofrequency ablation for incompetent great saphenous veins (VeClose). J Vasc Surg. 2015;61(4):985-94.
24. Rivlin S. The surgical cure of primary varicose veins. Br J Surg. 1975;62:913-17.
25. MacKenzie RK, Paisley A, Allan PL, et al. The effect of long saphenous vein stripping on quality of life. J Vasc Surg. 2002;35(6):1197-203.
26. Christenson JT, Gueddi S, Gemayel G, Bounameaux H. Prospective randomized trial comparing endovenous laser ablation and surgery for treatment of primary great saphenous varicose veins with a 2-year follow-up. J Vasc Surg. 2010;52(5):1234-41.
27. Darwood RJ, Theivacumar N, Dellagrammaticas D, et al. Randomized clinical trial comparing endovenous laser ablation with surgery for the treatment of primary great saphenous varicose veins. Br J Surg. 2008;95(3):294-301.
28. Gloviczki P, Bergan JJ, Rhodes JM, et al. Mid-term results of endoscopic perforator vein interruption for chronic venous insufficiency: lessons learned from the North American subfascial endoscopic perforator surgery registry. The North American Study Group. J Vasc Surg. 1999;29(3):489-502.
29. Sybrandy JEM, van Gent WB, Pierik EGJM, Wittens CHA. Endoscopic versus open subfascial division of incompetent perforating veins in the treatment of venous leg ulceration: Long-term follow-up. J Vasc Surg. 2001;33(5):1028-32.
30. Escribano JM, Juan J, Bofill R, et al. Durability of reflux-elimination by a minimal invasive CHIVA procedure on patients with varicose veins. A 3-year prospective case study. Eur J Vasc Endovasc Surg. 2003;25(2):159-63.
31. Carandina S, Mari C, De Palma MG, et al. Varicose vein stripping vs haemodynamic Correction (CHIVA): A long term randomised trial. Eur J Vasc Endovasc Surg. 2008;35(2):230-7.
32. Shamiyeh A, Schrenk, P, Huber E, et al. Transilluminated powered phlebectomy: advantages and disadvantages of a new technique. Dermatol Surg. 2003;29(6):616-9.
33. Chetter IC, Mylankal KJ, Hughes H, Fitridge R. Randomized clinical trial comparing multiple stab incision phlebectomy and transilluminated powered phlebectomy for varicose veins. Br J Surg. 2006;93(2):169-74.
34. Deisenhofer I, Zrenner B, Yin YH, et al. Cryoablation versus radiofrequency energy for the ablation of atrioventricular nodal reentrant tachycardia (the CYRANO Study): results from a large multicenter prospective randomized trial. Circulation. 2010;122(22):2239-45.

Chapter 52

Sclerotherapy

S Sacchidanand, TS Nagesh, Sujala S Aradhya

Key Messages

- Sclerotherapy refers to the introduction of a sclerosing solution into the lumen of a vessel producing endothelial damage and subsequent fibrosis.
- Sclerotherapy consists of liquid sclerotherapy and foam sclerotherapy.
- Indications include varicose veins, telangiectasia and cysts.
- Smaller veins respond better to sclerotherapy.

INTRODUCTION

Sclerotherapy refers to the introduction of a foreign substance (sclerosing solution) into the lumen of a vessel producing endothelial damage, which leads to thrombosis and subsequent fibrosis. The extent of damage to the blood vessel wall determines the effectiveness of the solution. Sclerotherapy has been extensively used by dermatosurgeons in the management of superficial varicose veins and other venous abnormalities.[1,2]

HISTORY

Historical methods for causing venous endothelial damage include a slender rod of iron, reportedly used by Hippocrates himself; absolute alcohol, introduced by Monteggio and Lerpy D'Etoilles in the 1840s; and ferric chloride, introduced by Charles Gabriel Pravaz in 1851.[3] The idea of injecting irritant substances into the vein for purpose of obliteration appears frequently in the French literature of last century. The injections were made with strong caustic and toxic substances. In 1908 Beniamino Schiassi in Bologna, first used iodine as sclerosant. Linser, started the use of 20% sodium chloride solution. The French school under the leadership of Sicard has used sodium salicylate in 20–40% solutions. Nobl has tried injections of 50% dextrose and a mixture containing equal parts of dextrose and levulose with 4% sucrose. Meisen uses equal parts of 25% sodium salicylate and 10% sodium chloride.[4]

Foam sclerotherapy was first described in 1939 by S McAusland. Subsequently, in 1949, Sigg reported that the injection of foam into a vein was beneficial because it washed away less rapidly, thus introducing the concept that foam with greater viscosity has advantages over other contemporary sclerotherapy techniques. The following year, Orbach compared the efficacy of sodium tetradecyl sulfate (STS) foam with that of an injection of an equal amount of STS in liquid form. He found that the STS foam had 3.5–4 times the thrombogenic property of the solution. In 1953, the Norwegian doctor Arve Ree injected pure ethamolin foam into varicose veins and reported excellent results in a series of 50 patients. In 1956, Peter Fluckiger was the first to notice that the foam could be directed into regions other than the site of injection by manual manipulation. This concept is now widely practiced with ultrasound-guided foam sclerotherapy.

OBJECTIVES AND MECHANISM OF SCLEROTHERAPY

Varicose vein is one of the clinical manifestations of venous hypertension. It has been estimated that between 17% and 50% of persons with varicose veins have cutaneous findings. Patients with chronic venous insufficiency (CVI) and superficial venous insufficiency may benefit from sclerotherapy or surgical treatment of the superficial venous system.[5] The ultimate goal of sclerotherapy as an interventional procedure is to normalize venous physiology.

Box 1: Indications of sclerotherapy in varicose veins.

- Pain
- Major tributaries of greater and lesser saphenous veins
- Major perforator reflux
- Lateral venous system varicosities
- Complications of varicose veins like stasis dermatitis and venous ulcers
- Cosmetic—telangiectasias/spider webs

Sclerotherapy of incompetent perforators and/or varicose veins increases the efficacy of calf muscle pump, resulting in an improved clearance of extravascular fluid.[5] Sclerotherapy has shown to help in the healing of venous ulcers and stasis eczema.[6] Vascular fibrosis and obliteration occur in response to irreversible endothelial cellular damage and exposure of underlying subendothelial layer in a dose-dependent manner after sclerotherapy. If the sclerosant is too weak, it will not cause any endothelial injury; if little stronger, vessel is damaged but recanalization occurs forming an incompetent pathway; and if too strong, the endothelium is destroyed but the sclerosant flows into adjacent normal vessels causing extensive tissue necrosis. Hence, the key to successful outcome is to inject an appropriate amount and concentration of sclerosant which causes irreversible damage to the endothelium of the abnormal vessel, while leaving adjacent normal vessels untouched.[3] Injection of the sclerosant and its subsequent dilution with blood results in three zones. Zone 1 is the site of irreversible endothelial injury which scleroses completely and is replaced by fibrous tissue. Partial or complete thrombosis of the vessel takes place in Zone 2 which eventually recanalizes. In Zone 3, the sclerosant is diluted to below its injurious concentration, without causing any endothelial injury.[3] The extent of different zones depends on the concentration of the sclerosant used, vessel diameter and the position of the patient.

INDICATIONS OF SCLEROTHERAPY IN VARICOSE VEINS[7,8]

Indications for sclerotherapy in varicose veins are shown in Box 1.

CONTRAINDICATIONS[8,9]

Contraindications for selerotherapy are listed in Table 1.

Table 1: Contraindications for sclerotherapy.

Absolute contraindications	*Relative contraindications*
▪ Acute superficial or deep vein thrombosis	▪ Leg edema
▪ Local infection in the area of sclerotherapy or severe generalized infection	▪ Saphenofemoral junction incompetence
▪ Immobility, confinement to bed	▪ Thrombophilia with history of deep vein thrombosis
▪ Advanced peripheral arterial occlusive disease (stage 3 or 4)	▪ Long-standing diabetes
▪ Hyperthyroidism (in the case of sclerosants containing iodine)	▪ Peripheral arterial occlusive disease stage II
▪ Pregnancy in the first trimester and after the 36th week of gestation	▪ Poor general health
▪ Known allergy to the sclerosant	▪ Myocardial decompensation
▪ Severe systemic disease	▪ Migraine
	▪ Bronchial asthma
	▪ Marked allergic diathesis
	▪ Known hypercoagulability

SCLEROSING SOLUTIONS[7,10,11]

There are many sclerosing solutions available. Important parameters to be considered in selecting a sclerosant include:

- Vessel diameter
- Reflux considerations
- Patient allergy profile
- Pain tolerance
- Previous treatment response to a given agent
- Minimal sclerosing concentration
- Sclerosant complication profile.

Sclerosing solutions are classified into three groups, based on their mechanisms of destruction of the endothelium; detergent agents, osmotic agents and chemical irritants.

Detergent Agents

This group of sclerosants act by protein theft mechanism; these agents cause vascular injury by altering the surface tension around the endothelial cells. Structurally, they contain one pole that is hydrophilic and one pole that is hydrophobic. Rapid endothelial cell wall damage occurs when over hydration results from the hydrophilic pole, attracting water into the cell, while the hydrophobic pole attaches to the vein wall. Examples of detergent agents include sodium tetradecyl sulfate (STS), polidocanol, sodium morrhuate and ethanolamine oleate.[3,11]

Osmotic Agents

This group of sclerosants cause endothelial cell damage through dehydration. Examples of osmotic agents include hypertonic saline and hypertonic saline dextrose.[11]

Chemical Irritants

This group of sclerosants cause endothelial cell damage by their direct corrosive action. After injection, the endothelium near the site of injection is destroyed within seconds. The corrosive action is limited because of rapid inactivation by blood proteins. At the site of endothelial destruction the chemical can penetrate further and diffuse into deeper layers of the vessel wall causing further destruction. Examples of chemical irritants include chromate glycerin and polyiodinated iodine. These agents are not approved by the US Food and Drug Administration (FDA).

The current FDA approved sclerosing agents include STS, polidocanol, sodium morrhuate and hypertonic saline and are dealt in greater detail.

Table 2: Comparison of various sclerosants.[7,12-14]

Sclerosing solution	*Category*	*Advantages*	*Disadvantages*	*Vessels treated*	*Concentrations*	*Maximum volume/ dose of sclerosant*
Sodium tetradecyl sulfate	Detergent	▪ FDA approved ▪ Painless unless injected extravascularly	▪ May cause skin breakdown at higher concentrations	All sizes	▪ 0.1–0.2% telangiectasias ▪ 0.2–0.5% reticular ▪ 0.5–1.0% varicose ▪ 1.0–3.0% axial varicose	10 cc of 3%
Polidocanol	Detergent	▪ FDA approved ▪ Painless	▪ Ulcerogenic	Small to medium	▪ 0.25–0.5% Telangiectasias ▪ 0.5–1.0% reticular ▪ 1.0–3.0% Varicose	20 cc of 3%, not to exceed 2 mg/kg
Hypertonic saline	Hyperosmolar	▪ Low risk of allergic reactions	▪ Ulcerogenic ▪ Painful	Small	▪ 23.4–11.7% telangiectasias ▪ 23.4% Reticular	Maximum 20 cc per session, restrict volume in salt restricted diets
Hypertonic saline + dextrose	Hyperosmolar	▪ Low risk of allergic reaction ▪ Mild stinging ▪ Low ulcerogenic potential	▪ Not FDA approved ▪ Relatively weak sclerosant	Small	▪ Undiluted—telangiectasias ▪ Undiluted—reticular	10 cc
Sodium morrhuate	Detergent	▪ FDA approved	▪ Allergic reactions highest	Small	▪ Undiluted—telangiectasias ▪ Undiluted—reticular	2–5 cc of 5%, 50–250 mg depending on vein diameter
Chromated glycerin	Chemical irritant	▪ Low skin ulcer potential	▪ Not FDA approved ▪ Very weak sclerosant	Smallest	▪ Undiluted to half strength—telangiectasias	
Polyiodinated iodine	Chemical irritant	▪ Highly corrosive; allows treatment of largest veins	▪ Not FDA approved ▪ Avoid in iodine allergic patients	Largest	▪ 1–2% for up to 5 mm veins ▪ 2–6% for the largest veins	2–3 cc of 6%

Sodium Tetradecyl Sulfate

Sodium tetradecyl sulfate is a long chain fatty acid salt with strong detergent properties. It is a highly effective sclerosing solution used worldwide. Approved for use in the United States since 1946, it has been popular with vascular surgeons since the 1960s and was first described for use in telangiectasias in the 1970s. Appropriate concentrations for superficial telangiectasias are 0.1–0.2%. Other concentrations are 0.2–0.5% for reticular veins or small varicosities and 0.5–3% for larger varicosities related to major sites of valvular reflux. A relatively high incidence of postsclerosis pigmentation has been reported at high doses (1% STS).[11]

Polidocanol

The detergent-based polidocanol, a urethane compound, was originally developed as an anesthetic, but was found to have the property of sclerosing small diameter vessels after intradermal injection. Polidocanol contains hydroxylpolyethoxydodecane dissolved in distilled water with 5% ethanol as a stabilizer.

Hypertonic Saline

Although approved by FDA only for use as an abortifacient, it is a commonly employed solution in the United States of America. A theoretical advantage of hypertonic saline is its total lack of allergenicity when unadulterated.[11] It has been commonly used in various concentrations from 10% to 30%, with occasional addition of heparin, procaine or lidocaine. However, evidence for benefits of the additional agents is lacking and hence hypertonic saline is used either unadulterated or diluted to 11.7% with sterile water for smaller telangiectasias. With hypertonic saline, damage of tissue adjacent to injection sites may easily occur. Skin necrosis may be produced by extravasation at the injection site particularly when injecting very close to the skin surface. Injection of hyaluronidase into sites of extravasation may significantly reduce the risks of skin necrosis with hypertonic saline.

Sodium Morrhuate

Sodium morrhuate is a 5% solution of salts of saturated and unsaturated fatty acids in cod liver oil. Approximately, 10% of its fatty acid composition is unknown. This agent is preferred primarily for sclerosis of esophageal varices. Although it is approved by the FDA for sclerosis of varicose veins, use in treatment of telangiectasias is not common because of its caustic qualities, with potential for cutaneous necrosis and higher risk of allergy. Its use is limited by reports of fatalities secondary to anaphylaxis.

Table 2 shows comparison of different sclerosing agents.[7,12-14]

PRE-PROCEDURE ASSESSMENT[9]

Case Selection

A reasonable approach for treating an individual with varicose veins should consider the likely benefits of a particular intervention in three areas.

1. Cosmetic benefit
2. Symptomatic benefit

3. Prevention of progression of venous insufficiency and venous ulceration.

The correlation between symptoms and severity of varicose veins is so poor that it is very difficult to predict the likely outcome after intervention as far as symptoms are concerned. As a general observation, patients who obtain benefit from properly fitted graduated elastic hosiery are likely to benefit from intervention in appropriate cases. If the procedure is in a patient who has already developed signs of chronic venous insufficiency, positive outcome is assured. If the purpose of the intervention is cosmetic, it is reasonable to go ahead after careful discussion with the patients about the risks and benefits, as with any other cosmetic procedure.

History

A detailed history including general medical conditions, smoking, physical activity, pregnancy and intake of estrogens, hormone replacement therapy, oral contraceptives, aspirin and nonsteroidal anti-inflammatory drugs (NSAIDs) should be obtained. History of Raynaud's phenomenon, vascular insufficiency and systemic diseases such as diabetes mellitus, hypertension and schemic heart disease should be recorded. Results of previous treatment received for the condition and whether it is a primary or recurrent lesion are also noted.

Examination

Physical examination to assess the skin for evidence of stasis dermatitis, stasis ulcer, examination of the venous system for varicosity, small vessels and large vessels and status of perforators is essential. Examination should include looking for evidence of previous deep vein thrombosis. Arterial pulses should be checked properly. In case of vascular malformation, the extent of malformation, pulsations and whether a bruit is present to rule out an arteriovenous fistula is important.

Investigations

General investigations such as complete blood counts, bleeding and clotting time, blood sugar and ECG may be carried out. The duplex ultrasound (Doppler test) is the most useful tool for workup and has replaced many of the physical examination maneuvers and physiological tests previously used for diagnosis.

Duplex Doppler Ultrasonography[15]

The advent of color flow duplex scanning has revolutionized the assessment of venous disease. It is a valuable noninvasive tool, simple in application. This technique combines B-mode real-time ultrasonography with pulsed Doppler ultrasonography. The B-mode image allows visualization of the underlying vessels so that a pulsed Doppler signal can then be specifically targeted to assess flow in a particular vessel. Forward flow of venous blood toward the heart is augmented by a maneuver such as compression of the calf muscle; reverse flow of blood following this maneuver indicates that the vein is incompetent. The duplex scan provides the following information, which will have an effect on the decision to treat and the nature of the procedure.

- Patency and competence of the deep veins (obstruction and incompetence)
- Site and level of major incompetence (evaluation of perforator incompetence)
- Anatomy of the popliteal fossa can be identified accurately
- Anatomical abnormalities can be identified
- Duration and velocity of venous reflux

Duplex has become the modality of choice for the diagnosis before beginning a treatment protocol and allows to tailor treatment appropriately to individual cases. It has also been shown to be superior to venography (Fig. 1).

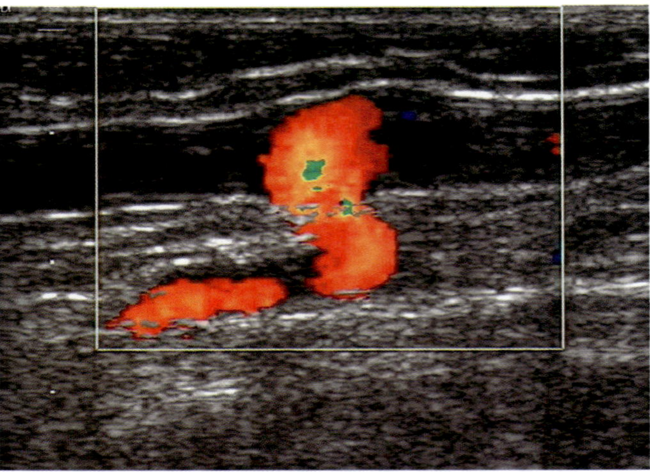

Fig. 1: Venous Doppler showing perforator incompetence. (*Source:* Dr HT Narayana, Professor and Head, Department of Radiodiagnosis, Sri Siddartha Medical College, Tumkur).

PROCEDURE

Materials Required[16] (Fig. 2)

- Cotton balls soaked in spirit
- Protective gloves
- Disposable syringes of 1 cc or 3 cc with 30 gauge disposable transparent hub needles
- Elastocrepe for compression
- Hypoallergenic tape
- Topical nitroglycerine ointment (2%)
- Sclerosing solutions (stored separately from injectables) diluted with normal saline
- Magnifying loupes or lenses.

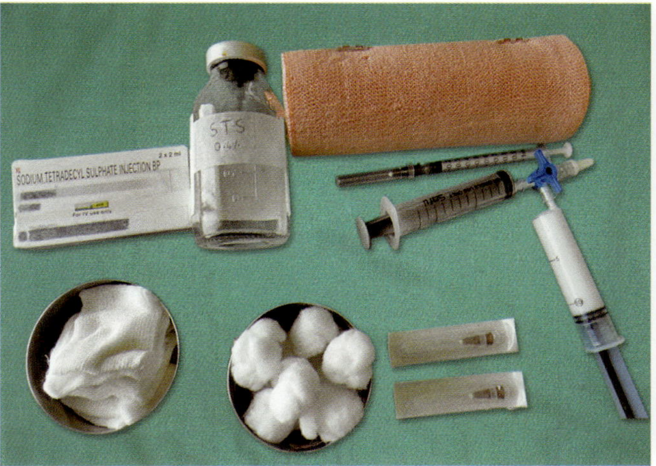

Fig. 2: Sclerotherapy tray.

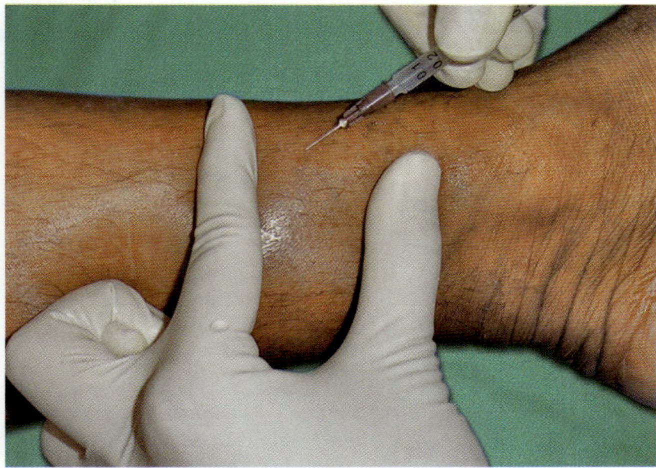

Fig. 3: Position of the hand while injecting.

Box 2: Indications for different concentrations.

Higher concentrations
- Younger patients
- Thick-walled vessels determined by palpation
- Hand/ feet/ pretibial veins
- Vessels >4 mm in diameter to compensate for dilution

Lower concentrations
- Age >60 years
- 0.6–0.9 mm in diameter elevated spider veins
- Thin-walled vessels
- Easy bruisability
- History of spontaneous bleeding following minor trauma

Sclerosant Concentrations[14]

Indications for different concentrations are shown in Box 2.

Principles of Varicose Vein Sclerotherapy[5]

- Always inject proximal to distal
- Inject the larger vein before smaller veins
- Vein must be emptied of blood by various maneuvers
- Exert direct finger pressure in spreading and compressing motion after injection
- Reflux points should be determined initially and treated specifically
- Immediate and adequate compression is important
- Ensure adequate ambulation immediately after treatment

Patient Preparation[16]

The patient should be in recumbent position that allows convenient access to the veins to be treated. Motorized table with height adjustment will facilitate easy access to all regions of the legs. Both the physician and the patient should be comfortable, and proper lighting should be available. The area to be treated is exposed adequately and cleaned thoroughly with spirit or povidone-iodine. Usually anesthesia, intralesional or topical, is not required. An anxious patient is counselled and an analgesic or antianxiety drug may be administered. The sclerosant is diluted to the required concentration (See Table 2) with distilled water or saline and loaded in a syringe.

TECHNIQUES

Techniques depend on the size of veins as follows:

Sclerotherapy Techniques for Large Veins

There are two common techniques employed: Fegan's technique and Sigg's technique.[5]

Fegan's Technique

The classic technique presently employed with minor modifications is that of Fegan. The patient sits at end of the examining table with the leg to be treated dependent. The bulging varicosity is cannulized with a needle, butterfly or angiocatheter (Figs. 3 and 4). The leg is elevated and supported by the physician above cardiac level for 1–2 minutes to allow drainage of blood. Before injection, a small amount of blood is drawn into the syringe to ensure that the needle remains in the varicosity lumen. Too much blood may cause dilution of the sclerosant. As the injection of approximately 0.5–1.0 mL occurs, finger pressure several centimeters above and below the injection point is applied to confine the action of the sclerosing solution to the affected site. Finger pressure is maintained for 30–60 seconds followed by immediate application of compression with a foam pad. The pad is secured by foam elastic tape or relatively inelastic wrap around bandage to maintain compression immediately.

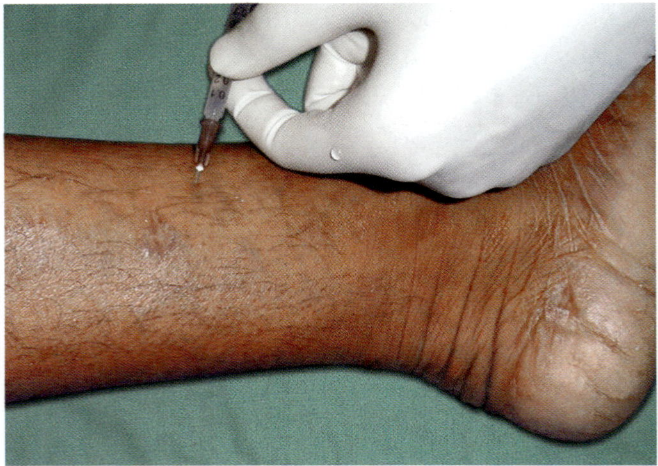

Fig. 4: Injection of sclerosant.

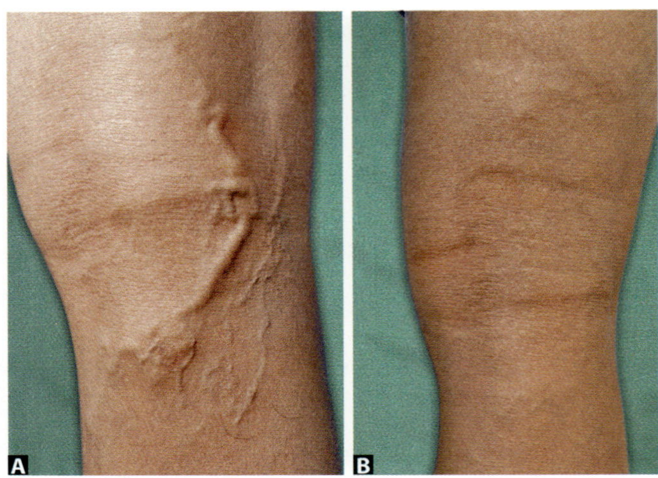

Figs. 5A and B: Before and after sclerotherapy.

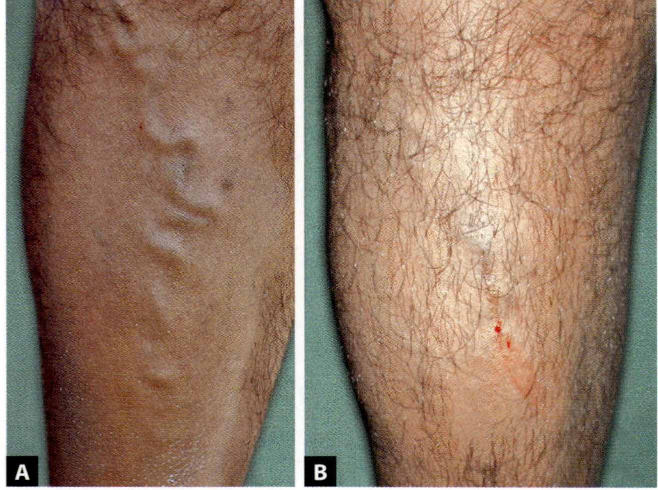

Figs. 6A and B: Before and after sclerotherapy.

Fegan's method is particularly effective for incompetent perforators. The fascial defects through which perforators course may be palpated and serve as the site of needle entry. The site of perforators can also be marked during the venous Doppler study.

A widely used variation of Fegan's technique is the marking of varicosities with the patient standing while needle insertion is done with the patient recumbent or in slight reverse Trendelenburg position. This minimizes the movement of the leg and the inserted needle. Immediately after injection, the leg can be elevated and compression applied. Cannulation of previously marked varicosity is straight forward with the patient supine and may greatly hasten the procedure and minimize loss of proper needle positioning by patient movement. Direct finger pressure and lateral movement outward from the injection site is often useful not only to spread the sclerosant, but also to promote contact with greater surface area of the varicosity by emptying the vessel.

Sigg's Technique

A method frequently used in Europe for sclerosing saphenous junctions is the use of an open needle, called the Sigg's technique. A needle (not attached to the syringe) is inserted into the skin and manipulated until blood drips from the hub, following which the sclerosant is injected.

Sclerotherapy of Reticular Veins

Treatment of reticular veins is similar to large varicose veins, although the concentration, strength, and volume of sclerosing solution are decreased.[5] Subdermal reticular veins are treated only after all sources of reflux have been treated by sclerotherapy or surgery. Doppler ultrasound may also be used as a guide to demonstrate reflux in the reticular veins and to locate those that require treatment. With the patient recumbent, a 3 mL syringe with a 30 gauge needle is inserted into the reticular vein which is usually superficial and visibly blue. When the sensation of piercing the vein is felt, the plunger is pulled back gently until blood is seen. Usually a volume of no more than 0.5 mL per injection site is injected. The sclerosing solution most commonly used is sodium tetradecyl sulfate in concentrations of 0.2–0.5%. The procedure may be done in multiple sittings. Treatment intervals may vary, but allowing 4–8 weeks between treatments helps to minimize the number of necessary sessions. Figures 5 and 6 show the results after sclerotherapy.

POST-SCLEROTHERAPY COMPRESSION[5,17,18]

Rapid, immediate and adequate compression after injection of the sclerosant is recommended. Graduated compression hoses (15–30 mm Hg) or cotton balls with elastocrepe can be used for adequate compression.

Post-sclerotherapy compression helps in:

- Limiting the flow of blood back into the varicosity, thereby decreasing both thrombus formation and the tendency for recanalization
- Improving the effectiveness with greater resolution of both small and large varicosities
- Complete mobility after treatment and enhances muscle pump function. This rapidly dilutes and removes any sclerosing solution that inadvertently entered deep system.

The duration of compression is still debated. Fegan recommended 6 weeks, but 3–5 days of compression has been suggested adequate. Walking may lessen the risk of deep vein thrombosis by avoiding stagnation of blood flow. Risks of deep vein thrombosis are also lessened by adhering to the principle of no more than 1.0 mL per injection site, with the usual volume being 0.5 mL.

SIDE EFFECTS AND COMPLICATIONS OF SCLEROTHERAPY

Post-Sclerotherapy Hyperpigmentation

It is the appearance of increased visible pigmentation along the course of a treated vein of any size. Initially, pigmentation is due to the perivascular hemosiderin deposition, but over time, the hemosiderin is replaced by melanin. The incidence of pigmentation is related to the dilution and type of sclerosant as well as size of the treating vessel. Incidence ranges from 11% to 30% for hypertonic saline and polidocanol and up to 30% with STS. Compression may help to prevent this side effect. Removal of postsclerotherapy coagula by a small incision using a 21 G needle and expressing it out may decrease the incidence of pigmentation. Pigmentation clears usually within 6 months and rarely persists for more than one year.

A study has shown that weekly subcutaneous administration of desferroxamine mesylate 500 mg reduces the time to depigmentation by 82% in patients with post-sclerotherapy cutaneous hyperpigmentation treated for telangiectasias and reticular veins and prolonged post-sclerotherapy hyperpigmentation in varicose veins.[19]

Matting

It is defined as the appearance of groups of new fine telangiectasias surrounding or replacing a previously treated area in blush-like manner. Resolution occurs spontaneously within a 3–12-month period with 70–80% spontaneous resolution within the first 6 months.

Cutaneous Necrosis

It may occur with all sclerosants if the solution spills outside the vessel into the skin. Studies have shown that extensive tissue necrosis following high concentration sclerotherapy may be rare, but its occurrence is serious and its treatment may be difficult.[20] In case of extravasation of the sclerosant, necrosis may be minimized by injecting normal saline in the ratio of 10:1 at the site. Application of 2% nitroglycerine paste at the extravasation site greatly reduces the risks of necrosis.

Superficial Thrombophlebitis

It is characterized by a very tender, indurated and linear erythematous swelling. Incidence is 0.01–1% following sclerotherapy. Administered transdermally, glyceryl trinitrate speeds the resolution of venous inflammation in patients with sclerotherapy-related thrombophlebitis. Nitric oxide released from glyceryl trinitrate may exert a direct anti-inflammatory action on the inflamed veins and surrounding tissues.[21]

Pulmonary Embolism

It probably occurs from extension of a superficial thrombus into the deep venous system. It is usually associated with injection of large quantities of sclerosant at a single site. There are reports of acute massive pulmonary embolism following high ligation combined with compression sclerotherapy when both procedures were done simultaneously in a patient with hypercoagulable state.[22]

Arterial Injection

This dreaded complication is extremely rare and can lead to large areas of skin necrosis and damage to the subcutaneous tissue and muscle, which may take months to heal. Emergency treatment involves immediate application of ice, attempts to flush the inadvertently injected artery with normal saline and heparin, injection of procaine 3% to inactivate STS and vascular surgery consultation for intravenous anticoagulation.

Allergic Reaction

Systemic allergic reactions to sclerotherapy treatment can occur rarely.[23] Anaphylaxis has been reported after sclerotherapy. However, very few reports of severe or fatal reaction have been reported. Hence, it is always recommended to make the patient stay in the hospital for about 30 minutes after the procedure before discharge. Also, emergency measures to manage anaphylaxis should be available at the place of treatment.

FOAM SCLEROTHERAPY

Foam sclerotherapy is often presented as a new method for the management of varicose veins. However, foam sclerotherapy was first described as early as 1939 by S McAusland. He injected froth, produced by shaking a rubber capped bottle filled with sodium morrhuate into spider veins. Further in 1944, Orbach demonstrated the use of air in sclerotherapy by airblock technique. In 1949, Sigg reported the benefit of foam as it washed away less rapidly, thus introducing the concept that foam with greater viscosity has advantages over other contemporary sclerotherapy techniques. Subsequently, in 1956, Peter Fluckiger was the first to notice that the foam could be directed into regions other than the site of injection by manual manipulation. Minor modifications in the way foam is produced, as well as the use of ultrasound to guide it to the sites of venous reflux, have resulted in a renewed interest in this technique.[24,25]

The detergent sclerosants like STS and POL can only produce foam.[11] Sclerosing foam is a mixture of gas bubbles in a liquid solution that contains surface-active molecules. The gas must be well tolerated by patients, physiologic, and the bubble size should be preferably under 100 μ. According to the bubble diameter, foams can be classified as froth, macrofoam, minifoam and microfoam. If the relative volume fraction of liquid is less than 5%, the foam is classified as dry, whereas if it is more than 5%, it is classified as wet. Wet foam (e.g. Tessari's foam) has the maximum stability. Uniform bubble diameter also provides more stability.[24]

Techniques of Foam Sclerotherapy[26]

- *Monfreux method:* Foam is produced in a glass syringe filled with 0.3 to 0.5 mL of sclerosant. Negative pressure is created by closing the tip of the syringe with sterile plug and holding tension on the piston until 2–3 mL of foam is generated. The consistency is low probably due to the large size of the bubbles and also this technique has a higher rate of side effects.
- *Cabrera method:* Juan Cabrera has used CO_2 for producing the foam.
- *Benigni-Sadoun method:* Plastic syringes are used with repeated and fast pulling and release of piston. The foam is very short lasting.
- *Lorenzo Tessari's Tourbillon technique:* Two plastic disposable syringes are connected by a three-way stopcock. The foam is formed by mixing the liquid sclerosant with 4 or 5 parts of air, through 20 passes between the two syringes with the hub at a 30° rotation. This rotation narrows the stopcock passage generating high turbulence, which produces high quality microfoam. This is one of the most frequently used technique.[27]
- *Modifications of Tessari:*
  - Two way female connector [28]
  - Automated foaming device turbofoam Kreussler Pharma, France[29]
- *Frullini method:* Mechanism of foam generation uses the same turbulence effect of Tessari method. Here a connecter is inserted in a vial of STS and the other end is connected to a syringe. The vial is positioned upside down and quick injection/aspiration of the solutions is performed.

Foam Stability

The stability of foam is affected by the injection technique, composition and volume of foam. The homogenecity of the bubble size, viscosity and temperature all influence the quality and longevity of foam.[29]

The bubble size is inversely related to the difference in density between a liquid and gas as shown in the below equation:[30]

d_p = bubble diameter
d_o = orifice diameter
σ = surface tension
$\Delta\rho$ = difference in density between a liquid and gas

The density of the air also determines the size of the bubbles in foam. Carbon dioxide being 1.5 times denser than room air produces smaller bubbles compared to room air. Also the foam bubbles produced by Tessari technique are smaller compared to other techniques. The smaller bubble size leads to increased suface area of the sclerosant as well as increased amount of sclerosant being delivered to the endothelial cells and hence more efficacious.[31,32]

Injection using ultrasound guidance and direct puncture technique are commonly used while performing foam sclerotherapy for large veins like great saphenous vein. Short and long catheters with balloon tips are used for the procedure. However, there is a possibility of deep vein thrombosis while using long catheters due to the passage through perforators.[33,34]

Advantages and Disadvantages of Foam Sclerotherapy

Foam preparations are considered to be three to four times more potent than equivalent oncentrations and volumes of liquid sclerosants. The advantages of foam sclerosants compared to conventional liquid sclerotherapy are:[13,24]

- Increase in the effective surface area of foams compared with liquid
- Displacement of blood from the treated vein which produces prolonged undiluted intimal contact
- Increased vasospasm and sclerosis of veins at a greater distance from the injection site than can liquid preparations
- Smaller volumes and concentrations
- Enhanced visibility on duplex imaging due to echogenicity of foams and hence greater efficacy.

The main disadvantage of foam is the difficulty in standardization. In patients with patent ductus arteriosus, foam can lodge in the lungs and produce pulmonary fibrosis. There are reports of deep vein thrombosis and superficial thrombophlebitis following foam sclerotherapy. There are four case reports of transient ischemic attack and stroke following foam sclerotherapy for varicose veins in a patient, who later was found to have patent foramen ovale and atrial septal defects.[29,35] Also pain and pigmentation is relatively more in patients treated with foam.[24]

However, various randomized controlled studies comparing the incidence of adverse events with foam and liquid sclerotherapy of the saphenous vein have shown no statistical difference between these techniques.[29]

LASER TREATMENT OF TELANGIECTASIAS AND RETICULAR VEINS

Laser therapy is mainly indicated for telangiectasia/venulectasia or reticular veins less than 3 mm in diameter. It is mainly used for patients with areas of neovascularization with telangiectatic matting, veins resistant to sclerotherapy and non-cannulizable vessels. The concept of selective photothermolysis by laser with hemoglobin as the chromophore is the principle behind using lasers for leg veins. Hemoglobin has an absorption spectrum which has broad peaks at 410 nm, 540 nm and 577 nm and smaller peaks at 920 nm and 940 nm. The various lasers used include pulsed dye (585–605 nm), KTP (532 nm) alexandrite (755 nm), diode (810 nm), Nd:YAG (1,064 nm) and intense pulse light (IPL). The important parameters which influence the treatment and management of individual vessels include the wavelength, pulse duration and spot size. The larger vessels respond to longer wavelengths or the ratio of vessel to epidermal heating increases the probability of achieving complete vessel coagulation. However, lasers and IPL may not be replacements for sclerotherapy, mainly because hydrostatic pressure considerations are not addressed by light endothelial interactions and also, it may be difficult to have sufficient penetration of photons safely through the thick epidermaldermal wall surrounding the lower extremity vessels.[36]

Endovenous Ablation

Both radiofrequency and endovenous laser ablations have been used to treat varicose veins[37,38] and have been dealt with in previous chapter.

SUMMARY

Sclerotherapy is a simple and effective procedure for the treatment of varicose veins. With experience, larger veins can also be treated effectively with sclerotherapy. It can prevent the complications of varicose veins if done in the initial stages. Sclerotherapy being an outpatient procedure, when done with adequate precautions is associated with very minimal morbidity, mortality and loss of work time compared to surgery. Sclerotherapy has emerged as a simple, safe and effective treatment modality for management of venous abnormalities, both therapeutically and esthetically. The advent of foam sclerotherapy has carried the field further forwards. New advances in laser ablation have opened new avenues for management of these common therapeutic and esthetic problems.

Tips and Tricks

- Using a bent needle to inject can help in keeping the injecting hand more stable
- Always withdraw to look for blood in the syringe before injection and avoid the urge to inject till the needle is in the vein
- Start with lower concentrations and lower volumes of injections in the initial days
- Not more than 0.5–1 cc of the sclerosant to be injected at each site
- Not more than 10 cc of the sclerosant injection per session
- Vessel size is the best prognostic indicator of treatment response and complications
- Patients can be asked to mark the vessels which they feel is most troublesome
- Selection of sclerosant concentration can be done on an individual basis.

REFERENCES

1. Goldman MP. Treatment of varicose and telangiectatic leg veins: double-blind prospective comparative trial between aethoxyskerol and sotradecol. Dermatol Surg. 2002;28:52-5.
2. Lorenz MB, Gkogkolou P, Goerge T. Sclerotherapy of varicose veins in dermatology. JDDG: Journal der Deutschen Dermatologischen Gesellschaft. 2014;12(5):391-3.
3. Feied C. Sclerosing solutions. In: Bergan JJ (Ed). The Vein Book. USA: Elsevier Academic Press; 2007. pp.125-31.
4. De Takas G. Varicose veins and their sequelae. JAMA. 1929;92:775-9.
5. Goldman MP, Weiss RA, Bergan JJ. Diagnosis and treatment of varicose veins: a review. J Am Acad Dermatol. 1994;31:393-413.
6. Subbarao NT, Aradhya SS, Veerabhadrappa NH. Sclerotherapy in the management of varicose veins and its dermatological complications. Indian J Dermatol Venereol Leprol. 2013;79:383-8.
7. Weiss RA, Weiss MA. Treatment of varicose and telangiectatic veins. In: Freedberg JM, Eisen AZ, Wolff K, et al. (Eds). Fitzpatrick's Dermatology in General Medicine. 6th edition. USA: McGrawHill Publishers; 2003. pp.2549-56.
8. Rabe E, Breu FX, Cavezzi A, et al. European guidelines for sclerotherapy in chronic venous disorders. Phlebology. 2014;29:338-54.
9. Khunger N, Sacchidanand S. Standard guidelines for care: sclerotherapy in dermatology. Indian J Dermatol Venereol Leprol. 2011;77:222-30.
10. Sadick N, Li C. Small vessel sclerotherapy. Dermatol Clinics. 2001;19:475-81.
11. Weiss MA, Hsu JT, Neuhaus I, et al. Consensus for sclerotherapy. Dermatologic Surgery. 2014;40(12):1309-18.
12. Breadon J. Sclerotherapy. In: Burgess MC (Ed). Cosmetic Dermatology. Germany: Springer Publications; 2005. p.147.

13. Weiss RA, Feied CF, Weiss MA. Treatment of large varicose veins. In: Weiss R, Feied C, Feied CF, Weiss M (Eds). Vein Diagnosis and Treatment: A Comprehensive Approach. USA: McGrawHill Publishers; 2001. p.102.
14. Duffy DM. Sclerotherapy. In: Dover JS, Alam M, Nguyen TH (Eds). Treatment of Leg Veins. USA: Elsevier Saunders; 2006. pp.71-105.
15. Labropoulos N, Landon P, Jay T. The impact of duplex scanning in phlebology. Dermatol Surg. 2002;28:1-5.
16. Weiss RA, Weiss MA. Sclerotherapy treatment of telangiectasias. In: Bergan JJ (Ed). The Vein Book. USA: Elsevier Academic Press; 2007. pp.133-8.
17. Goldman MP. How to utilize compression after sclerotherapy. Dermatol Surg. 2002;28:860-2.
18. Nootheti P, Cadag KM, Magpantay A, et al. Efficacy of graduated compression stockings for an additional 3 weeks after sclerotherapy treatment of reticular and telangiectatic leg veins. Dermatol Surg. 2009;35:53-8.
19. Lopez L, Dilley RB, Henriquez JA. Cutaneous hyperpigmentation following venous sclerotherapy treated with desferrioxamine mesylate. Dermatol Surg. 2001;27:795-8.
20. Bergan JJ, Weiss RA, Goldman MP. Extensive tissue necrosis following high concentration sclerotherapy for varicose veins. Dermatol Surg. 2000;26:535-42.
21. Berrazueta JR, Fleitas M, Salas E, et al. Local transdermal glyceryl trinitrate has an anti-inflammatory action on thrombophlebitis induced by sclerosis of leg veins. Angiology. 1994;45:347-51.
22. Yamaki T, Nozaki M, Sasaki K. Acute massive pulmonary embolism following high ligation combined with compression sclerotherapy for varicose veins. Dermatol Surg. 1999;25:321-5.
23. Goldman MP. Complications and adverse sequelae of sclerotherapy. In: Bergan JJ (Ed). The Vein Book. USA: Elsevier Academic Press; 2007. pp.149-53.
24. Geroulakos G. Foam sclerotherapy for the management of varicose veins: critical reappraisal. Phlebolymphology. 2006;13:202-6.
25. Orbach EJ. Sclerotherapy of varicose veins: utilization of intravenous air block. Am J Surg. 1944;362-6.
26. Frullini A, Cavezzi A. Sclerosing foam in the treatment of varicose veins and telangiectasias: history and analysis of complications. Dermatol Surg. 2002;28:11-5.
27. Tessari L, CavezziA, Frullini A. Premliminary experience with a new sclerosing foam in the treatment of varicose veins. Dermatol Surg. 2001;27:58-60.
28. Hamel-Desnos C, Desnos P, Wollmann JC, et al. Evaluation of the efficacity of polidocanol in the form of foam compared with liquid foam in sclerotherapy of the great saphenous vein: initial results. Dermatol Surg. 2003;29:1170-75.
29. Goldman MP, Jean-Jerome G, Weiss RA (Eds). Clinical methods for sclerotherapy of varicose veins. In: Sclerotherapy Treatment of Varicose and Telangiectatic Leg Veins, 5th edition. Saunders Elsevier, Edinburgh; 2011. pp.242-7.
30. Hu WS. Oxygen Transfer in Cell Culture Bioreactors. Cellular Bioprocess Technology; 2004. pp.1-14.
31. Frullini A, Cavezzi A. Sclerosing foam in the treatment of varicose veins and telangiectases: history and analysis of safety and complications. Dermatol Surg. 2002;28:11.
32. Redondo P, Cabrera J. Microfoam treatment of Klippel-Trénaunay syndrome and vascular malformations. J Am Acad Dermatol. 2008;59:355.
33. Breu FX, Guggenbichler S. European consensus meeting on foam sclerotherapy, April 4–6 2003, Tegernsee Germany. Dermatol Surg. 2004;30:709-17.
34. Cavezzi A, Tessari L. Foam sclerotherapy techniques: different gasses and methods of preparation, catheter versus direct injection. Phlebology. 2009;24:247.
35. Adatia S, Nambiar V, Kapadia R, et al. Acute ischemic stroke caused by paradoxical air embolism following injection sclerotherapy for varicose veins. Neurol India. 2013;61:431-3.
36. Sorhaindo SN. Laser treatment of telangiectasias and reticular veins. In: Bergan JJ (Ed). The Vein Book. USA: Elsevier Academic Press; 2007. pp.157-65.
37. Weiss R, Elston DM. Varicose veins treated with radiofrequency ablation therapy; 2016. [Online] Emedicine website. Available from: http://emedicine.medscape.com/article/ 1085800-overview [Accessed November 2016].
38. Khilnani NM, Elston DM. Varicose vein treatment with endovenous laser therapy; 2016. [Online] Emedicine website. Available from: http://emedicine.medscape.com/article/1815850-overview [Accessed November 2016].

Chapter 53

Sclerotherapy for Vascular Malformations

Sujay Khandpur

Key Messages

- Sclerotherapy is an important, simple, cheap, easy and minimally invasive technique for management of vascular malformation.
- Indications include hemorrhage, lesions located at life- or limb-threatening sites, lesions-threatening vital functions: seeing, hearing, eating, breathing, disabling pain, functional impairment secondary to swelling or pain, tissue loss or ulceration and severe cosmetic deformity.
- In particular, sclerotherapy is indicated for extratruncular diffuse infiltrative vascular malformations (VM), extratruncular localized vascular malformation or as adjunct to surgery.
- The success of sclerotherapy procedure depends upon the concentration of the sclerosant used and its dwell time.
- Complications depend on vascular malformation morphology, extent and depth of the lesion (superficial or deep) and the type of sclerosant used.

DEFINITION

Sclerotherapy is a technique which induces local endothelial cell damage by selective intraluminal delivery of endothelial-cidal agent/sclerosant into chosen abnormal intravascular space that exerts its injurious effect on endothelial cell by direct contact in dose-dependent manner.[1] It is an important therapeutic modality for treating venous malformations (VM) that occur with an incidence of 1–2 per 10,000 births and a prevalence of 1%.[2] VM not only produce a devastating cosmetic impact but may be associated with pain, bleeding, ulceration, secondary infection and even compress vital structures.

Management of VM may be conservative or interventional. It requires a multidisciplinary approach with participation of a general surgeon, plastic surgeon, orthopedician, head and neck surgeon, dermatologist, pediatrician, interventional radiologist, physiotherapist, nurse and a patient care coordinator.[3]

Conservative management is indicated when patient is either not wanting intervention or the symptoms are not meeting "intervention threshold".[4] Conservative therapy includes elevation of involved area during sleep, avoidance of activities producing symptoms, cessation of oral contraceptives, alleviation of paroxysmal pain due to localized intravascular coagulopathy with NSAIDs such as aspirin therapy, prophylactic administration of low molecular weight heparin for large VM in high-risk states and use of pressure garments/stockings.

Interventional management includes sclerotherapy, lasers and other technologies and surgery.[1] Of these, sclerotherapy is simple, cheap and relatively noninvasive.

INDICATIONS FOR INTERVENTIONAL MANAGEMENT

Indications for interventional management of VM include:[5]

Absolute Indications

- Hemorrhage
- Lesions located at life- or limb-threatening sites
- Lesions threatening vital functions: seeing, hearing, eating, breathing
- Disabling pain
- Functional impairment secondary to swelling or pain
- Tissue loss or ulceration
- Severe cosmetic deformity.

Relative Indications

- Vascular-bone syndrome
- Location at high risk of complications like hemarthrosis, deep venous thrombosis
- Recurrent infection
- Cosmetic deformity.

Surgical excision is indicated when it can be completely removed without recurrence, the lesion is focal and well-defined, thrombosed, confined to single or specialized muscle group, causing neurologic or compression symptoms, when there is good possibility of anatomic/functional restoration or for truncal VM.[1] However, surgical excision is difficult to perform when VMs occupy multiple anatomic spaces, multiple muscle groups/fascial planes or encase critical structures.[6]

SCLEROTHERAPY

This is indicated for extratruncular diffuse infiltrative VM, extratruncular localized VM or as adjunct to surgery.[6] The success of sclerotherapy procedure depends upon the concentration of the sclerosant used and its dwell time (time for which the sclerosing agent is in contact with endothelial cells).[7]

The commonly used sclerosing agents are:

- 100% ethanol
- 3% sodium tetradecyl sulfate
- 1% polidocanol
- 5% ethanolamine oleate alcoholic solution of zein (ethibloc)
- 5% sodium morrhuate
- Hypertonic 50% dextrose
- Hypertonic saline
- Acetic acid
- Methylmethacrylate
- Triamcinolone
- Bleomycin
- Tetracycline.

Table 1 shows the properties and relative advantages and disadvantages of commonly used sclerosing agents for VM.

PROCEDURE

Preoperative Preparation and Counseling

Prior to the procedure, a detailed history and a thorough physical examination is undertaken. This is followed by measurement of the lesion, a baseline photograph and imaging studies (color Doppler/Magnetic resonance imaging) to estimate the location, extent of the lesion and flow velocity (low flow or high flow). A preoperative counseling is done in which the patient is explained about the specific indication for this procedure, technique to be employed, possible complications, postoperative pain and swelling.

Table 1: Commonly used sclerosing agents.

Agent	*Mechanism of action*	*Advantages*	*Disadvantages*
Absolute ethanol[8,9]	▪ Dehydration of endothelial cells ▪ Precipitation of cytoplasm ▪ Sloughing and denudation of endothelial cells ▪ Vessel wall fracture ▪ Precipitation of blood proteins	▪ High response rate ▪ Cheap ▪ Easy to obtain ▪ Long shelf life	▪ Very toxic; use with caution ▪ Juxtalesional necrosis; skin necrosis ▪ Very painful; GA ▪ Nerve impairment ▪ Hemoglobinuria ▪ Pulmonary artery vasospasm/hypertension ▪ Intoxication, bronchospasm, hyperthermia, cardiopulmonary collapse, death
5% Ethanolamine oleate[10,11]	Vascular fibrosis and sclerosis by: ▪ Oleic portion: intimal and extravascular inflammation ▪ Ethanolamine: suppresses fibrin clot formation	▪ Wide safety margin due to low penetrance beyond vessel wall ▪ Low incidence of distal embolization; used in both HFL and LFL	▪ High dose: hemolysis, renal insufficiency, hepatotoxicity.
3% sodium tetradecyl sulfate (anionic surfactant; injectable form is soapy in consistency)[12,13]	▪ Sludging of RBCs ▪ Thrombosis ▪ Intimal necrosis, adventitial fibrosis, luminal collapse	▪ Less toxic ▪ Lower rates of skin necrosis, nerve impairment, systemic sideeffects	▪ Less effective in permanent closure in high-flow lesion ▪ Lower rate of permanent closure of venous malformations
1% polidocanol (non-ionic surfactant)[14]	▪ Endothelial cell overhydration ▪ Effects intrinsic coagulation pathway	▪ Painless due to anesthetic effect ▪ Low complications: skin necrosis, nerve impairment	▪ Systemic complications: hemolysis, hemoglobinuria, cardiac arrest

(HFL: High flow lesions; GA: Gallic acid; LFL: Low flow lesions).

Anesthesia

The procedure is performed under sedation or local, regional or general anesthesia in case of large and deep VM.[15] However, for treatment of localized and relatively small VM, no anesthesia is required.

Procedure

Sclerotherapy is performed in a room equipped with angiographic facilities, real-time ultrasonography and facility to review previous images. The patient is positioned to allow best access of lesion then draped, exposing all relevant access points. The instrument tray which includes labeled syringes, saline, iodinated contrast, sclerosants, 20–26 gauge needle with connector tubing or butterfly needle is kept ready. Some physicians perform a direct percutaneous phlebogram by injecting a contrast medium, prior to the procedure. In deep VM, butterfly needle is introduced into VM under real-time ultrasound, fluoroscopic or even magnetic resonance imaging guidance while in superficial lesions, it is entered by palpation alone. Syringe is gently aspirated until flashback of blood is observed signifying intraluminal position of needle followed by injecting of the sclerosing agent. The patient is continuously monitored to assess extravasation of the sclerosant, any resistance to injection, signs of patient distress or skin blanching (which indicates chemical toxicity or ischemia to skin). The lesion is continuously palpated for induration and administration of the sclerosant is limited as it becomes firm. The procedure is terminated when maximum allowable sclerosant dose is reached.

For smaller lesions, sclerotherapy can be undertaken without any anesthesia as an OPD procedure. Under aseptic conditions and by fixing the lesion between the thumb and index finger, the agent is injected into each lesion with insulin syringe and 26 gauge needle, initially withdrawing blood to confirm appropriate entry of needle into the vascular space and then injecting the agent to reach appropriate induration of lesion and blanching.

Post-procedure compression is applied to the lesion (for 3–4 hours for small lesions to 24 hours–3 to 7 days for large VM) to allow vascular wall apposition and reduce intralesional volume and dilution effects. Table 2 shows response to sclerotherapy in relation to morphology of VM.

Table 3 shows results after sclerotherapy in different studies.

IMMEDIATE POST-PROCEDURE MANAGEMENT

The patient is advised oral analgesics. Systemic steroids may be indicated after use of stronger sclerosants like ethanol, following sclerotherapy on large areas, when VM have proximity to vital structures or ethanol-treated head and neck lesions. Low molecular weight heparin may be administered if sclerotherapy is performed in conjunction with surgery. Doppler ultrasound is advised if there are concerns of deep vein thrombosis. Physiotherapy is indicated if the lesions are located on mobile regions as VM may form scars post-sclerotherapy.

Patient Follow-up

A repeat session may be undertaken after 3 weeks to 3 months. Lesion size is measured to look for shrinkage post-sclerotherapy and also a repeat photograph is taken for comparison. Figures 1 to 8 show the results after sclerotherapy in different vascular malformations. A radiological review is also undertaken post-therapy. Patient's disease status and expectations are also discussed and limitations of the procedure explained.

Table 2: Response to sclerotherapy in relation to venous malformation morphology.[16]

	Grade of venous malformation	*Definition*	*Size*	*Response to sclerotherapy*
Magnetic resonance imaging	Grade 1	Well-defined	< 5 cm diameter	71% excellent result 29% good result 0% poor result
	Grade 2A	Well-defined	> 5 cm diameter	22% excellent result 44% good result 33% poor result
	Grade 2B	Ill-defined	< 5 cm diameter	26% excellent result 15% good result 60% poor result
	Grade 3	Ill-defined	> 5 cm diameter	0% excellent result 43% good result 57% poor result
	Tissue layer involved ▪ Skin ▪ Subcutaneous ▪ Muscle ▪ Tendon ▪ Bony cortex			Risk of skin or nerve injury Muscular involvement: risk of contracture Bone or bone marrow involvement: risk of fracture

Table 3: Review of literature of sclerotherapy results.

S. No.	Author	Type of lesions	Number of patients	Agent used	Result	Complications
1.	Mahesh B, et al.[19]	Peripheral VM	40	Color Doppler ultrasound guided 3% SDS	HFLs, 81.25% regression; LFLs, 83.3% regression	
2.	Jain R, et al.[20]	VM, 9 Lymphangiomas, 3 Venous pseudoaneurysm, 1 AV malformation of pinna, 1	15	Ultrasound guided 1% polidocanol (1–20 injections)	Complete response ▪ VM, 7 (77.8%); ▪ Lymphangiomas, 3 (100%); ▪ AV malformation, 1 (100%) Partial response ▪ VM, 2 (22.2%) ▪ Venous pseudoaneurysm (100%)	Minor complications
3.	Rimon U, et al.[21]	VM: face, neck, chest, extremities	21	95% ethanol ↓ GA	Complete to partial improvement in 17 cases (81%) after 1–9 sessions	Five Cases: Skin ulcer, 2; Skin blister, 1; Pulmonary embolism, 1; Pulmonary hypertension with CVS collapse, 1.
4.	Berenguer B, et al.[22]	Craniofacial VM	18	Ethanol or SDS ↓ GA	Cured or marked improvement, 76%	Skin blisters, 50% Deep ulceration, 13% Nerve injury, 7.5% Hemoglobinuria, 28%
5.	O'Donovan JC, et al.[7]	VM (15), hemangioma (6)	13, sclerotherapy alone; 8, sclerotherapy surgery	3% SDS	Beneficial in 86%	Skin ulcers, 14.28%
6.	Tan KT, et al.[23]	Peripheral VM	72	3% STS (mean, 3.1 sessions)	Patients became asymptomatic, 15%; Good response, 28%; Improved, 24%; Unchanged, 28%; Worsened, 5.6%. Change in size by MRI; Decreased, 54%; No change, 31%; Increase, 14%.	Skin necrosis, 6.9%; Transient sensory deficit/urticaria, 1.4%; Venous thrombosis, one case
7.	Kuo HW, et al.[24]	Venous lake	2	1% polidocanol	Complete resolution after 2 sessions	Minimal scar
8.	Park CO, et al.[25]	Lymphangioma, Acq. digital arterio-venous malformation	1 each	STS	Near complete clearance after several sessions	
9.	Khandpur S, et al.[26]	VM, 13	13	3% STS	90–100% subsidence in 11 cases (84.6%) after mean 4 injections	Cutaneous blister formation, erosions, and crusting at injection site: 7 cases (53.8%); Atrophic scarring: 4 patients (30.8%)
10.	Jairath V, et al.[27]	Cherry angiomas	100 lesions in 20 patients	3% sodium tetradecyl sulfate	42 lesions responded with single dose, 44 lesions required two sessions, remaining 14 lesions required four sessions	Persistent crusting for >15 days in 17.2% of cherry angiomas. Other side effects were postinflammatory hyperpigmentation and ulceration, which eventually resolved with minimal scarring (n = 11). Scaring, which was temporary in 11 cases

contd...

contd...

S. No.	Author	Type of lesions	Number of patients	Agent used	Result	Complications
11.	Wang Y, et al.[28]	Angiolymphoid hyperplasia with eosinophilia	One patient	1% polidocanol solution	Bleeding and pruritus completely resolved after second treatment. Complete resolution after 7 sessions, each injection given every 10 days	Mild pain, bleeding
12.	Kupetsky EA, et al.[29]	Lymphangioma circumscriptum	One patient	1% sodium tetradecyl sulfate	After 4 treatment sessions (one every 4 weeks), 50% reduction in lesions	Not mentioned
13.	Deore GD, et al.[30]	Recurrent oral pyogenic granulomas in a case of port -wine stain	One patient with multiple lesions	3% sodium tetradecyl sulfate		

(AV: Arteriovenous; CVS: Cardiovascular system; GA: Gallic acid; HFLs: High flow lesions; LFLs: Low flow lesions; SDS: Sodium dodecyl sulfate; STS: Sodium tetradecyl sulfate; VM: Venous malformations).

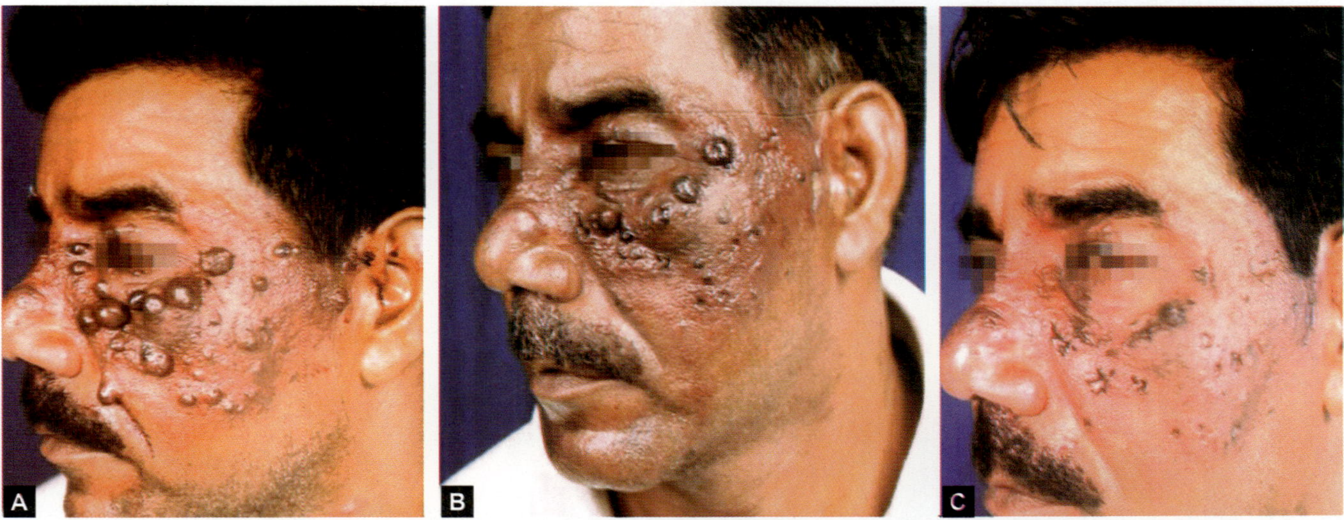

Figs. 1A to C: (A) Multiple nodules overlying port-wine stain left face. (B) Subsidence of majority of nodules after five sessions. (C) Resolution of all nodules after six sessions with atrophy at injection site.

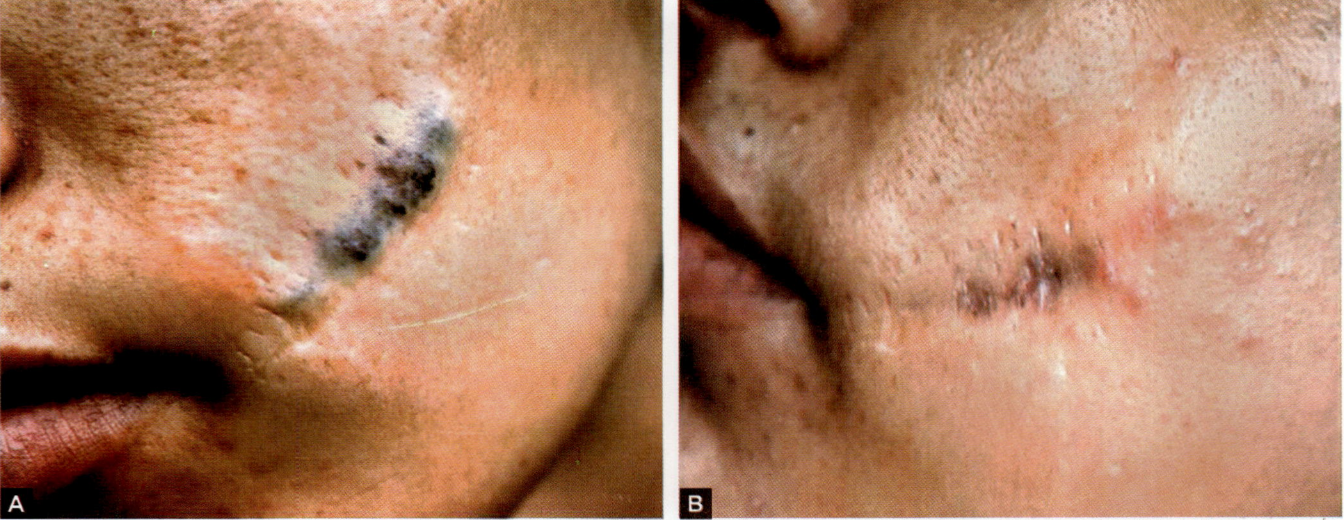

Figs. 2A and B: (A) Linear venous malformation of left face with post-excision scar. (B) Subsidence of lesion after three sessions.

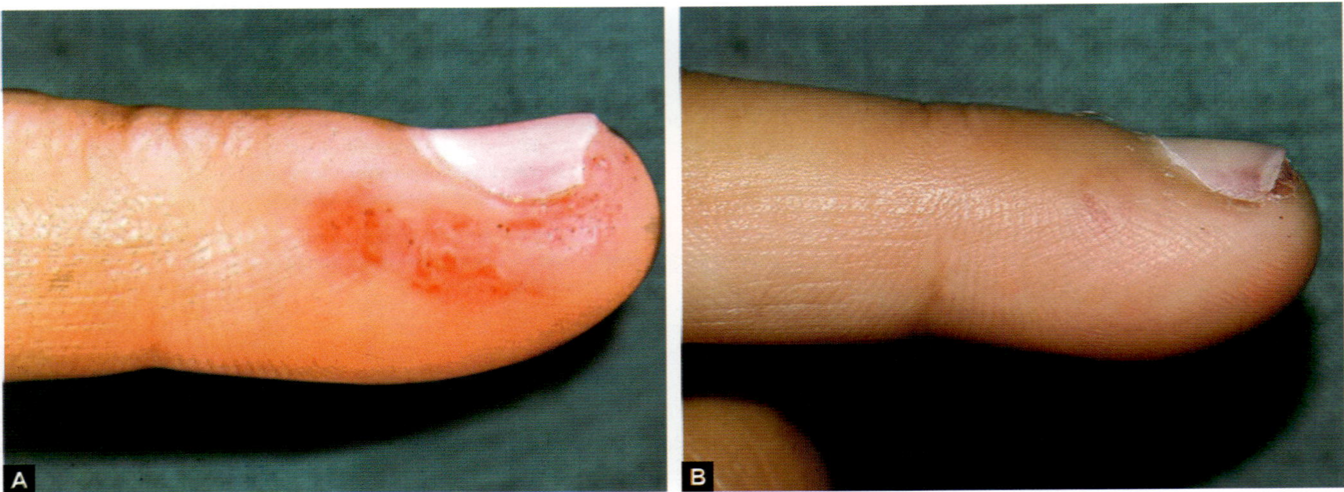
Figs. 3A and B: (A) Lesion over right middle finger. (B) More than 90% subsidence after one session.

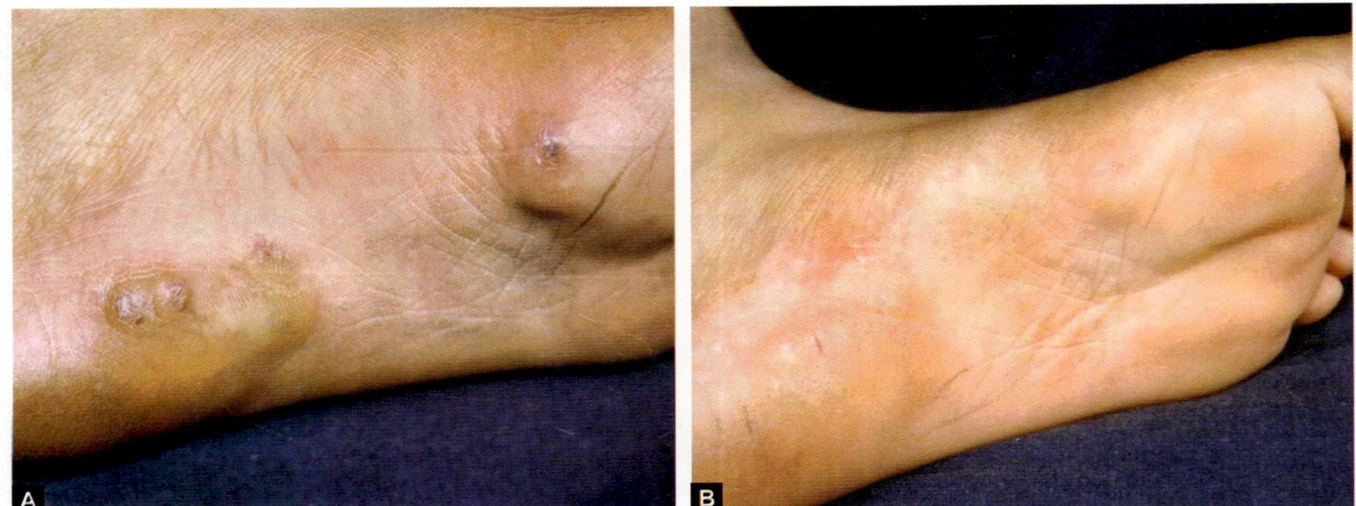
Figs. 4A and B: (A) Venous malformations—left sole. (B) Complete resolution after four sessions.

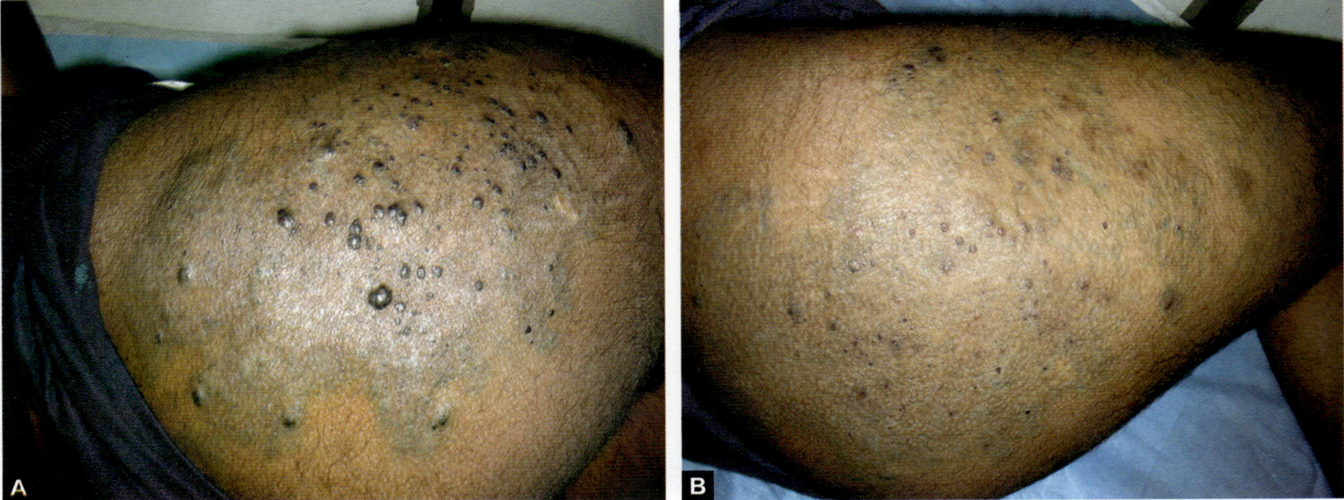
Figs. 5A and B: (A) Venous malformations over right thigh. (B) More than 90% regression after four sessions.

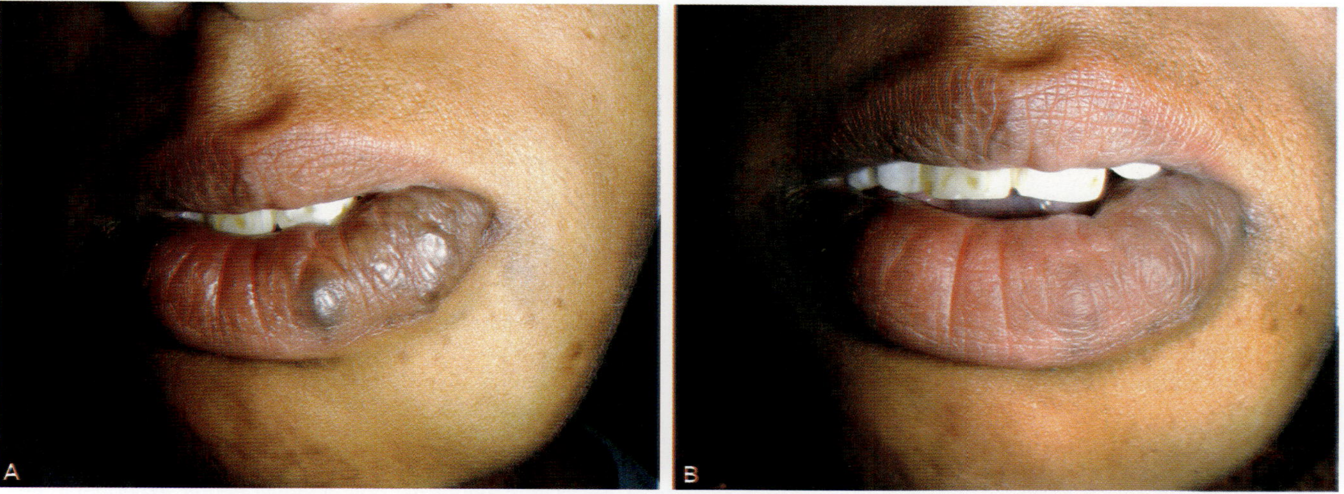

Figs. 6A and B: (A) Venous malformations over right lower lip. (B) More than 90% regression after two sessions.

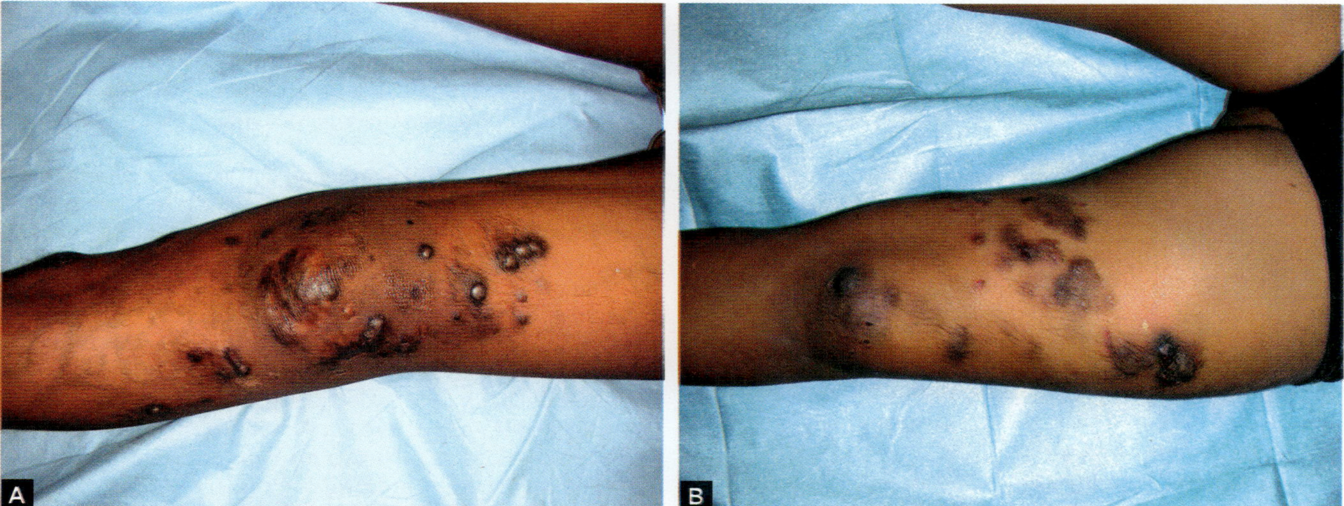

Figs. 7A and B: (A) Multiple venous malformations—left lower limb. (B) Significant subsidence after three injections.

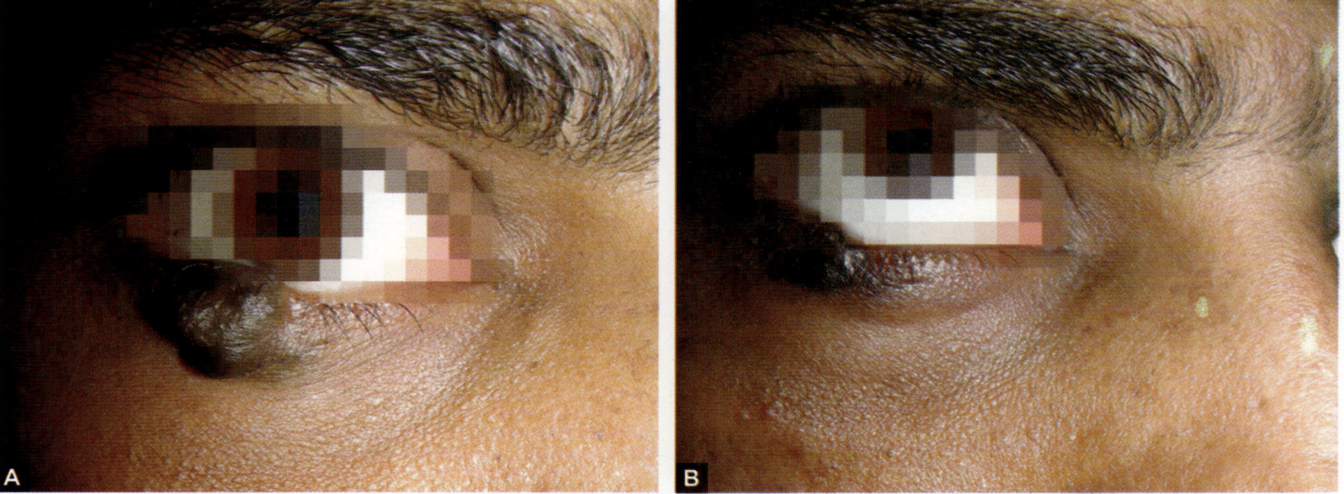

Figs. 8A and B: (A) Venous malformation—right lower eyelid. (B) Near complete resolution after one injection.

FOAM SCLEROTHERAPY

This modification of the sclerotherapy procedure has shown greater efficacy than liquid form since foam displaces blood from target vessel, remains undiluted and persists in the vessel to maximize its action.

This technique was originally conceived in 1944 by Orbach.[17] Cabrera and coworkers (1990s) used therapeutic foam of sodium tetradecyl sulfate or polidocanol for varicose veins.[18] In 2003, they used sclerosant in microfoam form to treat VM. In this technique, 0.25–4% polidocanol-carbon dioxide mixture or 3–6:1 room air to sclerosant using sodium tetradecyl sulfate or polidocanol is used.[31]

COMPLICATIONS

The complications depend on VM morphology, extent and depth of the lesion (superficial or deep) and the type of sclerosant used, e.g. ethanol is most toxic, complications are low with sodium tetradecyl sulfate, polidocanol and ethanolamine oleate.[32]

Complications include:

Minor Local Complications

- Erythema, swelling, pain and tenderness
- Skin blistering, hyperpigmentation, skin ulceration and necrosis.

Major Local Complications

- Transient or permanent nerve impairment or paralysis
- Thrombophlebitis, deep venous thrombosis
- Muscular contracture
- Compartment syndrome.

Major Systemic Complications

- Hemolysis
- Renal toxicity
- Pulmonary embolism
- Ocular disturbances
- Anaphylactic reactions
- Hypotension, bradyarrhythmia and cardiopulmonary collapse.

Specific tips for sclerotherapy according to type of venous malformations are shown in Box 1.

Box 1: Specific tips for sclerotherapy.

- In cases of slow-flow VM, direct sclerotherapy into nidus is preferred
- In cases of intermediate-flow VM, sclerotherapy controlled flow with balloon occlusion, tourniquet and coil are preferred. Cyanoacrylate embolization prior to sclerotherapy may also be used
- In cases of high-flow VM, a multidisciplinary approach should be used since there is rate of treatment failure, recurrence and complications

REFERENCES

1. Hein KD, Mulliken JB, Kozakewich HP, et al. Venous malformation of skeletal muscle. Plast Reconstr Surg. 2002; 110:1625-35.
2. Eifert S, Vyllavicencio JL, Kao TC, et al. Prevalence of deep venous anomalies in congenital vascular malformations of venous redominance. J Vasc Surg. 2000;31:462-71.
3. Nagy M, Brodsky L. Multidisciplinary approach to management of hemangiomas and vascular malformations. Facial Plast Surg Clin Morth Am. 2001;9:551-9.
4. Buckmiller LM. Update on hemangiomas and vascular malformations. Curr Opin Otolaryngol Head Neck Surg. 2004;12:476-87.
5. Lee BB. New approaches to the treatment of congenital vascular malformations: a single center experience. Eur J Vasc Endovasc Surg. 2005;30:184-97.
6. Lee BB, Bergan JJ. Advanced management of congenital vascular malformations: a multidisciplinary approach. Cardiovasc Surg. 2002;10:523-33.
7. O'Donovan JC, Donaldson JS, Morello FP, et al. Symptomatic hemangiomas and venous malformations in infants, children and young adults: treatment with percutaneous injection of sodium tetradecyl sulphate. Am J Roentgenol. 1997;169:723-9.
8. de Lorimier AA. Sclerotherapy for venous malformations. J Pediatr Surg. 1995;30:188-93.
9. Shin BS, Do YS, Lee BB, et al. Multistage ethanol sclerotherapy of soft-tissue arteriovenous malformations.effect on pulmonary artery pressure. Radiology. 2005;235:1072-7.
10. Johann AC, Aguiar MC, do Carmo MA, et al. Sclerotherapy of oral benign vascular lesion with ethanolamine oleate: an open clinical trial with 30 lesions. Oral Surg Oral Med Oral Pathol Oral Radiol Endod. 2005;100:579-84.
11. Hyodoh H, Fuita A, Hyodoh K, et al. High-flow arteriovenous malformation of the lower extremity: ethanolamine oleate sclerotherapy. Cardiovasc Intervent Radiol. 2001;24: 348-51.
12. Siniluoto TM, Svendsen PA, Wikholm GM, et al. Percutaneous sclerotherapy of venous malformations of the head and neck using sodium tetradecyl sulphate. Scand J Plast Reconstr Surg Hand Surg. 1997;31:145-50.
13. Anavi Y, Har-El G, Mintz S. The treatment of facial hemangioma by percutaneous injections of sodium tetradecyl sulphate. J Laryngol Otol. 1988;102:87-90.
14. Guex JJ. Indications for the sclerosing agent polidocanol. J Dermatol Surg Oncol. 1994;19:959-61.
15. Legiehn GM, Heran MKS. Venous malformations: classification, development, diagnosis and interventional radiological management. Radiol Clin North Am. 2008;46: 545-97.
16. Goyal M, Causer PA, Armstrong D. Venous vascular malformations in pediatric patients: comparison of results of alcohol sclerotherapy with proposed MR imaging classification. Radiology. 2002;223:639-44.
17. Orbach EJ. Sclerotherapy of varicose veins: utilization of intravenous air block. Am J Surg. 1944;66:362-6.
18. Cabrera J, Cabrera J Jr, Garcia-Olmedo MA, et al. Elargissement des limites de la sclerotherapie nouveaux produits sclerosants. Phlebologie. 1997;2:181-8.

19. Mahesh B, Joseph G, Khazanchi RK, et al. Colour duplex ultrasound-guided sclerotherapy: a new approach to the management of patients with peripheral vascular malformations. Clin Imaging. 2003;27:171-9.
20. Jain R, Bandhu S, Sawhney S, et al. Sonographically guided percutaneous sclerosis using 1% polidocanol in the treatment of vascular malformations. J Clin Ultrasound. 2002;30: 416-23.
21. Rimon U, Garniek A, Galili Y, et al. Ethanol sclerotherapy of peripheral venous malformations. Eur J Radiol. 2004;52: 283-7.
22. Berenguer B, Burrows PE, Zurakowski D, et al. Sclerotherapy of craniofacial venous malformations: complications and results. Plast Reconstr Surg. 1999;104:1-11.
23. Tan KT, Kirby J, Rajan DK, et al. Percutaneous sodium tetradecyl sulfate sclerotherapy for peripheral venous vascular malformations: a single-center experience. J Vasc Interv Radiol. 2007;18:343-51.
24. Kuo HW, Yang CH. Venous lake of the lip treated with a sclerosing agent: report of two cases. Dermatol Surg. 2003; 29:425-8.
25. Park CO, Lee MJ, Chung KY. Treatment of unusual vascular lesions: usefulness of sclerotherapy in lymphangioma circumscriptum and acquired digital arteriovenous malformation. Dermatol Surg. 2005;31:1451-3.
26. Khandpur S, Sharma VK. Utility of intralesional sclerotherapy with 3% sodium tetradecyl sulphate in cutaneous vascular malformations. Dermatol Surg. 2010;36:340-6.
27. Jairath V, Dayal S, Jain VK, et al. Is sclerotherapy useful for cherry angiomas? Dermatol Surg. 2014;40:1022-7.
28. Wang Y, Tu Y, Tao J, et al. Angiolymphoid hyperplasia with eosinophilia responsive to sclerotherapy. Dermatol Surg. 2014;40:1042-3.
29. Kupetsky EA, Pugliano-Mauro M. Lymphangioma circumscriptum: sodium tetradecyl sulfate 0.1% versus hypertonic saline. Dermatol Surg. 2014;40:928-30.
30. Deore GD, Gurav AN, Patil R, et al. Sclerotherapy: a novel bloodless approach to treat recurrent oral pyogenic granuloma associated with port-wine stain. Ann Vasc Surg. 2014;28:1564.e9-14.
31. Pascarella L, Bergan JJ, Yamada C, et al. Venous angiomata treatment with sclerosant foam. Ann Vasc Surg. 2005;19: 457-64.
32. Legiehn GM, Heran MKS. Classification, diagnosis and interventional radiological management of vascular malformations. Orthop Clin North Am. 2006;37:435-74.

Chapter

54

Leg Ulcers

Reena Rai, R Jayashree, CR Srinivas

Key Messages

- **Leg ulcers may be either acute or chronic.**
- Leg ulcers are commonly due to venous, arterial and neuropathic causes.
- Clinical presentation varies according to whether it is venous, arterial or neuropathic ulcer.
- Treatment should be aimed at treating the underlying cause.
- For venous ulcers, compression therapy is the mainstay of treatment, along with local wound care and periwound protection.
- For arterial ulcers, treatment is aimed at establishing adequate arterial supply.
- For neuropathic ulcers, treatment is aimed at minimizing pressure with aggressive debridement of dead tissue and callus.

INTRODUCTION

Ulcers of the lower extremities are a common cause for visits to the surgeon, vascular surgeon or dermatologist. Leg ulcers refer to full thickness skin loss on the leg or foot due to any cause. They occur in association with a range of disease processes and may be acute or chronic. Acute ulcers are those that follow the normal phases of healing; they are expected to show signs of healing in less than 4 weeks and include traumatic and postoperative wounds. Chronic ulcers are those that persist for longer than 6 weeks and are often of complex nature.[1] Of the various causes of leg ulcers, 70% are due to venous disease, 20% have mixed arterial and venous disease, and 10% result from other causes like neuropathy, infections, malignancy and inflammatory causes.[2]

CAUSES OF LEG ULCERS

The causes of leg ulcers are elaborated in Box 1.

CLINICAL FEATURES OF LEG ULCERS

The clinical feature of venous, arterial and neuropathic ulcers according to their characteristic are elaborated in Table 1.

VENOUS ULCERS

Pathophysiology of Venous Ulcers

Figure 1 shows normal anatomy of venous system of legs.

The venous system in the lower extremities comprises of three systems of veins: superficial veins, deep veins and communicating veins (Fig. 1). Blood flows from the superficial to deep veins through the communicating veins, then up from the foot to the thigh and thence to the abdomen, before venous blood returns to the heart. These veins contain valves which prevent backflow of blood and allow unidirectional flow. During muscular activity, a high pressure develops in the deep venous system allowing blood to flow from deep to the superficial veins. When the calf muscle relaxes, high pressure in the superficial veins allows blood to flow from superficial to deep veins.

This mechanism is called "calf muscle pump". Failure of this pump which could be due to incompetence of the valves, muscle weakness and distension of veins might lead to reflux of blood from deep to superficial veins causing high pressure in the superficial venous system and chronic venous insufficiency (CVI). Further detailed discussion on anatomy of venous system of legs can be found in the chapter on varicose veins.

Various theories have been postulated to explain the mechanism of cutaneous ulceration.

Box 1: Causes of leg ulcers.

1. **Vascular diseases**
   - *Venous*
   - *Arterial*
     - Atherosclerosis
     - Thromboangiitis obliterans
     - Arteriovenous malformation
     - Hypertensive ulcers (Martorell's ulcer)
     - Cholesterol embolism
   - *Mixed (arterial and venous)*
   - *Vasculitis*
     - Idiopathic
     - Small vessel vasculitis
       - Rheumatoid arthritis
       - Lupus erythematosus
       - Hypersensitivity vasculitis
       - Scleroderma
       - Behcet's disease
     - Medium and large vessel vasculitis
       - Polyarteritis nodosa
       - Wegener's granulomatosus
       - Nodular vasculitis
   - *Vaso-occlusive states*
     - Calciphylaxis
     - Cryofibrinogenemia
     - Cryoglobulinemia
   - *Hypercoagulable states*
     - Antiphospholipid antibody syndrome (APLA)
     - Protein C or S deficiency
   - Lymphatic's
     - Lymphedema
2. **Neuropathic diseases**
   - Diabetes mellitus
   - Leprosy
   - Tabes dorsalis
   - Syringomyelia
3. **Hematological diseases**
   - *Disorders of red blood cells*
     - Sickle cell anemia
     - Hereditary spherocytosis
     - Thrombocytosis
     - Thalassemia
   - *Disorders of white blood cells*
     - Leukemia
   - *Dysproteinemias*
     - Cryoglobulinemia
   - *Physical causes*
     - Trauma
     - Burns (thermal, chemical)
     - Cold injury (frostbite)
     - Radiation dermatitis
     - Factitial ulcers
   - *Infections*
     - *Bacterial*
       - Furuncle, ecthyma, gram negative infections, anaerobic infections
       - Mycobacterial, spirochetal infections, diphtheria, tropical ulcers
       - Septic emboli
     - *Fungal*

   Deep fungal infections, Majocchi's granuloma
   Protozoal
   Infestations and bites
4. **Skin diseases**
   - Pyoderma gangrenosum
   - Epidermolysis bullosa
5. **Neoplasm**
   - Squamous cell carcinoma (SCC)
   - Basal cell carcinoma (BCC)
   - Kaposi's sarcoma
   - Lymphomas
   - Metastatic tumors
6. **Metabolic diseases**
   - Diabetes mellitus
   - Gout
   - Prolidase deficiency
7. **Drugs**
   - Ergotism
   - Hydroxyurea
   - Halogenoderma
8. **Genetic**
   - Klinefelter's syndrome
   - Werner's syndrome

Table 1: Clinical features of leg ulcers.

	Venous ulcer	*Arterial ulcer*	*Neuropathic ulcer*
Complaints	Heaviness, pain and swelling of limbs which is aggravated on standing and relieved by limb elevation	Claudication pain in the calves upon walking relieved by rest Rest pain in advanced stages	Burning, numbness itching, pain or paresthesias of distal extremities
Location	Gaiter area of leg (Medial malleolar region)	Pressure sites such as toe, ankle, etc.	Pressure sites like plantar surface of first and fifth metatarsal heads, plantar surface of great toe (Fig. 4)
Morphology	Single or multiple ulcers with irregular borders, shallow depth and sloping edges (Fig. 2)	Round with sharp borders with dry necrotic base (Fig. 3)	Punched out with a thick rim of callus around
Surrounding skin	Pigmentation and lipodermatosclerosis	Shiny with loss of hair, cold limbs	Dryness and fissuring of skin with decreased or loss of sweating
Other features	Varicose veins, ankle edema, inverted champagne bottle appearance (stasis dermatitis)	Poor or absent peripheral pulses, pallor on limb elevation with rubor in dependent position	Features of peripheral neuropathy, deformities of foot

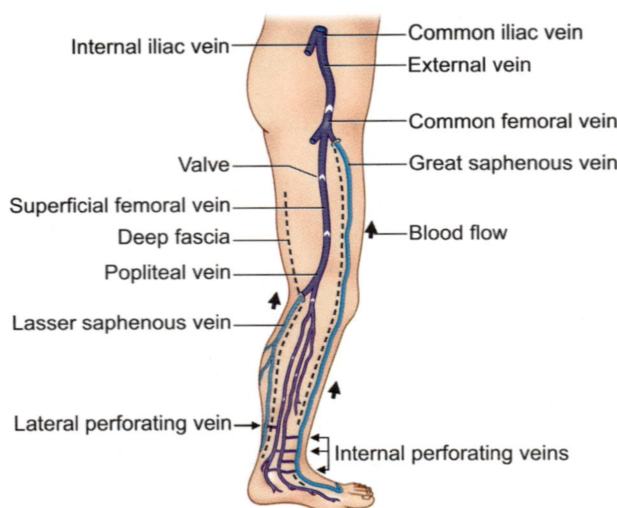

Fig. 1: Normal venous anatomy.

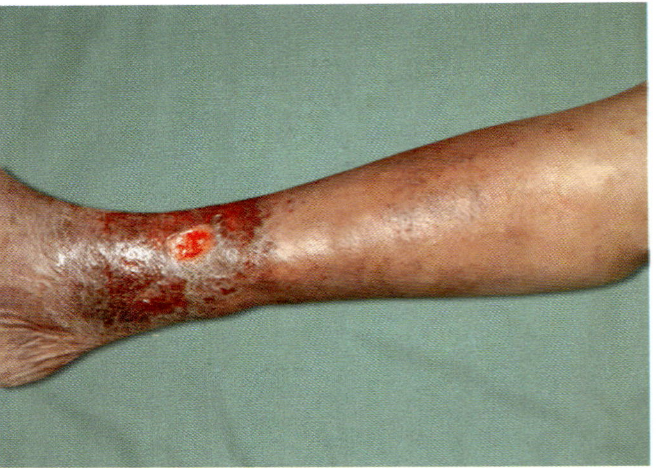

Fig. 2: Venous ulcer over the medial aspect of leg with varicose veins and surrounding pigmentation.

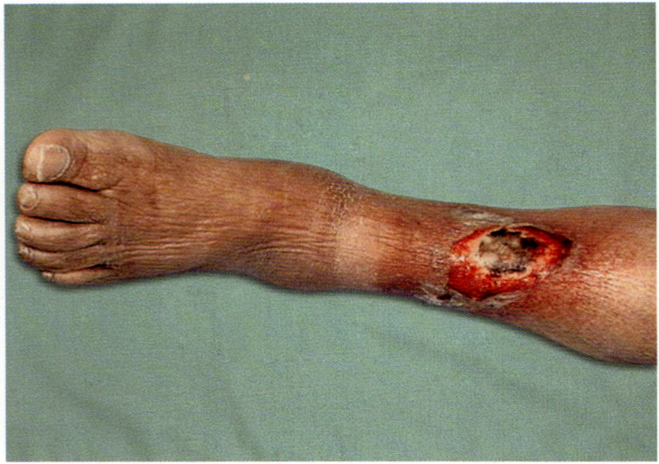

Fig. 3: Arterial ulcer with a necrotic slough at the base.

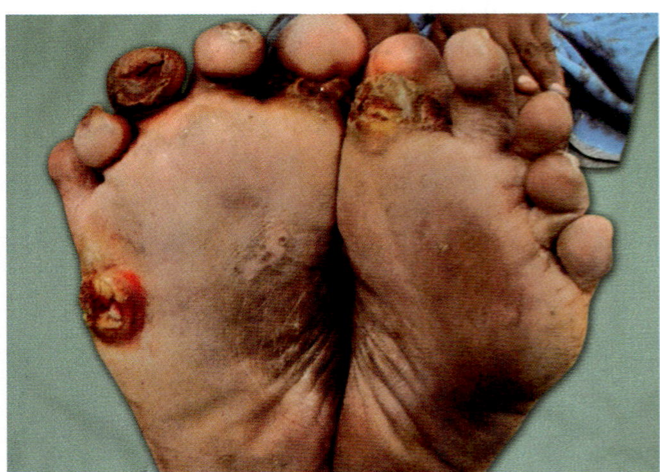

Fig. 4: Trophic ulcer on the plantar aspect of the toes and lateral aspect of right sole.

Homans stated that stasis of venous blood could lead to tissue anoxia leading to venous ulcers.[3] Brown and Burnard postulated that venous hypertension could lead to endothelial distension causing leakage of fibrinogen into the interstitial fluid which forms a pericapillary fibrin "cuff" that acts as a barrier to diffusion of oxygen causing ischemia and ulcer formation.[4] Coleridge Smith et al. thought that white blood cells disappear from the venous blood when the leg is in dependent position. These leukocytes might get trapped in the capillaries and obstruct the flow causing ulceration.[5] Adhesion molecules, like intercellular adhesion molecule-1 (ICAM-1) and vascular cell adhesion molecule-1 (VCAM-1), also become over expressed in CVI leading to continuous migration of leucocytes to the dermis.[6,7] Falanga and Eaglestein suggested that in patients with CVI, the pericapillary fibrin cuffs prevent the transfer of growth factors which leads to delayed wound healing.[8] Another theory suggests that elevated pressure on the venular side of capillaries leads to widening of interendothelial spaces and disintegration of collagen IV. This is laid down around capillaries leading to decreased availability of various growth factors required for wound healing.[9] Yes another theory suggests that fibroblasts present in chronic wounds may become senescent leading to impaired wound healing.[10]

Pathogenesis of Arterial Ulcers

Cigarette smoking, diabetes mellitus, hypertension and high lipid diet are thought to encourage the development of atheroma which leads to accumulation of cells, tissue debris and cholesterol plaques in the vessel intima leading to narrowing of arterial lumen of vessels of heart and lower limb.

Inadequate collaterals or occlusion from thrombosis before collaterals develop causes tissue infarction leading to ischemic ulceration of the skin.[11]

Pathogenesis of Neuropathic Ulcer

In neuropathy, there is loss of pain sensation so repetitive trauma, shearing and frictional forces leads to ulceration. Moreover autonomic neuropathy leads to hypohydrosis of foot causing dry skin and development of fissures and calluses leading to ulcers.[12]

LABORATORY EVALUATION OF LEG ULCERS

Leg ulcers need proper evaluation and often a battery of tests as mentioned below may be needed.

Complete blood count: To rule out infection, anemia and polycythemia

Blood sugars, Hb A1C for diabetic status

- Serum albumin, transferrin, ferritin, vitamin A, C, zinc, iron—to rule out nutritional deficiency
  - Vitamin A, C; iron and zinc are important in wound healing[11,13]
  - Serum homocysteine levels—increased in vitamin B6, B12 and folate deficiency
- Screening for lupus anticoagulant, anticardiolipin antibodies
- Antinuclear antibody (ANA), rheumatoid factor, anti-neutrophil cytoplasmic antibody (ANCA) (P and C), cryoglobulins.[14]

Protein C, protein S and antithrombin III, factor V

- Leiden[14]
- Wound swabs for bacterial culture and sensitivities[15] Tissue for mycobacterial and fungal cultures

Deep wedge biopsies including ulcer margin and bed— to rule out malignancy, vasculitides, panniculitis[15] Venous Doppler (color Doppler duplex ultrasound):

- For information on venous anatomy and reflux[16,17] Arterial Doppler (color Doppler duplex ultrasound):
- When peripheral pulses are impalpable, Doppler flow meter is used to hear the pulsation over the dorsalis pedis and posterior tibial arteries and ankle brachial pressure index (ABPI) is calculated as follows:

$$\text{ABPI} = \frac{\text{Systolic pressure in the ankle}}{\text{Higher of the two systolic pressure obtained from brachial arteries in both arms}} = 1.1$$

- ABPI: 0.5–0.8 indicates occlusive arterial disease and arteriography should be performed.
- ABPI <0.5 indicates severe arterial obstruction.[18]

Plain radiograph—To rule out osteomyelitis

- Patch testing—To rule out allergic contact dermatitis to medicaments and preservatives especially when patient has been applying topical medication for a long time. Common allergens that have been detected include neomycin, lanolin, bacitracin, formaldehyde and parabens.[15]

TREATMENT

Venous Ulcers

After arterial disease has been excluded, the primary aim of treatment of venous ulcers is to reduce venous hypertension, promote wound healing, prevent recurrences and to make the patient ambulant as early as possible.

Venous hypertension can be reduced by various ways. These include simple leg elevation and compression therapy. Simple leg elevation should be above the level of the heart and various compression devices.

Compression therapy: The aim of compression therapy is to achieve sustained graded compression of 30–40 mm Hg at the ankle thereby reducing the edema and improving the function of calf muscle pump and promoting ulcer healing.[19-21]

Various compression devices that can be used are elaborated in Table 2.

Wound Care for Leg Ulcers

Wound can be managed by dressings, debridement, topical, systemic treatment and biophysical treatment modalities.[22]

Dressings

Maintaining a moist environment, accelerates wound healing, is very important. This can be accomplished by frequent application of saline dressings over the wound which helps to keep the wound surface moist, debrides the wound and removes the surface bacteria.

Recent research on wound care has resulted in increased use of interactive and active dressings rather than passive dressings that cover and absorb. Active dressings deliver substances, such as growth factors, which are important in the healing cascade. Interactive dressings are occlusive dressings. They provide a favorable micro-environment for the growth of new tissue. Moist occlusive dressings control the exudates while epithelial cell migration is encouraged. Eschar is liquefied and fibrin is lysed to allow convenient debridement. Infection is managed through wound fluid rich in leukocytes. These dressings are also believed to provide symptomatic relief such as decreased pain and pruritus.

The various dressings, their advantages and disadvantages[21,25] are elaborated in Table 3.

Periwound protection: The skin surrounding the ulcer can be damaged due to excess moisture, wound fluid proteases and adhesives present in the dressings.[21,26] Barrier creams and ointments are available which protects the skin around the ulcer. These include:

- Vaseline petroleum jelly: Protects the periwound skin, but interferes with dressing adherence

Table 2: Compression devices.

Types	*Functions*
Unna's boot A preparation consisting of zinc oxide 5 parts, gelatin 5 parts, boric acid 1 part, glycerin 8 parts and water 6 parts. Ichthyol 1 or 2 parts is incorporated into it. Moist gauze impregnated with this paste is wrapped from behind the first metatarsal up to an inch below the knee, either in a figure-of-8 pattern or adding pleats while wrapping. It can be left in place for 7 days before changing	Protects against trauma and maintains the ambulatory status of the patient. But cannot be used in highly exudative wounds. Pressure variation can also occur
Graduated compression stockings Three classes are available depending on the desired degree of ankle pressure in mm of Hg. *Class-I* (18–21 mm Hg) Indicated in mild varicosis, early varicosis in pregnancy and heaviness of legs *Class-II* (23–32 mm Hg) Indicated in severe varicose veins, moderate edema, pronounced varicosis in pregnancy, posthealing minor ulcerations, superficial thrombophlebitis and postsclerotherapy *Class-III* (34–46 mm Hg) For severe chronic venous insufficiency, marked edema and induration of skin	Improves the venous return, raises the hydrostatic pressure and decreases the superficial venous pressure; therapy reducing the leak of solutes and fluid into the interstitial space also enhances release of plasminogen activator which helps in breakdown of pericapillary fibrin deposits and restores defective fibrinolysis
Orthotic devices	*Bulky*
Four-layered bandaging (Velfour™) High compression bandage system (sub-bandage pressure of 35–40 mm Hg at the ankle) that incorporates elastic layers to achieve sustained compression (Figs. 5 and 6)[23] Layer 1 is orthopedic wool Layer 2 is a cotton crepe bandage Layer 3 is a light weight class 3A* elastic compression bandage Layer 4 is a class 3B** cohesive compression bandage and it retains the bandage in position *Class 3A: Maintains low level of pressure up to 20 mm Hg at the ankle **Class 3B: Maintains a pressure of 30 mm Hg at the ankle	Promotes healing of ulcer in patients with superficial, deep venous incompetence and mixed ulcers (arterial and venous). Also used in lymphatic disorders
Intermittent pneumatic compression Used in those who do not respond to stockings or compression bandages[24]	Relieves edema and promotes healing in patients with venous ulcers, also used to treat lymph edema

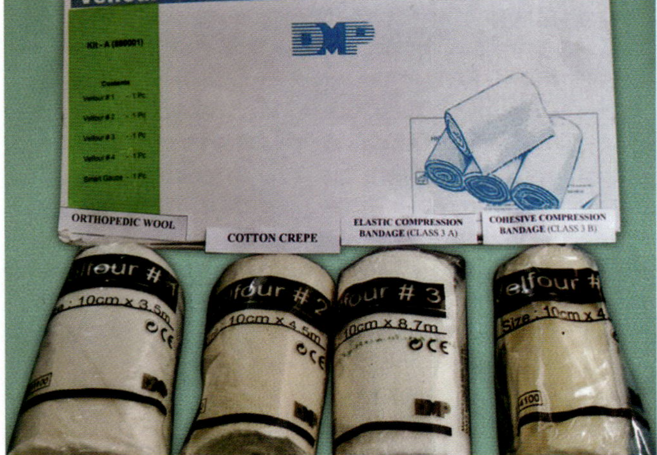

Fig. 5: Four-layered bandage.

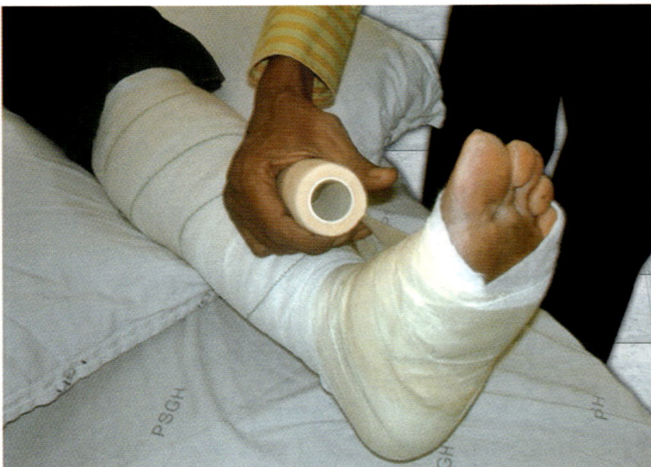

Fig. 6: Application of four-layered bandage.

- Unna's paste: It is a preparation containing zinc oxide 5 parts, gelatin 5 parts, boric acid 1 part, glycerin 8 parts and water 6 parts with ichthyol 1 or 2 parts. It protects the skin around the wound, and has anti-inflammatory effect and promotes healing. It can also interfere with dressing adherence.[27,28]

Debridement

Standard wound care consists of debridement which removes the necrotic debris and helps in formation of healthy granulation tissue.[21,29] Various methods of debridement include:

Table 3: Types of dressings.

Types of dressings	Availability	Indications and adverse effects
Films	Thin transparent adhesives, made of polyurethane to be changed every 12–24 hours, e.g. Tegaderm	Protects the wound from contamination but may strip away the newly forming granulation tissue. Used in wounds with moderate exudates
Hydrogels	Gel like sheets. Semitransparent and nonadhesive. To be changed every 1–3 days, e.g. restore hydrogel, Vigilion	Helps in desloughing the wound and can also be used as drug vehicles. Causes incarceration of skin around the ulcer
Hydrocolloids	Occlusive dressing composed of hydrocolloid with a polyurethane outer coating. Can be changed once a week, e.g. Duoderm	Cost effective. Traps the fluid under the dressing producing an offensive odor. Can be used in wounds with moderate exudates. Early removal strips off the newly formed epidermis
Alginates	Biodegradable. Derived from seaweeds Can be left in place until soaked with exudates, e.g. Sorbsan	Highly absorbent and hemostatic. Dries out the exudating wound making it more painful
Collagen	Available in particle and sheet form Obtained from human, porcine and bovine sources. Forms a biodegradable gel over the wound surface, e.g. Promogran	Promotes wound healing by laying down a matrix that leads to new tissue formation and depletion of free radicals and proteases that hinder the healing process

Surgical debridement: Surgical debridement is done using a curette and scissors where chronic wound is converted into an acute wound. Neutrophils and macrophages which are recruited to the area secrete growth factors and phagocytize the bacteria and nonviable tissue.[21,30]

Autolytic debridement: Autolytic debridement is the gentle separation of slough from wound bed that occurs slowly in a moist wound environment. It is accomplished by placing an occlusive dressing on a wound and allowing proteases within the wound space to liquefy the necrotic tissue. It is useful in patients with bleeding tendencies where surgical debridement is not feasible.[21,31]

Enzymatic debridement: It consists of application of topical protease preparation that targets the fibrin and collagen of necrotic tissue. These include papain urea preparations—papain obtained from papaya contains protease and urea is a protein denaturant.[26] Collagenase, derived from *Clostridium histolyticum,* targets collagen.[31,32]

Biodebridement: This is achieved by using maggots. They are the larvae of a species of fly (*Lucilia sericata*) also known as "green bottle" blow fly which selectively debride the dead tissue and tissue debris by secreting collagenase.[33]

Topical Treatment

Wound healing is impaired when bacterial colonization exceeds 10^5 organisms per gram of tissue.[34] As systemic antibiotics are reserved only for patients with evidence of cellulitis or systemic infection, topical antiseptics and antibiotics have been used to reduce the wound bioburden. The various preparations used are:

- Acetic acid: Acetic acid 0.25% is used in the treatment of wounds infected with *Pseudomonas aeruginosa*[35]
- Twenty percent benzoyl peroxide has antimicrobial properties when applied under occlusion[36,37]
- Silver compounds: Silver ions have proven efficacy against various gram negative bacteria. It is incorporated into various wound dressing products, creams and gels, and is used for its bactericidal properties[38] Iodosorb (cadexomer iodine): A complex of iodine with cadexomer (starch based polymer bead) promotes absorption of wound fluid, debris and bacteria from wound bed by controlled release of iodine.[39]

Other topicals: Metronidazole gel provides good anaerobic coverage. Retapamulin, the first drug in the class of pleuromutilin antibiotics, acts by inhibiting bacterial protein synthesis by interacting at a site on the 50S ribosome subunit of bacterial ribosome. When used as a topical antibiotic, it is effective against gram positive bacteria including methicillin resistant *Staphylococcus aureus* (MRSA).[40] Mupirocin ointment is effective against gram negative organisms including MRSA. Modified Dakin solution (hypochlorite) at a concentration of 0.025% elicits antimicrobial effects. Neomycin and bacitracin are avoided because of their potential to cause contact sensitivity.[41,42]

Systemic Treatment

Antibiotics are recommended only for patients with evidence of cellulitis or systemic infection.[43]

Fibrinolytics: Browse et al. have demonstrated that patients with lipodermatosclerosis have reduced fibrinolytic activity.[44] The commonly used fibrinolytics are stanozolol, an anabolic steroid in the dose of 2 mg twice daily reduces the pain and dermal thickness in acute lipodermatosclerosis.[45] Pentoxifylline, a substituted xanthine in a dose of 400 mg thrice a day also has fibrinolytic properties. It acts by decreasing blood viscosity, increases red blood cell deformability, inhibits platelet aggregation and production of proinflammatory cytokines.[46–48]

Other drugs which can be used as adjuvant to compression therapy are oral enteric coated aspirin (300 mg), micronized purified flavanoid fraction (Daflon 500), etc.

Biophysical Treatment Modalities

Electrical stimulation: It promotes wound healing by inhibiting bacterial growth, attracting fibroblasts towards the wound and expression of transforming growth factor on fibroblasts.[49–51]

Low frequency ultrasound: Continuous wave low frequency ultrasound of 34 KHz has a temporary stimulatory effect on microcirculation mainly due to improved oxygenation and improves wound healing.[52-54]

Topical negative pressure devices: It consists of a fenestrated evacuation tube embedded in a foam dressing covered with an airtight dressing. This tube is attached to a vacuum source and a subatmospheric pressure of 100–125 mm Hg is applied in a continuous or intermittent manner. Promotes wound healing by absorbing the exudates and promoting healthy granulation tissue formation.[55]

Hyperbaric oxygen therapy: It is based on the theory that tissue hypoxia results in failure of chronic wounds to heal, 100% oxygen is breathed in at superatmospheric pressure while inside a compression chamber to facilitate wound healing.[56]

Surgical Options for Covering the Wound

Skin grafting is indicated when there is slow epithelialization with nonsurgical measures.

Pinch grafts: Pinch grafts are useful for small nonhealing ulcers, provided the ulcer bed is clean with healthy granulation tissue (Fig. 7).[57]

Procedure: One percent lidocaine is injected into the anterior aspect of thigh (donor area) to raise a number of wheals. Skin around the wheal is stretched firmly so as to pinch up the wheals and grafts are harvested by shaving off the top of each wheal with a number 11 parker blade and placed on the ulcer bed with dermal side down. Multiple grafts are placed on the ulcer bed, spacing them few millimeters apart from one other and then both donor and recipient sites are covered with a dressing for a week.

Advantage: Simple technique can be done on outpatient basis.

Disadvantage: Cobble stoning of the ulcer site and scarring over the donor site.

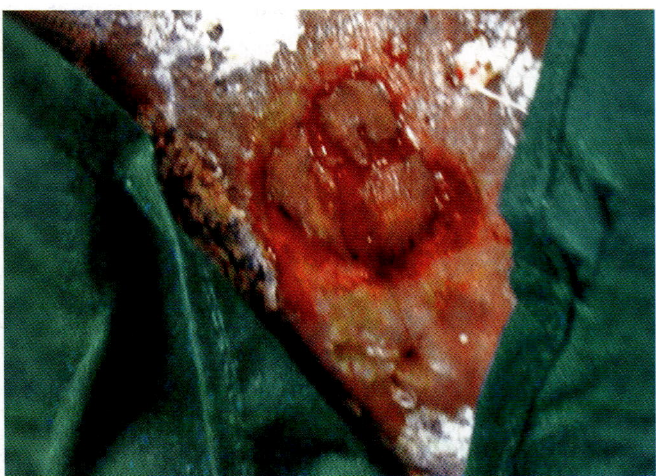

Fig. 7: Pinch graft over the ulcer.

Split thickness skin grafting: Split thickness skin grafting (SSG) consists of epidermis and a portion of the dermis, from the selected donor site and grafting on to the recipient site. The thickness of the graft may vary depending upon the amount of dermis included in the graft.

Preoperative preparation of recipient site: Ulcer is debrided to remove the necrotic tissue and a healthy granulating base is created before SSG.

Procedure: Done under local, spinal or general anesthesia. After cleansing the donor and recipient site with povidone iodine or surgical spirit, the skin over the donor area is stretched and the cutting edge of the knife or a razor blade is held at 15–30° angle to the skin surface and sunk to the desired depth. The blade is moved back and forth gently by sawing movement to obtain a translucent graft, which is then placed on the recipient site, with dermal side down and secured with sutures and covered with a nonadhesive pressure dressing. Sutures can be removed after a week.[58]

Advantage: Covers large defects.

Disadvantage: Less durable and might undergo contraction.

Skin Substitutes

Cultured epidermal grafts: Another approach in the treatment of leg ulcers secondary to CVI is the use of cultured epidermal cells (keratinocytes) as skin grafts which can be derived from patients own skin (autograft) or from an unrelated donor (allograft). Growth factors released by the skin keratinocytes promote wound healing.[59,60]

Dermal substitutes: Manufactured from human newborn foreskin fibroblast cells seeded on to a bioabsorbable mesh scaffold which when implanted on to the wound, secrete various growth factors and cytokines, persist in the wound for several months and are eventually replaced by host tissue.[61]

Composite graft: Apligraf (has both dermal and epidermal components).

Apligraf is a living bilayered skin substitute manufactured using neonatal foreskin keratinocytes and fibroblasts with bovine type-I collagen. As it contains living cells, it should be kept sealed in its nutrient medium and 10% CO_2 or air atmosphere under controlled temperature 68–88°F (20–31°C) and used within 15 minutes of opening. Used in leg ulcer due to venous insufficiency of more than 1 month duration along with standard compression therapy.[62]

LASER FOR LEG VEINS

Pulsed dye laser (PDL): At a wavelength of 585 nm and pulse duration 1–40 ms, PDL is capable of treating leg veins less than 0.2 mm in diameter. For larger veins up to 1.5 mm, long pulsed (595 mm) PDL can be used[63,64] *Diode laser (800 mm)*: Long pulsed Nd:YAG laser (1064 mm), long pulsed alexandrite laser (755 nm) intense pulsed light (515–1200 nm) are also used for treating leg telangiectasias.

Long pulsed Nd:YAG laser (1064 nm): Has maximum penetration of 3 mm, making it ideal for the destruction of large vessels of 0.5–3 mm diameter for the destruction of large vessels in the mid-dermis.[65]

Long pulsed alexandrite laser: With a wavelength of 755 nm and pulse duration of up to 20 ms or longer, alexandrite lasers penetrate 2–3 mm into the skin. Ideal for treating medium sized vessels (0.4–1 mm) and larger vessels (1–3 mm).[66]

Diode lasers: At 800–930 nm, the diode lasers can be used to treat deeper and larger reticular veins. More recently, 940 nm diode lasers has been found to be efficacious in the treatment of leg veins up to 1 mm in diameter.[67]

Intense pulsed light: It is a noncoherent, 515–1200 nm flash lamp pumped light source with a fluence of 90 J/cm^2 and pulse duration of 2–100 ms. To increase the selectivity, IPL uses filters that remove lower wave-lengths. Filters (550 and 570 nm) are useful for vascular lesions that deliver light of yellow and red wavelengths and some infrared light. Broadband source of 515–1200 nm helps in treating the smaller superficial vessels and large deeper vessels simultaneously.[68]

Endovenous Laser and Radiofrequency Treatment

Under duplex ultrasound guidance, a needle is inserted into the saphenous vein followed by a guide wire. Finally either radiofrequency energy or light from 810 nm diode, 940 nm diode or 1320 nm Nd:YAG laser is delivered into the incompetent saphenous vein using a fibrotic catheter. Ninety percent clearance has been reported after a single treatment.[69,70]

INDICATIONS FOR SURGICAL INTERVENTION IN LEG ULCERS SECONDARY TO CHRONIC VENOUS INSUFFICIENCY

- Recurrent episodes of hemorrhage
- Development of lipodermatosclerosis
- Recurrent, hard to heal ulcers despite conservative treatment.

Surgical options: Surgical options include surgical ligation, endoscopic perforator ligation combined with superficial vein ligation.[71,72] These are discussed in detail in the chapter on varicose veins.

Injection sclerotherapy and ultrasound-guided foam sclerotherapy[73] are discussed in detail in the chapter on sclerotherapy.

Ambulatory Phlebectomy

Removal of diseased venous segments by hook avulsion wherein incisions are made parallel to the diseased venous segments along the long axis. The vein is then exteriorized using a phlebectomy hook and avulsed after clamping both the proximal and distal aspect. This process is repeated at 3–5 cm intervals along the entire length of the vein until the diseased vein is removed. Patient can be ambulant after the procedure so that normal gait and calf muscle pump function returns quickly.[74]

Shave therapy: This is a simple and effective treatment for recalcitrant leg ulcer with deep venous insufficiency (Post-thrombotic type). Under General/Spinal anesthesia, the ulcer and the surrounding lipodermatosclerosis are removed or shaved off in horizontal layers followed by application of a meshed split-skin graft from the thigh on the (0.4–0.6 mm thick) wound area.[75]

Treatment of Arterial Ulcers

Aim of therapy is to establish adequate arterial supply[76] and wound care.

General Measures

Patient is advised to keep the extremities warm, quit smoking, to lose weight if obese, low cholesterol diet and to keep diabetes and hypertension under control.

Lipid lowering drugs like statins, antiplatelet drugs like aspirin, clopidogrel (inhibits ADP-induced platelet aggregation), and cilostazol (Phosphodiesterase III inhibitor) prevent ischemic events.[76,77]

Referral to vascular surgeon for assessment and revascularization by angioplasty, arterial bypass surgery may be necessary in selected cases.

Treatment of Neuropathic Ulcers

Patient is advised to the inspect the feet daily for any blisters, to moisturize the feet adequately but to keep the interdigital spaces dry and use proper footwear with offloading of pressure. Aggressive debridement of the dead tissue and the surrounding callus is followed by saline gauze dressings which is changed thrice a day.[78] Occlusive dressings like alginates which absorb the exudates and maintain a moist environment is also helpful.

Becaplermin Gel: A topical recombinant platelet derived growth factor has been approved by FDA as an adjunctive for treatment of diabetic neuropathic ulcers.[78,79] Vascular surgery to be considered if there is severe vascular impairment after confirming by arteriography or MRI of limb vessels.

Biological and Bioengineered Therapies

Biological therapies refer to tissue-based treatments (acellular and cellular), autologous platelet-rich plasma (PRP), as well as recombinant human growth factor, human platelet-derived growth factor (rhPDGF), fibroblast growth factor (rhFGF), and epidermal growth factor (rhEGF) therapies. Numerous other growth factors have been isolated and investigated, such as vascular endothelial growth factor (VEGF), keratinocyte growth factor-2, TGF-β, and granulocyte-macrophage colony-stimulating factor, but these currently are not approved for use in wound care.

rhEGF is perhaps the best studied growth factor for cutaneous ulcers and wounds Applied as a topical cream, or more commonly, by intralesional injections, EGF has been found also to expedite the healing of a variety of types of cutaneous wounds. Several small trials attest to the healing benefits of EGF compared with controls.[80]

rhEGF is considered a potent angiogenic growth factor, also has an isoform (FGF-10) commonly known as keratinocyte growth factor-2 or repifermin which is reported to accelerate wound healing.[81]

Platelet concentrates are a concentrated suspension of growth factors found in platelets, which act as bioactive surgical additives that are applied locally to induce wound healing. Platelet concenterates can be used as 1) platelet-rich plasma (PRP) and 2) platelet-rich fibrin (PRF). PRP (also referred to as platelet enriched plasma, platelet rich concentrate, autologous platelet gel and platelet releasate) is a volume of autologous plasma that has a platelet concentration above baseline, five times more than the normal.

The cocktail of growth factors (GFs) in PRP by virtue of platelets alone (stored as alpha granules in platelets) are platelet derived growth factor (αα, αβ, ββ), transforming growth factor β1, β2, vascular endothelial growth factor, epidermal growth factor, hepatocyte growth factor, fibroblast growth factor. These GFs are pivotal in modulation of tissue repair and regeneration. The plasma proteins in PRP, namely, fibrin, fibronectin and vitronectin act as scaffold for the bone, connective tissue and epithelial migration. Degranulation of the prepackaged GFs in platelets occurs upon "activation", i.e. on coming in contact with coagulation triggers. The secreted GFs in turn bind to their respective transmembrane receptors expressed over adult mesenchymal stem cells, osteoblasts, fibroblasts, endothelial cells, and epidermal cells. This further induces an internal signal transduction pathway, unlocking the expression of a normal gene sequence of a cell like cellular proliferation, matrix formation, osteoid production, collagen synthesis, angiogenesis, mesenchymal cell recruitment, proliferation and extracellular matrix synthesis, thereby augmenting the natural wound healing process.[82]

PRF is a second-generation platelet concentrate which contains platelets and growth factors in the form of fibrin membranes prepared from the patients own blood free of any anticoagulant or other artificial biochemical modifications. The PRF clot forms a strong natural fibrin matrix, which concentrates almost all the platelets and growth factors of the blood, harvest a complex architecture as a healing matrix with unique mechanical properties which makes it distinct from other platelet concentrates.[83] PRF is superior to other platelet concentrates like PRP due to its ease and inexpensive method of preparation and also it does not need any addition of exogenous compounds like bovine thrombin and calcium chloride. Thus, PRF has emerged as one of the promising regenerative materials for wound healing.

Acellular Therapies

The most common types of advanced biological therapies for chronic wounds are acellular therapies—those dermal, amniotic, or collagen-based tissues (human or animal) that have been decellularized during their processing. Often referred to as acellular and/or extra cellular matrix (ECMs), these biological products serve as substrates into which cells can migrate and initiate angiogenesis, thereby promoting granulation tissue development and tissue regeneration. Once considered only as inert structural collagen tissue providing a scaffold for cellular in growth, ECMs are now known to play an active part in tissue regeneration through a dynamic interaction with growth factors and host cells.[84] ECMs contain not only structural collagen but also glycosaminoglycans (including hyaluronan), proteoglycans, and glycoproteins—all essential components to replace the defective ECM of injured tissues. Human dermal allografts have become increasingly popular in recent years for augmenting tissue regeneration in chronic lower extremity wounds amd these are harvested from screened donors, and each is prepared with proprietary processes to decellularize and cryopreserve the dermis while maintaining the natural structure of the collagen and ECM. The dermal matrices serve as scaffolds for cellular repopulation and angiogenesis, with varying degrees of incorporation into the recipient wound.[85]

Amniotic membranes (AMs) and umbilical cord tissues have been used for many years for corneal ulcers and were actually the earliest reported biomaterials used for wound repair. In recent years, they have been tried for chronic wounds, likely due to the wide availability of placental tissues after cesarean deliveries. Due to their rich cellular content AMs contain a number of cytokines and growth factors bound to the ECM after decellularization and preparation that remain available to augment angiogenesis and tissue repair when implanted into chronic wounds.[86] AMs are available in the cryopreserved state or as dehydrated products for direct implantation.[87] Several products are also available in a micronized formulation that can be applied topically or hydrated for injection into wounds to augment healing.[88,89]

Stem Cell Therapies

The most recent advancements for wound care therapies are that of stem cell therapies, primarily bone marrow derived, and most recently, placental-derived stem cells. Both sources are considered as adult stem cells, and the cell lineage of interest are the mesenchymal stem cells (MSCs). They are multipotent progenitor cells that can directly differentiate into mesenchymal tissues, such as bone, tendon, and cartilage. Their ability to affect cutaneous repair, however, is through an indirect paracrine function (trophic activity), whereby they synthesize essential growth factors and cytokines that affect cell migration, proliferation, and metabolic activity of host cells and tissues. In this manner, MSCs play an active role in the inflammatory, proliferative, and remodeling phases of wound repair. SCs can respond to the host environment by upregulating anti-inflammatory cytokines in the presence of inflammation and respond to hypoxic environments by upregulating the release of VEGF to induce angiogenesis. During the remodeling phase, MSCs produce growth factors, such as TGF-β3, to limit excessive scarring as well as modulate the balance between matrix metalloproteinases and tissue inhibitors of metalloproteinases while regulating collagen deposition. Important for allogeneic implantation, MSCs are characterized as being immune privileged since they lack cell surface antigens that would typically engender a foreign body reaction.[90]

Bone marrow-derived stem cells (BMSCs) have been of interest for some time now and studies have indicated their ability to augment repair or regeneration of numerous tissues, including cardiac, bone, cartilage, blood vessels, and skin.[91]

Placental tissues—including the umbilical cord, the amnion, and the chorion—are a rich source of MSCs and are readily available without the ethical concerns of embryonic stem cells.[92] Placental-derived MSCs show minimal differences from those obtained from different sites, and yet retain all of the metabolic, paracrine, and immunomodulative properties previously described while maintaining their immune-privileged status.[91]

CONCLUSION

Chronic leg ulcer is a difficult to treat condition with 20% chance of recurrences. Hence, a methodical approach to identify and treat the factors influencing underlying wound healing would go a long way in preventing recurrences.

Tips and Pitfalls

Tips for better results and pitfalls to avoid

Compression is the main stay of treatment for venous ulcers. High compression is better than low compression

- Graduated sustained compression reduces pressure in the superficial venous system, aids venous return to the heart and promotes ulcer healing
- When peripheral pulses are impalpable, ABPI should be calculated and if ABPI is <0.5, compression is contraindicated
- Topical medicaments to be avoided as they may lead to contact sensitization
- Bilayered skin substitutes promote better wound healing when combined with standard compression therapy
- Surgery is indicated in ulcers secondary to CVI when there are recurrent episodes of hemorrhage, lipodermatosclerosis and when ulcers fail to heal with conservative treatment.

REFERENCES

1. Nelzen O, Bergqvist D, Lindhagen A, et al. Chronic leg ulcers: an underestimated problem in primary health care among elderly patients. J Epidemiol Commun Health. 1991;45:184-7.
2. Abbade LP, Lastoria S. Venous ulcer: Epidemiology physiopathology, diagnosis and treatment. Int J Dermatol. 2005;44:449-56.
3. Homan SJ. The etiology and treatment of varicose ulcer of the leg. Surg Gynecol Obstet. 1917;24:300-11.
4. Browse NL, Burnand KG. The cause of venous ulceration. Lancet. 1982;2:243-5.
5. Coleridge Smith PD, Thomas P, Scurr JH, et al. Causes of venous ulceration: a new hypothesis. Br Med J (Clin Res Ed). 1988;296:1726-7.
6. Peschen M, Lahaye T, Hennig B, et al. In: Maessen-Visch MB (Ed). Expression of the adhesion of molecules ICAM1, VCAM-1, LFA-1 and VLA-4 in the skin is modulated in progressing stages of chronic venous insufficiency with and without atrophie blanche. Atrophic Blanche (Thesis) Nijmegen: Drukkerij Hendrix Volharding 1999;77-87.
7. Veraart JC, Verhaegh ME, Neumann HA, et al. Molecule expression in venous leg ulcers. VASA. 1993;22:213-8.
8. Falanga V, Eaglestein WH. The 'trap' hypothesis of venous ulceration. Lancet. 1993;341:1006-8.
9. Neumaan HA, Van den Broek MJ. Increased Collagen IV layer in the basal membrane area of the capillaries in severe chronic venous insufficiency. VASA. 1991;20:26-9.
10. Mendez MV, Raffeto JD, Phillips TJ, et al. The proliferative capacity of neonatal skin fibroblasts is reduced after exposure to venous ulcer wound fluid; a potential mechanism for senescence in venous ulcers. J Vasc Surg. 1999;30:734-43.
11. Philips TJ, Dover JS. Leg ulcers. J Am Acad Dermatol. 1991;25:965-87.
12. Caputo GM, Cavanagh PR, Ulbrecht JS, et al. Assessment and management of foot disease in patients with diabetes. N Engl J Med. 1994;331:854-60.
13. Ruberg RL. Role of nutrition in wound healing. Surg Clin North Am. 1984;64:705-14.
14. Bello YM, Philips TJ. Management of venous ulcers. J Cutan Med Surg. 1998;3:6-12.

15. Ouahes N, Philips TJ. Leg ulcers. Curr Probl Dermatol. 1995;7:109-42.
16. Coleridge-Smith P, Labropoulos N, Partsch H, et al. Duplex ultrasound investigation of the veins in chronic venous disease of the lower limbs–UIP consensus document Part-1. Basic principles. Eur J Vasc Endovasc Surg. 2006;31:83-92.
17. Cavezzi A, Labropoulos N, Partsch H, et al. Duplex ultrasound investigation of the veins in chronic venous disease of the lower limbs-UIP consensus document (Part-II anatomy). Eur J Vasc Endovasc Surg. 2006;31:288-99.
18. Vowden K, Vowden P. Doppler and the ABPI; how good is our understanding? J Wound Care. 2001;10:197-202.
19. Partsch H. Compression therapy of the legs. A review. J Dermatol Sur Oncol. 1991;17:799-805.
20. Coleridge-Smith PD, Leg ulcer treatment. J Vasc Surg. 2009;49:804-8.
21. Fonder MA, Lazarus GS, Cowan DA, et al. Treating the chronic wound: A practical approach to the care of non healing wounds and wound care dressings. J Am Acad Dermatol. 2008;58:185-206.
22. Paquette D, Falanga V. Leg ulcers. Clin Geriatr Med. 2002;18: 77-88.
23. Blair SD, Wright DD, Backhouse CM, et al. Sustained compression and healing of chronic venous ulcers. BMJ. 1988;297:1159-61.
24. Philips TJ. Current approaches to venous ulcers and compression. Dermatol Surg. 2001;27:611-21.
25. Philips TJ. Current approaches to venous ulcers and compression. Dermatol Surg. 2001;27:611-21.
26. Bishop SM, Walker M, Roger AA, et al. Importance of moisture balance at the wound dressing interface. J wound Care. 2003;12:125-8.
27. Agren MS. Studies on zinc in wound healing. Acta Derm Venerol Suppl (Stockh). 1990;154:1-36. Stromberg HE, Agren MS. Topical zinc oxide treatment improves arterial and venous leg ulcers. Br J Dermatol. 1984;111:461-8.
28. Stromberg HE, Agren MS. Topical zinc oxide treatment improves arterial and venous leg ulcers. Br J Dermatol. 1984;111:461-8.
29. Steed DL. Debridement. Am J Surg. 2004;187:71S-4S.
30. Williams D, Enoch S, Miller D, et al. Effect of sharp debridement using curette on recalcitrant nonhealing venous leg ulcers: a concurrently controlled, prospective cohort study. Wound Repair Regen. 2005;13:131-7.
31. Konig M, Vanscheidt W, Augustin M, et al. Enzymatic versus autolytic debridement of chronic leg ulcers: a prospective randomised trial. J Wound Care. 2005;14:320-3.
32. Alvarez OM, Fernandez-Obregon A, Rogers RS, et al. A prospective, randomized, comparative study of collagenase and papain-urea for pressure ulcer debridement. Wounds. 2002;293-301.
33. Ziffren SE, Heist HE, May SC, et al. Secretion of collagenase by maggots and its implication. Ann Surg. 1953;138:932-4.
34. Robson MC, Stenberg BD, Heggers JP, et al. Wound healing alterations caused by infections. Clin Plast Surg. 1990;17: 485-92.
35. Lineweaver W, Howard R, Soucy D, et.al. Topical antimicrobial toxicity. Arch Surg. 1985;120:267-70.
36. Pace WE. Treatment of cutaneous ulcers with benzoyl peroxide. Can Med Assoc J. 1976;115:1101-6.
37. Alvarez OM, Mertz PM, Eaglstein WH. Benzoyl peroxide and epidermal wound healing. Arch Dermatol. 1983;119:222-5.
38. Ip M, Lvi SL, Poon VK, et al. Antimicrobial activities of silver an in vitro comparison. J Med Microbiol. 2006;59-63.
39. Zhou LH, Nahm WK, Badiavas E, et al. Slow release iodine preparation and wound healing: In vitro effects consistent with lack of in vivo toxicity in human chronic wounds. Br. J Dermatol. 2002;146:365-74.
40. Jones RN, Fritsche TR, Sader H, et al. Activity of retapamulin (SB-275833), a novel pleuromutilin, against selected resistant gram-positive cocci. Antimicrob Agents Chemother. 2006;50:2583-6.
41. Jones RN, Fritsche TR, Sader H, et al. Activity of retapamulin (SB-275833), a novel pleuromutilin, against selected resistant gram-positive cocci. Antimicrob Agents Chemother. 2006;50:2583-6.
42. Zaki I, Shall L, Dalziel KL. Bacitracin: a significant sensitizer in leg ulcer patients? Contact Dermatitis. 1994;31:92-4.
43. Valencia IC, Falabella A, Kirsner RS, et al. Chronic venous insufficiency and venous leg ulceration. J Am Acad Dermatol. 2001;44:401-21.
44. Browse NL, Gray L, Jarrett PE, et al. Blood and vein wall fibrinolytic activity in health and vascular disease. Br Med J. 1977;1:478-81.
45. Vesic S, Vukovic J, Mendenica LJ, et al. Acute lipodermatosclerosis: an open clinical trial of stanozolol in patient unable to sustain compression therapy. Dermatol online J. 2008;14:1.
46. Jarret PE, Moreland M, Browse NL. The effect of oxypentifylline (Trental) on fibrinolytic activity and plasma fibrinogen levels. Curr Med Res Opin. 1977;4:492-5.
47. Jarret PE, Moreland M, Browse NL. The effect of oxypentifylline (Trental) on fibrinolytic activity and plasma fibrinogen levels. Curr Med Res Opin. 1977;4:492-5.
48. Phillips TJ, Dover JS. Leg ulcers. J Am Acad Dermatol. 1991;25:965-87.
49. Gault WR, Gatens PF. Use of low intensity direct current in management of ischaemic skin ulcers. Phys Ther. 1976;56:265-9.
50. Barran SD, Spardaro JA, Berger TJ, et al. In vitro effects of a weak direct current on Staphylococcus aureus. Clin Orthop Rel Res. 1974;100:250-5.
51. Erickson CA, Nucitelli R. Embryonic fibroblast motility and orientation can be influenced by physiological electrical fields. J Cell Biol. 1984;98:296-307.
52. Ernst E. Ultrasound for cutaneous wound healing. Phlebology. 1995;10:2-4.
53. Johannsen F, Gam AN, Karlsmark T. Ultrasound therapy in chronic leg ulceration: a meta analysis. Wound Repaid Regen. 1998;6:121-6.
54. Wollina U, Heining B, Naumann G, et al. Effects of low frequency ultrasound on microcirculation in venous leg ulcers. Indian J Dermatol. 2011;56:174-9.
55. Shirakawa M, Isseroff RR. Topical negative pressure devices use for enhancement of healing chronic wounds. Arch Dermatol. 2005;141:1449-53.
56. Kranke P, Bennett M, Roec RI-Wiedmann I, et al. Hyperbaric oxygen therapy for chronic wounds. Cochrane Database Syst Rev. 2004;CD004123.
57. Ceilley RI, Rinck MA, Zuchlke RL. Pinch grafting for chronic ulcers on lower extremities. J Dermat Surg Oncol. 1977;3: 303-9.
58. Skouge JW. Techniques for split thickness skin grafting. J Dermatol Surg Oncol. 1987;13:841-9.

59. Kirsner RS, Falanga V, Kerdel FA, et al. Skin grafts as pharmacological agents: pre wounding of the donor site. Br J Dermatol. 1996;135:292-6.
60. Limova M. Active wound coverings: Bioengineered skin and dermal substitutes. Surg clin North Am. 2010;90:1237-55.
61. Harding KG, Moore K, Philips TJ. Wound chronicity and fibroblast senescence implications for treatment. Int Wound J. 2005;2:364-8.
62. Karr JC. Retrospective comparison of diabetic foot ulcer and venous stasis ulcer healing outcome between a dermal repair scaffold (Primatrix) and a bilayered living cell therapy (Apligraf). Adv Skin wound care. 2011;24:119-25.
63. Garden JM, Backus AD. Treatment of leg veins with high energy pulsed dye laser. Lasers Surg and Med. 1996;8:34.
64. Bernstein EF, Lee J, Lowery J, et al. Treatment of spider veins with the 595 nm pulsed dye laser. J Am Acad Dermatol. 1998;39:746-50.
65. Eremia S, Li CY. Treatment of leg and face veins with a cryogen spray variable pulse width 1064 nm Nd: YAG laser – a prospective study of 47 patients. J Cosmet Laser Ther. 2001;3:147-53.
66. Kauvar AN, Lou WW. Pulsed alexandrite laser for the treatment of leg telangiectasia and reticular veins. Arch Dermatol. 2000;136:1371-5.
67. Kaudewitz P, Klovekorn W, Rother W. Treatment of leg vein telangiectasis. 1- Year results with a new 940 nm diode laser. Dermatol Surg. 2002;28:1031-4.
68. Goldman MP, Eckhouse S. Photothermal sclerosis of leg veins ESC Medical Systems Ltd., Photoderm VL Cooperative Study Group. Dermatol surgery. 1996;22:323-30.
69. Goldman MP. Intravascular lasers in the treatment of varicose veins. J Cosmet Dermatol. 2004;3:162-6.
70. Weiss RA. Endovenous techniques for elimination of saphenous reflux; a valuable treatment modality. Dermatol Surg. 2001;27:902-5.
71. Padberg FT. Surgical intervention in venous ulceration. Cardiovasc Surg. 1999;7:83-90.
72. Van Gent WB, Hop WC, Van Praag, et al. Conservative versus surgical treatment of venous leg ulcers: a prospective, randomized multicenter trial. J Vasc Surg. 2006;44: 563-71.
73. Nijsten T, van den Bos RR, Goldman MP, et al. Minimally invasive techniques in the treatment of saphenous varicose veins. J Am Acad Dermatol. 2009;60:110-9.
74. Sadick NS. Multi-focal pull-through endovascular cannulation technique of ambulatory phlebectomy. Dermatol Surg. 2002;28:32-7.
75. Schmeller W, Gaber Y, Gehl HB. Shave therapy is a simple effective treatment of persistent venous ulcers. J Am Acad Dermatol. 1998;39:232-8.
76. William D, Enoch S, Miller D, et al. Effect of debridement using curette on recalcitrant nonhealing venous leg ulcers. A currently controlled prospective cohort study. Wound Repair Regen. 2005;13:131-7.
77. Hiatt WR. Medical treatment of peripheral arterial diseaseand claudication. N Eng J Med. 2001;344:1608-21.
78. Caputo GM, Cavanagh PR, Ulbrecht JS, et al. Assessment and management of foot disease in patients with Diabetes. N Eng J Med. 1994;331:854-60.
79. Choucair MM, Philips TJ. What is new in clinical research in wound healing. Dermatol Clinics. 1997;15:45-58.
80. Singla S, Garg R, Kumar, et al. Efficacy of topical application of beta urogastrone (recombinant human epidermal growth factor) in Wagner's Grade 1 and 2 diabetic foot ulcers: comparative analysis of 50 patients. J Nat Sci Biol Med 2014;5:273-7.
81. Ohura T, Nakajo T, Moriguchi T, et al. Clinical efficacy of basic fibroblast growth factor on pressure ulcers: case-control pairing study using a new evaluation method. Wound Repair Regen 2011;19:542-51.
82. Lacci KM, Dardik A. Platelet-rich plasma: Support for its use in wound healing. Yale J Biol Med 2010;83:1-9.
83. Dohan DM, Choukroun J, Diss A, et al. Platelet-rich fibrin (PRF): A second-generation platelet concentrate. Part II: Platelet-related biologic features. Oral Surg Oral Med Oral Pathol Oral Radiol Endod. 2006;101:e45–50.
84. Greaves NS, Iqbal SA, Baguneid M, et al. The role of skin substitutes in the management of chronic cutaneous wounds. Wound Repair Regen 2013;21:194-210.
85. Iorio ML, Shuck J, Attinger CE. Wound healing in the upper and lower extremities: a systematic review on the use of acellular dermal matrices. Plast Reconstr Surg 2012;130:232S-241S.
86. Litwiniuk M,Grzela T. Amniotic membrane: new concepts for an old dressing. Wound Repair Regen 2014;22:451-56 .
87. Koob TJ, Rennert R, Zabek N, et al. Biological properties of dehydrated human amnion/chorion composite graft: implications for chronic wound healing. Int Wound J 2013;10:493-500.
88. Fetterolf DE, Snyder RJ. Scientific and clinical support for the use of dehydrated amniotic membrane in wound management. WOUNDS 2012;24:299-307 .
89. Zelen CM, Gould L, Serena TE, et al. A prospective, randomised, controlled, multi-centre comparative effectiveness study of healing using dehydrated human amnion/chorion membrane allograft, bioengineered skin substitute or standard of care for treatment of chronic lower extremity diabetic ulcers. Int Wound J 2015;12:724-32.
90. Wu Y Huang S, Enhe J, Fu X. Insights into bone marrow-derived mesenchymal stem cells safety for cutaneous repair and regeneration. Int Wound J 2012;9:586-94.
91. Maxson S, Lopez EA, Yoo D, et al. Concise review: role of mesenchymal stem cells in wound repair. Stem Cells Transl Med 2012;1:142-49.
92. Gu C, Huang S, Gao D, et al. Angiogenic effect of mesenchymal stem cells as a therapeutic target for enhancing diabetic wound healing. Int J Low Extrem Wounds 2014;13: 88-93.

Chapter 55

Surgery of Nails

Sushil Tahiliani, Harsh Tahiliani, Manjit Sandhu Tahiliani

Key Messages

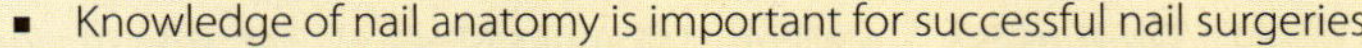

- Knowledge of nail anatomy is important for successful nail surgeries.
- Conservative surgical approach leads to less downtime and morbidity.
- Nail plate is formed essentially by matrix and hence it should be handled with utmost care.
- Knowledge of clinical conditions leads to planning of nail surgeries in an appropriate manner.
- Most of basic nail surgeries can be performed using proximal or distal digital block.

INTRODUCTION

Interest in field of nail surgery is recent. It has already been introduced in core curriculum of US dermatology residents and books devoted to the subject have been published in western world more than a decade ago.[1-3] In our country, it still remains a 'poor cousin' and a dermatology resident can pass the postgraduate exam without bothering to touch the subject. It is an 'orphan' that needs to be adopted by us, and doing so leads to job satisfaction and earning gratitude of a relieved patient.

Nail surgeries could be classified in one of the following two ways:

A. **Basic/Advanced**:
   - **Basic surgeries** include nail avulsion and nail plate, nail bed biopsy
   - **Advanced surgeries** include matrixectomy, matrix biopsy, nail fold surgeries and nail unit tumor surgeries.

B. **Diagnostic (biopsy of nail unit)/Therapeutic surgeries.**

Basic nail surgery is in domain of general dermatologist and can safely be performed as office procedure under local anesthesia. More advanced nail surgeries require collaboration between an orthopedic or plastic surgeon and the dermatologist and should be performed in a standard surgical facility.[1]

RELEVANT AND APPLIED ANATOMY

The nail unit (nail complex) consists of proximal nail fold (PNF), lateral nail fold (LNF), nail matrix, nail bed, nail plate and hyponychium (Figs. 1 and 2).

Nail Plate

It is a flat, translucent, rectangular, convex and hard structure that consists of closely packed adherent, interdigitating cells without nuclei and organelles. It is formed almost exclusively by nail matrix. Proximal matrix forms the dorsal part and distal matrix forms the ventral part of nail plate.[4] There is a small contribution of cells by nail bed to under surface of nail plate. Longitudinal brown to black bands seen throughout the length of the nail plate may be a normal finding in Fitzpatrick type IV, V and VI people.[4-6] The part of nail plate in relation to nail bed is thicker and firmly attached whereas the part over lunula is thinner and loosely attached.[7,8]

Nail Matrix

The nail matrix is the germinative portion of the nail complex, giving rise to the nail plate[4,5,7,8]. The matrix is at the most proximal point of the nail bed and is seated deep beneath the PNF; it is separated from the distal phalanx by only a few millimetres. The proximal matrix continues

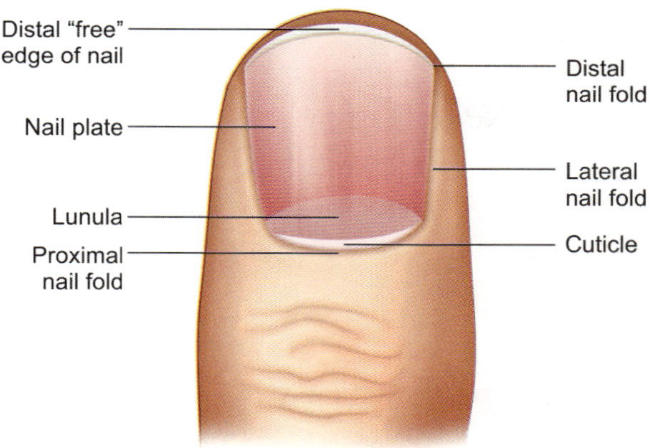

Fig. 1: Nail unit.

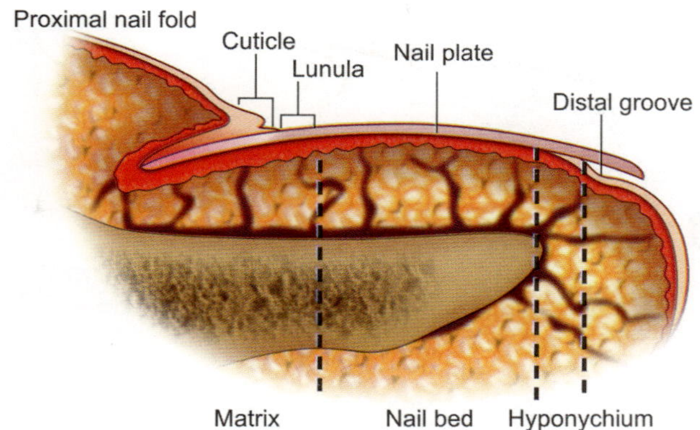

Fig. 2: Sagittal section through nail unit.

proximally and laterally to form the lateral matrix horn. The nail surgeon should be cognizant that the lateral matrix horn may be extensive. The lunula is usually seen through the transparent nail plate, especially on the thumbs and great toes, as the visible distal component of the nail matrix. Several reasons exist why the nail surgeon must attempt to leave the structural and functional boundaries of the nail matrix intact when performing nail surgery,[1,9-11] some of them mentioned below:

- The matrix is the center of nail formation and the source of the nail plate.
- Nail growth is a direct function of the rate of turnover of matrix cells.
- Nail thickness is directly related to the length or the size of the nail matrix.
- The shape of the distal border of the lunula determines the shape of the nail. If this border is convex, the distal free edge of the plate will also be convex.

Nail Bed

The nail bed extends from the distal lunula to the point of origin of the hyponychium. LNF mark the lateral border of nail bed. The epidermis of the nail bed is relatively thin, with a dimensional thickness of only 1-2 cells[7]. Like matrix, it has no granular layer. The epidermal surface of the bed has parallel longitudinal ridges that interlock with similar folds on the ventral surface of the nail plate. There is a corresponding unique, longitudinal, tongue-in-groove spatial arrangement of dermal papillae and epidermal rete ridges.[5,7,12] The dermis has a wealth of glomus bodies and rich network of longitudinally oriented capillaries. It lacks an underlying subcutaneous layer of adipose tissue. As a result, nothing separates the dermis from the periosteum of the distal phalanx. Melanocytes are not found in the nail bed.

Hyponychium

The hyponychium is the anatomical area that begins at the onychodermal band, where the nail bed ends, and terminates at the distal groove. The distal groove is a transverse demarcation extending across the distal digit that divides the hyponychium from the volar epidermis of the digit. This groove is the first component of the nail unit to be recognized during the embryologic period, and it is the origin point of the volar epidermis.

Proximal Nail Fold

The PNF is a continuation of the dorsal skin of the digit that folds back on itself at the nail root to create two epithelial surfaces: a superficial dorsal layer and a deep ventral layer.[5,7,10,11] The ventral layer travels to the base of the nail plate to create the nail matrix. Where the two epithelial surfaces meet, the cuticle converges onto the distal nail plate.

The PNF is contiguous with the lateral nail folds (LNFs) that border the nail plate.

Proximal and Lateral Nail Grooves

These are potential spaces created by overlap of PNF and LNF over the nail plate.

Blood Supply[1,13,14]

Blood supply is derived from lateral digital arteries which supply the nail unit through formation of superficial, proximal and distal arcades (Figs. 3A and B).

Venous drainage follows arterial vasculature, the only difference being that it combines proximally forming two digital veins on either side.

Vascular structure of nail bed is unique in that it must supply a vascular structure between two hard surfaces, the nail plate and distal phalanx.[1]

Large AV anastomoses including glomus bodies are found at the level of the anastomotic arteries and the deep venous circulation in all the areas of nail unit except the PNF.

Nerve Supply[15]

Innervation of the nail unit is through two laterally positioned sensory nerves—dorsal and ventral. Nail unit is richly innervated (Fig. 4).

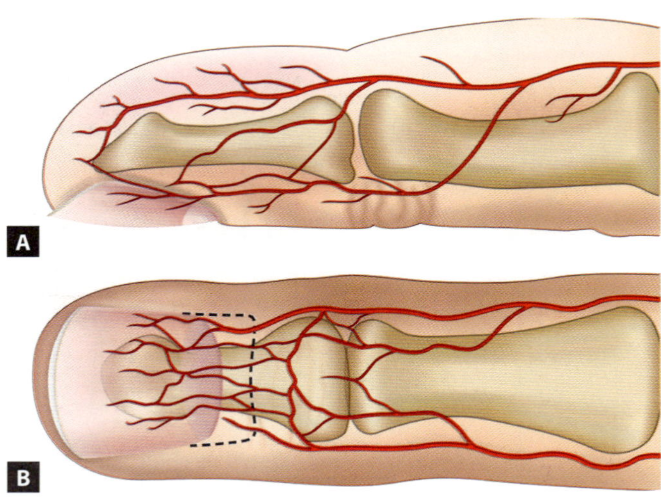

Figs. 3A and B: Vasculature of nail: (A) Laterat view; (B) Dorsal view.

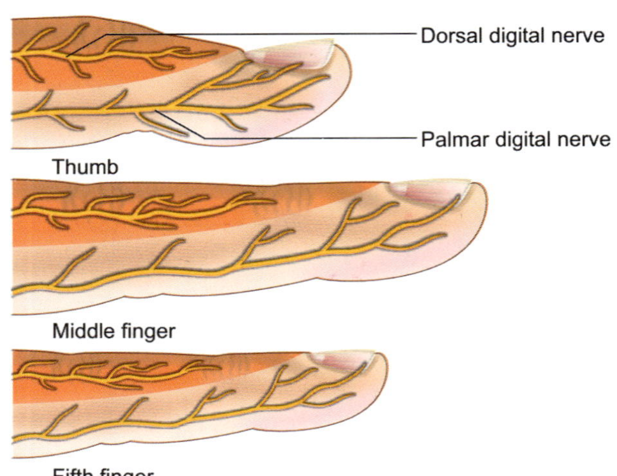

Fig. 4: Nerve supply of nail.

INDICATIONS FOR NAIL SURGERY[1,16,17]

1. Diagnostic dilemmas: To differentiate between infective and non-infective disorders, accurate diagnosis of 'Twenty nail' syndrome, differentiate between sub-ungual hematomas and malignant melanoma are some examples.
2. Onychocryptosis.
3. Acute paronychia and sub-ungual abscess.
4. Trauma: E.g. subungual hematoma.
5. Myxoid cyst.
6. Benign and malignant growths involving the nail unit: warts, pyogenic granuloma, glomus tumor, Koenen's tumor, subungual exostosis, malignant melanoma, BCC, SCC, Bowen's disease[18].

CONTRAINDICATIONS[17]

With refinement of technique and availability of better medical care, the contraindications are 'relative'.

1. Established peripheral vascular disease.
2. Collagen vascular disease.
3. Uncontrolled diabetes mellitus.
4. Disorders of hemostasis.
5. Very acute infections/inflammation of nail unit.

Preoperative Evaluation

- To rule out local infection, vasculopathies
- To rule out drug allergies
- To rule out significant systemic disorders and to control existing disorders
- To rule out intake of agents that may interfere with hemostasis
- To evaluate and discuss with the patient, duration of functional impairment and risk of short-term and long-term nail dystrophy
- To take a good clinical photograph
- To take informed consent.

Surgical Setting

Nail avulsions, biopsies and simple excisions can safely be performed in dermatologist's office under same conditions as basic skin surgery procedures. Advanced nail surgical procedures should be performed in operation theatre.[1]

Anesthesia

Depending on procedure, indication, and personal preference, we have a choice of various types of digital (local) anesthesia techniques as well as variety of regional blocks. Surgeries done in a dermatologist's office require only a distal or proximal digital block.

Syringe: Dental syringe/2 mL Luer lock syringe for distal nail blocks.

Needle: 27/30 gauge needle.

Anesthetic agent: Plain Lidocaine (2% preferred over 1%). Lidocaine with adrenaline is safe for digital anesthesia[19-22] but not very useful as exsanguination is still necessary.[1]

Ropivacaine and Bupivacaine are preferred for regional blocks.[23]

I. Digital anesthesia:

A. Distal nail blocks:
- Distal digital block (wing block)
- Distal anesthesia through PNF
- Distal anesthesia through hyponychium.

B. Proximal digital block.

C. Transthecal digital anesthesia.

II. Regional blocks:

A. Wrist block.

B. Median nerve block at wrist.

C. Ulnar nerve block.

D. Nerve blocks for posterior tibial, deep peroneal, sural nerves.[24]

Table 1: Advantages and disadvantages of distal digital block.

Advantages	*Disadvantages and contraindications*
Immediate effect (in less than 1minute)	Injection relatively painful
Low risk of neurovascular compromise	Local infection
Induces compression hemostasis	Vasculopathies (e.g. systemic sclerosis)
	May cause inadequate coverage and swelling of surgical field in large surgeries

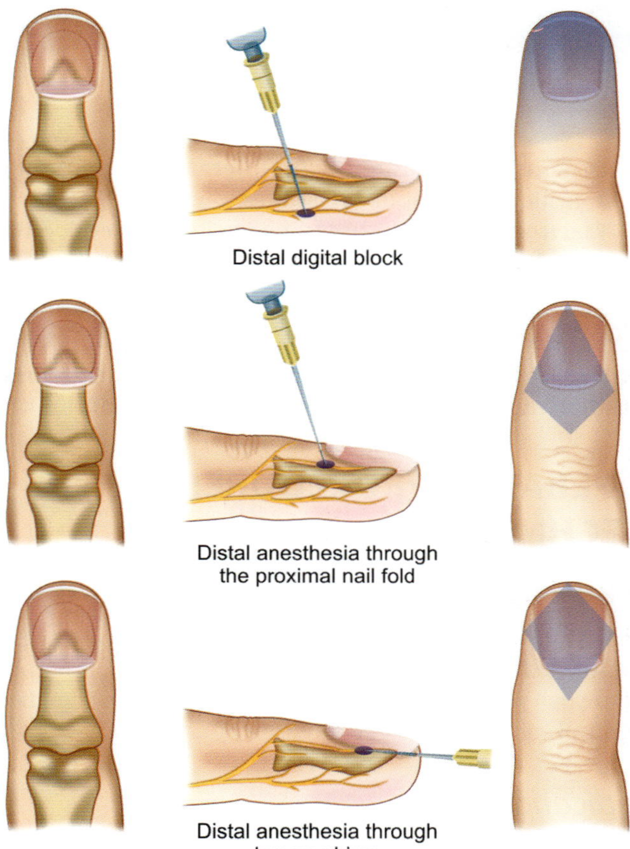

Fig. 5: The 3 types of distal digital anesthesia with area covered. (*Source:* Abimelec P, Dumontier C, Basic and advanced nail surgery. In: Scher RK, Daniel CR (Eds). Nails: Diagnosis Therapy, Surgery, 3rd ed. Saunders, 2005:267).

Digital blocks offer total nail unit anesthesia and are hence the preferred methods. These would be discussed in further detail.

Distal Digital Block (Figs. 5 and 6)

Needle is inserted 2–3 mm proximal to the junction of PNF and LNF. After raising a wheal- to minimize pain, the needle in inserted vertically down towards ventral aspect. While doing so, 0.5–1 ml of anesthetic agent is injected to cover the dorsal and ventral digital nerves. Both sides of digit are injected. Advantages and disadvantages of distal digital block are summarized in Table 1.

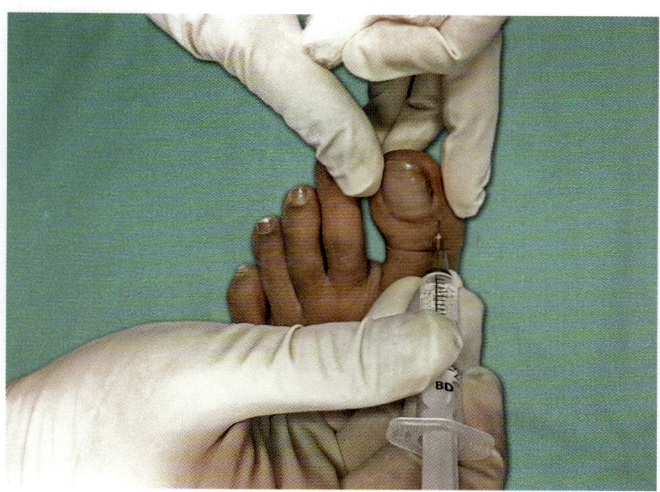

Fig. 6: Distal digital block – given at a point 2-3 mm proximal to junction of PNF and LNF.

Proximal Digital Block (Fig. 7)

Needle is introduced at the base of digit and a wheal raised. The needle is then pushed gently in ventral direction injecting a larger amount near the dorsal and ventral digital nerve (1 mL for each nerve for thumb and 2 mL for toe). It takes 10 to 15 minutes for full effect to take place. It is not a ring block which should be avoided.

Transthecal Digital Block

At the level of the palmar flexion crease, 2 mL lidocaine is injected into the potential space of the flexor tendon sheath with a syringe and 26 gauge hypodermic needle. The digit is anesthetized through centrifugal diffusion.[25]

INSTRUMENTS

Most instruments used for nail surgery are not specific.

General Instruments (Fig. 8)

- Binocular magnifying loupe that magnifies 2.5 to 3.5 times at a distance of 35 to 45 cm
- Delicate Adson's forceps with one by two teeth/ Castroviejo forceps
- Biopsy punch
- Double prong Guthrie retractors
- Delicate needle holder
- Stevens/Graddle scissors
- Straight mosquito forceps
- Curette
- Digital tourniquet.

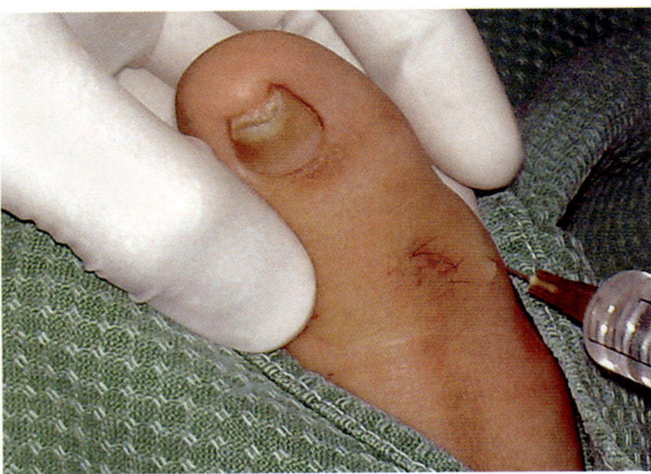

Fig. 7: Proximal digital block.

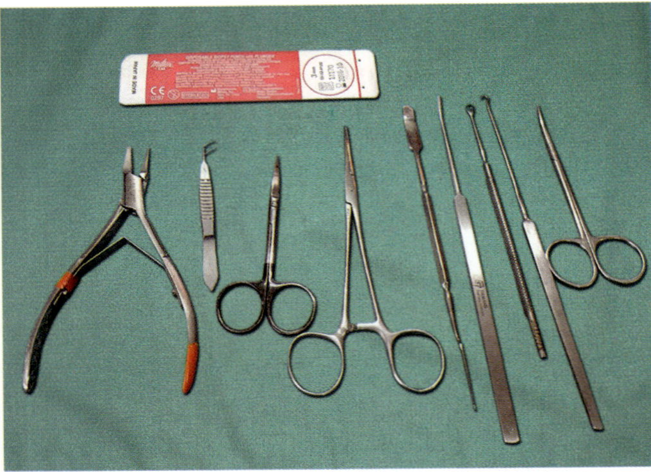

Fig. 8: Nail instruments.

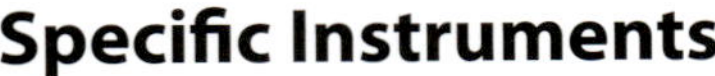

Specific Instruments

- Nail elevator: Lempert (2-3 mm wide)/Freer septum elevator/ dental spatula
- English anvil-action nail splitter
- Nail nipper.

SUTURES

- Biopsies and excisions with a diameter ≤3 mm do not require suturing
- PNF/LNF: Absorbable suture (Vicryl Rapide: 4–0 for toes, 5-0 for fingers)
- Nonabsorbable suture like Ethilon/Prolene can also be used
- Nail matrix: Absorbable suture (Vicryl 6-0)
- Nail bed: Absorbable suture (Vicryl 5-0).

HEMOSTASIS

Intraoperative

A bloodless field is mandatory for optimal results.

i. Pressure applied to lateral digital arteries—by an assistant—suffices for simple avulsions and biopsies.
ii. Digital tourniquet at the base of finger is used most commonly. Various agents like penrose drain, rubber band, urinary catheter and a rolled rubber glove finger whose tip has been removed, have been used. For finger nail surgery, the whole glove (patient's glove size) is a better alternative as it provides adequate (not excessive) and reliable pressure while providing a sterile surgical field.[26] A tourniquet should not be applied for more than 15 minutes at a stretch.[27]
iii. Pneumatic tourniquet: It is applied to upper arm/ forearm after exsanguination. It is used in cases with a digital infection or a distal vascular compromise. A conscious patient can tolerate a pneumatic tourniquet for about 30 minutes.

Electrocoagulation should be avoided to reduce the risk of nail tissue scarring and permanent nail dystrophy.

Postoperative

Bulky dressing, gentle pressure and overhead limb positioning are sufficient measures in majority of cases.

OPERATIVE PROCEDURES/ TECHNIQUES

Nail Plate Avulsion

Nail avulsion is the most common surgical procedure performed on the nail unit. It is the excision of the body of the nail plate from its primary attachments, the nail bed ventrally and the PNF dorsally.

Indications

i. To treat recalcitrant onychocryptosis.
ii. To excise tumors of the nail unit.
iii. To allow full examination and exploration of the nail bed, the nail matrix, the PNF and the LNF, and the nail grooves for the presence of pathology.
iv. To use as a preliminary step before performing biopsy on the nail bed and the nail matrix.
v. Avulsion of the nail plate is frequently used as a therapeutic adjunct in long-standing fungal infections of the nail, such as chronic onychomycosis, and in acute bacterial infections.
vi. In traumatic nail injuries, avulsion may be used to evaluate the stability of the nail bed or to release a subungual hematoma after failed puncture aspiration.

Nail plate avulsion is done as partial or total. Total avulsion could be chemical (40% urea) or surgical.

Surgical Avulsion[1,28,29]

Steps

1. Nail plate, PNF separation (Fig. 9): Dental spatula/Freer septum elevator is pushed back towards the cuticle and gently introduced under the PNF. The instrument is moved laterally in gliding movement to separate the remaining part of PNF from nail plate.
2. Nail plate, nail bed separation (Fig. 10): The same instrument is introduced under the nail plate at the level of hyponychium and pushed towards lunula. There is lesser resistance to the movement of spatula underneath lunula. The instrument is withdrawn and reintroduced in the adjoining region till the entire area to be avulsed is separated. The spatula must not be swept laterally to respect the longitudinal orientation of the ridges and grooves in this region.
3. In case of complete nail avulsion, the separated nail plate is grasped with a hemostat and avulsed by twisting the hemostat around it's long axis.
4. In partial nail plate avulsion (Fig. 11), the most commonly performed technique is longitudinal avulsion. The part to be avulsed is sectioned using English anvil nail splitter till the distal most part of PNF. Stevens' scissor is then introduced under the PNF with its blades closed. The blades are next opened and the part of nail plate under the PNF is sectioned. The separated part of nail plate is then avulsed using previously described technique (Fig. 12).

The partial nail plate avulsions could be also be done as proximal (for nail matrix exposure), distal, circular in less common indications.

In proximal approach (Figs. 13A and B), the spatula is inserted under the detached PNF and pushed proximally till one feels the proximal edge of the nail plate. It is then flipped and rotated to go under the proximal part of nail plate. The tip of spatula would now be facing the hyponychium. It is gently pushed in that direction to cause separation of nail plate from nail bed.

Complications

- Bleeding
- Pain
- Distorted curvature or hypertrophy of newly grown nail due to trauma to nail matrix and/or nail bed.

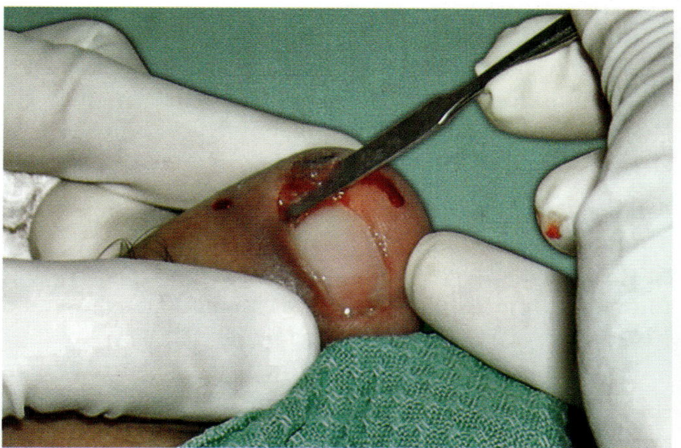

Fig. 9: Separation of nail plate from PNF.

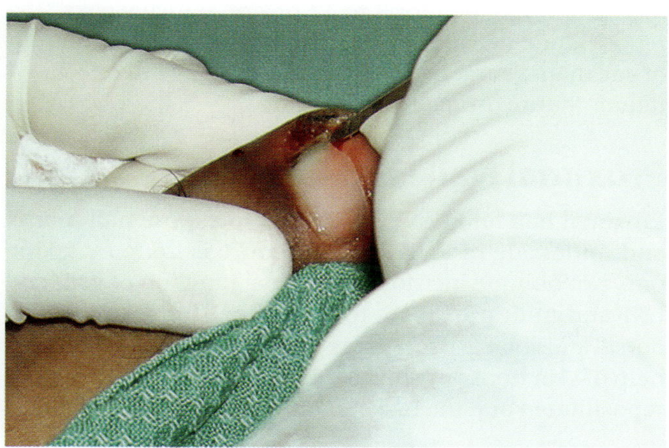

Fig. 10: Separation of nail plate from nail bed.

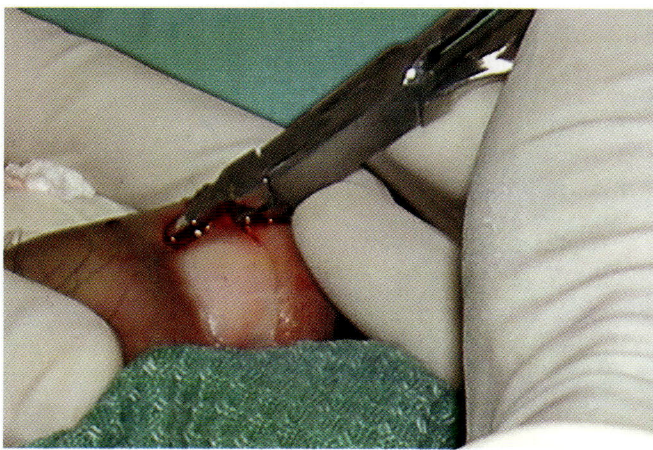

Fig. 11: Sectioning of nail plate with nail splitter.

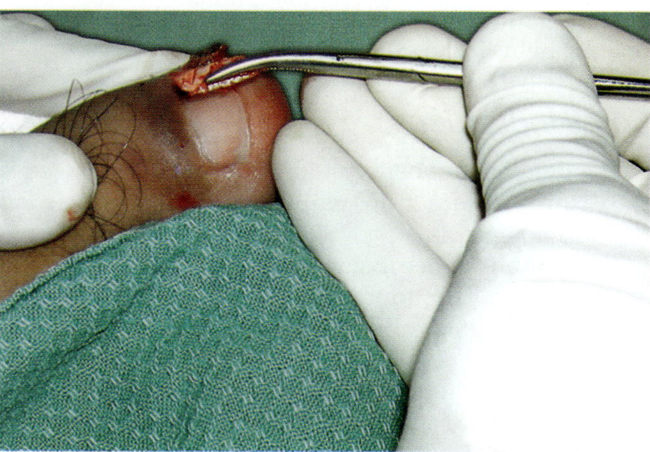

Fig. 12: Avulsion of separated and sectioned part of nail plate.

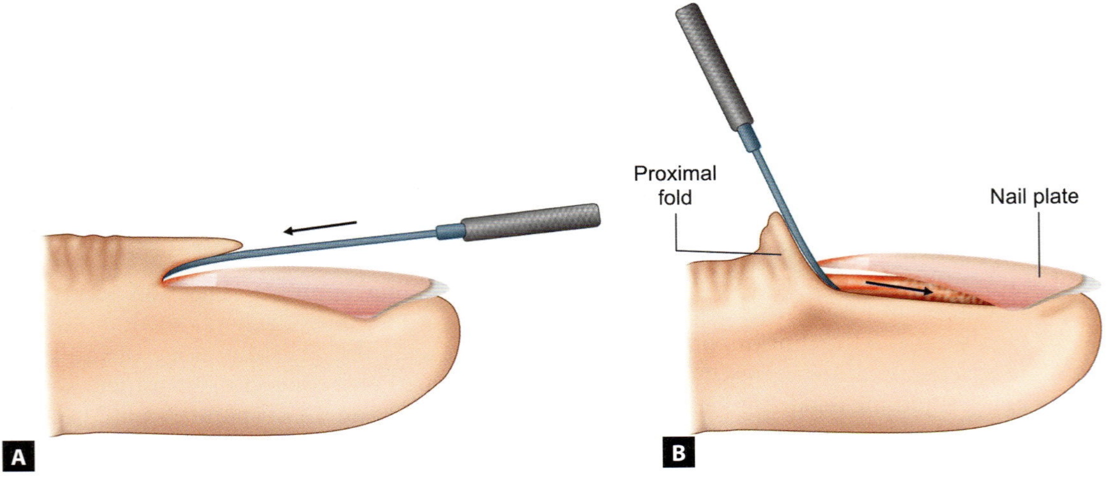

Figs. 13A and B: Proximal approach for nail avulsion.
(*Source:* Salasche SJ. Nail unit surgery. In: Robinson JK, Arndt KA, LeBoit PE, Wintroub BU (Eds). Atlas of Cutaneous Surgery (1st ed). Philadelphia, Saunders,1996:193.)

Nail Plate Repositioning[1]

After some surgeries like nail matrix biopsy, nail bed tumor removal, the avulsed nail plate is repositioned as this gives a natural and effective protection to the wound, nail matrix and nail bed for 3 to 12 postoperative weeks. The repositioned nail also prevents pterygium unguis in event of nail matrix surgeries. It is secured to LNF with one Vicryl Rapide suture on each side.

Proximal Nail Fold Reflection

Proximal nail fold (PNF) is needed to expose nail matrix and underside of PNF. The procedure is done by taking one/two oblique incisions starting at junction of PNF and LNF and going proximally towards the DIP crease between dorsal and volar aspect. The separated PNF is reflected with help of skin hooks or sutures. After the surgery, the PNF is repositioned and the incisions are closed using Vicryl 5-0.

Biopsy (Figs. 14 to 16)

Biopsy is useful for diagnosis of various skin diseases when careful medical history, clinical examination and other investigations fail to establish a precise diagnosis.

Some Indications[30]

1. To differentiate between inflammatory and infective disorders affecting nail unit, e.g. psoriasis *vs.* onychomycosis.
2. To establish the diagnosis in cases with one nail/ 'twenty nail' dystrophy.
3. To establish the cause of longitudinal pigmented streaks.
4. To differentiate between subungual hematoma and malignant melanoma.
5. To differentiate between benign and malignant tumors.
6. To identify the cause of pain (e.g. glomus tumor).

Types

Nail bed, nail plate, nail matrix, nail fold, nail unit (combined biopsy of LNF, lateral nail matrix and PNF).

Technique[1,30]

Nail plate: Distal part with a nail nipper, other areas with 3 or 4 mm biopsy punch (Fig. 14). The nail plate may get stuck in the punch thus causing confusion and scare. It should be looked for and removed from there.

Nail bed: Done after partial nail plate avulsion with a 4 mm punch or nail plate lifting. A 3 mm punch is used to take the sample. Punch is moved deeper gently till it touches the periosteum. The base is separated using small iris scissors or 11 number scalpel blade (Fig. 15).

For larger sample size, elliptical excision with a maximum width of 3 mm should be taken with long axis of incision being along long axis of nail. The wound thus created would have to be undermined and sutured.

Nail matrix: Proximal avulsion of the nail plate has to be performed initially to visualize the matrix. The matrix sample is taken using a 3 mm punch or a longitudinal elliptical sample oriented horizontally or along long axis of digit. The elliptical wounds have to be undermined and closed with absorbable suture material.

Matrixectomy[1,16,17]

Destruction of nail matrix to prevent regrowth of nail plate in conditions like onychogryphosis, pincer nails, onychocryptosis and permanently split nails. It may involve entire matrix or part of it (total or partial).

Modalities

i. Chemical (Fig. 17): Done by applying fully saturated (88%) liquefied phenol or 10% NaOH directly to

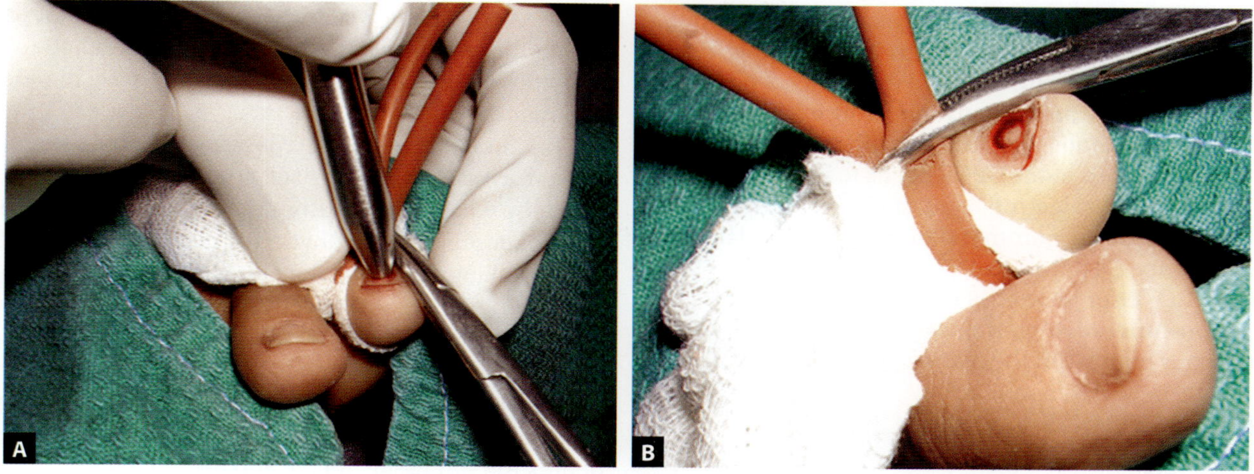

Figs. 14A and B: Nail plate biopsy with subsequent exposure of nail bed.

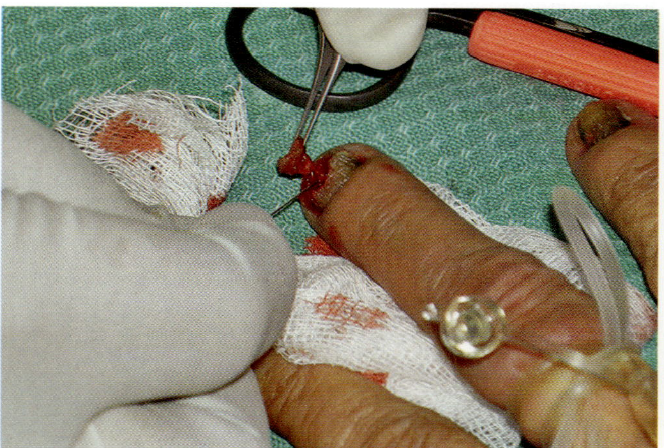

Fig. 15: Nail bed biopsy with a 11 no. blade.

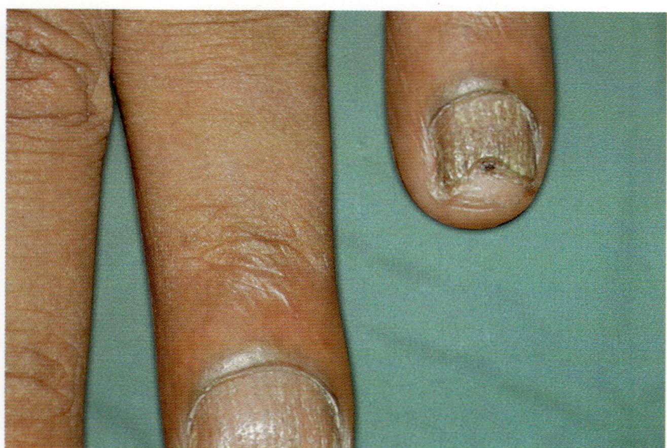

Fig. 16: Healing of the biopsied nail plate, circular defect grows out.

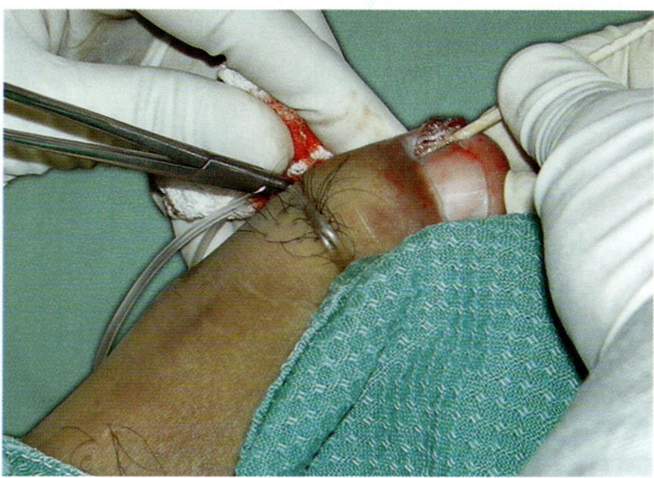

Fig. 17: Application of phenol after securing tourniquet.

exposed matrix. Phenolization as a method for partial destruction of nail matrix has been in use for more than 50 years and is the most commonly used method. It is by far the simplest, least traumatic and most successful of all methods. A recent review in Cochrane Library has endorsed the same and shown that it carries the least rate of recurrence postoperatively at 6 months and above.[31] Phenol has the added advantage of being an antimicrobial agent and of causing damage to nerve endings thus reducing postoperative pain. It should be applied with help of cotton tipped tooth-picks, though other methods have been described. Phenol should be kept for 2 to 3 minutes. Duration of contact for 10% NaOH is 1 minute.[32] The duration of postoperative drainage is shorter for NaOH (avg 9 days vs 17 days). Oozing period has been shown to be reduced by using lignocaine and adrenaline combination for anesthesia[33] and by using Monsel's solution postoperatively.[34] Both these chemicals are safe in diabetics and children. In only one series, 100% Trichloracetic acid was used with results comparable with previously mentioned chemical but with a healing time of 2 weeks.[35]

ii. Surgical (removal of matrix, lateral matrix horns, under surface of PNF). PNF needs to be reflected. A more extensive surgery (wedge excision) is popular with orthopedic surgeons but in view of higher risk of infection, pain, recurrence and deformity of nail plate, it should not be performed for treating ingrowing nails.

iii. CO_2 laser (ablation with focussed mode or vaporization with defocused mode). PNF needs to be reflected.

iv. Radiosurgery/electrocoagulation (insulated matrix electrode set is commercially available – H9 from Ellman Inc.).

Both CO_2 laser as well as radiosurgery carry a higher risk of postoperative pain as well as periostitis due to overzealous removal of the matrix.

Complications

- Pain
- Bleeding
- Infection
- Failure to prevent regrowth
- Growth of nail spicules due to inadequate damage to matrix
- Nail plate disfigurement.

Onychocryptosis (Ingrown Nail)

Management: It is a very painful commonly seen condition due to impacting of the nail plate in periungual soft tissue. The most common variant is seen due to piercing of lateral nail sulcus by the nail plate due to trimming the nail plate too short or wearing shoes with a narrow toe box. Less commonly seen variants are due to increased transverse curvature of nail plate or due to swelling of periungual tissue. In the latter condition distal embedding of the nail plate happens due to lack of counter-pressure of nail plate on distal part of pulp.

1. **Prophylaxis:**
   - Avoidance of overaggressive trimming of nail plate
   - Cutting the distal edge of nail plate straight and not in a curvilinear shape
   - Avoidance of narrow, closed footwear.
2. **Conservative management**
   Works in cases with tenderness but no granulation tissue/severe discharge. Splinting of nail plate border using a flexible plastic tube,[36] introducing cotton wisp/dental floss between the nail plate and distal part of nail groove;[37] and use of adhesive tape to pull the LNF away from nail plate[38] are some of the methods that have been described as innovative office-based procedures to successfully treat such cases.
3. **Surgical management**
   Indicated in cases where conservative measures have failed or the condition is extremely painful/recurrent.

Approaches

A. Narrowing of the nail plate (partial nail plate avulsion).

B. Debulking the soft tissues.

A. Partial nail plate avulsion with matrixectomy: For lateral ingrowing nail, vertical avulsion of involved part of nail plate followed by destruction of relevant part of matrix chemically is a very successful method to treat more severe cases and cases where above mentioned methods fail to work.

The procedure has been described under headings of nail avulsion and matrixectomy.

B. Debulking of periungual soft tissue: For distal embedding and very hypertrophic and exuberant LNF, debulking with secondary intention/primary intention healing is the most effective and easy to perform, with great results.[39]

Howard-Dubois procedure, VandenBos' procedure, Super U, Noel's procedure, Tweedle and Ranger's transposition flap are some of the methods described to debulk the soft tissue in PNF and the nail pulp.

A detailed knowledge of anatomy is essential before doing these surgeries. One should also train to acquire commensurate surgical skills. These surgeries need a proper operation theatre with facilities matching orthopedic surgery standards.

Surgery for Subungual Hemorrhage

An acute painful reddish hematoma occupying 25% of nail bed needs to be evacuated to cause instant relief from pain and a chance of salvaging the nail. It is done with no.18 needle, a pointed scalpel blade, a drill or electrosurgical apparatus.[40] One should rule out a fracture to distal phalanx and presence of malignant melanoma.[41] Old asymptomatic bluish hematoma should be left untouched.

Nail Unit Infections (Pyogenic)

Acute pyogenic abscesses involving the nail folds should be drained in conjunction with the use of appropriate antibiotics. The incision should be parallel to the nail fold length. Baran and Bureau recommend incising the site of maximum pain rather than the site of maximum soft tissue induration.[42] Formed septa in the abscess base are destroyed by using the tip of a curved hemostat.[43] In case of nail bed abscess, the methods described for subungual hematoma may be used (Figs. 18 to 20).

POSTOPERATIVE DRESSING AND CARE

A non-adherent gauze coated with petrolatum or an antibiotic is used to cover the operated area. This is then covered by many layers of absorbent gauze. A roller bandage is next used to secure the gauze and put some pressure. The limb may have to be elevated and immobilized in case of major surgeries. The dressing is changed after 48 hours and operated area examined to look for complications like infection, hematoma and dehiscence. Smaller dressing is used in place, the bulky dressing applied on surgery day. The dressings may be necessary for 10 to 30 days.[1]

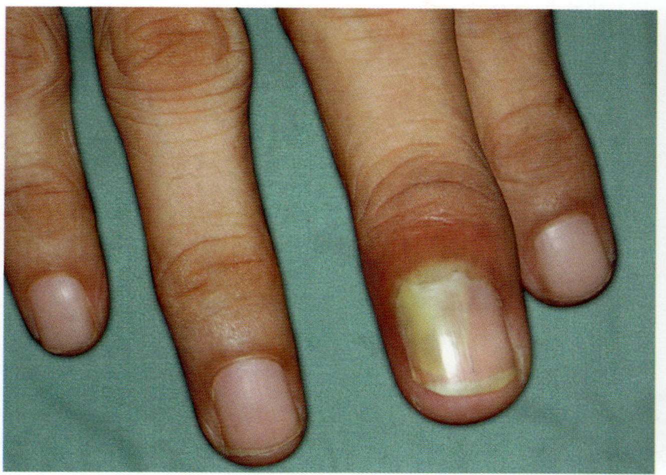

Fig. 18: Subungual abscess.

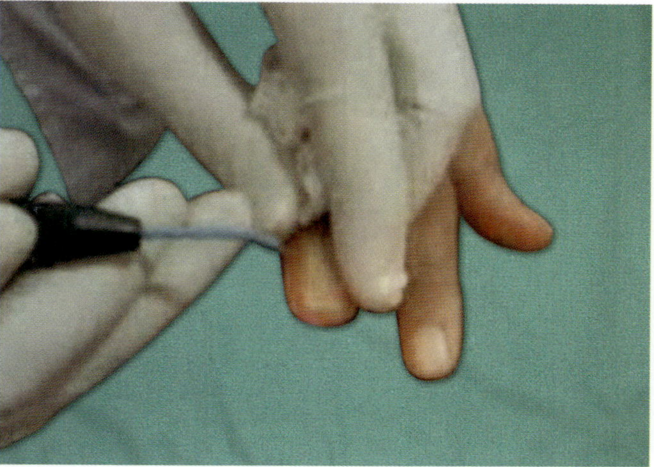

Fig. 19: Ellman RF equipment used to drain a subungual abscess.

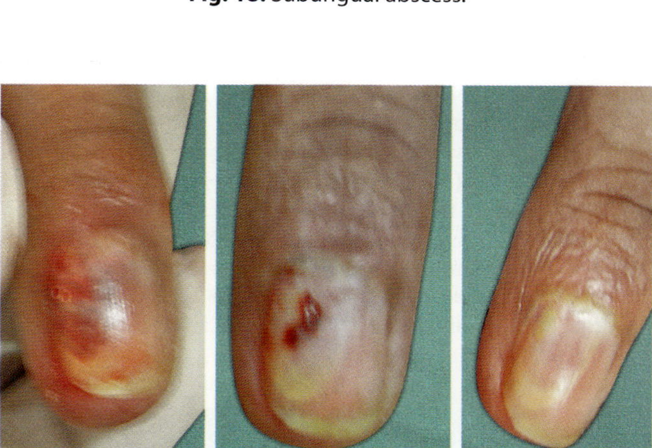

Fig. 20: Results after drainage of subungual abscess.

Lasers and the Nail Unit

Multiple laser wavelengths and techniques have shown utility in the treatment of various nail disorders. In particular CO_2 laser has been used for different purposes; (a) Incisional mode for incising nail plate to expose underlying tissue (b) Vapourization mode for matricectomy and periungal and subungal verrucae.[44]

Advantages

- Hemostasis
- Visualization
- Less traumatic with higher precision
- Sterilization and sealing of tissue leading to non-inoculation
- Helps to avoid blotting of surgical site, tourniquet and bulky dressings
- Improved functional and cosmetic outcomes.

Disadvantages

- Cost factor (equipment, training, operational and setup time)
- Lack of robust evidence.

Lasers can be used for the management of following disorders of the nail apparatus:

- Subungual hematoma
- Nail fold and plate dystrophies
- Onychomycosis
- Periungual/subungual verrucae
- Matricectomy
- For making incisions
- Laser-assisted drug delivery.

Onychomycosis

Laser treatment in onychomycosis have been approved by FDA, however doubts still exist over the fungicidal effect of lasers. There is a lack of literature of high methodological quality or evidence through randomized placebo controlled studies comparing their efficacy with systemic therapy in onychomycosis.

Lasers may be considered due to:

1. Poor penetration of topical drugs through the non-porous nail plate.
2. Long-term systemic therapy.
3. Pain, discomfort and prolonged nail regrowth time post operatively.

Fractional CO_2 laser has been used to aid the delivery of topical antifungal agents[45,46] (Figs. 21A and B) and Fractional CO_2 laser associated with photodynamic therapy[47] have been used for the management of onychomycosis.

Long pulsed Nd: YAG laser delivers extremely brief micro-second bursts of energy resulting in ablative thermal destruction of the fungi with minimal damage to the

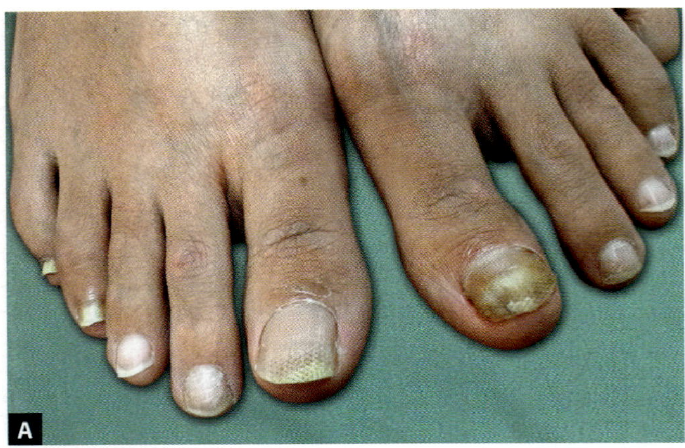

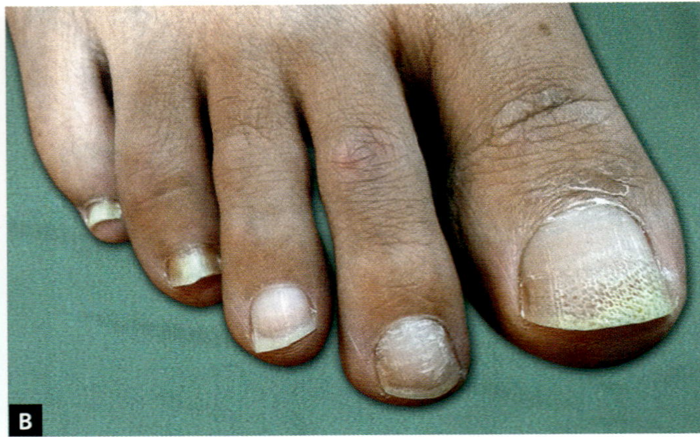

Figs. 21A and B: Fractional CO_2 laser-assisted drug delivery.

surrounding epidermal tissue.[48] Toenails have a higher cure rate as compared to fingernails with this laser.[49]

Diode laser at 870 nm and 930 nm has also been used but questions have been raised over the mechanism of action and effectiveness of this laser.

Tips and Tricks

- Learn your anatomy, be a good clinician.
- Nail surgery is not difficult to master, take a plunge.
- Anesthesia: Distal/proximal digital anesthesia should be used. Ring block must be avoided. Though 1-2% lignocaine is the agent of choice, bupivacaine could be injected postoperatively to prolong pain free period.
- There is no need to routinely exsanguinate the digit.
- Tourniquet is not needed in all cases. When reuired, it should not be put for >15 minutes. Pressure on digital vessels by an assistant is sufficient to get a 'bloodless' field.
- During a punch biopsy of nail bed through the nail plate, a 4 mm punch should be used for nail plate and a 3 mm punch should be used for nail bed. The nail plate gets separated from nail bed and may get embedded in punch.
- One should combine technologies to get optimum results.
- One should be innovative and adapt to available facilities.
- One should be conservative as reduced operative trauma leads to lesser downtime.
- One should accept the limitations and take the help of orthopedic/plastic surgeons wherever needed.

REFERENCES

1. Abimelec P, Dumontier C. Basic and advanced nail surgery. In: Scher RK, Daniel CR (eds). Nails: Diagnosis Therapy, Surgery, 3rd eds. Philadelphia: Saunders. 2005:265-306.
2. Dumontier C. L'Ongle. Paris: Elsevier; 2000.
3. Krull EA, Zook EG, Baran R, Haneke E. Nail surgery: A text and atlas. Philadelphia: Lippincott, Williams and Wilkins; 2001.
4. Zaias N. The Nail in Health and Disease. Norwalk, Conn: Appleton & Lange; 1990.
5. Ditre CM, Howe NR. Surgical anatomy of the nail unit. J Dermatol Surg Oncol. 1992;18(8):665-71.
6. Fleegler EJ. A surgical approach to melanonychia striata. J Dermatol Surg Oncol. 1992;18(8):708-14.
7. Dawber RP, Baran R, Berker D. Science of the nail: gross anatomy. In: Baran R, Dawber RP, (eds). Diseases of the Nails and their Management. Oxford, England: Blackwell Science; 1994:1-34.
8. Gonzalez-Serva A. Structure and function. In: Scher RK, Daniel CR, (eds). Nails: Therapy, Diagnosis, Surgery. Philadelphia, Pa: WB Saunders; 2005:12-31.
9. Scher RK. The nail. In: Roenigk RK, Roenigk HH, Ratz JL, (eds). Dermatologic Surgery-Principles and Practice. New York, NY: Marcel Dekker; 2006:281-88.
10. Siegle RJ, Swanson NA. Nail surgery: a review. J Dermatol Surg Oncol. 1982;8(8):659-66.
11. Samman PD. Tumors producing nail disorders: benign tumours. In: The Nails in Disease. Boston, Mass: Butterworth-Heinemann; 1994:169-82.
12. Fleckman P. Basic science of the nail unit. In: Scher RK, Daniel CR, (eds). Nails: Therapy, Diagnosis, Surgery. Philadelphia, Pa: WB Saunders; 2005:37-54.
13. Flint MH. Some observations on the vascular supply of the nail bed and terminal segments of the finger. Br J Plast Surg. 19955;8:186-95.
14. Samman PD. Human toe nail: is genesis and blood supply. Br J Dermatol. 1959;71:296-302.
15. Fleckman P, Allan C. Surgical anatomy of the nail unit. Dermatol Surg. 2001;27:257-60.
16. Salasche SJ. Nail unit surgery. In: Robinson JK, Arndt KA, LeBoit PE, Wintroub BU (eds). Atlas of cutaneous surgery, (1st edn). Philadelphia: Saunders,1996:189-200.
17. Onumah N, Scher RK. Nail surgery. In Elston DM chief (eds). Medscape ref, 2009.
18. Pardo-Castello V, Pardo O. Diseases of the Nails. Springfield, Ill: Charles C Thomas; 1960.
19. Denkler K. A comprehensive review of epinephrine in the finger: to do or not to do. Plast Reconstr Surg. 2001;108(1):114-24.
20. Krunic AL, Wang LC, Soltani K, Weitzul S, Taylor RS. Digital anesthesia with epinephrine: an old myth revisited. J Am Acad Dermatol. 2004;51(5):755-9.
21. Wilhelmi BJ, Blackwell SJ, Miller J, Mancoll JS, Phillips LG. Epinephrine in digital blocks: revisited. Ann Plast Surg. 1998;41(4):410-4.
22. Sylaidis P, Logan A. Digital blocks with adrenaline. An old dogma refuted. J Hand Surg [Br]. 1998;23(1):17-9.

23. Salam GA. Regional anaesthesia for office procedures: Part II, Extremity and inguinal area surgeries. Am Fam Physician. 2004;69(4):896-900.
24. Cohen SJ, Roenigk RK. Nerve blocks for cutaneous surgery on the foot. J Dermatol Surg Oncol. 1991;17(6):527-34.
25. Chiu DTW. Transthecal digital block: flexor tendon sheath used for anaesthetic infusion. J Hand Surg. 1990;15A:471-3.
26. Hixson FP, Shafiroff BB, Werner FW, Palmer AK. Digital tourniquets: a pressure study with clinical relevance. J Hand Surg (Am). 1986;11(6):865-68.
27. Richert B. Basic nail surgery. Dermatol Clin. 2006;24(3): 313-22.
28. Abimelec P. Nail surgery made easy,can it be true? In: American Academy of Dermatology. New Orleans; 1999.
29. Abimelec P. Tricks and tips of nail surgery: nail symposium. In: American Academy of Dermatology Annual Meeting. Orlando FL; 1998.
30. Rich P. Nail biopsy: indications and methods. Dermatol Surg. 2001;27(3):229-34.
31. Rounding C, Bloomfield F. Surgical treatments for ingrown toenails. Cochrane Database Syst Rev, 2005;2:CD001541.
32. Oxdemir E, Bostanci S, Ekmekci P, Gurgey E. Chemical matricectomy with 10% sodium hydroxide for the treatment of ingrowing toenails. Dermatol Surg. 2004;30(1):26-31.
33. Altinyazar HC, Demirel CB, Koca R, Hosnuter M. Digital block with and without epinephrine during chemical matricectomy with phenol. Dermatol Surg. 2010;36(10): 1568-71.
34. Aksakal AB, Atahan C, Oztas P, Oruk S. Minimizing postoperative drainage with 20% ferric chloride after chemical matricectomy with phenol. Dermatol Surg 2001: 27(2): 158-60.
35. Kim S-H, Ko H-C, Oh C-K, Kwon K-S, Kim M-B. Trichloroacetic acid matricectomy in the treatment of ingrowing toenails. Dermatol Surg. 2009:35(6):973-9.
36. Schulte KW, Neumann NJ, Ruzicka T. Surgical pearl: nail splinting by flexible tube--a new noninvasive treatment for ingrown toenails. J Am Acad Dermatol. 1998;39(4 Pt 1): 629-30
37. Heidelbaugh JJ, Lee H. Management of the Ingrown Toenail. Am Fam Physician. 2009;79(4):303-8.
38. Haneke E. Nail Surgery. In: Rusciani L, Robins P (Eds). Textbook of Dermatologic Surgery. Piccin. 2008:300-1.
39. Richert B. Surgical management of ingrown toe nails-an update overdue. Dermatol Therapy. 2012;25:498-509.
40. Herndon JH, Myers SR, Akelman E. Advanced surgery. In: Scher RK, Daniel CR (Eds). Nails: Therapy, Diagnosis, Surgery. Philadelphia, Pa: WB Saunders; 2005:350-62.
41. Clark RE, Madani S, Bettencourt MS. Nail surgery. Dermatol Clin. 1998;16(1):145-64.
42. Baran R, Bureau H. Surgical treatment of recalcitrant chronic paronychias of the fingers. J Dermatol Surg Oncol. 1981;7(2):106-7
43. Salasche SJ. Surgery. In: Scher RK, Daniel CR, eds. Nails: Therapy, Diagnosis, Surgery. Philadelphia, Pa: WB Saunders; 2005:326-49.
44. Lim JT, Goh CL. Carbon dioxide laser treatment of periungual and subungual viral warts. Australas J Dermatol. 1992;33(2):87-91.
45. Bhatta AK, Keyal U, Huang X, Zhao JJ. Fractional carbon-dioxide (CO_2) laser-assisted topical therapy for the treatment of onychomycosis. J Am Acad Dermatol. 2016;74 (5):916-23.
46. Lim EH, Kim HR, Park YO, Lee Y, Seo YJ, Kim CD, Lee JH, Im M. Toenail onychomycosis treated with a fractional carbon-dioxide laser and topical antifungal cream. J Am Acad Dermatol. 2014;70(5):918-23.
47. de Oliveira GB, Antonio JR, Antonio CR, Tomé FA. The association of fractional CO_2 laser 10.600nm and photodynamic therapy in the treatment of onychomycosis. An Bras Dermatol. 2015;90(4):468-71.
48. Moon SH, Hur H, Oh YJ, Choi KH, Kim JE, Ko JY, Ro YS. Treatment of onychomycosis with a 1,064 nm long-pulsed Nd:YAG laser. J Cosmet Laser Ther. 2014;16(4):165-70.
49. Li Y, Yu S, Xu J, Zhang R, Zhao J. Comparison of the efficacy of long-pulsed Nd:YAG laser intervention for treatment of onychomycosis of toenails or fingernails. J Drugs Dermatol. 2014;13(10):1258-63.

Chapter

56

Surgery and Cosmetic Procedures of Nails: Excision of Subungual Tumors

Chander Grover, Archana Singal

Key Messages

- Nail unit is the site of origin for many benign and malignant tumors of varied origin.
- The tumors arising in the nail unit may be difficult to diagnose as the presenting features may be different from those arising elsewhere.
- Imaging studies are an absolute must before considering any surgical intervention.
- In general, benign growths present with local swelling whereas local destruction signifies a malignant potential.
- Glomus tumors are commonly seen in the nail unit and are characterized by intense, localized pain with cold sensitivity.

INTRODUCTION

A tumor refers to a circumscribed swelling. Evidently, these may or may not be of neoplastic origin. A number of cellular proliferations, degenerative lesions, reactive lesions and true neoplasms are referred to as "tumors". This chapter deals with the common nail unit tumors (NUT) and their management.

The nail unit is the site of involvement with various tumors and clinical manifestations tend to overlap. These are frequently diagnosed late because of covering by the nail plate. Interestingly, they are difficult to diagnose clinically in the nail area and supportive investigations (imaging and histopathology) are routinely recommended and required. Surgical management depends on the tumor type, size or location within the nail.

NAIL UNIT TUMORS

Nail unit comprises of six components (*germinal portion*: matrix; *product portion*: nail plate; *ensheathing portion*: eponychium and hyponychium; *framing portion*: nail folds; *supporting system*—nail bed mesenchyme and phalanx; and *anchoring ligaments*). Hence, tumors could arise from any of these components. A variety of tumors have been described in the nail unit;[1] including, but not restricted to, the following (Table 1).[2] This chapter focuses on surgical management of the most commonly seen nail tumors.

PATIENT EVALUATION: HISTORY, COUNSELING, PHOTOGRAPHY, IMAGING

Patients with NUT generally present with a *growth* or *swelling* in the subungual or periungual location.[3] Owing to innocuous and asymptomatic nature, the duration is generally long (many years). Presence of significant pain (or cold sensitivity) points towards a glomus tumor whereas significant destruction of the nail plate points towards a possible malignancy. Many lesions commonly present as pressure changes with secondary distortion of nail plate.

Any lesion in the subungual or periungual location should be promptly imaged.[4] A routine skiagram may show evidence of bony outgrowth (exostosis) or distortion/depression of bone (due to larger subungual tumors like the glomus). High frequency ultrasound can help delineate the size, location or type of lesion. However, the investigation of choice is magnetic resonance imaging (MRI) which can pick up even very small lesions.[4]

Table 1: Classification of nail unit tumors.

Epithelial tumors	*Soft tissue tumors*	*Melanocytic tumors*	*Others*
Benign ▪ Wart ▪ Syringoma ▪ Eccrine poroma ▪ Distal keratoacanthoma ▪ Onychopapilloma ▪ Onychomatricoma ▪ Keratin cysts	*Fibrous tumors* ▪ Koenen's tumors ▪ Acquired digital fibrokeratoma ▪ Infantile digital fibromatosis ▪ Keloid	*Benign* ▪ Longitudinal melanonychia ▪ Benign melanocytic hyperplasia ▪ Lentigo simplex ▪ Blue nevus	*Pseudotumors* ▪ Myxoid pseudocyst ▪ Primary osteoma cutis ▪ Subungual calcifications ▪ Foreign body granuloma ▪ Gout
Malignant ▪ Squamous cell carcinoma ▪ Epithelioma cuniculatum ▪ Sebaceous gland carcinoma	*Vascular tumors* ▪ Hemangiomas ▪ AV malformation ▪ ALHE ▪ Pyogenic granuloma ▪ Glomus tumor ▪ Lymphangioma circumscriptum	*Atypical* melanocytic hyperplasia	*Histiocytic and lymphomatous tumors*
	Osteocartilaginous tumors ▪ Exostosis ▪ Osteochondroma ▪ Enchondroma ▪ Osteoid osteoma ▪ Giant cell tumor of bone	*Nail melanoma*	*Metastatic tumors*
	▪ Tumors of peripheral nerves ▪ Synovial tumors ▪ Lipomatous/myxomatous ▪ Sarcomas		

(AV: Arteriovenous; ALHE: Angiolymphoid hyperplasia with eosinophilia).

SURGICAL MANAGEMENT OF NAIL UNIT TUMOR

Basic Anatomy

Thorough knowledge of nail unit anatomy helps to minimize potential scarring and adverse surgical outcomes associated with nail surgery. The details have been incorporated in the previous chapter. This chapter deals with surgical management of commonly observed nail tumors, including warts (periungual or subungual), glomus tumor, acquired fibrokeratomas, and digital myxoid cysts.

Ungual Verrucae (Periungual and Subungual)

Warts arising in the subungual or periungual location are often difficult to treat because of hindrance by overlying nail plate and potential of damage to underlying nail matrix.[5] Routine topical treatments may not be practical requiring removal of nail plate to expose the wart in its totality. The same holds true for destructive options like electrosurgery, radiofrequency destruction or lasers. Here, procedure of choice may be intralesional bleomycin which is safe as well as effective.

Details About the Procedure

Bleomycin is a glycopeptide which is used as an antimitotic drug.[6,7] It acts by causing DNA strand scission preventing cell replication. The intralesional use of bleomycin is not Food and Drug Administration (FDA) approved but multiple clinical studies have described its use, documenting beneficial response[8] as well as adverse events.[9] Intralesional bleomycin is commonly used for viral warts in difficult-to-treat sites like subungual, periungual and palmoplantar mosaic warts. Reported cure rates in ungual warts range from 76% to 94%.[10]

Preoperative Workup or Preparation

It is imperative to comprehend the extent and number of warts in the subungual and periungual location before treating with intralesional bleomycin. Warts in the proximal nail fold (PNF) area need to be treated carefully to avoid inadvertent damage to underlying matrix. The patient also needs to be assessed for signs of digital ischemia which may be further worsened by such injections.

Bleomycin is available as a dry powder which is to be reconstituted to prepare a 5 mL stock solution of 3 U/mL. The stock solution has to be stored at 4°C and is stable for 30–60 days.

Procedure Itself Step by Step

- Generally no digital anesthesia is required. However, a proximal digital block is advisable for very apprehensive patient with multiple warts over a digit. This is because the process of infiltration may be painful.

- The warts to be injected may be debulked prior to injection, by paring with a scalpel blade. This eases penetration into the substance of the wart.
- The stock solution can be injected in strength varying from 1 U/mL to 3 U/mL. Authors prefer using the higher strength. If dilution is required, it may be done with normal saline or 1% lignocaine without adrenaline.
- It is injected into the substance of the wart with an aim to produce blanching. The injection is preferably given with 1 mL tuberculin syringe with inbuilt 30 G needle. This eases penetration into thick warts, minimizes pain, and prevents backsplash.
- Repeated punctures may be needed to infiltrate the substance of the wart depending on its size. Though there are no clear data available, the usual injected volume should generally not exceed 1–2 mL per session.

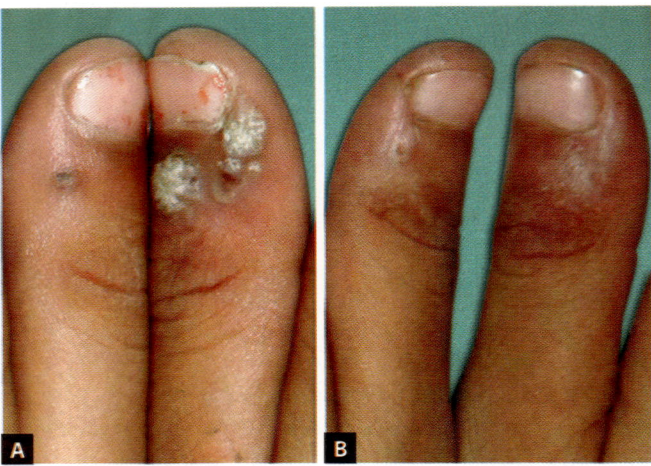

Figs. 1A and B: A 19-year-old girl with multiple periungual and digital warts. The result seen after three sessions of intralesional bleomycin (3 U/mL) administered at 2 week intervals. There is complete resolution without any scarring or pigmentary changes.

- Following treatment, the patients are advised to use heavy emollients like petrolatum which help in softening the lesion and eases symptoms associated with appearance of necrotic eschar or hemorrhagic bullae. No oral antibiotics or pain killers are required.
- The wart is reassessed in 2–3 weeks by which time most of the eschar would have fallen off revealing any residual lesions. This may be further injected. The average number of injections per wart varies from 1–4 (Figs. 1 and 2).

Ungual warts can also be dealt with nail avulsion (partial or complete depending on the extent of the wart) followed by use of destructive methods like radiofrequency cautery, electrocautery or ablative lasers. However, there is a low success rate as well as high risk of recurrence in author's personal experience.

Glomus Tumor

Glomus tumors are vascular tumors common in the subungual location. These are hamartomas of the neuromyoarterial glomus body, which is responsible for thermoregulation.[11] Diagnosis is mainly on clinical grounds although imaging may be useful in localizing the lesion and determining its size. Surgical excision is the treatment of choice.

A diagnosis of glomus tumors is largely based on clinical signs and symptoms in the form of spontaneous pain, sensitivity to touch, and cold sensitivity with an area of blue-reddish discoloration.[11] Some cases may have associated nail deformity. Pain may be severe and paroxysmal, often radiating to the shoulder. Love's sign and Hildreth's test are helpful in achieving the diagnosis.[12] Love's sign refers to severe localized tenderness elicited on applying pressure with a pinhead, along with relief of pain when the pressure is removed. Hildreth's test involves reduction or abolition of lesional pain and tenderness on

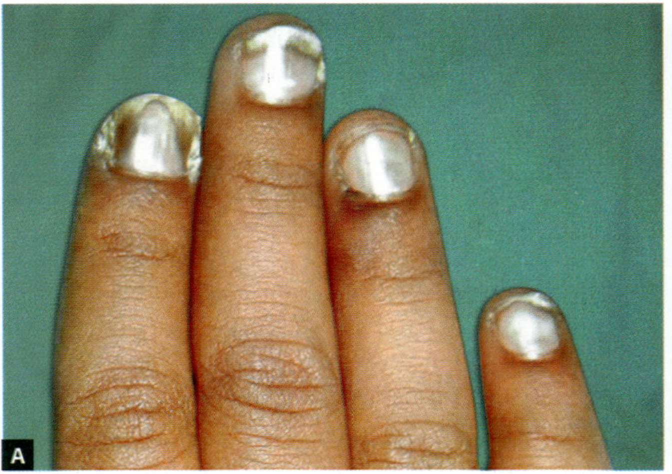

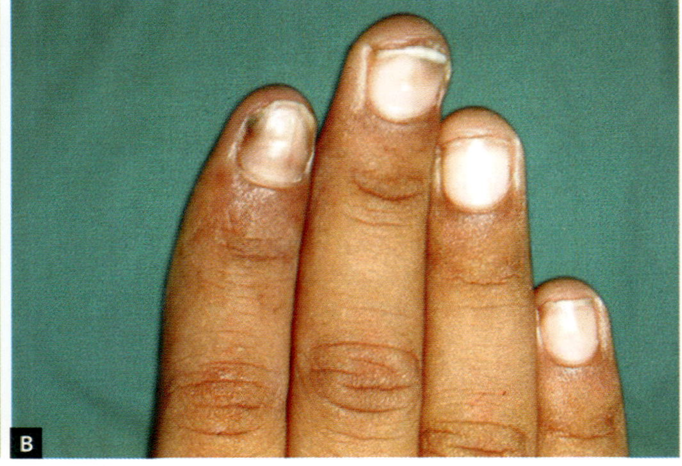

Figs. 2A and B: A 16-year-old boy with extensive periungual and subungual warts treated with intralesional bleomycin. These warts required four sessions (2 weeks apart) to clear. Secondary nail surface irregularities can be seen.

elevating the patient's arm and inflating the blood pressure cuff. Releasing the cuff then causes a sudden return of pain.

Details About the Procedure

Treatment of glomus tumors is purely surgical, the major concerns being the risk of nail deformity and risk of recurrence. Incomplete surgical removal and preexisting synchronous satellite lesions are associated with persistent or recurring pain. There are two possible approaches for surgical excision of glomus tumor: (1) transungual[11] and (2) lateral.[13] The former is preferred and routinely resorted to by authors because of a better visualization of the subungual region and easier exploration. If the lesion is believed to be involving the nail matrix, an eponychial flap has to be raised to ensure complete removal. Careful handling of tissues during surgery and meticulous repair of the defect created by excision can prevent scarring. Postoperatively, repositioning the avulsed nail plate helps prevent adhesions of the eponychium to the matrix; favors repair of nail bed and reduces pain.

Preoperative Workup or Preparation

Clinical confirmation of diagnosis requires careful history and clinical examination including bedside tests as mentioned earlier. The lesion can mostly be localized on the basis of clinical signs in the form of point of maximal tenderness (Love's test); the point of visible erythema of the nail plate; or the painful base of an erythronychial band.

Plain radiographs should be done, although diagnostic yield is low. Changes may be seen only with very large tumors producing a bony depression, erosion or cortical thinning seen in 30–60% cases. It may be useful for differentiating glomus tumors from subungual exostoses. Ultrasonography can also localize and assess the size of the tumor preoperatively. These are seen as well-circumscribed hypoechoic masses. Doppler ultrasonography can identify low signals within the hypoechoic mass and is preferred over standard ultrasonography.

Magnetic resonance imaging is the investigation of choice as it can detect lesions as small as 2 mm in size. The classical findings include marked hyperintensity seen on T2-weighted images with a strong enhancement with gadolinium-based contrast.[11] MR angiography also shows a typical appearance of strong arterial enhancement and tumor blush in delayed phase.[14] MRI is also useful for assessment of patients with recurrence or incomplete resolution of symptoms following surgery.

Procedure Itself Step by Step (Figs. 3A to H)

- The digit to be operated is anesthetized with proximal nerve block using 2% lignocaine hydrochloride with epinephrine (1:2,00,000) solution.
- Digital exsanguination followed by tourniquet at the base helps in achieving a relatively avascular operating field helping in localization of the tumor (Fig. 3A).
- The nail plate overlying the tumor is carefully avulsed either distally or proximally, depending on the location of the tumor (Fig. 3B). Thus, prelocalization of the possible location of the tumor is very useful. As far as possible, partial nail plate removal should be attempted. Conservative nail plate avulsion followed by repositioning of the avulsed nail plate postsurgery helps improve postsurgical outcomes in the short term as well as in long term.
- If the glomus tumor is in the nail matrix location, it would require additional retraction of the PNF and raising an eponychial flap (lateral release incisions and stay sutures) to ensure adequate exposure.
- Once the area of nail bed or matrix is exposed, blunt dissection with fine forceps is used to enable separation of the tumor from surrounding tissue (Fig. 3C). This takes a few minutes but helps in removal of the lesion in toto. Punch excision can also be attempted for very small lesions. For larger lesions, there is a risk of incomplete excision with a punch.
- Resultant defect is primarily repaired with 6-0 absorbable sutures, if possible (Figs. 3D and E). For very large tumors (more than 7–8 mm), this may not be possible.
- The avulsed nail plate can be trimmed and repositioned whenever and wherever possible (Figs. 3F and G).
- The eponychial flap, if raised, is allowed to fall back and sutured in place with 4-0 nonabsorbable suture.
- Postoperative dressing is done using antibiotic cream and gauze.
- Patient is prescribed postoperative oral antibiotics and analgesics. They are reviewed at 1 week, or are asked to report back earlier if there is severe pain in the operated digit (suggestive of tight dressing).
- Any nonabsorbable sutures used are removed at the end of the 1st week (Fig. 3H).

Acquired Digital Fibrokeratoma

It is an uncommon acquired growth, in the digits, which resembles cutaneous horn. On the basis of distinctive histopathology, the lesions were named acquired digital fibrokeratoma (ADFK).[15,16] Subsequently, similar lesions were reported on the proximal hand, toes, sole, etc. hence renamed acral fibrokeratomas. In the ungual or periungual location, they are also known as garlic-clove fibromas (Fig. 4A), owing to their clinical presentation in the form of skin colored asymptomatic nodule with hyperkeratotic tip. Mostly, it originates from under the PNF, placing itself on top of nail plate. The pressure on the underlying matrix can results in a grooved nail plate surface. Less common sites of origin may be nail matrix (intraungual fibrokeratoma) or nail bed (subungual fibrokeratoma). Multiple such lesions seen in a patient with tuberous sclerosis are known as Koenen's tumors.

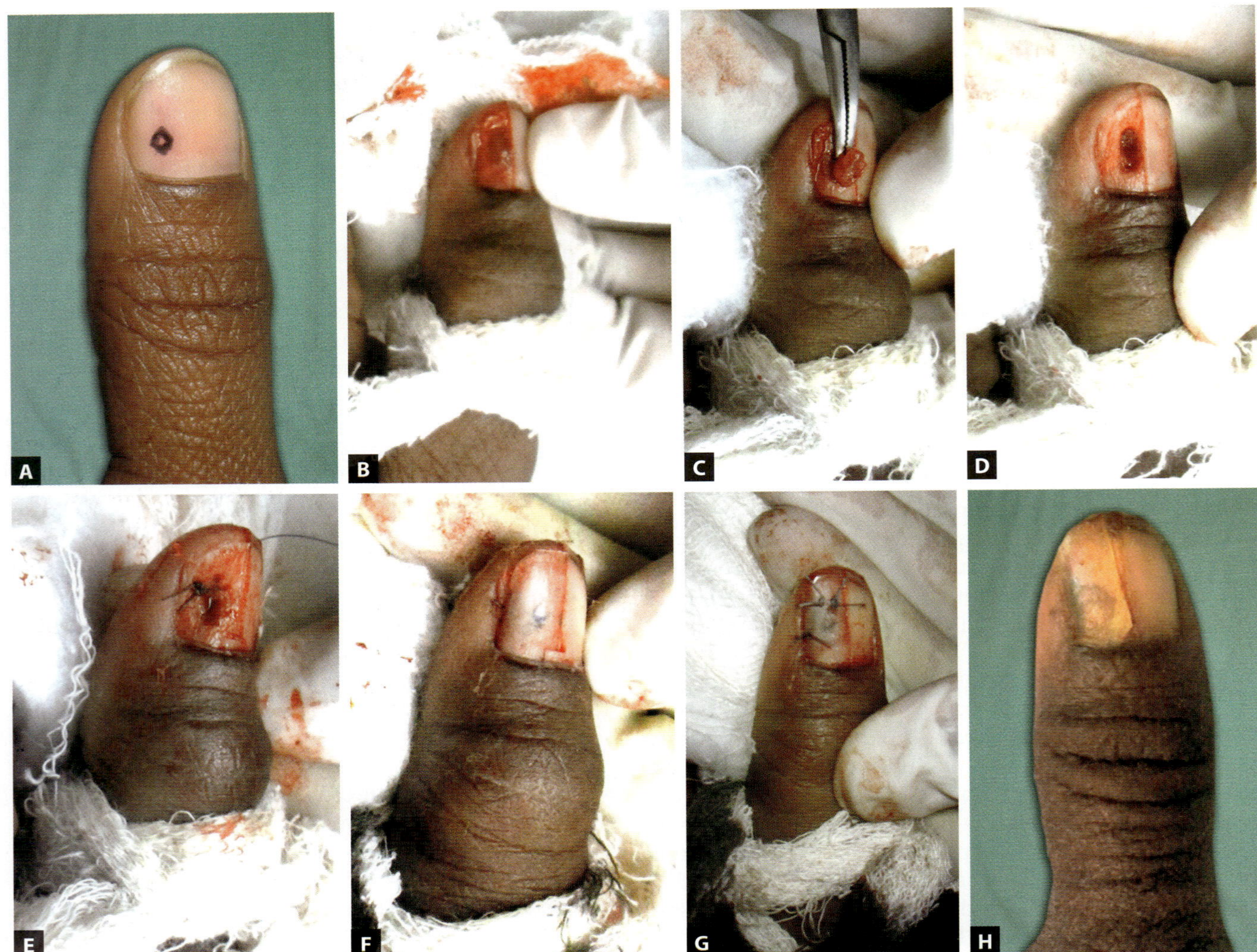

Figs. 3A to H: Surgical management of glomus tumor. (A) An extremely painful area of reddish discoloration in the nail bed of 4 years duration. The point of maximum tenderness is marked before administering anesthesia. This helps in localization of the tumor intraoperatively; (B) After anesthesia, digital exsanguinations and tourniquet, a lateral partial avulsion of the nail plate has been done using a distal approach. This reveals the longitudinally oriented bluish swelling in the nail bed; (C) The lesion is gently separated from the surrounding nail bed using blunt dissection. It is advisable to remove the lesion in toto; (D) The resultant linear defect after the glomus tumor has been removed; (E) Primary closure of the defect after mobilizing nail bed tissue by undermining; (F) The nail plate is trimmed (made shorter) and repositioned over the surgical wound; (G) It is held in situ with stay sutures; and (H) The stay sutures are removed after a week. The nail plate sheds off subsequently.

Details About the Procedure

The procedure involves removal of the tumor from its most proximal origin in the most proximal part of the ventral surface of PNF.[17] For intraungual fibrokeratomas, the lesion has a matrix origin; and for subungual ones, the nail bed origin is to be delineated. The origin has to be removed in toto, without any margin, to prevent recurrences. The removal can be less complete in Koenen's tumors because of the high chances of recurrence anyways.

Preoperative Workup or Preparation

Preoperative workup involves routine precautions similar to those for any nail or digital surgery. In case of multiple lesions, tuberous sclerosis should be ruled out. Preoperative imaging helps delineate the extent, if any, of the bone involvement.

Procedure Itself Step by Step

- The digit to be operated is anesthetized with proximal nerve block using 2% lignocaine hydrochloride with epinephrine (1:2,00,000) solution.
- Digital exsanguination followed by tourniquet at the base helps in achieving a relatively avascular operating field helping in localization of the tumor.
- For tumors overlying the thinned nail plate, no nail plate avulsion is needed. Instead the PNF needs to be retracted fully to visualize the origin of the tumor from

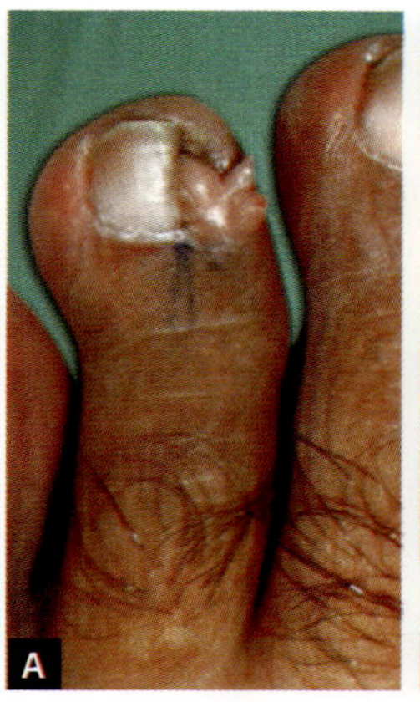
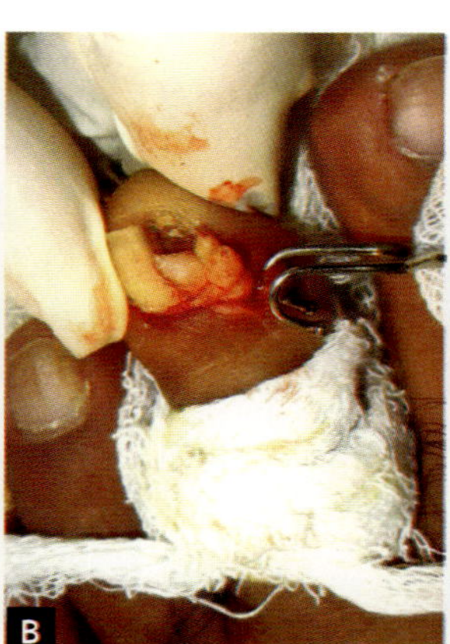
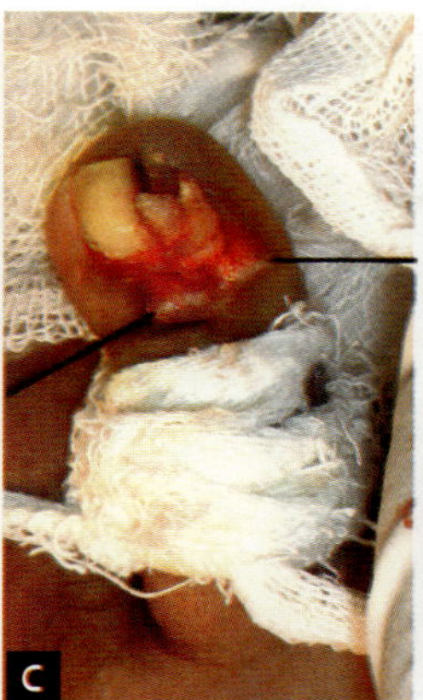
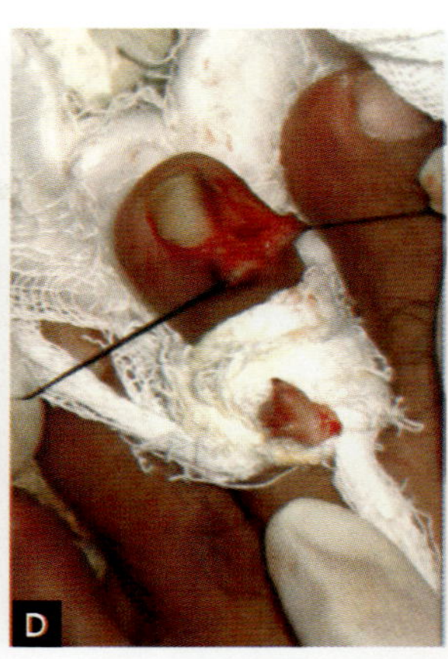
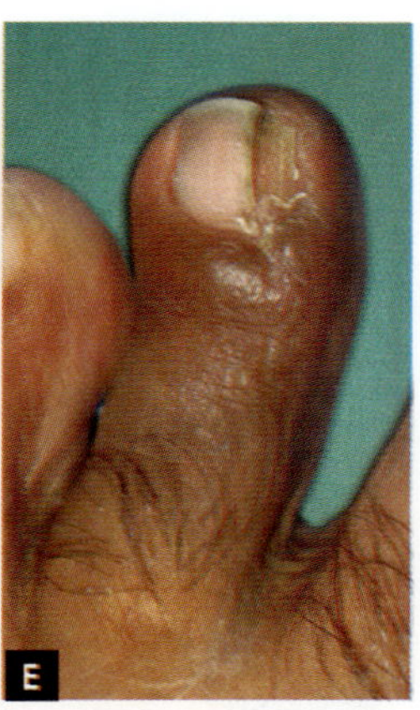

Figs. 4A to E: Surgical management of acquired digital fibrokeratoma. (A) Third toenail of a 40-year-old male showing a fleshy growth for the past 2 years. The lesion has typical "garlic clove" morphology. The underlying nail plate is very much thinned out due to the pressure of the lesion; (B) After administering digital block, exsanguinating and tying tourniquet; an incision is given at lateral and proximal nail fold junction, overlying the tumor and extend laterally as far back as possible to expose the origin; (C) Both the nail folds are retracted with stay sutures. This helps in severing the tumor from its base; (D) The tumor has been removed from its origin. The nail folds are then sutured back preventing any damage to underlying bed or matrix; (E) The surgical wound after 3 weeks.

the most proximal part of the ventral surface of the PNF (Fig. 4B). For nail bed lesions, partial nail plate avulsion (the part lying above the tumor) is needed.

- For more laterally placed lesions, a lateral release incision at the junction of the PNF and lateral nail fold (LNF) helps locate the origin. The separated nail folds are held back with stay sutures (Fig. 4C).
- For more centrally placed lesions, the PNF is gently separated from the nail plate surface. Then two lateral incisions are needed to fully retract the nail fold.
- The fibrokeratoma is dissected from its ventral aspect down to its base where it is severed from the PNF (Fig. 4D).
- The nail folds are then allowed to fall back and are sutured in place.
- For nail bed lesions, similar technique is followed after avulsing or laterally curling the nail plate. The resultant nail bed defect can then be primarily repaired with 6-0 absorbable sutures.
- The nail plate, if it had been avulsed, can be trimmed and repositioned whenever and wherever possible.
- Postoperative dressing is done using antibiotic cream and gauze.
- Patient is prescribed postoperative oral antibiotics and analgesics. They are reviewed at 1 week, or are asked to report back earlier if there is severe pain in the operated digit (suggestive of tight dressing).
- Any nonabsorbable sutures used are removed at the end of the 1st week (Fig. 4E).

Digital Myxoid Pseudocyst

It is a benign ganglion cyst of the digit which mostly presents over the distal interphalangeal (DIP) joint in the area of PNF. They are more common on the hands. Etiologically, they are a result of mucoid degeneration and are mostly asymptomatic, not requiring treatment. If large in size, they can produce a cosmetic disfigurement and secondary pressure changes on the nail plate and nail deformity (Fig. 5A).[18] Both medical and surgical interventions are worth attempting. This chapter will describe the surgical removal of an organized cyst.

Details About the Procedure

Pseudomyxoid cysts are a result of mucoid degeneration of connective tissue. They may or may not have a communication with the adjacent DIP joint with or without osteoarthritis.[18] Digital mucous cysts have a good prognosis, though recurrence is common. Radical surgery carries low recurrence but significant associated morbidity. Several different treatment options exist but recurrence is high. If asymptomatic, the lesion can be left untreated with a possibility of spontaneous resolution. Other treatment options include repeated drainage of cyst fluid, cryotherapy, etc. More destructive modalities to be attempted under local anesthesia include curettage, cauterization, or even isolation of the origin of leakage from joint space by injection of a dye, and subsequent ligation.[19,20] This section describes method of cyst excision.

Preoperative Workup or Preparation

Digital X-ray is must to rule out extensive involvement of the joint space or osteoarthritis. In *cases with an organized cyst with no bony abnormalities, cyst excision can be attempted.*

Procedure Itself Step by Step

- The digit to be operated is anesthetized with proximal nerve block using 2% lignocaine hydrochloride with epinephrine (1:2,00,000) solution.

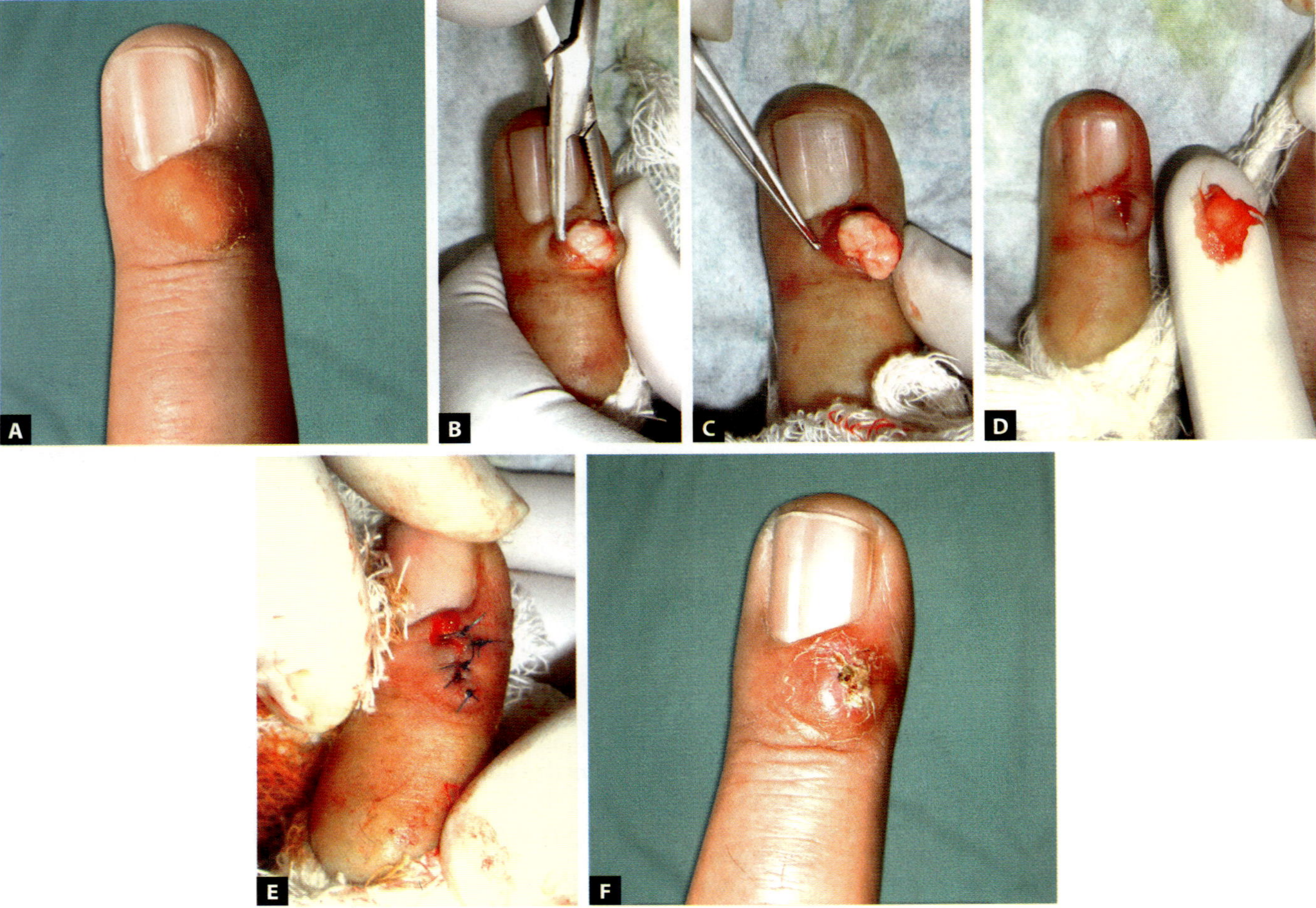

Figs. 5A to F: Surgical management of digital myxoid pseudocyst. (A) A myxoid pseudocyst in the proximal periungual location. Note the pressure effects of the cyst producing a linear depression on nail plate; (B) The cyst is exposed through a longitudinally oriented incision in the proximal nail fold area; (C) The cyst is dissected from its attachment and extracted. It generally does not have a defined cyst wall; (D) The resultant defect is shown along with the removed myxoid material; (E) The defect is sutured primarily; (F) Postoperative period. Healing wound at 2 weeks.

- Digital exsanguination followed by tourniquet at the base helps in achieving a relatively avascular operating field helping in localization of the tumor.
- For cysts in the PNF area, longitudinal incision is oriented over the most prominent part of the cyst (Fig. 5B).
- This is followed by the use of fine artery forceps (mosquito forceps) to carefully separate the cyst from the overlying skin and the underlying structures (Fig. 5C).
- The separated cyst is removed in toto (Fig. 5D), followed by primary closure of the PNF incision (Fig. 5E).
- Postoperative dressing is done using antibiotic cream and gauze.
- Patient is prescribed postoperative oral antibiotics and analgesics. They are reviewed at 1 week, or are asked to report back earlier if there is severe pain in the operated digit (suggestive of tight dressing).
- Nonabsorbable sutures used are removed at the end of the 1st week (Fig. 5F).

Tips

For ensuring good results

- It is important to preoperatively localize the tumor so as to plan the approach and extent of nail plate removal.
- Preoperative imaging is must to rule out underlying bone involvement.
- Nail bed incisions should be oriented longitudinally while nail matrix incisions should be oriented horizontally.
- Nail bed or matrix defects can be sutured with fine absorbable suture whereas for the nail fold, nonabsorbable sutures are preferred.
- As far as possible, an attempt should be made to reposition the avulsed nail plate after suitably trimming it.

SUMMARY

- Tumors tend to behave differently in the nail as compared to other sites and presentation depends on the site of origin within the nail unit, rather than on the histological type

- Radiological investigation to assess type and extent of involvement of underlying bone is an absolute must before any surgical intervention.
- Generally, a deformity of nail plate suggests benign disease whereas active destruction suggests possible malignancy
- Glomus tumors are common in subungual location and are characterized by pain and cold sensitivity.

REFERENCES

1. Domínguez-Cherit J, Chanussot-Deprez C, Maria-Sarti H, et al. Nail unit tumors: A study of 234 patients in the dermatology department of the "Dr Manuel Gea González" general hospital in Mexico City. Dermatol Surg. 2008; 34(10):1363-71.
2. Tosti A, Richert B, Pazzaglia M. Tumors of the nail apparatus. In: Scher RK, Daniel IIICR (Eds). Nails: Therapy Diagnosis, Surgery, 3rd Edition, China, Elsevier Saunders 2005; 195-204.
3. Grover C, Khurana A. Nail tumors. In: Sacchidanand S, Savitha AS (Eds). Nail and its Disorders, 1st edition, Jaypee Brothers Med Publishers, Delhi, India, 2013;169-81.
4. Baek HJ, Lee SJ, Cho KH, et al. Subungual tumors: clinicopathologic correlation with US and MR imaging findings 1. Radiographics. 2010;30(6):1621-36.
5. Tosti A, Piraccini BM. Warts of the nail unit: surgical and nonsurgical approaches. Dermatologic Surgery. 2001; 27(3): 235-9.
6. Cordero AA, Guglielmi HA, Woscoff A. The common wart: intralesional treatment with bleomycin sulfate. Cutis. 1980;26(3):319-20.
7. Saitta P, Krishnamurthy K, Brown LH. Bleomycin in dermatology: a review of intralesional applications. Dermatologic Surgery. 2008;34(10):1299-313.
8. Soni P, Khandelwal K, Aara N, et al. Efficacy of intralesional bleomycin in palmo-plantar and periungual warts. Journal of Cutaneous and Aesthetic Surgery. 2011;4(3):188.
9. Miller RA. Nail dystrophy following intralesional injections of bleomycin for a periungual wart. Archives of Dermatology. 1984;120(7):963-4.
10. Shumer SM, O'Keefe EJ. Bleomycin in the treatment of recalcitrant warts. Journal of the American Academy of Dermatology. 1983;9(1):91-6.
11. Grover C, Khurana A, Jain R, et al. Transungual surgical excision of subungual glomus tumour. Journal of Cutaneous and Aesthetic Surgery. 2013;6(4):196.
12. Bhaskaranand K, Navadgi BC. Glomus tumour of the hand. Journal of Hand Surgery (British and European Volume). 2002;27(3):229-31.
13. Vasisht B, Watson HK, Joseph E, et al. Digital glomus tumors: a 29-year experience with a lateral subperiosteal approach. Plastic and Reconstructive Surgery. 2004;114(6):1486-9.
14. Theumann NH, Goettmann S, Le Viet D, et al. Recurrent glomus tumors of fingertips: MR imaging evaluation 1. Radiology. 2002;223(1):143-51.
15. Bart RS, Andrade R, Kopf AW, et al. Acquired digital fibrokeratomas. Arch Dermatol. 1968;97(2):120-9.
16. Kint A, Baran R, De Keyser H. Acquired (digital) fibrokeratoma. Journal of the American Academy of Dermatology. 1985;12(5):816-21.
17. Haneke E, Richert B, DiChiacchio N. Surgery of the proximal nail fold. In: Richert B, Chiacchio D, Haneke E (Eds). Nail Surgery, 1st edition. Informa Healthcare, London, UK, 2011;42-54.
18. Lin YC, Wu YH, Scher RK. Nail changes and association of osteoarthritis in digital myxoid cyst. Dermatologic Surgery. 2008;34(3):364-9.
19. Salasche SJ. Myxoid cysts of the proximal nail fold: a surgical approach. The Journal of Dermatologic Surgery and Oncology. 1984;10(1):35-9.
20. de Berker D, Lawrence C. Ganglion of the distal interphalangeal joint (myxoid cyst): Therapy by identification and repair of the leak of joint fluid. Archives of Dermatology. 2001;137(5):607-10.

Chapter 57

Eyelid Surgery

Manas Chatterjee, Dipali Rathod,
Krishan Mehra, Harish Prasad

Key Messages 

- Majority of the eyelid surgeries are office procedures and therefore dermatosurgeons need to be fully aware of them and include them in their armamentarium.
- Proper planning and execution of these procedures require good understanding and knowledge of eyelid anatomy, vascular and nerve supply which would aid in preventing serious surgical events.
- Various procedures undertaken for the common correctable eyelid disorders in dermatology such as simple excision and suturing, tarsorrhaphy, blepharoplasty, vitiligo surgeries, ocular leprosy surgeries and few others would be discussed in detail in this chapter.
- Eyelash transplantation has created a new ray of hope in vitiligo patients with leukotrichia of the eyelashes.
- The eyelid procedures should be meticulously performed as inappropriate techniques may result in scarring and may further cause ectroprion.

I shut my eyes and all the world drops dead; I lift my eyes and all is born again.

—**Sylvia Plath**

INTRODUCTION

Our eyes are used as an important landmark on the face, hence the knowledge and understanding of the anatomy and dynamics of eyelids is of vital importance for the treating dermatologist and the aesthetic surgeon in order to avoid any injury to the underlying structures. Also, a regular assessment of the eyes during the general physical examination may help in appropriate diagnosis and treatment of many systemic diseases. The eyelids consist of a complex structure with multiple subunits mainly the palpebral (pretarsal and preseptal subunits) and orbital (encircling the eyebrow and extending to the junction of the cheek). The three primary causes of aging which play an influential role and affect the periorbital area include photoaging (affecting the skin), gravitational aging (causing ptosis of all soft tissues) and volumetric aging (atrophy of soft tissues and, with advanced age of bone).

This chapter is intended to give a comprehensive account of all the common diseases that affect the eyelids, for which a dermatologist needs to be alerted and if need be, advice an urgent referral to an ophthalmologist.

HISTORY

Since the time of ancient Greeks and Romans, surgical procedures of eyelid were penned down. Aulus Cornelius Celsus, a first-century Roman, has described about an incision in the skin to relax the eyelids in his book "De Medicina".

In 1817 Beer first published medical illustration of the aging eyelid. It was during this time period that many in Europe first began to advocate the removal of the upper eyelid skin to correct associated functional problems. In 1844, Sichel described "ptosis adiposa" as a condition in which the excessive upper eyelid skin fold was filled with fat. He theorized that the disproportionate adipose tissue caused the skin to hang down over the lid. However, Fuchs later correctly recognized the role of the fascia attachments between skin, orbicularis, tarsus and the levator in the development of the supratarsal skin fold and the importance of its recreation in blepharoplasty.

EMBRYOLOGY

The eye and skin share a common embryological origin. The anatomy of the eyelid is shown in Figure 1. The structure of the lid, conjunctiva, the lacrimal gland, and associated drainage are derived from the surface ectoderm

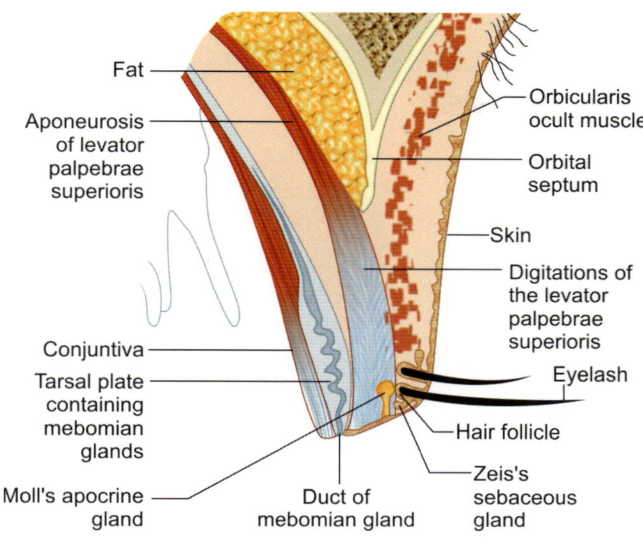

Fig. 1: Eyelid anatomy.

whereas the remaining structures of the eye arise from the epithelium of ectodermal neural plate. The myoblasts of the extraocular muscles are the only mesodermal contribution to the eye apparatus.

ANATOMY OF EYELID

The contour of the eyelid is highly dependent on the race, gender, and age of the individual. The lateral canthus of a typical eyelid is approximately 2 mm superior to the medial one. In Asians, this vertical elevation may be slightly higher and this is referred to as the "Mongoloid slant".

The palpebral fissure in the adult measures 10–12 mm vertically and 28–30 mm horizontally.

In adults, about 1–2 mm of the superior cornea is covered by the upper eyelid margin and the apex of the upper lid margin is found nasal to a vertical line drawn through the center of the pupil.

The vertical palpebral fissure and position of the upper eyelid crease varies among different ethnic groups. This finding has important implications in both ptosis and upper eyelid blepharoplasty surgery.

The upper eyelid crease (formed by attachment of the levator aponeurosis to skin) in Caucasians is situated 7–8 mm above the lid margin in men and 10–12 mm in women. In Asians, the crease is lower and the upper sulcus is more full. This occurs because the orbital septum and levator aponeurosis fuse lower on the lid, below the superior tarsal border. However, a recent study by Kakizaki et al. showed that this fusion occurred above the tarsal border.[1]

In either case, the preaponeurotic fat pad (PFP) descends and prevents a higher insertion of the levator aponeurosis to the upper lid skin.[2] These variations result in an inferiorly positioned or absent upper eyelid crease in Asians.

The skin of the eyelids is the thinnest (0.05 mm) as compared to the other parts of the body. The subcutaneous tissue consists of loose connective tissue. Fat is absent from the pretarsal skin and very sparse in the preseptal and preorbital skin. Also the medial and lateral palpebral ligaments show absence of subcutaneous tissue and therefore the skin here adheres directly to the underlying fibrous tissue. Relaxed skin tension lines (RSTLs) around the eyes can be used easily as they follow the lid creases. Upper eyelid can be excised without any deformity as it has more elastic skin.

The prime most important function of the eyelid is to protect the eyeball. It contains fine hair (cilia) at its outer margin (eyelashes), both apocrine and eccrine sweat glands and sebaceous glands. About 300 eyelashes are arranged in two rows along the lid margin, two thirds of which are in the upper lid. The lids lack the arrector muscles. The tarsal plate of each eyelid gives the palpebral aperture to its shape and stability. Additional components of the eyelid include the superior palpebral fold, the palpebral fissure, the medial limbus, and the medial canthus. Just lateral to the bony orbital margins, the thin and smooth eyelid skin transforms into a coarse and thicker skin with numerous sebaceous glands. Significance of this transition is the different manner in which each of them recovers from a surgical incision. The distinct anatomical layers of the eyelids comprise of the skin, subcutaneous tissue, tarsal plate and conjunctiva and striated muscles which affect the movement of the eyelids.

The eyelid is made up of four layers:

1. Skin layer—it consists of the epidermis and the dermis
2. Muscle layer
3. Tarsus layer
4. Mucous layer

Skin Layer

Epidermis

The epidermis of the eyelid is lined by four layers of keratinocytes. Apart from these cells it also consists of melanocytes, Langerhans cells and Merkel cells.

Dermis

The dermis is much thicker than the epidermis. It is composed of connective tissue and contains blood vessels, lymphatics and nerve fibers in addition to fibroblasts, macrophages and mast cells. In the eyelid the dermis lies directly on the orbicularis muscle. Skin appendages (adnexae) lie deep in the dermis or within the tarsal plates.

- *Sebaceous glands*: These are located in the caruncle and within the hair of eyebrow. Tiny sebaceous glands are associated with the thin (vellus) hair covering periocular skin.
- *Eccrine sweat glands*: These are distributed throughout the eyelid skin and are not confined to the lid margin, unlike glands of Moll.
- *Pilosebaceous units*: These comprise of hair follicles together with their sebaceous glands.

- *Glands of Zeis*: These are modified sebaceous glands developed as outgrowth of the hair follicles of the eyelashes.
- *Glands of Moll*: These are modified apocrine sweat glands. They are more numerous in the lower lid. The ducts of Zeis and Moll glands open both into the lash follicles and directly onto the anterior lid margin between the lashes.
- *Meibomian glands*: These are modified sebaceous glands located in the tarsal plates. They empty through a single row of vertically arranged ducts, about 30 openings into each lid. A gland consists of a central duct with multiple acini, the cells of which synthesize lipids (meibum-oily secretion) that pass into the duct and form the outer layer of the precorneal tear film.

Muscle Layer

It consists of the following:

- The horizontal concentric fibers of orbicularis oculi which are supplied by the facial nerve
- The levator palpebral superioris which ends in an aponeurosis which is inserted
  - To the skin of the upper lid
  - Upper border of the tarsus
  - Conjunctiva at the fornix.

  It is supplied by the third cranial nerve. The levator aponeurosis is supplanted by the preaponeurotic fat compartments (pockets) of the eyelids (Fig. 2).
- Müller's muscle, also known as superior tarsal muscle is supplied by the sympathetic nerve.

The striated levator palpebrae superioris opens the eye and the striated orbicularis oculi muscle closes it. Both are innervated by the facial nerve. Two divisions of the trigeminal nerve supply sensation to the eyelids; the upper lid and medial canthus are supplied by the ophthalmic division and the remainder of the lower lid by the maxillary division.

The upper lid margin is positioned over the upper cornea at midpoint between the upper edge and the pupillary border. Sometimes in a normal eye, there is visible sclera below the cornea. The lateral and medial angles of the palpebral aperture lie along a single horizontal plane.

The superior palpebral sulcus in upper eyelid results from insertion of the levator aponeurosis into the lid skin. This insertion varies considerably in different persons. Measured from the lid margin, the fold or sulcus may be as high as 12 mm in eyes that have a high prominent, supraorbital rim. Conversely, the lid fold may be as low as 5–6 mm above the lid margin in an eyelid that usually appears to be heavy and full. The inferior palpebral sulcus marks the lower margin of the inferior lid tarsus.

Tarsus Layer

It consists of the tarsal plates. The tarsi (tarsal plates) are two comparatively thick, elongated plates of dense connective tissue, about 2.5 cm (1.0 inch) in length; one is found in each eyelid, and contributes to its form and support. They are located directly above the lid margins. Embedded in it are enormously developed sebaceous glands—the meibomian glands.

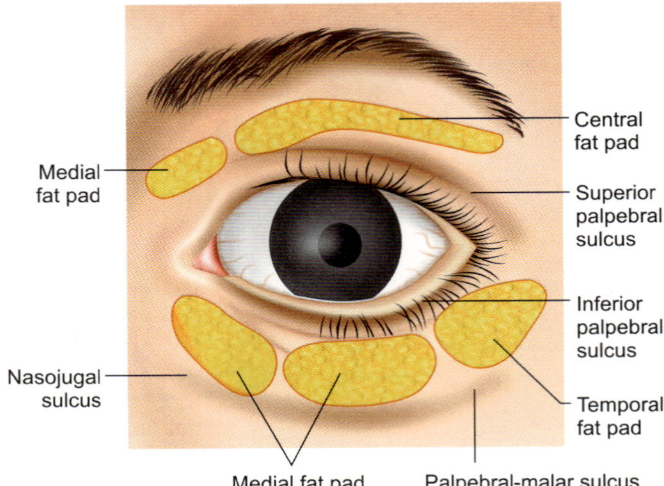

Fig. 2: Fat pockets and sulci.

Mucous Layer

It is formed by the palpebral conjunctiva. The lid margin consists of the following:

- Eyelashes—arranged in 2–3 rows anteriorly. The normal eyelashes point forwards.
- Opening of the ducts of the meibomian gland posteriorly.
- Glands of Zies and Moll.

The upper and lower eyelid layers are classically divided into the anterior (skin and orbicularis oculi muscle of upper eyelid), middle (orbital septum) and posterior lamellae (tarsal plate, eyelid retractors and conjunctiva). The gray line is a darker line in the middle of the lid margin that is between the anterior and middle lamellae of the lid. Any lesion extending beyond the gray line or if there is a possibility of malignancy, a full-thickness lid excision is required.

BLOOD SUPPLY

The eyelid has a rich blood supply, mainly through the medial and lateral palpebral arteries, which are branches of the ophthalmic artery. There is also a rich anastomosis between adjacent arteries arising from the internal and external carotid arteries. The blood drains through a network of veins to the facial and orbital veins and the cavernous sinus.

This good blood supply is responsible for rapid healing of eyelid wounds with relative lack of infection.

NERVE SUPPLY

Motor

The facial nerve [cranial nerve (CN) VII] innervates the orbicularis oculi, frontalis, procerus, and corrugator supercilii muscles and supports eyelid protraction. The temporal and zygomatic branches of the facial nerve supply the orbicularis oculi, the main eyelid protractor. The facial nerve also supplies the corrugator supercilii and the procerus, both of which secondarily contribute to upper eyelid protraction.

The oculomotor nerve (CN III) innervates the main upper eyelid retractor and the levator palpebrae superioris via its superior branch. Sympathetic fibers contribute to upper eyelid retraction by innervation of the superior tarsal muscle, also known as Müller's muscle. Sympathetic fibers also innervate the inferior tarsal muscle, contributing to lower lid retraction.

Sensory

Trigeminal Nerve (CN V) supplies somatosensory innervation to the eyelid via its ophthalmic (V1) and maxillary (V2) divisions. Terminal branches of the ophthalmic division supply the upper eyelid as the lacrimal, supraorbital and supratrochlear nerves (lateral to medial) and the medial aspect of both upper and lower lids as the infratrochlear nerve. Terminal branches of the maxillary division supply the lower eyelid as the zygomaticofacial and infraorbital nerves. The zygomaticofacial nerve supplies the lateral lower lid and the infraorbital nerve supplies the lower eyelid proper.

Lymphatic Drainage

The eyelid consists of superficial and deep lymphatic system with respect to the orbicularis oculi muscle. Also, there are lymphatic channels interconnecting the superficial and deep lymphatic systems and the conjunctival lymphatic network draining through the tarsal plate to the deep lymphatic system.[3]

The superficial lymphatic channels travel in the subcutaneous fat within the nasolabial and lateral orbital fat compartments. The lateral deep lymphatic channels travel beneath the orbicularis oculi muscle, then through the superficial orbicularis retaining ligament, travel further into the suborbicularis oculi fat in the roof of the prezygomatic space. Further, these vessels descend to the preperiosteal fat at the level of zygomaticocutaneous ligaments to reach adjacent to the facial nerve and then into the preauricular nodes. The lymphatic pathways finally drain laterally to the parotid nodes and medially to submandibular nodes.

Incisions and dissections in the infraorbital area make the superficial system vulnerable to damage while dissection around the orbicularis retaining ligament and the zygomaticocutaneous ligaments damages the deep system. Therefore, concurrent damage to both the lymphatic systems, especially laterally, may be responsible for postoperative chemosis and edema.

OPHTHALMIC PATHOLOGICAL TERMS AND THEIR DEFINITION

Different ophthalmic pathological terms with their definitions are as follows:

- *Anophthalmia*: Absence of eye
- *Atrichiasis*: Absence of lashes
- *Blepharitis*: Inflammation of the eyelid margin
- *Blepharochalasis*: Elastic tissue atrophy causing loose eyelid skin
- *Coloboma*: Congenital cleft created by failure of development of a portion of the eye or adnexal structures
- *Dermatochalasis*: Laxness of the skin of the eyelids
- *Distichiasis*: Accessory row of eyelashes
- *Ectropion*: Eversion of the eyelid
- *Entropion*: Inversion of the eyelid
- *Epicanthal fold*: Accessory fold of skin at the inner canthal region of the eye
- *Epicanthus inversus*: Lower lid fold larger than upper lid fold
- *Epiphora*: Excess tearing
- *Episcleritis*: Inflammation of the superficial scleral tissues
- *Hypertelorism*: Increased distance between the two eyes measured radiologically
- *Hypopyon*: The presence of pus in the anterior chamber
- *Keratitis*: Inflammation of the cornea
- *Keratoconjunctivitis sicca*: Corneal and conjunctival inflammation associated with impaired tear secretion and ocular dryness
- *Keratoconus*: Conical distortion of the central cornea as a result of a degenerative process in the stroma
- *Keratopathy*: Corneal abnormalities including—*exposure keratopathy*—from corneal exposure and drying of the cornea
- *Lagophthalmos*: Persistent exposure of the eyeball despite closure of the eyelid
- *Limbus*: Boundary between the cornea and sclera
- *Madarosis*: Loss of the eyelashes, sometimes eyebrow
- *Preseptal cellulitis*: Cellulitis of the eyelids that has not penetrated through the orbital septum to involve the orbit
- *Symblepharon*: Adhesions between the bulbar and palpebral conjunctiva resulting in complete or partial obliteration of the eyelid fornices
- *Telecanthus*: Increased distance between the inner canthi

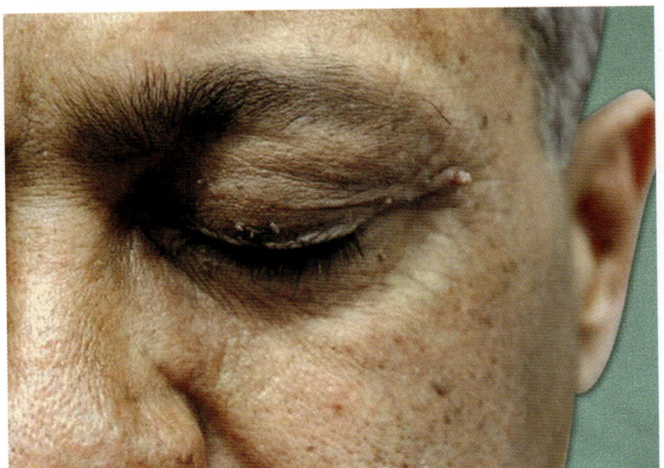

Fig. 3: Acrochordons of upper eyelid.

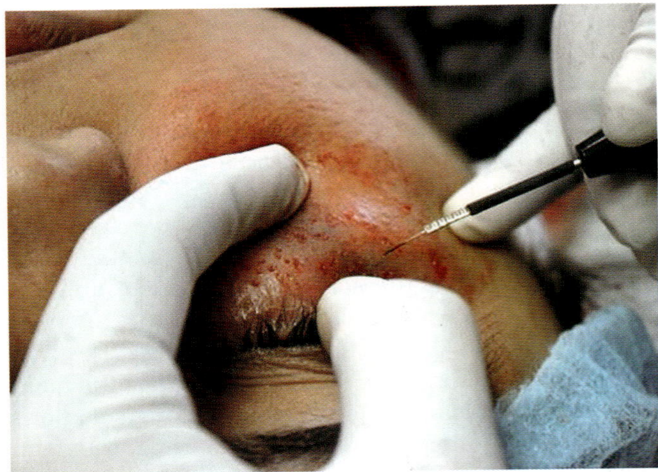

Fig. 4: Extensive milia being treated with radiofrequency needle electrode.

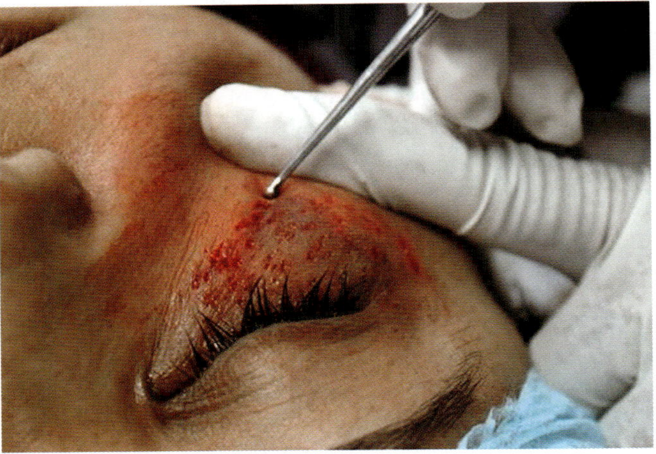

Fig. 5: Extensive milia being curetted post RF.

- *Trichiasis*: Lashes that turn inward toward the cornea usually as a result of entropion
- *Uveitis*: Inflammation of the uveal tract

CLASSIFICATION OF COMMON EYELID AND EYELASH DISORDERS

Disorders of Eyelids

Dermatological Conditions

Various dermatological conditions include:

- Infections:
  - Molluscum contagiosum
  - Verruca (filiform)
  - Leprosy (ocular complications-madarosis, conjunctivitis, episcleritis or scleritis, keratitis, lagophthalmos, trichiasis, uveitis and secondary infection)
- Benign tumors:
  - Epidermal: Papilloma (squamous or basal cell), pigmented nevi, neurofibroma, acrochordons (Fig. 3), seborrheic keratoses, actinic keratoses, dermatosis papulosa nigra melanoacanthoma, keratoacanthoma
  - Dermal: Hemangioma (capillary hemangioma, port-wine stain), pyogenic granuloma, dermatofibroma[4,5]
  - Adnexal tumors: Syringomas, milia (Figs. 4 and 5.), pilomatricoma, eccrine hidrocystoma, trichoepitheliomas, tricholemmomas
  - Miscellaneous: Xanthelasma palpebrarum, juvenile xanthogranuloma, pilonidal sinus,[6] etc.
- Malignant tumors: Basal cell carcinoma (BCC) (rodent ulcer), squamous cell carcinoma, melanoma, meibomian gland carcinoma, sebaceous gland carcinoma, eccrine carcinoma, epithelioma, Merkel cell carcinoma, kaposi sarcoma, etc.
- Premalignant: Cutaneous horn
- Autoimmune conditions:
  - Vitiligo
  - Alopecia areata

Structural Abnormalities

- Lagophthalmos
- Entropion
- Ectropion
- Epicanthal fold
- Tear trough or nasojugal groove
- Dermatochalasis
- Blepharochalasis
- Lid laxity
- Ptosis

Disorders of Eyelashes

- Trichiasis
  - Congenital districhiasis
  - Acquired districhiasis
- Eyelash ptosis
- Trichomegaly

- Madarosis
- Leukotrichia
- Poliosis

GENERAL PRINCIPLES OF THE EYELID SURGERY

One should possess a thorough knowledge regarding the vascular and nerve supply of eyelid in order to prevent serious surgical events during the operation.

- Local anesthesia using a mix of lidocaine 2% with epinephrine (1:100,000) is commonly used.
- As blood supply of the eyelid is good, always use adrenaline 1/100,000 along with the local anesthetic agent.
- In case the patient is anxious, sedation is advised and avoid adrenaline in hypertensive patients.
- A newer agent that has been tried is ropivacaine, which produces less intraoperative or postoperative bleeding and swelling with epinephrine 1:100,000.[7]
- During the surgery, if the eyelid is fixed and kept taut, it becomes much easier to perform the procedure. This can be done with a lid guard or a clamp. The exercise of holding the lid steady and secure also helps to protect the cornea from accidental damage anytime during the operation. Because of the pressure, the guard or the clamp lessens the bleeding. However, they should be applied just tight enough to occlude the marginal arteries, as too much of pressure may permanently damage the tissues.
- Avoid placing the knots on the inner conjunctival surface which may otherwise irritate the cornea. The suture generally used during eye surgeries is 5-0 polypropylene (prolene), which is a nonabsorbable monofilament suture.
- Always try to approximate the skin and conjunctiva so as to avoid any "bare areas". In case a bare area is left, it may fill up with granulation tissue, which may eventually get converted to fibrous tissue causing lid deformity few months later.
- Ensure good hemostasis from the marginal arteries at the medial and lateral margins of the tarsal plates and try to avoid excessively tight padding of the eye postoperatively.
- As the eyelid skin heals very quickly, sutures may be removed early (4–5 days). However, mattress sutures used to rotate or to alter the position of some tissue should be left in for about 2 weeks to ensure a permanent correction. In case the patient cannot return in 2 weeks, then absorbable mattress sutures should be used. Buried sutures ideally should be absorbable but may be nonabsorbable. However, the buried suture technique in double-eyelid blepharoplasty, which is a popular aesthetic surgery, is associated with complications related to the suture thread implantation. This complication can be addressed with a suture removal surgery.[8]

Preoperative Evaluation

It should include proper history and examination of the patient to rule out any local infection, significant systemic disorders, drug allergies, and intake of agents that may interfere with the hemostasis while operating.

Proper clinical photographs and informed consent are mandatory.

INDIVIDUAL PROCEDURES OF COMMON CORRECTABLE EYELID DISORDERS IN DERMATOLOGY

Excisions and Destructive Procedures

Most of the excisions can be done as an outpatient procedure under topical or injectable anesthesia. The skin lesions may be removed using various modalities depending upon the type of lesion.

Indications

- *Benign growths*: Warts, molluscum contagiosum, nevus, acrochordons, dermatosis papulosa nigra, seborrheic keratosis, actinic keratosis, neurofibroma, syringoma, pilomatricoma, eccrine hidrocystoma, milia, etc.
- *Malignant growths*: Squamous cell carcinoma, basal cell carcinoma (BCC), melanoma, etc.
- *Other conditions*: Xanthelasma palpebrarum.

Procedures

The following procedures can be utilized depending upon the pathology:

- Simple scissor excision
- Shave excision
- *Skin excision and suturing*: Full-thickness skin excision involving the growth is carried out. This technique involves removing the entire skin lesion up to the deeper levels of the skin with the help of 15 no. surgical blade mounted on a no. 3 Bard-Parker handle (down up to the fatty layer) in order to get rid of the entire affected area (Figs. 6 to 8). In an attempt to ensure that the excised tissue (skin cancer) is clear of any possible cancer cells (clear margins) a small amount of the surrounding normal tissue (3–4 mm) may be removed. Most often, an elliptical incision is taken and the growth excised, as this makes it easier to stitch the gap with sutures. In case a large area is removed, a skin graft or flap may be required to cover the defect.
- *Cryotherapy*: It may be used to destroy or remove warts, actinic keratoses, seborrheic keratosis, milia, dermatosis papulosa nigra, molluscum contagiosum,

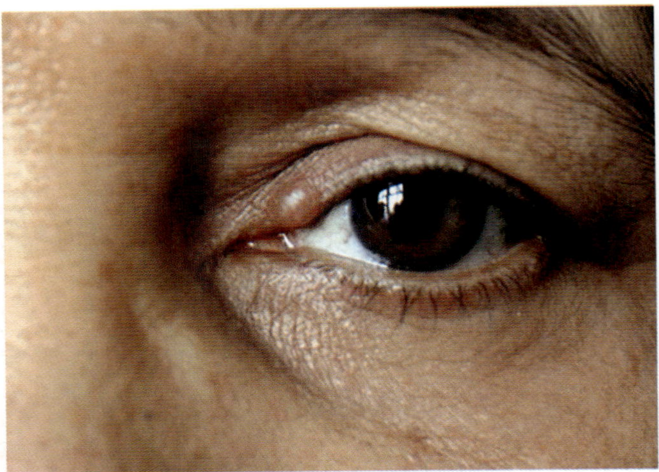

Fig. 6: Neurofibroma (biopsy proven) of upper eyelid margin.

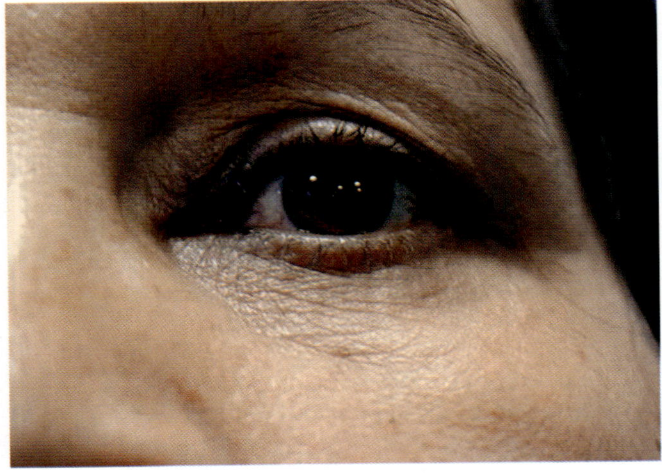

Fig. 7: Immediate post-excision of neurofibroma of upper lid margin.

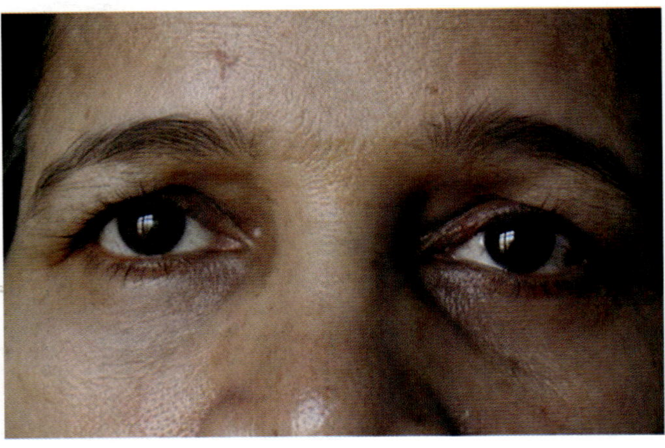

Fig. 8: 10 days postoperative following excision of neurofibroma upper eyelid margin.

etc. The disadvantage of using cryotherapy around the eyes is the thin skin reducing safety and possibility of ocular damage by contiguous spread or spillage.

Various Methods: Cryotherapy is done using a cotton swab that has been dipped into liquid nitrogen or a probe that has liquid nitrogen flowing through it. If a thermocouple is available, a temperature of –20°C is to be reached twice in two freeze-thaw cycles. If no thermocouple is available a standard cryosurgical unit with nitrous oxide or carbon dioxide gas can be used as carbon dioxide gas would achieve a tissue temperature of –20°C in 30 seconds. Therefore, freeze for 30 seconds, thaw and refreeze for 30 seconds. They are very effective for cryoepilation of eyelashes.

Cryoepilation of eyelashes: Use of a chalazion clamp is recommended while performing cryoepilation as it facilitates exposure of the surgical field and supports cryodestruction of the follicle by reducing blood flow to the gland, thereby speeding the freeze and slowing the thaw.

It is a least risky procedure, where the cryoprobe is applied over base of the affected Meibomian gland on the palpebral conjunctiva (3-4 mm behind the eyelid margin).

A double freeze–thaw (–25°C) cycle spares adjacent normal tissue, but destroys the affected follicles.

- *Electrosurgery*: The principle of this machine is to modify the alternating current (240 V) to achieve high voltage (550 V), high frequency and low amperage to generate oscillating waves which cause tissue destruction.
- *Radiofrequency (RF) excision*: This is a form of electrosurgery with the same principle, only advantage it has is that the unwanted frequencies are not produced as a result of which there is a better control of the procedure with lesser tissue destruction. The frequency ranges between 500 kHz and 4,000 kHz. It has been used in pyogenic granuloma, acrochordons, xanthelasma palpebrarum, BCC, seborrheic keratosis, milia, molluscum contagiosum, squamous cell carcinoma, hemangiomas, nevi (Figs. 9 and 10), etc.
- *Moh's micrographic surgery*: It is used to treat and cure certain skin cancers. Surgeons need to be trained for this procedure to do this surgery. It is a skin-sparing technique that allows skin cancer to be removed with less damage to the healthy skin around it.
- *Laser excision*: Laser can be used to excise benign or premalignant skin lesions. Ablative lasers are used, predominantly the carbon dioxide laser.

Tarsorrhaphy[9]

Procedure of joining a part or the entire upper and lower eyelids so as to attempt partial or complete closure of the eye.

The term tarsorrhaphy is most commonly used in the western countries, whereas in Russia the term—blepharorrhaphy is widely accepted. The latter seems to be a more appropriate term as the sutures are passed through all the palpebral layers and not just the cartilage.

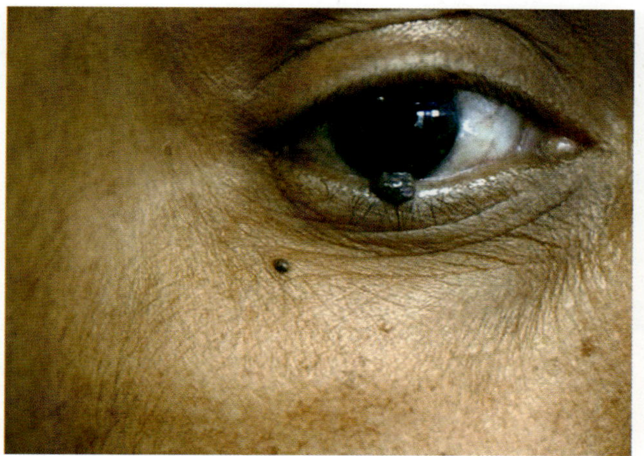

Fig. 9: Melanocytic nevus of lower eyelid.

Fig. 10: Immediate postoperative after radiofrequency excision of melanocytic nevus.

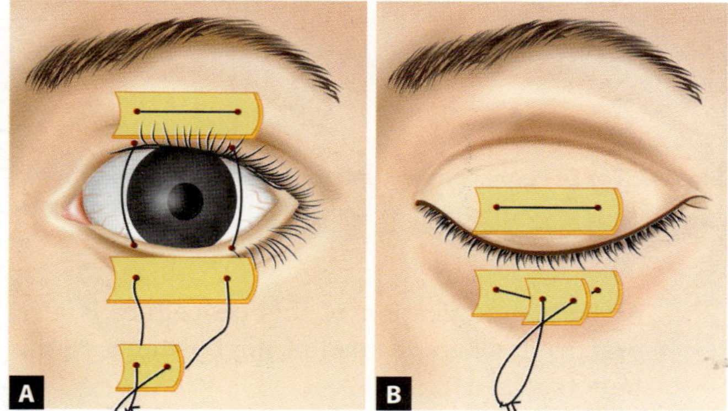

Figs. 11A and B: Temporary tarsorrhaphy procedure: (A) Alignment and threading of bolster; (B) Using sutures and bolster to close the eye.

Blepharorrhaphy may be temporary or permanent. Temporary procedure implies use of only sutures to bring the eyelids together and therefore, should be called simple blepharorrhaphy. As in the permanent procedure, the goal is to cause ankyloblepharon, hence ankylosing blepharorrhaphy is recommended, instead of permanent.

Indications

- To protect the cornea when there is inadequate closure of the eyelids as in:
  - Facial nerve palsy, ocular leprosy, post-burns scarring, proptosis, infrequent blinking as in intensive care unit (ICU) patients or those with severe brain injuries, protection of the anesthetic cornea from the risk of damage and infection, etc.
- To promote healing of the cornea in patients of corneal ulcer
- Exposure after ocular surgery to retain a conformer or other device, e.g. in children with anophthalmia or adults after evisceration or enucleation

Procedure

- *Temporary tarsorrhaphy*: It can be performed by using a drawstring, botulinum toxin (the upper lid levator muscle is paralyzed with the toxin), or by using cyanoacrylate glue to appose the lids.
  - After cleaning and dressing of the operation site, local infiltration is given. The procedure of temporary central tarsorrhaphy using a drawstring is as described (Figs. 11A and B).
  - After cleaning the area with 5% povidone iodine, anesthetize central part of both the eyelids with lidocaine and adrenaline. For each eye, prepare three bolsters (e.g. small cotton wool balls or plastic tubing), two with size 2 cm × 2 cm each and one of 1 cm × 1 cm size. The sutures are passed and tied over the bolsters to prevent them from cutting the skin. A double-armed nonabsorbable suture (e.g. silk, prolene or nylon 4-0, 5-0 or 6-0) is passed straight through one of the 2 cm bolsters, 2 mm from the end. After aligning the bolster in the middle of the upper lid, pass the same needle 3–4 mm above the upper eyelid margin, through the tarsal plate and come out of the gray line of the lid margin. Pass the same needle into the gray line of the lower lid, then into the tarsal plate and out of the skin 2–3 mm below the lower eyelid margin. After aligning the lower lid bolster centrally, pass the needle through it a few millimeters from one end. Similarly, then pass the suture through the other end of the upper bolster → upper lid → lower lid → lower bolster in the same fashion as the previous step.
  - The needles should be passed through the shorter length of bolster, 2 mm from each bolster end. Slide the two lower lid bolsters upwards to close the eye. The smaller bolster "locks" and closes the lid. To separate the lids, the smaller bolster should be pulled down and the lids will open up easily.

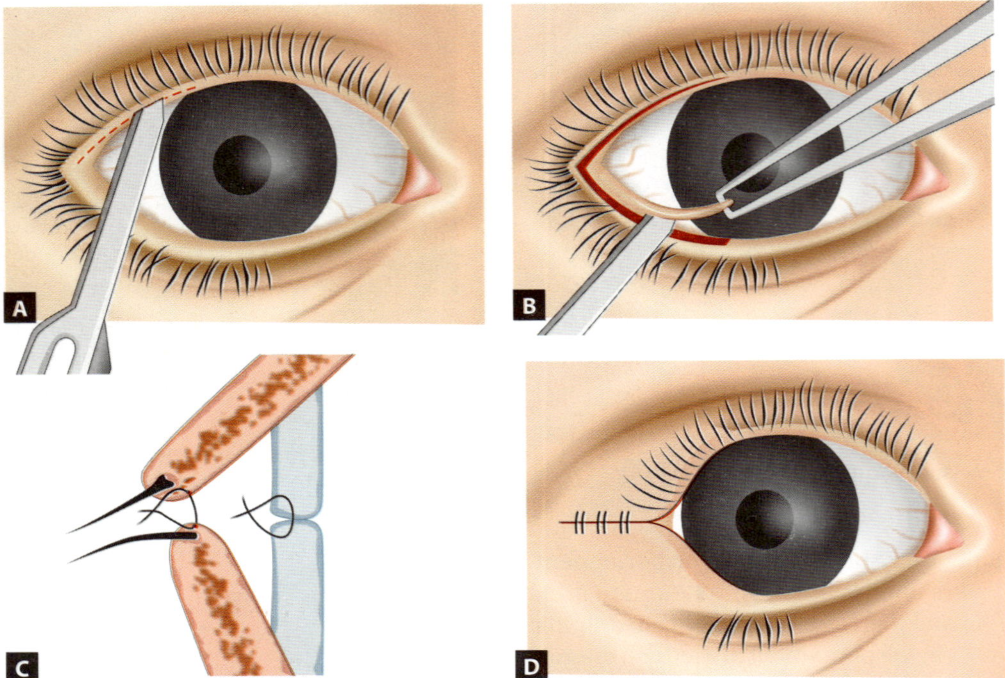

Figs. 12A to D: Permanent tarsorrhaphy: (A) Splitting the anterior and posterior lamella; (B) Excising 1 mm of the posterior lamella; (C) Closing the anterior and posterior lamella; (D) After the pocedure.

- A slight modification of this procedure is also practiced, where instead of the bolster, a sterile button is used.

- *Permanent tarsorrhaphy:* In this procedure, the lid margin is debrided which allows the lids to stick together as they heal. It is almost always restricted only to the lateral part of the eyelids, so that the patient is able to see through the central eyelid opening and therefore, the eye can still be examined. It may last at least 3 months (sometimes lifelong). In this technique the anterior and posterior lamellae of the lateral third of the upper and lower lids is split along the gray line using a no. 11 blade (no. 15 blade may also do) up to a depth of 2 mm.
  - The split should be continued over the lid for about 5 mm with the same blade or spring scissors. Care should be taken to keep the split parallel to the tarsal plate so that the eyelid separates into anterior and posterior lamellae neatly. In order to remove the epithelium of the eyelid, excise 1 mm of the posterior lamella which is then closed using 5-0 or 6-0 absorbable suture. This is followed by closure of the anterior lamella (eyelid skin) by 4-0 to 6-0 sized nonabsorbable suture (Figs. 12A to D).
  - These tarsorrhaphies almost often last forever, but if they need to be divided this can be done by cutting the sutures under the effect of a local anesthetic agent and the lids look perfectly normal.

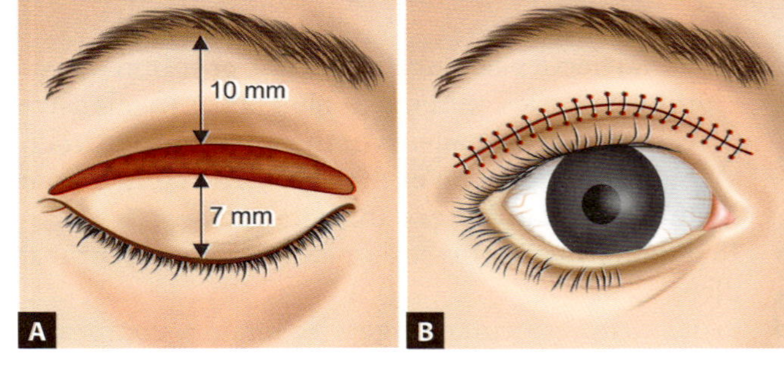

Figs. 13A and B: Upper eyelid blepharoplasty.

Blepharoplasty

The term blepharoplasty was coined by Karl Ferdinand von Gräfe[10] in 1818, where the technique was used for repairing deformities caused by eyelid cancer. Upper blepharoplasty improves the palpebral fissure (Figs. 13A and B).

Indications

The indications involved are as follows:

- Redundant and lax eyelid skin (dermatochalasis) causing double-eyelid fold creation
- Preaponeurotic fat herniation (steatoblepharon) that may result in either functional visual symptoms or cosmetic concerns in the affected patients
- Periorbital rejuvenation

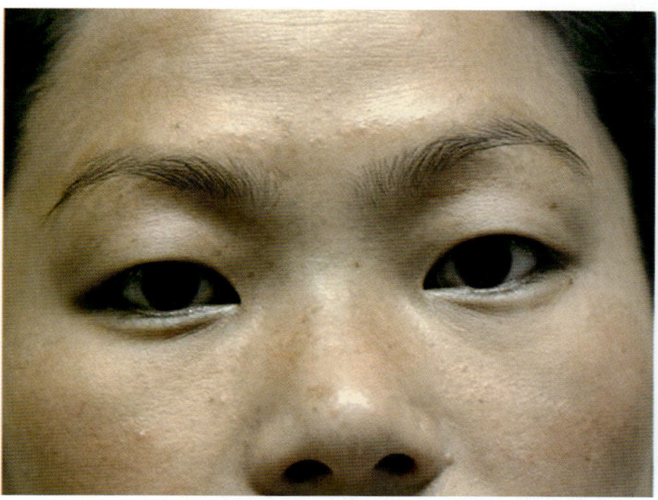

Fig. 14: Asian blepharoplasty preoperative.

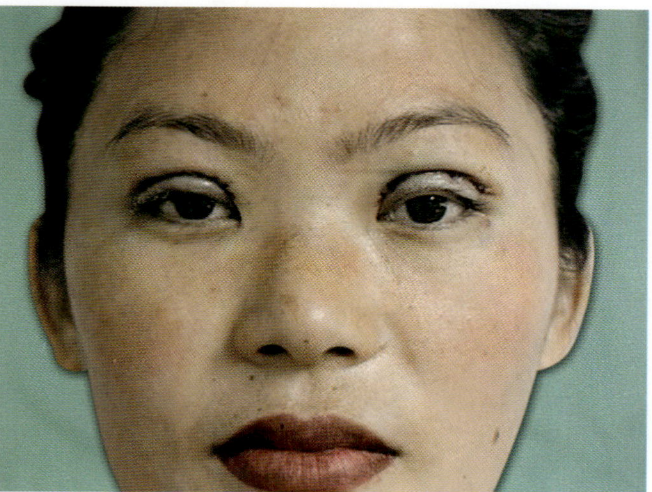

Fig. 15: Asian blepharoplasty immediate postoperative.

The goal of blepharoplasty should be to achieve the eyebrows at an appropriate level, neat looking eyelids with well-hidden scar, correction of fat bulges without too much excision or creating a sunken eye.

Situations where it can be combined with other procedures:[11]

- Blepharoplasty with skin excision may be indicated for patients with upper eyelid-skin redundancy and prominent double eyelids.
- Blepharoplasty with skin excision and nonburied suture fixation may be indicated for patients with upper lid skin redundancy and weak double eyelids.
- Blepharoplasty with skin excision and buried suture fixation may be indicated for patients with upper lid skin redundancy but no double-eyelid folds.
- Blepharoplasty with simultaneous ptosis (lid or lacrimal) correction may be indicated for patients with senile or subclinical ptosis requesting upper blepharoplasty.

Procedure of Asian Blepharoplasty (Figs.14 and 15)

It may be performed effectively under local anesthesia with or without sedation. Infiltration with 2% xylocaine with adrenaline mixed with 0.25% sensorcaine gives a very good anesthesia.[12]

The marking of the required skin to be excised should be done preoperatively in a sitting position. A curved line 9–10 mm above the lid margin in the mid-pupillary line is marked which corresponds to the supratarsal fold. The line should gently curve down to 7 mm above the lid margin at the medial and lateral ends. The excessive skin is thereafter marked by pinching it with a non-toothed forceps or marking the upper line 10 mm below the inferior margin of the eyebrow.

A scalpel or RF electrosurgical device may be used to make the incisions after cleaning and local infiltration. After excising the desired amount of eyelid skin, the orbicularis oculi fibers are excised. The preaponeurotic fat is made to protrude by a gentle pressure on the globe and also to help in identifying the septum and incising it. The septum is incised along its entire length to expose the levator aponeurosis lying under it. The fat pads are excised if in excess. Avoid giving traction to the fat pads and to the superior oblique tendon while dissecting the medial fat pad. The excessive skin and muscle are resected with scissors. Correction of the lid ptosis and lacrimal gland ptosis may be carried out. Hemostasis may be achieved with pressure or cautery and the incision is closed with interrupted 5-0 or 6-0 nylon or prolene sutures. The hitching suture should include the aponeurosis, orbicularis muscle and the skin so that when the patient blinks the eyelid moves with the contraction of the muscle and so that the upper eyelid crease is created. At last the cutaneous sutures are taken in a simple interrupted manner.

With upper lid blepharoplasty, the degree of lash ptosis was found to be reduced thereby improving the visual quality.[13]

The brow position does not seem to change in patients who undergo upper eyelid blepharoplasty for simple dermatochalasis.[14]

In the Asian population, too high eyelid folds after blepharoplasty may cause an unsatisfactory aesthetic outcome which is difficult and challenging to correct.

It may be attempted to correct with a procedure called "secondary blepharoplasty", wherein the levator is advanced and intervened between the levator aponeurosis and the overlying skin by in situ tissue or fat grafting.[15]

Postoperative Care

Ocular pad dressing should be given. Patient should be asked to apply antibiotic ointment two to three times

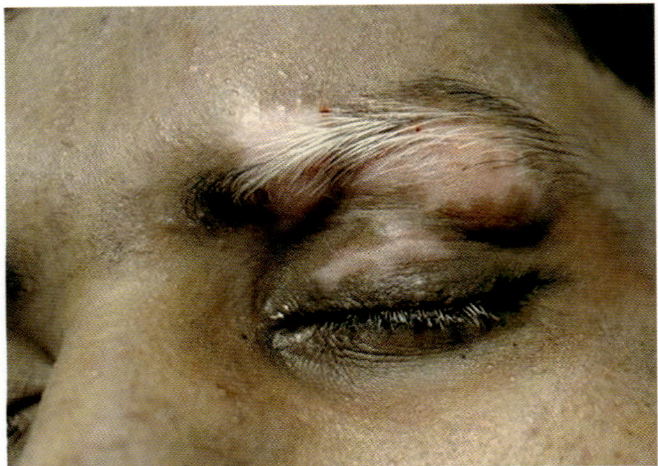

Fig. 16: Upper eyelid vitiligo.

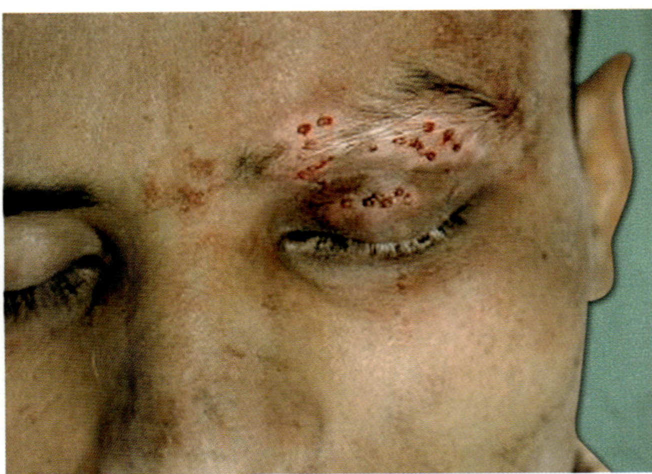

Fig. 17: Upper eyelid vitiligo immediately following minipunch grafting.

a day over the suture line. Artificial tear drops may be prescribed. Oral antibiotics and analgesics should be given for 5 days. Pain is usually very minimal which subsides with analgesics. If the pain still continues despite analgesics; rule out retrobulbar hemorrhage, which is a dreaded complication. Cold packs during the first 48 hours may be advised to reduce the edema. Patient must be advised to wait for 6 weeks for the swelling to resolve before judging the final results. The sutures are removed after 6 or 7 days. Patients should be advised to avoid the use of contact lenses and bending and lifting heavy weights for at least 2 weeks.

Lower lid blepharoplasty: The aim of lower eyelid blepharoplasty is to remove the pseudo-herniated fat via skin incision. However, the approach to this procedure remains controversial. Two approaches have been tried, the transconjunctival and the transcutaneous approach.

Transconjunctival lower lid blepharoplasty is performed through an incision made 4-6 mm below the lid margin through the conjunctiva with lower eyelid retractors. This approach has reduced chances of eyelid retraction, scleral show and postoperative ectropion.

Transcutaneous approach is performed through a subciliary incision with the skin elevated off the orbicularis oculi muscle. This approach is preferred in patients who have hypertrophy of this muscle and therefore requires excision of the muscle.

VITILIGO SURGERIES

Vitiligo is a common autoimmune disease seen approximately in 1% of the general population and is characterized by the presence of depigmented macules and patches,[16] which results in psychosocial morbidity. Surgical methods come into picture when the medical therapy fails to cause repigmentation of the affected skin or in cases of segmental vitiligo where the response is excellent post-surgery. Involvement of the head and neck area is associated with leukotrichia of the eyelashes and eyebrows.[17] In many cases, the surgical management of vitiligo may cause repigmentation of leukotrichia;[18] however, eyelash leukotrichia involving periocular region is generally resistant to medical or surgical therapy.[19]

Various factors to be kept in mind before conducting the surgeries on the eyelids are:

- Age of the patient
- Type of vitiligo (segmental vitiligo or vitiligo vulgaris)
- Size of the depigmented area
- Assessment of stability of vitiligo
- Patient expectation.

Various operations recommended for eyelid vitiligo are:

- Suction blister roof grafting
- Minipunch skin grafting (Figs. 16 and 17)
- Ultrathin or split-thickness skin grafting
- Autologous non-cultured melanocyte transplantation
- Cultured melanocyte transplantation
- Hair follicle grafting (Figs. 18 and 19).

Contraindications to the above surgeries are:

- Patients with unrealistic expectation
- Unstable vitiligo
- Children
- Keloidal tendency

Various grafting methods have been so far described elsewhere in the book including tissue and cellular grafts. The following methods of repigmentation have so far given good results and are recommended for vitiligo patches involving the eyelids.

Skin Grafting

Preparation of the Recipient Site

Dermabrasion of the recipient area can be carried out with Manekha's manual dermabrader or motorized dermabraders with a diamond fraise tip. Dermabrasion

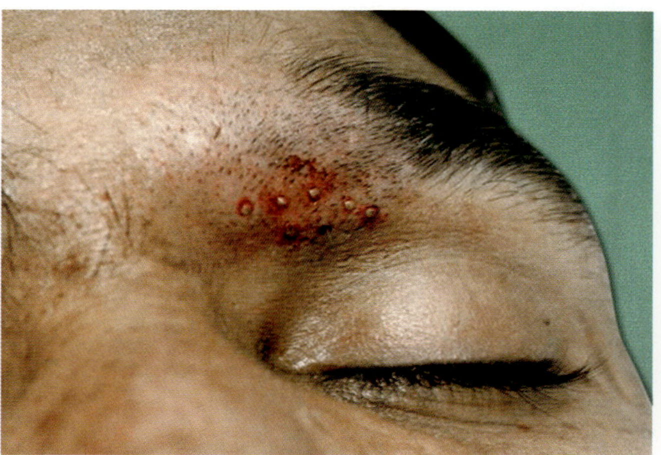

Fig. 18: Immediate post-follicular unit extraction and hair follicle grafting onto vitiliginous macule.

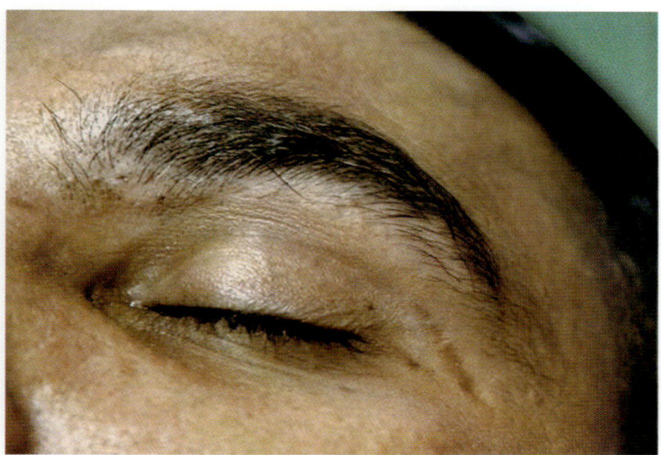

Fig. 19: Hair follicle graft: 1 month postoperative.

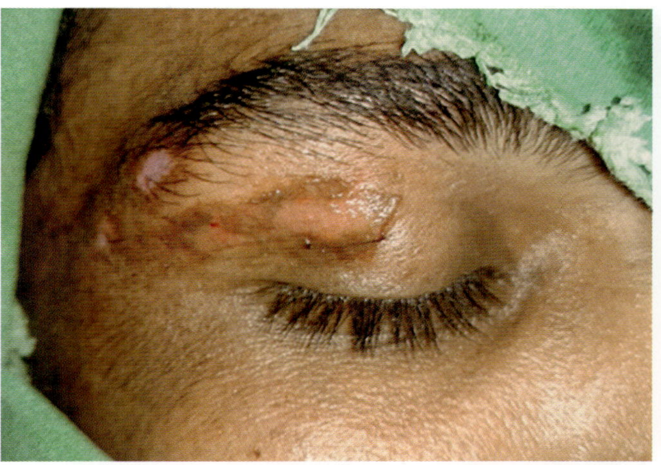

Fig. 20: Thin Thiersch's graft for vitiligo upper eyelid.

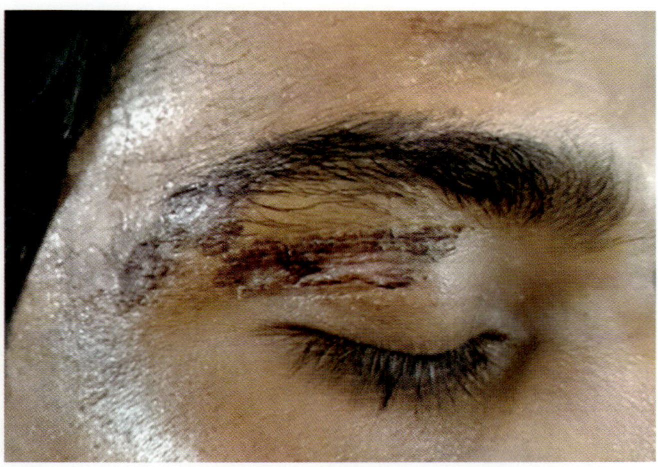

Fig. 21: One week after thin Thiersch's grafting over upper eyelid.

not only prepares the recipient area during grafting, but it also stimulates proliferation and migration of melanocytes.

Split skin grafts can be harvested from the donor area using Humby's knife or Silver's knife or dermatomes (disposable harvesting devices).

Suction Blister Grafting

The donor skin is split-thickness skin grafts containing only the epidermis produced due to a split at the dermoepidermal junction by prolonged suction at a negative pressure to the donor site. Repigmentation is achieved by melanocyte transplant and by securing the obtained epidermal sheet to the dermabraded or laser ablated depigmented patch.

Thin Thiersch's Split-thickness Skin Grafting

Very thin split-thickness grafts consisting of the epidermis and part of the upper papillary dermis are grafted on the dermabraded part of the stable vitiligo patch (Figs. 20 and 21). In very thin grafts, just like suction blister grafts, the graft itself sheds in a week or two, sometimes earlier.

Noncultured Epidermal Cell Suspension

Noncultured epidermal cell suspensions containing a mixture of melanocytes and keratinocytes are best for obtaining cosmetically pleasing results in the management of vitiligo of the eyelids (Figs. 22 to 26).

EYELASH TRANSPLANTATION (FOLLICULAR UNIT TRANSPLANTATION)

Eyelash transplantation is a procedure in which the hair follicles from hair-bearing areas are transplanted in the eyelashes. It has been used as a therapeutic option for:

- The loss of eyelash as a result of the following diverse etiologies such as:

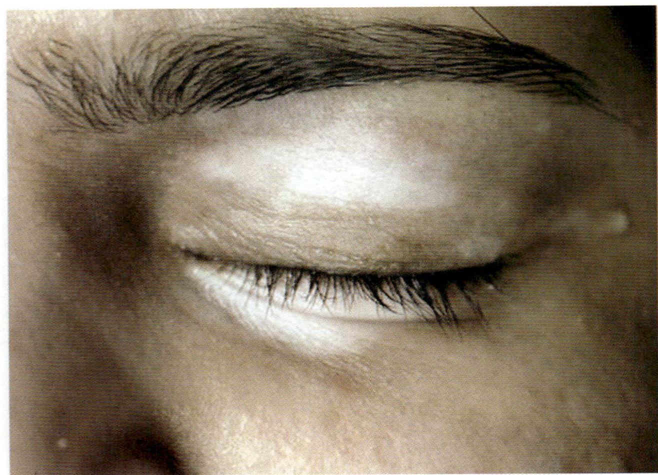

Fig. 22: Upper eyelid vitiligo.

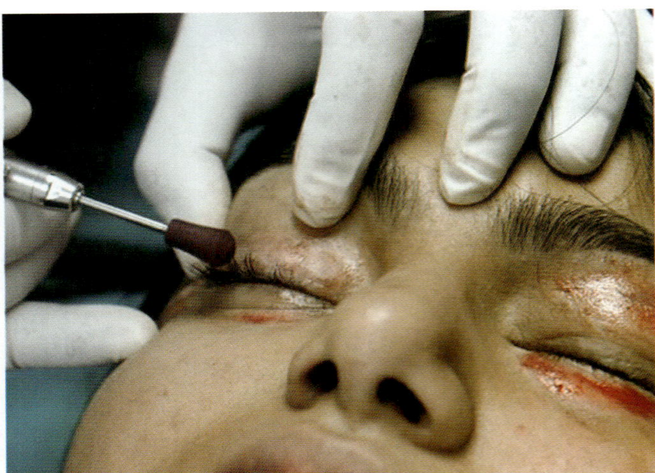

Fig. 23: Dermabrasion of recipient area.

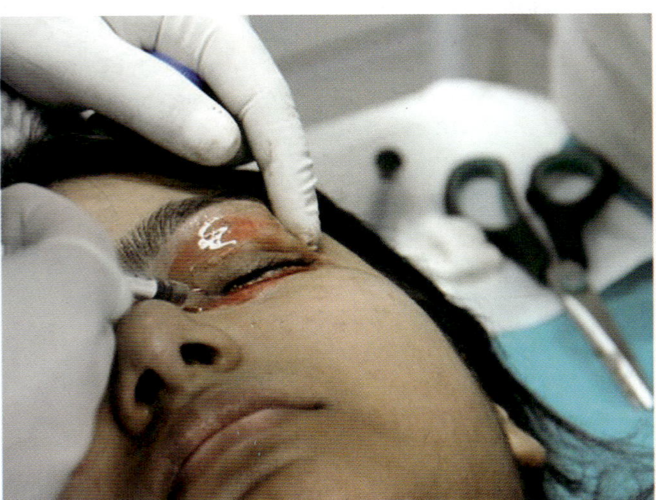

Fig. 24: Application of melanocyte-keratinocyte suspension.

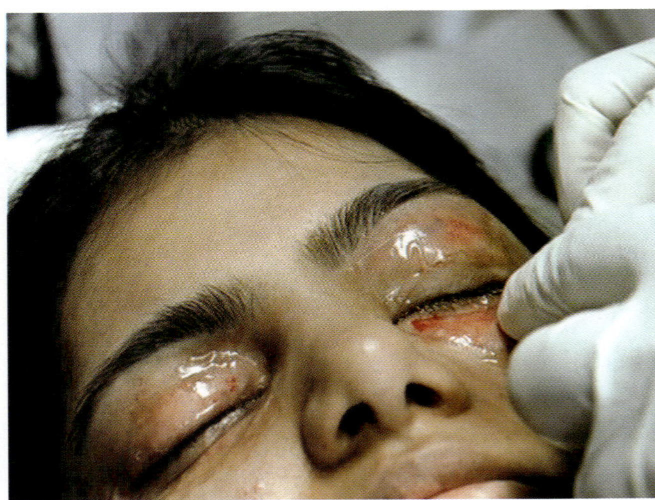

Fig. 25: Application of dry collagen sheet dressing.

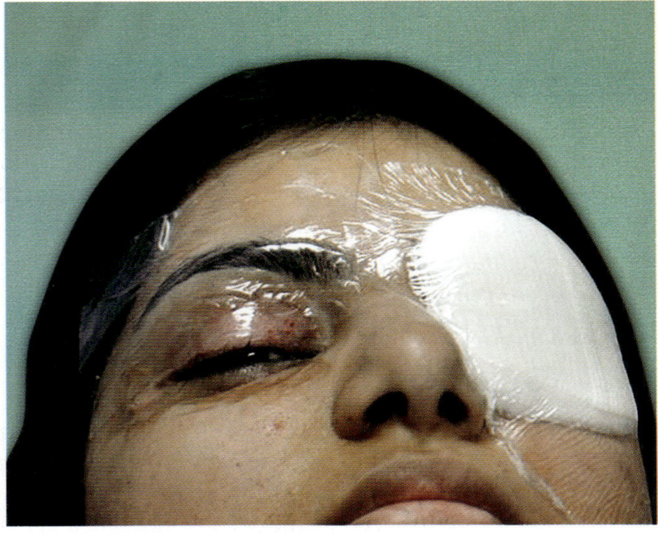

Fig. 26: Application of eye-pad dressing with eyes closed.

  - Trauma
  - Trichotillomania
  - Alopecia areata
- May also be performed for aesthetic purposes in situations such as:
  - Patients who demand denser eyelashes
  - Vitiligo associated leukotrichia (Figs. 27 and 28).

Procedure

Half an hour prior to the procedure, mild sedation can be achieved by giving the patient, tablet diazepam 10 mg orally. Corneal eye shield should be applied after topical anesthesia with lignocaine eye drops. Local anesthesia is achieved by infiltration of 2% lignocaine with adrenaline in the donor and recipient site.

The donor area is prepared by clipping the hair of the temporal area. Only single hair follicles are harvested

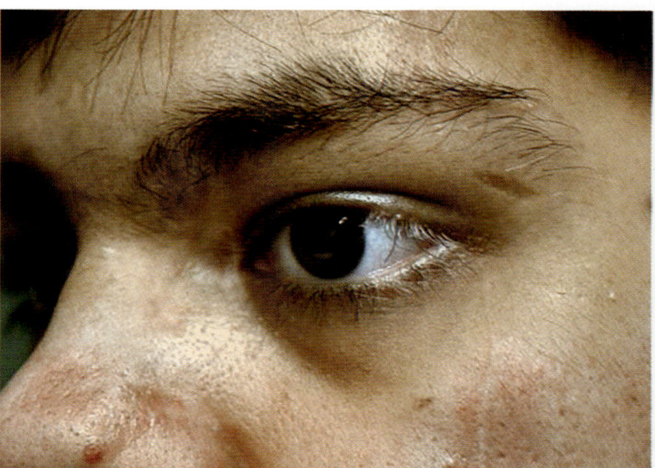

Fig. 27: Residual eyelash leukotrichia following vitiligo treatment.

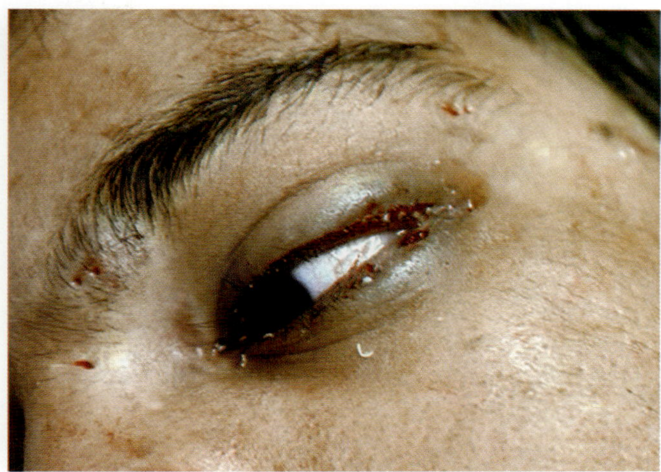

Fig. 28: Immediately following eyelash transplantation.

using 0.8 mm punch with the help of follicle unit extraction motor. The involved eyelashes of recipient area are removed with 20-gauge needle. The hair obtained are harvested in a similar way as in hair transplant surgery and the single hair follicles are grafted, using fine jeweler's forceps or implanters into the chambers created. Implantation can be carried out in one row in a fan-shaped manner. In a single sitting, 15–20 hair can be transplanted in each eyelid. Thereafter, the donor lashes are trimmed to the size of other eyelashes and the operated eye is padded with a bandage for a week. Few patients may need two to three sittings at the interval of 4 weeks. The surgery takes about 2–3 hours.

The procedure of eyelash transplantation can be performed by various other methods. It can be performed using Choi and Kim hair transplanter,[20] with single hair grafts or by strip composite eyebrow graft as described by Kasai.[21] It can also be performed using the "pluck and sew technique" as described by Caputy and Flowers.[22]

The present first author has harvested single unit grafts using motorized punches of 0.8 mm similar to hair transplantation and implanted them in the chambers created after removal of leukotrichic eyelash using forceps or implanter with excellent repigmentation of the leukotrichic eyelashes. Use of the implanter makes the procedure simpler and faster as compared to the manual forceps technique.

Post-procedure, the author observed that, the transplanted eyelashes matched closely with natural eyelashes and were cosmetically elegant.

Post-procedure Care

Capsule amoxicillin clavulanic acid 625 mg and tablet ibuprofen 400 mg 8 hourly are advised for 5 days. Protective goggles are advised for 4–6 weeks. The curvature of the eyelashes may be maintained with the regular use of mascara or a curling device.

Post-procedure, there is scab formation around the transplanted follicle and the transplanted hair which falls off by 2–3 weeks and regrowth of the eyelashes are first noticed by 8–10 weeks. The results are assessed at the end of 6 months. Surgery is most of the time free from major complications and most common complications noticed are swelling and bruising of eyelids and blepharitis. As the scalp hair grow faster, the patient should be advised to trim these lashes at regular intervals.

SURGERIES IN LEPROSY

Involvement of the eye in leprosy may lead to following mentioned conditions:

- Lagophthalmos
- Trichiasis
- Ectropion
- Entropion

Lagophthalmos

Both paucibacillary and multibacillary leprosies may affect the eyelids. Lagophthalmos is the common complication seen in these patients, where there is a visible lid gap due to incomplete closure of the eyelids. This condition puts the eye at risk of exposure and external injuries further giving rise to sequelae of exposure keratitis, secondary infection, corneal ulcer and finally vision loss. At times, the infection may involve the deeper tissues causing panophthalmitis.

It may be aggravated by anesthesia of the cornea due to fifth nerve involvement.

Medical Management

Role of medical management is usually limited. It is neither cost-effective, nor permanent and therefore the results are not satisfactory. However, if the condition is left untreated, there is every possible way by which the patient

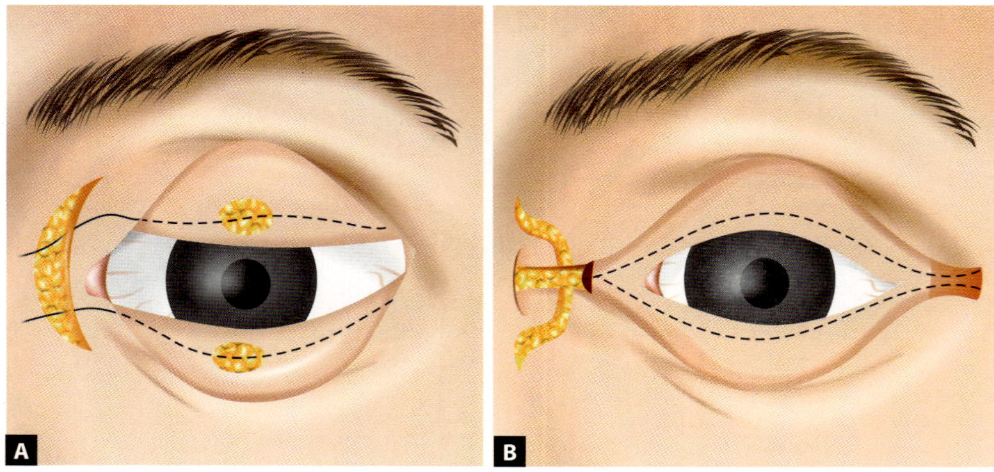

Figs. 29A and B: Temporalis muscle transfer (TMT) through eyelids to medial canthal ligaments and tarsal plates.

may develop fulminating corneal complications. Few measures to address the situation at the earliest include:

- In early phase or during presence of facial patches without lagophthalmos, prompt initiation of systemic steroids (tablet prednisolone 40–60 mg daily dose for 4–6 weeks)
- Artificial tear substitutes (carboxy methyl cellulose solution)
- Stimulation of muscle (electrostimulation)
- Physiotherapy: Exercises (active and passive) to close the eye.

The patient is observed for 6 months; if the lid gap persists for more than 5 mm then surgery is often required, however, spontaneous recovery has been reported even after 1 year.[23]

Surgical Management[24]

- *Dynamic Procedures:* Gillie's and Johnson's temporalis muscle transfer (TMT) procedures are commonly carried out. However, in the Indian subcontinent, Johnson's TMT procedure (Figs. 29A and B) is considered the surgery of choice. The procedure has few limitations which include prolonged admissions, well-motivated patient, well-trained oculoplastic surgeon, good corneal sensitivity and postoperative intensive physiotherapy. In this procedure strips of the temporalis muscle are tunneled through the tarsal plates and anchored to the medial canthal ligaments.
- *Static Procedures*: Various procedures have been carried out which include the canthopexies, palpabroplasties, slings, springs, gold implants, ear cartilage grafts, etc. Two procedures that are effective in corneal blindness are tarsal strip (Kuhnt-Szymanowski) and tarsorrhaphy (discussed earlier in this chapter).

Trichiasis

The term trichiasis means that some of the eyelashes point backwards and hence rub against the cornea. Usually every patient with entropion will have trichiasis. However, sometimes the misdirected lashes may turn inwards without the turning in of the whole eyelid (i.e. trichiasis without entropion). Treatment of this condition is removal of the incriminating eyelashes.

Removal of the Lashes

Recommended only if there is trichiasis. Various methods tried to remove the lashes are as follows:

- Epilation
- Cutting the lashes
- Excision and suturing of small clumps of lashes or lash follicles
- Electrolysis
- Cryotherapy.

- *Epilation*: The offending lashes are plucked out with the epilation forceps after which the patient may temporarily heave a sigh of relief. The symptoms usually recur as the lash nearly always grows again. This procedure requires repeated epilation to keep the eyes comfortable and therefore patients with only slight trichiasis are the ideal candidates.
- *Cutting the lashes:* Scissors are used to cut off the offending lashes which also gives temporary relief. But at times it may be worse as after cutting, the eyelash end becomes sharper and therefore it may be an irritant.
- *Excision of misdirected lashes*: This procedure in undertaken in patients who present with just one or two small tufts of abnormal eyelashes. It involves excision of the affected lashes along with their roots without affecting the eyelid. This procedure may be an alternative to electrolysis or cryotherapy (described later) in milder cases of trichiasis.
- *Electrolysis:* The principle of electrolysis is to pass a low voltage current through a fine needle along the eyelash up to the root of the lash causing a localized burn enough to destroy the lash root. It is an ideal procedure in patients with few ingrowing eyelashes.

- *Procedure*: After infiltrating the eyelid with local anesthesia, insert the electrolysis needle along the direction of the eyelash into the lash follicle up to a depth of 3 mm. The current is passed for at least 5 seconds. Tiny bubbles may appear on the surface of the eyelid at the entry point of the needle. Even when the local anesthesia effect is adequate, patient may feel some discomfort with the passage of current. In order to check the adequacy of the procedure, lift the lash out of the tissues with an epilation forceps; if the lash root has been destroyed, the lash can be lifted out without any resistance and in case there is some resistance, the procedure should be repeated. Continue the procedure until each ingrowing eyelash has been treated. Repeated treatment may be required.

- *Cryotherapy:*
  - *Principle:* The hair follicles are destroyed permanently if the lid margin is frozen to –20°C with a cryoprobe. It is the temperature of the tissues that is important and not that of the probe. The tissue temperature can be measured with a fine needle thermocouple inserted into the roots of the lashes. However, it is thought that freezing twice is more effective than freezing once.

Advantage of electrolysis and cryotherapy is that no surgery is performed. However, the disadvantages are as follows:

- Painful procedure
- Erythema
- Edema
- Depigmentation of skin
- Scarring
- Trichiasis
- Atrophy
- Expensive equipment required
- Recurrence
- Multiple sittings

To minimize the above complications, cryotherapy may be combined with an anterior lamellar resection to help destroy the lash roots effectively.

Surgery

A treatment of choice in the management of trichiasis and cicatricial entropion of the upper or lower eyelid is orbicularis oculi fibers shortening.

Ectropion and Entropion

Ectropion (eversion) and entropion (inversion) of the eyelid are most commonly seen in old cases of leprosy who have thin tarsal plate and orbicularis oculi. Both the conditions may be associated with trichiasis.

Better results are seen in patients with entropion operated with tarsal plate fracture with rotation.

Ectropion surgery: Lateral tarsorrhaphy, electrosurgery and suture repair can be done.

The surgical outcome after the tarsal strip procedure for lower eyelid ectropion was similar with both the absorbable and nonabsorbable sutures.[25]

MISCELLANEOUS SURGERIES

Xanthelasma Palpebrarum

The term "xanthelasma" is derived from the Greek words "*xanthos*" which means "yellow" and "*elasma*" which means beaten metal plate. Xanthelasma palpebrarum are yellowish plaques that occur most commonly near the inner canthus of the eyelid, more often on the upper eyelids than the lower. The plaques frequently have symmetrical distribution and may be soft, semisolid or calcareous. Most of the individuals with xanthelasma have a lipid disorder; however, it may occur in normolipemic individuals as well who have low levels of high-density lipoprotein cholesterol or other lipoprotein abnormalities. They have a tendency to progress, coalesce and become permanent.

Treatment

- *Medical management:* In patients having dyslipidemia—advice strict dietary restriction and pharmacologic reduction of serum lipids. However, this may yield only limited response.
- *Surgical management:* Various options are available for the removal of xanthelasma palpebrarum, ranging from chemical cauterization, electrodessication, cryotherapy, surgical excision to argon and carbon dioxide laser ablation. However, one should always keep in mind that if the xanthelasma extends deep into the orbicularis muscle, it may not respond to the surface ablation techniques.
  - *Chemical cauterization*: Use of chlorinated acetic acids has been found to be effective in the removal of xanthelasma. Monochloroacetic acid, dichloroacetic acid and trichloroacetic acid (TCA) have been used with good results. They dissolve the lipids and precipitate and coagulate the proteins. Dichloroacetic acid (100%) has been used with excellent results and minimal scarring.
  - *Electrodessication/radiofrequency and cryotherapy*: Xanthelasma may be destroyed with the above methods when they are superficial but may require repeated treatments. Cryotherapy may cause hypopigmentation and scarring. In comparison to the TCA application, RF ablation required fewer sessions in order to achieve more than 75% clearance of lesions; however, TCA applications were associated with fewer complications.[26]
  - *Surgical excision*: Smaller lesions may be removed with incision and dissection (uncapping), followed

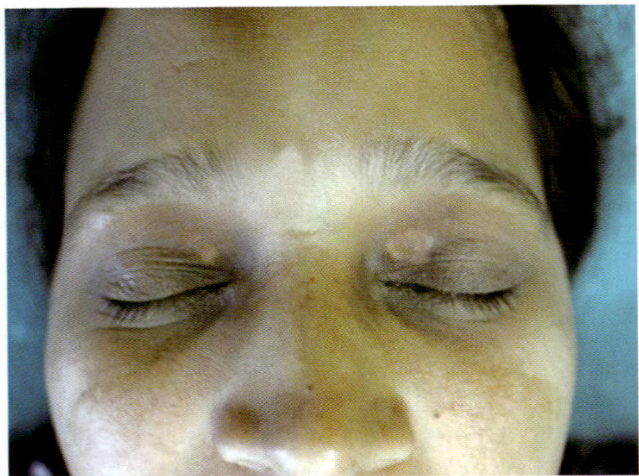

Fig. 30: Xanthelasma with depigmentation post 50% trichloroacetic acid application.

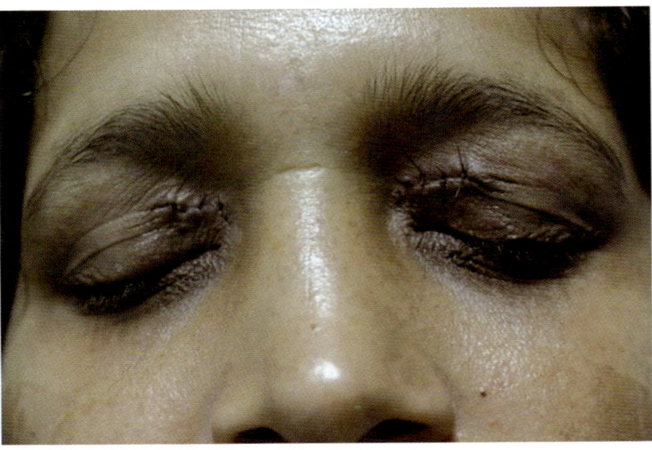

Fig. 31: Post-surgical excision of xanthelasma and depigmented area.

by replacement and suturing of the flap. In case there are small linear lesions, total excision is recommended, as the scarring would blend along with the surrounding eyelid tissue. Sometimes, excision of xanthelasma along with depigmentation caused by previous TCA application may need to be done (Figs. 30 and 31). In case of full-thickness excisions, the lower lid is more prone for development of prominent scarring, as the tissue here tends to be thicker. Simple excision of larger lesions increases the risk of eyelid retraction, ectropion and need for more complicated reconstructive procedures. Incorporation of xanthelasma removal into routine blepharoplasty may increase the risk of ectropion formation by extending the incisional limits.

- *Carbon dioxide and argon laser ablation*: Better visualization, lack of suturing, enhanced hemostasis and speed have been cited as the reasons to use this technique; however, scarring and pigmentary alterations are inevitable. A couple of case reports have shown conflicting results in the context of using Q-switched Nd:YAG (neodymium-doped yttrium aluminum garnet) in the treatment of xanthelasma.[27,28]

Basal Cell Carcinoma

Basal cell carcinoma (BCC), also called rodent ulcer, is most common in whites; however, it is not rare in the darker population.[29]

Outdoor occupations with increased sun exposure and sunburns, ionizing radiation are important risk factors. It may also arise in burn scars nevus sebaceous, and melanocytic nevus. Most commonly, it is seen on the eyelid, inner canthus and behind the ear; uncommon on limbs and back, rare on vermilion of lips, palms and soles. It starts as a small papule which later ulcerates to give rise to rolled-up edges with a crusted base and easily bleeds on slight touch.

Various modalities are useful for the treatment of BCC. For the superficial lesions, excision remains the treatment of choice. Other modalities can be used in patient where surgery is contraindicated. Excision by RF, with mild curettage has been done, which has been proved effective and yielded satisfactory therapeutic results.[30]

The procedure is described as follows:
After local infiltration, the ulcer is excised with RF kept in the cutting mode. The incision is taken in an elliptical fashion. Approximately 5 mm of the normal skin margins may also be included in the excision. After excision, the base should be gently curetted and bleeding points cauterized. Wound is then closed after undermining it with 5-0 prolene and pressure dressing should be given.

Sometimes, an extensive procedure in the form of eyelid reconstructive surgery is required. This procedure has triple objective of tumor removal, functionality and an aesthetic outcome. Problems may arise when treating BCC, due to their local growth and therefore curative excision remains the preferred choice every time. BCC of the eyelids has a high risk of recurrence. Recurrences have a considerably poorer rate of cure than the primary tumors and are more severe, aggressive, infiltrative and destructive.

Moh's Micrographic Surgery

This procedure involves complete excision of the tumors with predetermined margins in different sized BCCs.

In BCCs less than 2 cm with well-defined clinical margins, a 3-mm margin will clear the tumor in 85% of cases and a 4–5-mm margin in 95% of cases.[31-33] Large BCCs (>2 cm), with poorly defined clinical margins have high chances of recurrence due to subclinical extension. In the absence of either frozen section control or Moh's surgery, these tumors will require large predetermined margins;

even a 5-mm margin will only give complete excision of 82% of morphoeic BCCs.[31]

Patients who undergo Moh's micrographic excision for the indication of an eyelid cancer may present with a full-thickness defect of the lower lid. Hughes flap (tarsal-conjunctival flap), is a common procedure performed to address this defect. The disadvantages of this procedure is that the edge of the flap is often edematous (eye is closed) and erythematous postoperatively and a second stage is often required. Lateral stabilization of the posterior lamella with a periosteal strip and myocutaneous advancement flap is a one-step excellent procedure that avoids the complications seen with the Hughes procedure performed for the reconstruction of large full-thickness defects of the lower lid.[34]

Ex vivo confocal microscopy, a recent imaging technique is being used for assessing the tumor margins after excision of the carcinoma perioperatively.[35] Its reflectance mode with an "en face" scanning can control tumor margins of eyelid and optimize the surgical management. The advantage of this procedure in the fluorescent mode is that it does not need any contrast agent.

Grafting

The periorbital region requires different and special care in terms of reconstruction, because of its complex anatomy and important structures. Here we describe simple full-thickness grafting over eyelids.

Indications: Soft-tissue defects such as trauma, tumors, burns, radiation, infection and congenital anomalies.

Method: The method includes the following steps:

1. Prepare the bed for the graft. Incise along the edge of the scar so as to free the tissues completely. Make sure there is no bleeding from the bed once the graft is placed, because hemorrhage will separate the graft from its bed and may cause graft failure. The other common cause for graft failure is infection of the bed.
2. A piece of sterile silver paper or similar material is cut to match the shape of the area to be grafted. This is used to make sure that the donor skin is of the right shape and size. The donor skin will shrink by 10% and so should be cut slightly larger than the defect.
3. The best donor site is the upper lid as there is enough skin to spare. If the lower lid is being grafted with skin from the upper lid on the same side, it is wiser to make a small pedicle which ensures that the blood supply of the graft remains intact. If for any reason the skin from the upper lid cannot be used, the next best donor site is the area immediately behind the ear which gives a free graft. Having cut the graft using a scalpel and scissors make sure there is no fat on its undersurface; keep the graft moist in normal saline and close up the defect in the donor site. For very large defects, a split-thickness skin graft from the arm or thigh may be needed if there is not enough skin behind the ear.
4. Place graft over the bed and suture it in place. Keep some stitches long and use them to tie a bolster of sterile cotton moistened with antibiotic ointment or vaseline gauze over the graft. This keeps the graft in place resting tightly on the bed. Make two or three small holes in the graft to drain any possible hematoma.
5. Apply a bandage and leave it for at least 7 days. Systemic antibiotics should be prescribed to prevent the graft from becoming infected. Remove the bandage and the bolster with very great care after 7 days.

Chalazion Excision

Chalazion is one of the most common eyelid lesion requiring surgical excision. When the lesion presents on the anterior lid, the chalazion clamp is placed encircling the lesion and a horizontal incision is made over the mass. The cyst is evacuated, necrotic debris is curetted and fibrous tissue is excised. The skin is closed with 5-0 or 6-0 prolene. The horizontal scar blends well with the normal skin crease.

When the lesion presents on the posterior lid surface, a chalazion clamp is applied and the lid is everted. A vertical incision is then made over the mass. The procedure is then repeated as mentioned earlier. Suturing is not necessary here and bleeding can be controlled with a cautery which is usually very minimal. The advantage of using the chalazion clamp is that it provides a bloodless field while operating.

Sclerotherapy

Using sclerotherapy, smaller hemangiomas and small visible periocular veins can be safely treated with sodium tetradecyl sulfate (STD) in 1:4 dilution. However, one should be careful while injecting making sure that adequate protection of cornea is achieved as sclerosant can damage the cornea and cause ulcerations. It is always advisable to direct the injection away from the cornea and mid-face as much as possible to avoid untoward complications. Recently, a series of 50 adult female patients underwent successful sclerosing of their visible periocular veins without experiencing any ophthalmological or neurological sequelae.[36]

Medial Canthus Reconstruction

At this site, simple defects should be closed in a diamond-shaped manner. To restore the normal canthal angle in all types of medial canthus reconstruction; whether allowing it to heal with secondary intention or by using full-thickness skin graft or glabella flap,[37] the edge of the lid remnants must be attached to the posterior reflection of the medial canthal tendon.

Table 1: Showing the common complications and treatment for the same.

S. No.	Common complications	Treatment
1	Due to infiltration of anesthesia	
	▪ Local injection site reactions: swelling, bruising, pain, and pruritus	Proper technique including slow and precise injections, injecting small quantities of anesthesia using small-gauge needles, minimizing the number of needle punctures, immediate application of cold compresses or pressure to the area post-injection. Analgesics may be given
	▪ Systemic – Vasovagal syncope – Hypersensitivity reaction – Anaphylaxis	Elevate the leg end and lower the head end and monitor the vitals, intervene accordingly. Intravenous hydrocortisone, adrenaline subcutaneously, bronchodilator (nasal or oral spray) Emergency tracheotomy or Cricothyroidotomy may be required To prevent such an occurrence perform an intradermal test for lidocaine sensitivity before the procedure
2	Due to procedure. ▪ Early: Hematoma, bleeding, bruises, nerve damage causing sensory or motor loss ▪ Late: – Bacterial infection – Viral infection (reactivation of herpes simplex virus) – Dyschromia, scarring, distortion of the eyelid anatomy, permanent blindness, sepsis, secondary hemorrhage, nonhealing or delayed healing of the wound, ocular irritation, epiphora, symblepharon or loss of eyelid due to failure of healing – Exposure keratopathy – Ectropion and entropion – Trichiasis ▪ Post-blepharoplasty – Retrobulbar hemorrhage – Bulbar hematoma – Diplopia – Lagophthalmos – Scarring of conjunctiva, symblepharon – Pyogenic granuloma	Use of small-gauge needles, minimizing the number of needle punctures, immediate application of cold compresses or pressure to the area post-injection and stopping the use of alcohol, aspirin or other blood-thinning agents 7–10 days before injections. Proper skin preparation with antiseptic solution. Infection of danger zones of the face—hospital admission for intravenous antibiotics. If nidus of infection present—purulent collections should be removed either through aspiration or incision and drainage and sent for bacterial culture and sensitivity before initiating empiric antibiotic therapy (e.g. cephalosporin or doxycycline). Antiviral prophylaxis—tablet valacyclovir 500 mg twice daily to start 2–3 days before and 7 days post-procedure. To be managed with respective specialists/dermatological management Tarsorrhaphy, artificial tear drops, goggles Corrective surgeries Epilation, electrolysis, cutting the lashes, excision and suturing, etc. Referral to an ophthalmologist for appropriate management. Corrective surgeries mentioned above Corrective surgeries Excision with RF/EF

This may be achieved by placing a strong permanent suture such as 5-0 prolene through the tarsal remnant of both upper and lower lids and then attaching it to the posterior reflection of the medial canthal tendon. In most situations, the best result is obtained by allowing defects of the medial canthus that are equal above and below the caruncle to heal by secondary intention.

COMMON COMPLICATIONS AND MISTAKES TO AVOID

Complications are bound to occur in the hands of an astute and experienced dermatosurgeon, despite most of these being simple and reliable outpatient-based procedures. The risks may be minimized by careful patient selection, performing the surgeries meticulously by a trained personnel, early recognition, treatment of complications and appropriate keep pre and postoperative skin care (Table 1).

CONCLUSION

To conclude, most of the above-mentioned procedures are within the reach of an eminent dermatosurgeon provided they are done meticulously in a set-up well equipped with all the required materials and instruments.

Thus, the expectations of a digitally savvy patient of today's era of having a perfect outcome, rapid postoperative recovery with no complications can be addressed.

Tips and Pearls

Surgical tips and pearls

- Local anesthetic infiltration in the sublesional plane lifts the lesion away as a result of "ballooning" effect which protects the tarsal plate during a destructive surgery.
- While performing surgeries which necessitate the eyes to be open, use a corneal eye shield after topical anesthesia to prevent damage to the cornea.
- A 27-gauge needle and a 26-gauge-filling cannula, may be utilized to give anesthesia, which reduces the number of punctures and thereby decreases the incidence of postoperative hematomas and bruising.[38]
- As the skin of the eyelids is extremely thin and at the free margin continues with the conjunctiva, precaution should be taken to maintain the borders of the margin to prevent asymmetry due to contractures postoperatively (e.g. ectropion post-biopsy or excisional surgery around the eyes).
- During grafting, attempt should be made to harvest thin grafts in order to maintain the proper functioning and contour of the eyelids.
- Graft may be rejected in the eyelid area because of the increased folds and rugosity. In order to prevent this and corneal xerosis, a pad dressing must always be given keeping the eye in the closed position with stay sutures or proper taping.
- Cyanoacrylate glue has been successfully used in stabilizing the skin grafts and flaps in the immediate postoperative period.[39]
- While padding the eye, care should be taken to avoid inward upper eyelid push on the lower eyelid which may otherwise result in an involutional lower eyelid entropion.[40]

REFERENCES

1. Kakizaki H, Leibovitch I, Selva D, et al. Orbital septum attachment on the levator aponeurosis in Asians: in vivo and cadaver study. Ophthalmology. 2009;116(10):2031-5.
2. Chen WP. Asian blepharoplasty: update on anatomy and techniques. Ophthal Plast Reconstr Surg. 1987;3(3):135-40.
3. Shoukath S, Taylor GI, Mendelson BC, et al. The lymphatic anatomy of the lower eyelid and conjunctiva and correlation with postoperative chemosis and edema. Plast Reconstr Surg. 2017;139(3):628e-37e.
4. Jakobiec FA, Zakka FR, Tu Y, et al. Dermatofibroma of the Eyelid: Immunohistochemical Diagnosis. Ophthal Plast Reconstr Surg. Feb. 2017.
5. Betharia SM, Ramakrishna K, Sen S, et al. Dermatofibroma of the eyelid: a case report. Orbit. 2000;19(3):161-4.
6. Ovhal A. Pilonidal sinus of eyelids: A rare presentation. Indian J Dermatol Venereol Leprol. 2013;79(1):113-5.
7. Ensat F, Heinrich K, Kholosy HM, et al. A double-blind randomized prospective study comparing prilocaine versus ropivacaine in upper blepharoplasty. J Plast Reconstr Aesthet Surg. 2017;70(3):375-9.
8. Mizuno T. Treatment of suture-related complications of buried-suture double-eyelid blepharoplasty in Asians. Plast Reconstr Surg Glob Open. 2016;4(8):839.
9. Boiko EV, Chernysh VF. Medical terminology: Blepharorhaphy. Vestn Oftalmol. 2016;132(5):93-5.
10. Rees TD. Aesthetic Plastic Surgery. Philadelphia: WB Saunders Company; 1980. p. 459.
11. Park KS, Park D. Objective outcome measurement after upper blepharoplasty: An analysis of different operative techniques. Aesthetic Plast Surg. 2017;41(1):64-72.
12. Subramanian N. Blepharoplasty. Indian J Plast Surg. 2008;41(Suppl):S88-92.
13. An SH, Jin SW, Kwon YH, et al. Effects of upper lid blepharoplasty on visual quality in patients with lash ptosis and dermatochalasis. Int J Ophthalmol. 2016;9(9):1320-4.
14. Nakra T, Modjtahedi S, Vrcek I, et al. The effect of upper eyelid blepharoplasty on eyelid and brow position. Orbit. 2016;35(6):324-7.
15. Wattanakrai K, Chiemchaisri N, Wattanakrai P. Secondary blepharoplasty: Correction of the high fold. Aesthetic Plast Surg. 2016;40(6):914-20.
16. Ezzedine K, Eleftheriadou V, Whitton M, et al. Vitiligo. Lancet. 2015;386(9988):74-84.
17. Lee DY, Park JH, Lee JH, et al. Is segmental vitiligo always associated with leukotrichia? Examination with a digital portable microscope. Int J Dermatol. 2009;48(11):1262.
18. Gan EY, van Geel N, Goh BK. Repigmentation of leucotrichia in vitiligo with noncultured cellular grafting. Br J Dermatol. 2012;166(1):196-9.
19. Lee DY, Kim CR, Park JH, et al. The incidence of leukotrichia in segmental vitiligo: Implication of poor response to medical treatment. Int J Dermatol. 2011;50(8):925-7.
20. Choi YC, Kim JC. Single hair transplantation using the Choi hair transplanter. J Dermatol Surg Oncol. 1992;18(11):945-8.
21. Kasai K. Eyelash reconstruction with strip composite eyebrow graft. Ann Plast Surg. 2008;60(6):649-51.
22. Caputy GG, Flowers RS. The "pluck and sew" technique of individual hair follicle placement. Plast Reconstr Surg. 1994;93(3):615-20.
23. Rajan MA. The Eye in Leprosy 1980 to 2005: A Study of 30, 121 patients. Kolkata, India: Proceedings of the First International Symposium on Ocular Leprosy; 2005. pp. 86-9.
24. Joshua J. Surgical Management of Lagophthalmos in Leprosy. Kolkata, India: Proceedings of the First International Symposium on Ocular Leprosy; 2005. pp. 125-35.
25. Sommer F. Surgery of lower eyelid ectropion with the tarsal strip procedure, using absorbable or non-absorbable sutures for periosteal fixation. Klin Monbl Augenheilkd. 2017;234(1):59-63.
26. Reddy PK, Kunneth ST, Lakshminarayana SP, et al. Comparative study to evaluate the efficacy of radiofrequency ablation versus trichloroacetic acid in the treatment of xanthelasma palpebrarum. J Cutan Aesthet Surg. 2016;9(4):236-40.
27. Fusade T. Treatment of xanthelasma palpebrarum by 1,064-nm Q-switched Nd:YAG laser: A study of 11 cases. Br J Dermatol. 2008;158:84-7.
28. Karsai S, Schmitt L, Raulin C. Is Q-switched neodymium-doped yttrium aluminium garnet laser an effective approach to treat xanthelasma palpebrarum? Results from a clinical study of 76 cases. Dermatol Surg. 2009;35(12):1962-9.
29. Wolff K, Johnson RA, Suurmond D (Eds). Color Atlas and Synopsis of Clinical Dermatology. London: McGraw-Hill; 2005. pp. 282-9.
30. Savant SS. Radiosurgery. In: Savant SS, Shah RA, Gore D (Eds). Textbook and Atlas of Dermatosurgery and Cosmetology. Mumbai: ASCAD; 2005. pp. 305-14.
31. Breuninger H, Dietz K. Prediction of subclinical tumor infiltration in basal cell carcinoma. J Dermatol Surg Oncol. 1991;17(7):574-8.

32. Wolf DJ, Zitelli JA. Surgical margins for basal cell carcinoma. Arch Dermatol. 1987;123(3):340-4.
33. Kimyai-Asadi A, Alam M, Goldberg LH, et al. Efficacy of narrow-margin excision of well-demarcated primary facial basal cell carcinomas. J Am Acad Dermatol. 2005;53(3):464-8.
34. Perry CB, Allen RC. Repair of 50–75% full-thickness lower eyelid defects: Lateral stabilization as a guiding principle. Indian J Ophthalmol. 2016;64(8):563-7.
35. Espinasse M, Cinotti E, Grivet D, et al. "En face" ex vivo reflectance confocal microscopy to help the surgery of basal cell carcinoma of the eyelid. Clin Exp Ophthalmol. Dec. 2016.
36. Green D. Removal of periocular veins by sclerotherapy. Ophthalmology. 2001;108(3):442-8.
37. Meadows AE, Manners RM. A simple modification of the glabellar flap in medial canthal reconstruction. Ophthalmol Plast Reconstr Surg. 2003;19(4):313-5.
38. Trapasso M, Veneroso A. Local anesthesia for surgical procedures of the upper eyelid using filling cannula: our technique. Plast Reconstr Surg Glob Open. 2014;2(5):e143.
39. Jackson CM, Nguyen M, Mancini R. Use of cyanoacrylate glue casting for stabilization of periocular skin grafts and flaps. Ophthal Plast Reconstr Surg. Nov. 2016.
40. Sun MT, O'Connor AJ, Wood J, et al. Tissue engineering in ophthalmology: Implications for eyelid reconstruction. Ophthal Plast Reconstr Surg. Oct. 2016.

SUGGESTED READING

1. Collin JRO A Manual of Systematic Eyelid Surgery, 3rd edition. Oxford: Elsevier Butterworth-Heinemann; 2006.
2. Saw V, Leonard J. Dermatoses of the eye, eyelids and eyebrows. In: Griffiths C, Barker J, Bleiker T, Chalmers R, Creamer D (Eds). Rook's Texbook of Dermatology, 9th edition. New Jersey, United States: Wiley Blackwell; 2016. pp. 109.1-109.51.
3. WHO. Trichiasis Surgery for Trachoma—the Bilamellar Tarsal Rotation Procedure. Geneva: WHO; 1993.

Chapter

58

Dermatologic Surgery of the Lips

Raghunatha RR, Shashikumar BM, Savitha AS

Key Messages

- The vermilion border is a very important structure for esthetic appearance of lips and it should not be distorted during procedures.
- Incisions should be vertical all around except at the commissures.
- Dehiscence and notching of the lip can occur because of the high mobility of the area. If this occurs, conservative management may be all that is necessary; notch formation will require surgical revision.
- Lip contracture with elevation of the vermilion border may require a Z-plasty.

INTRODUCTION

The lips are graceful structures that symmetrically occupy the lower third of the facial profile. Lips represent the anterior border of the mouth. The skin of the lips contains hair, sebaceous glands, and eccrine glands. In the male, the skin of upper lip and central portion of the lower lip are hair-bearing. The vermilion border is the mucocutaneous junction between the skin and the dry mucosa of lip; lips are red in color because of lack of keratinization and the underlying capillary plexus (Fig. 1). Sebaceous glands are found in normal vermilion tissue 50% of the time, although no hair follicles are seen. The dry vermilion becomes a wet mucous membrane proximally in the oral cavity. The bulk of the tissue comprising the lips consists of striated muscle, primarily the orbicularis oris. The vasculature of the lips consists mainly of the inferior and superior labial arteries, which are the main branches of the facial artery (Fig. 2).[1]

Commonly procedures performed by dermatologists are enumerated in Table 1.

This chapter deals with surgical procedures performed on lips. Reader is also referred to the chapter on "Lip Augmentation".

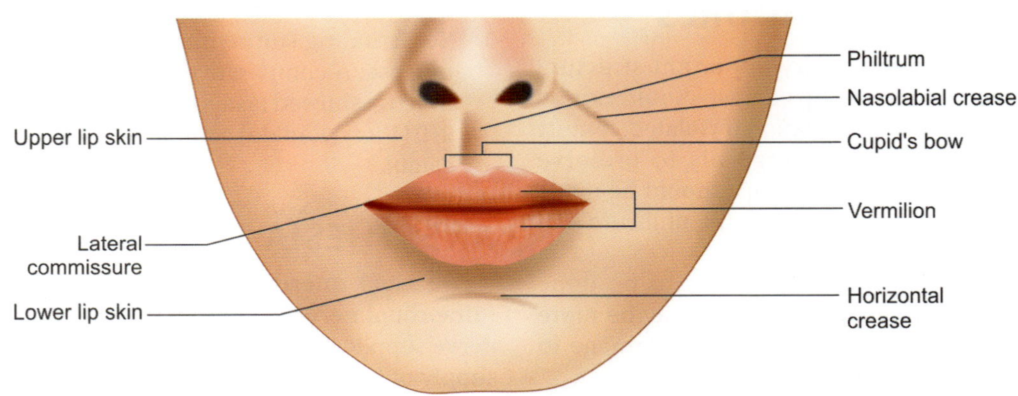

Fig. 1: Lip anatomy.

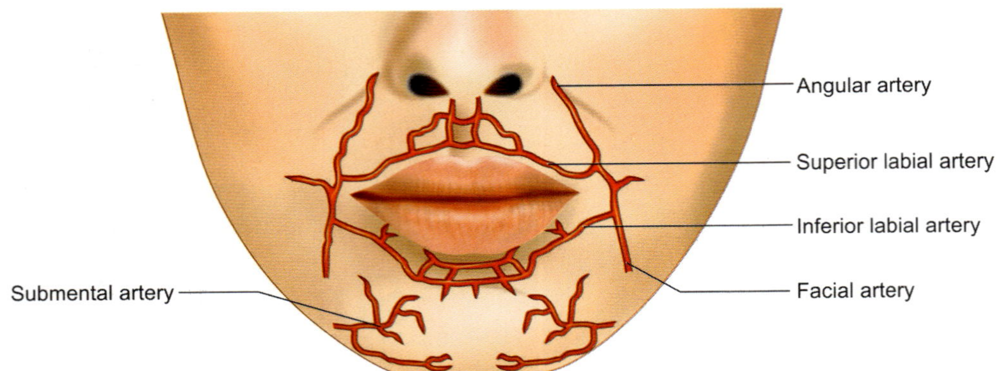

Fig. 2: Blood supply of lip.

Table 1: Commonly performed procedures by dermatologists.

Sl. No.	Conditions	Surgical methods
1.	Lip biopsy	▪ Diagnostic ▪ Therapeutic
2.	Lip vitiligo	▪ Mini-punch grafting ▪ Suction blister grafts ▪ Simple excision and closure ▪ Ultrathin split skin graft ▪ Mucosal advancement flap ▪ Noncultured epidermal cell suspension
3.	Mucous cyst	▪ Simple excision ▪ Radiofrequency ▪ Deroofing and removal ▪ Sclerotherapy
4.	Benign lesions, premalignant and malignant lesions	▪ Simple excision and closure ▪ Shave excision ▪ Flap surgery
5.	Lip enhancement surgery	▪ Autologous fat graft ▪ Fillers ▪ Dermal graft ▪ Vermilion advancement ▪ Lip implants ▪ Surgical lip lift
6.	Hair transplantation	▪ For scars on lips: post-traumatic or postsurgery cleft lips

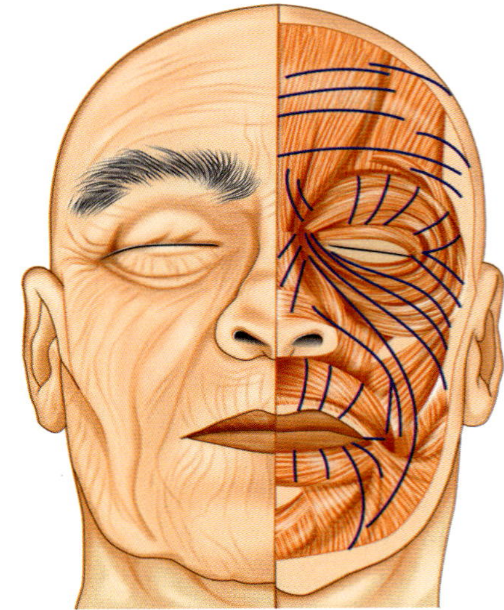

Fig. 3: Relaxed skin tension lines around the lips.

PRINCIPLES OF PROCEDURES

1. The vermilion border is a very important structure for esthetic appearance of lips and it should not be distorted. In an inevitable situation if violated, it must be precisely reconstructed surgically to preserve normal lip symmetry. Every attempt should be made to retain the normal contours, with the philtrum and Cupid's bow.
2. Undermining in the philtral area has to be done superficial to underlying muscle, and may be more difficult. Care should be taken to avoid damage to subdermal hair bulbs in male patients.
3. Incisions around lips should follow skin tension lines. Incisions should be vertical all around except at the commissures. Figure 3 illustrates the relaxed skin tension lines (RSTLs) over the face. Incisions should be made at the junction of natural boundaries to hide their placement (i.e. vermilion border, nasolabial fold, and chin horizontal crease).
4. Defects involving up to one-third of the upper or lower lip can be closed primarily in a layered fashion. Larger defects may require local or pedicle flap closure.
5. Nonirritating suture materials are preferred over the mucosa. A comparative study of suture material over mucosa showed faster wound healing with polyglactin 910 (Vicryl Rapide) compared to polyglycolic acid and catgut.[2]

ANESTHESIA

Nerve block anesthesia is better tolerated by patients. Infraorbital nerve supplies the upper lip and the mental nerve supplies the lower lip. Figure 4 illustrates the nerve supply of lips. Local infiltration of either local anesthetic or tumescent anesthetic agent may then be added for hemostasis. For details on the nerve blocks, please refer to the chapter on "Nerve Blocks".

> **Tips**
> - Marking lip margins with marker pen, methylene blue, 7-0 silk suture, or with scalpel nicks prior to administering local anesthesia can help to identify the border during closure.
> - For excision of smaller lesions, use of chalazion ring forceps helps to stabilize the lesion on the lip/tongue during biopsy/excision. The ring of the forceps also helps to achieve circumferential pressure and hemostasis providing a bloodless field during surgery. As the instrument is self-retaining, need of the assistant is eliminated.
> - Stabilization of the lip may also be achieved with dental rolls (or rolled gauze) between the lip and gums, suture ligatures temporarily placed, or instruments like long artery forceps.
> - Airway maintenance is of utmost importance both during and after surgical procedures. Postoperative edema may impair the airway.

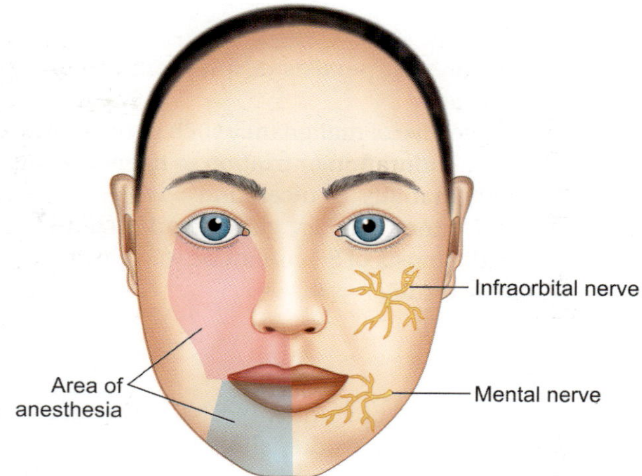

Fig. 4: Nerve supply of lip.

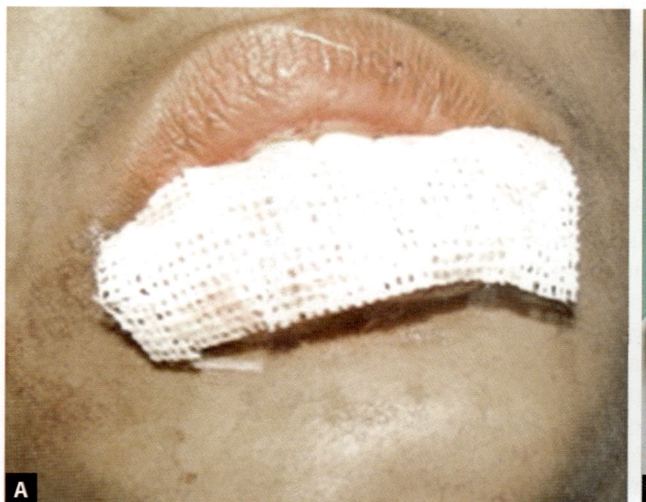

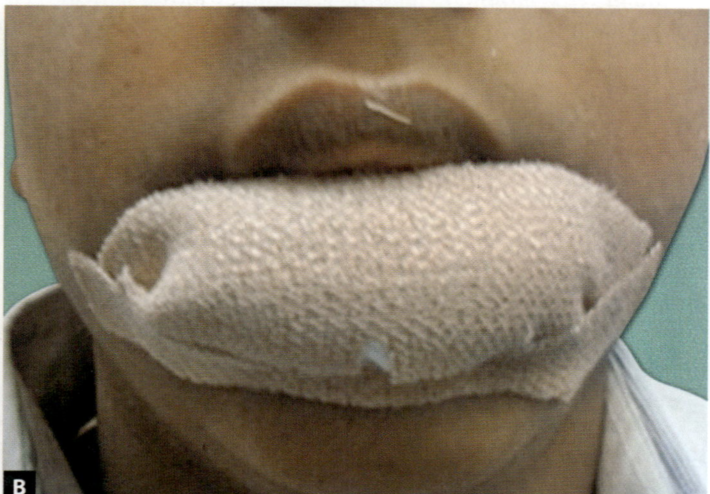

Figs. 5A and B: Postoperative dressing in layers.

COMMON PREOPERATIVE AND POSTOPERATIVE INSTRUCTIONS AND CARE

- Rule out any foci of infection at the site of surgery
- Take an informed consent including for photographs
- Lignocaine test dose to be given prior to procedure
- Surgical preparation with povidone-iodine and spirit.

Postoperative Dressing and Care

Dressing is to be applied in layers, first topical antibiotic followed by sterile vaseline gauze, cotton gauze and cotton pad in that order (Figs. 5A and B).

Antibiotics and analgesics are prescribed for 5–7 days. Patient is advised liquid diet on the day of procedure followed by soft food to be taken for few days carefully with a spoon and liquids with a straw to prevent wetting of the dressing. Dressing to be changed once in 2–3 days after surgery and may be left open after 7 days depending on the healing. For small lesions of the lip, no dressing is needed.

Dehiscence and notching of the lip can occur because of the high mobility of the area. If this occurs, conservative management may be all that is necessary; notch formation will require surgical revision. Lip contracture with elevation of the vermilion border may require a Z-plasty. In females, the use of lip color may provide the finishing touch to conceal scars and give a more pleasing appearance.

Lip Biopsy

Lip biopsy is performed to identify the histopathology of a visible oral lesion or to assist in the diagnosis of a systemic disorder like Sjögren syndrome (SS) or sarcoidosis. Like any other skin biopsy either a punch biopsy, incisional or excisional biopsy can be performed on the lip with a scalpel. Using a chalazion forceps helps to stabilize the biopsy site as well as helps to achieve hemostasis.

Indications

- Any oral lesion that persists despite removal of any irritative stimulus
- Findings suggestive of malignancy such as red or white discoloration, induration or fixation to deeper tissues, rapid growth, friability, or ulceration
- Submucosal minor salivary gland biopsy should be done if the diagnosis of SS cannot be made by history and serologic testing.

Anesthesia

Lip biopsy is typically done under local anesthesia, using 1% lidocaine with 1:100,000 adrenaline. Topical anesthetic sprays are not usually sufficient for anesthesia in the case of biopsies. Inject the lip at the desired biopsy location using a 27- or 30-gauge needle and a 1- to 3-mL syringe.

Ensure that adequate lighting is available either a head mirror, headlight, or surgical light.

Procedure

After surgical preparation, plan and mark the elliptical incision before infiltration. Orientation of the ellipse should take into account the vascular and neural structures in the area, as well as any functional or cosmetic concerns. The incision should parallel the long axis of the lip to most easily allow the recommended 3:1 length: width ratio. In large resections, the vermilion of the lip may be reduced or the white roll at the vermilion junction may be retracted. Incisions perpendicular to the long axis cause less of this distortion but may require extension beyond the vermilion border or onto gingival tissue to maintain the 3:1 ratio. After infiltration, the incision is done along the markings. Delicately grasp the edge of the ellipse with fine forceps. Dissect beneath the ellipse with fine sharp scissors. The depth of dissection should be determined by the lesion characteristics. In most mucosal lesions, the plane of dissection is in the layer that contains the minor salivary glands, leaving the orbicularis oris muscle intact. Alternately, a punch of optimum size can be used to take a biopsy. The specimen is sent to the pathology laboratory in the appropriate tissue media. Obtain hemostasis via manual pressure, silver nitrate cautery, or electrocautery. Closure of the wound may be aided by circumferential undermining, depending on the size of the resultant defect. Suture the mucosa to reapproximate the edges. Postoperative dressing is not required usually.

VITILIGO SURGERY OVER LIP MUCOSA

Lip vitiligo has much more impact on the social and psychological well-being of the individual compared to localized vitiligo elsewhere, however, small it may be. Repigmentation of lip is slower with medical lines of management due to the lack of hair follicles, thus surgical treatments become essential in most of the cases of lip vitiligo.

Miniature Punch Grafts

Extraction of punch grafts from the donor area is similar to standard procedure. The 1 mm punches are used for both donor and recipient areas. Uniform wells are created using 1 mm punches at an average distance of 0.5–1 mm. Grafts should be placed along the margins to prevent perigraft halo. Application of glue is optional, if needed, should be applied after hemostasis is achieved, to prevent the glue getting entry to the punch thereby causing graft rejection (Figs. 6A and B). Bleeding is controlled by applying pressure with wet gauze. Dressing and postoperative care as mentioned earlier. Phototherapy is advised once the dressing is removed. Cobblestone appearance is the most common complication noticed.

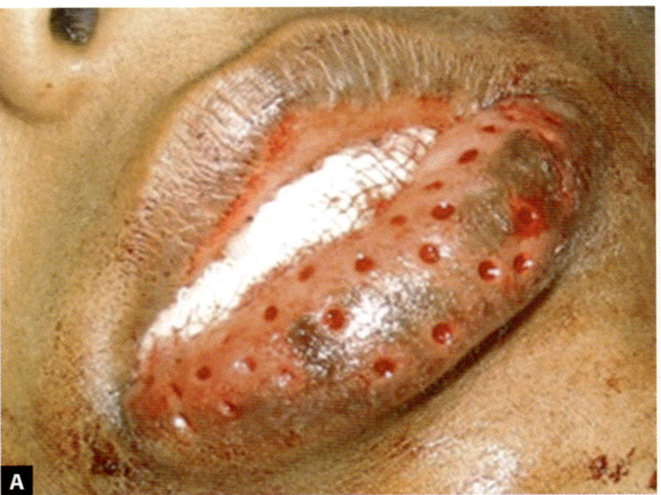

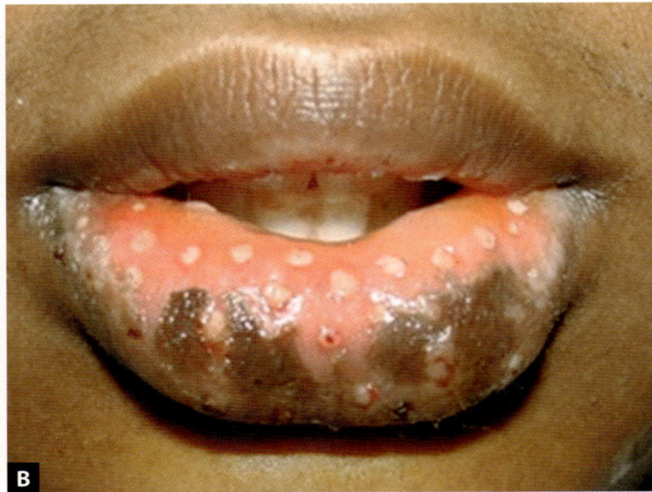

Figs. 6A and B: (A) Uniform wells created using 1 mm punch at the recipient area; (B) Grafts in place and taken up 5 days after grafting without glue.

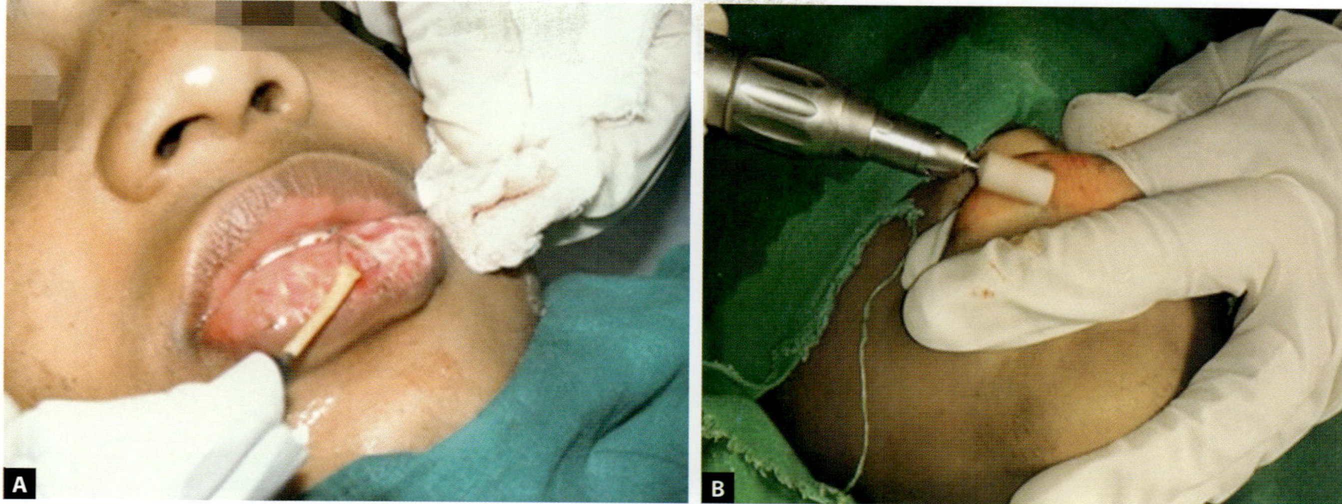

Figs. 7A and B: De-epithelialization of lip. (A) Triangular loop of radiofrequency; (B) Motor dermabrasion.

Suction Blister Graft

Induction of blister and removal of graft from donor area are similar to standard procedure of harvesting suction blister. The lip as a recipient bed can be prepared either with triangular probe of radiofrequency in cut-coagulation mode with low energy and with a gentle and fast movement of the probe very superficially (Fig. 7A), erbium:yttrium-aluminum-garnet (Er:YAG) or carbon dioxide laser by superficially deepithelializing the tough epidermal layer followed by superficial dermabrasion by either manual or motor dermabrader (Fig. 7B). The dermabrasion should always be superficial and optimal for graft uptake, to prevent possibility of hematoma formation and for faster healing. The graft is then gently placed on the lip with dermal side down (Figs. 8A and B). Ensure that the edges are smoothened out to avoid folds and incurvings of borders, otherwise there will be thickening of the graft due to rolling of edges (Fig. 8C). The grafts should be placed to cover the entire depigmented area and also about 2–3 mm from the margins (Fig. 8D).

The grafts can be secured in place by application of glue to the edges, or by stay sutures with 5-0 or 4-0 suture material of choice. A hypodermic needle can be fixed to the glue for easier and nonmessy application (Fig. 9).

Dressing and postoperative care as discussed earlier.

Known complications are irregular, uneven pigmentation and thickening of grafts (Fig. 10).

Excision and Closure for Small Depigmented Areas

The borders of the area to be excised have to be marked before infiltrating the lesion or giving the block (Fig. 11A). This procedure is ideal only for smaller or linear lesions which can be excised and sutured without distorting the shape of the lip. A sponge holding forceps can be used to achieve homeostasis during the procedure. Care should be taken not to crush and traumatize the lips. Incision is put along the premarked lines and the vitiliginous area excised (Figs. 11B and C). Wound edges are approximated with running sutures or percutaneous interrupted sutures (Fig. 11D). Undermining to be done where deemed necessary. Caution to be exercised to prevent lip inversion or distortion of the shape by undermining.

Ultrathin Graft

Conventional thin split-thickness skin grafting technique continues to be the most commonly practiced and also the most successful amongst all methods of vitiligo surgery.[3] With ultrathin grafts without any dermal component present, excellent results can be achieved at both the recipient as well as donor sites (Fig. 12). Ultrathin grafts are harvested either with a dermatome or Silver's knife. It needs a properly trained person to do the procedure. The quality of the grafts can be gauged by means of their translucent nature and by their ability to float on isotonic saline. The edges should not be rolled upon itself.[4] The graft placement and follow-up are similar to that of suction blister grafting, however, the graft has to be fixed with sutures, preferably 5-0 absorbable.

Mucosal Advancement Flap[5]

The mucosal advancement flap is a novel procedure practiced as a therapeutic modality to cover excised lip lesions of varying etiologies. This principle has been applied to treat lip vitiligo as an innovative surgical technique by the author. The principle of mucosal advancement flap is shown in Figure 13.

After the standard surgical precautions and preparation of the part, the depigmented patch is marked. Two

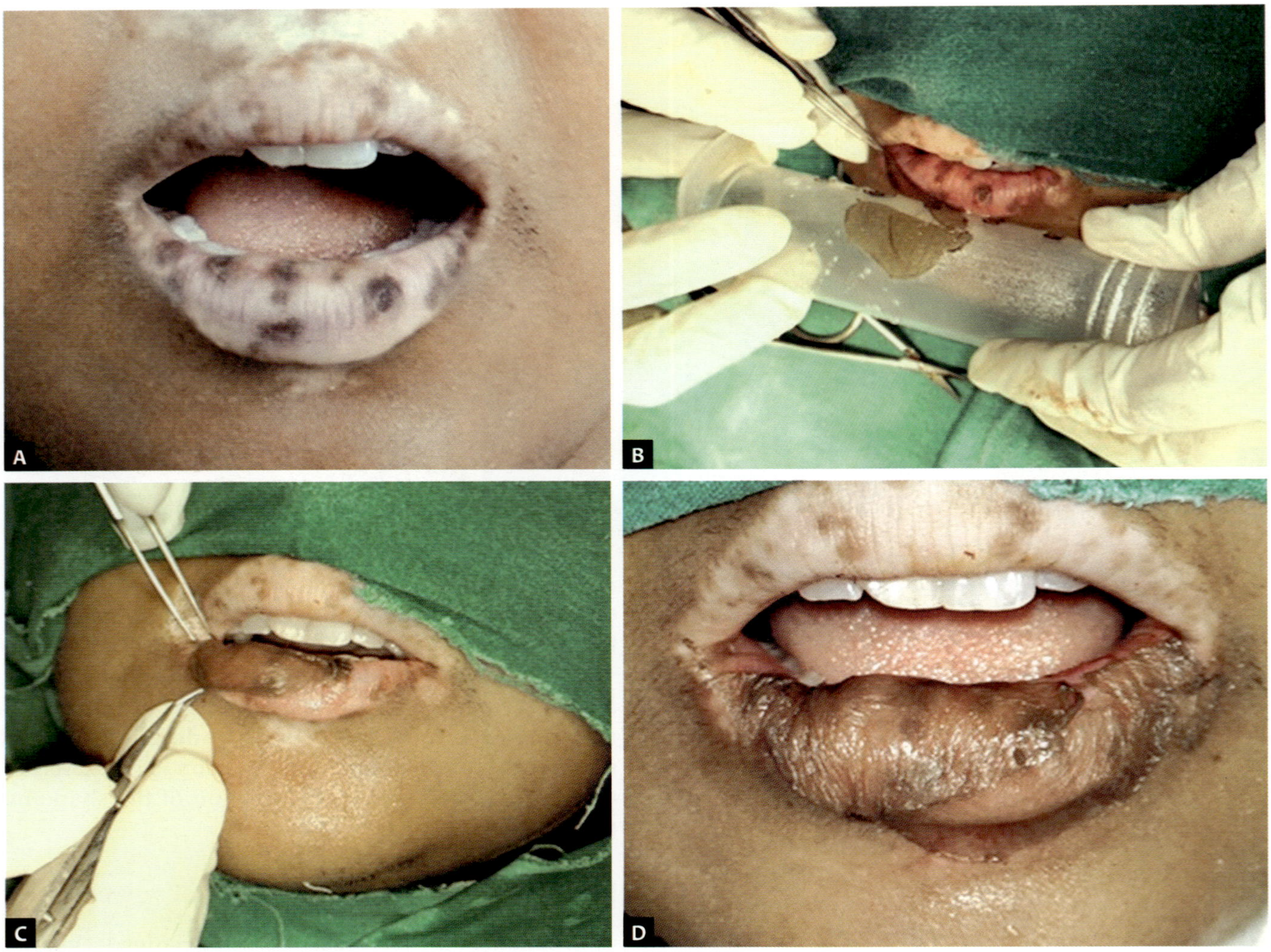

Figs. 8A to D: (A) Preprocedure; (B) Placing graft on prepared lip; (C) Smoothening out the edges; (D) Immediately postprocedure.

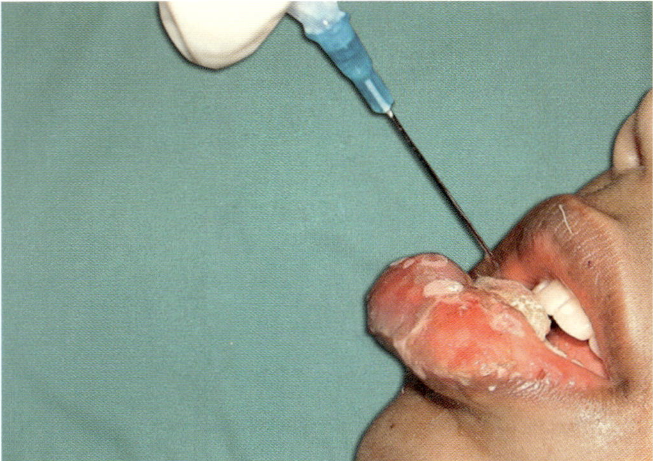

Fig. 9: Securing with glue.

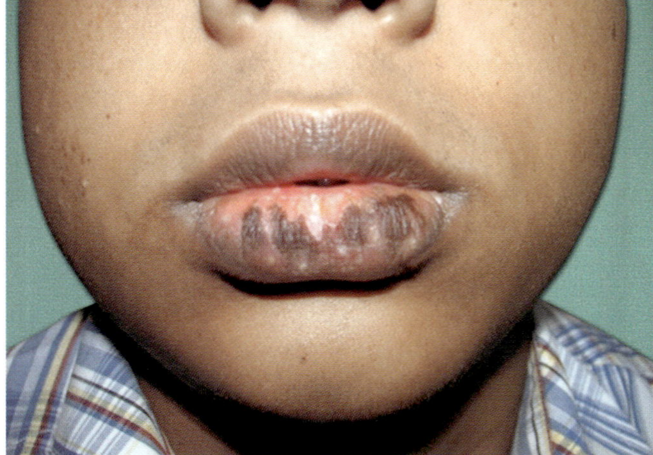

Fig. 10: Irregular and uneven pigmentation in postblister graft.

perpendicular lines are drawn from the lateral edges of the depigmented lesion over the lower lip, extending downward up to 1 cm above the junction of gingivolabial sulcus. Burrows triangles are marked on either side at the lower end of the marking, 2 cm above the anterior sulcus (Fig. 14). The area is infiltrated with 2% xylocaine

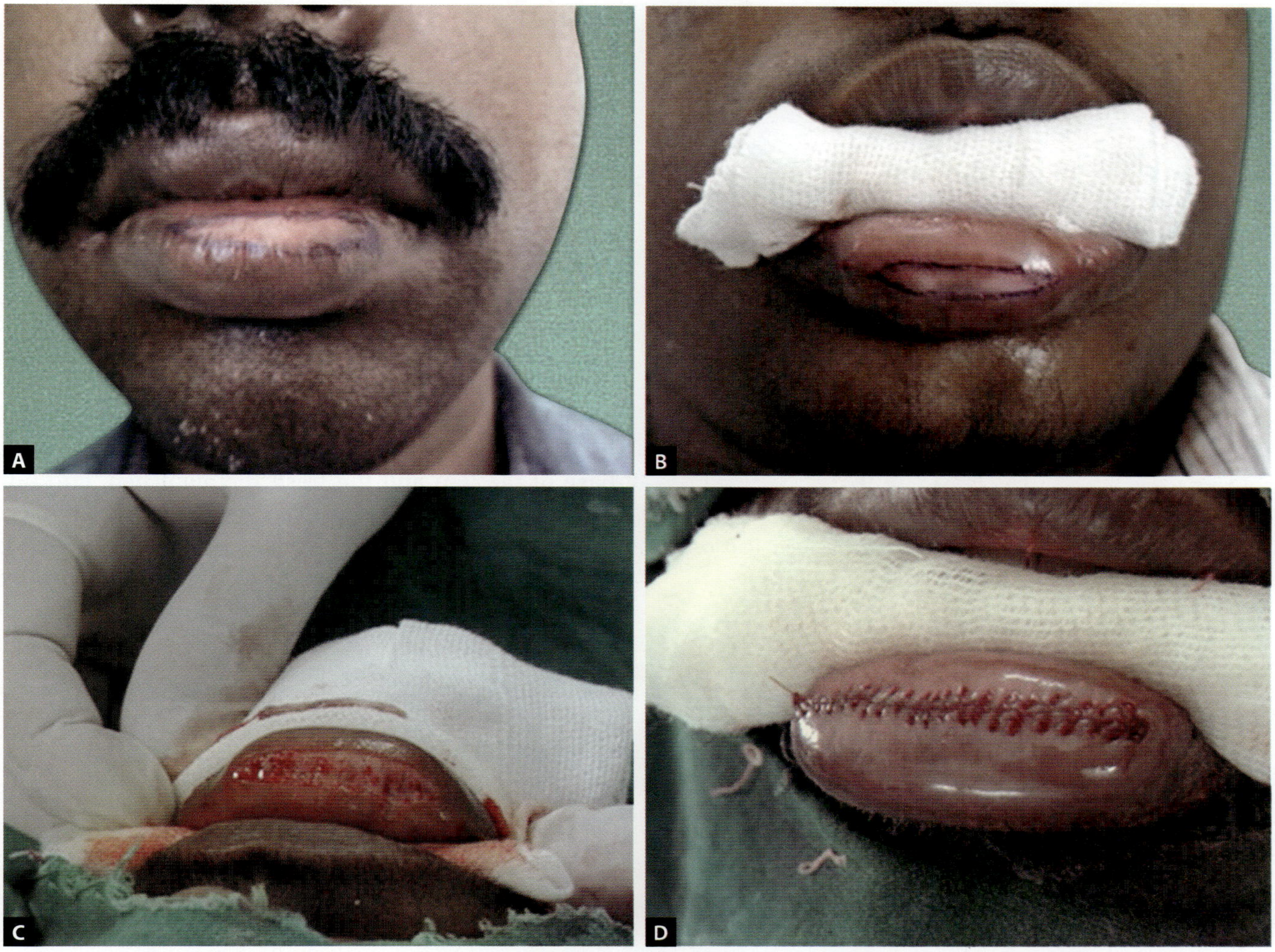

Figs. 11A to D: (A) Marking the area before infiltration; (B) Local infiltration; (C) Vitiliginous area excised; (D) Primary closure with continuous sutures.

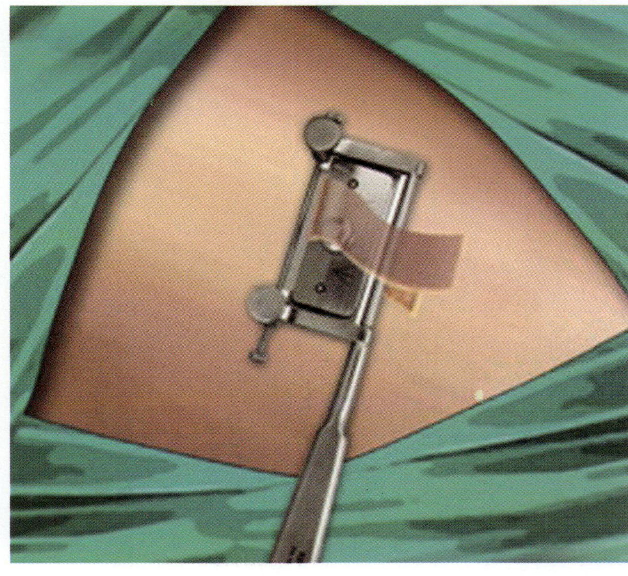

Fig. 12: Ultrathin split-thickness graft obtained from the upper thigh.

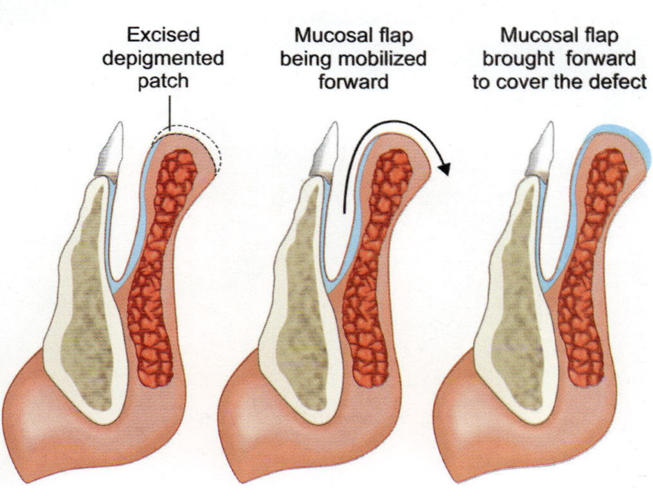

Fig. 13: Principle of mucosal advancement flap.

hydrochloride, and an incision is made along the markings. Depigmented mucosa is excised (Figs. 15A and B). The flap is dissected in the submucosal plane up to 2 cm above the gingivolabial sulcus (Fig. 15C). A Burrow's triangle is excised to prevent possible dog ear deformity as a result of mucosal advancement. The dissected mucosal flap with the intact attachment at the lower end is advanced and mobilized forward to cover the excised defect and sutured with preferably absorbable sutures (Figs. 15C and D).

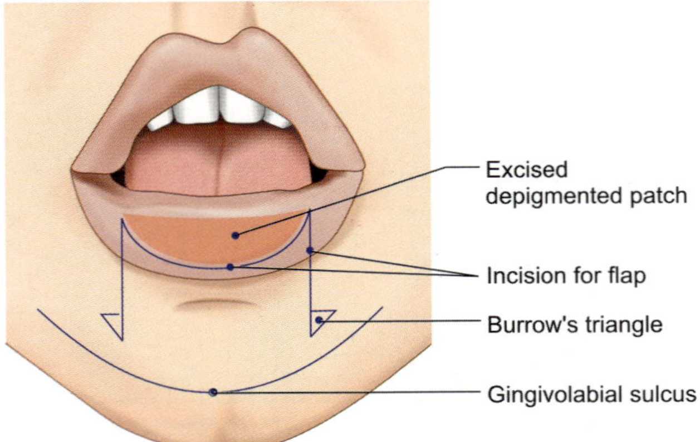

Fig. 14: Surgical markings for mucosal advancement flap inside the oral cavity.

The possible complications of the mucosal advancement flap are lip inversion, flap necrosis, rounded appearance of the vermilion, and decreased anterior-posterior dimensions of the lip. These complications can be avoided by taking the following steps: sufficient length of flap mobilization with a Burrow's triangle and proper undermining in the subcutaneous plane to avoid lip inversion, ensuring sufficient blood supply from the base of the flap and the fresh recipient bed, and not disturbing the vermilion and excising the lesion of the lip clearly away from the vermilion. This procedure being an innovative and skilled-surgical procedure, it may be

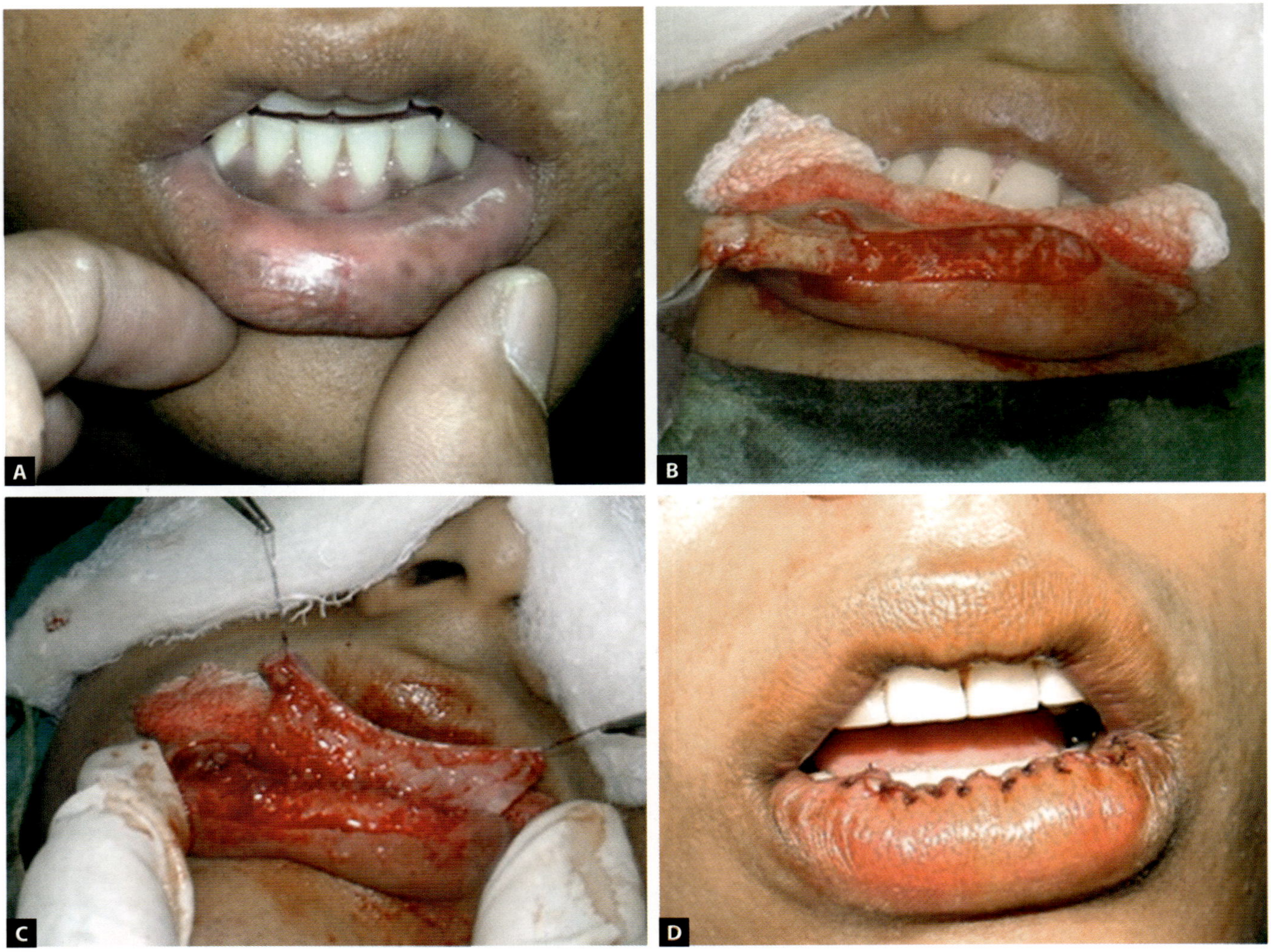

Figs. 15A to D: (A) Vitiligo patch on lower lip mucosa; (B) Excision of depigmented mucosa; (C) Mobilized mucosal flap; (D) The defect is sutured with 5-0 Vicryl interrupted sutures.

Table 2: List of transplantation procedures commonly used for lip vitiligo with their advantages, disadvantages, and outcome in various studies.[6]

Type of grafts for lip leukoderma	*Advantages*	*Disadvantages*	*Summary of the outcome of literature analysis for surgical treatment of lip vitiligo [Successful/total (%)]*
Thin and ultrathin split-thickness skin grafts (STSGs)	High success rates with immediate results, but not a best choice	Color and texture mismatch, donor area scarring, recipient area contracture, occurrence of dermatological diseases, such as psoriasis, malignant transformation, expertise skill needed. Lip may look heavy with stuck on appearance	2/2 (100%)
Suction blister grafting (SBG)	The ease of procedure, the high success rate, and the excellent cosmetic results. No scarring at donor site as the graft consists of only epidermis	Time-consuming, hyperpigmentation at the recipient site and donor site, unsuitable for larger areas. Lip should not be covered partially. Even if the lesion is small grafting should be done for the entire lip to have uniformity in color	40/45 (88.88%)
Miniature punch grafting	Easy to perform and can take care of a relatively larger vitiligo area	Cobblestone appearance, polka-dot appearance, depigmentation of the grafts, perigraft halo, graft rejection, hypertrophic scarring, and variegated appearance with color mismatch at the recipient sites, scarring at the donor site. Usually requires postsurgical medical management	102/132 (77.21%)
Noncultured melanocyte grafting of epidermal suspensions	Larger area can be treated with a smaller size of donor graft. Excellent color match	Time-consuming, need for specialized equipment, such as centrifuge, incubator, and reagents, training and experience to obtain standardized uniform results and hence there is an initial learning curve. The epidermal cell suspension may run away and produce irregular pigmentation. Not a best procedure for the lip compared to other sites	6/14 (42.9%)
Cultured "pure" melanocytes (CM) and epithelial grafts (CE)	Large area can be treated in a single session	Time-consuming and labor intensive technique, requires a sophisticated laboratory setup for cell culture	Not available at all places except in specialized centers
Micropigmentation	Relatively inexpensive, simple office procedure with instant results may be performed for vitiligo of the angle of the mouth where graft placement is difficult	Difficult to adjust or homogenize tone of skin color, pigment migration, bluish discoloration due to Tyndall effect. It is almost an obsolete procedure	100%. However, the author's experience does not recommend this since the long-term results are poor with undesirable results such as color change of pigmentation. It should be discouraged due to availability of much better procedures
Mucosal advancement flap	Single-case report. Best and suitable graft to replace the excised mucosa due to various causes, since it is a natural replacement of lip mucosa with oral mucosal tissue	If performed in a suitable case where the patch is small, the results are excellent with complete natural appearance and function. Is a skilled procedure and requires surgical expertise	Though a single-case report in published literature, author's experience is good with 8 cases performed in a situation where other grafting techniques have failed

practiced only in special situations where other methods have failed or not suitable (Table 2).

PROCEDURES FOR MUCOUS CYST

Mucous cyst arises either due to extravasation of mucus from the damaged salivary gland duct or due to obstruction of the duct. Lower lip is the most common site for mucous cyst. High rate of recurrences are common as feeding mucous glands are left behind. Modalities of treatment include the following:

Excision and Closure

There are various modalities of excision of mucous cyst as explained below.

Deroofing the Cyst

It is always better to mark the margins of the cyst before infiltration of anesthesia. After infiltration, the mucocele can be stabilized with chalazion forceps. The cyst roof is deroofed with scissors or scalpel blade and all contents removed. Then the base of the cyst is electrofulgrated. After removal of chalazion forceps, the wound is left open to heal by secondary intention. The risk of recurrence is slightly higher with this method.

Simple Excision and Closure

After marking the margins of the cyst and infiltrating the surrounding skin with lignocaine 1% with adrenaline (Fig. 16A). A linear or elliptical incision is placed over

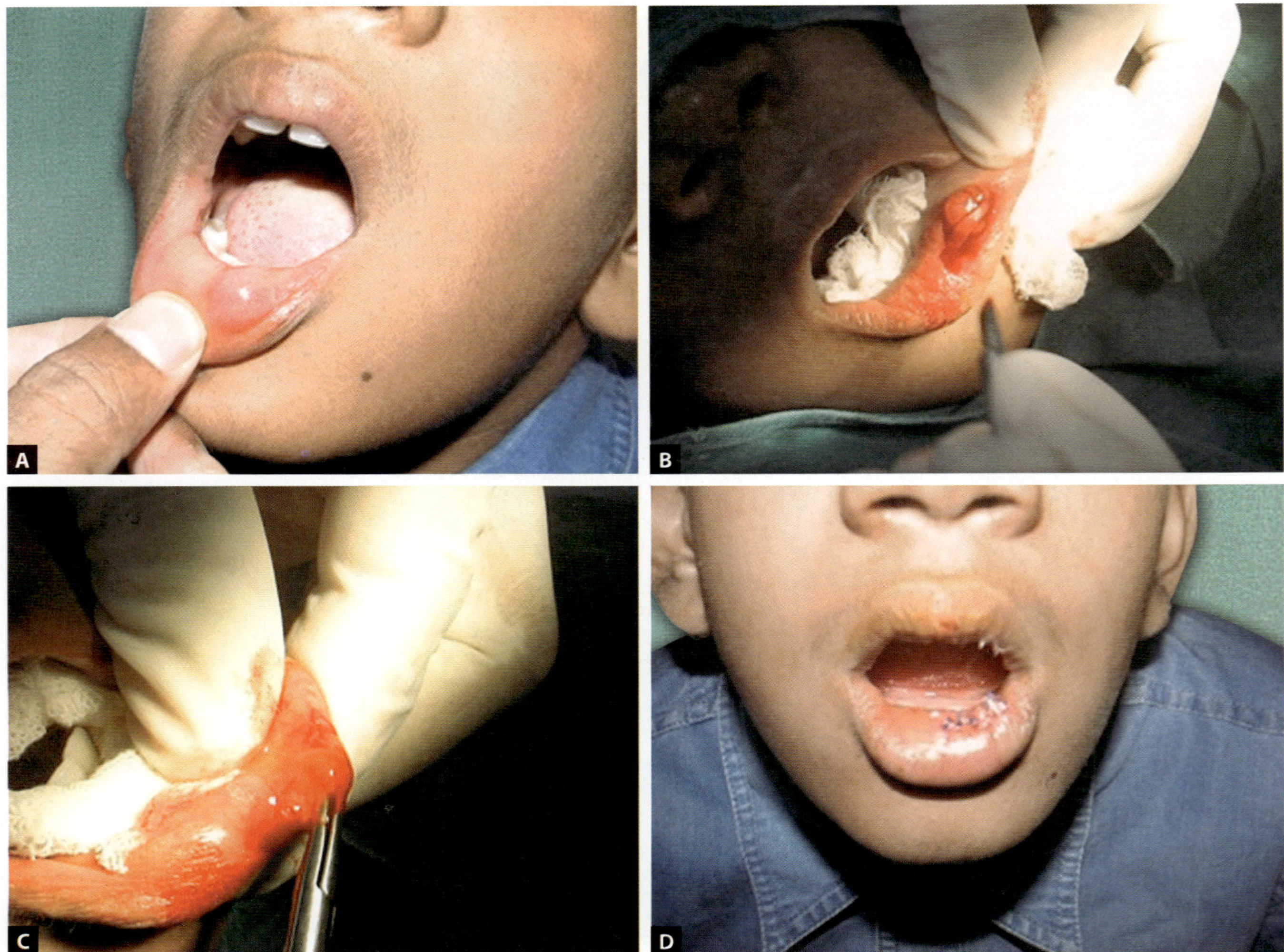

Figs. 16A to D: (A) Mucous cyst over lower lip; (B) The cyst pops out when the mucosa is incised; (C) If the cyst ruptures remove the cyst wall and sack in total; (D) Mucosa sutured with prolene 5-0 with simple interrupted sutures.

the cyst superficially taking care not to rupture the cyst preferably. When the mucosa is incised, the cyst pops out (Fig. 16B) or dissect it carefully to excise it in total. If the cyst ruptures remove the cyst wall and sack in total (Fig. 16C). The cyst is removed and mucosa sutured with prolene 5-0 with simple interrupted sutures or with absorbable sutures (Fig. 16D). Healing is complete in a week without any scar (Figs. 17A and B).

Complete Excision

Mucous cysts can be completely excised and sutured. The rate of recurrence will be almost nil with this method. After marking the margins of the cyst and infiltrating the surrounding skin with lignocaine 1% with adrenaline. An elliptical incision is placed around the mucous cyst and the cyst is dissected from the surrounding tissue to be removed in total. After achieving hemostasis by compression, sutures are placed (Figs. 18A to D).

Application of Caustic Chemicals

The caustic agents like phenol can be used to treat mucoceles. No local anesthesia is required. Under aseptic precautions, a very small quantity of 88% phenol is injected into the cyst cavity using insulin syringes. No dressing is given afterwards. Patients are given analgesics post-procedure for 1 day (Fig. 19).[7]

Sclerotherapy

Sclerosing agents like polidocanol or sodium tetradecyl sulfate can also be injected into the mucous cysts. The minimum concentration required to produce desired results with least complications is 1.5%. In those patients who show partial response in initial sittings, concentration can be increased to 2%. Common complications include pain on injection, erythema and healing with post-inflammatory hyperpigmentation (Figs. 20A and B).

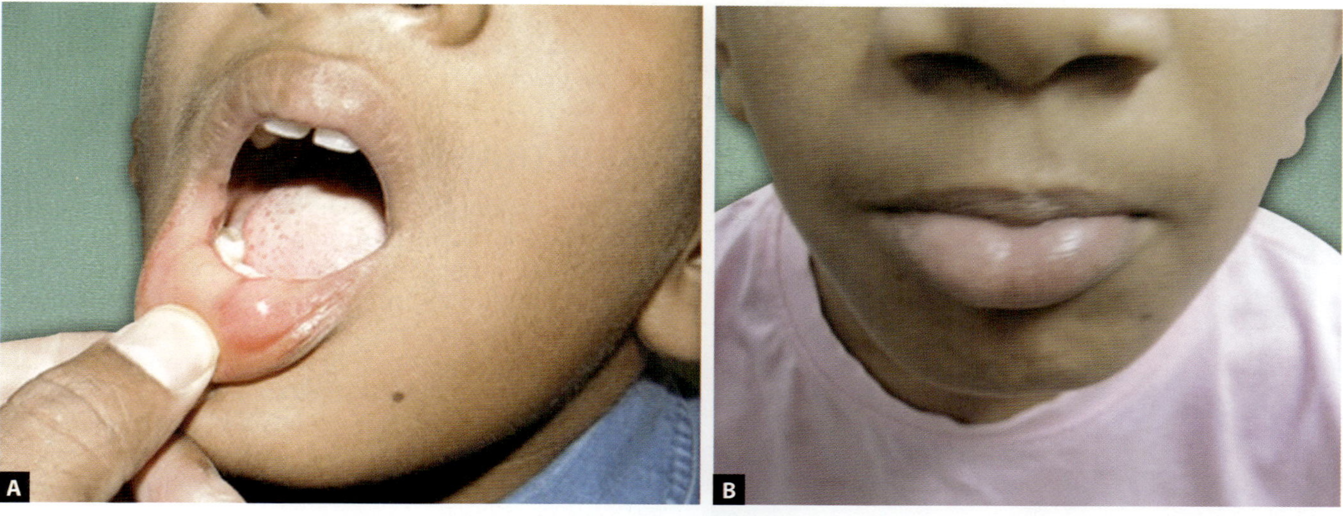

Figs. 17A and B: Healing is complete in a week without any scar.

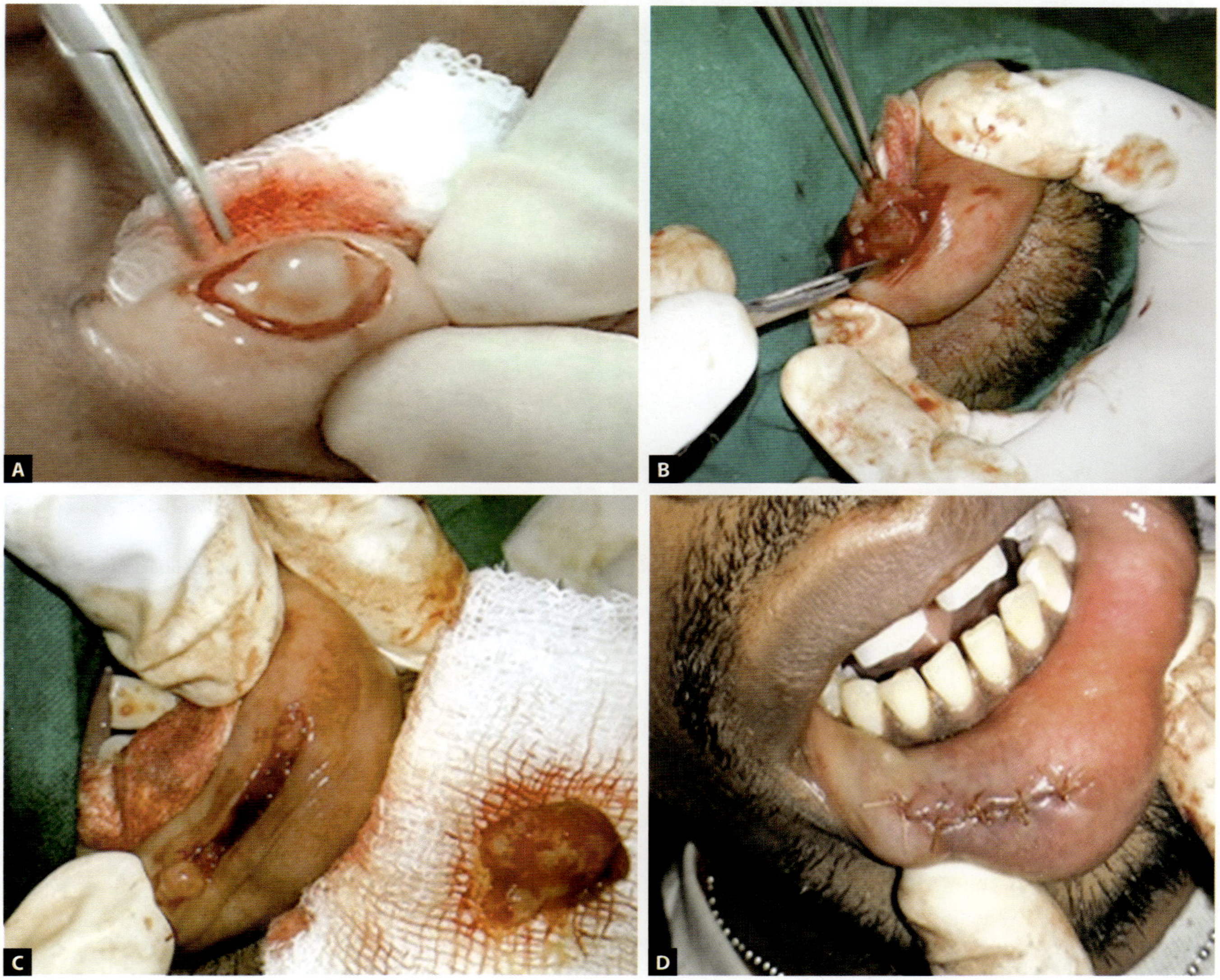

Figs. 18A to D: (A) Elliptical incision is placed around the mucous cyst; (B) The cyst is dissected from the surrounding tissue; (C) The cyst is removed in total; (D) Wound closed with interrupted sutures.

Removal of Superficial Growths

Small superficial lesions around the lip removed by shave excision with a number 15 blade heal well by secondary intention with excellent cosmetic results (Fig. 21). Small excision or punch biopsy also will heal satisfactorily by secondary intention but may heal more rapidly by simple primary closure.

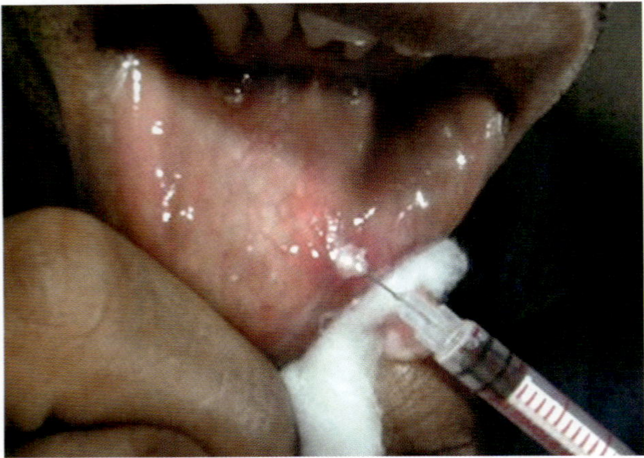

Fig. 19: Injection of phenol into the mucous cyst.

HAIR TRANSPLANTATION

Hair transplantation on upper lip is frequently requested by patients for scars: post-traumatic or postsurgical (due to cleft lip surgery). Occasionally, patients seek hair transplantation for moustache enhancement. While a detailed discussion is out of scope of this chapter, the following salient points need to be kept in mind:

- Donor hair can be obtained from scalp or beard since the number of grafts needed is small, extraction method is preferred for harvesting.
- Direction of hairs varies according to location; in the center of the lip, hairs grow vertically down, but grow downwards and laterally in the lateral parts of the lip.
- Only single-hair units are preferred.
- Lip is a mobile and vascular area and hence graft placement and stabilization cause challenges.

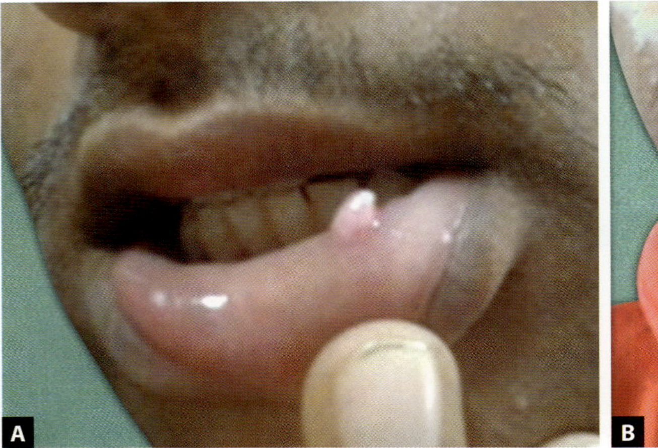

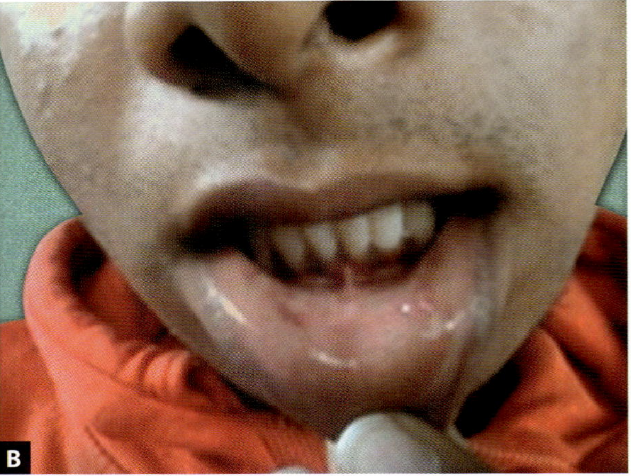

Figs. 20A and B: Before and 1 week after sclerosant injection.
Source: Courtesy of Dr Shruthi C, Department of Dermatology, Bangalore Medical College and Research Institute, Bengaluru.

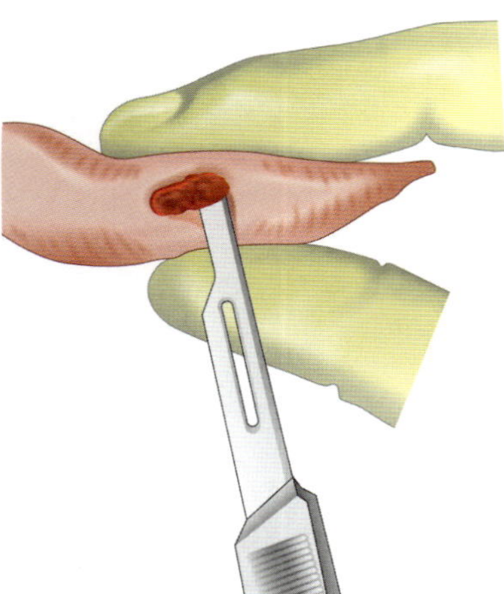

Fig. 21: Schematic diagram of shave excision.

- Patient should be advised to avoid undue movements of the lips for 5 days till grafts get stabilized.
- Postoperative edema may occur.

Despite these challenges, results are satisfying.

PEARLS

- Lips are an important component of facial aesthetics. While performing procedures the shape of the lip and vermilion border should be maintained.
- Nerve blocks are better tolerated by patients.
- Use of chalazion ring forceps helps to stabilize the lesion on the lip/tongue during biopsy/excision and provides adequate hemostasis.
- Airway maintenance is of utmost importance both during and after surgical procedures.
- Marking lip margins with marker pen, methylene blue, 7-0 silk suture, or with scalpel nicks prior to administering local anesthesia can help identify the border during closure.

REFERENCES

1. Greenway HT. The lips and oral cavity. In: Roenigk RK, Ratz JL, Roenigk HH (Eds). Roenigk's Dermatologic Surgery: Current Techniques in Procedural Dermatology, 3rd edition. New York: Informa Healthcare; 2007. pp. 231-8.
2. Mirković S, Durdević-Mirković T, Branislav B, et al. Choice of surgical suture material used in oral cavity-clinical study. Med Pregl. 2010;63(7-8):497-501.
3. Khunger N. Recent advances in the surgical treatment of vitiligo. In: Ghosh S (Ed). Recent Advances in Dermatology. India: Jaypee Brothers Medical Publishers (P) Ltd; 2007. pp. 319-40.
4. Majid I, Imran S. Ultrathin split-thickness skin grafting followed by narrowband UVB therapy for stable vitiligo: an effective and cosmetically satisfying treatment option. Indian J Dermatol Venereol Leprol. 2012;78:159-64.
5. Reddy RR, Basavapura SM, Chandramouli GA. Mucosal advancement flap: an innovative surgical technique for treatment of lip vitiligo. Dermatol Surg. 2013;39(2):334-7.
6. Shilpa K, Sacchidanand S, Savitha S, et al. A study of the outcome of primary excision and closure technique in the management of lip leukoderma in 30 patients. J Cutan Aesthet Surg. 2016;9(1):20-6.
7. Sacchidanand S, Sujaya SN, Purohit V. Phenolisation as a mode of treatment of mucosal cysts. J Cutan Aesthet Surg. 2012;5(3):210-1.

Chapter 59

Surgery on the Ear

Raghunatha Reddy, Savitha AS, Shashikumar BM

Key Messages

- Repair of cleft ear lobe and keloid surgeries are the commonly performed procedures on the ear.
- Dermatologists with basic surgical skills and regular dermatosurgical practice can safely perform these procedures.
- Nonsurgical closure techniques are better avoided in earlobe repair due to the weak scar, high recurrence rates and ugly scar following non-surgical closure.
- It is preferable to avoid simple closure techniques and advisable to practice complex closure techniques like unilateral Z-plasty and lower border advancement flap repair to prevent recurrences and to avoid lower border notching.
- Recurrence rate of earlobe keloid is much less after surgery and postsurgical preventive measures compared to other sites, making it more amenable for surgical reduction and management by dermatologists.

EAR ANATOMY

The parts of the ear are depicted in Figure 1.

Most of the auricle has a cartilaginous framework, with the lobule being the only part not supported by cartilage.

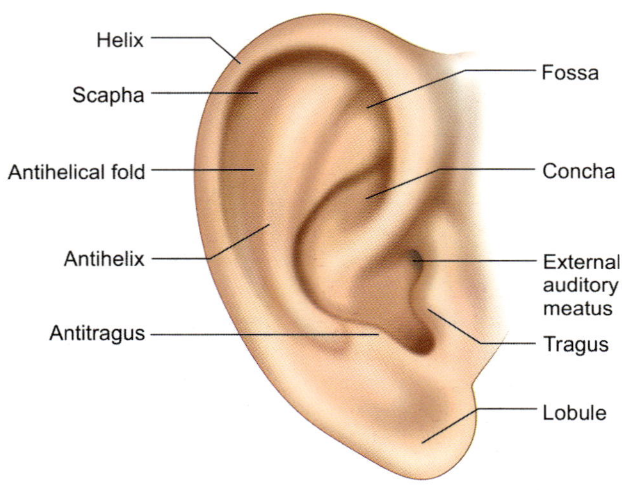

Fig. 1: Anatomy of external ear.

Sensory Innervation of External Ear (Figs. 2 and 3)

The sensory innervation of the external ear is composed of the following:

- The greater auricular nerve supplies the lower two-thirds of the anterior and posterior external ear

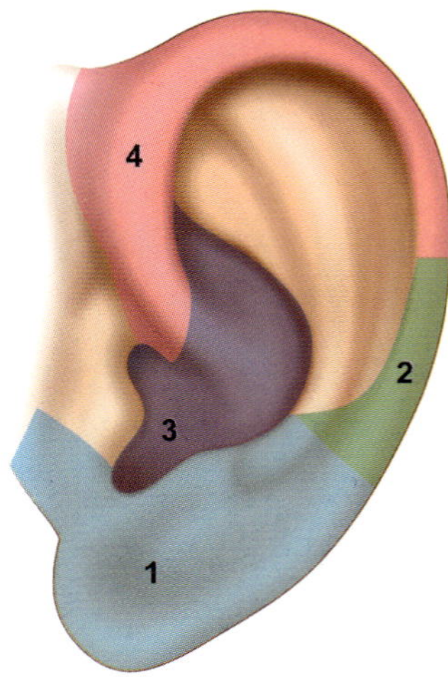

Fig. 2: Sensory supply of external ear: (1) Greater auricular nerve; (2) Lesser occipital nerve; (3) Auricular branch of vagus nerve; (4) Auricular culotemporal nerve.

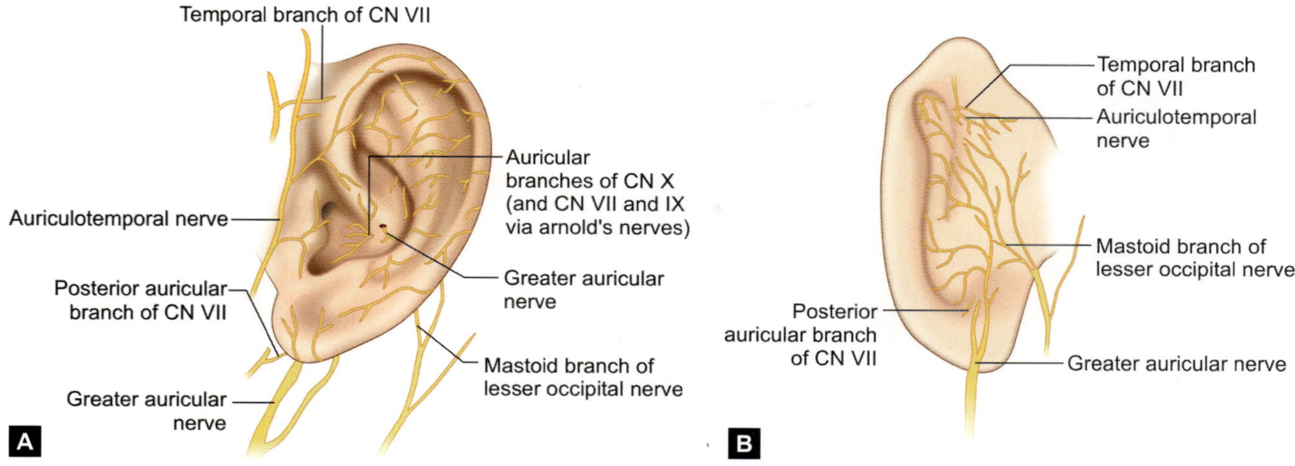

Figs. 3A and B: Innervations of the ear.

- The auriculotemporal nerve supplies anterior superior one-third
- The lesser occipital nerve supplies the posterior surface of the superior one-third
- The auricular branch of vagus nerve innervates the external auditory canal floor and concha.

Vascular Supply

The earlobe is supplied by a rich plexus of perforators from both the superficial temporal and posterior auricular arteries, which are the branches of external carotid artery. Venous drainage is from the accompanying vein.[1] Rich vascularity of the earlobe is an advantage for all ear lobe surgeries as it helps in better and faster healing, due to which flap necrosis following the earlobe repair is uncommon.

The auricle develops from six mesenchymal proliferations located at the dorsal ends of the first and second pharyngeal arches. These swellings are called *auricular hillocks*. Congenital earlobe cleft is probably the result of failure of fusion between the first and sixth hillocks, the tragus and lobule, respectively.[2]

ANESTHESIA

Ring Block Technique

The ring block, shown in Figures 4A and B, provides anesthesia to the entire ear, excluding the concha and external auditory canal.

- The needle is inserted into the skin just inferior to the attachment of the earlobe to the head. ***Do not insert the needle into the earlobe itself.*** Advance the needle just anterior to the tragus. Aspirate and then inject 2–3 mL of anesthetic while withdrawing the needle slowly back toward the puncture site without removing it.

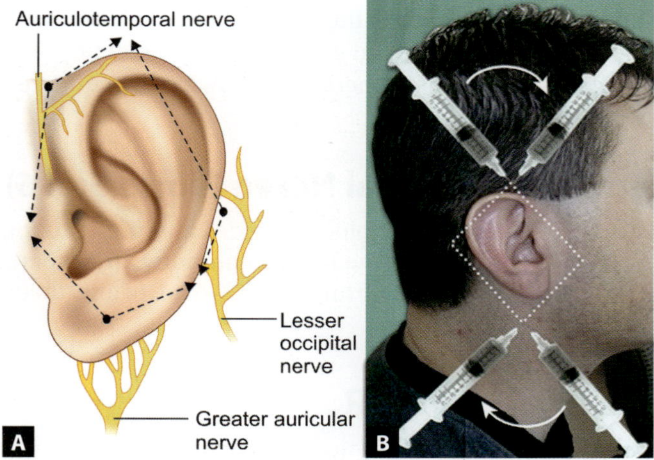

Figs. 4A and B: Ring block.

- Redirect and advance the needle posteriorly along the inferior posterior auricular sulcus, aspirate and inject 2–3 mL of anesthetic while withdrawing the needle.
- Remove the needle and reinsert it just superior to the attachment of the helix to the scalp. Direct and advance the needle just anterior to the tragus, aspirate and inject 2–3 mL of anesthetic while withdrawing the needle toward the puncture site.
- Redirect and advance the needle posteriorly along the superior posterior auricular sulcus, aspirate and inject 2–3 mL of anesthetic while withdrawing the needle.
- Be aware that the superficial temporal artery, located medial to the ear, crosses over the zygomatic arch. If the artery is cannulated by accident, maintain firm pressure with gauze for at least 20–30 minutes.

Field Block Technique

The field block, depicted in Figure 5, provides anesthesia to the earlobe and lateral helix (greater auricular and lesser occipital nerve branches). Insert the needle just posterior to

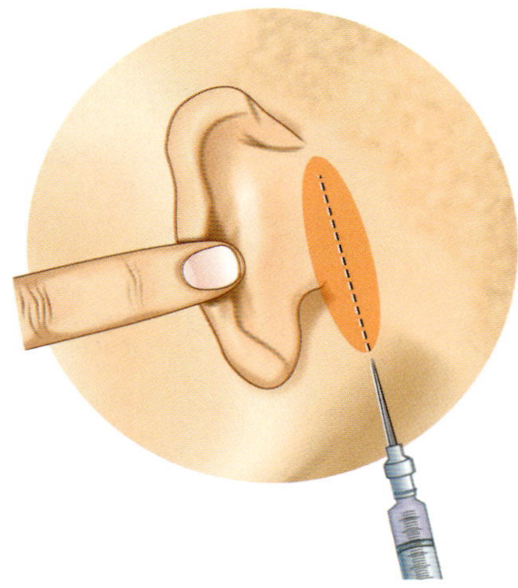

Fig. 5: Field block.

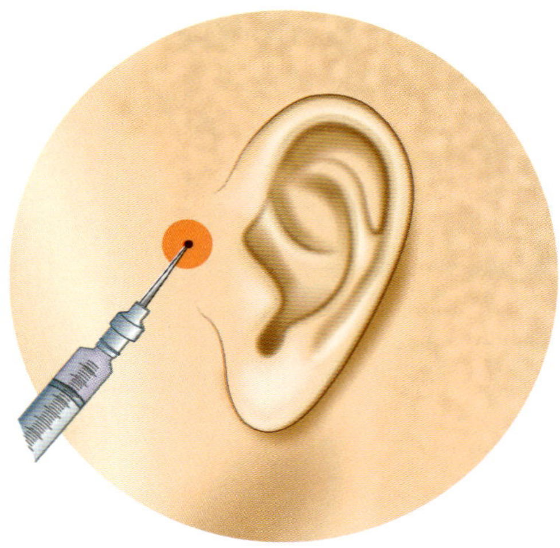

Fig. 6: Auriculotemporal nerve block.

the inferior attachment of the auricle (behind the earlobe). Aspirate and inject a total of 3–4 mL of anesthetic while advancing the needle superiorly, following the curvature of the posterior sulcus.

Auriculotemporal Nerve Block (Fig. 6)

Auriculotemporal nerve block provides anesthesia to the helix and tragus. Insert the needle anteriorly and superiorly to the tragus. Aspirate and inject 3–4 mL of anesthetic (Fig. 6).

EARLOBE REPAIR

Ear piercing has been practiced across the globe irrespective of race, religion and region, to adorn the ear with ear rings and ornaments. It has also been practiced during religious customs since time immemorial. However, many patients present with complications as a result of wearing heavy ear rings or due to sudden or prolonged pull. Partial or complete tears or enlarged ostium are the common complaints. Torn earlobes or cleft earlobes, may be classified as either a complete or partial cleft. A complete cleft usually occurs when the earring is pulled suddenly, forming a divided medial and lateral limb. A partial cleft occurs when piercing canal is elongated or deformed, due to the practice of wearing heavy ear rings or due to persistent and prolonged pulling habits, but has not severed through the earlobe.[3]

The pathology of the tear concerns around the torn edges of the lobe becoming epithelialized, thus forming a fistula or cleft. All methods of earlobe repair are aimed at removal of the scar epithelium and approximation of the fresh edges by various methods.[4]

Causes for Cleft Earlobe

Congenital earlobe clefts show a wide range of severity from simple notching to extensive tissue deficiency. These variable forms have been subtyped by several authors. Kitayama et al. described four subtypes as longitudinal, transverse, triple lobe and defective types. Yamada et al., classified them as anterior, posterior and double lobe types. Usually, a congenital earlobe cleft has soft tissue deficiency and curved cleft margin.

Acquired cleft of the earlobe is usually due to tear through the lobe by a sudden pull on an earring or by prolonged pull of a heavy earring or because of direct trauma. Factors influencing the clefting of the earlobe are congenital alterations, local trauma, facial aging, keloids, earlobe tumors and as a result of the treatment for the same. Several retrospective studies have reported a 1–2% incidence rate of torn earlobes in patients wearing earrings.[3] Pierced earlobes may encounter trauma due to the following causes:[4]

- Heavy earrings
- Poor piercing technique
- A sudden pull on the earring by babies or spouses
- Chronic friction from headgear or telephone
- Entanglement in telephone cords, hair brushes and clothing.

Earlobe Repair Techniques

Torn ear lobes can be repaired either by surgical or non-surgical methods.

Nonsurgical Methods

Epithelium around the cleft is de-epithelialized by various non-surgical method and the cleft is closed by applying a glue and a tubular bandage, allowing the de-epithelialized edges to be united, thus closing the cleft. But the resultant closure will be a weak scar, and the recurrence is almost invariable following wearing of ear-rings, post non surgical repair.

Incomplete earlobe cleft repair can be done by using various methods to de-epithelialize the tissue by:

- Trichloroacetic acid (TCA) 90%
- 88% phenol solution
- Ablative laser or radiofrequency de epithelialization
- Dermabrasion by manual or motorized dermabraders followed by applying surgical glue or tubular dressing to unite the de-epithelized edges.

Surgical Methods

Partial cleft repair

- Excision followed by simple repair
- Punch excision (for defects <4 mm in length) with simple closure
- Parallel opposed flaps
- Purse string repair
- Wedge excision with Z-plasty

Complete cleft repair

- Without preservation of piercing site
  - Excision and closure
  - Z-plasty
  - L-plasty
  - Interlocking V-incisions
  - Partially incised V-plasty
  - Rotation flap
  - Z-plasty and advancement flap
- With preservation of piercing site
  - Pardue technique
  - Z-plasty

Nonsurgical Techniques for Cleft Earlobe Repair

Various nonsurgical techniques have been described in the literature and are being practiced. Most of the nonsurgical methods for the earlobe repair are practiced by dermatologists since the surgical techniques require proper training and certain degree of surgical skills.

Freshening of the edges for de-epithelialization and application of surgical glue with dressing is the simplest procedure. De-epithelialization of the cleft is done by various chemical agents like trichloroacetic acid and phenol, dermabrasion and lasers.

Maria Christina Cardoso De Mendonca et al.[5] have reported a nonsurgical technique for incomplete earlobe cleft repair. Selected patients were subjected to a noninvasive incomplete earlobe cleft repair consisting of application of TCA 90% inside the cleft with nonsurgical incisions until frosting was achieved. No acid neutralization was needed. The cleft was then occluded with micropore tape until complete cicatricial adhesion of the cleft borders was achieved. The complete coagulation of the cleft borders may require several TCA 90% applications and the patients were advised to return weekly for evaluation of the cicatricial process.The major disadvantage of the nonsurgical technique without suturing or other advanced repair techniques is that, the scar following the nonsurgical correction is weak and prone for recurrences after reuse of earrings. Hence, surgical techniques are preferred.

Instruments and Materials Required

Skin marking pen, Inj. lignocaine hydrochloride 1–2%, sterile wooden tongue blades, skin hooks, No. 15 blade, No. 3 B.P. handle, Adson's toothed forceps, iris scissors, Castroviejo's needle holders and 5-0 or 6-0 prolene or ethilon.

Informed consent should be taken in all patients and necessary preoperative medications administered.

Preoperative Preparation

The entire area is prepared by standard methods of sterilization. After the anesthesia either a field block or ring block, a small quantity of anesthetic may be injected along the slit with the extension beyond the margins.

Surgical Technique

Various surgical techniques have been advocated for both complete and partial cleft earlobe repair to provide a good, cosmetically acceptable and stronger scar with less possibility of recurrences. If the cleft is partial with a significant portion of the earlobe being intact, the deformity may be corrected without cutting through the intact portion to convert into a complete cleft. But it is always preferable to convert a partial cleft into a complete tear-through, if the cleft is large with remaining portion of the intact skin minimal.

Reiter and Alford, in a study involving 68 earlobe clefts, suggested that lobe thickness is also an important factor to be considered before choosing the technique to repair the clefts. Lobes measuring less than 4 mm at their greatest thickness have the greatest likelihood of developing elongation of the piercing site or complete clefting. Patient should be informed about this before repiercing the repaired earlobe.[6]

Partial Cleft Repair

Partial cleft repair methods include excision followed by simple repair, punch excision with simple closure, parallel opposed flaps, purse string repair, and wedge excision with Z-plasty.

- *Simple excision and closure (McLaren Side-to-Side Closure):*[7] Excision of the skin margins of the cleft with No. 15 blade on anterior and posterior margins was first described by McLaren. Suture from side-to-side the opposing edges with simple interrupted sutures using 5-0 or 6-0 prolene and suture similarly on the opposing posterior sides. Hemostasis may be achieved by application of pressure and dress with antibiotic ointment (Figs. 7 and 8).
- *Punch excision with simple closure: Tan's technique*[8] Punch excision for defects less than 4 mm in length is done after stabilizing the ear with chalazion forceps

followed by punch excision of the elongated slit and simple closure of the wound. The punch, one millimeter larger than the cleft, is positioned perpendicular to the lobe, and its rotation movement de-epidermises the cleft from its front to the back side, i.e. throughout its length. The skin should be pulled by the tip of the lobe during the punch action, which results in an incision and consequent transverse suture in relation to the lobe (Fig. 9). Re-piercing should be done six months after complete healing. Though this method

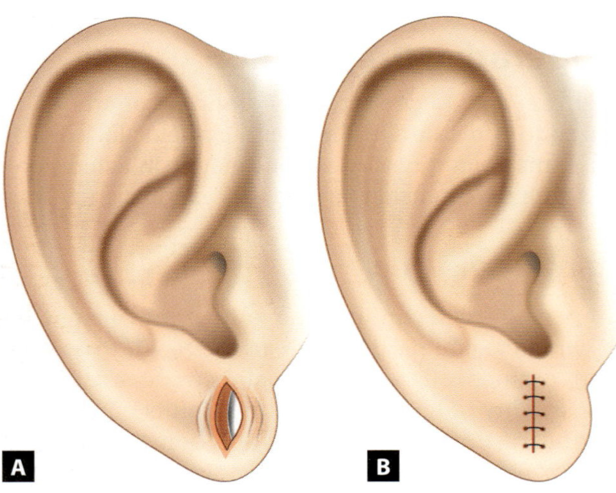

Figs. 7A and B: Schematic of side-to-side repair.

has been described in the literature, in the opinion of the authors, it is not a satisfactory method. It would be difficult to cut the margins by using punches even after fixing it with chalazion clamp. Hence, the authors' recommend that cutting the free margins of the cleft with a No. 11 surgical blade is better than cutting by using the punches. One shortcoming of a side-to-side partial cleft closure is the resultant elongation of the inferior lobule. In the instance of small tears, this may be negligible; however, in a longer partial tear, this resultant elongation may look unsightly.

- *Parallel opposed flaps (Reiter and Alford technique):*[6] Here flaps are created with pedicles along the edge of the slit, one in front at the right side and another in the back at the left side of the lobe. The flaps are rotated as saloon doors (each flap is pulled through the cleft) trimmed at the end, and closed in the form of a "C" on each side of the lobule. Each one will cover the raw area of the other when sutured, making the cleft disappear. While this elegant repair preserves the inferior contour of the lobule, it is time consuming in comparison to a simple side-to-side closure (Fig. 10).
- *Repair of partial earlobe cleft using a "Purse-String" repair was described by Justin Vujevich and Suzan Obagi:*[3] Using a No. 15 blade, a full thickness elliptical incision is made around the partial cleft, hemostasis is obtained, a running 5-0 Prolene or 5-0 Ethilon suture is placed in a purse-string manner through the intradermal tissue. After encircling the defect, the free

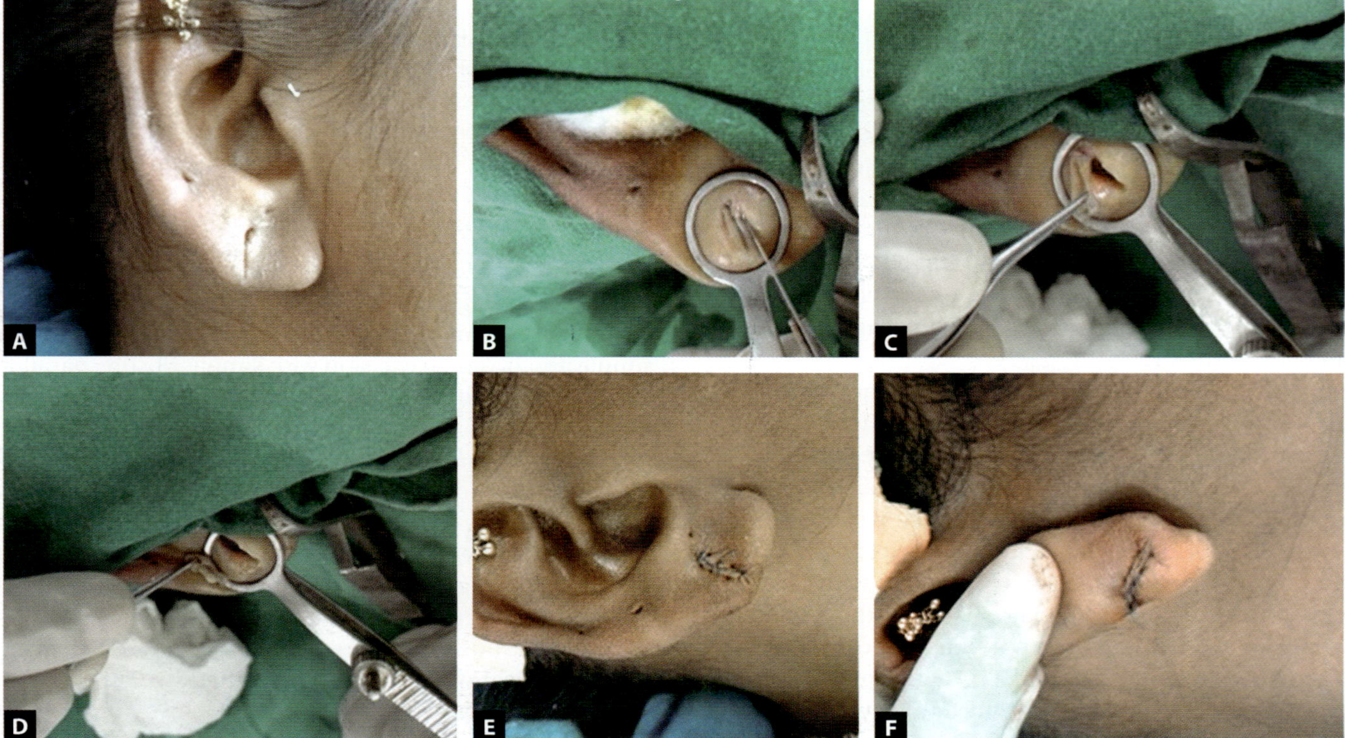

Figs. 8A to F: Side to side closure of partial cleft: (A) Partial tear, (B) Chalazion clamp applied for pressure and hemsostasis, freshening of edges with scalpel, (C and D) Epithelized portion removed from the cleft, (E and F) edges opposed with simple interrupted sutures.

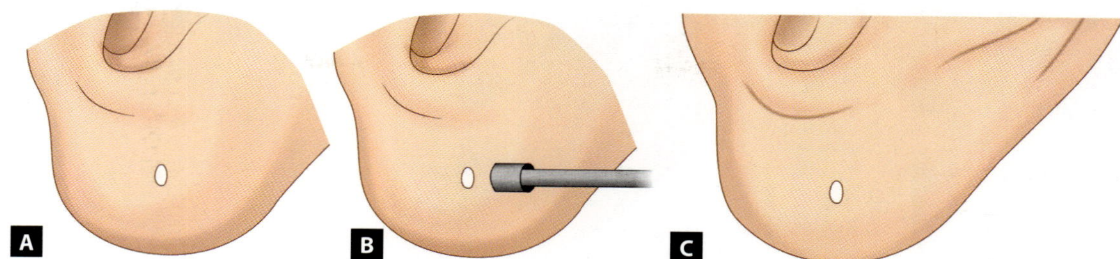

Figs. 9A to C: Schematic of punch excision.

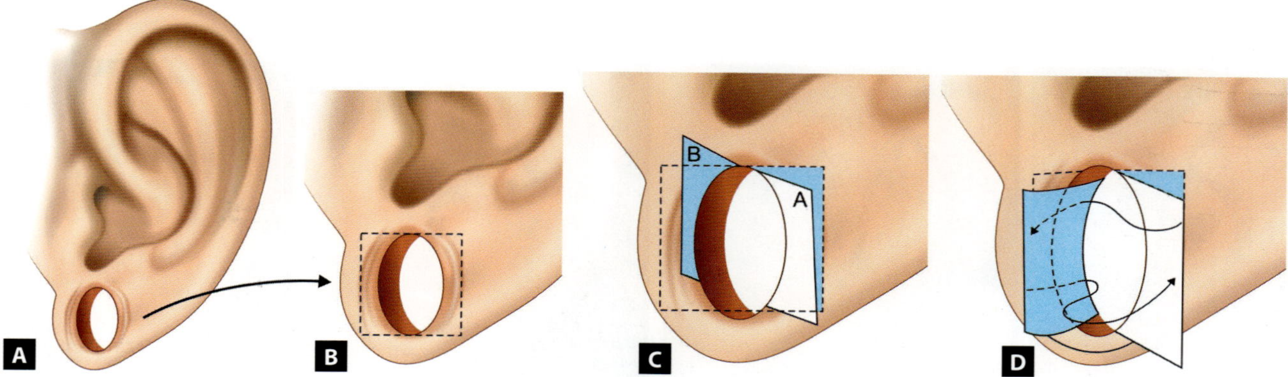

Figs. 10A to D: Reiter and Alford technique (parallel opposing flaps): Frontal flap and Dorsal flap.

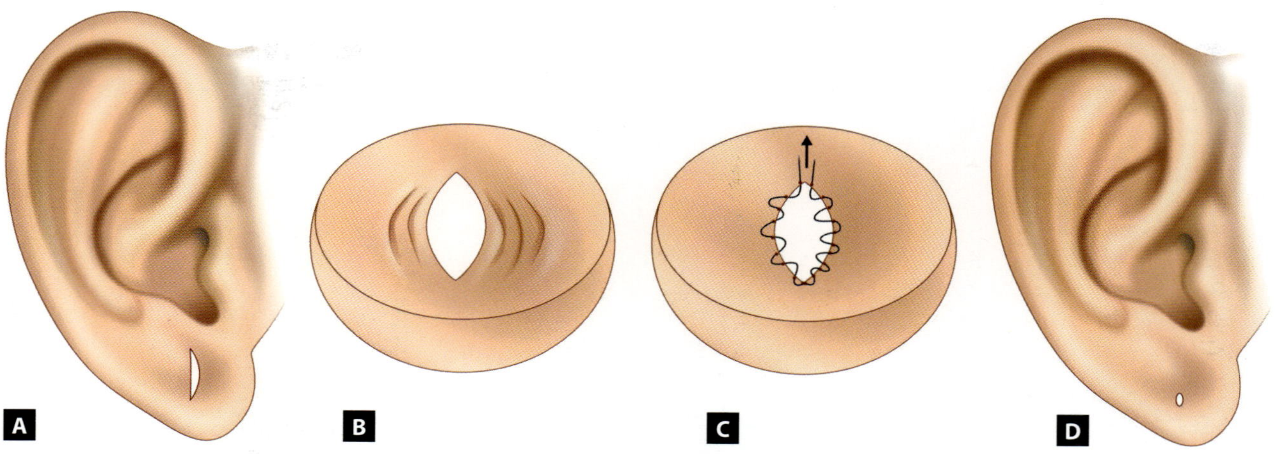

Figs. 11A to D: Illustration of purse string repair.

ends of the suture are pulled together and knotted from the anterior, superior edge of the lobule. Any scar that remains is easily camouflaged when the earlobe is subsequently repierced. The sutures are removed after 7 days (Figs. 11A to D).

- *Side-to-side closure with half Z-plasty:* Abenavoli described a side-to-side closure incorporating a half-Z-plasty (Figs. 12A to C). Once the limbs of the Z-plasty are made, the inferior margins of the cleft are freshened, and the flaps are transposed onto one another. This technique allows preservation of the earring canal and a staggered suture line away from the line of gravity.[9] Unilateral Z-plasty and partial advancement flap can also be done (Figs. 13A to D).

Complete Cleft Repair Methods without Preservation of Piercing Site

Different methods have been employed as below:

- **Side-to-side closure:** The simplest way to repair a complete cleft earlobe is to incise the cleft with an inverted V-shaped excision as described by Apesos and Kane. Once excised, the anterior and posterior edges of skin are undermined to about approximately 1 cm and the wound edges are reapproximated with a straight line closure. While this repair is quick and simple, the ensuring scar may contract, resulting in a groove or notch at the inferior earlobe border (Figs. 14 and 15). Vertical or horizontal mattress sutures placed in the inferior rim of the earlobe may prevent this notching

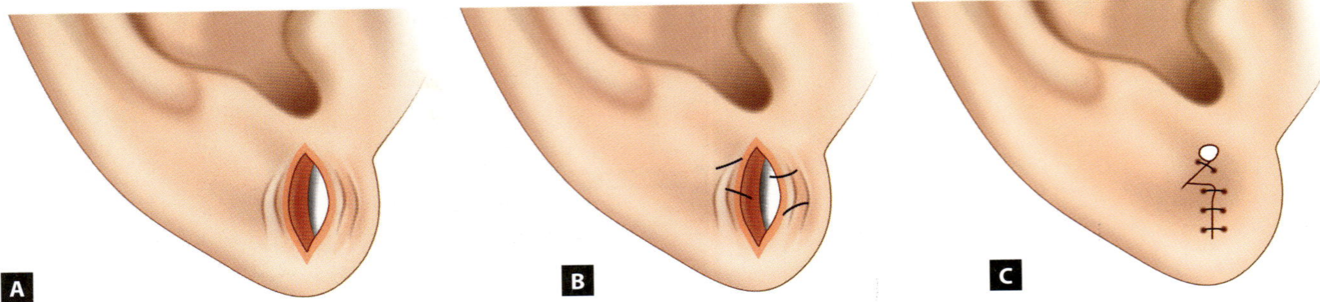

Figs. 12A to C: Illustration of side-to-side closure with half Z-plasty.

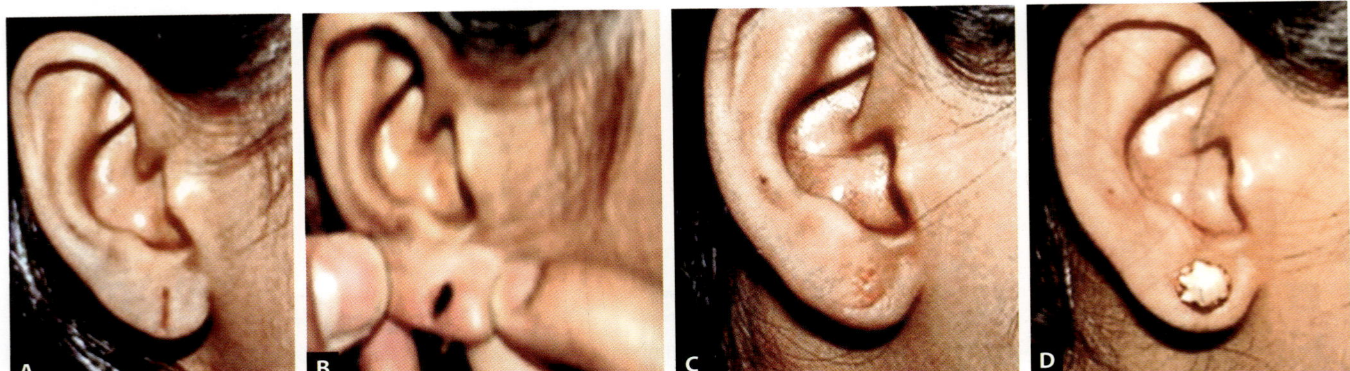

Figs. 13A to D: Unilateral Z-plasty and advancement flap for partial cleft.

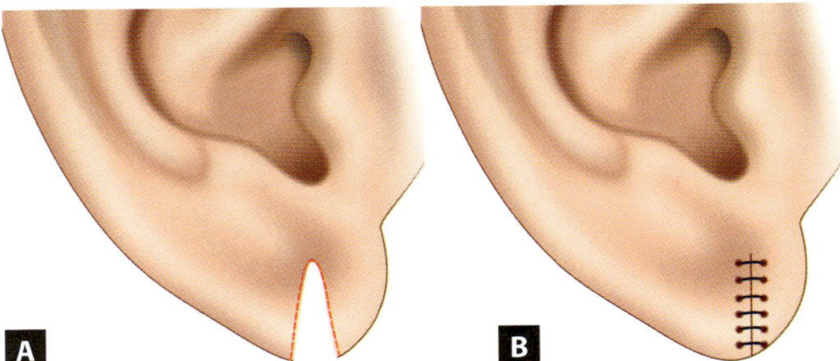

Figs. 14A and B: Schematic of side-to-side closure of complete tear.

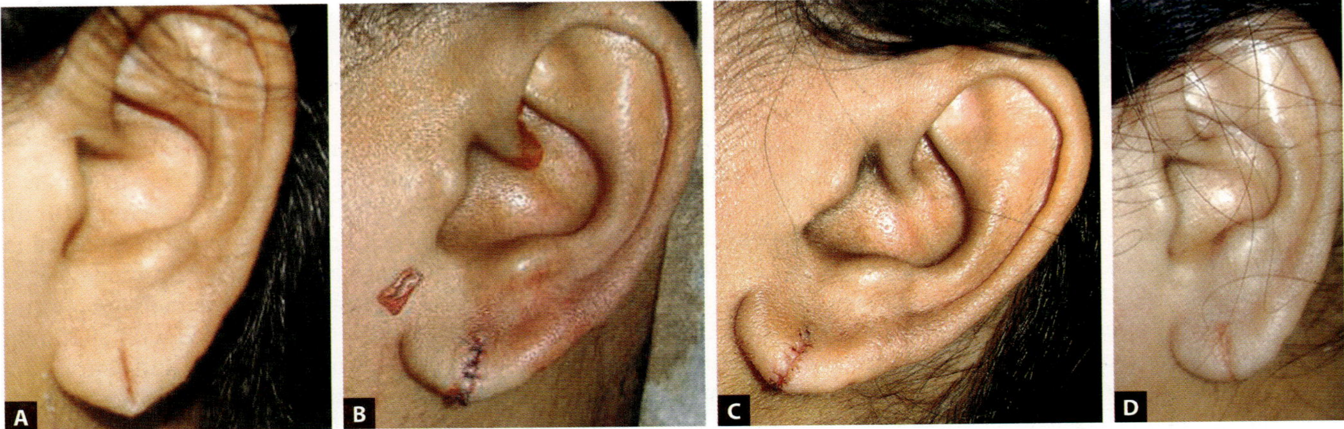

Figs. 15A to D: Simple excision and closure: (A) Acquired partial ear lobe defect (p.e surgical); (B) Simple excision and closure with simple interrupted sutures; (C) Immediately after suture removal; (D) Notching following repair with simple excision and closure.

(Figs. 16A to F).[10] Another modification to prevent notching is to create a Z-plasty incision on the inferior margin of the lobule and transpose the resultant flaps over each other and closed with interrupted sutures (Figs. 17A to F).[11]

- Reiter and Alford described utilizing a full thickness Z-plasty for complete cleft earlobes thicker than 4 mm (Figs. 18 and 19). Alternatively for earlobe less than 4 mm thickness, the same author advocated the use of partial thickness Z-plasty on the lateral surface of the earlobe, and a linear closure on the medial sides of the lobe (Figs. 20A to C). One disadvantage of utilizing a Z-plasty, however, is the requirement of a precisely angled small incision on a small amount of skin on the lobe.[6]
- *Side-to-side closure with L-plasty:* Fatah MF described the creation of an L-shaped flap on the medial or lateral side of excised cleft and a complementary L-shaped defect on the other side of the ear lobe. The lateral flaps are inserted onto one another and sutured together and the medial flaps are inserted onto one another and sutured together (Figs. 21A to C).[12]

A modification of L-plasty is to create a L-shaped flap on the anterior and posterior sides of the lobule, then a partial incision is made on the anterior and posterior surface lobule, the flaps are inserted with a Z in the lower end (Figs. 22A to C).[13]

- *Side-to-side closure with a V-flap:* Two small 3 mm incisions are made in the shape of a V on the free margin of the inferior lobe. The V-flap is then inserted together and the superior portion is sutured together in a straight-line fashion. The advantages of using this flap are the prevention of notching at the earlobe rim, and the utilization of a simpler flap than the Z-plasty (Figs. 23A to C).[14]
- *Side-to-side closure with a rotational flap:* After the edges of the cleft are split, a short segment of posterior edge of the cleft is de-epithelialized and curled back into the cleft. This technique, however, may produce a "trap door" deformity in the vertical and horizontal planes, resulting in notching of the rim (Figs. 24A to C).[15]

Complete Cleft Repair with Preservation of Piercing Site

- **Side-to-side closure with preservation of apical skin:** This is performed by excising 80% of the lining epithelium leaving an intact superior lining edge. The anterior and posterior opposing edges are then

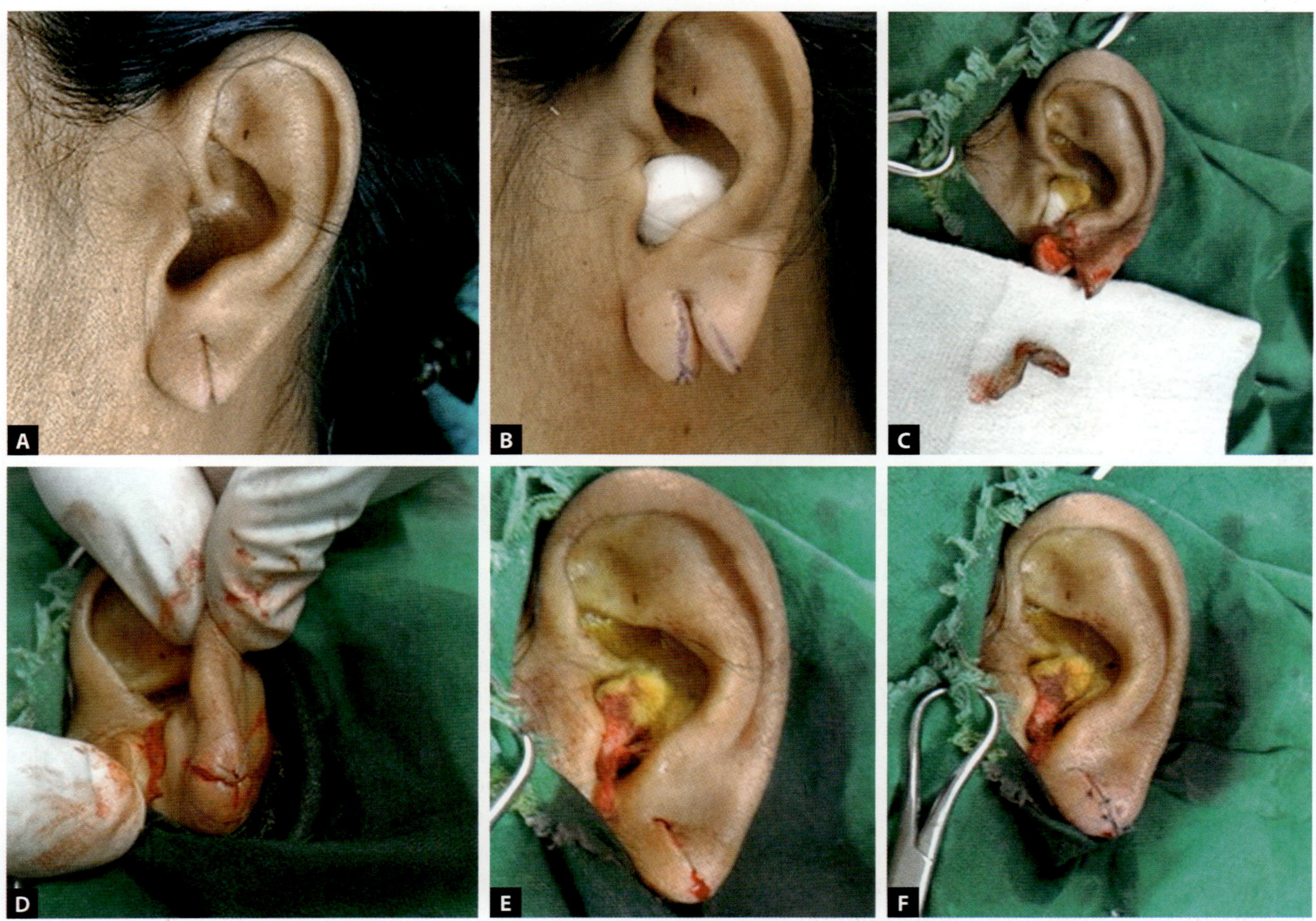

Figs. 16A to F: Simple excision and closure. The mattress suture at the lobule prevents notching.

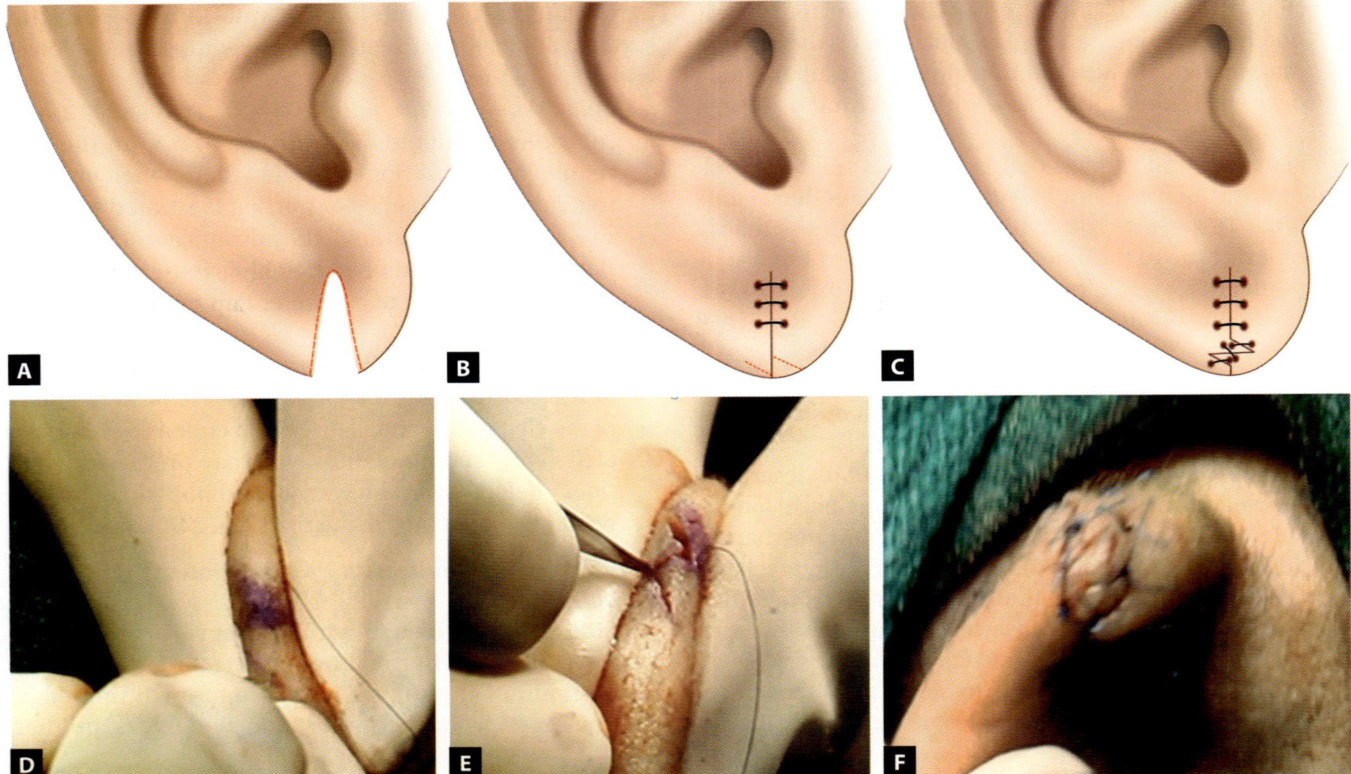

Figs. 17A to F: Z-plasty at the edge of the lobule: (A to C) Schematic diagram (D) Marking of the Z; (E) incisions along the Z at the tip; (F) Z-plasty sutured.
(*Courtesy*: Dr Madura C, Cutis Academy of Cutaneous Sciences)

Figs. 18A to C: Schematic for full thickness Z-plasty.

sutured side-to-side retaining a small ostium at the superior pole of the sutured linear tract. The ostium is maintained by passing a light gold wire or silk suture at same sitting. While this technique is relatively easy to perform, the resulting earring canal is typically unable to withstand the weight of the earring, leading to cleft recurrence (Figs. 25A to C).

If patients insist on retaining the aperture inspite of counselling, an IV cannula or a small wire can be placed in the aperture during the procedure, and a suture can be passed through it after surgery (Figs. 26A to D).

- **Side-to-side closure with apical-lateral flap:** This technique was described by AM Pardue. The flap is based superiorly to one side of the upper end of the cleft. The width of the flap is the width of the inner surface of the cleft near its superior end. The flap is approximately 3 mm long and 1 mm thick.[1]

Operative technique: The procedure starts with outlining the flap and the area to be excised. The margins of the cleft are excised, and a small flap is raised on one side at the upper end of the cleft. The distal edge of the flap is sutured to the opposite side so that the suture line is not at the dependent area of the perforation. The raw surfaces of the cleft are approximated with two or three sutures 5-0 vicryl, and the skin margins are closed with 6-0 prolene. A Z-plasty may be used to interrupt the

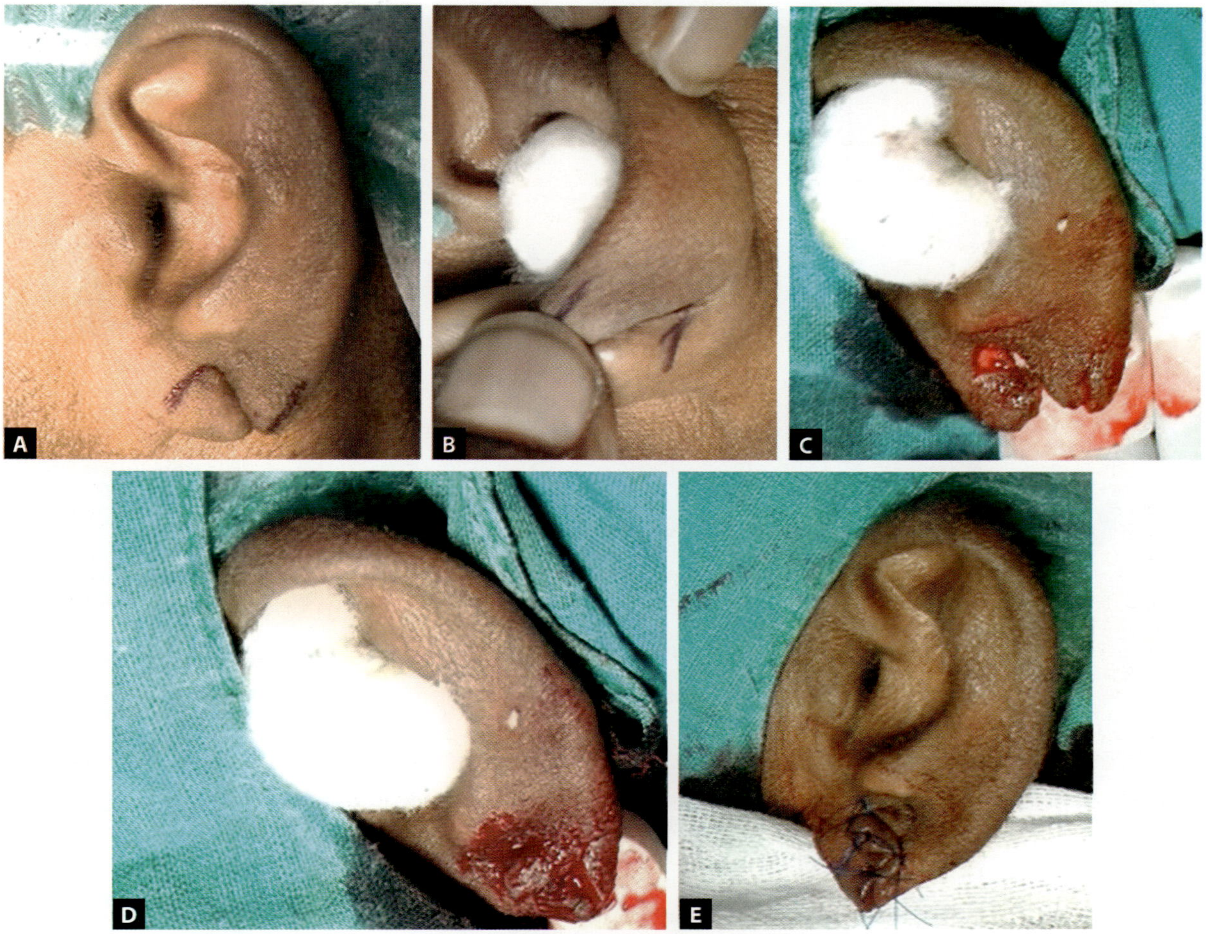

Figs. 19A to E: Z-plasty for ear-lobe repair.

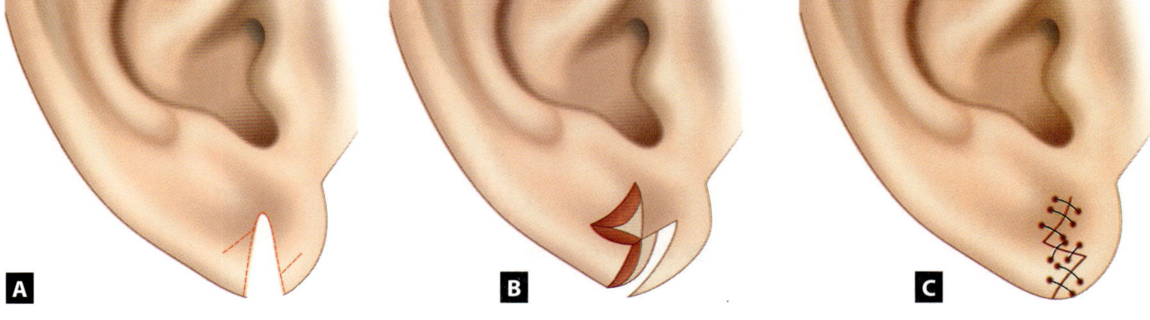

Figs. 20A to C: Schematic of partial thickness Z-plasty.

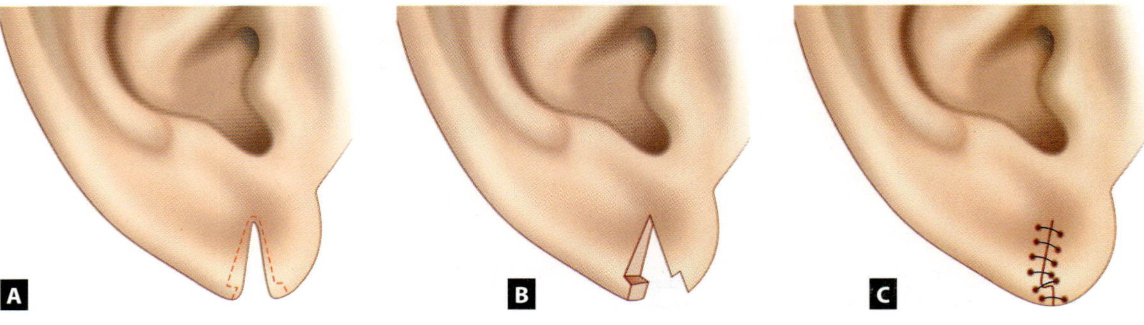

Figs. 21A to C: L-plasty.

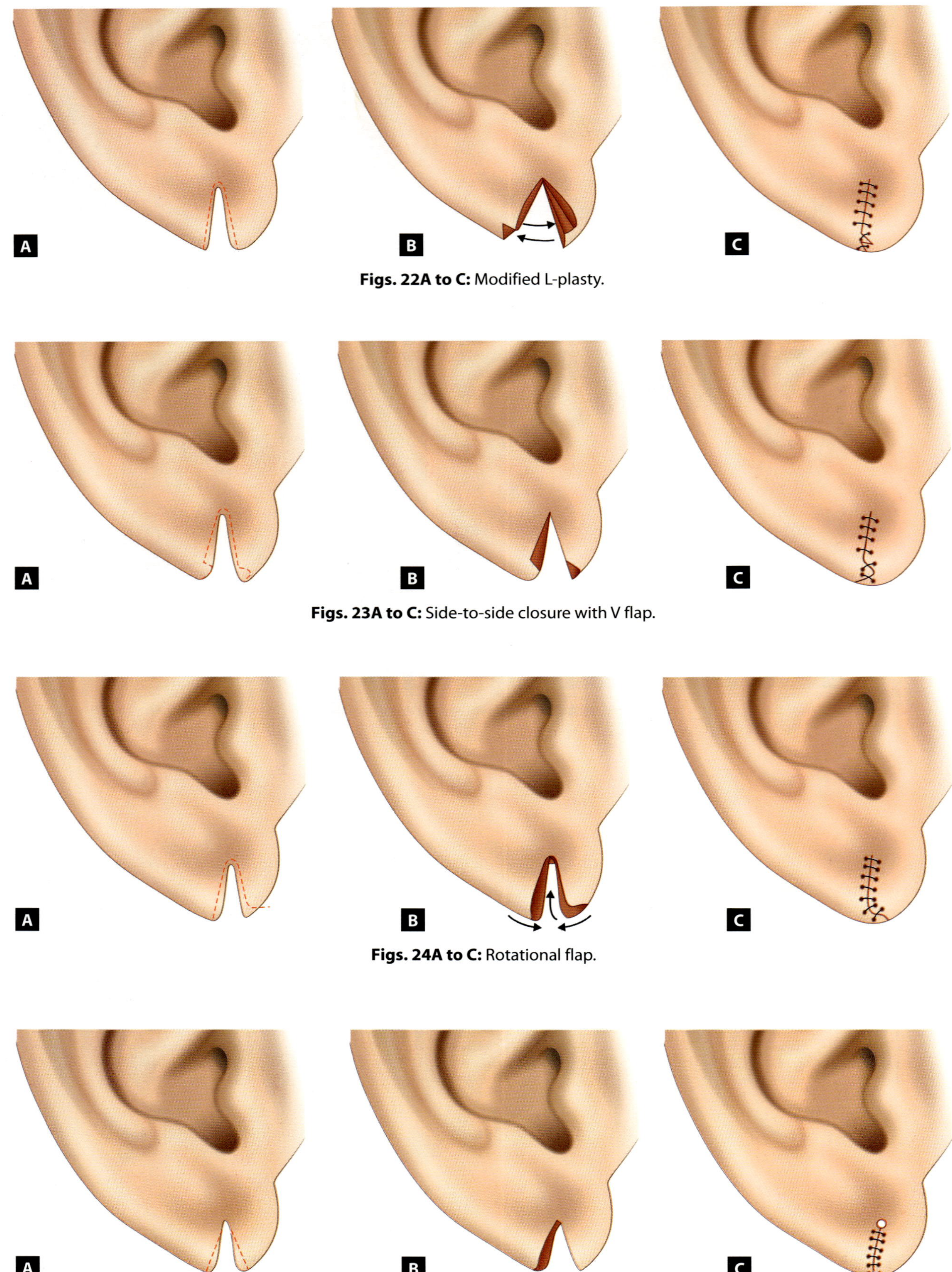

Figs. 22A to C: Modified L-plasty.

Figs. 23A to C: Side-to-side closure with V flap.

Figs. 24A to C: Rotational flap.

Figs. 25A to C: Side-to-side closure with preservation of apical piercing site.

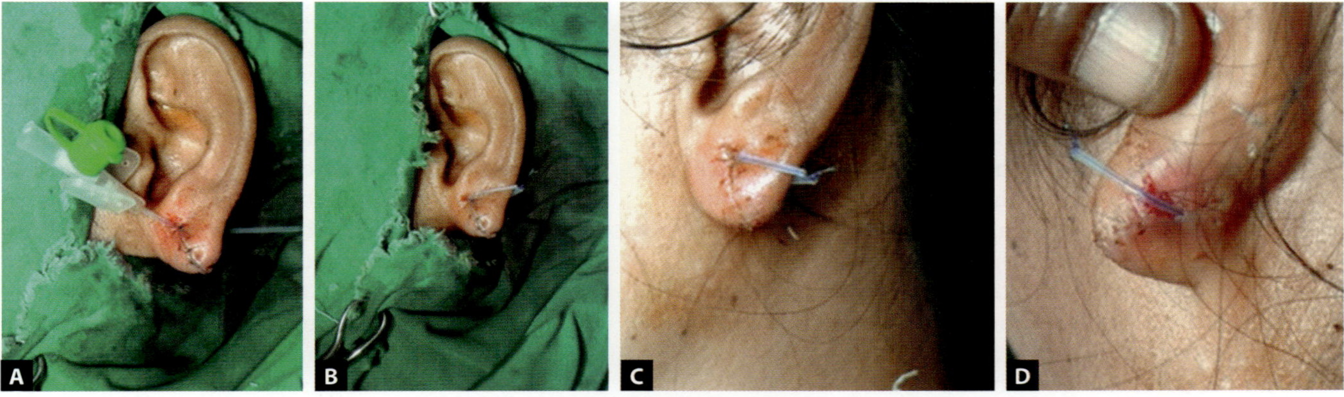

Figs. 26A to D: Maintaining the aperture during procedure.

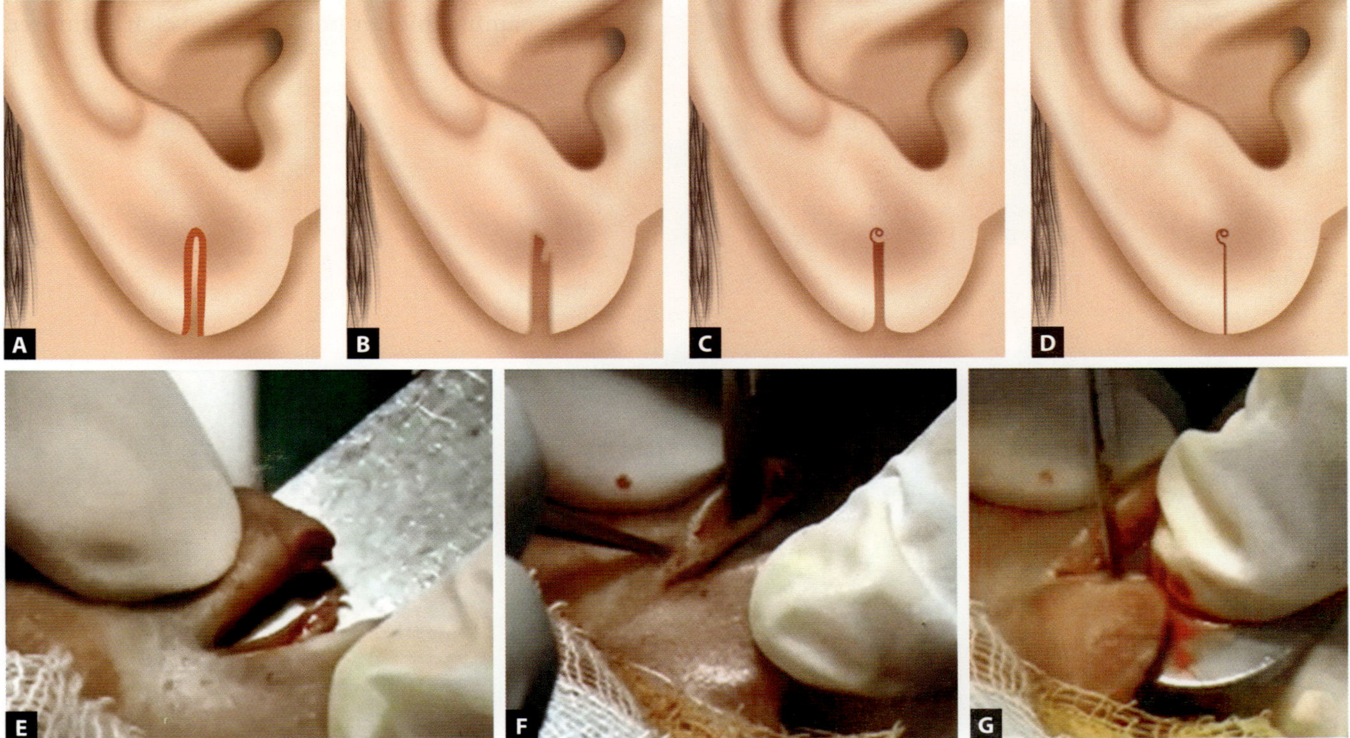

Figs. 27A to G: (A to D) Pardue technique; (E to G) A and B- flaps raised on the torn edges.

suture line on the curve of the earlobe. A single loop of 2-0 clear nylon suture is left within the perforation for 4–6 weeks and then is replaced with an earring. The technique is simple and is readily done with the patient under local anesthesia (Figs. 27A to D).

The drawback are this repair requires small tedious incisions to recreate the flap. In addition, the flap is composed of thin, already scarred skin, which may lead to cleft recurrence.

***Clinical results*:** Results with this technique have been uniformly good for both complete and incomplete clefts. There have been no reports of failures of the flap. The patient should be instructed not to wear heavy earrings again or ones that might be snagged easily, thereby retearing the earlobe.

This technique is further modified by doing a Z-plasty at the inferior rim of the lobule.

The Z-plasty serves to prevent notching and creates a more aesthetic nonlinear scar at the inferior lobule (Figs. 27E to G).[11]

- A different technique using a posterior transposition flap has been reported, but the design of this flap requires excising more normal skin from one side of the cleft, with possible distortion of the flap as it is transposed and twisted into the perforation canal.[16] The cleft is excised leaving the apical part of the cleft intact.

Subsequently, a 2 mm flap of skin on the posterior side cleft is created, turned on its axis, and drawn through the cleft to form the floor of the canal (Figs. 28A to E). The remainder of the cleft is then straight-line sutured with a Z-plasty at the inferior lobule.

- **Side-to-side closure with lap-joint flap:**[17] The cleft edges are first pared leaving an intact apical portion of the cleft. Then, each half of the lobule is split into 2 triangular flaps overlapped onto one another and sutured together. This method reconstructs the apical earring canal, avoids the formation of a notch, staggers the scar on the lobule, and allows the surgeon to create a thinner or thicker lobule based on the construction of the flaps (Figs. 29A to C).
- **Modification of lap-joint flap with Pardue's flap:** This method combines a small apical-lateral flap, similar to Pardue's flap, with L-flap to repair the split lobe (Figs. 30A to C).
- **Side-to-side closure with rectangular flap:** Once the cleft is excised leaving the apical portion intact, rectangular flaps are created on the anterior and posterior aspects of the cleft. Each flap is half the thickness of the lobule and extends up to the apical earring canal. The flaps are then overlapped onto one another and sutured together (Figs. 31A to C).[18]
- **Side-to-side closure with superior-based flap:** Parallel incisions are placed on both sides of the cleft to create hanging flaps (Figs. 32A to D). The upper ends of the superior-based flaps are sutured together to create an earring tract. A nylon loop is then passed through the canal. The remaining parts of the hanging flaps are excised and the edges of the cleft are sutured together. Alternately the first flap can be sutured to the tip of the split to recreate the earring hole. The second flap is sutured to the raw surface of the first flap. Finally, the remaining inferior portion of the cleft is sutured

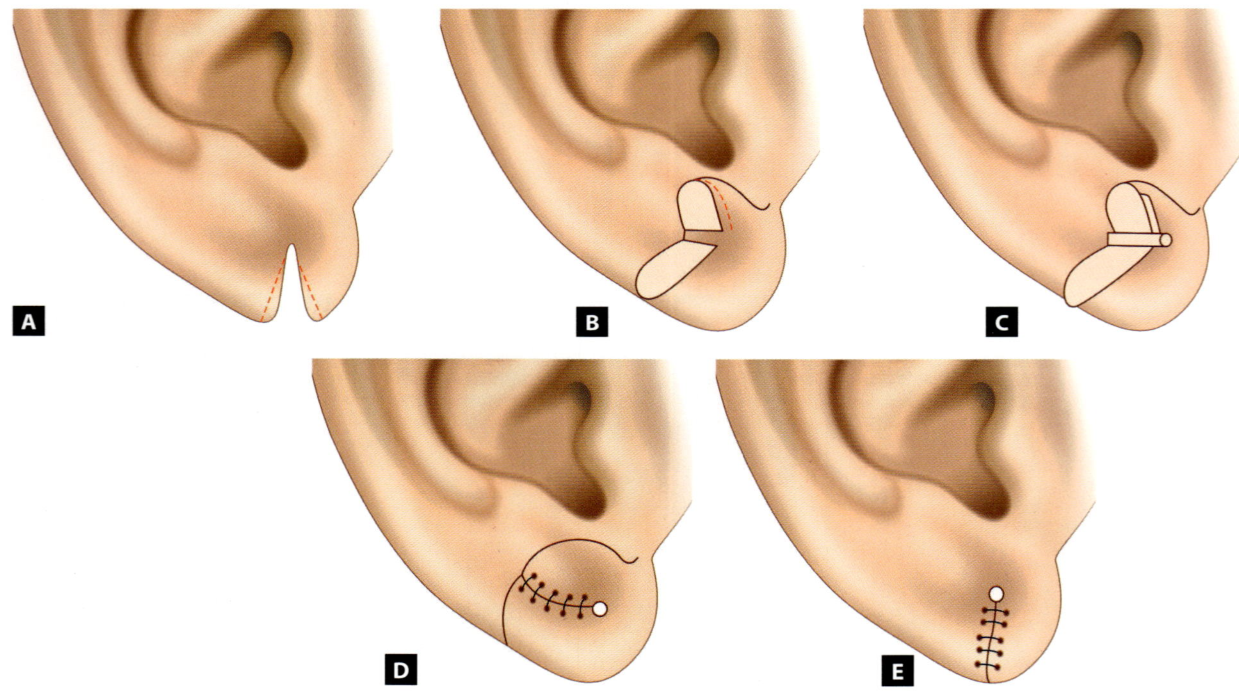

Figs. 28A to E: Posterior transposition flap.

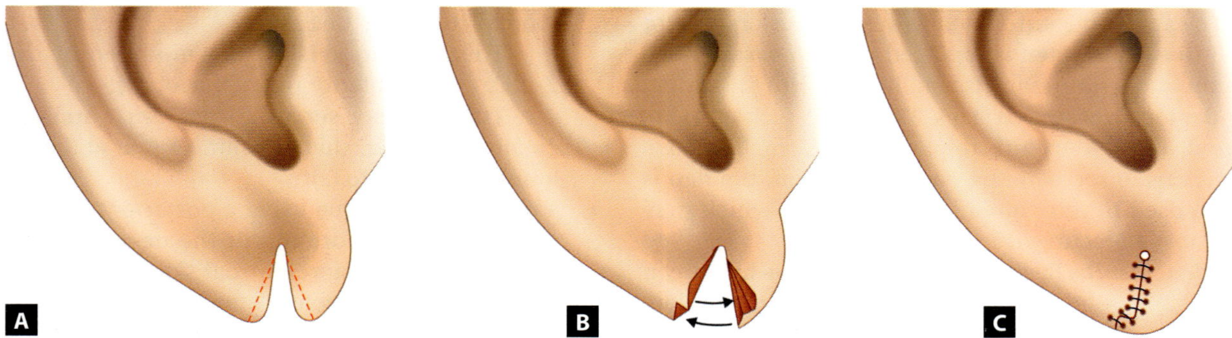

Figs. 29A to C: Schematic representation of lap joint repair.

together. The authors state that the use of 2 flaps produces a stronger "cradle" of tissue for the new earring to rest. This technique, however, is rather complicated and requires a fair amount of time and suturing of tiny strands of tissue (Figs. 32E to H).

- **Excision followed by unilateral Z-plasty and advancement flap (Figs. 33 and 34):**[2] The two unequal, unilateral Z-plasties are transposed in a superior direction. An incision on posterior limb of the cleft bisects this limb, using the lower third as the

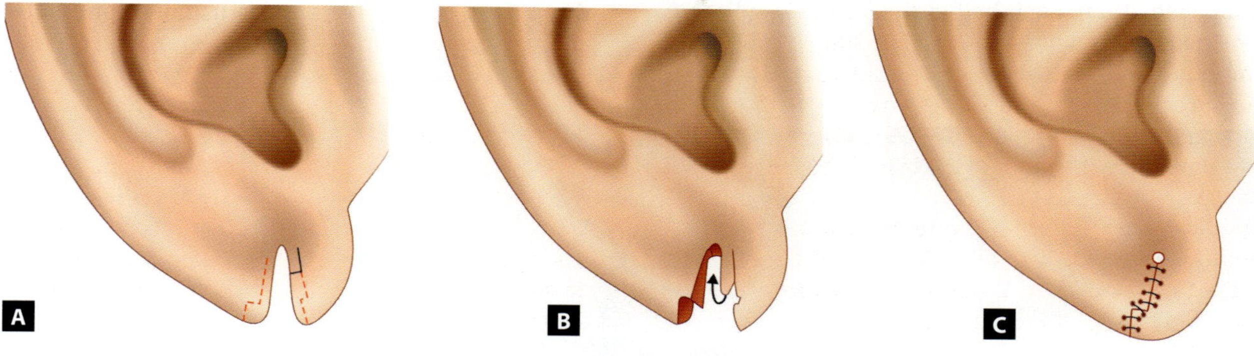

Figs. 30A to C: Lap-joint flap with Pardue's flap.

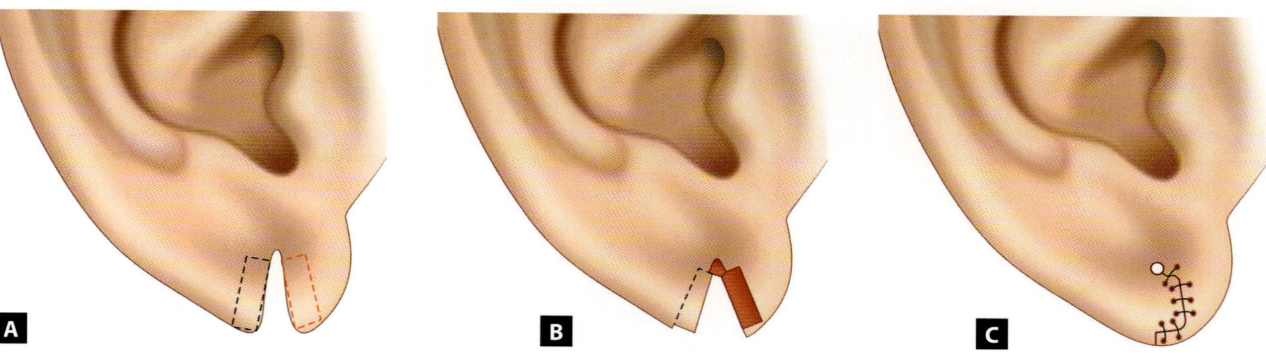

Figs. 31A to C: Side-to-side closure with rectangular flap.

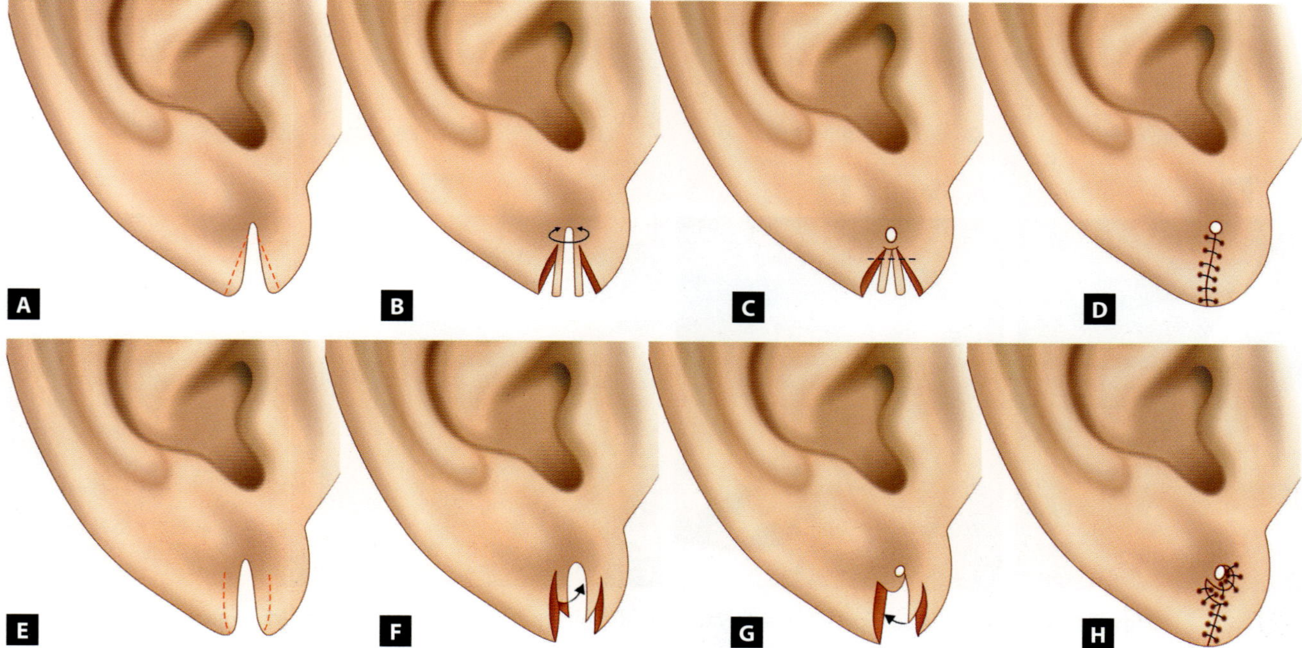

Figs. 32A to H: Superior-based flap side-to-side closure.

advancement flap and the upper two-thirds becomes the lower unilateral Z-plasty. An incision on the anterior limb of the cleft creates the second unilateral Z-plasty. Inferior border of the anterior limb of the cleft is de-epithelialized to accept the advancement flap.

An advancement flap from the posterior limb of the cleft provides the rounded contour of the lower edge of the lobule. The inferior limb of the cleft is de-epithelialized to accept the advancement flap. Two unequal, unilateral Z-plasties are transposed in a superior direction (Figs. 33 and 34).

Postoperative Precautions and Instructions

Appropriate systemic antibiotics for 7–10 days and NSAIDs for 2–3 days. Suture removal is usually done between

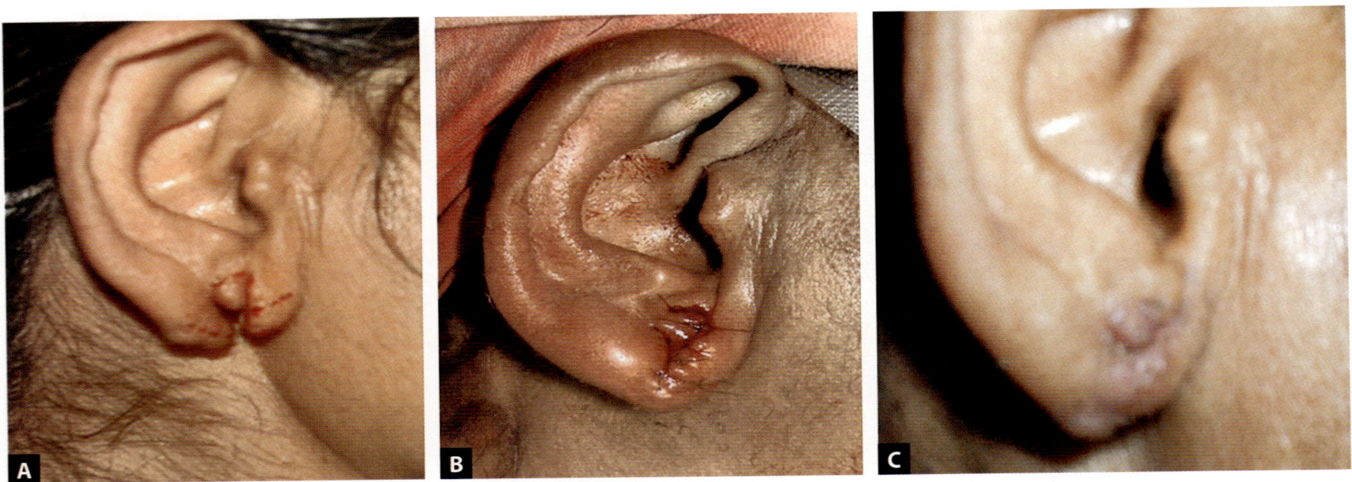

Figs. 33A to C: Excision followed by unilateral Z-plasty and lower end advancement flap for incomplete cleft earlobe.

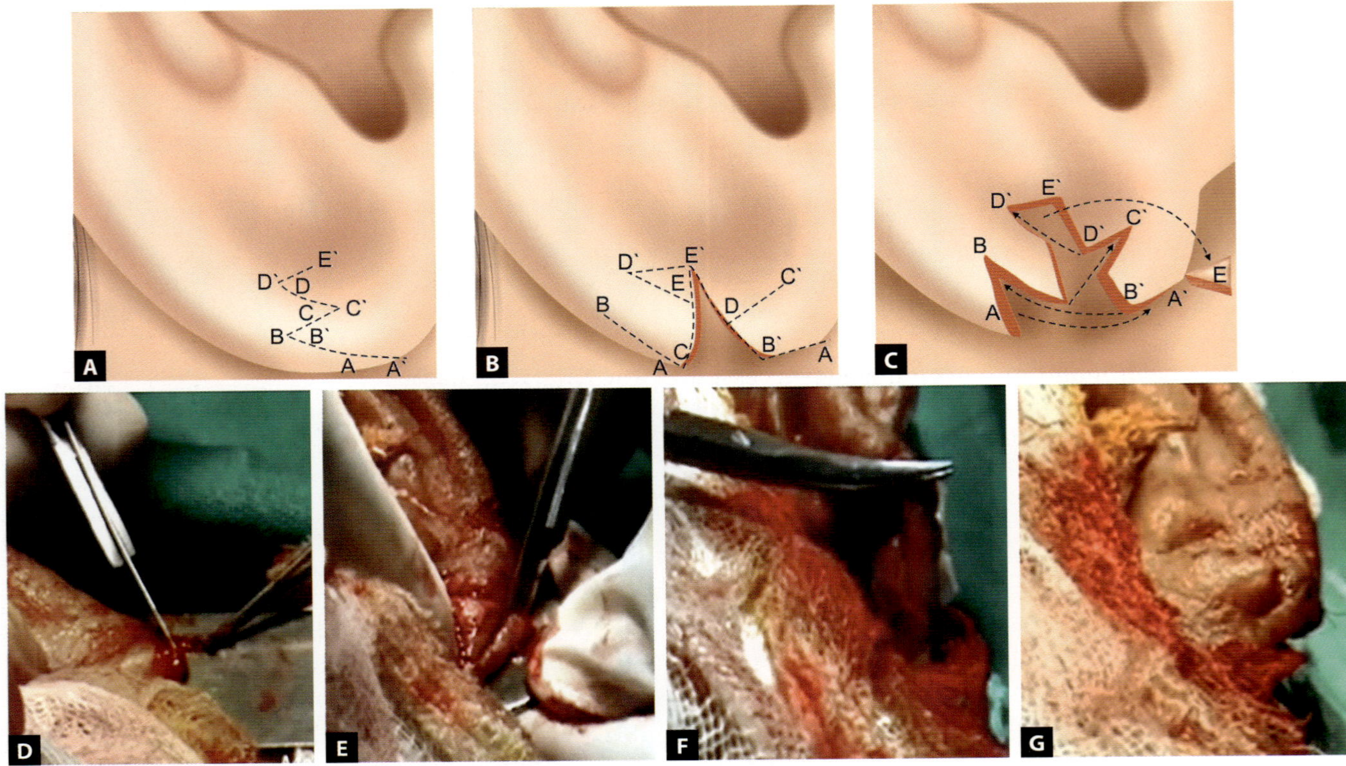

Figs. 34A to G: (A to C) Excision followed by unilateral Z-plasty and advancement flap—diagrammatic design of the flap; (D) Tissue excised from the lateral limb od cleft; (E) Flap raised from the medial end of cleft; (F and G) The flap advanced laterally and sutured.

5 and 7 days. Patient is advised to wait for minimum of 3 months before undertaking ear piercing and discouraged to wear heavy earrings further.

Complications and Their Prevention

Complications are infrequent with earlobe repair. The most common complications are depressed linear scar and inferior margin notching of lobe. Everting the edges by placing one or two deep sutures and a single key suture, and maintaining the everted edges while closing the edges are helpful to prevent the depressed linear scar. A depressed linear scar usually spontaneously improves over several months and patients are encouraged to wait. If the linear scar is persistent and bothers the patient, it may be treated by resurfacing with CO_2 laser. Three to four passes with moderate fluence and energy will gradually ablate the area and gives a good cosmetic acceptance.

Inferior margin notching results from improper alignment of the inferior lobe or from scar retraction, and is more commonly seen with simple linear closure without Z-plasty or advancement flap. It can be prevented by performing advancement flap repair at the lower margin.

Postoperative infection is infrequent, healing is quick and flap necrosis is uncommon due to the rich vascularity of the earlobe and is one of the major advantages for healing and scar remodeling. The possibility of keloid formation is minimal if there is no infection, unless the patient is genetically predisposed for the formation of keloids. Keloid formation is rare if the surgery is done before puberty.

EAR KELOID MANAGEMENT

External ear is one of the commonest site for keloid formation, more common after puberty due to hormonal influences. External ear keloids occur commonly after ear piercing. The incidence is about 2.5% after ear piercing.[19] Due to its location, ear keloids are cosmetically disfiguring and treatment is also challenging. There are various modalities of treatment of keloids, however no single method has been found to be completely successful. Combination of techniques offers better results. Surgical excision of keloids alone has a poor success with a high recurrence rate of 55%.[20] Simple excision is thought to promote additional collagen synthesis, resulting in fast regrowth and frequently an even larger keloid.[21] A study by Akoz et al. found combination of surgery, intralesional injection and silicone gel sheets to be effective.[22]

If keloid is smaller in size, intralesional injections of various medications like intralesional triamcinolone acetonide 10–40%, 5-fluorouracil (5-FU), bleomycin either alone or in combination, can be used. However, combination of triamcinolone acetonide and 5-FU is best studied.

Liquid nitrogen cryotherapy is one of the important modalities of treatment either given alone or with various intralesional medications. If the keloid is small and flat, surface cryotherapy with intralesional medication of above mentioned agents work in synergy and yield superior results compared to either of them used alone. If keloids are bulky, intralesional cryotherapy is the best option.

Intralesional Cryotherapy

After local anesthesia, depending upon the size of the keloid, an 18 G hypodermic needle or spinal needle is inserted through the summit of the keloid from one side to another. Either single or multiple needles depending upon the size of the keloid can be used. Padding with cotton gauge to be done at the exit point of the needle to protect the surrounding skin. Liquid nitrogen is sprayed from the hand held cryo gun either directly into the hub of the needle or with a modified rubber tubing fitted to the spray tip of hand held cryo gun. Freezing is done till the entire keloid mass is frozen from within the core of the keloid without freezing the surface of the skin. Freeze time may vary depending upon the size of the keloid from 1 minutes to 3 minutes. Complete thawing to be allowed which is usually 2–3 times that of freezing. Two freeze thaw cycles to be done depending upon the size and bulk of keloid. Patient is advised to take analgesics for 2–3 days. The procedure may be repeated after 2–4 weeks depending on the response. Intralesional cryo has been reported to give good results with lesser complications compared to surface cryo. Intralesional steroid or combination with 5-FU may be given 10–15 minutes after complete thawing.

Surgical Excision

Surgical excision is one of the commonly practised treatment for earlobe keloids. Excision should be performed gently and atraumatically so that the borders of the wound can be approximated without tension. Intrakeloidal excision, without traumatizing the normal skin and excising the keloid with incision within the keloid is ideal.

Fillet Technique

Fillet technique involves strict intramarginal keloid excision in which the keloid scar is sharply dissected from the covering skin and the keloid mass is completely removed. Skin over the keloid is termed a "keloid fillet flap". Subcutaneous sutures are not used, and the keloid fillet flaps are closed with 6-0 nylon sutures after trimming. The keloid mass functions as an endogenous expander of the skin, and removal results in an excess of skin soas to adapt the wound edges without tension. According to Kim et al, the "5 As and one B" (Asepsis, atraumatic technique, absence of raw surface, avoidance of tension, accurate approximation of wound margin, and complete bleeding control) are important factors in reducing the recurrence rate of earlobe keloids in surgical excision.[23] The flap is marked so that the pedicle is toward the free edge of the earlobe and the line of incision close to the retroauricular crease, if the keloid is on the posterior aspect of earlobe, since it would be more cosmetically acceptable. If the keloid is on the anterior aspect of the earlobe, the flap is marked so that the pedicle is in the posterior position. Marking the incision and flap is very important and it varies depending on the type, size and location of keloid. Marking should always be done before injecting the local anesthetic agent. A local anesthetic (2% lidocaine with 1:100,000 epinephrine) is infiltrated at the surgical site, after delineation of the line of incision so that borders of the mass are not obscured. Then, the cutaneous compartment is separated from the main keloidal mass using a curved blunt iris scissor until the keloid mass was completely separated, with normal skin all around. A sharp tipped scissor is used to separate the mass from its bed without perforating normal skin on either side. The thickness of the flap should be not too thin to prevent necrosis. If perforation occurred, it is closed using nylon 5-0 interrupted sutures. Bleeding is controlled by pressure.[24] Care should be taken not to overzealously excise the keloid mass. Sufficient tissue should be left attached to the earlobe all around to enable primary closure of the flaps after removing the core keloid tissue at the base. The thickness of the flaps should not be too thin to prevent necrosis considering the less vascularity of keloid tissue (Figs. 35 and 36).

If keloids are involving the undersurface or lower border of ear lobe altering the normal anatomy, flaps has to be raised posteriorly and the core of the keloid to be debulked from behind and the flap sutured on posterior aspect maintaining the near normal rounded anatomy of the earlobe. Incision of the skin at lower margin to be avoided (Figs. 37A to C).

Keloids which reach the other skin side, at the site of ear piercing, i.e. dumbell keloid, can be excised both anteriorly and posteriorly leaving behind a sufficient skin flap for primary closure ensuring the core of the keloid tissue which is connecting both the sides is removed completly. The skin flaps harvested are closed with primary closure using 5-0/6-0 suture similar to core fillet. Before proceeding to wound closure, meticulous palpation of the wound all around and also the bed is done to make sure that there is no residual fibrous tissue. A pressure dressing is applied and sutures are removed 7 to 10 days later.

In contrast, extramarginal keloid excision, which is defined as an incision of physiological skin and removal of the entire lesion, produces a linear scar. The disadvantage occurs in maintaining tension in the suture. Particularly after resection of larger keloids, skin grafts or local flaps often are required to perform the primary wound closure.

If the keloid is a pedunculated mass, mark the incision leaving behind a pedicle which will be sufficient for primary closure. Excise the mass leaving behind a pedicle, debulk the keloidal tissue from within the left out base with No. 15 surgical blade carefully without nicking or cutting the flaps, leaving behind bulky flaps

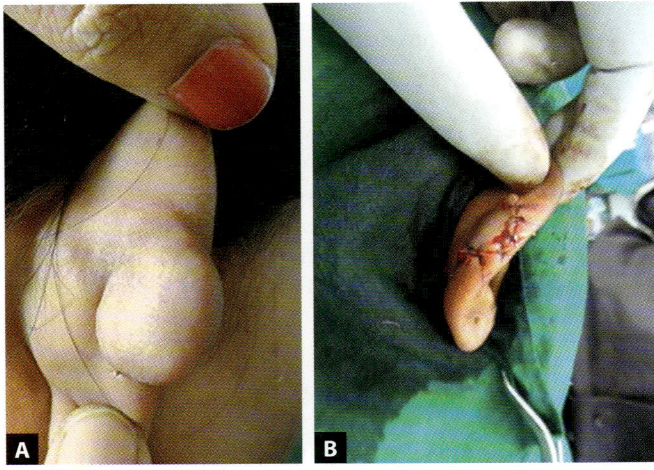

Figs. 35A and B: Excision of intrakeloidal tissue and closure with C flap.

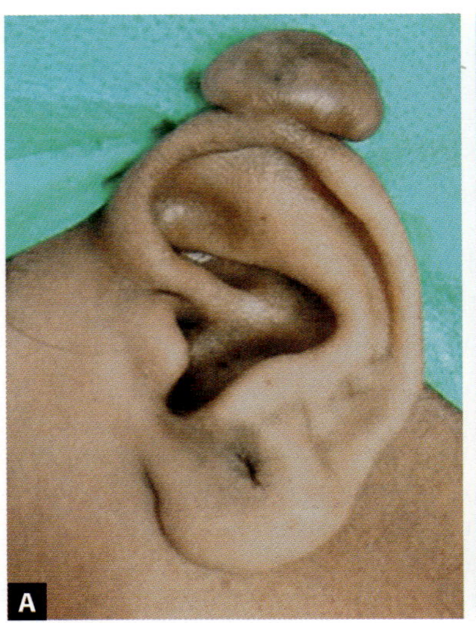

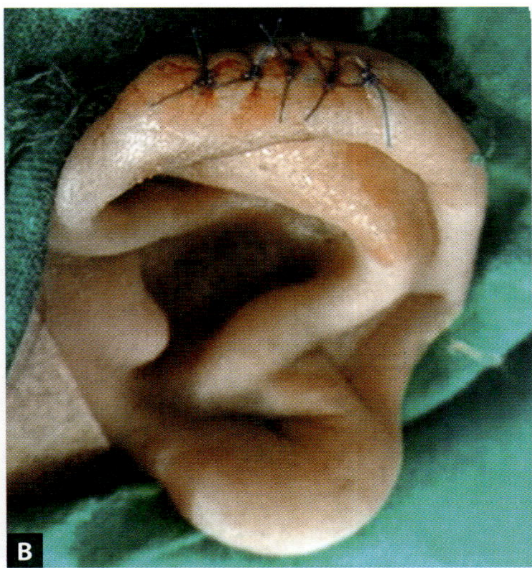

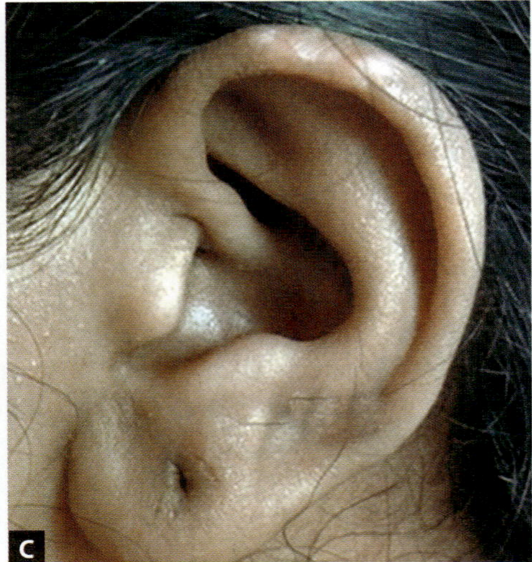

Figs. 36A to C: Keloid excision and closure.

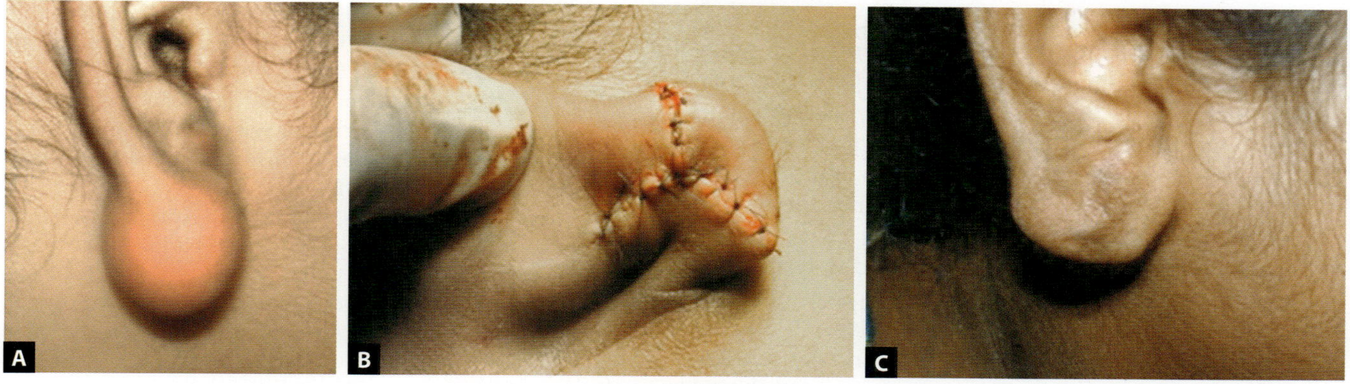

Figs. 37A to C: Excision of keloid over lobule, debulking of keloid with flaps on posterior aspect, sutures applied posteriorly.

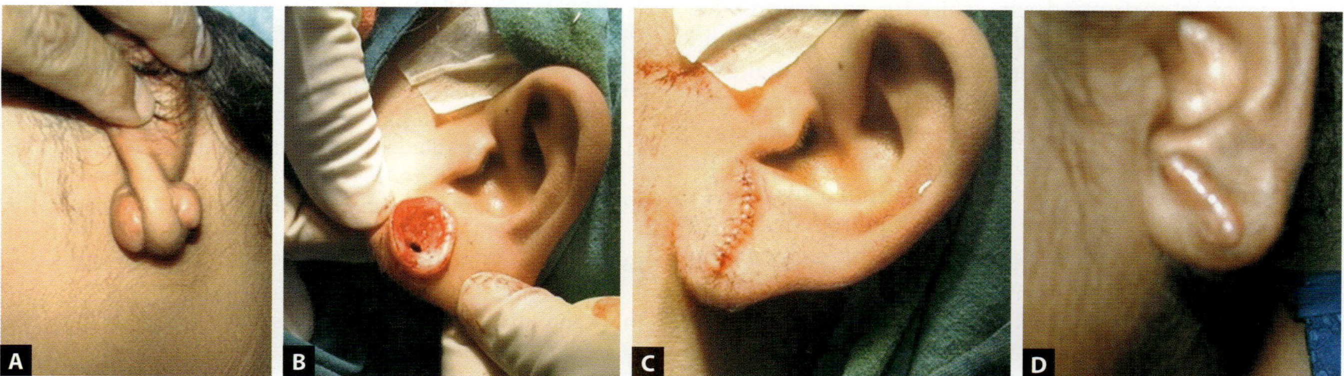

Figs. 38A to D: Intrakeloidal surgical debulking of dumbbell keloid on both anterior and posterior.

on either side at the base and closure of the flaps with primary closure without dead space. Pressure bandage is applied. Suture removal to be done 7 to 10 days later (Figs. 38A to D).

Various surgical methods are available for debulking of keloids tissue with primary intention of reducing the size of keloid without cutting the normal tissue, however surgery alone leads to high rate of recurrences, hence post surgical preventive strategies are most important for prevention of recurrences of earlobe keloids.

LASERS

Role of lasers have been described in the literature in the management of earlobe keloids. Photothermal effect of lasers produce collagen denaturation. The heat energy ruptures collagen stabilizing intermolecular and molecular cross links. In addition, the concurrent superheating of collagen fibers could also dissociate disulfide bonds with a subsequent realignment of these fibers.[25] However, lasers have limited role in the authors experience. Flash lamp pulsed dye laser (FPDL) has been used for the treatment of keloids with achievement of promising results, however, the treatment by FPDL alone is suitable only for small keloids with a limited volume.[26] Nd:Yag, carbon dioxide and diode laser have been used to treat earlobe keloids.[27,28]

However, the role of lasers in keloids is limited in a large bulky keloids, which are firm and hard with less vascularity.

To reduce recurrence rates, surgery is often combined with adjuvant treatment

- *Corticosteroid injections.* In addition to their anti-inflammatory effect, corticosteroids reduce collagen and glycosaminoglycan synthesis and the proliferation of fibroblasts. Triamcinolone acetonide, 10 to 40 mg, is often used as an active ingredient in intralesional injections. Injection at the correct depth in the mid-dermis is important to prevent undesired adverse effects, such as atrophy of the skin, telangiectasia, or pigmentary abnormalities. Steroids can be either first line or adjuvant to surgery. Injections are given perioperatively and then every three weeks.
- *Corticosteroid injection* in association with 5-fluorouracil, pulsed dye laser, and cryotherapy has been reported to be more efficient than corticosteroid alone.[29]
- *Verapamil hydrochloride* is a widely used calcium channel antagonist which inhibits the synthesis/

secretion of extracellular matrix molecules including collagen, glycosaminoglycans and fibronectin while increasing collagenase. It can be injected locally, intraoperatively before application of the pressure dressing, then postoperatively every 2 weeks for 1 month, then monthly for 3 months. The injection is given along suture lines and also into the wound bed.[24]

- Topical controlled pressure is reported to reduce the capillary perfusion that causes local hypoxia and leads to a decrease of myofibroblasts and collagen synthesis, acceleration of collagen maturation, and consequent flattening of the keloid.[30] The pressure exerted should be at least 24 mm Hg, in order to exceed the inherent capillary pressure, but must be < 30 mm Hg, otherwise it diminishes the peripheral blood circulation. This therapy is performed especially for ear keloids, for which pressure is applied at the front and back to build an abutment.[31] Making an auricle splint is demanding due to complex anatomy of external ears. To overcome this custom made devices have been tried.

  Custom made methyl methacrylate stent can be used as pressure devices. This is applied two weeks post excision to ensure primary healing. Since, the fabricated pressure device is unique for each ear, the natural folds of the ear are not compromised during application, enhancing its usage as postoperative pressure therapy.[32] Pressure devices should be used up to 20 hours per day during 12 months; and then 12 hours per day for another 6 months. Other modification to this is U-shaped screw-and-pin system which helps to adjust auricle pressure. [33]
- *Cryotherapy:* The freeze induces vascular damage that may lead to anoxia and ultimately tissue necrosis. Fikrle reported good results using cryotherapy alone for ear keloids in young patients.[34]
- *Other adjuvant therapies* are silicon gel sheets, radiation therapy, imiquimod.

CONCLUSION

Earlobe cleft and keloids present commonly to dermatologists.

A proper knowledge of various techniques for the earlobe repair and keloid surgery followed by proper postsurgical preventive methods are essential. These procedures can be very well-handled by dermatologists with surgical skills. Each procedure has its own advantages which a surgeon can make use of, depending on the type of earlobe deformity and type, site and size of ear lobe keloid.

REFERENCES

1. Pardue AM. Repair of torn earlobe with preservation of the perforation for an earring. Plast Reconstr Surg. 1973;51: 472-3.
2. Strauch B, Keyes-Ford M. Repair of the cleft earlobe with an advancement flap and two unilateral Z-plasties. Plastic Reconstr Surg. 1997;99:924-6.
3. Vujevich J, Obagi S. Repair of partial earlobe cleft using "purse string" repair. Dermatol Surg. 2006;32:969-7.
4. Niamtu J 3rd. Eleven pearls for cosmetic earlobe repair Dermatol Surg. 2002;28:180-5.
5. deMendonça MC, de Oliveira AR, Araújo JM, et al. Nonsurgical technique for incomplete earlobe cleft repair. Dermatol Surg 2009;35:446-50.
6. Reiter D, Alford EL. Torn earlobe: a new approach to management with a review of 68 cases. Ann OtolRhinolLaryngol. 1994;103:879-84.
7. McLaren LR. Cleft earlobe: a hazard of wearing earrings. Br J Plast Surg. 1954;7:162-5.
8. Tan EC. Punch technique: an alternative approach to the repair of pierced earlobe deformities. J Dermatol Surg Oncol. 1989;15:270-2.
9. Avenavoli FM. Split earlobe: repair using a half Z-plasty technique. Plast Reconstr Surg. 1996:98:372-3.
10. Apesos J, Kane M. Treatment of traumatic earlobe clefts. Aesthetic Plast Surg. 1993;17:253-5.
11. LaRossa D, Hamilton R. Method for repair of cleft earlobes. Plast Reconstr Surg. 1973;51:472-3.
12. Fatah MF. L-plasty technique in the repair of split earlobe. Br J Plast Surg. 1985;38:410-4.
13. Harahap M. Repair of split earlobes. A review and a new technique. J Dermatol Surg Oncol. 1982;8:187-91.
14. Kalimuthu R, Larson BJ, Lewis N. Earlobe repair: a new technique. Plast Reconstr Surg. 1984;74:299-300.
15. Effendi SH. Reconstruction of the middle-aged torn earlobe: a new method. Br J Plast Surg. 1988;41:174-6.
16. Buchan NG. The cleft ear lobe: a method of repair with preservation of the earring canal. Br J Plast Surg. 1975;28: 296.
17. Argamaso RV. The lap-joint principle in the repair of the cleft ear-lobe. Br J Plast Surg. 1978;31:337-8.
18. Zoltie N. Spilt earlobes: a method of repair preserving the hole. Plast Reconstr Surg. 1987;80:619-21.
19. Simplot TC, Hoffman HT. Comparison between cartilage and soft tissue ear piercing complications. Am J Otolaryngol. 1998:19:305-10.
20. Cosman B, Wolff M. Correlation of keloid recurrence with completeness of local excision. A negative report. Plast Reconstr Surg. 1972;50:163.
21. Niessen FB, Spauwen PH, Schalkwijk J, Kon M. On the nature of hypertrophic scars and keloids: a review. Plast Reconstr Surg. 1999:104:1435-58.
22. Aköz T, Gideroǫluk, Akan M. Combination of different techniques for the treatment of earlobe keloids. Aesth. Plast. Surg. 2002;26:184-18.
23. Kim DY, Kim ES, Eo SR, et al. A surgical approach for earlobe keloid: keloid fillet flap. Plast Reconstr Surg. 2004;113(6):1668-74.
24. El-Kamel MF, Selim MK, Alghobary MF. Keloidectomy with core fillet flap and intralesional verapamil injection for recurrent earlobe keloids. Indian J Dermatol Venereol Leprol. 2016;82:659-65.
25. Alster TS. Laser scar revision: comparison study of 585 nm pulsed dye laser with and without intralesional corticosteroids. Dermatol Surg. 2003;29(1):25-29.

26. Dierickx C, Goldmann MP, Fitzpatrick RE. Laser treatment of erythematous/hypertrophic and pigmented scars in 26 patients. Plast Reconstr Surg. 1995;95(1):84-90.
27. Norris JE. The effect of carbon dioxide laser surgery on the recurrence of keloids. Plast Reconstr Surg. 1991;87:44-9.
28. Kassab AN, Kharbotly AEl. Management of ear lobule keloids using 980-nm diode laser. Eur Arch Otorhinolaryngol. 2012; 269:419-23.
29. Sobec R, Dobreanu C, Fodor L, Comcutean A, Cichil I, Cosgarea M. Ear keloids: A review and update of treatment options. Clujul Medical. 2013;86(4):313-17.
30. Macintyre L, Baird M. Pressure garments for use in the treatment of hypertrophic scars. Burns. 2006;32(1):10-5.
31. Bran GM, Brom J, Hörmann K, et al. Auricular keloids: combined therapy with a new pressure device. Arch Facial Plast Surg. 2012;14(1):20-6.
32. Kadouch DJ, van der Veer WM, Delavary BM, et al. An alternative adjuvant treatment after ear keloid excision using a custom-made methyl methacrylate stent. Dermatologic Therapy. 2010;23:686-92.
33. Tanaydin V, Colla C, Piatkowski A, et al. Management of ear keloids using custom-molded pressure clips: a preliminary study. Eur J Plast Surg. 2014; 37:259-66.
34. Fikrle T, Pizinger K. Cryosurgery in the treatment of ear lobe keloids: report of seven cases. Dermatol Surg. 2005; 1:1728-31.

Chapter 60

Hidradenitis Suppurativa

M Kumaresan

Key Messages

- Hidradenitis suppurativa is a chronic disorder which can lead to severe morbidity.
- There is no satisfactory medical or surgical treatment available.
- Medical treatments include antibiotics, dapsone, retinoids, intralesional steroids and biologics.
- Lasers (CO_2 laser, Nd:YAG laser) have been tried with variable success.
- Surgery is needed in most cases and consists of deroofing, limited local excision and wide excision.

INTRODUCTION

Hidradenitis suppurativa (HS, derived from the Greek word "hidros" meaning sweat and "aden" meaning glands), is also known as Verneuil's disease, acne inversa or smokers boils. HS is a chronic, recurrent, debilitating disease that presents usually after puberty with painful, deep seated, inflammatory lesions in the apocrine glands of the body. HS is seen usually after puberty during the second and third decade of life and onset after menopause is rare.[1] HS in prepubertal age group is associated with premature adrenarche.[2,3] It is seen more commonly in females than the males.[1] Autosomal dominant type of inheritance has been reported in families.[1,4]

PATHOGENESIS

The pathogenesis of HS is not clearly understood. Initially it was thought to be a disorder of apocrine origin, but recent evidence states that HS is caused primarily by follicular occlusion with secondary involvement of the apocrine glands.[5] Follicular plugging leads to occlusion and dilation of the pilosebaceous unit, with subsequent rupture.[1] Extrusion of follicular contents, primarily consisting of corneocytes, bacteria, sebum products, and hair into the dermis produce a chemotactic inflammatory response.[1] The resulting influx of neutrophils, lymphocytes, and histiocytes lead to abscess formation.[6] This facilitates infection with further suppuration. With recurrence, sinuous and fistulous tracts evolve.[6,7] The role of hormones in HS is controversial and it is likely that hyperandrogenism does not play a role in the pathogenesis.[1] Some investigators postulate that there may be an underlying immunologic aberration involved in the pathogenesis of HS.[1]

The bacterial species isolated from HS include *Streptococcus viridans*, *Staphylococcus aureus*, *S. milleri*, anaerobes (*Peptostreptococcus species*, *Bacteroides melaninogenicus*, and *B. corrodens*), coryneform bacteria, gram-negative rods, gram-negative bacteria such as *Escherichia coli*, *Klebsiella*, and *Proteus.* No single bacterial species predominated in the culture, and this indicates that the bacteria are secondary colonizer rather than a primary agent. The most common bacteria isolated are *S. epidermidis* and *S. aureus*.[8] Increased prevalence of smoking has been found among patients with HS, suggesting that tobacco is a potential trigger for HS.[9,10] A significant association with obesity has been reported in HS.[11] Obesity aggravates disease through sweat retention, maceration, shearing of follicular or ductal outlets.[12]

CLINICAL FEATURES

Hidradenitis suppurativa is insidious in onset and usually seen in postpubertal males and females who are otherwise healthy.[13] Lesions are most frequently seen in the intertriginous apocrine glands as the axillary, inguinal, perianal, perineal, mammary, inframammary, buttock, pubic, chest, scalp, retroauricular, and eyelid areas.[14] This distribution pattern corresponds for the most part with the "milk line" distribution of apocrine-related mammary tissue in mammals.[1] The sites affected in HS correspond not only to the location of apocrine glands in the body but also to that of terminal hair follicles dependent on low androgen concentrations.[7] Lesions begins usually in axillae and anogenital regions, but as the disease progresses, new lesions develop in areas of friction including the submammary region, nape of the neck, waistband area, and in the inner thighs.[6] Perineal HS is associated with higher recurrence and poor prognosis than axillary HS.[15] Hidradenitis suppurativa lesions are characterized by tender subcutaneous nodules. With time, nodules rupture spontaneously or coalesce to form painful, deep dermal abscesses. These abscesses are rounded without central necrosis or pus pointing and exude a purulent foul smelling discharge. Double comedone is a blackhead with multiple apertures that communicate below the skin and is typical for HS.[16] Early symptoms include burning, pruritus, local warmth, hyperhidrosis, and pain. HS may be divided into acute and chronic forms. Acute HS presents with a few deep-seated nodules, which may coalesce developing into cord-like red-to-bluish red structures.[1] Chronic HS is characterized by multiple abscesses, internetworking sinus tracts, foul exudate from draining sinuses, inflammation, both atrophic and hypertrophic scars, ulceration, and infection which may extend deep into the fascia.[1] Hurley separated patients into three groups based largely on the presence and extent of cicatrization and sinuses (Table 1). Over time, sinus tracts can coalesce into large regions of subcutaneous honeycombing.[17] They can potentially dissect into deep structures including muscle, fascia, lymph nodes, the urethra, and the bowels.[6,14] They release a serous to purulent malodorous discharge, resulting in ulceration[18] soiling of clothes and social embarrassment. The ulcers characteristically present with rolled, boggy, ragged edges and clean granulating bases.[18] Patients with anogenital HS may also have disease in the anal canal.[19] The severity of disease varies considerably. The diagnosis of HS is made clinically by the following features chronicity, recurrence of disease, failure to completely clear with antibiotics, characteristic multifocal lesion distribution, sinus formation, scarring, dermal contracture, presence of double comedones, multiple open comedones, nodules, papules, tenderness of lesions, and malodorous discharge.[1]

PROGNOSIS AND COMPLICATIONS

Contractures, strictures, serious infection, and anemia are also potential sequelae of HS.[1] Risk of SCC is increased in those with HS.[1] The ratio of SCC in HS favors males (4:1).[20] Majority of SCC occurred in perineum or buttocks.[20]

Table 1: Hurley staging system for hidradenitis suppurativa.

Hurley stage	*Extent of disease in tissue*
I	Abscess formation (single or multiple) without sinus tracts and cicatrization
II	One or more widely separated recurrent abscesses with tract formation and scars
III	Multiple interconnected tracts and abscesses throughout an entire area

DISEASE ASSOCIATION

Hidradenitis suppurativa has been associated with many disorders. The other disorders of follicular occlusion (acne conglobata, dissecting cellulitis of the scalp, and pilonidal cyst) are well-known associations with HS, and make up the so-called follicular occlusion tetrad.[21] Acne vulgaris and Crohn's disease are the other common associations.[1]

TREATMENT

There is no single effective therapy for HS. Treatment modality depends on the disease severity. Treatment for HS is classified as either medical or surgical (Flowchart 1).

Medical Treatment

Conservative Measures

Conservative measures include warm baths, avoidance of shaving if irritation occurs, avoiding prolonged exposure to heat, humidity, hydrotherapy, weight loss, and use of topical cleansing agents to reduce bacterial load. Nonsteroidal anti-inflammatory drugs (NSAiDs) can be used to alleviate pain as well as inflammation. Antibiotics either topical or systemic agents are used as the first-line agents or in Hurley's stage 1 disease. Though, antibiotics are used to improve HS, complete remission is rarely achieved with antibiotics. The only topical antibiotic that has been proven effective in a randomized controlled trial is clindamycin. Topical 1% clindamycin phosphate applied twice daily for a period of minimum 3 months has been shown to be effective in Hurley stage 1 & 2 disease.[22] Combination of rifampicin (600 mg) and clindamycin (300 mg twice daily) for 10 weeks has been shown to be effective in moderate-to severe HS.[23,24] Dapsone had been reported to be an effective and safe alternative therapeutic option for HS at a dose of 25–150 mg/day (4–12 weeks) and may be particularly useful for women in the reproductive age group.[25] The other combination reported to improve refractory HS is rifampicin, moxifloxacin and metronidazole.[26] Antistaphylococcal agents are best for axillary disease, and more broad-spectrum coverage is preferred for perineal disease.[27] There is no evidence that chronic suppressive antibiotic therapy alters the natural history of HS. Oral retinoids work by inhibiting sebaceous gland function and abnormal keratinization. Pretreatment with isotretinoin at a dosage of 0.5–1.0 mg per kg daily for a few months before surgery has been recommended to reduce the inflammatory components.[27] Acitretin appears to be an effective treatment for refractory HS, leading to reduction of pain from painful nodules and reducing the extent of the disease for a prolonged period.[28] Hormonal therapy should be considered in females presenting

Flowchart 1: Treatment algorithm.[55]

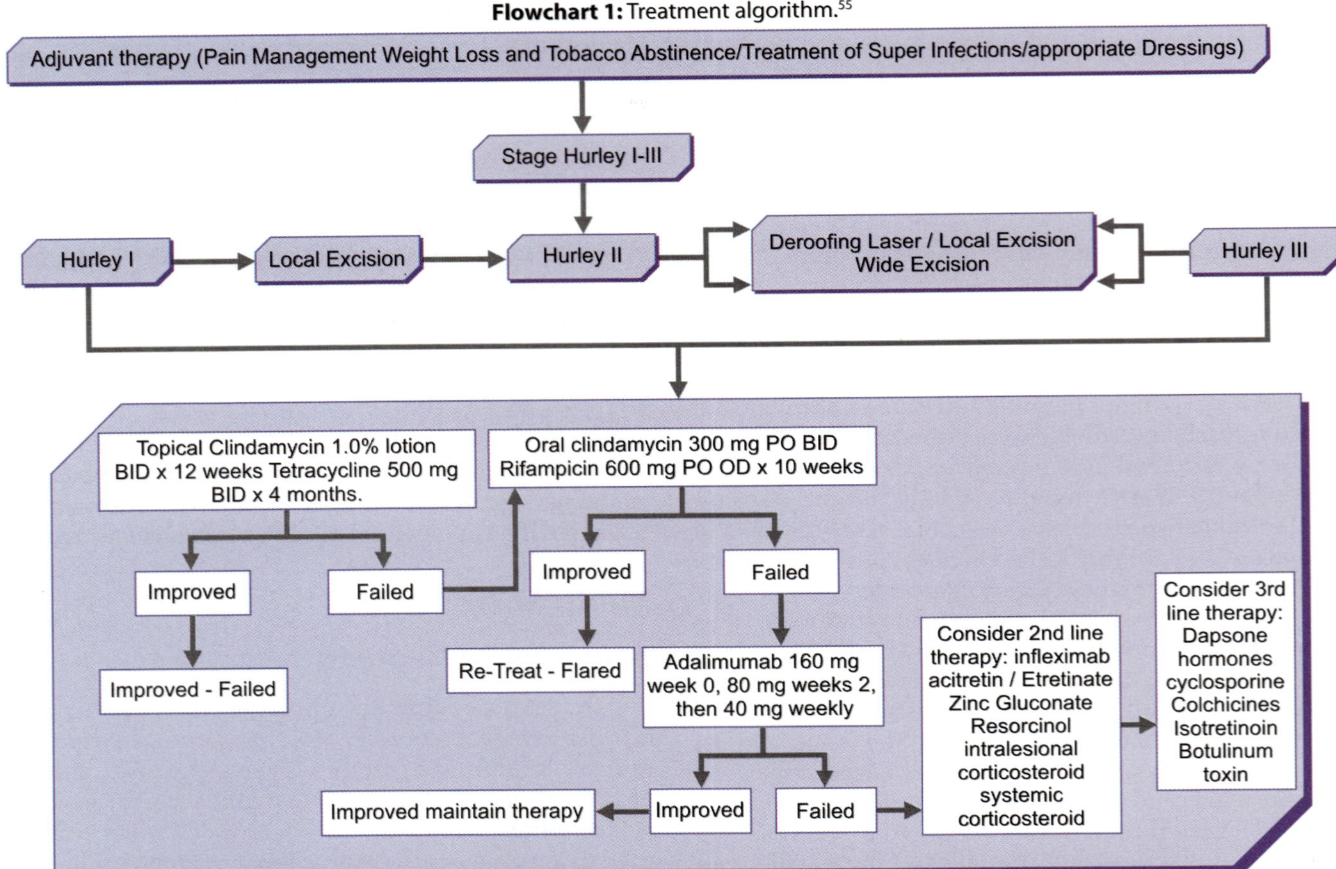

with HS.[29] Oral contraceptive agents that contain a high estrogen-to-progesterone ratio and low androgenicity of progesterone, finasteride at a dosage of 5 mg daily and cyproterone acetate have been reported to be effective in HS.[27] Immunosuppressive drugs such as cyclosporine, azathioprine and prednisone are occasionally successful.[30] The use of biologic drugs for the treatment of HS has variable long-term results and is laden with significant adverse effects.[31] Among the biological agents, infliximab, etanercept and adalimumab has been reported to be effective in HS.[31]

Botulinum Toxin

Botulinum toxin has been reported to be effective in HS by decreasing apocrine gland sweat secretion and limiting tendency towards follicular rupture.[32] Prepubertal HS has been successfully treated with botulinum toxin.[33] Dose ranges from 50–100 units, injected intradermally as in hyperhidrosis. Botulinum toxin treatment appears to be suppressive with the effect lasting for 6 months.

Radiotherapy

Radiotherapy has been suggested as efficacious for early lesions of HS but not for sinuses.[34] Hair follicle destruction is the suggested mechanism of action.[34] When more radical and invasive surgical options fail, radiotherapy is a viable option.[35] Doses of 7.5 Gy at 2.5 Gy per fraction has been reported to be beneficial in refractory cases.[35] Caution should be exercised when offering this therapy to younger atients.

Cryotherapy

Cryosurgery has been studied as a potential HS treatment. Complications like pain, ulceration, secondary infection and prolonged healing limits its routine use in HS.[36]

LASERS AND LIGHT DEVICES

Laser and light devices acts in two main ways, selective and ablative. IPL and lasers such as Nd:YAG, Alexandrite and Diode act in a selective manner and are useful in Hurley stage I or II to reduce the number of hair follicles and sebaceous glands and thereby bacterial load in the treated areas, deocclusion of the follicle followed by drainage of the inflammatory lesion and destruction of the follicular unit while the CO_2 laser debulks the diseased tissue and established sinus tracts and hence more useful in stage II to III disease. Laser offers a safe, effective, alternative treatment for moderate stage HS.[37]

Nd:YAG Laser

Prospective randomized controlled studies has shown that long pulse Nd:YAG lasers are effective in controlling the existing lesions and preventing the new lesions of HS.[38,39] As the inflammatory lesions of HS are located in the mid-reticular dermis and the subcutaneous tissue, a longer wavelength device like Nd:YAG would increase the efficacy of treatment. Treatment with Nd:YAG laser in patients with HS is characterized by rupture of nodules, abscesses, and sinus tracts with relative increase in the discharge in the initial few days followed by a rapid healing of HS lesions.[3] Areas with dark coarse terminal hair such as the axilla shows faster and greater degrees of improvement than areas with fine vellus hair, such as the inframammary region.[39] Improvement in the inframammary areas can be explained by nonspecific thermal damage of the laser on the skin with water being the likely chromophore.[39] Excessive scarring present in chronic stages of the disease leads to decreased penetration of the laser beam and hence results in lesser efficacy in patients with long-standing disease with extensive scarring.[39] The parameters for skin types IV to VI is, fluence: 25–35 J/cm^2, pulse duration: 35 milliseconds and spot size of 10 mm.[39]

Carbon Dioxide Laser

CO_2 lasers offer a promising treatment option in HS, advantages are, good hemostasis, excellent operative field visualization and reduced risk of postoperative scar contractures, infection, and recurrence.[40] CO_2 laser ablation is also termed as carbon dioxide laser stripping (CLS). CLS can also be performed as a office procedure, offering rapid recovery, and reduced patient costs.[40]

CO_2 laser treatment aims at focal radical vaporization of all nodules, abscesses and fistulas, leaving healthy tissues in between the pathological lesions. The lesions are vaporized under local anesthesia from "inside and out" until surrounding healthy tissues is reached, superficially and deep. In this way the technique can be tissue sparing and at the same time radical. Usually the vaporization reaches the deep subcutaneous fat or fascia. In the axillary and inguinal region, major vessels and the nerve plexus must be protected, but this depth is seldom reached in Hurley stage II lesions. The smaller blood vessels are coagulated by the laser, but bleeding from vessels larger than 0.5–1 mm in diameter is usually controlled with electrocoagulation or ligation. Carbon dioxide laser can also be used to excise smaller or larger skin areas en bloc with or without laser coagulation of remnants (marsupialisation) in the deep tissues, with less bleeding and better visualization than in standard excisions (Figs. 1 and 2).[41,42]

Wound Healing[43]

The wound is generally left to heal by secondary intention. The wound is immediately covered with dry dressings or ointment-impregnated dressings and a covering bandage attached with surgical adhesive tape or gauze underwear. The dressings are initially left on for 2 or 3 days without changing to prevent early bleeding. Thereafter, the wound is cleaned, and the bandage is changed as often as necessary, sometimes daily, pending complete healing. Healing time ranges from 6–8 weeks. CO_2 laser excision followed by split skin grafting has been reported to accelerate wound healing (Fig. 3).[44]

Complications

The common complications encountered are secondary infection, prolonged healing time, scarring and scar contracture. Fractional CO_2 laser has been reported to reduce the scar contracture and improve the healing of chronic ulcers in cases, who had undergone CO_2 laser excision earlier.[45]

Internal Pulsed Light (IPL) and Diode Laser

IPL and diode laser works on the same principle as Nd:YAG. IPL has also been shown to have anti-inflammatory effect

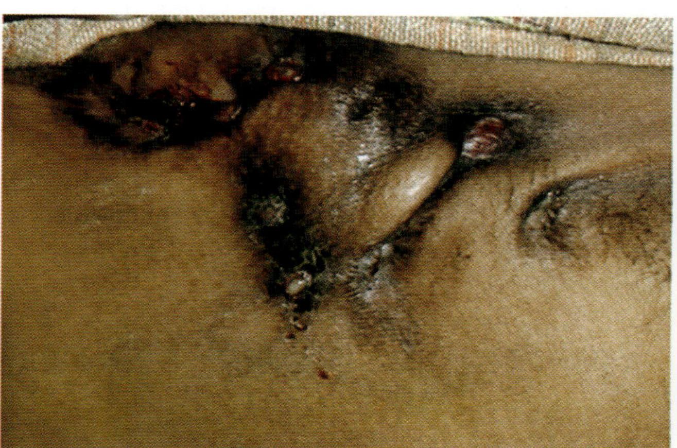

Fig. 1: HS before CO_2 laser surgery.

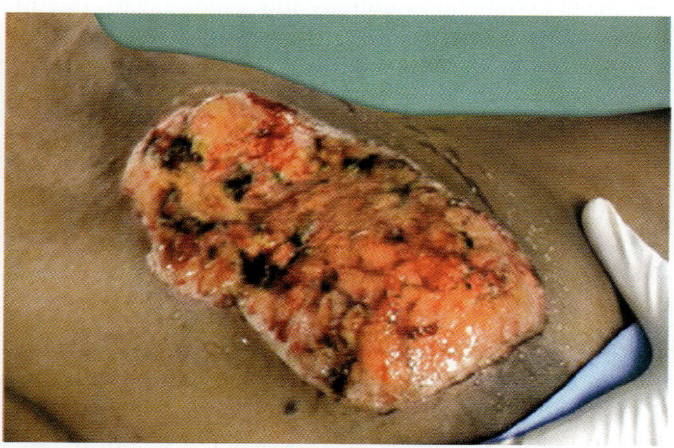

Fig. 2: Post CO_2 laser excision of the affected tissue.

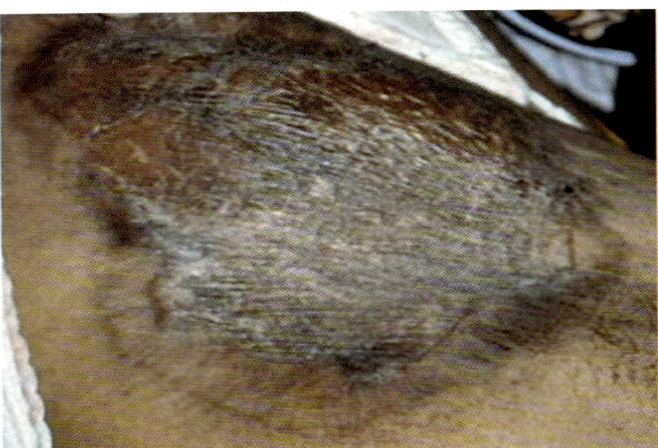

Fig. 3: Postoperative image following skin grafting at the end of 12 months.

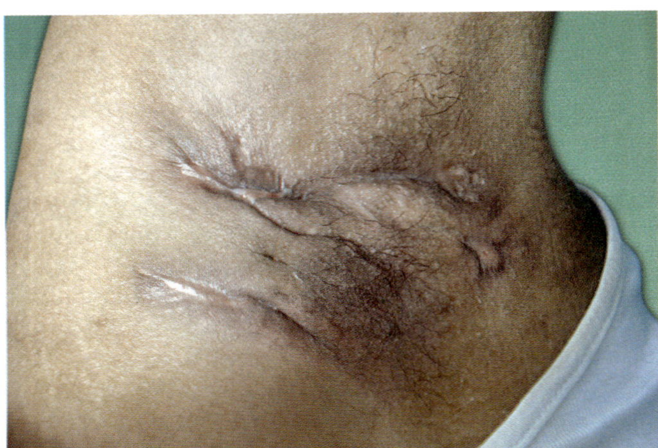

Fig. 4: Axillary HS with sinus tracts before deroofing.
Courtesy: Dr Venkataram Mysore and Dr Anita.

and has the ability to eliminate the chronic inflammation within the diseased tissue.[46]

Photodynamic Therapy

The mechanism of action of photodynamic therapy (PDT) in HS treatment is the cytotoxic effects, which cause selective cell necrosis, immunomodulatory effects and the ability of 5-aminolevulinic acid (PDT-ALA) or its methyl ester (PDT-MAL) to break up the bio-film produced by coagulase negative *Staphylococcus* (CONS) and other antibacterial effects in patients in whom bio-film plays a pivotal part of their pathogenesis.[47] PDT is not a first line treatment for HS but in some cases could be added as an adjuvant. More studies are needed to establish the role of PDT treatment in HS.

INTRALESIONAL CORTICOSTEROIDS

The use of intralesional triamcinolone acetonide 5-10 mg/mL has been advocated for the rapid reduction of inflammation associated with acute flares and for management of recalcitrant nodules and sinus tracts.[48] It is utilized as both monotherapy and an adjunct to systemic therapies. When effective, clinical response (flattening, resolution or spontaneous discharge of nodules) is seen within 48-72 hours. Therapy is contraindicated if clinical suspicion of bacterial infection exists. Local complications include atrophy, infection, pigmentary change and telangiectasia.

Surgical

Surgery is largely regarded as one of the most effective treatment for intractable HS.[1] Patients should be advised that surgery treats only the disease that is present at the site of the excision and a recurrence at a new site is possible. Incision and drainage of abscesses is not recommended because it is only transiently beneficial and does nothing to halt progression of the disease.[27] On an individual basis, however, incision and drainage might be indicated to relieve excessive lesional pain.[27] Single nodules may be injected with intralesional triamcinolone (3–5 mg/mL) to decrease inflammation.[49] The efficacy of the surgical treatment depends upon the number of lesions and the disease duration. A better outcome is seen with fewer lesions and shorter duration. Deroofing, limited local excision and wide excision are the routine surgical modalities practiced in HS.

Deroofing

The deroofing technique was first described by Mullins et al. in 1959.[50] The deroofing technique is an effective, simple, minimally invasive, tissue-saving surgical intervention for the treatment of mild-to-moderate HS lesions at fixed locations and it is suitable as an office procedure.[50] This technique converts, with limited surgery and maximal preservation of the surrounding healthy tissue, painful recurrent lesions into cosmetically acceptable scars.[50] The lesions to be deroofed are marked with an ink. After cleansing the target area, local anesthesia should be infiltrated into the lesion and the surrounding area. The discharging sinus tracts should be explored with the help of a blunt probe introduced into the sinus through the opening, if there are no openings detectable, incisions are done over the sinus tract to introduce the probe. The roof of the tract is surgically removed leaving the floor open. The purulent discharge and other exudates on the floor of the tracts are curetted out and the ulcer allowed to heal by secondary intention. The defects heals with cosmetically acceptable scars (Figs. 4 to 8).

EXCISION

Limited local excision is associated with more recurrence.[51] Wide excision is done by removing all of the apocrine glands from hair bearing skin to the deep underlying fascia

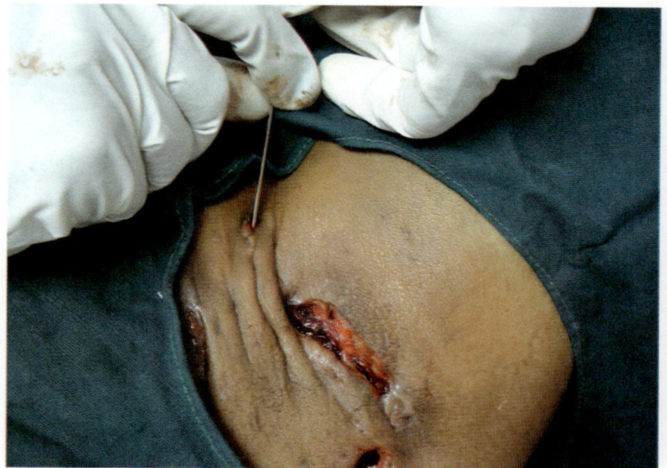

Fig. 5: Blunt probe to visualize the sinus tract.
Courtesy: Dr Venkataram Mysore and Dr Anita.

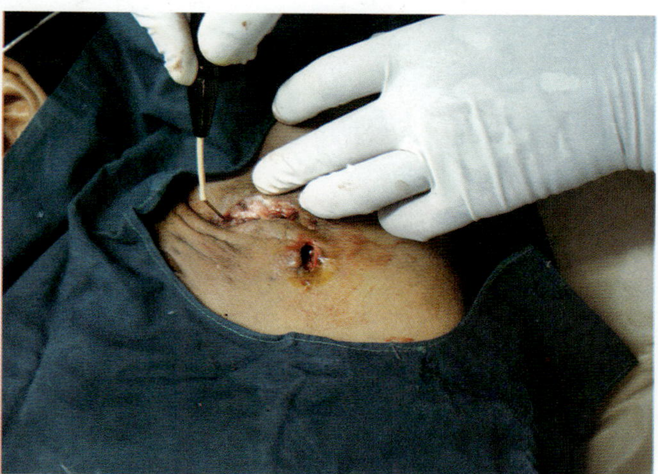

Fig. 6: Deroofing the sinus tract.
Courtesy: Dr Venkataram Mysore and Dr Anita.

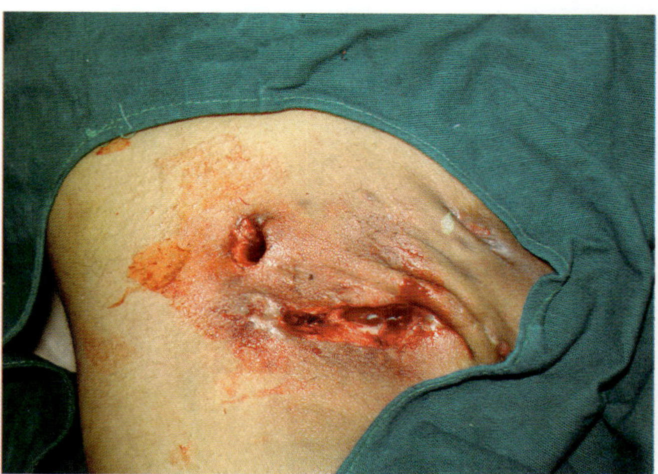

Fig. 7: Wound after deroofing.
Courtesy: Dr Venkataram Mysore and Dr Anita.

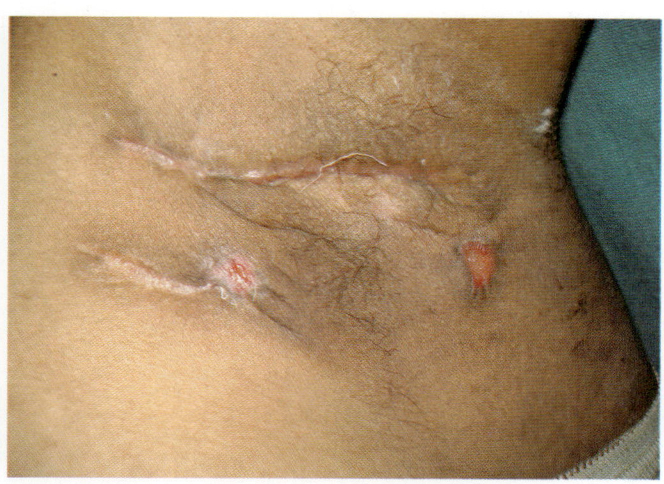

Fig. 8: Complete healing of wound by secondary intention after deroofing.
Courtesy: Dr Venkataram Mysore and Dr Anita.

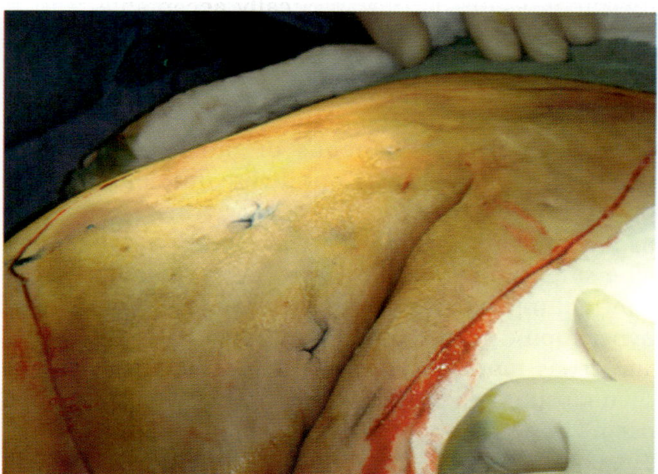

Fig. 9: Perianal HS before wide surgical excision.
Courtesy: Uwe Wollina, MD, Department of Dermatology & Allergology, Hospital Dresden-Friedrichstadt, Academic Teaching Hospital of the Technical University of Dresden, Friedrichstrasse, Dresden, Germany.

(Fig. 9).[52] Reconstruction after wide excision is important in terms of wound healing time and cosmetic results, the methods commonly practiced are primary closure, secondary intention healing, graft and flap closure.[53] Primary closure is appropriate in minor defects surrounded by lax skin.[51] High recurrence rate have been associated with primary closure, which may be due to inadequate excision.[54] The usual purse string suture frequently leads to premature suture extrusion and wound dehiscence.[51] Secondary intention healing gives satisfactory results in wounds up to 20 cm (Figs. 9 to 13).[51] New granulation tissue in secondary healing eliminates the risk of recurrence because it does not include apocrine glands.[53] Major drawback in secondary healing is long duration for healing (6–12 weeks) and need for supervision by a physician.[51] Closure of wounds with split thickness graft is associated with low recurrence rates.[53] Bacterial contamination

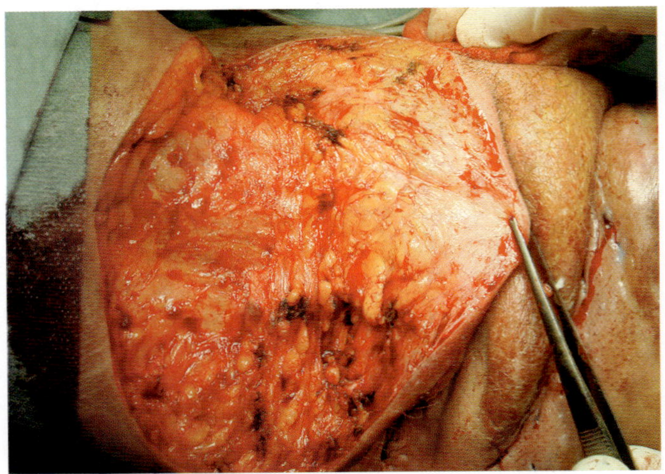

Fig. 10: Surgical removal of the inflamed subcutaneous tissue, sinus tract and fistula.
Courtesy: Uwe Wollina, MD, Department of Dermatology & Allergology, Hospital Dresden-Friedrichstadt, Academic Teaching Hospital of the Technical University of Dresden, Friedrichstrasse, Dresden, Germany.

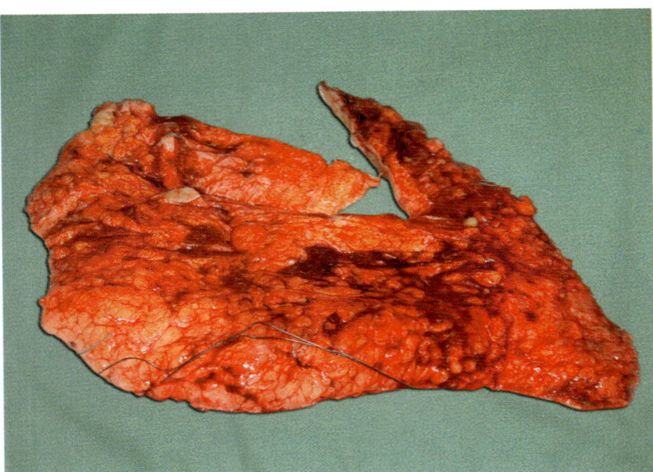

Fig. 12: Excised tissue from the groin.
Courtesy: Uwe Wollina, MD, Department of Dermatology & Allergology, Hospital Dresden-Friedrichstadt, Academic Teaching Hospital of the Technical University of Dresden, Friedrichstrasse, Dresden, Germany.

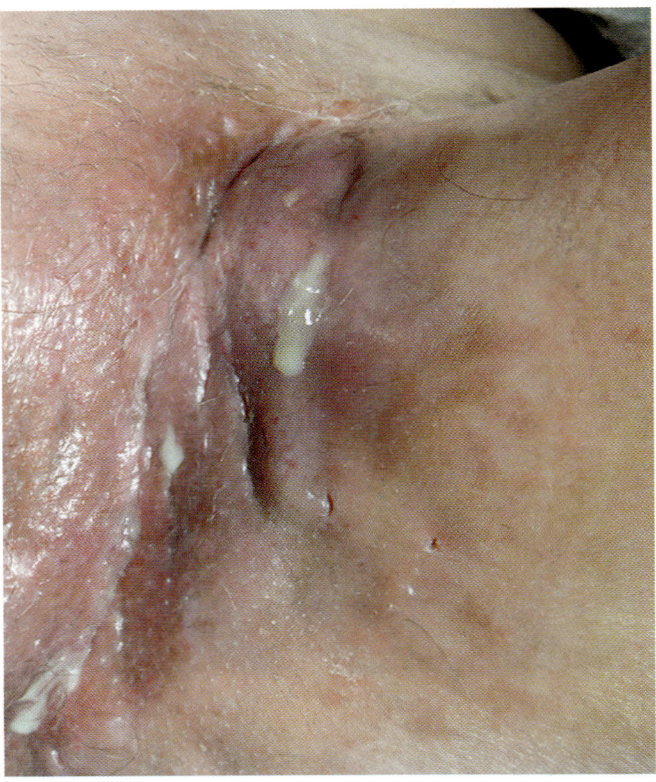

Fig. 11: Hidradenitis suppurativa on the groin before surgical excision.
Courtesy: Uwe Wollina, MD, Department of Dermatology & Allergology, Hospital Dresden-Friedrichstadt, Academic Teaching Hospital of the Technical University of Dresden, Friedrichstrasse, Dresden, Germany.

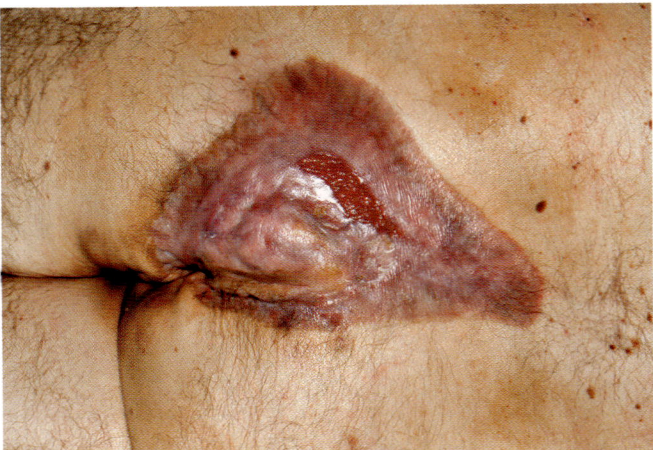

Fig. 13: Healed wound at the end of 3 months.
Courtesy: Uwe Wollina, MD, Department of Dermatology & Allergology, Hospital Dresden-Friedrichstadt, Academic Teaching Hospital of the Technical University of Dresden, Friedrichstrasse 41, 01067 Dresden, Germany.

of skin in the axillary, perineal and perianal region may lead to graft loss.[53] Other shortcomings of surgery include contracture development and limitation of movement.[53] Flap techniques described for the closure of defects in HS are lipocutaneous, fasciocutaneous, myocutaneous and free flaps. In axillary, perineal and perianal regions repair with fasciocutaneous or musculocutaneous flaps are recommended. Contracture development and limitation of movement are observed less frequently in flap repair methods. The common complications after surgical methods in HS are pain, wound infection, contracture, bleeding and excessive proliferation of hypertrophic granulation tissue.[51] Recurrence following surgery is more likely related to insufficient excision than closure technique.[53] Great majority of recurrence occurs in perineal, perianal, gluteal and inguinal sites.[53] The use of MRI and ultrasound will help in preoperative assessment of the extension of the lesions and planning of radical surgery.[51] The lesions at the scrotum, gluteal region, perianal and perineum should be treated surgically because the lesions in this area are more painful, cause

Table 2: Category of evidence/strength of recommendation rating scale.[55]

Treatment modality	*Category of evidence*	*Strength of recommendation*
Excision or curettage of individual lesions	III	C
Total excision of lesions and the surrounding hair-bearing skin	IIb	B
Secondary intention healing	IIb	B
Primary closure	III	C
Reconstruction with skin grafting	III	C
Reconstruction with skin flap plasty	1a/IIa	A/B
Deroofing	IV	D
CO_2 laser	Ib	A
Nd:YAG laser	Ib	A
IPL	IV	D
Intralesional steroids	IV	D
Botox	IV	D

movement restriction, and carry the risk of urethral fistula. In the perianal, perineal and gluteal area, colostomy helps in control of postoperative infection and contributes to the success of radical surgical excision.[51]

CONCLUSION

Though there are numerous options available for treatment of HS, there is no universally effective single therapy. Therefore, the treating physician must weigh the risks and benefits of each option based on the patient's disease severity and personal circumstances and manage accordingly.

Category of evidence/strength of recommendation rating scale[55] are shown in Table 2.

REFERENCES

1. Alikhan A, Lynch PJ, Eisen DB. Hidradenitis suppurativa: a comprehensive review. J Am Acad Dermatol. 2009;60:539-61.
2. Lewis F, Messenger AG, Wales JK. Hidradenitis suppurativa as a presenting feature of premature adrenarche. Br J Dermatol. 1993;129:447-8.
3. Mengesha YM, Holcombe TC, Hansen RC. Prepubertal hidradenitis suppurativa: two case reports and review of the literature. Pediatr Dermatol. 1999;16:292-6.
4. Gao M, Wang PG, Cui Y, et al. Inversa acne (hidradenitis suppurativa): a case report and identification of the locus at chromosome 1p21.1-1q25.3. J Invest Dermatol. 2006;126:1302-6.
5. Pironi D, Caruso F, Panarese A, et al. Chronic hidradenitis suppurativa in the inguinal, perineal and scrotal regions: A case report and review of the literature. Ann Ital Chir. 2010;81:465-70.
6. Mortimer PS, Lunniss PJ. Hidradenitis suppurativa. J R Soc Med. 2000;93:420-2.
7. Yu CC, Cook MG. Hidradenitis suppurativa: A disease of follicular epithelium, rather than apocrine glands. Br J Dermatol. 1990;122:763-9.
8. Jemec GB, Faber M, Gutschik E, et al. The bacteriology of hidradenitis suppurativa. Dermatol. 1996;193:203-6.
9. Rompel R, Petres J. Long-term results of wide surgical excision in 106 patients with hidradenitis suppurativa. Dermatol Surg. 2000;26:638-43.
10. Freiman A, Bird G, Metelitsa AI, et al. Cutaneous effects of smoking. J Cutan Med Surg. 2004;8:415-23.
11. Revuz JE, Canoui-Poitrine F, Wolkenstein P, et al. Prevalence and factors associated with hidradenitis suppurativa: results from two case-control studies. J Am Acad Dermatol. 2008;59:596-601.
12. Edlich RF, Silloway KA, Rodeheaver GT, et al. Epidemiology, pathology, and treatment of axillary hidradenitis suppurativa. J Emerg Med. 1986;4:369-78.
13. Wiseman MC. Hidradenitis suppurativa: A review. Dermatol Ther. 2004;17:50-4.
14. Slade DE, Powell BW, Mortimer PS. Hidradenitis suppurativa: pathogenesis and management. Br J Plast Surg. 2003;56:451-61.
15. Williams ST, Busby RC, DeMuth RJ, et al. Perineal hidradenitis suppurativa: presentation of two unusual complications and a review. Ann Plast Surg. 1991;26:456-62.
16. Larralde M, Abad ME, Munoz AS, et al. Childhood flexural comedones: a new entity. Arch Dermatol. 2007;143:909-11.
17. Brown TJ, Rosen T, Orengo IF. Hidradenitis suppurativa. South Med J. 1998;91:1107-14.
18. Anderson MJ, Dockerty MB. Perianal hidradenitis suppurativa: a clinical and pathologic study. Dis Colon Rectum. 1958;1:23-31.
19. Culp CE. Chronic hidradenitis suppurativa of the anal canal. A surgical skin disease. Dis Colon Rectum. 1983;26:669-76.
20. Maclean GM, Coleman DJ. Three fatal cases of squamous cell carcinoma arising in chronic perineal hidradenitis suppurativa. Ann R Coll Surg Engl. 2007;89:709-12.
21. Scheinfeld NS. A case of dissecting cellulitis and a review of the literature. Dermatol Online J. 2003;9:8.
22. Jemec GB, Wendelboe P. Topical clindamycin versus systemic tetracycline in the treatment of hidradenitis suppurativa. J Am Acad Dermatol. 1998;39:971-4.
23. Van der Zee HH, Boer J, Prens EP, et al. The effect of combined treatment with oral clindamycin and oral rifampicin in patients with hidradenitis suppurativa. Dermatol. 2009;219:143-7.
24. Gener G, Canoui-Poitrine F, Revuz JE, et al. Combination therapy with clindamycin and rifampicin for hidradenitis suppurativa: a series of 116 consecutive patients. Dermatol. 2009;219:148-54.
25. Kaur MR, Lewis HM. Hidradenitis suppurativa treated with dapsone: A case series of five patients. J Dermatolog Treat. 2006;17:211-3.
26. Join-Lambert O, Coignard H, Jais JP, et al. Efficacy of rifampin-moxifloxacin-metronidazole combination therapy in hidradenitis suppurativa. Dermatol. 2011;222:49-58.
27. Shah N. Hidradenitis suppurativa: a treatment challenge. Am Fam Physician. 2005;72:1547-52.

28. Boer J, Nazary M. Long-term results of acitretin therapy for hidradenitis suppurativa. Is acne inversa also a misnomer? Br J Dermatol. 2011;164:170-5.
29. Kraft JN, Searles GE. Hidradenitis suppurativa in 64 female patients: retrospective study comparing oral antibiotics and antiandrogen therapy. J Cutan Med Surg. 2007;11:125-31.
30. Mitchell KM, Beck DE. Hidradenitis suppurativa. Surg Clin North Am. 2002;82:1187-97.
31. Shuja F, Chan CS, Rosen T. Biologic drugs for the treatment of hidradenitis suppurativa: an evidence-based review. Dermatol Clin. 2010;28:511-21.
32. O'Reilly DJ, Pleat JM, Richards AM. Treatment of hidradenitis suppurativa with botulinum toxin A. Plast Reconstr Surg. 2005;116:1575-6.
33. Feito-Rodríguez M, Sendagorta-Cudós E, Herranz-Pinto P, et al. Prepubertal hidradenitis suppurativa successfully treated with botulinum toxin A. Dermatol Surg. 2009;35:1300-2.
34. Zeligman I. Temporary X-ray epilation therapy of chronic axillary hidradenitis suppurativa. Arch Dermatol. 1965;92:690-4.
35. Trombetta M, Werts ED, Parda D. The role of radiotherapy in the treatment of hidradenitis suppurativa: case report and review of the literature. Dermatol Online J. 2010;15:16.
36. Bong JL, Shalders K, Saihan E. Treatment of persistent painful nodules of hidradenitis suppurativa with cryotherapy. Clin Exp Dermatol. 2003;28:241-4.
37. Mahmoud BH, Tierney E, Hexsel CL, et al. P controlled clinical and histopathologic study of hidradenitis suppurativa treated with the long-pulsed neodymium:yttrium aluminium-garnet laser. J Am Acad Dermatol. 2010;62:637-45.
38. Tierney E, Mahmoud BH, Hexsel C, et al. Randomized control trial for the treatment of hidradenitis suppurativa with a neodymium-doped yttrium aluminium garnet laser. Dermatol Surg. 2009;35:1188-98.
39. Mahmoud BH, Tierney E, Hexsel CL, et al. Prospective controlled clinical and histopathologic study of hidradenitis suppurativa treated with the long-pulsed neodymium:yttrium aluminium-garnet laser. J Am Acad Dermatol. 2010;62:637-45.
40. Crocco EI, Dalapicola MC, Suzuki NM, Alves RO. Surgical Treatment of Chronic Hidradenitis Suppurativa: CO_2 Laser Stripping—Second Intention Technique. Dermatol Surg. 2016;42:429-31.
41. Finley EM, Ratz JL. Treatment of hidradenitis suppurativa with carbon dioxide laser excision and second-intention healing. J Am Acad Dermatol. 1996;34:465-9.
42. Hazen PG, Hazen BP. Hidradenitis suppurativa: successful treatment using carbon dioxide laser excision and marsupialization. Dermatol Surg. 2010;36:208-13.
43. Zouboulis CC1, Desai N, Emtestam L, et al. European S1 guideline for the treatment of hidradenitis suppurativa/acne inversa. J Eur Acad Dermatol Venereol. 2015;29:619-44.
44. Natarajan K, Srinivas CR, Thomas M, et al. Hidradenitis suppurativa treated with carbon dioxide laser followed by split skin thickness graft. Indian J Dermatol Venereol Leprol. 2014;80:376-8.
45. Nicholson CL, Hamzavi I, Ozog DM. Rapid healing of chronic ulcerations and improvement in range of motion after fractional carbon dioxide (CO_2) treatment after CO_2 excision of hidradenitis suppurativa axillary lesions: A case report. J Am Acad Dermatol. 2016;2:4-6.
46. Jain V, Jain A. Use of lasers for the management of refractory cases of hidradenitis suppurativa and pilonidal sinus. J Cutan Aesthet Surg. 2012;5:190e2.
47. Scheinfeld N. The use of photodynamic therapy to treat hidradenitis suppurativa a review and critical analysis. Dermatol Online J. 2015;15:21.
48. Jemec GBE, Revuz J, Leyden J. Hidradenitis suppurativa. Berlin, Heidelberg: Springer. 2006.pp.138-140.
49. Krbec AC. Current understanding and management of hidradenitis suppurativa. J Am Acad Nurse Pract. 2007;19:228-34.
50. van der Zee HH, Prens EP, Boer J. Deroofing: a tissue-saving surgical technique for the treatment of mild to moderate hidradenitis suppurativa lesions. J Am Acad Dermatol. 2010;63:475-80.
51. Büyükaik O, Hasdemir AO, Kahramansoy N, et al. Surgical approach to extensive hidradenitis suppurativa. Dermatol Surg. 2011;37:835-42.
52. Parks RW, Parks TG. Pathogenesis, clinical features and management of hidradenitis suppurativa. Ann R Coll Surg Engl. 1997;79:83-9.
53. Bieniek A, Matusiak L, Okulewicz-Gojlik D, et al. Surgical treatment of hidradenitis suppurativa: experiences and recommendations. Dermatol Surg. 2010;36:1998-2004.
54. Watson JD. Hidradenitis suppurativa—a clinical review. Br J Plast Surg. 1985;38:567-9.
55. Gulliver W, Zouboulis CC, Prens E, et al. Evidence-based approach to the treatment of hidradenitis suppurativa/acne in versa, based on the European guidelines for hidradenitis suppurativa. Rev Endocr Metab Disord. Feb 1,2016 published onlineDOI10.1007/s11154-016-9328-5.

Chapter 61

Circumcision

Aniketh Venkataram, SDN Guptha, Vishal Chugh

Key Messages 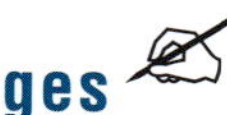

- Circumcision is one of the world's oldest surgical procedures. It is performed for a variety of reasons, some justified, others less so.
- The most common indications are phimosis and paraphimosis.
- It is usually performed under local anesthesia—either penile or ring block.
- The most common technique is the dorsal slit technique.
- Postoperative care is important to reduce discomfort.
- Meticulous technique and understanding of anatomy are needed to avoid complications.

INTRODUCTION

Circumcision is the surgical removal in part or the entire foreskin (prepuce) from the penis. The word 'circumcision' comes from Latin *circum* meaning 'around' and *cædere* meaning 'to cut.' Circumcision is performed extensively for religious and cultural factors in Muslims and Jews.[1]

HISTORY

Circumcision is one of the world's oldest surgical procedures. It was performed in ancient Egypt, and more famously in the Jewish religion and is described in Genesis.[2] Circumcision in the West is performed very commonly for religious purposes with 20% of all men worldwide circumcised, and 84% of white men.[3] In India, the proportion of medical circumcision is higher as compared to religious but exact figures are lacking.

PHYSIOLOGY

The skin of the penile shaft develops during the 8th week of gestation, and the preputium develops from this ectoderm. At first, the glands penis and inner surface of the prepuce are adherent. The prepuce can be retracted in 4 percent of newborns, 90% at 3 years, and 87% at 17 years of age.[4] This separation occurs due to desquamation of epithelial cells forming smegma. In some cases, this physiological phimosis might not be resolved due to adhesions between the glans and the prepuce. The prepuce was classified into 5 types based on retractability by Kabaya et al.[5]

1. Type I: preputium cannot be retracted.
2. Type II: only the urethral meatus can be exposed.
3. Type III: preputium can be retracted to expose half of the glans.
4. Type IV: the corona cannot be exposed because of preputial adhesions to the corona.
5. Type V: no adhesions. The entire glans can be exposed.

INDICATIONS

Several Indications have been Quoted, Some of them Controversial and discussed below.

Urinary Tract Infections

Several studies have documented the increased risk for UTIs in uncircumcised infants. In a study published in 1998 on 58,000 children from Canada, who were less than a year of age and diagnosed with UTI, the risk for UTI was found to be 1.88/1000 in circumcised children and 7.02/1000 in uncircumcised ones.[6] Another study showed that the risk for UTI in similar subjects was reported to be 1.4 and 0.19% in uncircumcised and circumcised children respectively.[7] However, this data should be taken with a pinch of salt as there is lack of standardization in urine collection methods, and the patient groups were dissimilar. Moreover the effect of other factors such as breastfeeding was not taken into account. As a result of this, the risk of UTI has not been found high enough to recommend routine circumcision.

Sexual Function

The role of the prepuce in sexual function is debated. Many groups who object to circumcision argue that the procedure reduces sensation and reduces function. Circumcision reduces the protection to the glans and leads to keratinization. Masters and Johnson[8] found no differences in glanular tactile sensation in circumcised men. They did not study, however, alterations in fine touch that may be affected by circumcision.

Malignancy

Circumcision during infancy appears to decrease the risk for penile cancer whereas later surgery does not.[9]

STDs

Prevention of sexually transmitted diseases (STDs) has long been thought to be one of the advantages of circumcision. However one large review found no evidence in favor of this.[10] Other individual studies are conflicting. Hence, this is not a strong enough reason to advocate circumcision.

Medical Indications

These are less controversial than the above mentioned indications.[11,12]

- Phimosis
- Paraphimosis
- Balanoposthitis
- Balanitis xerotica obliterans
- Zoon's balanitis
- Preputium cysts, penile lymphedema
- Ammonia dermatitis
- Clean intermittent catheterization.

The common indications for circumcision, from a dermatosurgeon's perspective, are summarized in Box 1.

Contraindications for circumcision include:

- Premature infants
- Hypospadias
- Epispadias
- Chordee
- Penile webbing
- Concealed penis
- Blood dyscrasias.

Box 1: Common indications for circumcision.

- *Congenital*: True phimosis obstructing meatus
- Phimosis and paraphimosis[2,3]
- *Infectious*: Chronic or recurrent balanoposthitis (candidial, herpetic)[4]
- *Inflammatory*: Balanitis xerotica obliterans, erythroplasia of Queyrat, Zoon's balanitis[5]
- *Religious*: Jews and Muslims

INSTRUMENTS REQUIRED

Artery forceps, scissors, Adson's toothed forceps, needle holder, absorbable sutures 3-0/4-0.

PREOPERATIVE INVESTIGATIONS

Preoperative investigations include routine blood tests as for any surgery. Specific investigations as per the requirement of each case, such as biopsy, serological tests may be performed. Patient should be explained about the procedure, complications, benefits, possible outcome prior to the procedure. Informed written consent is mandatory in all cases. Stilbesterol (5 mg) three times a day Stilbesterol can be started 3 days prior to the surgery and to be continued at least for 5 days after surgery to prevent erection of penis. Surgeons differ in their recommendation for Stilbesterol.

ANESTHESIA[13-15]

Circumcision is often performed in children without anesthesia. However, the American Association of Pediatricians (AAP) recommends that anesthesia be used in all cases, not only adults.

Penile Block

- This is the most common form of anesthesia used for circumcision surgery. It blocks the dorsal nerves of the penis.
- The penis is gently pulled downward. This increases the space between the pubic bone and the root of the penis and makes injection of the anesthetic secure.
- The two injection points 0.5–1 cm lateral to the lower end of the pubic bone are then marked. A small gauge needle is used to inject bupivacaine 0.1 mg/kg on each side. Lignocaine can also be used but is shorter acting.
- The needle is injected perpendicular to the skin till the sub-pubic space is reached. When the deep membraneous layer of the superficial fascia is breached, an elastic recoil is felt.
- Both sides are injected the same way. It is preferable to use two injection points rather than one to reduce the chance of injuring the dorsal penile artery and causing hematoma.

Ring Block

- This can be used to reinforce the penile block. It consists of infiltration of lidocaine at the base of the penis.

Other Options Include

- Caudal block: This is regional nerve block to be administered by an anesthesiologist.
- General anesthesia—Preferred in small children.

PROCEDURE[16-20]

The three common techniques of performing circumcision are: the dorsal slit, the guided forceps and the sleeve resection.

Dorsal Slit Technique

This technique is most preferred for use in patients with phimosis or paraphimosis and as an emergency procedure in phagedena.

1. Prepare the surgical site with a povidone-iodine scrub of the genital area. Use sterile drape to identify the surgical area.
2. Accomplish anesthesia by dorsal penile nerve block or a ring block as mentioned earlier.
3. Three small artery forceps are applied to the edge of the prepuce, one in midline ventrally at 6'o clock position; two are placed on either side of the mid-dorsal line of the prepuce, one at 3'o clock and the other at 9'o clock.

   A circumferential mark is made around the foreskin at about 75% distance from meatus to the corona glans. Any adhesions between the glans and the prepucial sac are released by blunt dissection with hemostatic forceps. The prepuce in the mid-dorsal line is slit between two dorsally placed artery forceps until the marking area. The redundant parts of the prepuce on either side of the dorsal slit are cut off circumferentially parallel to the corona. The underlying inner layer of the prepuce is trimmed in the same way leaving it about 0.5 cm longer than the skin (Fig. 1).
4. Excess bleeding is controlled with direct pressure and electrocautery. All bleeding vessels are ligated with 3-0 absorbable sutures. The frenular artery is secured with figure of eight suture at the frenulum.
5. The cut edge of the skin is sutured to the cut edge of the inner layer of the prepuce with multiple interrupted stitches using 3-0 absorbable sutures.
6. A sterile dressing of gauze dipped in betadine is secured under the frenular artery suture and circumferentially around the raw area with the help of stay sutures at regular intervals. A paraffin gauze dressing is then applied over the area and antibiotic ointment applied to glans and meatus to prevent drying.

The advantages and disadvantages of dorsal slit technique are given in Box 2.

Guided Forceps Technique

The foreskin is pulled forward using clamps, the extent of the traction determining the tightness of the resulting circumcision. A large pair of artery forceps is then clamped across the foreskin at the place where the cut is to be made. Optionally, the smaller clamps are then removed before a sharp scissor is run across the top of the big forceps. The cut edges of inner and outer skin are then normally brought together and held by stitches (Fig. 2). The advantages and disadvantages of guided forceps technique are given in Box 3.

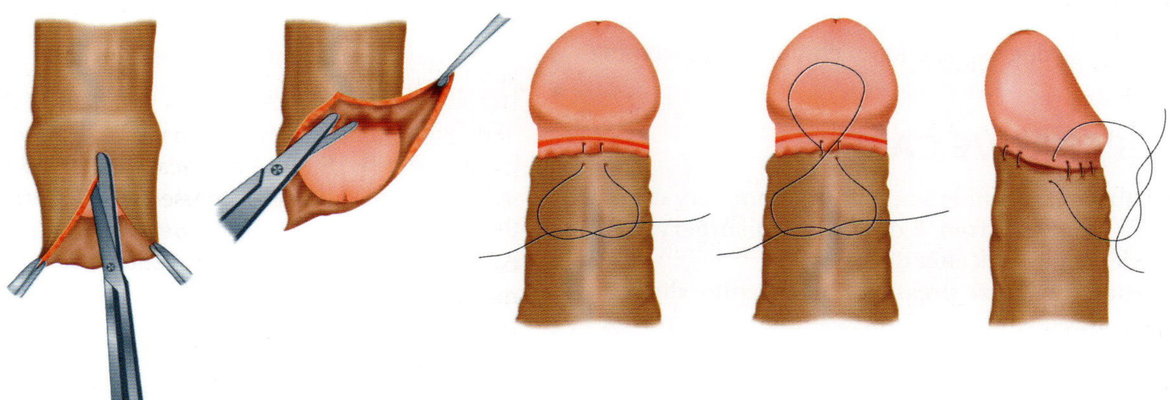

Fig. 1: Circumcision (dorsal slit technique).

Box 2: Advantages and disadvantages of dorsal slit technique.

Advantages
- Useful in emergency situations
- Simple technique and does not require high surgical skills

Disadvantages
- Possibility of excess bleeding, if frenular artery is not secured properly

Box 3: Advantages and disadvantages of guided forceps technique.

Advantages
- Technique can be easily learned by beginners
- Ideal for use in limited resource settings
- Can be done without a surgical assistant

Disadvantages
- Cosmetic effect may be less satisfying
- It leaves 0.5–1 cm of mucosa proximal to corona
- One has to be careful to avoid clamping glans which can be disastrous.

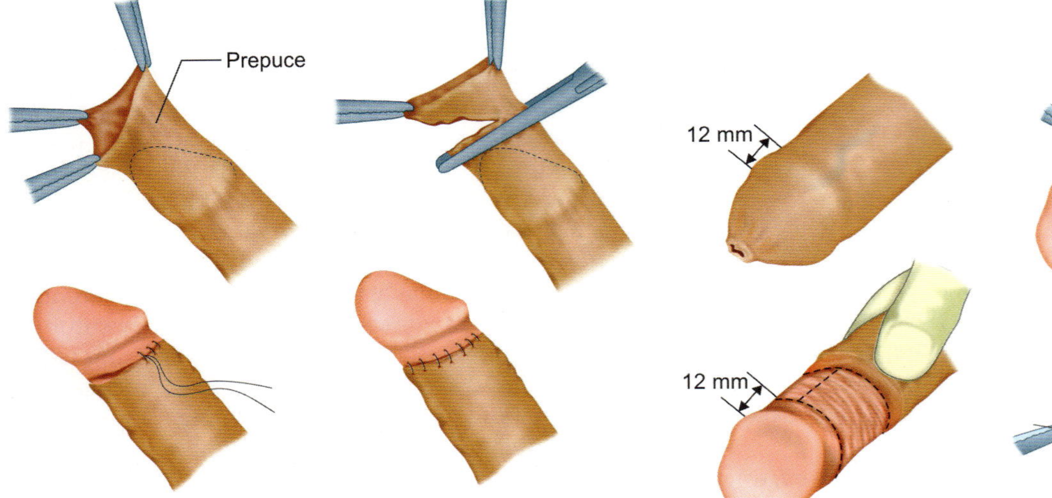

Fig. 2: Guided forceps technique.

Fig. 3: Sleeve resection technique.

Sleeve Resection Technique

The sleeve resection method of circumcision, though more complicated, is often preferred when there is a risk for excessive bleeding. In this procedure, two parallel cuts are made along the shaft of the penis, resulting in a thin band or sleeve of detached foreskin. When this is removed, the top and bottom portions of the foreskin are attached with dissolving sutures. It differs from the dorsal slit procedure described above; in that, the foreskin is removed from its retracted position [i.e. the foreskin is not pulled back over the glans before circumcision (Fig. 3)]. The advantages and disadvantages of sleeve resection technique are given in Box 4.

POSTOPERATIVE CARE

1. Broad-spectrum antibiotics, anti-inflammatory drugs and analgesics started 1 day prior to surgery, are continued for a week after the surgery.
2. The petroleum gauze dressing and betadine dipped gauze secured with stay sutures should be removed 72 hours after surgery, following which no further dressing is necessary and the patient can then shower regularly.
3. Patient should be instructed to wear loose fitting briefs and refrain himself from intercourse and masturbation for 4–6 weeks after the procedure to prevent breakdown of the wound.

Box 4: Advantages and disadvantages of sleeve resection technique.

Advantages
- The technique provides best cosmetic results
- Provides better control of bleeding in patients with large subcutaneous veins

Disadvantages
- Technique requires good surgical skill
- It requires an assistant

POSTOPERATIVE MANAGEMENT

- A ring block or penile block is reinforced at the end of surgery for longer pain relief. In children, suppositories are used while in adults, oral analgesics are used.
- Perioperative oral antibiotics are given for 3 days.
- The dressing is changed on the second postoperative day. Any crusts are cleaned.
- After 2 days topical antibiotic cream is sufficient.
- The most distressing problem for the patient is hypersensitivity of the exposed glans, which lasts till keratinization is complete. We have found that the use of briefs instead of boxers which restrict movement of the penis give better relief to the patient.
- Patient is advised to refrain from intercourse or masturbation for 4–6 weeks.
- The use of stilbestrol after surgery to prevent erection is controversial but it can be given for 5 days. In our experience the tenderness of the sutures prevents erections.

CIRCUMCISION IN INFANTS

In infants and young boys, circumcision is usually performed at the request of the parents for social and religious reasons. Other indications include phimosis obstructing the meatus causing difficulty in passing urine leading to recurrent infection. The circumcision in infants may also be done for removal of retention underneath the prepuce which cannot be drained easily. The operation is performed under general anesthesia with the child supine.

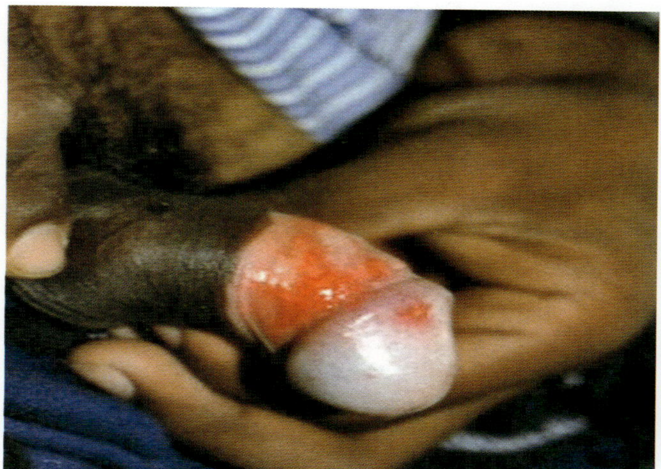

Fig. 4: Excess prepuce remnant causing recurrent balanoposthitis.

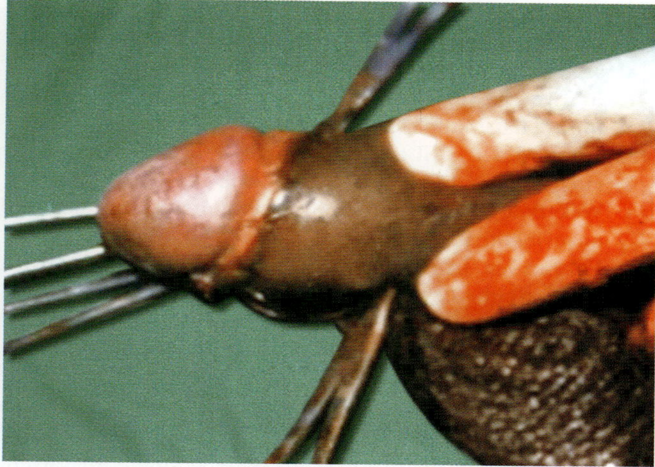

Fig. 5: Skin sutured to inner layer of prepuce with interrupted sutures.

A number of devices such as the Gomco clamp, Plastibell clamp and Morgan clamp, of which the Hollister Plastibell is the best known, are available for circumcising the infant and they make the operation simpler and quicker. The Plastibell is pushed into the space between the glans and prepuce and the ligature, supplied with kit is applied around the lip of the bell. The prepuce is cut off with the scissors and the plastic device extruded.

COMPLICATIONS[21,22]

Bleeding—The most common complication is bleeding from the frenular artery. It is ideal to ligate the artery in all cases and not rely on pressure or cautery hemostasis alone.

- *Infections*—This is infrequent due to the excellent blood flow to the penis. Wound hygiene and topical antibiotics are usually adequate.
- Glans or shaft amputations are rare but the most serious. If it occurs the amputated part must immediately be taken to a microsurgical unit for reattachment.
- Sometimes, the frenulum might be too short and it can pull the glans ventrally. This is solved by incising it horizontally and suturing it vertically.
- *Trapped penis*—This is seen in obese patients with excessive prepubic fat, where too much skin is resected leading to penile retraction and cicatricial scar formation. When mild, it is treated by topical application of betamethasone 0.05%.
- *Residual skin*—If not done symmetrically areas of excess skin can be excised and sutured.
- As with any other surgical procedure, bleeding and infection are the most common complications of circumcision in adult patients. Other complications being hematoma formation, wound dehiscence, poor esthetic result, diffuse swelling and edema postoperatively. Excess prepuce remnant may lead to recurrent balanoposthitis (Fig. 4).

The practical tips for circumcision are given in Box 5.

Box 5: Practical tips for circumcision.

- Circumcision should be performed meticulously in chronic balanoposthitis with due consideration given to excising the mucus surface completely (Fig. 5) or else the recurrent balanitis will persist starting on uncircumcised mucous membrane (author's personal observation)
- Sufficient skin on the penile shaft must be retained to allow an erection without skin tension and it is helpful to mark the intended site of the circumferential skin incision before commencing the operation[9]
- Never use monopolar diathermy when performing circumcision in infants as the point of maximal electrical resistance may be at the base of penis, particularly if the penis is under any traction, with the risk of coagulation and loss of whole penis.[11]

REFERENCES

1. Rizvi SA, Naqvi SA, Hussain M, et al. Religious circumcision: a Muslim view. BJU Int. 1999;83:13-6.
2. Niku SD, Stock JA, Kaplan GW. Neonatal circumcision. Urol Clin North Am 1995;22:57-65.
3. Burgu B, Aydogdu O, Tangal S, Soygur T. Circumcision: pros and cons. Indian J Urol. 2010;26(1):12-5. doi: 10.4103/0970-1591.60437
4. Bopyce WT. Care of the foreskin. Pediatr Rev 1983;5.26-30.
5. Kayaba H, Tamura H, Kitazima S, et al. Analysis of shape and retractability of the prepuce in 603 Japanese boys. J Urol. 1996;156:1813-15.
6. Nelson JD, Peters PC. Suprapubic aspiration of urine in premature and term infants. Pediatrics. 1965;36:132-4.
7. Pryles CV. Percutaneous bladder aspiration and other methods of urine collection for bacteriologic study. Pediatrics. 1965;36:128-31
8. Masters WH, Johnson VE. Human sexual response. Boston: Little Brown; 1966.
9. Bissada NK, Morcos RR, el-Senoussi M. Postcircumcision carcinoma of the penis. I. Clinical aspects. J Urol. 1986;135:283-5

10. Laumann EO, Masi CM, Zuckerman EW. Circumcision in the United States: prevalence, prophylactic effects, and sexual practice. JAMA. 1997;277:1052–7.
11. Rickwood AMK. Medical indications for circumcision. BJU Int. 1999;83(Suppl 1):45–51.
12. Ferrándiz C, Ribera M. Zoon's balanitis treated by circumcision. J Dermatol Surg Oncol. 1984;10:622-5.
13. Wakefield SE, Elewa AA. Adult circumcision under local anaesthetic. Br J Urol. 1995;75:96.
14. Fernandez JA, Kimrey SS, LaMay DM, et al. Adult plasticylinder circumcision. Mil Med. 1987;152:200-1.
15. Szmuk P, Ezri T, Ben Hur H, et al. Regional anaesthesia for circumcision in adults: a comparative study. Can J Anaesth. 1994;41:1181-4.
16. Holman JR, Stuessi KA. Adult circumcision. Am Fam Physician. 1999;59:1514-8.
17. Savant SS. Dermatosurgery for male genitalia. In: Savant SS (Ed). Textbook and Atlas of Dermatosurgery and Cosmetology, 2nd edition. Mumbai: ASCAD Publishers; 2005;275-81.
18. Farquharson M, Moran B. Male urethra and genital organs. In: Farquharson M (Ed). Farquharson's Textbook of Operative General Surgery, 9th edition. London: Edward Arnold Publishers. 2005;475-7.
19. Das S. Operations on the penis. In: Das S (Ed). A Practical Guide to Operative Surgery, 3rd edition. Calcutta; 1988;3659.
20. Fowler C. The urethra and penis. In: Williams NS, Bulstrode CJK, O'Connell PR (Eds). Bailey and Love's Short Practice of Surgery, 25th edition. London: Edward Arnold Publishers; 2008;1371-3.
21. Kaplan GW. Complications of circumcision. Urol Clin North Am. 1983;10:543-9.
22. Williams N, Kapila L. Complications of circumcision. Br J Surg. 1993;80:1231-6.

Chapter

62

Leprosy Surgery

Sanjay Sane

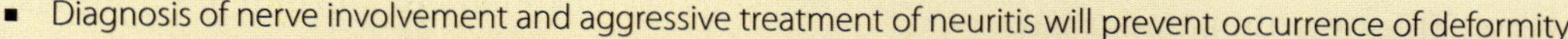

Key Messages

- Diagnosis of nerve involvement and aggressive treatment of neuritis will prevent occurrence of deformity.
- Perineural steroid injection and nerve decompression plays an important role in prevention of deformities.
- Patient to be referred for surgery should be medically stabilized/cured by multidrug therapy (MDT).
- Protective footwear plays an important role in management of neuropathic plantar ulcers.
- High plantar pressures, precursors of neuropathic plantar ulceration, can be diagnosed by foot pressure measurement system.

INTRODUCTION

Hansen's disease patients, even after the medical cure with multidrug therapy (MDT) are stigmatized due to the disability and deformity left by the disease. This needs intervention by a leprosy reconstructive surgeon and correction of the deformities, giving the patient the cosmesis and functional hands and feet. Surgeon has an important role in prevention of neural damage, if diagnosed early and further deformities by timely nerve decompression surgery.

In prevention of deformities, the primary role is of the dermatologists to diagnose and treat neuritis, by medication, adequate rest and physiotherapy. Surgeon may be called for either giving perineural steroid injection or perform surgical nerve decompression.

In established deformities, primary role is of the surgeon to reconstruct the paralyzed limb by reconstructive surgical procedures. Cosmetic surgery is resorted to correct the loss of eyebrows, depression of nose and other deformities. The physiotherapist has an important role to prepare the hand or foot for reconstructive surgery by splinting, exercises, etc.

Surgery can be considered only for patients who are medically stabilized or cured. Lepromatous cases should have completed the required MDT and should not have history of reaction for 12–18 months prior to surgical intervention.

INDICATIONS FOR SURGICAL INTERVENTION IN A CASE OF HANSEN'S DISEASE PATIENT

Indications for surgical intervention are shown in Box 1. Out of these indications, nerve biopsy has been explained in a separate chapter.

Nerve Decompression Surgery

To understand the role of nerve decompression surgery, it is important to understand the pathophysiology of nerve damage (Fig. 1).

Hansen's neuritis causes nerve damage by two mechanisms. First is *internal nerve compression* caused by the disease inflammatory process progressing in a closed compartment of thickened epineurium, leading to increased intraneural pressure. In situ destruction of nerve tissue leads to development of intraneural abscess due to caseation necrosis. Second is the external compression on the inflamed nerve because of the nerve and the adjoined

Box 1: Indications for surgical intervention in a case of Hansen's disease.

- Nerve biopsy, skin biopsy for diagnostic purposes
- Nerve decompression surgery
- Reconstructive surgery for claw fingers and thumb, foot drop
- Cosmetic surgery for facial deformities, viz. depressed nose, loss of eyebrows, lagophthalmos and gynecomastia
- Surgery for the neuropathic trophic ulcers

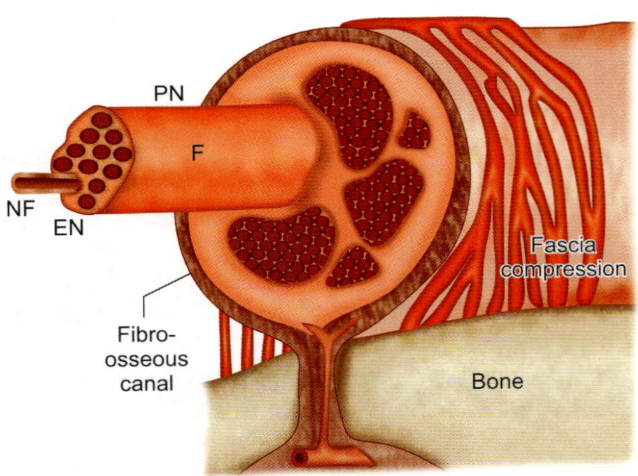

Fig. 1: Pathophysiology of nerve damage in Hansen's disease.

morphological structures in the anatomical compartments through which nerves traverse. Thus, the inflamed ulnar nerve traversing through the fibro-osseous canal behind the medial epicondyle is subjected to external compression.

Treatment of neuritis, thus aims at reducing the internal compression by anti-inflammatory medicines systemic steroids, rest and proper splintage of the limb and managing external compression by surgery.

Management of Internal Compression

Medical management of neuritis: Hansen's neuritis pain is one of the worst pains to suffer and requires rest to the affected limb in form of splint, anti-inflammatory analgesics and judicious use of steroids to control intraneural inflammation. Steroids form an important part of drug regime to combat the neuritis, aid in decompressing the nerve to relieve the intraneural pressures and save the axons from damage. Giving systemic steroids for a long time either orally or parenterally invites gastrointestinal and systemic side effects. Hence, giving perineural or paraneural steroids by injection is an excellent way to administer maximum steroid dose at the specific site with minimal systemic side effects.

Long-acting steroids like, dexamethasone or triamcinolone is administered, diluted with distilled water. One has to be certain that the injection is given by the side of the nerve and not intraneurally. Intraneural injection destroys the already damaged nerve. The whole procedure has to be done with total aseptic precautions preferably in an operation theater. During the treatment, physiotherapy plays an important role in splinting the fingers, electrical stimulation of the weakened muscles and joint mobilization.

Procedure of perineural injection: The steroid injection is given peri- or paraneurally and never intraneurally. The drug has to be diluted with saline or distilled water and is given along the whole length of clinically thickened nerve. One has to use a long thin needle, e.g. 23 or 24 spinal needle. Needle has to remain subcutaneous. Needle is first advanced the whole length and after confirming that needle is not in a vessel, withdraw the needle slowly injecting the drug.

Common complications: Intraneural injection and injury to adjoining vessel.

Splinting of the affected limb: The splinting is done across the joint along which the nerve traverses, e.g. for ulnar nerve, above elbow posterior slab is given. If fingers show early paralysis, splints to prevent clawing are given.

Management of External Compression

Surgical management of neuritis: If there is predominantly external compression, it can only be tackled by surgical decompression and freeing the nerve from the fibro-osseous canal. External compression is surgically treated by external neurolysis and division of fibro-osseous canal, and the internal compression treated by epineurotomy, partial excision of thickened epineurium and interfascicular nerve decompression under magnification. In practice, both procedures are performed together. Additionally, procedures like medial epicondylectomy and anterior transposition of ulnar nerve may be required to relieve external compressive forces.

Patient with neuritis should be referred to a surgeon in the following instances:

a. Occurrence of nerve abscess, absolute indication for surgical intervention.
b. Neuritis not responding to the medical line of treatment.
c. Intractable pain and progressive motor loss in the muscles supplied by the nerve.

If patient is on steroids, it is advisable to taper oral steroids before surgery.

The nerves that are amenable for surgical decompression are:

- Ulnar nerve, at medial epicondyle of elbow (Figs. 2A and B)
- Median nerve, in carpal tunnel
- Posterior tibial nerve, in the tarsal tunnel
- Lateral popliteal nerve, around neck of fibula.

Reconstructive Surgery

Patients may be referred for reconstruction provided:

- There is no active neuritis and disease is stabilized. Patient is medically released from treatment, i.e. cured.
- Deformity is established, at the same time, is mobile and surgically correctable.
- Patient must have taken adequate preoperative physiotherapy.

Preoperative physiotherapy involves wax therapy and oil massage to soften the skin and mobilize the joints, plaster and dynamic splints to passively mobilize and correct the deformities, isolation and strengthening the muscle to be transferred is mandatory for good surgical correction. Physiotherapy time duration may vary from 3 to 10 weeks depending on the duration of the deformity.

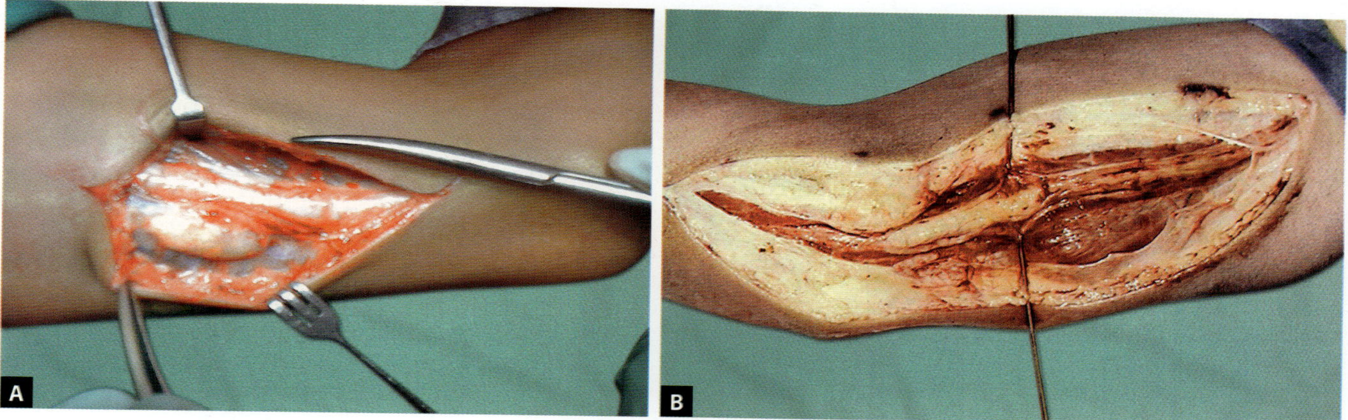

Figs. 2A and B: (A) Ulnar nerve single paraneural abscess and thickened nerve; (B) Ulnar nerve decompression at medial epicondyle of elbow, note inflamed nerve partially decompressed above the medial epicondyle and near normal nerve below the epicondyle.

Reconstructive Surgery of the Hand

Hand: Hand is involved following the involvement of the ulnar nerve at the elbow and/or median nerve at the wrist, leading to ulnar claw hand and clawed thumb or inability to oppose the thumb against the palm respectively. This is due to the paralysis of intrinsic muscles of fingers and the thumb leading to hyperextension of the metacarpophalangeal (MCP) joints and flexion of interphalangeal (IP) joints. In a normal hand, the fingers function due to the action of long extensors and the finger flexors, and are kept straight in all functional positions by the stabilizing action of the intrinsic muscles. Intrinsics strike a delicate balance between the extensors and flexors, while they act on the triple joint chain of fingers. Once the intrinsics are paralyzed, there is unopposed action of the extensors at the MCP joint and the unopposed action of flexors at the IP joints.

The reconstructive surgery either involves the correction of the deformity by dynamic procedures such as, intrinsic muscle power replacement by another muscle; tendon transfers, or by passive procedures such as, mechanical correction of MCP hyperextension, e.g. MCP joint volar capsulorrhaphy.

Ulnar claw hand or the claw fingers can be corrected by using different motor tendons, e.g. flexor digitorum sublimis of one of the fingers, palmaris longus, extensor carpi radialis longus and distribute the muscle power by four tendon strips to all clawed fingers. There are many variants in the procedures and surgical details are beyond the purview of this chapter.

Thumb correction surgery: Thumb paralysis is a result of loss of action of the thenar muscles and surgery aims at restoring the action by tendon transfer. Muscles of choice are: flexor digitorum sublimis from ring finger, extensor indicis or palmaris longus with a fascia extensor graft. The aim is to restore the lost abduction and opposition function (Figs. 3A and B).

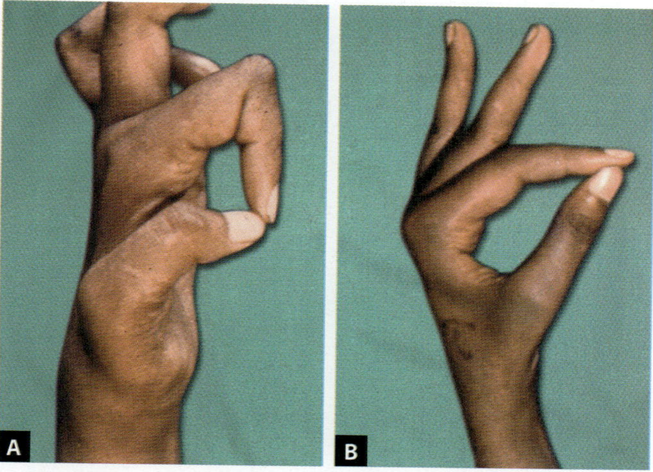

Figs. 3A and B: (A) Preoperative deformity; (B) Postoperative result after opponens plasty.

Surgery for the Foot Drop Correction

Involvement of the lateral popliteal nerve leads to first, the paresis and later total irreversible paralysis of anterolateral group of leg muscles, i.e. the ankle and toe dorsiflexors and the evertors of the foot. Paralysis leads to the foot drop, i.e. loss of foot and toe dorsiflexion and foot eversion. The anesthetic foot is liable to strike on the forefoot and the lateral border at each step, making the foot prone to forefoot high plantar pressure injury and instability. Long standing foot drop is complicated by the tendo-Achilles contracture, which first has to be addressed by preoperative physiotherapy and at times by surgical tendo-Achilles lengthening.

Reconstruction of the foot drop is done by transferring the tibialis posterior tendon to the dorsum of the foot, either by circumtibial or trans interosseous membrane approach, and suturing by two slips, one to the insertion of paralyzed tibialis anterior and the extensor hallucis longus and second slip to the toe extensors. The transferred slips have to be balanced delicately, so that the foot is held in dorsiflexion and eversion. Position is maintained with below-knee (BK) plaster for 5–6 weeks. After removal of plaster, graded supervised physiotherapy is necessary for 4 weeks to teach the patient to use the transferred tendon for foot dorsiflexion, to walk again.

Surgery for Correction of Facial Deformities

Following deformities are amenable for correction: depressed nose (Figs. 4A and B), lagophthalmos or inability to close the eyes, loss of eyebrows, partial or total facelift operation to remove the facial wrinkles, and correction of elongated ear lobules.

Eyelid closure is restored by static procedure such as, lateral tarsorrhaphy, where the palpebral fissure is permanently reduced from lateral side by suturing the two eyelids. Dynamic procedure uses part of temporalis muscle tendon unit, extending it with a fascia graft, and used to achieve dynamic eyelid closure when person mildly clenches his teeth (Figs. 5A to C).

Neuropathic Foot Ulcers

To understand the mechanism of how foot ulcers are caused, one needs to understand the walking cycle.

Each walking cycle comprises of three phases:

1. *Heel strike*: Foot in dorsiflexion, comes in contact with the ground, also called as heel contact phase. Heel structures bear maximum weight-bearing stress (Fig. 6).
2. *Mid stance phase*: Whole foot in contact with the ground.
3. *Push off phase* (Fig. 7): This is the propulsive phase, forefoot bears maximum body weight and is under tremendous pressure, almost total body weight from above and the ground reaction from below. These high plantar pressures in neuropathic foot are responsible for tissue injury in neuropathic foot. These ulcers occur on the sole of the foot, on the areas where the metatarsal heads and the heel bone bear the maximum body weight to the ground (Fig. 8).

The ulcers occurring on the sole of the feet in Hansen's disease are due to tissue injury following trauma (such as cuts, nail prick, footwear injury) on the sole of the foot. Ulcers occurring due to nail prick, shoe bite, etc. occur from skin to the deeper tissues, whereas ulcers due to high plantar pressures occur from within outside (Fig. 9). Weakening of the foot occurs due to loss of sensation, the intrinsic muscle paralysis and resultant weakening of the

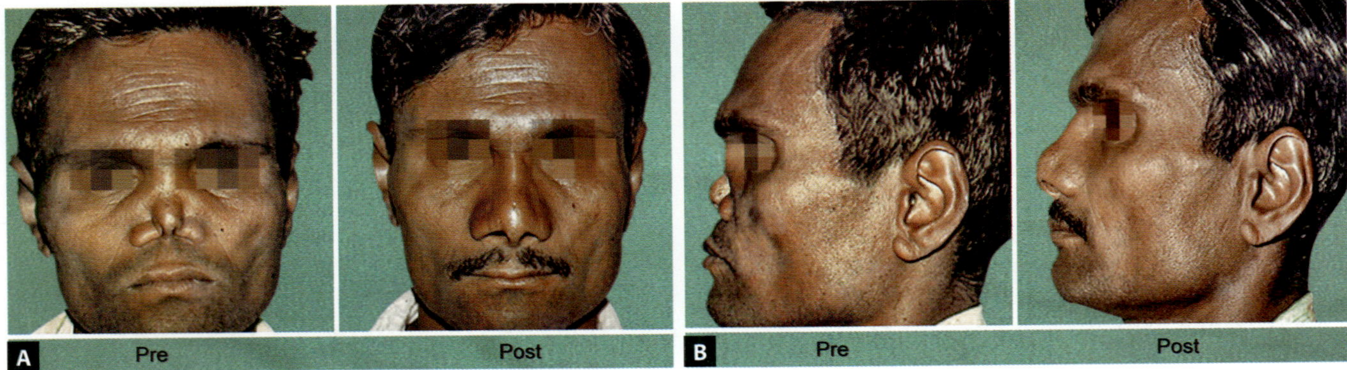

Figs. 4A and B: Nose reconstruction: preoperative and postoperative.

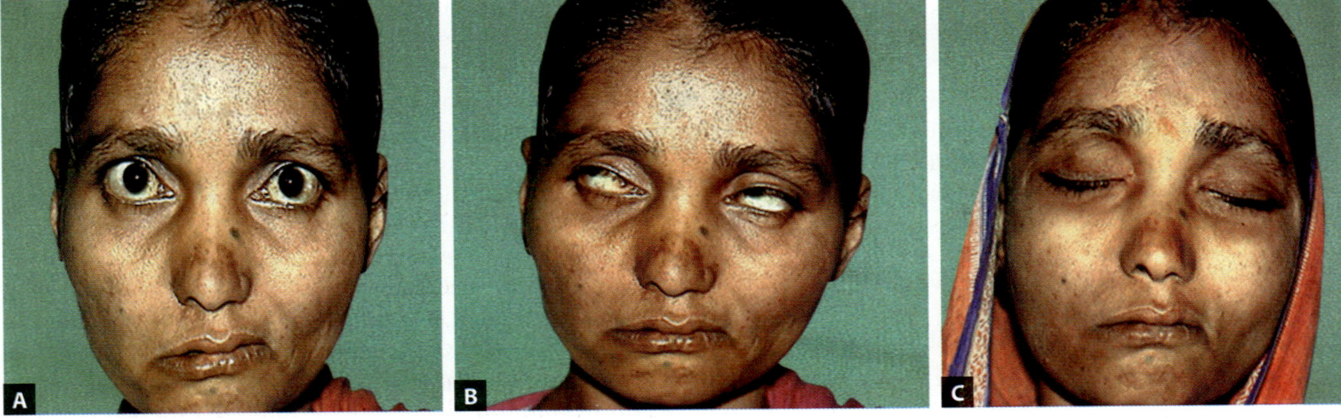

Figs. 5A to C: Lagophthalmos surgical correction: (A) Eyes open before surgery; (B) Eyes closed before surgery; (C) Eyes closed after surgery.

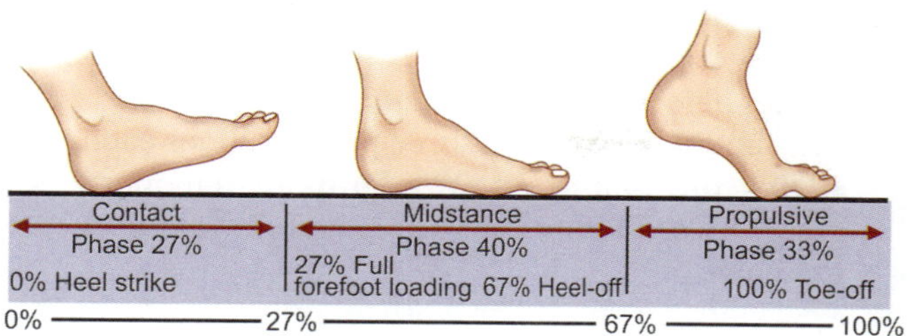

Fig. 6: Phases of walking cycle.

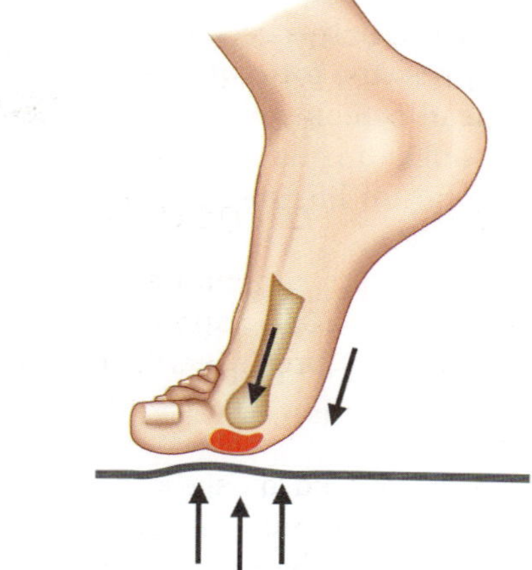

Fig. 7: Propulsive phase.

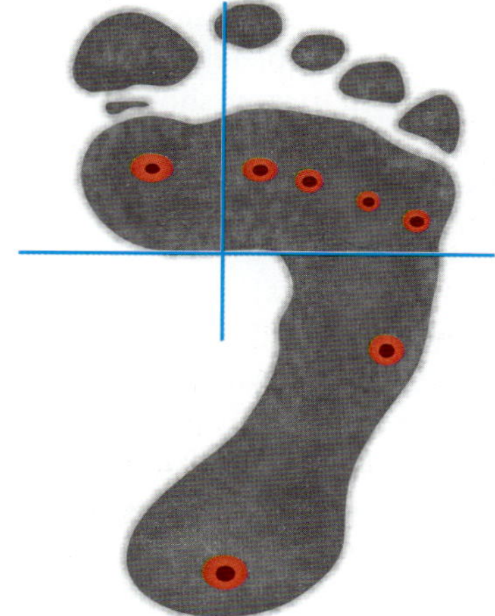

Fig. 8: Location of foot ulcers.

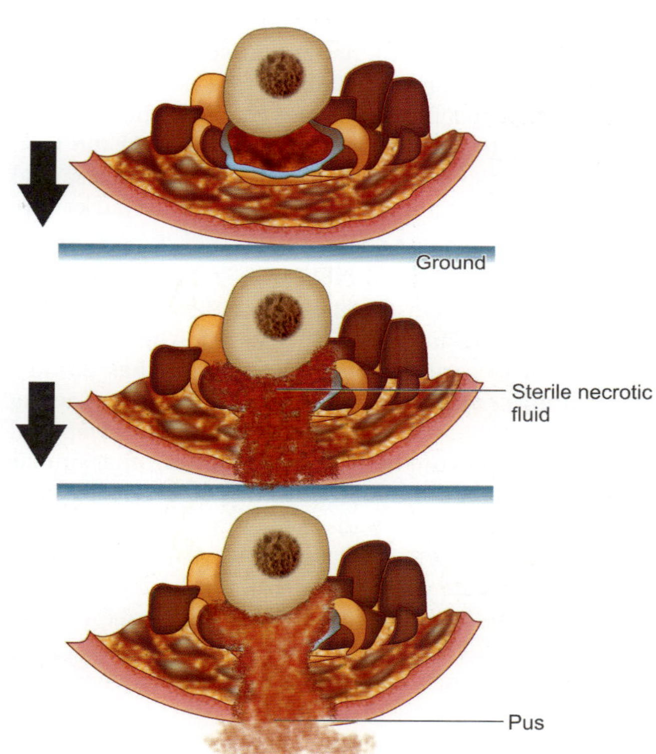

Fig. 9: Ulcers due to high plantar pressures occur from within outside.

foot architecture. This trauma, coupled with the walking stresses and strains exerted on the weakened neuropathic foot leads to foot ulcers.

Autonomic neuropathy leads to dry plantar skin, excessive fissures and cracks which make sole vulnerable to ulceration. Perceived trauma is the causative factor in about 20% of cases. In 80% of cases, unperceived trauma during normal daily walking on neuropathic weakened foot is responsible for foot ulceration.

The tissue injury starts deepest below the bony points and aseptic tissue necrosis starts. Person unaware of the damage due to neuropathy continues to walk and compounds the damage. As a result, the damage reaches the plantar skin and opens on the plantar skin as ulcer.

Ulcers are frequently preceded and underlie a pre-existing corn or callus, frequently indicative of high plantar pressure. Trauma from heat, cold, shoe bite or penetration by a sharp object are also potential causes. Neuropathy allows the lesions to develop because the normal warning sense of pain has been lost and they go unrecognized. Continued pressure or walking on the injured skin creates even further damage and the ulcer will worsen. The open sore will frequently become infected and may even penetrate to bone.

Ulcer Management

Neuropathic foot with ulceration needs constant expert attention, X-rays to rule out osteomyelitis, antibiotics and at times, surgical interventions. Proper protective footwear in the form of microcellular rubber (MCR) sandals and use of orthotic supports to aid offloading are needed.

Ulcers are categorized as acute and chronic.

Acute ulcers: Acute ulcer requires rest to the foot with elevation, at times, admission if infection is severe and use of antibiotics. Once infection is under control, adequate rest and offloading of the foot will achieve tissue healing. If not cared for, ulcers turn chronic and nonhealing and will need more aggressive treatment. Foot X-ray to rule out osteomyelitis of bones is necessary.

Chronic ulcers: Osteomyelitis is commonest cause of nonhealing of ulcers. Such ulcers require in addition, surgical intervention in the form of wound debridement and removal of dead osteomyelitic bone. Postoperative care involves rest, offloading till ulcer heals. Constant use of protective footwear for lifetime is always necessary to keep the foot ulcer-free.

Footwear as a therapy: Once we understand that high pressures on the sole of the feet of Hansen's disease patients are responsible for majority of foot problems, it will not be an exaggeration, if we say that protective footwear protects the foot, just as a helmet protects the head while driving a two wheeler. While standing on our feet, footwear is the only interface between the sole of the foot and the ground below which we can suitably alter and use it to counteract the bad effects of pressures on the sole of the foot. The footwear should be made according to individual measurements, sewed or glued, without any nails or rivets, and with a hard outer sole for protection. It is used with cotton socks. Most of the neuropathic feet have lost the capacity to hold the chappal while walking and can lead to friction between the sole and the foot, leading to injuries and ulceration. In these cases, a sandal pattern is ideal as it holds the footwear with the back strap.

Microcellular rubber: MCR is the material available in India which is soft, comfortable, gives a good cushioning effect and helps in redistribution of plantar pressures from area of high pressure prone to ulceration to the whole area of foot in contact with the ground. It has 25–30% shore hardness and reduces ground reaction forces acting on the sole of the foot. It has been tested and compared favorably with polyurethane, sorbothane and other similar materials available abroad. It is used as an insole material and to fabricate orthotic pads.

Shoes, when prescribed must always fit comfortably and have adequate width and depth for the toes. Canvas shoes and good quality leather shoes easily adapt to the shape of your feet and allow them to "breathe". Athletic shoes, jogging shoes, and sneakers are usually excellent choices, if they are well fitted and provide adequate cushioning. "Extra-depth" shoes or custom-molded shoes may be required to adapt to patient's particular needs, or orthoses to provide cushioning and support.

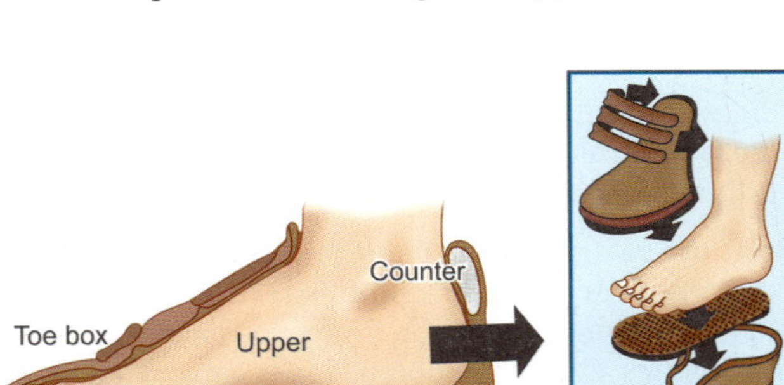

Fig. 10: Insole, the important part in the footwear.

Patient should be given the following instructions:

a. Always check your shoes for foreign objects or torn linings before putting them on.
b. You should have two or three pairs of shoes each day, so that, one pair is not worn for more than four to six hours. This will minimize the possibility of injury due to footwear.
c. New footwear should be worn for only a few hours at a time and you should take care to inspect your feet for any points of irritation.
d. Socks should be well-fitted without seams or folds. They should not be so tight as to interfere with circulation.
e. Well-padded socks can be very protective, if there is an abundance of room in your shoes.
f. Avoid wearing open-toed shoes or sandals, until you have discussed this with your surgeon.
g. Above all, do not walk with barefoot.

Insole/orthotic modifications (Fig. 10): These are to be worn inside protective footwear. These are the devices which support the weakened foot, help to redistribute the plantar pressures, and help to take off the high plantar pressures from an area of ulceration and give rest to the part, at the same time, allow the patient to carry out the daily routine.

- Offloading: In simple terms, it can be defined as avoidance of all mechanical stress on the injured weakened extremity, while maintaining necessary ambulation. This is achieved by crutches, walker, wheel chair, use of total contact cast (TCC),or a walking window plaster, depending on the severity of the ailment. Footwear modifications like protective shoes or sandals, fixed ankle brace can be used.
- Orthotic supports (Fig. 11): These are insole modifications, used in shoes or sandals, which help to redistribute the plantar pressures and help to take off the high plantar pressures from an area of ulceration, support the weakened neuropathic foot, give rest to the part, at the same time, allow the patient to carry out the daily routine.

Foot care: Important aspects of foot care are shown in Box 2.

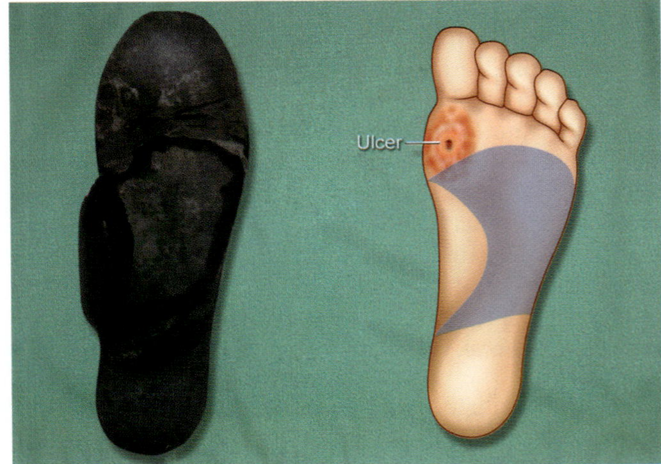

Fig. 11: Orthotic support.

Box 2: Important aspects of foot care.

- Examine the feet daily
- Soak both the feet in water daily for 10–15 minutes
- Mop dry especially between the toes and apply white soft paraffin or petroleum jelly
- Use well-fitting sandals or canvas shoes with cotton socks
- Do not walk barefoot
- Avoid walking long distances
- Do not treat your foot yourself
- Report to doctor for the slightest foot complaint

NEWER INVESTIGATIONS TO DIAGNOSE HIGH PLANTAR PRESSURES

It is now well known that the normal walking and standing can generate high plantar pressures sufficient to damage the insensitive and weakened foot. These pressures, if diagnosed before their pathological manifestations, can be effectively managed by scientific footwear and external foot supports to be used inside the shoes (orthotic supports).

In footscan plate, patient puts a single step on the platform and pressures below the sole of the foot are recorded instantly, and with the help of a unique software information is transformed into a multicolored picture. Each color represents a different pressure; red and pink areas denote highest pressures (Fig. 12).

Based on these foot pressure records, external foot supports to be used inside the shoes, are prepared with the help of a special microcellular rubber. They are called as orthotic supports. They help to correct the foot stance, posture and support the weakened arch of the foot. It also helps in giving rest to the painful foot, keeping the patient ambulatory.

CONCLUSION

It is important for the physician to diagnose and treat the Hansen's disease in early stage, to prevent the occurrence of disability and deformities. Perineural steroid injection, nerve decompression resorted before the onset of deformity can prevent the occurrence of deformities and social stigmatization and segregation. Physicians treating the disease should learn to perform diagnostic nerve biopsy, give perineural steroid injection and play an important role in prevention of deformities.

Treatment of plantar ulceration needs rest, antibiotic cover, and if complicated by osteomyelitis, good surgical debridement needs to be done. This can be done by any qualified surgeon. Important feature which is lacking is prescription of a protective footwear, which should be done on a priority basis. Foot pressure measurement or foot scan is an important investigation to diagnose and prevent plantar ulceration due to high plantar pressures.

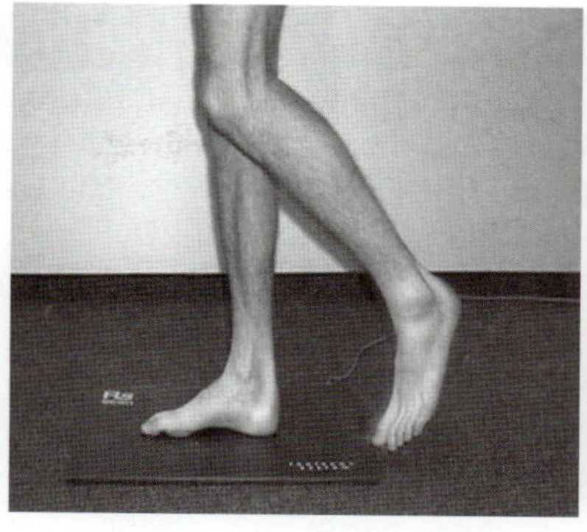

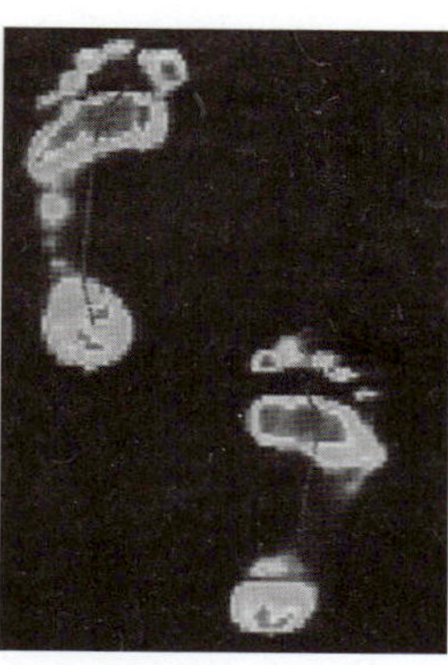

Fig. 12: Footscan plate and scan report.

BIBLIOGRAPHY

1. Anderson GA. The surgical management of deformities of the hand in leprosy. J Bone Joint Surg Br. 2006;88: 290-4.
2. Dandapat MC, Sahu DM, Mukherjee LM, et al. Treatment of leprous neuritis by neurolysis combined with perineural corticosteroid injection. Lepr Rev. 1991;62:27-34.
3. Duerksen F, Schwarz R. Ulnar nerve palsy. In: Schwarz R, Brandsma W (Eds). Surgical Reconstruction & Rehabilitation in Leprosy and other Neuropathies, 1st edition. Kathmandu: Ekta Books Distributors Pvt. Ltd; 2004;47-64.
4. Gore D, Atal-Shah R. Surgery in leprosy. In: Savant SS (Ed). Textbook of Dermatosurgery and Cosmetology, 2nd edition. Mumbai: ASCAD; 2005;289-96.
5. Jopling WH, McDougall. Handbook of Leprosy, 5th edition. New Delhi: CBS Publishers and Distributors; 2005.
6. Margery I, Joyce P, Job CK. Role of nerve biopsies in the diagnosis of leprosy in the post multidrug therapy era. Indian J Lepr. 2008;80:279-82.
7. Nilsen R, Mengistu G, Reddy BB. The role of nerve biopsies in the diagnosis and management of leprosy. Lepr Rev. 1989;60:2832.
8. Parkes AR. Paralytic claw fingers—a graft tenodesis operation. Hand. 1973:5;192.
9. Ramaratnam S. Neurologic Manifestations of Leprosy. [online] Available from emedicine.medscape.com/ article/1165419. [Accessed March, 2012].
10. Reddy RR, Singh G, Sacchidanand S, et al. A comparative evaluation of skin and nerve histopathology in single skin lesion leprosy. Indian J Dermatol Venereol Leprol 2005;71:401-5.
11. Richard B. Surgical management of neuritis. In: Schwarz R Brandsma W(Eds). Surgical Reconstruction & Rehabilitation in Leprosy and other Neuropathies, 1st edition. Kathmandu: Ekta Books Distributors Pvt. Ltd; 2004;25-32.
12. Ruth A, Schulmeyer FJ, Roesch M. Diagnostic and therapeutic value due to suspected diagnosis, long-term complications, and indication for sural nerve biopsy. Clin Neurol Neurosurg. 2005;107:214-7.
13. Schwarz R. General principles of reconstructive surgery for leprosy and other peripheral neuropathies. In: Schwarz R, Brandsma W (Eds). Surgical Reconstruction & Rehabilitation in Leprosy and other Neuropathies, 1st edition. Kathmandu: Ekta Books Distributors Pvt. Ltd; 2004;1-10.

14. Sharma VK, Malhotra AK. Leprosy: classification and clinical aspects. In: Valia RG, Valia AR (Eds). Textbook and Atlas of Dermatology, 3rd edition. Mumbai: Bhalani Publishing House; 2008;2032-69.
15. Srinivasan H, Palande DD. Essential surgery in leprosy: Techniques for district hospitals. Available at http://whqlibdoc.who.int/hq/1996/WHO_LEP_96.2.pdf (accessed on 15-3-2012).
16. Srinivasan H. Leprosy: disablement—its prevention and manage-ment. In: Valia RG, Valia AR (Eds). Textbook and Atlas of Dermatology, 3rd edition. Mumbai: Bhalani Publishing House; 2008;2119-38.
17. Srinivasan H. Prevention of disabilities in patients with leprosy: A practical guide, WHO, Geneva; 1993.
18. Warren G, Schwarz R. Surgery of the nose and other aesthetic surgery. In: Schwarz R, Brandsma W (Eds). Surgical Reconstruction & Rehabilitation in Leprosy and other Neuropathies, 1st edition. Kathmandu: Ekta Books Distributors Pvt. Ltd; 2004;271-301.
19. Warren G. Neuropathic feet. In: Schwarz R, Brandsma W (Eds). Surgical Reconstruction and Rehabilitation in Leprosy and other Neuropathies, 1st edition. Kathmandu: Ekta Books Distributors Pvt. Ltd; 2004;148-74.

Chapter 63

Nerve Biopsy: Technique and Role in Dermatology

Raghunatha Reddy R, Shashikumar BM, Savitha AS

Key Messages

- Nerve biopsy is a key diagnostic procedure to definitely diagnose pure neuritic leprosy in a situation of diagnostic dilemma either to confirm or to rule out neuritic leprosy.
- Commonly performed on a pure cutaneous nerve like sural nerve and radial cutaneous nerve. Biopsy of mixed or motor nerve is done very rarely in special circumstances.
- Complete circumference of the nerve taken for biopsy is better than taking a few fascicles. However, partial thickness nerve biopsy may be done if the cutaneous nerve trunk is grossly thickened.
- Nerve biopsy can also be done for the diagnosis of vasculitis, inflammatory, congenital, and metabolic disorder.

INTRODUCTION

Nerve biopsy is an invasive procedure where a nerve is sectioned either fully or partially to identify potentially treatable causes of neuropathy. The evaluation of a nerve biopsy is often the final step in the diagnostic workup of a neuropathy of unknown origin.[1] Etiology of a peripheral neuropathy is difficult to ascertain in many cases and nerve biopsy may be essential to confirm diagnosis when all other available diagnostic methods fail to establish the diagnosis.

INDICATIONS

Being an invasive procedure, a nerve biopsy is recommended when:

- The neuropathy is progressive
- Threatens to become debilitating
- Other tests fail to identify a cause.

Common indications for nerve biopsy is enumerated in Table 1.[1-3]

PREPARATION

Before considering nerve biopsy other less invasive investigations should be considered to know the cause of pathology. In a situation of thickened nerve with infective etiology like Hansen's disease even fine needle aspiration cytology (FNAC) of the affected nerve can offer some diagnostic help, but negative aspiration findings cannot rule out the diagnosis. Electromyography and nerve conduction studies should be carried out along with other investigations for vasculitis screening, genetics, diabetes, erythrocyte sedimentation rate (ESR), vitamin deficiency, autoimmune disease (e.g. rheumatoid arthritis or systemic lupus erythematosus), renal and liver function tests.[4] All patients should have a full blood count with or without clotting studies depending on the hematological history preoperatively.

Informed consent for the surgery should be obtained, clearly indicating the possible clinical diagnoses, the need for the biopsy, the procedure involved and the possible consequences. All preoperative evaluations, preoperative and postoperative instructions and medications are similar to other minor surgical procedures.

SELECTION OF BIOPSY SITE

Nerve biopsy is performed most often on a pure cutaneous nerve trunk. Rarely the biopsy of combined nerve and muscle biopsy or nerve supplying to muscle which is either suspected to be affected or located nearer to the site of affection on the body can be biopsied. Partial fascicular biopsy of a mixed cutaneous and motor nerve trunk is practiced very rarely in special and unavoidable situations.

Table 1: Common indications for nerve biopsy.

Genetic	▪ Charcot-Marie-Tooth (CMT) diseases ▪ Hereditary motor and sensory neuropathies ▪ Familial amyloid neuropathy ▪ Giant axonal neuropathy ▪ Infantile and juvenile neuroaxonal dystrophy (Seitelberger disease)
Vasculitides	▪ Polyarteritis nodosa ▪ Microscopic polyangiitis ▪ Churg-Strauss syndrome ▪ Rheumatoid arthritis
Infectious neuropathies	▪ Leprosy ▪ Herpes zoster and simplex ▪ Human immunodeficiency virus (HIV) ▪ Lyme disease or borrelia neuropathy
Inflammatory and immune alterations	▪ Sarcoidosis ▪ Ganglionitis ▪ Chronic inflammatory demyelinating polyradiculoneuropathy (CIDP) ▪ Monoclonal gammopathy
Storage disorders	▪ Amyloidosis ▪ Glycogen storage disorders
Metabolic disorders	▪ Diabetic uremic, nutritional neuropathies
Toxic neuropathies	▪ Amiodarone ▪ Chloroquine ▪ Antiretroviral drugs ▪ Industrial agents like n-hexane, methyl n-butyl ketone, acrylamide
Tumors	▪ Primary and secondary nerve tumors: Schwannomas, neurofibromas ▪ Malignant peripheral nerve sheath tumors ▪ Paraneoplastic neuropathy
Ischemic injury of nerve	▪ Chronic nerve compression
Others	

Nerve biopsy should target a cutaneous nerve that is constant in anatomical location and readily accessible. In comparison with full thickness nerve biopsy, fascicular biopsy causes fewer complications or less sensory deficit, but provides less tissue for analysis. This is especially important if focally accentuated lesions including inflammatory processes are looked for. Such foci are less likely to be detected if just a portion of the nerve is examined. Therefore, biopsy of the complete cross section of the nerve is recommended where ever possible.[5] The minimum recommended length of the biopsied nerve segment should be 5 cm.[2] Less than minimum may give unsatisfactory results. Table 2 summarizes the common nerve biopsied along with site and indication.

Combined nerve and muscle biopsies can be obtained by the same skin incision, but in separate pieces. The possibility of detecting inflammatory changes, in particular vasculitis, is significantly higher in a combined biopsy compared to either nerve or muscle biopsy alone. In addition, other disorders that can affect both nerve and muscle such as amyloidosis and certain hereditary diseases including neuropathy and myopathies can benefit by combined biopsy. In patient with pure motor neuropathy, biopsying nerve supplying a muscle with little functional importance (e.g. the nerve to gracilis) needs to be preferred.

BIOPSY SAMPLE HANDLING[2]

The biopsy nerve samples are prepared in three different ways to fully assess the tissue for diagnostic purposes (Table 3).

Table 2: Site of nerve biopsy.[2-4]

Nerve	Site of incision	Indication	Remarks
Distal sural nerve	Behind the lateral malleolus	Vasculitis, Hansen's disease	With minimal postoperative problems or complications
Superficial peroneal (fibular nerve)	Junction of the middle and distal thirds of leg on lateral aspects	Vasculitis	Access to the peroneus brevis muscle through the same incision
Medial sural nerve	Junction of the gastrocnemius muscle bellies	Vasculitis	Concomitant gastrocnemius muscle biopsy can be done. Very minimal sensory loss
Distal superficial radial nerve (radial cutaneous nerve)	Anatomical snuff box	Upper limb neuropathy, including Hansen's disease	Visible scar, neuroma common, no major postprocedure complications
Dorsal cutaneous branch of the ulnar nerve	Wrist	Upper limb neuropathy, including Hansen's disease	
Obturator nerve biopsy	4 inches distal to the pubis bone over medial aspect of thigh	Useful to differentiate motor neuropathies and lower motor neuron diseases like motor neuron disease, Guillain-Barré syndrome, and mixed neuropathy with prominent motor symptoms	Very rarely done. Concomitant gracilis muscle biopsy is taken
Greater auricular nerve	Sternocleidomastoid muscle at the upper and lateral aspect of the neck	Hansen's disease	Considered rarely for biopsy

Table 3: Biopsy sample handling.

Segment	Length	Method of fixation or processing	Uses
1st piece	0.5 cm	Formalin-fixed, paraffin-embedded	H&E and special stain is useful in diagnosing vasculitis, amyloidosis, sarcoidosis, leprosy, lymphoma
2nd piece	0.5 cm	Transported in Michel's medium and frozen	Staining of light chains is useful in diagnosis of amyloidosis
3rd piece	2–2.5 cm	Glutaraldehyde fixed for transverse semithin plastic sections	Useful for analysis of myelinated fibers

Table 4: Complications of nerve biopsy and its prevention.[2-4,6-8]

Complication	Prevention
Hematoma	Hemostasis, postoperative compression dressing, limb elevation and stopping anticoagulants at least 1 week prior to surgery
Muscle herniation (only if motor nerves deep to muscles are biopsied)	Proper closer of fascia
Wound dehiscence	Adequate rest and support
Wound infection	Adequate antibiotics
Neuroma	Transected nerve can be sutured into the surrounding muscle
Pain, dysesthesia, paresthesia	Immobilizing the leg in plaster cast for 7–10 days

COMPLICATIONS

The rate of complications varies from centers and with expertise of surgeon. Surgery-related complications are persistent pain, dysesthesia, paresthesia, allodynia, sensory impairment, and neuroma (Table 4). In case of pure cutaneous nerves biopsy like sural or radial cutaneous nerves, except for paresthesia or anesthesia over the small area supplied by the respective nerve biopsied, no major side or adverse effects are reported. Many a times, it has been reported that the nerve trunks get reunited and may reestablish the sensations.

SURAL NERVE BIOPSY

Nerve biopsy has been a well-established diagnostic procedure for the investigation of peripheral neuropathies. Leprosy is one of the most common treatable causes of peripheral neuropathy but diagnosing leprosy in the absence of typical dermatological features is challenging. Despite the availability of many diagnostic tools like, nerve conduction studies, electromyelogram, ultrasound examination, imaging techniques, etc. the best diagnosis of Hansen's disease is by clinical examination. In a situation where both clinical examination and other diagnostic tests cannot either confirm or rule out Hansen's disease, the nerve biopsy becomes crucial which is the most conclusive diagnostic test. Thus, the nerve biopsy may give useful information in diagnosing pure neuritic form of Hansen's disease.

The sural nerve is most often biopsied because:[6]

- Sural nerve is pure sensory nerve and no motor loss on biopsy.
- Resulting sensory loss is confined to a small area on the dorsolateral aspect of the foot.
- It is usually readily accessible at the level of the lateral malleolus.
- Its structure has been studied extensively in health and disease.

Anatomy of Sural Nerve[4] (Fig. 1)

Sural nerve is pure sensory nerve and supplies sensation to dorsolateral aspect of the foot and ankle region. Distal sural nerve is formed by joining of medial sural nerve (branch of the tibial nerve that is found approximately 6 cm proximal to the fibular head) and the lateral cutaneous sural nerve (branch of common peroneal nerve). The two branches meet in the distal third of the leg at approximately 11–20 cm proximal to the lateral malleolus. Distally, it courses subcutaneously in a fascial sling between the deep crural fascia and superficial fascia adjacent to the short saphenous vein and lateral to the Achilles tendon.

Anatomical Variation

Amalgamation of medial and lateral sural nerve may occur in the popliteal fossa in 12% cases rather distally.[8] Anatomical variations include early union or nonunion of the medial or lateral cutaneous sural nerves or very rarely the sural nerve may be completely absent.[9]

Procedure (Figs. 2 and 3)

After obtaining informed consent, the skin is prepared, draped and anesthetized with infiltration of local anesthetic agent. The leg is flexed at the knee to 30° with a soft bolster and the ankle slightly everted at 90° to keep the sural nerve under slight tension and to aid localization. Surface marking is done along the course of the nerve. A superficial, vertical incision is made halfway between the Achilles tendon and the lateral border of fibula, commencing at the lateral malleolus and extending 5 cm upwards along the course of nerve following Langer's lines. With sharp dissection and careful undermining of tissues, proceed through the superficial fascia until the lesser

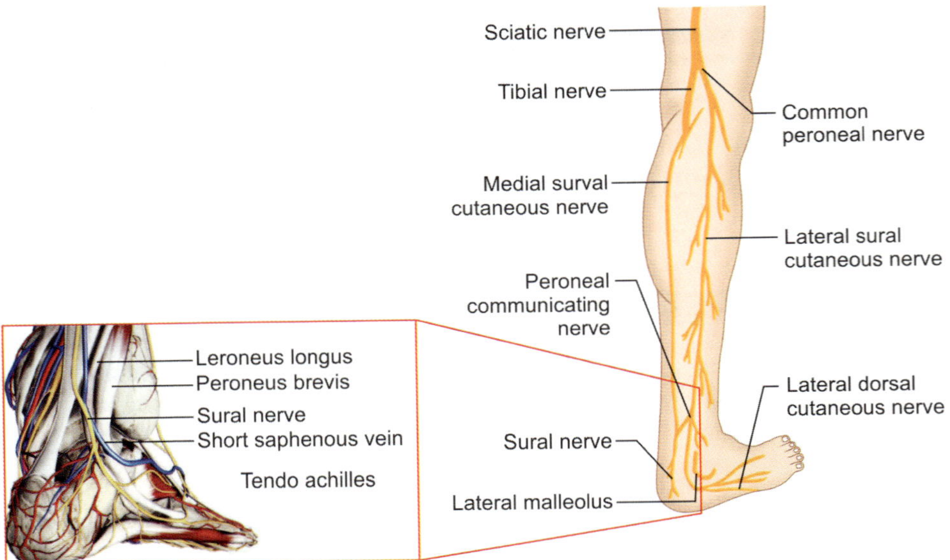

Fig. 1: Anatomy of sural nerve.

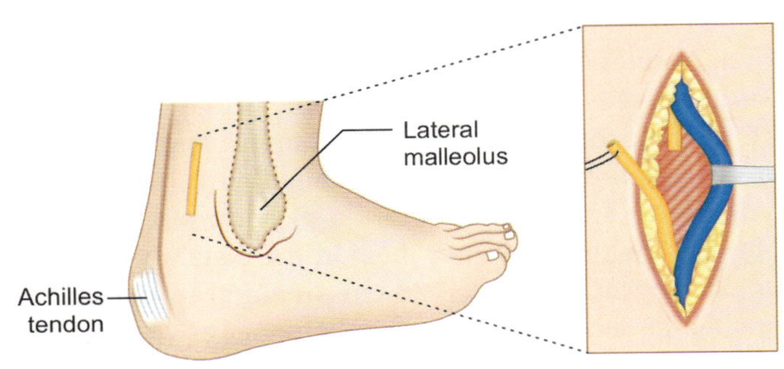

Fig. 2: Distal sural nerve biopsy technique. A superficial, vertical incision is made halfway between the Achilles tendon and the lateral border of fibula, commencing at the lateral malleolus and extending 5 cm upward along the course of nerve.

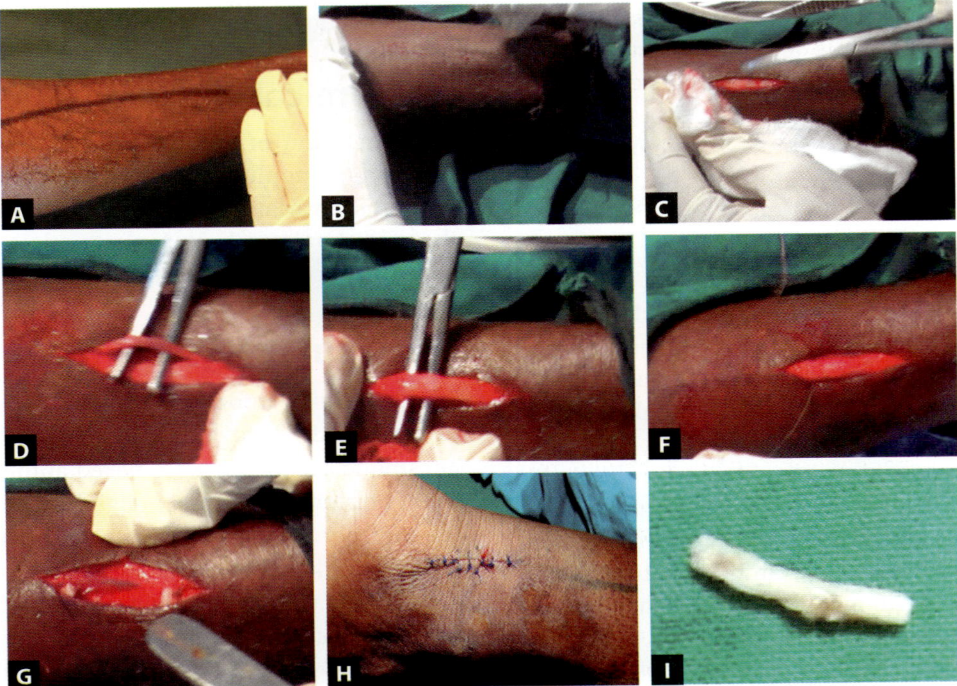

Figs. 3A to I: (A) Sural nerve course is marked; (B) Superficial vertical incision; (C) Sharp dissection and careful undermining of tissues; (D) Identifying and retracting lesser saphenous vein; (E) Separating of sural nerve; (F) Proximal nerve is ligated cut with sharp blade; (G) Hemostasis achieved; (H) Wound is sutured; (I) Cut section is sent for histopathology.

Box 1: Differentiating nerve from vessel.[6]

- Nerve is glistening white and solid in appearance, if examined carefully, fascicles can be visualized
- Vessels will have true lumen and tributaries
- Nerve has pattern of alternating longitudinal lighter and darker bands

saphenous vein is identified and retracted posteriorly to reveal the sural nerve immediately medial to it.[10] Care should be taken to preserve saphenous vein. Prior to nerve section a small bolus of local anesthetic can be injected into the proximal nerve as sectioning of nerve is painful (but not necessary always). A single 3.0 nylon suture is placed proximally through the nerve: it is important that the nerve is only minimally manipulated using the proximal suture for moving it (Fig. 2). The nerve is sharply cut with a scalpel (scissors will produce compression trauma artifact) proximally first to prevent pain when the distal end is subsequently sectioned. The nerve is left alone or buried into the adjacent muscle. In case of fascicular biopsy, a few fascicles are separated and sectioned (Box 1). The wound is sutured in layers. The specimen is processed as mentioned in Table 3.

Postoperative Care

Immediate postoperatively look for appropriate hemostasis and possibility of hematoma if any. They are advised to keep the wound dry for 48 hours and avoid strenuous activity for 2 weeks. Optionally leg can be immobilized in a plaster cast for 7–10 days. Skin sutures may be removed after 10 days. Appropriate antibiotics and anti-inflammatory drugs are to be given for a required duration.

DISTAL SUPERFICIAL RADIAL NERVE BIOPSY[4]

Anatomy

The distal superficial radial nerve is a direct continuation of the radial nerve. It travels under the brachioradialis along the anterolateral aspect of the forearm. It pierces the deep fascia in the distal forearm and lies subcutaneously. The nerve can usually be palpated directly over the distal radius or in the anatomical snuff box laterally over the extensor carpi radialis longus, which aids in planning the approach. The boundaries of the anatomical snuff box include posteriorly the extensor pollicis longus tendon, anteriorly the tendons of the extensor pollicis brevis and abductor pollicis longus and proximally the styloid process of the radius, while the floor consists of both the trapezium and scaphoid.

Procedure (Figs. 4 and 5)

Preoperative preparations are same as described earlier. Region around anatomical snuff box is cleaned and draped. The operating field is then infiltrated with 1% lignocaine. Identify and mark the course of radial artery to avoid injury or inadvertent cutting anterior-laterally, a longitudinal or a transverse incision is placed over the distal radius or anatomical snuff box. The cephalic veins lying medially are retracted to visualize the nerve lying superficial to the extensor retinaculum. The nerve is ligated proximally to 3–5 cm of nerve and is resected mostly in total thickness or partial thickness if it is grossly thickened. After achieving hemostasis, wound is closed in layers. Postoperative care is done as described earlier.

Tips

For surgery

- Sural nerve is the most common nerve biopsied by a dermatologist, mainly to rule out Hansen's disease.
- Knowing proper anatomy and variation is crucial before planning surgery.
- Gentle handling of nerve with blunt dissection is crucial.
- Sharp section of nerve is important.

CONCLUSION

Nerve biopsy is the confirmatory test in pure neuritic leprosy. Knowledge of the anatomy of the nerve is important. If performed by a experienced surgeon, it is a safe procedure without any sequelae.

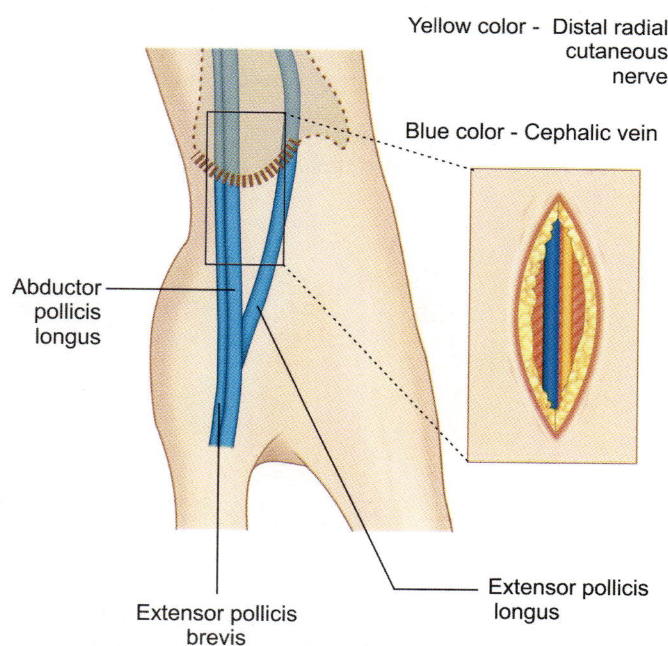

Fig. 4: Distal radial nerve biopsy anatomy technique.

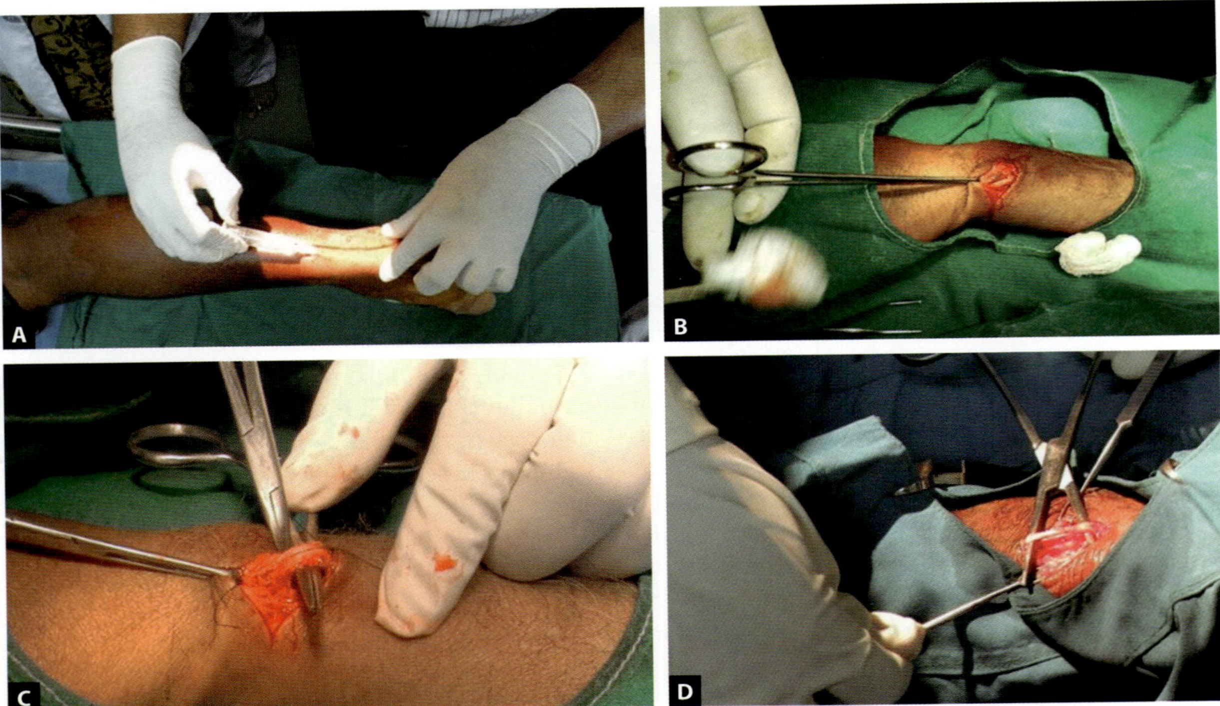

Figs. 5A to D: Distal radial nerve biopsy technique. (A) Local anesthesia infiltration; (B) Incision and blunt dissection; (C) Identification of nerve; (D) Separation and ligation of nerve.

REFERENCES

1. Sommer C, Brandner S, Dyck PJ, et al. 147th ENMC international workshop: guideline on processing and evaluation of sural nerve biopsies, 15–17 December 2006, Naarden, The Netherlands. Neuromuscul Disord. 2008;18(1):90-6.
2. Weis J, Brandner S, Lammens M, et al. Processing of nerve biopsies: a practical guide for neuropathologists. Clin Neuropathol. 2012;31(1):7-23.
3. Vallat JM, Funalot B, Magy L. Nerve biopsy: requirements for diagnosis and clinical value. Acta Neuropathol. 2011;121:313-26.
4. Hart MG, Santarius T, Trivedi RA. Muscle and nerve biopsy for the neurosurgical trainee. Br J Neurosurg. 2013;27:727-34.
5. Pollock M, Nukada H, Taylor P, et al. Comparison between fascicular and whole sural nerve biopsy. Ann Neurol. 1983;13:65-8.
6. Ginsberg L, King RH, Orrell RW. Nerve biopsy: how to do it. Pract Neurol. 2003;3:306-13.
7. Mellgren SI, Lindal S. Nerve biopsy—some comments on procedures and indications. Acta Neurol Scand Suppl. 2011;(191):64-70.
8. Ducic I, West J. A modified approach to sural nerve biopsy: minimizing complications. Ann Plast Surg. 2009;62:220-2.
9. Devi SK, Sharmila BP, Susan PJ, et al. Variant formation of sural nerve and its distribution at the dorsum of the foot. Int J AnatomVar. 2009;1:33-4.
10. Bevilacqua NJ, Rogers LC, Malik RA, et al. Technique of the sural nerve biopsy. J Foot Ankle Surg. 2007;46(2):139-42.